9th Edition

DARBY'S

# COMPREHENSIVE REVIEW OF DENTAL HYGIENE

**CHRISTINE M. BLUE**, BSDH, MS, DHSc
Associate Professor
Assistant Dean for Faculty Development
School of Dentistry
University of Minnesota
Minneapolis, Minnesota

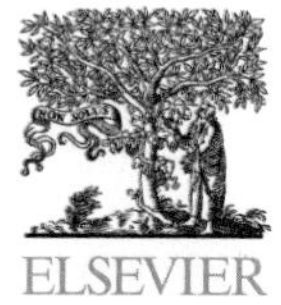

Elsevier
3251 Riverport Lane
St. Louis, Missouri 63043

DARBY'S COMPREHENSIVE REVIEW OF DENTAL HYGIENE, NINTH EDITION ISBN: 9780323679480


ISBN: 9780323679480

*Content Strategist*: Joslyn Dumas/Kelly Skelton
*Director, Content Development*: Ellen Wurm-Cutter
*Senior Content Development Specialist*: Laura Klein
*Publishing Services Manager*: Shereen Jameel
*Project Manager*: Nadhiya Sekar
*Design Direction*: Renee Duenow

Printed in India

Last digit is the print number: 9 8 7 6 5 4 3 2

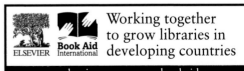

# CONTRIBUTORS

**Michelle C. Arnett, RDH, BS, MS**
Assistant Professor
Department of Primary Dental Care
University of Minnesota
Minneapolis, Minnesota

**Jessica N. August, RDH, MSDH**
Associate Professor
Quinsigamond Community College
Worcester, Massachusetts

**Stephen C. Bayne, MS, PhD**
Active Emeritus Professor
Cariology, Restorative Sciences, and Endodontics
School of Dentistry, University of Michigan
Ann Arbor, Michigan

**Christine French Beatty, RDH, BS, MS, PhD**
Professor Emeritus
Dental Hygiene Program
Texas Woman's University
Denton, Texas

**Christine M. Blue, BSDH, MS, DHSc**
Associate Professor
Assistant Dean for Faculty Development
School of Dentistry
University of Minnesota
Minneapolis, Minnesota

**Cristina Casa-Levine, RDH, EdD**
Associate Professor
Dental Hygiene
Farmingdale State College of New York
Farmingdale, New York

**Alison F. Doubleday, PhD**
Associate Professor
Oral Medicine and Diagnostic Sciences
University of Illinois at Chicago, College of Dentistry
Chicago, Illinois

**Miranda A. Drake, RDH, RF, MSDH**
Interim Division Director of Dental Hygiene
Clinical Associate Professor
Department of Primary Dental Care
Division of Dental Hygiene
University of Minnesota
Minneapolis, Minnesota

**Margaret J. Fehrenbach, RDH, MS**
Oral Biologist and Dental Hygienist
Educational Consultant and Oral Biology Writer
Seattle, Washington
Adjunct Instructor
Dental Hygiene Program
Seattle Central College
Seattle, Washington

**JoAnn R. Gurenlian, RDH, MS, PhD, AFAAOM**
Professor and Graduate Program Director
Dental Hygiene
Idaho State University
Pocatello, Idaho

**Elena Bablenis Haveles, BS Pharmacy, PharmD**
Adjunct Associate Professor of Pharmacology
School of Dental Hygiene
Old Dominion University
Norfolk, Virginia

**Laura Jansen Howerton, RDH, MS**
Three-Dimensional Software Technologist
Carolina OMF Imaging
Franklinton, North Carolina

**Kim T. Isringhausen, BSDH, MPH**
Associate Dean, Risk and Compliance
Virginia Commonwealth University School of Dentistry
Richmond, Virginia

**Vickie Kimbrough, RDH, MBA, PhD**
Director
Dental Hygiene Program
Taft College
Taft, California

**Janet Kinney, RDH, MS**
Associate Clinical Professor and Director of Dental Hygiene
Periodontics and Oral Medicine
University of Michigan
Ann Arbor, Michigan

**Leslie Koberna, BSDH, MPH/HSA, PhD**
Clinical Professor
Department of Communication Sciences and Oral Health
Texas Woman's University
Denton, Texas

**Demetra Daskalos Logothetis, RDH, MS**
Professor Emeritus
Department of Dental Medicine
University of New Mexico
Albuquerque, New Mexico

**Lisa F. Mallonee, MPH, RDH, RD, LD**
Professor and Graduate Program Director
Codirector for Dental Hygiene, Master of Science in Education for Health Care Professionals Program
Texas A&M University College of Dentistry, Caruth School of Dental Hygiene
Dallas, Texas

**Jill Mason, RDH, MPH, EPP**
Associate Professor
Community Dentistry
Oregon Health & Science University
Portland, Oregon

**Laura Mueller-Joseph, BSDH, MS, EdD**
Vice President for Academic Affairs and Professor
Department of Dental Hygiene
State University of New York at Farmingdale
Farmingdale, New York

**Sandra L. Myers, RDH, DMD**
Associate Professor
Diagnostic & Biological Sciences
University of Minnesota School of Dentistry
Minneapolis, Minnesota

**Joanne Pacheco, RDH, MAOB**
Program Director
Dental Hygiene
Fresno City College
Fresno, California

**Darnyl M. Palmer, RDH, MS**
Clinical Instructor
Dental Hygiene
Georgia State University's Perimeter College
Dunwoody, Georgia

**John M. Powers, PhD**
Volunteer Faculty
Restorative Dentistry and Prosthodontics
University of Texas School of Dentistry at Houston
Houston, Texas
President
Dental Advisor
Dental Consultants, Inc.
Ann Arbor, Michigan

**Danielle Rulli, RDH, MS, DHSc**
Director, Graduate Dental Hygiene Program
Periodontics & Oral Medicine, Division of Dental Hygiene
University of Michigan School of Dentistry
Ann Arbor, Michigan

**Jessica Peek Scott, RDH, DHSc**
Oral Health Coordinator
Oral Health Section
North Carolina Department of Health and Human Services, Division of Public Health
Raleigh, North Carolina

**Susan Lynn Tolle, BSDH, MS**
Professor, University Professor
Dental Hygiene
Old Dominion University
Norfolk, Virginia

## SUBJECT MATTER EXPERT (EVOLVE)

**Elizabeth M. Kostas, RDH, MS**
Assistant Professor, Dental Hygiene Program
Southwestern College
San Diego, California

# PREFACE

An interdisciplinary approach to health care, research advancements, and the need for evidence-based education and practice serve as the prime forces guiding the development of the 9th edition of *Darby's Comprehensive Review of Dental Hygiene*. Publishing a book that comprehensively reviews the foundation for dental hygiene competencies is a challenge. Demographic, societal, and educational trends require dental hygienists to possess competence in the biological, social, behavioral, and dental hygiene sciences and in general education. The book and the accompanying Evolve website offer a complete learning package to:

- assist individuals in reviewing the theory, skills, and judgments required on national, regional, and state dental hygiene board examinations;
- prepare dental hygienists for reentry into professional dental hygiene roles—clinician, educator, advocate, researcher, and administrator/manager;
- provide educators with salient information used for course and curriculum development and outcomes assessment.

A special effort was made to design testlets for the community oral health content and case-based questions that include patient health; dental, pharmacologic, and cultural history; and dental charts, radiographs, and photographs.

## ORGANIZATION

The 9th edition of *Darby's Comprehensive Review of Dental Hygiene* is divided into 22 independent, interrelated chapters. Chapter 1 provides guidance on how to use the text effectively to prepare for written and clinical board examinations, including test-taking strategies and trends in standardized board examinations. Each subsequent chapter focuses on different content areas, emphasizing the knowledge and skills necessary for dental hygiene practice. At the end of each chapter are review questions that mimic the various types used on the actual National Board Dental Hygiene Examination.

The rationales for the correct and incorrect answers, in Evolve, provide an additional strategy for efficient board preparation by requiring decision making and judgment in integrating professional knowledge, and facilitates mastery of each chapter's content, further increasing the likelihood of success on examination day.

Internet links and a comprehensive index that enables users to locate information quickly and easily are included. Illustrations and the appendices minimize the need to search alternative sources; however, reference lists and website resources are provided for those who desire more in-depth study or enrichment.

## SIMULATED NATIONAL BOARD DENTAL HYGIENE EXAMINATIONS/ELECTRONIC RESOURCES

### Resources for Students and Faculty

Providing four simulated National Board Dental Hygiene Examination-style exams provides the practice opportunities needed to ensure test-taking confidence and exam-day success. The examinations are located on the Evolve companion site (see inside front cover for access information), and students have the ability to take each exam in practice and study modes. Practice mode displays the answer and rationale after the student answers each question, whereas exam mode mimics a realistic testing experience with timer functionality and end-of-exam results and feedback. Questions are scrambled each time, and students can take them as many times as they want. In addition, faculty members who have adopted this text can enroll students into their class to monitor progress, publish class syllabi and lecture notes, and enable communication with and among students.

# ACKNOWLEDGMENTS

I would like to express my sincere appreciation to those who helped make the 9th edition of *Darby's Comprehensive Review of Dental Hygiene* a reality. Detailed outlines, review questions, answers, and rationales were developed by renowned experts identified in the table of contents. I am inspired by these individuals—all have shaped our discipline and advanced the profession of dental hygiene. Additionally, comments and suggestions from students, faculty, and returning dental hygienists who have used the book are embodied in this edition. The exemplary work of these contributors has made *Darby's Comprehensive Review of Dental Hygiene* a board preparation experience that is second to none.

My special thanks go to Joslyn Dumas and Kelly Skelton, Content Strategists; Laura Klein, Senior Content Development Specialist; Ellen Wurm-Cutter, Director, Content Development; and Nadhiya Sekar, Project Manager, who facilitated the many steps of the publication process at Elsevier. Also acknowledged are the authors, corporations, and publishers who granted permission to use quotes, concepts, photographs, figures, and tables.

The work of those who contributed to the earlier editions remains central to this revision, and I want to gratefully acknowledge their efforts. Without the earlier contributions of these talented people, the current edition of *Darby's Comprehensive Review of Dental Hygiene* would not be possible.

As always, the 9th edition of *Darby's Comprehensive Review of Dental Hygiene* is dedicated to Michele Darby—a person who continues to inspire me.

Dr. Christine Blue

1

# Preparing for Dental Hygiene Board Examinations

*Jill Mason*

Licensure of dental hygienists is a means of regulation to protect the public from unsafe practice of the profession and unqualified individuals. The expected dental hygiene foundational knowledge and competencies are similar in the United States and Canada. The examination and licensure processes have both similarities and differences. This section will review the general processes for each country. It is always best to contact the regulatory entity for the area in which you plan to practice for any specific requirements.

The board exam process that leads to licensure eligibility is a complex mosaic of test development organizations, testing organizations, and state board, provincial, or territory acceptance of exams for licensure. Preparing for board examinations requires deliberate planning, study and review, time management, organization of information and schedules, and a positive confident attitude. Conscientious dental hygienists will organize a plan for success well in advance and will be well prepared to satisfy board requirements with confidence in their professional knowledge and skills. This book is a guide through the evidence-based knowledge on which dental hygiene practice is based. Systematic use of this book enables one to reinforce professional education, integrate concepts and ideas from many dental hygiene educators, and identify subject areas in which additional study is warranted.

The introductory chapter is a primer in navigating the examination and licensure system—whether a new graduate, a practicing dental hygienist who is moving to another licensing jurisdiction, or a dental hygienist returning to practice after a lapse of activity—to prepare for both written and clinical board examinations. A dental hygienist must master all subject matter and skills necessary for practice; therefore, each subsequent chapter focuses on different content areas of such knowledge and skills. In addition, success on board examinations also relies on being psychologically, emotionally, and physically prepared to demonstrate competence. It is essential to become thoroughly familiar with the format, logistics, and requirements of any preparatory examination for licensure.

This chapter discusses the multifaceted licensure structure and explains the roles and interactions of the numerous organizations within the system. Information on the US National Board Dental Hygiene Examination (NBDHE), the Canadian National Dental Hygiene Certification Exam (NDHCE) and clinical board examinations is provided. The chapter concludes with an overview of this review book, including its purpose and organization, as well as instructions on how to use the text effectively.

## DENTAL HYGIENE LICENSURE IN THE UNITED STATES

In the United States, licensure falls under the authority of an individual state or jurisdiction. Each state has a *state dental practice act* that defines the practice of dental hygiene, establishes educational and testing requirements for licensure, sets parameters for enforcement of the law within that jurisdiction, and creates a state board of dentistry or dental hygiene to serve in accordance with the statute. A certificate for successful completion of an examination is *not* authorization to practice. Beginning practice without a license is illegal. Dental hygiene licensure requirements vary from state to state, but virtually every state has the following three requirements:

- Educational: graduation from a dental hygiene program accredited by the Commission on Dental Accreditation (CODA) or, based on reciprocity, by the Commission on Dental Accreditation of Canada (CDAC)
- Written examination: successful completion of the NBDHE
- Clinical examination: successful completion of an accepted clinical board examination

Recognition of an accrediting agency is a governmental function. In health care fields with a domain of specialized education, accreditation is conducted by a dedicated agency within the profession. In dentistry, the US Department of Education (USDE) has recognized the Commission on Dental Accreditation (CODA) as the official accrediting body for schools of dentistry, dental hygiene, dental assisting, dental laboratory technology, and dental therapy. The CODA is also listed in the publications of accreditation agencies by the Council for Higher Education Accreditation (CHEA). A diploma, certificate, associate degree, or baccalaureate degree in dental hygiene indicating graduation from an accredited program is an essential component for licensure that is based on the accreditation system carried out under the auspices of the CODA. States that provide for licensure of a dental hygienist from a nonaccredited school generally require evidence of an educational program approved by the state board. The written NBDHE is developed and administered by the Joint Commission on National Dental Examinations (JCNDE).

**BOX 1.1 Regional Clinical Testing Agencies and Contact Information[1]**

**Central Regional Dental Testing Service, Inc. (CRDTS)**
Central Regional Dental Testing Service, Inc.
1725 SW Gage Boulevard
Topeka, KS 66604-3333
Phone: 785-273-0380
Fax: 785-273-5015
www.crdts.org

**Commission on Dental Competency Assessments (CDCA)**
1304 Concourse Dr., Suite 100
Linthicum, MD 21090
Phone: 301-563-3300
Fax: 301-563-3307
http://www.cdcaexams.org

**Council of Interstate Testing Agencies (CITA)**
1518 Elm St Suite A
Sanford, NC 27330
Phone: 919-460-7750
1-866-678-9795
Fax: 919-460-7715
http://www.citaexam.com

**Southern Regional Testing Agency, Inc. (SRTA)**
4698 Honeygrove Road, Suite 2
Virginia Beach, VA 23455
Phone: 757-318-9082
Fax: 757-318-9085
http://www.srta.org

**Western Regional Examining Board (WREB)**
23460 North 19th Avenue, Suite 210
Phoenix, AZ 85027
Phone: 623-209-5400
Fax: 602-371-8131
www.wreb.org

[1]Current information about examination policies, procedures, criteria, locations, dates, registration, and frequently asked questions can be accessed at the respective agency's website.

Patient-based clinical examinations are conducted by five regional testing agencies. Box 1.1 provides contact information for the regional testing agencies, and Box 1.2 indicates the member states for each agency. Currently some regional testing agencies administer the American Board of Dental Examiners (ADEX) dental hygiene licensure examination. ADEX is strictly a *test development* corporation; it does not administer any examinations. Some state boards administer independent examinations, created by the board. Clinical examinations accepted for initial dental hygiene licensure are shown in Fig. 1.1.

A license is applicable only within the geographic boundaries of the issuing state. However, most states have provisions for granting dental hygiene licensure by credentials or reciprocity. Requirements generally include an active license in good standing, recent practice experience, graduation from an accredited program, successful completion of the NBDHE, and successful completion of a clinical examination. Specific requirements

**BOX 1.2 Membership in the Five Regional Clinical Testing Agencies in the United States[2]**

**CITA (Uses ADEX Exam)**
Alabama
Arkansas
Louisiana
North Carolina
Tennessee
Utah
US Virgin Islands
West Virginia
Puerto Rico

**CRDTS**
Alabama
Arkansas
California
Georgia
Hawaii (dental hygiene only)
Illinois
Iowa
Kansas
Minnesota
Missouri
Nebraska
New Mexico
North Dakota
Oklahoma
South Carolina
South Dakota
Texas
Washington
West Virginia
Wisconsin
Wyoming

**CDCA (Uses ADEX Exam)**
Arizona
Arkansas
Connecticut
District of Columbia
Florida
Hawaii
Illinois
Indiana
Kentucky
Maine
Maryland
Massachusetts
Michigan
Minnesota
Mississippi
Missouri
Nevada
New Hampshire
New Jersey
New Mexico
New York
Ohio
Oregon
Pennsylvania
Rhode Island
Utah
Vermont
Washington
West Virginia
Wisconsin
Wyoming
Commonwealth of Jamaica
Puerto Rico?

**SRTA**
Arkansas
Alabama
South Carolina
Tennessee
Virginia
West Virginia

**WREB**
Alaska
Arizona
California (dental only)
Hawaii (dental hygiene only)
Idaho
Illinois
Iowa
Kansas
Kentucky
Minnesota
Mississippi
Missouri
Montana
Nevada
New Mexico
North Dakota
Ohio
Oklahoma
Oregon
Texas
Utah
Washington
West Virginia
Wisconsin
Wyoming

[2]*CITA,* Council of Interstate Testing Agencies; *CRDTS,* Central Regional Dental Testing Service, Inc.; *CDCA,* Commission on Dental Competency Assessments; *SRTA,* Southern Regional Testing Agency, Inc.; *WREB,* Western Regional Examining Board.
A state may be a member of multiple testing agencies. Membership in a testing agency denotes acceptance of the exam, however multiple exams may be accepted by a state for licensure, regardless of membership with a testing agency. Membership/Exam acceptance is continuously changing, and the state dental board should be contacted for current information.

**Clinical Examinations Accepted for Initial Dental Hygiene Licensure***

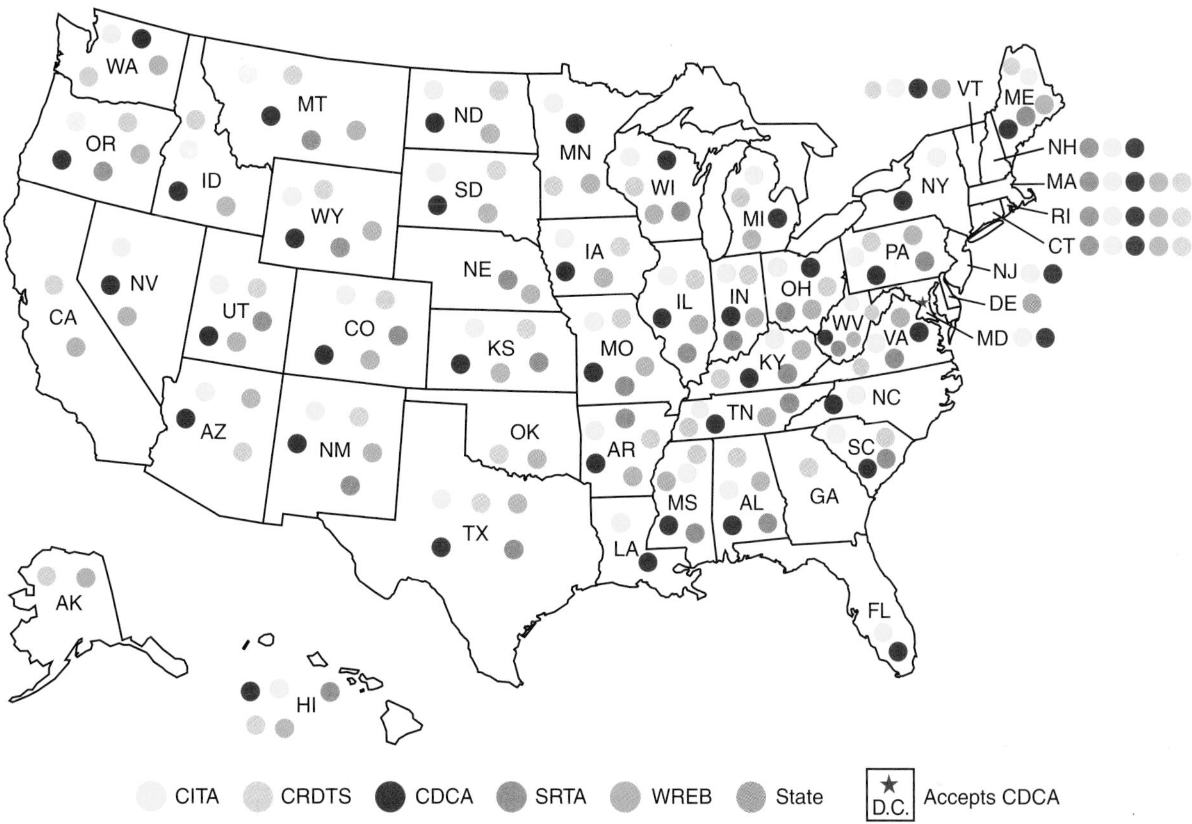

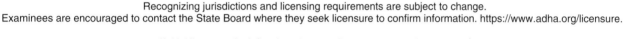

Recognizing jurisdictions and licensing requirements are subject to change.
Examinees are encouraged to contact the State Board where they seek licensure to confirm information. https://www.adha.org/licensure.

*Initial licensure is defined as the state licensure sought immediately following graduation from an accredited dental hygiene program.

**Fig. 1.1** Clinical examinations accepted for initial dental hygiene licensure.

differ from state to state and are subject to change. Applicants for dental hygiene licensure must contact the individual state licensing board for current requirements and information. The American Association of Dental Boards (AADB) website (http://www.dentalboards.org) features a list of the states with direct links to state board offices. State board websites are also readily accessible through an online search listing the state and "dental/dental hygiene board."

## STATE BOARDS OF DENTISTRY OR DENTAL HYGIENE AND PROFESSIONAL ASSOCIATIONS

State boards of dentistry or dental hygiene are governmental agencies that control and manage dental hygiene licensure in accordance with laws adopted by the legislature of the respective states. Boards have the power or influence to grant, deny, and revoke licenses. Board members are charged with the following duties:

- Enforcing the state practice act and its rules and regulations
- Conducting or recognizing examinations for competence
- Reviewing and investigating complaints concerning unlawful or unprofessional conduct by licensees

Significant variations exist from jurisdiction to jurisdiction in regulatory board organizational structure, scope of power and authority, and agency title. For the purpose of clarity in this text, the term *state board* is used to refer to the *regulatory body* in a respective legal jurisdiction that is empowered to determine prerequisites for licensure and issue licenses to practice dental hygiene.

Frequently, licensure candidates and even licensed practitioners confuse the state board with the state professional association. Although strong ties may exist between a state board and the state professional association, distinct legal differences exist between these two bodies. The state board of dentistry/dental hygiene is a *governmental agency,* established by law, which functions as an arm of state government to regulate the practice of dentistry, dental therapy, and/or dental hygiene. Its sole purpose is to protect the public from incompetent or unethical practitioners. In contrast, a state dental hygiene or dental association is a *voluntary membership organization* of practitioners, who join together to advance the profession and promote the oral health of the public.

Practitioners need to understand both this distinction and the interaction between state boards and professional associations. Professional associations *do not* determine requirements for licensure or regulate practice; this is founded by law and implemented through state boards. Professional associations do, however, initiate programs and research projects, and propose legislative changes that may ultimately be incorporated into the legal requirements for practice. In most states, state board members are appointed by the governor. In a few states, board members are designated through election by members of the profession or through appointment by another governmental body. Professional associations may nominate and/or influence board appointments.

All states have some form of dental hygiene representation on the board. Recent years have seen a trend toward self-regulation, with the establishment of separate dental hygiene state boards and advisory committees. The legislative and political arenas in dentistry are constantly changing, as are technologic advancements in health. As a result, revision to state practice acts—including the definitions of dental hygiene and the scope of practice—is ongoing. Likewise, as the standards of competence in dental hygiene are redefined in terms of requisite professional skills and knowledge, examinations undergo continual revision. State practice acts charge the state board with conducting or sanctioning both didactic and clinical examinations to determine competence for entry into the profession. The majority of practice acts authorize the state board to recognize multiple examinations (see Fig. 1.1). Although other agencies are part of the licensure process, the fundamental authorization to recognize qualifications for licensure lies with the individual state regulatory board.

## JOINT COMMISSION ON NATIONAL DENTAL EXAMINATIONS (JCNDE)

The JCNDE is the organization responsible for the development and administration of the NBDHE. It includes a 15-member panel of representatives, as follows:

- American Dental Association, ADA (3)
- American Dental Education Association, ADEA (3)
- American Association of Dental Boards, AADB (6)
- American Dental Hygienists' Association, ADHA (1)
- Public Member (1)
- American Student Dental Association, ASDA (1)

A standing committee of the JCNDE, the Committee on Dental Hygiene (CDH), consists of five dental hygienists (including the ADHA Commissioner)—two educators and two practitioners and a dental hygiene student representative appointed by the ADHA—plus one Commissioner from the ADA, the ADEA, and the AADB. The CDH's responsibilities relate primarily to the NBDHE and include the following:

- Examination content and specifications
- Test construction procedures, including nomination of test constructors
- Information to publicize or explain the testing program
- Examination regulations that affect dental hygiene examinees
- Matters pertaining to finances, the ADA and the Joint Commission Bylaws, and the Joint Commission Standing Rules that affect the NBDHE

The Commission has final authority to act on committee recommendations, but historically, the CDH has been the guiding force of the dental hygiene examination program.

## NATIONAL BOARD DENTAL HYGIENE EXAMINATION

### Examination Format

The NBDHE is designed to "assess the ability of an examinee to understand important information from biomedical, dental, and dental hygiene sciences, and the ability to apply such information in a problem-solving context."[1] All US licensing jurisdictions recognize NBDHE results. This includes all 50 states, the District of Columbia, Puerto Rico, Guam, and the Virgin Islands of the United States. The examination is computer-based and includes approximately 350 multiple-choice items in independent, case-based, and testlet formats. The NBDHE is a comprehensive examination with two components. Component A presents 200 discipline-based items in three major areas, as follows:

- Scientific basis for dental hygiene practice
- Provision of clinical dental hygiene services
- Community health/research principles

Component B presents 150 case-based items, which relate to 12 to 15 dental hygiene patient cases. Case material includes dental and health histories, dental charting, radiographs, and clinical photographs. Every examination includes one or more of the following patient types: geriatric, adult–periodontitis, pediatric, special needs, and medically compromised. The case-based items address knowledge, skills, and judgments necessary for the following:

- Assessing client characteristics
- Obtaining and interpreting radiographs
- Planning and managing dental hygiene care
- Performing periodontal procedures
- Using preventive agents
- Providing supportive treatment services
- Professional responsibility

The NBDHE tests the examinee's ability to apply the essential knowledge and skills as a beginning safe practitioner to solve oral health care problems and answer questions related to dental hygiene care. The examination is based on practice competencies underlying entry-level dental hygiene practice as defined by the ADEA, the ADHA, the *Accreditation Standards* published by the CODA, and other communities of interest. As part of its validity analyses to verify that the examination content supports these competencies, the JCNDE conducts a nationwide practice survey every 5 years. Test specifications, included in the *National Board Dental Hygiene Examination Candidate Guide,*[1] are the blueprint for test development. The outline lists the specific categories of subject matter included in the examination, with an itemization of the number of items devoted to each area. It should be referenced as a guide for study and review.

Examination items are written and selected by test construction committees in accordance with the NBDHE Dental Hygiene Test Specifications. The test construction committees are composed of individuals who represent geographic areas across the country and are selected on the basis of their expertise in six areas: (1) basic sciences, (2) radiology, (3) periodontics, (4) dental hygiene curriculum, (5) clinical dental hygiene, and (6) community dental health. Test construction committees author new examination items and develop new cases, revise and clone test items, create multiple versions of the examination, and review examination drafts before publishing. Committees strive toward higher cognitive levels—understanding, application, and reasoning—in test development.

## NBDHE Item Formats

The multiple-choice items on the NBDHE consist of a stem, which poses a problem, and a list of three to five possible responses. The stem is usually either a question or an incomplete statement. Key words in the stem such as *best, most, first, not, except,* or *least* are capitalized. Only one response is correct or clearly the best choice by universally accepted standards of care.

A variety of item formats are used in the NBDHE. Descriptions of formats as well as sample items from the *National Board Dental Hygiene Examination Candidate Guide*[1] are provided next.

### Completion

As indicated by the name, *completion* items necessitate the correct completion of a theory or idea. For example:

The sensation of touch, pain, pressure, or temperature is determined by the:

a. Specific nerve fiber stimulated
b. Method of stimulation of a nerve fiber
c. Degree of myelinization of a nerve fiber
d. Strength of the stimulation to a nerve fiber
e. Frequency of the stimulation to a nerve fiber

### Question

A *question* item poses a problem or set of circumstances. Response choices include only one best answer. For example:

Which of the following is innervated by the phrenic nerve?

a. Diaphragm
b. Abdominal muscles
c. Sternocleidomastoid muscle
d. Internal intercostal muscles
e. External intercostal muscles

### Negative

A *negative* item is characterized with words such as *except* or *not* in the stem. These key words are emphasized by capitalization. For example:

Each of the following is affected by saliva EXCEPT one. Which one is the EXCEPTION?

a. Swallowing
b. Dental caries
c. Oral microflora
d. Protein digestion
e. Carbohydrate breakdown

### Paired True-False

In a *paired true-false* item, the stem consists of two sentences on the same topic. The examinee is asked to determine whether the statements are true or false. For example:

Protection from excessive exposure to radiation is aided by the use of aluminum filters and a lead diaphragm. The filters reduce the amount of soft radiation reaching the patient's face, and the diaphragm controls the area exposed.

a. Both statements are true.
b. Both statements are false.
c. The first statement is true, the second is false.
d. The first statement is false, the second is true.

### Testlet

*Testlet* items are used for testing knowledge and application of community health and research principles; they are also used in the case-based section of the examination. A short scenario describing a situation, event, or problem is followed by a set of associated multiple-choice items. For example:

A dental hygienist employed at a public health clinic in a rural county of the United States is assigned the project of developing a preventive dental health program for a subgroup of the population.

***Community Profile.*** The primary employers in this county have been coal-mining companies. The unemployment rate in the county has increased by 32% since the closing of the coal mines.

The median age of the population is 46 years. In the county, there are five general dentists, three dental hygienists, and one public health–centered dental clinic. The clinic employs a full-time dentist and dental hygienist. The public health clinic sees low-income children and senior citizens on a sliding-fee schedule.

The dental hygienist employed by the public health clinic conducts dental screenings for the kindergarten (K) students each year. The mean deft (decayed, extracted, filled teeth) scores for the K students for the last 3 years are $d = 1.02$, $e = 0.87$, and $f = 4.22$.

The community does not have water fluoridation because of multiple water sources. The state funds a 0.2% sodium fluoride rinse program in grades K through 5. The state mandates that a dentist or a dental hygienist perform deft/dmft (decayed, missing, filled teeth)/DMFT and Gingival Index (GI) scoring on all students in grades 1, 2, 3, 5, 7, and 10. On a yearly basis, all pathology is brought to the parent's attention and referred to a dental professional.

1. Which population group is dentally underserved in this community?
   a. Adult age
   b. Geriatric age
   c. Adolescent age
   d. Early-childhood age
   e. Elementary school age
2. What would be the next step for the dental hygienist to take in program planning after selecting the target population?
   a. Appraise the program
   b. Define goals for the program
   c. Compile data on the target group population
   d. Develop educational components
   e. Identify manpower resources in the community

3. Each of the following is perceived as a barrier to dental care for this community EXCEPT one. Which one is the EXCEPTION?
   a. Geographic isolation
   b. Lack of water fluoridation
   c. Maldistribution of providers
   d. Lack of affordable services
   e. Loss of income and insurance
4. What can be stated about the deft scores of the kindergarten students?
   a. Early exfoliation
   b. High decay rate
   c. Increased referrals
   d. Late eruption pattern
   e. Treatment needs are being met.
5. How often should the fluoride rinse for grades K through 5 be performed?
   a. Daily
   b. Weekly
   c. Monthly
   d. Three times a week
   e. Based on the caries rate of the child

### Case-Based

The *case-based* portion of the examination includes 150 items and presents 12 to 15 dental hygiene patient cases, including social, medical, and dental histories; a chief complaint; dental and periodontal charting; radiographs; and clinical photographs. Items based on observations and judgments about the client's clinical conditions and needs follow. These items may be presented in any of the test formats previously described.

Examples of cases and other items are provided in the NBDHE samples at the end of this book and on the Evolve website. Sample examination items can also be accessed from the ADA/JCNDE website.

## National Board Dental Hygiene Examination Eligibility and Application

Eligibility for the NBDHE requires qualification through one of the following stipulations:

- A student in an accredited dental hygiene program is eligible when certified by the program director to be prepared for the examination.
- A graduate of an accredited dental hygiene program is eligible following the JCNDE's receipt of evidence of graduation.
- A graduate of a nonaccredited program is eligible only if the program is deemed equivalent to an accredited program by an independent auditing agency (e.g., length of study, curriculum content, and hours of clinical instruction).

Applications must be submitted electronically to the Joint Commission. The steps involved in the application process include the following:

- Read the *NBDHE Guide* before applying.
- Obtain a Dental Personal Identifier Number (DENTPIN) from the ADA. The DENTPIN is a unique number to identify students and examinees for secure reporting, transmission of test scores, and tracking of academic data in the educational system of the United States.
- Apply for the examination. Confirm and agree to the rules and regulations. Include requests for score reporting to state boards where seeking licensure. If applicable, submit appropriate documentation of a disability to support an appeal for testing accommodation. Also, indicate whether the NBDHE was previously taken.
- After processing the application, the Joint Commission will send notification of eligibility, which lasts for a 6-month period.
- Schedule an appointment to take the examination at a Pearson VUE Testing Center. The computer-delivered NBDHE is scheduled and administered on an individual basis year-round.

## Examination Day

Candidates for the NBDHE must present two original, current forms of identification (ID) to the testing center, as follows.

- One government-issued ID with a photograph, name, and signature
- One secondary ID with a name and signature
- Any needed testing accommodations must be arranged well in advance.

Very strict examination regulations and rules of conduct are followed, by both the NBDHE and the testing centers. Review these in your candidate guide to avoid any surprises. Misconduct may be reported to school or licensing authorities. Unethical conduct carries a risk of delay, denial, or loss of licensure.

No personal items (e.g., cell phones, study materials, backpacks or purses, watches, "good luck charms," food, or water bottles) are allowed in the secure testing area. The testing schedule begins with an optional 15-minute tutorial. Three and one-half hours are allowed for the first session, Component A (200 discipline-based items), and 4 hours are allowed for the second session, Component B (150 patient case-based items). An optional 30 minute break is scheduled between the sessions.

## Examination Results

The examinee's total score is calculated by the number of correct answers selected. The total score is converted to a scale score, ranging from 49 to 99, which adjusts for any minor differences in difficulty across NBDHE forms. A score of 75 represents the minimum passing score. The NBDHE is "criterion referenced," that is, the minimum passing score is determined by experts through standard setting activities to ensure that scores accurately and fairly reflect the entry-level practitioner's ability to solve oral health care problems and to answer items relating to dental hygiene practice on the examination. Results on the NBDHE are reported as pass/fail only. The status of "pass" is reported if a standard score of 75 or higher is achieved. The status of "fail" is reported if a standard score below 75 is achieved. For remediation purposes, examinees who fail receive numerical scores for each of the major subject areas covered on the test. The examinee receives an individual score report, and by virtue of signing the NBDHE application, express permission is granted to give the dental hygiene program director a score report as well. Reports are sent directly to state licensing boards specified on the examinee's application.

## CANADIAN NATIONAL DENTAL HYGIENE CERTIFICATION EXAM (NDHCE)

In Canada, each province or territory has a dental hygiene regulatory body that sets parameters for licensure and practice. Jurisdictional requirements may vary and include differences in educational requirements, clinical competencies, continuing education requirements, language competencies, and written and practical examinations. Regulatory authorities in all provinces except Quebec require the National Dental Hygiene Certificate as one essential requirement for registration or licensure.

The National Dental Hygiene Certification Board (NDHCB) was established in response to a priority for licensure portability for Canadian dental hygienists. It follows a rigorous process in developing the NDHCE, a written national licensure exam that ensures that those who are certified possess sufficient knowledge and skills to safely perform the activities of their profession. The blueprint includes the competencies and domains that reflect entry-level dental hygiene. The competencies are based on the Dental Hygiene Process of Care Model: Assessment and Diagnosis; Planning; Implementation; Evaluation. Examination items are developed by subject matter experts (SME) throughout the country, who are trained in item writing. The items are reviewed and refined in several steps, prior to final approval and addition to the test bank.

The examination consists of 200 multiple choice items, 170 of which are scored for the results. The items are stand-alone independent questions or case study format. The case study format includes a scenario from clinical practice, community health, and health education with a series of five to seven multiple-choice questions based on the scenario.

The examination is computer-based and administered in both English and French three times per year at testing centers throughout Canada. Very strict examination regulations and rules of conduct are followed by the testing centers and the NDHCB. There are two 2-hour sessions, with a 15 minute break in between. A passing score is statistically determined on a scaled range from 200–800 with a passing score of 550. The metric and international tooth numbering systems are used.

Examination information can be obtained directly from the NDHCB using the following contact information:

National Dental Hygiene Certification Board
1929 Russell Road, Suite 322
Ottawa, Ontario K1G 4G3
Canada
Phone: 613-260-8156
Fax: 613-260-8511
General inquiries: exam@ndhcb.ca; http://www.ndhcb.ca/en/about.php
Regulatory Authorities in Canada: https://www.ndhcb.ca/regulatory-authorities

## PREPARING FOR NATIONAL BOARD DENTAL HYGIENE EXAMS

Studying for a comprehensive, high-stakes licensure examination is intensive and unique from studying for other tests. The following are suggested steps in preparing for the NBDHE or NDHCE:

1. Organize a study plan 4 to 6 months in advance to allow an orderly, progressive review without undue pressure.
2. Obtain the NBDHE or NDHCE guide and application materials provided by the respective organization. Study the information thoroughly to gain a clear understanding of the examination's format, design, and administration. View any online tutorials or practice exams provided.
3. Released examinations are valuable as examples. However, retired examinations may contain out-of-date subject material and should not be relied on as the sole study activity. Simulated board examinations, such as the ones in this text and on the Evolve website, may also prove beneficial during review.
4. Outline areas of weakness. Be guided by school experience, as indicated by grades or difficulty in certain subjects and by the items from the released or simulated examinations missed or marked as questionable. Dental hygienists who have been out of school or practice for some period should focus on basic science material and any developments in dental technology or procedures that have expanded or changed evidence-based practice since graduation.
5. Gather a personal resource library for reference throughout the review process. Properly used, this book should be the mainstay study guide; directions for its use are included at the end of this chapter. This book is designed to direct a comprehensive review of dental hygiene, provide questions to assess mastery of the subject material, and offer documentation for correct and incorrect responses. This review book may be supplemented with textbooks, class notes, pertinent journal articles, and websites for further study in focused areas. Ensure all textbooks and reference materials are current resources. The JCNDE does not approve or recommend any particular texts or review courses. The NDHCB lists texts that may be useful for study. Programs or conferences that profess to be "National Board Review Courses" are not affiliated in any way with the JCNDE or NDHCE.
6. If considering a study club, recruit three to five colleagues whose study habits, personal style, and self-discipline complement group efforts for collaboration. Otherwise, study alone.
7. If a study group is formed, do not rely exclusively on someone else for your preparation for the examination. Organize a schedule and procedures for the group. Content areas can be assigned to individuals for specific study and research, and then members of the group can pool information and notes. Discussion of items or content areas can contribute to the review process.
8. Create an orderly system to guide the review, and establish target dates to complete each area. Set deadlines for the review of each chapter in this book. Alternatively, organize review around the NBDHE/NDHCE test specifications. Another option is to assess and prioritize perceived needs. The point is to plan a system of review with goals and deadlines to monitor progress.
9. Launch, and then stay with the plan. If progress slows, assess the obstacles and make modifications to continue

**BOX 1.3 Tips for Managing Examination Anxiety**

- Be well prepared. Nothing boosts confidence like good advance preparation.
- Visit your campus counseling center for individualized tips on study strategies, time management, and relaxation techniques
- Study over several weeks. Follow your plan. Do not rely on last-minute cramming.
- Maintain a positive attitude when preparing for the examination.
- Get physical exercise prior to the test day—it will help reduce stress.
- Eat nutritious foods, and get plenty of rest in the days leading up to the examination.
- Avoid negative thoughts and messages. Anxiety is contagious.
- Plan a relaxing activity the evening before the examination.

*On the day of the examination:*

- Arrive early. Allow plenty of time for traffic, parking challenges, and bad weather.
- Dress comfortably according to exam standards, and layer clothing in case the room temperature is too hot or too cold.
- Bring the admission card and proper identification to the examination site.
- Leave study materials and cell phones at home or outside the examination center.
- Stay relaxed. If nervous, take a few deep breaths, and keep focused.
- Read the directions slowly and carefully. Follow all instructions.

comprehensive review. Aim to complete study at least 3 to 5 days before the examination date.

10. Take positive steps to manage examination anxiety (Box 1.3). Your school's counseling center or student resource center are good resources for reducing test anxiety or developing individualized study skills and test taking skills.

## FUNDAMENTAL GUIDELINES FOR TAKING MULTIPLE-CHOICE TESTS

A system for reading and responding to test items facilitates performance. Some general strategies for dealing with multiple-choice examination items follow:

A. Read the stem of the item carefully and completely before looking at the responses.
   1. Determine what the item is asking; identify key words; and try to formulate the answer before looking at the responses.
   2. Consider each response carefully, and determine whether the response is appropriate and complete.
   3. Immediately eliminate responses that are obviously incorrect; attempt to narrow the choices to no more than two.
   4. For combination items, consider only those choices confidently known to be correct.
   5. When the choices have been narrowed as much as possible and the correct answer is still not clear, make an educated guess.

B. Exercise caution in selecting any response that contains words such as *always, never, none, all,* or *every.* Unconditional responses are frequently incorrect.

C. Look for the answer that *best* applies to the conditions presented in the item.
   1. Avoid selecting responses based on isolated rules, are applicable only to certain locales or regions, or refer to procedures and techniques not universally accepted.
   2. If the item asks for an immediate action, such as the *first* thing one would do, all the options may be correct. The *best* answer would be based on identified priorities and conditions stipulated in the item.

D. The approach to case-based items encompasses a slightly different strategy.
   1. Case-based items require time to read and assimilate pertinent information; good time management is of critical importance. Before beginning a case-based section, estimate a reasonable amount of time that can be dedicated to each case and still complete the entire examination (divide the total time allowed by the number of cases in the section). If a case requires extra time, confidently answer as many items as possible, then flag remaining items and return to them when the other cases have been finished.
   2. When beginning a case, review *all* of the case material—client history; health, dental, and pharmacologic histories; chief complaint; clinical charts; radiographs; and photographs. Make a mental note of significant findings, and begin formulating a concept of specific problems or concerns about the case before attempting to answer the test items. Answering items *before* reviewing all the case material will result in overlooking important aspects of the case and subsequent incorrect responses.
   3. A well-constructed case *requires* referencing the case material to make clinical decisions and respond to the items. Superfluous information is not included in a case. Hence, all information is there for a reason. Before marking a response, consider what information is essential to answer an item correctly and where that information is documented in the case. For example, an item on an artifact in a radiograph may require looking only at a specific radiograph to determine the nature of the artifact. In contrast, an item on clinical attachment loss may necessitate review of periodontal probing depths, radiographs, and perhaps clinical photographs or client history. Items asking for disease classification or appropriate care plans are more likely to require consideration of *all* available information before responding.

E. Watch for grammatical clues. A well-edited item will offer responses that are grammatically consistent with the stem. If the item indicates a plural response, all the options should be in plural form. Any response that is incompatible with the flow of the question may be an indication of an incorrect response.

F. Take heed of the words *not, least,* and *except* in the item's stem. Read the stem carefully.

G. Carefully review questions that include "all of the above" or "none of the above." These responses impose broadly inclusive and exclusive conditions.

H. Avoid becoming upset over challenging items. Negativity and obsessing over a past difficult item affect the ability to concentrate on the current item. Also, remember, on any given test, up to 10% of the items are "seeded" or pretest items that will not count toward the final score.

## CLINICAL TESTING IN THE UNITED STATES

In the United States, clinical testing is integral to the process leading to licensure. In Canada, clinical testing is only used for licensure applicants who graduated from a nonaccredited program. The emphasis of the examinations conducted by regional and state clinical boards is on evaluating entry-level clinical competence. The methodology for assessing clinical ability involves hands-on clinical treatment of patients. In addition, some testing agencies include a computer-delivered clinical simulation component. Testing agencies are obliged to adhere to published psychometric guidelines such as those from the AADB, the American Psychological Association (APA), the National Council on Measurement in Education (NCME), the American Educational Research Association (AERA), and others in the development and administration of their examinations. Committees of examiners and educators collaborate to determine the appropriate criteria, standards, and technical aspects of clinical testing. Examination content and format are similar among clinical board examinations. An examinee's performance on the examination is reported to any of the regulatory state boards accepting that particular examination (see Fig. 1.1.) Every state has a practice act, which delineates all provisions for licensure, including the authority for approval of performance on an examination as meeting its requirements for licensure to practice. A license *must* be obtained before beginning practice.

Regional examining boards are corporate entities composed of individual dental and dental hygiene state boards. Regional agencies have no authority over state boards and cannot implement policy that supersedes the statutory powers of its member state boards. The state dental board makes the determination to accept the results of the clinical board as partial satisfaction of its requirements for licensure. A regional agency consists of states that have opted to standardize clinical testing requirements and pool resources to develop and administer reliable clinical examinations. Regional examinations are developed with the consensus of the member states (see Box 1.2).

The membership of regional testing agencies fluctuates as states join or withdraw. Many states belong to more than one regional board, whereas other states belong to a single regional board but accept the examination results of one or more of the others (see Box 1.2 and Fig. 1.1). The five existing regional testing agencies are similar in their organization and structure. Each maintains an office and employs staff separate from any of its member state board headquarters (see Box 1.1). A board of directors, steering committee, or general membership is responsible for determining agency policies and managing finances. A second key organizational element is an examination review committee or panel. Each member of a state board is represented in this group, which may include a dental hygiene program director or faculty member representing the region's educational institutions. The examination review committee oversees analysis, development, and administration. Some regional testing agencies do not develop their own exam, but administer the ADEX dental hygiene examination. As an organization whose exclusive purpose is examination development, ADEX formulates examination content, scoring, and criteria for the testing agencies that elect to administer it. Member state boards participate in ADEX examination development and approval. A list of member state boards, information on governance, and an overview of the dental and dental hygiene examinations are available on the ADEX website (http://www.adex.org). However, specific inquiries about administration of the ADEX examination are directed to the administering testing agencies. For jurisdictions conducting an independent examination, the state board is the testing agency.

### Examiner Selection and Training

Typically, state board member dental hygienists and dentists serve as examiners. The pool of examiners for regional testing agencies comes primarily from its member state boards. Most state boards also have the authority to designate additional examiners; these appointed examiners are licensed practitioners who meet the testing agency's defined requirements. The number of examiners assigned to an examination is based on the examination agency's administrative protocols. Testing dates and sites are scheduled in advance by the examining agency. Training programs for examiners vary but typically emphasize standardization and grading exercises to calibrate examiners in the evaluation of examination criteria. Examiners do not use their personal criteria to assess examinee performance. Most testing agencies have some type of *examiner performance review system* to monitor scoring and ensure compliance with the agency's standards. The objective is to achieve an accurate and uniform assessment of clinical competence.

### Examination Administration

Most clinical board examinations are administered anonymously or in a double-blind manner. Examinees are identified only by a number and are kept segregated from examiners. Patients are brought to the examiners' clinics; examinees are not present when the examiners conduct their evaluations. The purpose of this practice is to eliminate any potential for examiner bias based on an examinee's personality, race, gender, religion, or personal background. Evaluations are focused solely on clinical performance. Curious examinees might be tempted to seek information from their patients for perceived outcomes about the grading assessments. Examiners typically are prohibited from sharing any information on scoring, so making assumptions based on the reports of patients, who generally understand little about the examination process, will only lead to misinformation and erroneous conclusions.

### Clinical Facilities

Testing agencies use school clinical facilities to administer board examinations. Schools release their facilities for the days of the examination. Accommodating examination requirements entails scheduling adjustments, loss of clinic income, and increased demands on faculty and staff. Most schools charge a "school use fee" for services and supplies. This cost is added to the examination fee.

If testing will take place in an unfamiliar facility, visit the site before the testing date, if possible. Most testing agencies schedule an orientation session and clinic tour before the day of examination. The clinical facility is *not* under the management and control of the board examiners, and the school may have its own institutional requirements, or record keeping, for which the examinee is responsible. After an examination application has been processed, most testing agencies will mail examination-related documents as well as an information package from the school that includes a description of the clinic facilities, a list of provided supplies, emergency and infection control protocols, compatibility of handpieces, instrument rental policies, etc. Equipment rental is handled through the testing site. Concerns must be directed to the appropriate source. The testing site, or school, deals with questions about the facilities; the testing agency addresses questions about the examination itself; and the state board attends to jurisprudence and licensure applications.

## Examination Instruments

Because examiners are calibrated with select instruments, testing agencies are likely to require specific instruments for the examination. Although such requirements may present some inconvenience, they are vital to help ensure standardization in the examination process. Typically, instrument requirements pertain only to the examining instruments (e.g., mirror, explorer, periodontal probe). Handpiece and instrument selection for performing treatment are left to the examinee's discretion. Most clinical examinations allow the use of power scaling devices. If the required instruments are unfamiliar, obtain them and practice with them in advance. Reference the instrument's task analysis, seek guidance in correct adaptation and usage, or do both. Instruments should be in excellent condition and *sharp*. Examiners may request replacements if instruments are incorrect or defective. Have extra sets of sterile instruments in case a client is not accepted or an instrument is dropped.

## Examination Forms

Forms are an important consideration in charting, record keeping, and documentation required for the examination. Numerous systems for charting and for taking client histories exist. Obtain examination forms (or facsimiles) in advance, and study them carefully. Practice using them. If forms are not available prior to the examination, take the time to read and review them at the examination site to understand how to use the forms *before* beginning any charting procedures. When charting procedures are part of the examination, their function is to measure an examinee's ability to recognize and record oral conditions; copying from previous notes is considered an exam violation and may be grounds for dismissal. Familiarity with examination forms will help avoid confusion and facilitate recording of data on clinical judgments in the appropriate places. Follow exact instructions on *how* and *when* to complete the forms.

## Selection and Recruitment of Examination Patients

The selection of a board patient is the single most important factor in preparing for and successfully completing a clinical examination. Testing agencies develop and maintain highly defined and precise criteria in an effort to equalize difficulty in the examination. The agencies detail specific oral conditions as criteria for patient acceptability, including the number of teeth and surfaces that must have subgingival calculus, and acceptable ranges of sulcular probing depths. Most examinations require a patient with "moderate" to "heavy" subgingival calculus deposits. Patients exhibiting only plaque biofilm or supragingival deposits are probably inadequate to present a valid test of the examinee's skills. A patient with grossly heavy calculus or severe periodontal disease is likely too difficult for the purposes of a clinical examination.

Testing agencies do not provide patients. This responsibility belongs to the examinee. Some schools assist their students in patient recruitment and may allow examinees who are not students to screen patients before a board examination. Ultimately, however, *it is the responsibility of the examinee to present an appropriate patient.* Examiners make the final decision regarding acceptability. Dental hygiene educators and other licensed practitioners are not calibrated to testing agency standards. Patient selection is integral to the examination; it is part of the test. Success or failure on the examination often hinges on submitting a patient who meets the criteria—this crucial decision must not be delegated to an instructor or other licensed dental professionals. It is risky to present a marginally qualifying patient or to *design* the treatment selection by prescaling in hopes of an "easier" examination. Having a patient rejected results in enormous stress on the examinee, grading penalties or failure of the examination, the loss of treatment time, or all these consequences.

Historically, examinees have exhibited incredible resourcefulness in recruiting patients. Family and friends are primary sources. The college campus or one's personal dentist or dental hygienist also serves as a potential patient source. Students and staff at hospitals are frequently recruited. Many examinees have contacted local police and fire stations. Sometimes, graduating classes organize a collective effort to recruit patients, as well as backup patients, for the entire class. Examinees have been known to advertise online or in local newspapers to obtain patients. Follow any institutional policies relating to advertising and recruiting patients. Some schools have strict guidelines regarding this.

Stress can be avoided by beginning a search for patients well in advance of the examination. Maintain professionalism in all contacts with potential patients. The pressures of a high-stakes board examination do not supersede ethical considerations. A patient's personal, oral, and systemic health needs extend beyond the day of the examination and therefore must be given due consideration. Most testing agencies require some type of "continuing care" form to advise the patient of additional treatment that may be necessary but not provided during the examination.

Patient selection is dictated by the testing agency's defined criteria. Criteria may stipulate requirements for age; systemic health status; minimum number of teeth; combination of molars, premolars, and incisors; calculus deposits; periodontal conditions; radiographs; and more. The requirements also include informed consent from the patient for treatment, confidentiality, and adherence to universal precautions for infection control. Carefully review *all* prerequisites before recruiting patients.

In addition to published criteria, take into consideration the attitude and cooperativeness of the patient. Ascertain the patient's pain threshold and tolerance to treatment procedures. Advise the patient of the time commitment. Clinical examinations usually require long treatment sessions, waiting periods, and evaluation and instrumentation by multiple examiners. If patients are not adequately prepared for the demands of the examination, difficult situations can develop. Refusing to cooperate, threatening to leave, and actually leaving the examination are potential scenarios that must be circumvented. Advise the patient of the purposes of the examination, its importance to your future career, the treatment that will be provided, the examiners' role, the examination schedule, and delays that may arise. When patients understand the purpose and format of the board examination, most are supportive of the profession's efforts to ensure the competence of practitioners and are appreciative of the dental hygiene care to be received.

Finding the "perfect" patient who satisfies all criteria is challenging. It is prudent to recruit more than one patient for backup purposes. Inform these patients that they may not be needed for the examination, but if willing, they may be able to sit for another examinee. Stay in contact with any patients who have been recruited. Confirm the time and date, transportation or parking arrangements, and exact meeting locations.

## Clinical Examination Formats

Clinical examinations provide a reliable third-party assessment of examinees' patient-focused skills and judgments. Each testing program has distinct examination protocols, procedures, requirements, and forms. Examinees preparing to take a clinical examination *must contact the testing agency responsible for administering the examination* to obtain its test specifications (see Box 1.1). This chapter provides only a general overview.

Four basic categories of clinical competencies are typically included in regional and state clinical examinations: (1) appropriate patient and treatment selection, (2) calculus detection and removal, (3) oral and head and neck assessment, and (4) tissue management. Components within these areas may include dental and periodontal charting, extraoral and intraoral examination, charting the location of subgingival deposits, and removal of extrinsic stain, plaque, and supragingival calculus. Root debridement and removal of subgingival calculus are universal requirements. As previously noted, specific requirements for case acceptance vary among examinations. All regional examinations mandate a treatment submission of a minimum of six teeth; some require the teeth to be in one quadrant but allow for a limited number of additional teeth. Patient acceptability criteria also include a specific number of "qualifying" subgingival deposits. Typically, the number of anterior teeth that may be included in the treatment submission is limited, and a certain number of posterior teeth in proximal contact must be included. Examiners evaluate the treatment selection. If the patient does not meet the criteria, at a minimum, points are deducted; at a maximum, patient rejection results in failure of the examination.

Some examination requirements, although potentially affecting the examination outcome, are not actually scored. Acceptable client age and health criteria are prime examples of "nongraded" requirements. Acceptable probing depths are another such requirement. Diagnostic-quality radiographs must be submitted with the patient, although the radiographs may not be a graded feature. Some agencies require a full-mouth series, or panograph, and bitewing radiographs, both exposed within a prescribed time frame. Others require only periapicals and bitewings of the teeth in the treatment submission. Radiographs of "nondiagnostic quality" will result in point deductions, negative impact on patient acceptance and the ability to continue the examination, or both.

Allotted clinic time is another variable factor. Most board examinations place specific time limits for the completion of assignments. If an examinee has one or more treatment selections rejected, it is likely that a point deduction, loss of treatment time, failure of the examination, or all these consequences will be incurred. Pain management for the patient is addressed by various means. Most testing agencies permit administration of local anesthetic agents by the examinee in compliance with the host school's state practice act. Testing agency protocols range from confirmation of formal education in administration of local anesthesia to successful completion of an examination on local anesthesia delivery. Some agencies also have provisions for "qualified" licensed practitioners to administer the local anesthesia. Verify the authorization for the delivery of local anesthetics with the testing agency and the regulatory board *before* the examination.

In addition to patient-based testing in the clinic, some regional testing agencies utilize assessment on simulated patient cases at computer testing centers or at school testing sites. The knowledge, skills, and judgments necessary to provide competent entry-level dental hygiene care are evaluated in a standardized examination. Both the physical patient-based section and the simulation section must be passed for successful completion of the examination. Testing agencies may also provide written or clinical examinations for expanded function procedures, such as local anesthesia, nitrous oxide, or restorative procedures. These are administered separately and require a separate registration and fee.

## Examination Results

No uniform scoring system for regional or state board clinical examinations exists. Scoring is linked to the content and design of each examination. In general, clinical board examinations use a system of "weighting" to emphasize the importance or recognize the complexity of certain skills sets and treatment procedures. For example, dental hygiene practice surveys show that competency in scaling and root planing is more critical than competency in stain removal. Consequently, in examination development, when both components are measured, scaling and root planing are weighted with more point value than is stain removal. An examinee should strive to demonstrate competence in all skills that are evaluated in an examination but may choose to concentrate time and effort on each area in proportion to the weighted significance built into the examination.

The testing agency must be contacted for all performance criteria and the defined cutoff point separating acceptable performance from unacceptable performance (see Box 1.1).

### Ethical and Legal Issues

Because professional conduct and ethical behavior are central to the practice of dental hygiene, all testing agencies have stipulations for penalties, such as point deduction or immediate failure of the examination for infractions. Examples of improper and/or unethical conduct include, but are not limited to, the following:

- Violating standards as defined in the *Examination Guide*
- Evidence of dishonesty or misrepresentation during the application or course of the examination
- Misappropriation or damage of equipment during the examination
- Treatment of teeth other than those approved or assigned by examiners
- Receiving assistance from another practitioner or using unauthorized aids
- Altering examination records or radiographs
- Improper record keeping or failure to properly document anesthetic use
- Breach of infection control standards
- Causing excessive tissue trauma
- Rude or abusive behavior
- Continuing to work after the established cutoff time
- Disregard for patient welfare or comfort
- Use of cell phones, cameras, or electronic devices

Examinees found to have engaged in improper or unethical conduct may be denied reexamination for 1 full year. Testing agencies reserve the right to take other reasonable actions as deemed appropriate. Infractions are reportable to all state licensing jurisdictions, the examinee's school, other testing agencies, and professional organizations. Examinees failed for dishonesty may be permanently ineligible for licensue.

## PREPARING FOR CLINICAL BOARD EXAMINATIONS

Contact the state board office to obtain a licensure application. Note all requirements, including which board examinations are accepted and any related conditions or restrictions. Consult the current state dental practice act as well as the rules and regulations for this information. Some jurisdictions require successful completion of local anesthesia, nitrous oxide, and restorative examinations in addition to the dental hygiene examination. Prepare a scheduled timeline for satisfying all licensure requirements. List pertinent examination dates, as well as the testing agency's published time frame for releasing examination results.

1. Obtain the testing agency's examination schedule, application forms, *Examination Guide*, and any official information pertaining to the examination. Most testing agencies have this information available online. Review the information carefully well in advance of the examination.
2. Review all the application material, and flag the desired examination's application deadline. Note examination requirements, including eligibility and documentation that must be provided, client requirements, instruments, and supplies.
3. Assemble the credentials necessary to sit for the examination. These credentials may include school transcripts, the NBDHE score, a copy of the diploma, current cardiopulmonary resuscitation (CPR) certification, evidence of malpractice or liability insurance, and a passport-quality photograph. Retain copies of everything.
4. Check the testing agency's website for *Frequently Asked Questions*. This section can provide insights and coping strategies to enhance confident preparation.
5. Begin searching for eligible patients. Present prospective patients with a clear and professional explanation of the patient's role as well as your own in the examination.
6. For examinees still in school, many dental hygiene programs conduct "mock boards" as a trial practice run. Additional clinical experience with patients whose difficulty level is commensurate with board requirements is likely to be helpful as well.
7. Practicing dental hygienists can set up clinical simulations of board requirements using the examination's specified oral conditions and time constraints to evaluate clinical skills through critical self-assessment.
8. For dental hygienists who have been out of practice, many dental and dental hygiene schools offer continuing education programs. Review courses need to be investigated and pursued well before the examination date.
9. Obtain the required examination instruments, and practice using them.
10. Obtain examination forms before the test, and become familiar with them. If unavailable, study the Forms section of the *Examination Guide.*
11. Be observant of the tooth-numbering system used in the examination—it must be applied accurately. Noncompliance can result in charting errors or incorrectly identifying which teeth are assigned by examiners.
12. A few days before the examination, prepare your clinic attire, and organize instruments and supplies. Confirm arrangements with the patient(s) regarding time, date, location, and relevant directions. Check in with the patient again the night before the examination.
13. If taking the examination at an unfamiliar testing site, tour the clinical facilities before the examination.
14. Plan to arrive at the testing site on time, taking into consideration traffic and parking difficulties as well as the time required for locating the operatory, setting up, and orienting to the clinic. Avoid starting the day feeling rushed and distracted.

15. At the examination, listen closely to instructions, and read thoroughly all materials provided. Failure to read and follow instructions is a common denominator in problems experienced by examinees.
16. *Relax,* and concentrate on the high-quality dental hygiene care that you are able to provide because of your professional education and experience. Test-coping mechanisms are provided in Box 1.3.

## FUTURE TRENDS IN CLINICAL EXAMINATIONS AND LICENSURE

In response to a growing demand for greater portability of credentials in dental hygiene and dentistry, most states long ago implemented licensure by credentials for active practitioners. Increasingly, many states now not only accept results of multiple clinical examinations for initial licensure (see Fig. 1.1), but also are members of multiple testing agencies (see Box 1.2). An outcome of this overlap is increased competition for the market share among the testing agencies. In states where more than one examination is accepted for initial licensure, schools have a choice of which examination to host. This competition may result in enhancements to the examination process and, with the cross-pollination of examiners, who examine for multiple agencies, could result in an exchange of best practices and more standardized exam procedures. This may eventually lead to a single clinical exam accepted by all jurisdictions.

Debate continues on the appropriateness of the use of humans in clinical examinations. A cohort of educators, students, and some state boards advocate discontinuation of the use of humans, citing both ethical and practical reasons. Some examination agencies have incorporated computer-delivered "simulation exercises," in addition to patient-based testing, for the evaluation of clinical skills. The future will most likely see the patient-based examination disappear, in favor of other methodologies such as portfolios or Objective Structured Clinical Examinations (OSCE). It is generally agreed that a dental hygiene examination constructed, directed, and administered by dental hygienists, based on current and relevant scientific evidence, both benefits the dental hygiene community and provides protection of the public.

Most testing agencies utilize electronic scoring systems to augment efficiency in compiling and releasing examination scores, thus facilitating obtaining licensure in a timely manner. Software tracking of statistical data on examiner scoring and validation can be used to improve examiner training and standardization.

## INTERNATIONAL REQUIREMENTS

In our global culture, interest in working outside our own country is increasingly appealing. International licensure requirements vary significantly. A dental hygienist contemplating employment in another country should contact the ADHA, the ADA, the Canadian Dental Hygienists Association (CDHA), and the International Federation of Dental Hygienists (IFDH) for pertinent information and potential connections. The IFDH has compiled a database with detailed requirements for working as a dental hygienist in many countries. The information is available by clicking the "Working Abroad" tab and then the country of choice on the IFDH website (http://www.ifdh.org/work_abroad.html). Individual resources or personal contacts within the country of destination should also be pursued.

As a starting point, collect documentation of all credentials, including passports or visas, school transcripts, diplomas, licenses, board examination scores, and employment history. Some countries require language proficiency before certification is granted; others require an employment contract before issuing a work permit. Most countries require proof of graduation from an accredited school and successful completion of cognitive and clinical or case-based board examinations, while other countries may request additional information.

## CONTENT AND ORGANIZATION OF THIS REVIEW BOOK

This book presents a review, in outline form, of basic, dental, dental hygiene, and clinical sciences. Each review outline is followed by related questions that test the reader's knowledge of concepts, principles, and theories underlying the practice of dental hygiene. Each chapter contains a section on Evolve entitled "Answers and Rationales," which provides justification for the correct answer and every response in the review questions covering the subject matter. The rationale supporting the correct answer and explanations for incorrect responses are specified. By reviewing these rationales, the reader will be able to confirm facts and reinforce knowledge.

### CASE A

| Synopsis of Patient History<br>Case A | Age: 38<br>Sex : F<br>Height: 5′5″<br>Weight: 295 lb | VITAL SIGNS<br>Blood pressure: 138/86<br>Pulse Rate: 64, regular and steady<br>Respirations: 16 regular, easy |
|---|---|---|

1. Under Care of Physician
   X Yes ☐ No Condition: hypertension, fibrocystic ovaries, pregnancy 2nd term, depression, thyroid replacement medication
2. Hospitalized within the last 5 years
   ☐ Yes X No Reason:
3. Has or had the following conditions:
   hypertension, fibrocystic ovaries, pregnancy, depression, gestational diabetes, low thyroid (thyroid removed at age 18)
4. Current medications: levothyroxine .088 mg, Zoloft 50 mg, Nifedipine 30 mg, insulin, pregnancy vitamins Smokes or uses tobacco products

Continued

## CASE A—CONT'D

5. Is pregnant
   X Yes ☐ No

MEDICAL HISTORY: the patient has a history of hypertension, which began 5 years ago. The patient reports feeling fine and her hypertension is well controlled with medication. The patient is being treated for depression and reports it is also well controlled with medication. Her thyroid was removed at the age of 18 due to early thyroid cancer. The patient has a history of fibrocystic ovaries and used in vitro fertilization for her pregnancy. The patient reports she is in her 6th month of pregnancy with her first child and was recently diagnosed with gestational diabetes. She is currently taking insulin by injection and is able to maintain a healthy range of blood sugar levels (which she checks daily).

DENTAL HISTORY: she grew up with regular dental visits but has had a lapse of care for the past 3 years dependent on her income and lapse of dental insurance.

SOCIAL HISTORY: Caucasian, active 38 year old single woman who lives in Milwaukie, Oregon. She is a CNA working in a local hospital maternal/child department. She drinks diet soda or carbonated soda daily.

CHIEF COMPLAINT: "I need a dental cleaning and I have lost a portion of a filling on the lower right molar. The tooth does not hurt but is sensitive if sweets get stuck in it. My mouth is dryer than it used to be."

CURRENT ORAL HYGIENE STATUS: brushes twice daily with a manual toothbrush. Flosses daily with floss-piks.

**PERIO CHART**

| | 1 | 2 | 3 | 4 | 5 | 6 | 7 | 8 | 9 | 10 | 11 | 12 | 13 | 14 | 15 | 16 |
|---|---|---|---|---|---|---|---|---|---|---|---|---|---|---|---|---|
| F | | 323 | 333 | 323 | 323 | 323 | 323 | 323 | 323 | 223 | 323 | 323 | 323 | 323 | 433 | |
| L | | 323 | 323 | 323 | 322 | 223 | 222 | 323 | 322 | 222 | 222 | 323 | 333 | 323 | 323 | |
| | | | | | | | | | | | | | | | | |
| L | | 323 | 323 | 323 | 323 | 322 | 222 | 222 | 323 | 333 | 223 | 323 | 323 | 323 | 323 | |
| F | | 323 | 323 | 323 | 323 | 323 | 323 | 323 | 323 | 323 | 323 | 323 | 323 | 323 | 333 | |
| | **32** | **31** | **30** | **29** | **28** | **27** | **26** | **25** | **24** | **23** | **22** | **21** | **20** | **19** | **18** | **17** |

Light BOP on # 2, 4, 6, 7, 8, 13, 14, 18, 19, 20, 21, 25, 29 and 30.

### Supplemental Oral Examination Findings

- Short lingual frenum
- Mild attrition on maxillary and mandibular anteriors.
- Gingival description: generalized healthy with mild interproximal inflammation characterized by light bleeding.
- Plaque description: generalized very light plaque interproximals, and light plaque on the facial of 2 and 15
- Occlusion: class I, tendency to III, edge to edge bite on # 6–11.
- Decalcification # 19B, 20D, 2B
- No new carious lesions were detected.

### Radiographs

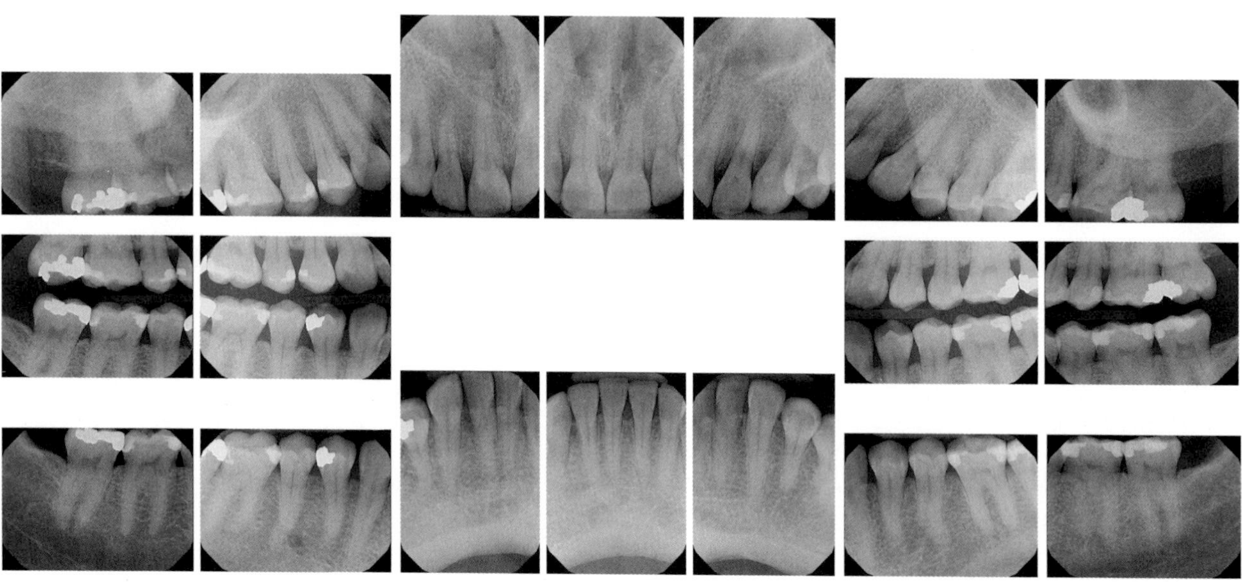

*Use Case A to answer questions 1 to 8.*

1. Based on the radiographs and the assessment findings, the patient's AAP would be classified as:
   a. Healthy
   b. Gingivitis
   c. Periodontitis, Stage I
   d. Periodontitis, Stage 2
   e. Periodontitis, Stage 3
2. Caries risk for this patient would be classified as:
   a. High
   b. Moderate
   c. Low
3. The radiographs indicate which of the following conditions for tooth #20 and #29?
   a. Dilaceration
   b. Abscess
   c. Concrescence
   d. Taurodontism
   e. Gemination
4. The maxillary right premolar PA is elongated. To correct this error, the vertical angulation should be decreased.
   a. Both statements are TRUE
   b. Both statements are FALSE
   c. First statement is TRUE, the second is FALSE
   d. First statement is FALSE, the second is TRUE
5. Treatment alterations for this patient should be?
   a. Morning appointment is recommended
   b. The patient would require premedication
   c. Avoid laying the patient back
   d. No alterations are necessary
6. Do the radiographs meet the requirements for a diagnostic full mouth set of films?
   a. Yes
   b. No
7. Which of her medications may be contributing to her symptoms of dry mouth?
   a. Levothyroxine
   b. Zoloft
   c. Nifedipine
   d. A & B
   e. B & C
8. Which of the following may be contributing to the wear on her anterior teeth?
   a. Medications
   b. Bruxism
   c. Occlusion
   d. A and B
   e. All of the above

## CASE B

| Synopsis of Patient History<br>Case B | Age: 62<br>Sex : F<br>Height: 5′4″<br>Weight: 175 lb | Vital Signs<br>Blood pressure: 132/84<br>Pulse Rate: 78 BPM, regular and weak<br>Respirations: 12 RPM, steady and deep |
|---|---|---|

1. Under Care of Physician
   X Yes ☐ No Condition: hypertension, rheumatoid arthritis, depression, migraines, hypothyroid
2. Hospitalized within the last 5 years
   X Yes ☐ No Reason: kidney infection caused by an antibiotic–resistant bacteria (1 year ago) and broken right leg (3 years ago)
3. Has or had the following conditions: hypertension, depression, low thyroid, kidney infection, gestational diabetes, basal and squamous cell skin lesions on face, chest, and head (have been treated and receives yearly screening), endometriosis
4. Current Medications: levothyroxine .075 mg, citalopram 20 mg, propranolol 10 mg for BP and migraines, hydroxychloroquine sulfate (Plaquenil) 400 mg, leflunomide 10 mg daily for rheumatoid arthritis, Excedrin Migraine, Zantac, folic acid, vitamin D
5. Smokes or uses tobacco products
   ☐ Yes X No
6. Is pregnant
   ☐ Yes X No
7. Allergies noted to Penicillin and Sulfa

MEDICAL HISTORY: the patient has a history of hypertension, which began 2 years ago. All conditions have or are being successfully managed with medications. The patient states she is experiencing headaches at least 5 times per week and believes they are related to stress.

DENTAL HISTORY: regular dental visits as an adult. As a child she did not go to the dentist. All restorations were placed in her twenties with crowns being placed as restorations wore out. Currently wears a night guard to help with recession, grinding, and headaches. Her last crown was placed over 10 years ago. She had a composite filling replaced last year on #18 occlusal due to a defective margin.

SOCIAL HISTORY: she is an active 62-year-old, married woman who lives in Seattle, WA. She is a college professor in a community college. No history of alcohol or tobacco use.

CHIEF COMPLAINT: "I need a dental cleaning and have sensitivity to brushing on the lingual of #18. My mouth is very dry."

CURRENT ORAL HYGIENE STATUS: brushes twice daily with a power toothbrush, ultrasoft head, and Crest toothpaste. Flosses daily. Rinses with Act several times per week.

*Continued*

## CASE B—CONT'D

**PERIO CHART**

| | 1 | 2 | 3 | 4 | 5 | 6 | 7 | 8 | 9 | 10 | 11 | 12 | 13 | 14 | 15 | 16 |
|---|---|---|---|---|---|---|---|---|---|---|---|---|---|---|---|---|
| CAL | | | 343 | 332 | 223 | 323 | 322 | 222 | 222 | 223 | 323 | 332 | 333 | 445 | 545 | |
| Rec | | | 2 | 1 | | | | | | | | 1 | 11 | 222 | 222 | |
| F | | | 323 | 322 | 223 | 323 | 322 | 222 | 222 | 223 | 323 | 322 | 322 | 223 | 323 | |
| L | | | 323 | 223 | 323 | 223 | 322 | 222 | 222 | 222 | 222 | 323 | 323 | 223 | 324 | |
| Rec | | | 2 | 2 | | | | | | | 1 | 2 | | 3 | 1 | |
| CAL | | | 343 | 343 | 323 | 223 | 322 | 222 | 222 | 222 | 232 | 343 | 323 | 253 | 334 | |
| | | | | | | | | | | | | | | | | |
| CAL | | | 343 | 342 | 232 | 223 | 332 | 222 | 222 | 222 | 222 | 232 | 333 | 443 | 443 | |
| Rec | | | 2 | 2 | 1 | | 1 | 1 | | | | 1 | 1 | 2 | 2 | |
| L | | | 323 | 322 | 222 | 223 | 322 | 222 | 222 | 222 | 222 | 222 | 323 | 423 | 423 | |
| F | | | 433 | 324 | 323 | 323 | 322 | 322 | 222 | 323 | 323 | 322 | 323 | 424 | 324 | |
| Rec | | | 2 | 1 | 1 | | | | | | | 1 | 1 | 2 | 2 | |
| CAL | | | 453 | 334 | 333 | 323 | 322 | 322 | 222 | 323 | 323 | 332 | 333 | 444 | 344 | |
| | 32 | 31 | 30 | 29 | 28 | 27 | 26 | 25 | 24 | 23 | 22 | 21 | 20 | 19 | 18 | 17 |

**Supplemental Oral Examination Findings**

Generalized recession, maxillary tori, aphthous ulcer measuring 2 mm x 3 mm on buccal mucosa across from #2. Class II furcations located on #19 and #30. Implant #8 was solid with no inflammation present.

No mobility, fremitus, bleeding on probing, or suppuration noted.

**Radiographs**

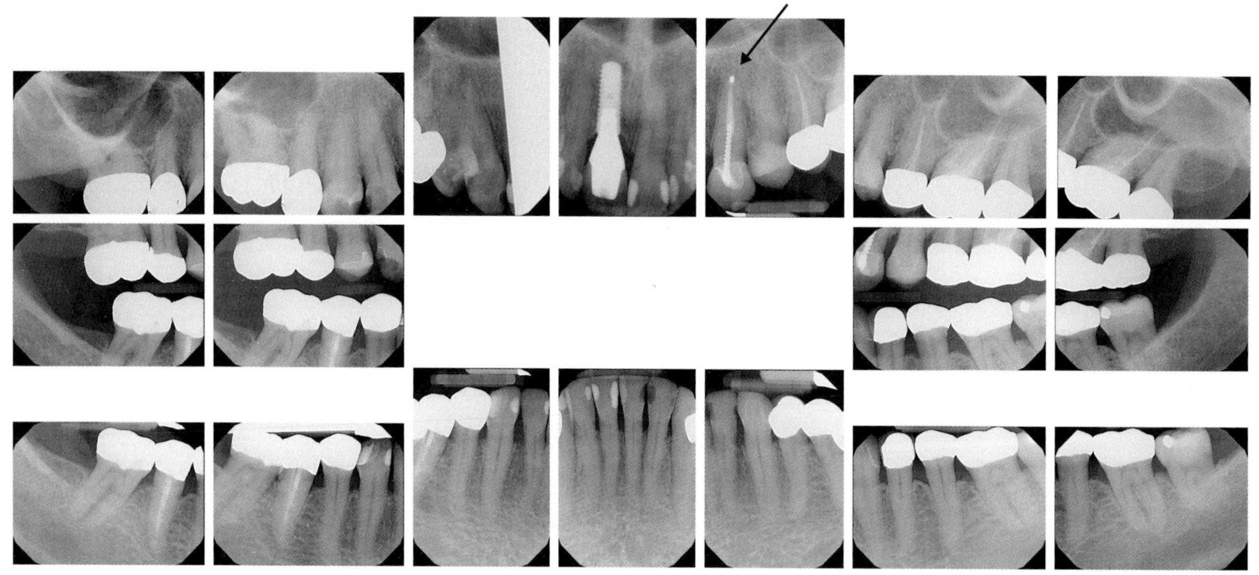

**Intraoral Photos**

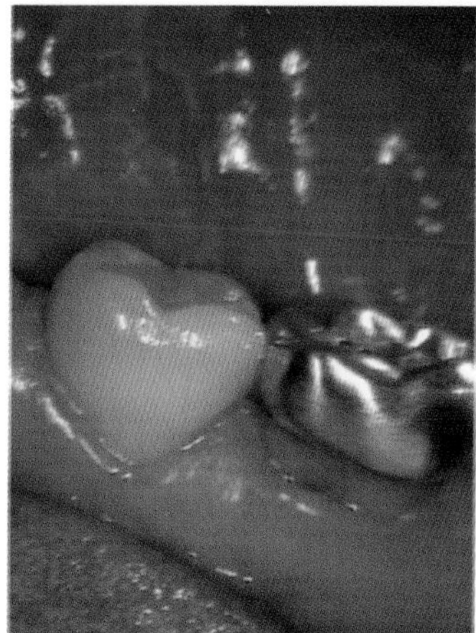

***Use Case B to answer questions 9 to 15.***

9. Sensitivity on #18 is most likely related to which of the following conditions:
   a. Age
   b. Brushing
   c. Recession
   d. Restoration
   e. Periodontal disease
10. The patient's AAP based on the radiographs and CAL would be classified as:
   a. Healthy
   b. Gingivitis
   c. Periodontitis, Stage I
   d. Periodontitis, Stage 2
   e. Periodontitis, Stage 3
11. The implant was a result of a fractured root. Do the assessment records show evidence of peri-implantitis?
   a. Yes
   b. No
12. What is MOST likely contributing to her dry mouth?
   a. Rheumatoid arthritis
   b. Medications
   c. Mouth breathing
   d. Hypertension
13. The arrow is pointing to a radiopaque dot on #11. Based on the radiographic appearance, what type of material is this?
   a. Amalgam
   b. Gutta percha
   c. Composite
   d. Calcium hydroxide
14. All of the following are likely sequela to this patient's teeth condition, except one. Which one is the exception?
   a. Abrasion
   b. Attrition
   c. Sensitivity
   d. Erosion
15. Which oral hygiene aide would be most appropriate to recommend for plaque removal at the gingival margin of #19 lingual?
   a. Toothbrush
   b. Proxabrush
   c. Perio-Aid
   d. Tuft Toothbrush
   e. Stimudent

## CASE C

| Synopsis of Patient History<br>Case C | Age: 8<br>Sex: M<br>Height: 4'5"<br>Weight: 65 lbs. | VITAL SIGNS<br>Blood pressure: 80/40<br>Pulse Rate: 78 BPM<br>Respirations: 16 RPM |
|---|---|---|

1. Under Care of Physician
   ☐ Yes X No
2. Hospitalized within the last 5 years
   ☐ Yes X No
3. Has or had the following conditions: strep throat 6 mo. ago
   Current Medications: none
4. Smokes or uses tobacco products
   ☐ Yes X No

*Continued*

## CASE C—CONT'D

5. Is pregnant
☐ Yes X No

MEDICAL HISTORY: the patient is a healthy child.

DENTAL HISTORY: this is the second time in his life he has been to a dentist for a dental exam. His last visit was 2 years ago when he had some fillings done. He currently has dental coverage under the Oregon Health Plan.

SOCIAL HISTORY: he is a third-grade Latino student who speaks both English and Spanish. His parents do not speak English.

CHIEF COMPLAINT: "Nothing."

CURRENT ORAL HYGIENE STATUS: states that he brushes almost every day with a toothpaste with fluoride in it but does not know how long he brushes. Does not clean interproximally. He just moved into a fluoridated area of the state.

PERIO CHART: there were no pockets over 3 mm, no recession, no suppuration, no bleeding.

**Supplemental Oral Examination Findings**

Decay noted on #3 lingual, A mesial, B distal, I mesial & distal, J mesial, L distal, T mesial, and 30 buccal. Moderate plaque at the gingival margin and interproximal. Mild marginal inflammation characterized by redness and mild puffiness.

**Radiographs**

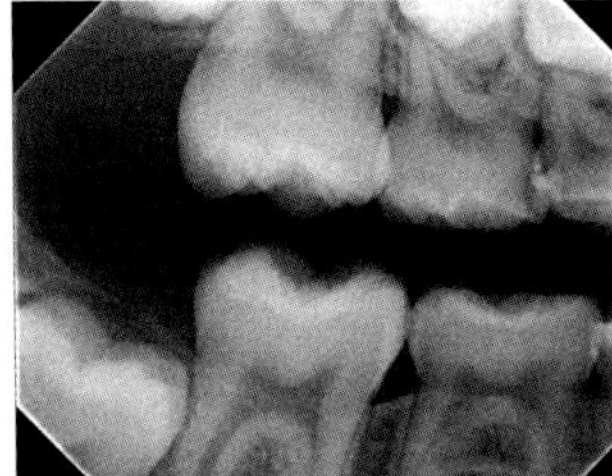
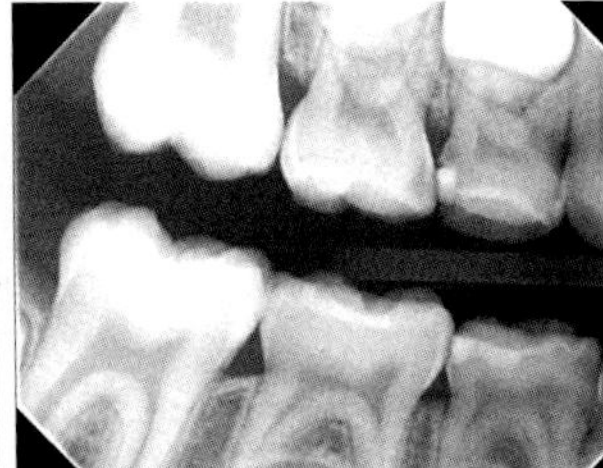
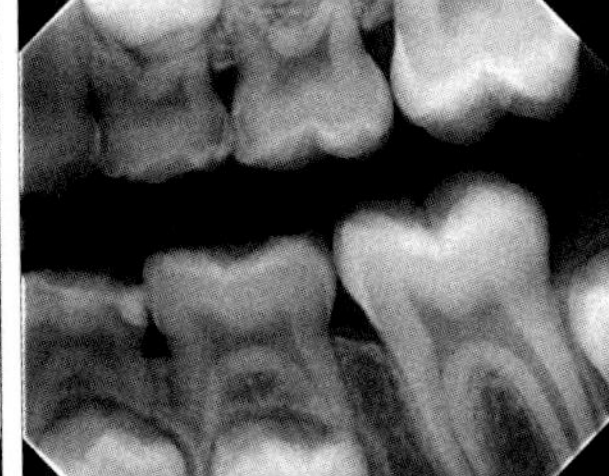
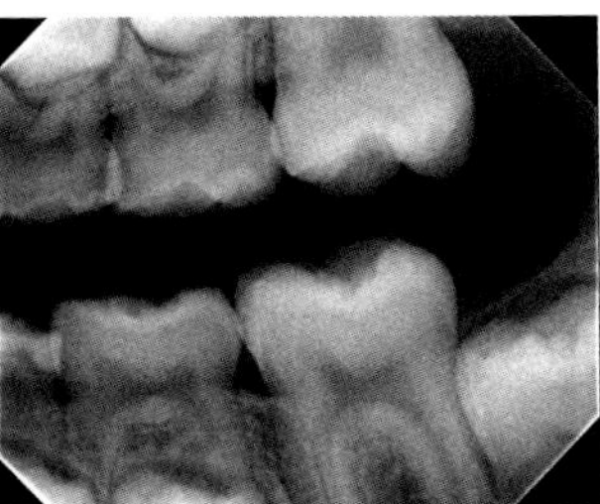

***Use Case C to answer questions 16 to 20***

16. The mother would like #J removed rather than restored. What is the BEST reason the tooth should be restored rather than extracted?
    a. A restoration will be more cost-effective.
    b. Jaw development will not be delayed
    c. Discomfort will be lessened for the child
    d. Its permanent replacement is years from erupting
17. What professional plaque removal method is BEST for this patient?
    a. Toothbrush
    b. Rubber cup polish
    c. Ultrasonic scaler
    d. Fluoride mouthrinse
18. What is the most likely cause of his decay?
    a. Diet
    b. Lack of fluoride
    c. Lack of knowledge about the decay process
    d. Lack of interproximal plaque removal
19. Earlier this year, the patient had a high fever. Which of the teeth are MOST likely to show enamel disruption upon eruption?
    a. Maxillary 2nd premolar
    b. Maxillary canines
    c. Mandibular canines
    d. Mandibular 3rd molar
20. Should a translator be present during care for this patient?
    a. No, the child is able to understand directions from the dental hygienist
    b. No, there is no requirement for a translator with children
    c. Yes, it would help with communication with the child
    d. Yes, it will be necessary to gain consent for treatment

## CASE D

Synopsis of Patient History
Case D

Age: 48
Sex: M
Height: 5′5″
Weight: 180 lb

VITAL SIGNS
Blood pressure: 126/96
Pulse Rate: 75 BPM
Respirations: 16 RPM

1. Under Care of Physician
   X Yes ☐No Condition: ADD
2. Hospitalized within the last 5 years
   ☐ Yes X No Reason:
3. Has or had the following conditions: Attention Deficit Disorder
4. Current Medications: Adderall 25 mg 2x/day but does not take it regularly
5. Smokes or uses tobacco products
   X Yes ☐No
6. Is pregnant
   ☐ Yes X No

MEDICAL HISTORY: the patient has a history of ADD, states his BP is only high at the dental office.

DENTAL HISTORY: he grew up with irregular dental visits. He has had a lapse of care for the past 15 years due to high dental anxiety. His last visit was for urgent dental care and #15 was extracted. Has had three separate injuries to the jaw. He has a history of clenching and grinding of his teeth.

SOCIAL HISTORY: currently self-employed as a handyman.

CHIEF COMPLAINT: pain on upper anteriors, stating the teeth do not hurt but are sensitive to sweets. General sensitively to hot and cold. "My mouth is dry".

**Current oral hygiene status:**

*Perio Chart*

| | 1 | 2 | 3 | 4 | 5 | 6 | 7 | 8 | 9 | 10 | 11 | 12 | 13 | 14 | 15 | 16 |
|---|---|---|---|---|---|---|---|---|---|---|---|---|---|---|---|---|
| F | | | | | | 447 | 644 | 343 | 445 | 343 | 434 | | 433 | | | |
| L | | | | | | 448 | 654 | 333 | 535 | 333 | 535 | | 433 | | | |
| | | | | | | | | | | | | | | | | |
| L | | 455 | 545 | 555 | 445 | 544 | | | 444 | 446 | 445 | 457 | | 665 | 556 | |
| F | | 454 | 546 | 434 | 644 | 545 | | | 333 | 447 | 444 | 515 | | 576 | 556 | |
| | 32 | 31 | 30 | 29 | 28 | 27 | 26 | 25 | 24 | 23 | 22 | 21 | 20 | 19 | 18 | 17 |

- Gingival description: generalized severe inflammation characterized by red rolled margins and bulbous papilla and bleeding on probing
- Plaque description: generalized light plaque present on all surfaces
- #13 class II mobility

**Supplemental Oral Examination Findings**

- Frequent intake of simple carbs throughout the day
- New carious lesions: #6 F, #7 MFD, # 9D, #10 fractured at the gumline, #13 F, #19 fractured MOFL restoration, #20 retained root tip, #21 F, #28 recurrent decay MFD, #30 B, #31 B
- Smokes less than 10 cigarettes per day
- History of prior periodontal disease and has not been stabilized
- Visible plaque
- Bridge from 24–27
- Heavy calculus
- Prior tooth loss has been due to decay and/or loss of bone
- Thyroid was large and firm on palpation

## CASE D—CONT'D

**Radiographs**

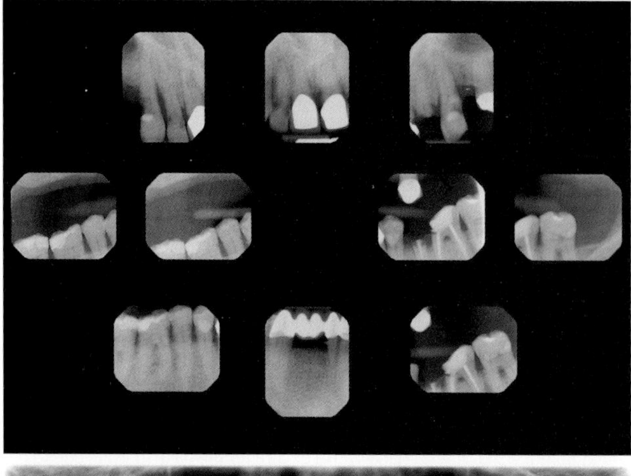

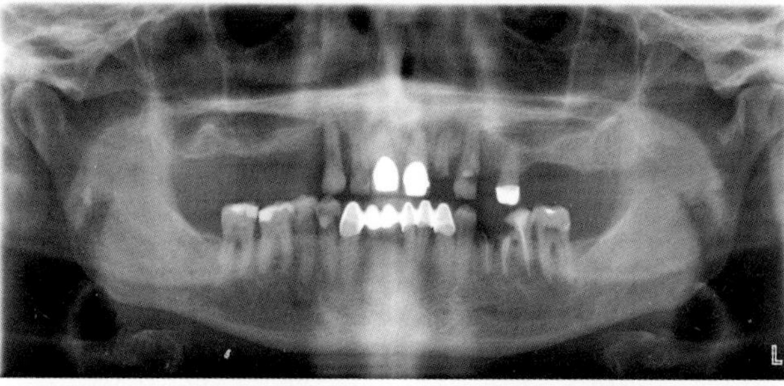


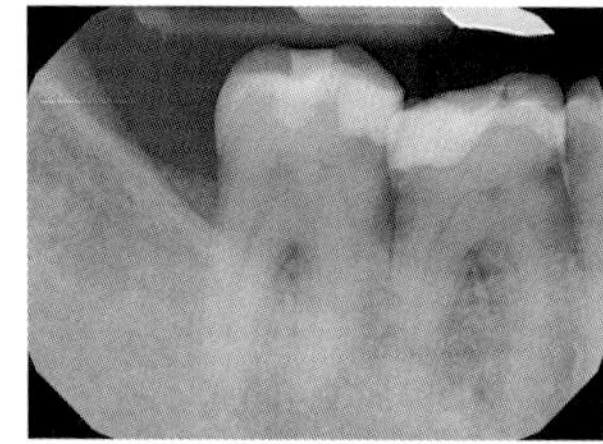

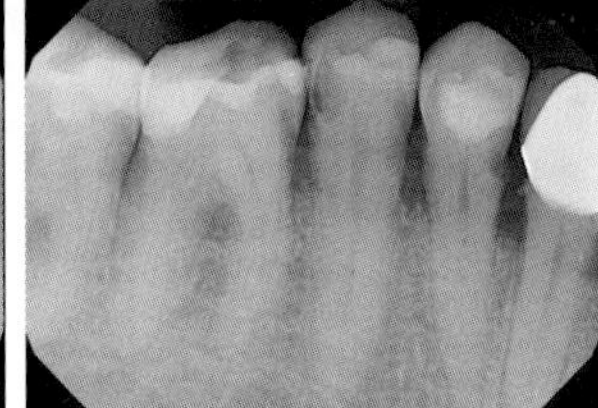

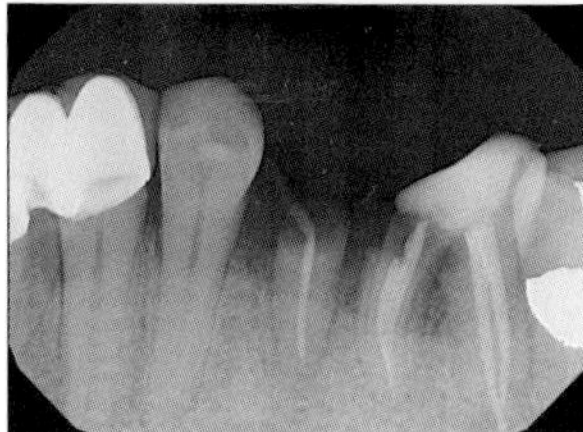

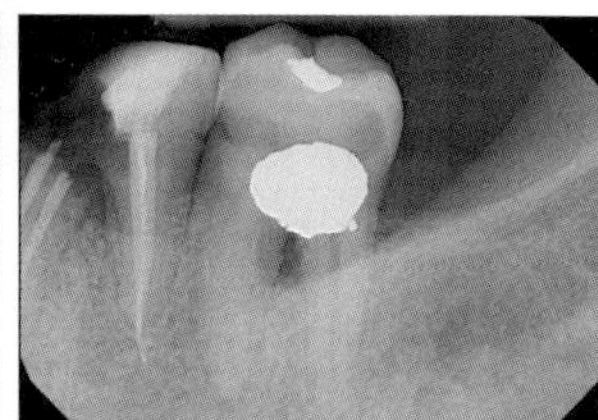

***Use Case D to answer questions 21 to 27***

21. Class III furcations are evident on which teeth?
    a. 31
    b. 18 and 19
    c. 30 and 31
    d. 18, 19, and 31
    e. 18, 19, 30, and 31
22. Calculus buildup would be considered:
    a. Light
    b. Moderate
    c. Heavy
23. His AAP classification would be considered:
    a. Healthy
    b. Gingivitis
    c. Periodontitis, Stage I
    d. Periodontitis, Stage 2
    e. Periodontitis, Stage 3
24. Which of the following would be the BEST option to help with the patient's anxiety?
    a. Morning appointment
    b. Nitrous oxide
    c. Motivational interviewing
    d. Local anesthesia
25. All of the following would be appropriate referrals EXCEPT:
    a. Periodontist
    b. Physician
    c. Endodontist
    d. Prosthodontist
    e. Orthodontist
26. The patient's complaint of sensitivity is most likely related to:
    a. Bone loss
    b. Furcation
    c. Fractured restoration
    d. Decay
    e. Broken tooth

27. During treatment, the patient complains of pain in his chest and left shoulder. What is the MOST likely explanation for the pain?
    a. Anxiety attack
    b. Myocardial infarction
    c. Angina attack
    d. Stroke

## HOW TO USE THIS BOOK IN STUDYING

A. Review one section of the content at a time. Study the material outlined in the section. Refer to other textbooks, websites, and references to research additional details if any area is unclear.
B. After reviewing the content, answer the review questions that immediately follow. As each question is answered, write a few words about why that response is correct; justify the response selected. If your response is a guess, make a special mark to identify it as such. This will enable ready identification of areas that need further review and clarification. Remember to analyze a question, narrow the choices, and select the correct or best answer.
C. Score yourself using the answers provided on the Evolve website. If the item was answered correctly, compare the reason noted for selecting that answer with the listed rationales. For each item answered incorrectly, review the correct answer and its rationale. Go back to the chapter pertaining to that subject, and research information in your reference material. Carefully review all the questions and rationales for the items identified as guesses to ensure mastery of the material.
D. After an interval of several days or weeks, review the chapters and answer the questions again. If the same items are missed, further study of that content material is necessary.

## COMPLETION OF THE REVIEW PROCESS

Board examinations can be attempted with confidence and success after completing the comprehensive review presented in this book; assessing areas of strength and weaknesses with the aid of the chapter review questions; reinforcing concentrated study of particular material pinpointed by the review; becoming familiar with the board examination process, protocol, and purpose; and following instructions for preparation. Preparation for board examinations actually begins with the accredited dental hygiene program's first class and continues throughout the educational process. This book is designed to present a cohesive, comprehensive review of that professional educational base, to reinforce existing knowledge, and to provide guidance for areas requiring more concentrated study.

## REFERENCES


1. American Dental Association. *National Board Dental Hygiene Examination (NBDHE) 2021 Candidate Guide*. Chicago: American Dental Association; 2021. Joint Commission on National Board Dental Examinations https://www.ada.org/en/jcnde/examinations/nb-guides.
2. National Dental Hygiene Certification Board. *National Dental Hygiene Certification Board Examination (NDHCE) Candidate Guide*. Ottawa: ON Canada; 2019.

# 2

# Histology and Embryology

*Joanne Pacheco*

During the intraoral examination, a dental hygienist must distinguish normal structures, variants of normal structures, and developmental abnormalities from pathology. A clear sense of developmental processes and tissue histology provides the background for competent assessment and evaluation.

Knowledge of tissue components and embryologic tissue origin supports an understanding of the physiologic changes that take place during the course of disease progression. This knowledge also provides insight into how tissue is capable of responding to a pathologic condition. This chapter contains basic general histologic information, with a focus on oral tissue components and oral and facial development. A dental hygienist uses this information to formulate a dental hygiene care plan, evaluate the outcomes of treatment, and make appropriate referrals to health care professionals as needed.

## GENERAL HISTOLOGY

### Cells

A. Smallest structures and functionally self-contained units in the body; they vary in size, shape, and surface, depending on functional specialization (Fig. 2.1)
B. Cells possess similar common physiologic properties that permit:
   1. Excitability
      a. Change in the environment stimulates the cell to bring about a response to adapt to a change
      b. Example—nerve cells conduct impulses
   2. Synthesis
      a. Cells must have the ability to form substances that produce products to aid in the body's function
      b. Example—glands synthesize and secrete products to aid bodily functions
   3. Membrane transport
      a. Fluids, chemical elements, and compounds must have the ability to move both in and out of cells
      b. Example—nutrients are transported across the epithelial lining of the gastrointestinal tract
   4. Reproduction
      a. Cells must have the ability to preserve the species by giving rise to offspring
      b. Example—union of a sperm and ovum can lead to the formation of an offspring
C. The building blocks of tissues in the body are attached to each other and to noncellular surfaces by cell junctions; the structures of various types of cell junctions depend on location and function; the types of junctions are:
   1. Desmosomes—cell-to-cell attachments; this type of attachment is found between ameloblasts (enamel-forming cells) and cells of the stratified squamous epithelium that lines the oral cavity
   2. Tight junctions—cells attach to each other by fusion of their cell membranes; adjacent odontoblasts (dentin-forming cells) form tight junctions that prevent substances in the pulp from passing into the dentin
   3. Gap junctions—contain a channel that runs between cells for communication of cell electrical impulses and passage of molecules; this type of junction is present among some odontoblasts, allowing them to coordinate their activity
   4. Hemidesmosome—the attachment of a cell to a noncellular surface; the basal layer cells of stratified squamous epithelium attach to the basement membrane by hemidesmosomes; this attachment mechanism is present in the epithelial attachment to the tooth; the epithelial attachment refers to the basal lamina and hemidesmosomes that connect the junctional epithelium of the soft tissue to the tooth surface
D. Cells are surrounded by a cell membrane that separates them from the extracellular environment; cell membrane encloses all components of the cell:
   1. Cytoplasm
   2. Organelles
   3. Inclusions
   4. Nucleus

#### Specialization

A. Differentiation
   1. Cells that recognize one another will group together
   2. Cancer cells do not recognize each other
B. Organization of chemicals
   1. Chemicals appear early in the development of the embryo
   2. Endocrine substances are produced by one type of cell and can affect other types of cells
C. Cells → tissues → organs → organ systems

#### Cell Membrane

A. Referred to as plasma membrane or plasmalemma; usually too thin to be seen with a light microscope; average width is approximately 7 nanometers (nm); considered selectively permeable because it controls passage of materials into and out of the cell

1. It surrounds the cell and is semipermeable, allowing some substances to pass through it and others to be excluded
2. Its permeability may vary selectively by porous openings
3. Selective permeability characteristics
   a. Protecting cell from external environment
   b. Permitting entrance and exit of selected substrates

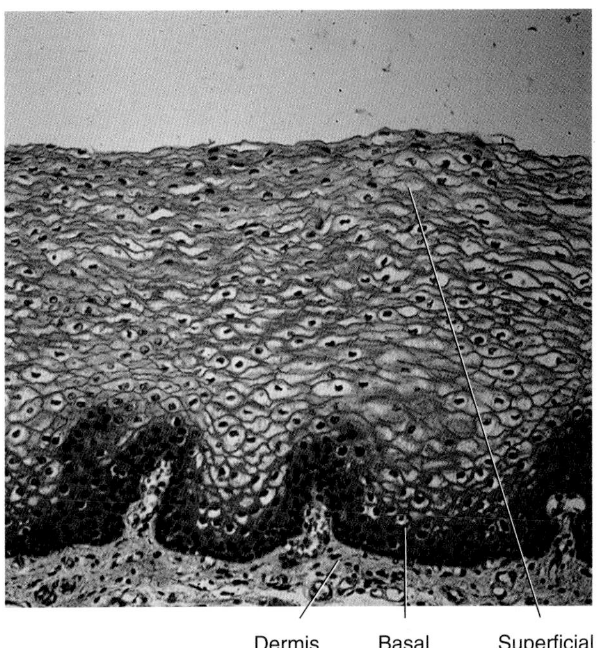


**Fig. 2.1** Typical cell. (From Chiego D. *Essentials of Oral Histology and Embryology, a Clinical Approach.* 4th ed. St. Louis: Elsevier; 2014.)

   c. Using active transport, passive transport, or facilitated diffusion
4. Its composition is a 3:2 ratio of proteins to lipids; lipids and proteins are the major components
5. Its structure is trilaminar, with a bipolar membrane and a central core of lipids between two layers of protein
6. The 0.8-nm pores in the surface allow diffusion of small, lipid-insoluble substances

B. Trilaminar structure composed of two facing layers of lipid molecules, into which large globular proteins are inserted (Fig. 2.2)

## Cytoplasm

A. Translucent, aqueous, homogeneous gel enclosed in the cell by the cell membrane; organelles and inclusions are suspended in the cytoplasmic gel
B. All metabolic activities of the cell occur in the cytoplasm, including:
   1. Assimilation (digestion)
   2. Synthesis of substances such as proteins, proteoglycans, and glycoproteins
   3. A transport medium in which all nutrients and metabolites are carried from one organelle to another
   4. Presence of enzymes and electrolytes, in which specific metabolic reactions take place (e.g., glycolysis)

## Nucleus

A. Controls the two major functions of the cell
   1. Chemical reactions—synthesizing activities; determines nutrient needs
   2. Stores genetic information of the cell

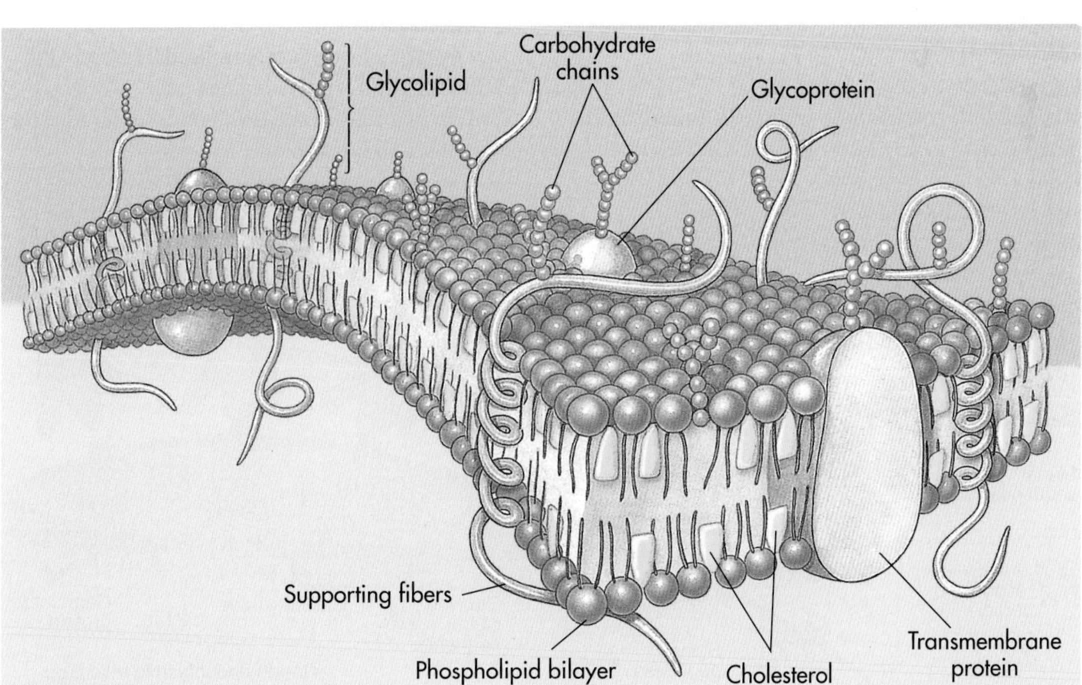


**Fig. 2.2** Fluid mosaic model. Schematic, three-dimensional view of the fluid mosaic model of membrane structure. The lipid bilayer provides the basic structure and serves as a relatively impermeable barrier to most water-soluble molecules. (Modified from Patton KT, Thibodeau GA. *Structure and Function of the Human Body.* 15th ed. St. Louis: Elsevier; 2016.)

B. Genetic information stored in chromosomes for cell duplication; chromosomal deoxyribonucleic acid (DNA); the human nucleus contains 46 chromosomes
C. Chromosomes are visible only during cell division, when they become long, coiled strands; at other times, chromosomal material is dispersed in granular clumps of material called *chromatin*
D. Each nucleus contains one or more round, dense structures referred to as the *nucleolus* (plural, *nucleoli*); these produce ribosomal ribonucleic acid (RNA)—protein plus RNA; the nucleus also is surrounded by a nuclear membrane and contains nuclear matrix with chromosomes

### Synthesis Activities

A. Three types of RNA are necessary for protein synthesis:
   1. Messenger RNA (mRNA) complementary copies of distinct DNA, the genetic code
      a. mRNA can be compared with a tape that contains all the genetic information of proteins, but it must pass through the ribosomes attached to the endoplasmic reticulum (ER)
      b. As the tape passes through the ribosomes, transfer RNA (tRNA) adds the exact amino acid to the newly forming proteins (Fig. 2.3)
   2. tRNA transporter of specific amino acids (building blocks of proteins)
   3. Ribosomal RNA (rRNA)—found floating freely in the cytoplasm (polyribosomes) or attached to the ER
B. Protein synthesis also can occur on polyribosomes floating freely in the cytoplasm; proteins synthesized on the free polyribosomes are used in cellular metabolic processes; proteins synthesized on the ribosomes attached to the ER are transported out of the cell

## Inclusions

A. Transitory, nonliving metabolic byproducts found in the cytoplasm of the cell
B. May appear as lipid droplets, carbohydrate accumulations (e.g., mucopolysaccharides), or engulfed foreign substances

### Lysosomes

A. Membrane-bound organelles responsible for the breakdown of foreign substances that are engulfed by the cell by the process of phagocytosis or pinocytosis
B. Produced by a budding process from the Golgi complex, lysosomes form spherical vesicles containing powerful degradative or hydrolytic enzymes; enzymes are first produced by the ER and then transported to the Golgi complex
C. During phagocytosis, lysosomes fuse with engulfed substances to form a secondary vesicle; the vesicle with digestive materials may remain in the cell as a residual body or may be discharged outside of the cell
D. Vitamins A and E and zinc are important stabilizers for the lysosome's membrane

### Golgi Complex

A. The structure consists of stacks of closely spaced membranous sacs, in which newly formed proteins are concentrated and prepared for export out of the cell (Fig. 2.4)
   1. Small membrane-bound vesicles pinch off from the Golgi complex and form secretory granules (newly formed proteins)
   2. Secretory granules attach to the inside of the cell membrane and are then discharged outside of the cell
B. Responsible for secreting to the external environment a variety of proteins synthesized on the ER.
C. Major site of membrane formation and recycling
D. Storage site for newly synthesized proteins
E. Site for packaging and transporting many cell products (e.g., polysaccharides, proteins, lipids)
F. Synthesis site for lysosomes
G. Also involved in the production of large carbohydrate molecules and lysosomes

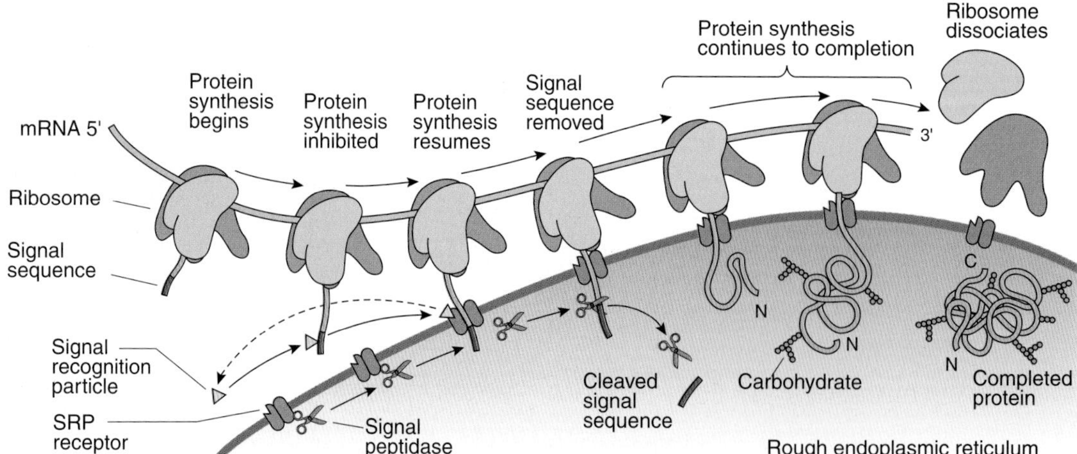


**Fig. 2.3** Ribosomes showing protein synthesis on rough endoplasmic reticulum. Messenger RNA is being passed through ribosomes on endoplasmic reticulum, where transfer RNA becomes incorporated in protein (being formed) that is assembled in the ribosome. (From Gartner LP, Hiatt JL. *Color Textbook of Histology*. 3rd ed. St. Louis: Saunders; 2007.)

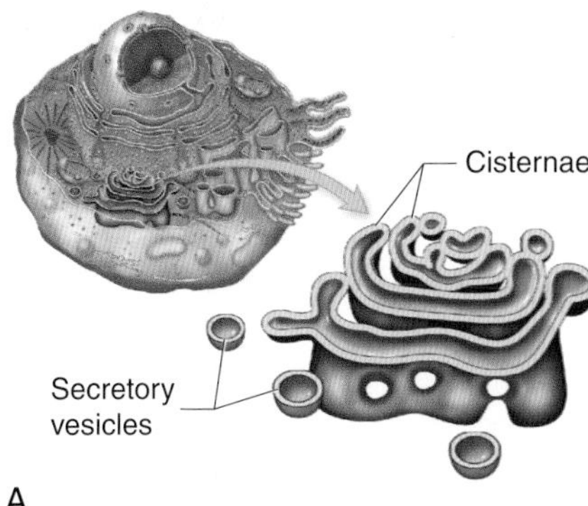


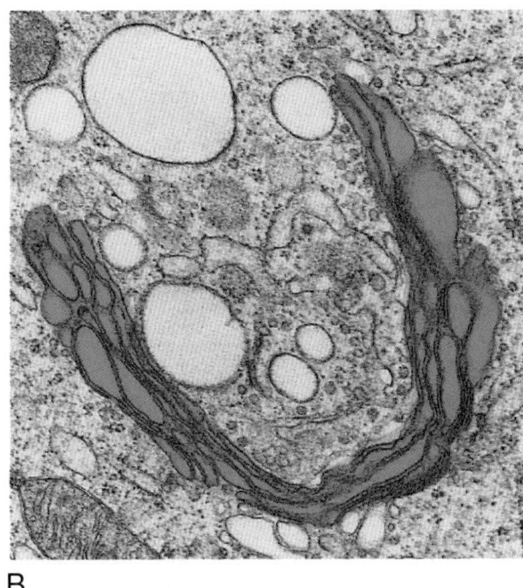


**Fig. 2.4** Golgi complex. (A) Schematic representation of the Golgi complex showing a stack of flattened sacs, or cisternae, and numerous small membranous bubbles, or secretory vesicles. (B) Transmission electron micrograph showing the Golgi complex highlighted with color. (From Patton KT. *Anatomy and Physiology*. 9th ed. St. Louis: Elsevier; 2016.)

## Mitochondria

A. Membranous structure bounded by inner and outer cell membranes; the membranes contain enzyme complexes in a particular array (e.g., tricarboxylic acid cycle enzymes)
   1. The inner part is formed into folds (cristae) that extend, like shelves, inside the mitochondria to provide an additional work surface area for the organelle
   2. More than one mitochondrion is usually present in a cell; the number depends on the amount of energy required by the cell

B. This structure provides the chief source of energy for the cell ("powerhouse of the cell" by oxidation of nutrients) through enzymatic breakdown of fats, amino acids, and carbohydrates; transforms the chemical energy bond of nutrients into the high-energy phosphate bonds of adenosine triphosphate (ATP)

C. A single cell may contain 50 to 2500 mitochondria, depending on the cell's energy needs (Figure 2.5)

## Endoplasmic Reticulum (ER)

A. Extensive membranous system found throughout the cytoplasm of the cell; composed of lipoprotein membranes existing in the form of connecting tubules and broad, flattened sacs (cisternae); the outer membrane may or may not be covered with ribosomes; the two types are:
   1. Granular or rough-surfaced endoplasmic reticulum (RER)
      a. Contains ribosomes that are attached to the cytoplasmic side of the membrane
      b. Site of protein synthesis
   2. Agranular or smooth-surfaced endoplasmic reticulum (SER)
      a. No ribosomes are present
      b. Site of steroid synthesis

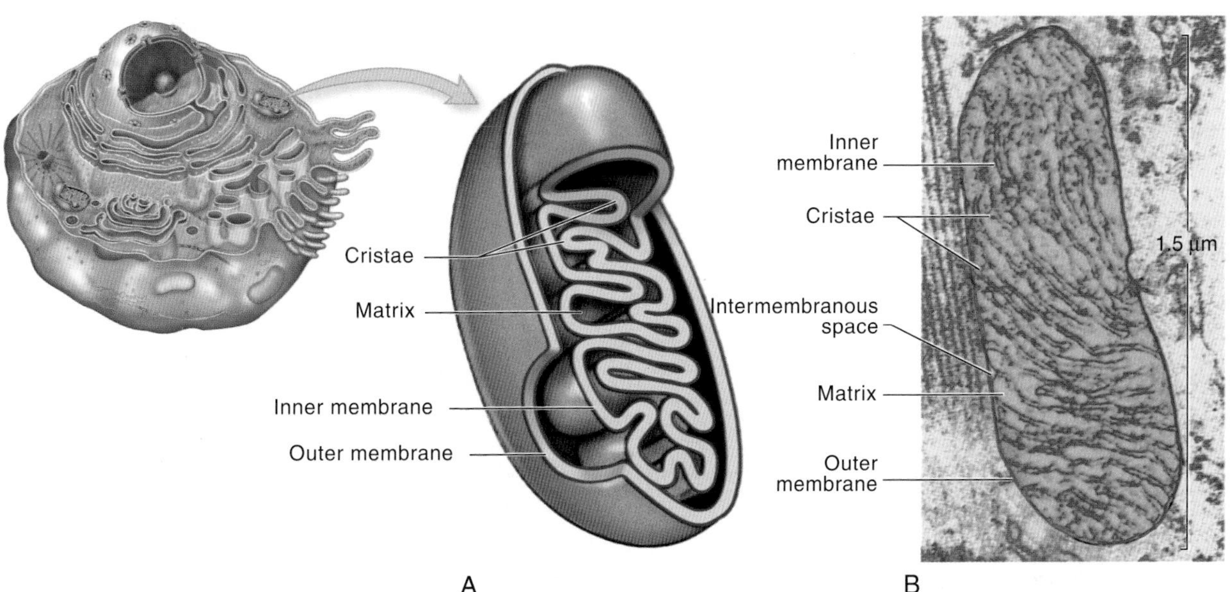


**Fig. 2.5** Mitochondrion. (A) Cutaway sketch showing outer and inner membranes. Note the many folds (cristae) of the inner membrane. (B) Transmission electron micrograph of a mitochondrion. Although some mitochondria have the capsule shape shown here, many are round or oval. (From Patton KT. *Anatomy and Physiology*. 9th ed. St. Louis: Elsevier; 2016.)

B. The membrane system functions to synthesize, circulate, and package intracellular and extracellular materials
C. Proteins are synthesized on ribosomes attached to the ER and are transported to the Golgi complex for packaging
D. The system contains enzymes involved in a variety of metabolic activities (e.g., lipogenesis, glycogenesis)
E. SER has a number of diverse roles and is found in a variety of cell types

### Filaments and Tubules

A. Thread-like structures approximately 7 to 10 nm thick; thicker filaments are the same as those seen in muscle (protein myosin strands) and have been associated with contractility in cells
B. Microfilaments act as a support system for the cell cytoskeleton
C. Bundles of microfilaments form tonofibrils and become part of the attachment apparatus (desmosomes) between cells

### Microtubules

A. Delicate tubes, 20 to 27 nm wide, found in cells that are undergoing mitosis and alterations in cell shape (cell morphology)
B. Microtubules have an internal support function, particularly in long cellular processes such as neurites or odontoblastic processes
C. Microtubules have the capacity to direct intracellular transport through the cytoplasm

### Centrioles

A. Cylindrical structures composed of microtubule-like components
B. Centrioles function in cell replication and the formation of cellular extensions

### Internal Environment and Homeostasis

A. Extracellular fluid
   1. Fluid mass that circulates outside and between cells
   2. Extracellular fluid composition must be regulated exactly:

$$[Na^+] = 142\frac{mEq}{L}$$

$$[K^+] = 5\frac{mEq}{L}$$

$$[Cl^-] = 103\frac{mEq}{L}$$

$$\left[Ca^{+2}\right] = 5\frac{mEq}{L}$$

$$pH = 7.4$$

B. Intracellular fluid
   1. Fluid located inside the cells of the body
   2. Intracellular fluid composition must be regulated exactly:

$$[Na^+] = 10\frac{mEq}{L}$$

$$[K^+] = 141\frac{mEq}{L}$$

$$[Cl^-] = 4\frac{mEq}{L}$$

$$\left[Ca^{+2}\right] = < 1\frac{mEq}{L}$$

$$pH = 7.0$$

C. Homeostasis—the delicate balance maintained between the two fluid compositions

### Transport through the Cell Membrane

A. Diffusion
   1. Definition—continuous movement of molecules among one another in liquids or gases
   2. Molecules may move across a membrane
   3. Direction of diffusion of a substance is from a region of high concentration to a region of low concentration, which is the *diffusion gradient*
   4. If equal amounts of a substance are placed at either end of a chamber such as a cell, they diffuse toward each other, and the net rate of diffusion equals zero
B. Osmosis
   1. Definition—process of net diffusion of water through a semi-permeable membrane caused by a concentration difference
   2. Osmotic pressure—pressure that develops in a solution as a result of the net osmosis into that solution; pressure is affected by the number of dissolved particles per unit volume of fluid
   3. Isotonic solution—when placed on the outside of a cell, will not cause osmosis (e.g., 0.9% sodium chloride)
   4. Hypertonic solution—when placed on the outside of a cell, will cause osmosis out of the cell (e.g., greater than 0.9% sodium chloride) and lead to crenation (shrinking) of the cell
   5. Hypotonic solution—when placed on the outside of a cell, will cause osmosis into the cell (e.g., less than 0.9% sodium chloride) and lead to cell lysis
C. Active transport
   1. Process used by a cell when large quantities of a substance are needed inside the cell and only a small amount of the substance is present in the extracellular fluid
   2. Involves pumping the substance against its concentration gradient

3. Uses a carrier system and energy (ATP)
4. Keeps sodium extra-cellularly (sodium pump) and potassium intra-cellularly; important for the transmission of nerve impulses
5. Almost all monosaccharides are actively transported into the body

D. Phagocytosis—movement of a solid particle into the cell
1. Cell wall invaginates around the particle
2. Pinches off from the rest of the membrane and floats inward

E. Pinocytosis—movement of fluid into a cell; similar to phagocytosis, except that the cell invaginates around fluid

## CELL REPLICATION

A. Mitosis—process of cell replication (Fig. 2.6)
1. Interphase
   a. The genetic material of each chromosome replicates
   b. Chromosomes are dispersed as chromatin material in the nucleus
2. Prophase
   a. Chromosomes coil and contract; each chromosome consists of a pair of strands called *chromatids*, which are held together by a centromere
   b. The nuclear envelope disappears
   c. The centriole divides, and the two centrioles move to opposite poles of the cell
   d. Spindle fibers develop
3. Metaphase
   a. Chromatids line up at the center
   b. Spindle fibers attach at the centromere
   c. The centromere replicates, allowing the separation of chromatids
4. Anaphase
   a. Spindle fibers pull the new chromosomes to opposite poles of the cell
5. Telophase
   a. A nuclear membrane forms around each set of chromosomes
   b. Centrioles replicate in each cell

### Concepts Relating to Dental Tissues

A. All calcified dental tissues are produced by secretory cells that require a great amount of energy in producing their organic matrices, which become calcified; organelles such as mitochondria play an important role in providing energy

B. Mitochondria have been associated with the calcification (mineralization) process that occurs in dental tissues

C. Cell organelles help maintain tissues after the initial formation by the cell; fibroblasts (i.e., connective tissue cells that are present in all tooth tissues except enamel) contain increased numbers of cell organelles; these additional organelles aid fibroblasts in their synthesizing and secretory functions

### Basic Tissues

A. At the beginning of human development, individual cells multiply and differentiate to perform specialized functions; groups of cells with similar morphologic characteristics and functions come together and form tissues

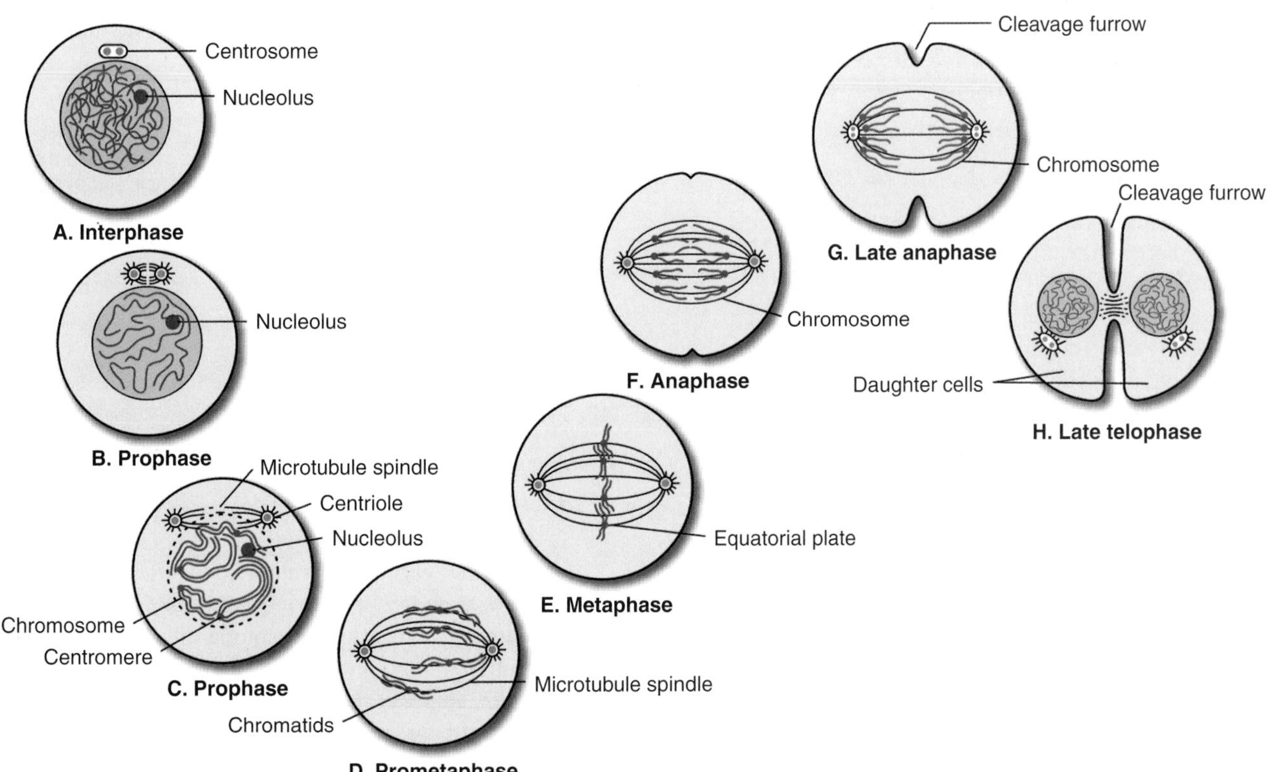


**Fig. 2.6** Phases of mitosis. (From Chiego D. *Essentials of Oral Histology and Embryology, a Clinical Approach.* 4th ed. St. Louis: Elsevier; 2014.)

B. Tissue components
  1. Cells
  2. Intercellular substance—a product of living cells; a medium for the passage of nutrients and waste within the tissue; the amount of substance varies with different tissues
  3. Tissue fluid—blood plasma that diffuses through capillary walls; the fluid carries nutrients to the intercellular substance and waste materials to capillaries
C. Tissues in the human body can be classified into four types:
  1. Epithelial tissue
  2. Connective tissue
  3. Nerve tissue
  4. Muscle tissue
D. Each of the four basic tissues may be further subdivided into several variations

## Epithelial Tissue

A. Main categories
  1. Surface epithelia
  2. Glandular tissue
B. The epithelium consists exclusively of cells held together by specialized cell junctions (minimal intercellular material is present between cells); cells rest on an underlying connective tissue, the *basement membrane*
C. Epithelial cells (keratinocytes) form continuous sheets (tissues) and perform the following functions:
  1. Protection—covering all outer surfaces of the body (e.g., skin)
  2. Absorption—forming the lining of all inner surfaces of the body (e.g., digestive tract)
  3. Secretion—forming glands (glandular tissue)
D. Epithelial tissue varies, depending on function—it may have surface specializations on its free surfaces
  1. Microvilli—for absorption
  2. Cilia—for surface transportation
E. Replicates through mitosis

### *Surface Epithelia*

A. The epithelium is classified according to:
  1. The shape of the most superficial cells
    a. Squamous (flat)
    b. Cuboidal (cubical)
    c. Columnar (tall, narrow—cylindrical or prismatic)
  2. Number of cell layers present
    a. One cell layer—simple; found in areas of little or no friction (e.g., lining of blood vessels)
    b. Several cell layers—stratified; capable of withstanding more functional use (e.g., mucous membranes)
B. Combined characteristics allow for six different types of epithelia (Fig. 2.7) and locations:
  1. Simple squamous—found in the walls of vessels
  2. Simple cuboidal—lines the ovaries
  3. Simple columnar—lines the intestines and the cervix of the uterus
  4. Stratified squamous—lines the oral cavity
  5. Stratified cuboidal and
  6. Stratified columnar—line the large ducts of the major salivary glands
C. Other, intermediate forms of epithelium
  1. Pseudo-stratified columnar (e.g., trachea)—appears stratified but is, in fact, only one layer
  2. Transitional (e.g., urinary tract)—resembles both stratified squamous and stratified cuboidal epithelia
D. Other cell types found in the epithelium
  1. Melanocytes—produce melanin (pigmentation); intensity of brown skin color is not caused by the difference in the number of melanocytes present but by the difference in the rate of melanin production, the size of pigment granules, and the length of time of their preservation
  2. Inflammatory cells—transient cells usually associated with inflammation
  3. Langerhans cells—antigen-presenting cells
  4. Merkel cells—mechano-receptors
E. The epithelium lining the oral cavity (oral mucosa) and the skin (dermis) is an example of stratified squamous epithelium

## Glandular Tissue

A. Most glands develop from the epithelium; the epithelial basal cell grows downward into the underlying connective tissue
B. Types
  1. Exocrine
    a. Serous; mucous or seromucous secretions
    b. Ducts carry secretions
      (1) Simple—nonbranching duct
      (2) Compound—branching duct
  2. Endocrine
    a. Hormone secretions directly into the bloodstream
    b. The bloodstream carries secretions; no ducts

## Connective Tissue

### *Connective Tissue Proper*

A. All connective tissue proper develops from the embryonic mesenchyme; contains large amounts and various types of intercellular material and few cells; highly vascular; has two main functions:
  1. Provides mechanical and biologic support (supports organs and other structures)
  2. Provides pathways for metabolic substances and thus aids in the distribution of nutrients
B. Types of connective tissue
  1. Bone—hard and calcified; serves supportive and protective functions
  2. Cartilage—firm but flexible; serves a supportive function
  3. Reticular—network of branching fibers; acts as a filter; loose and elastic; provides a connection between structures
  4. Bone marrow—site where blood cells are manufactured
  5. Lymphoid tissue (tonsils and lymph nodes)
  6. Fat or adipose (special type of connective tissue composed of fat cells)—located under the skin; provides insulation
  7. Dental tissues
    a. Pulp

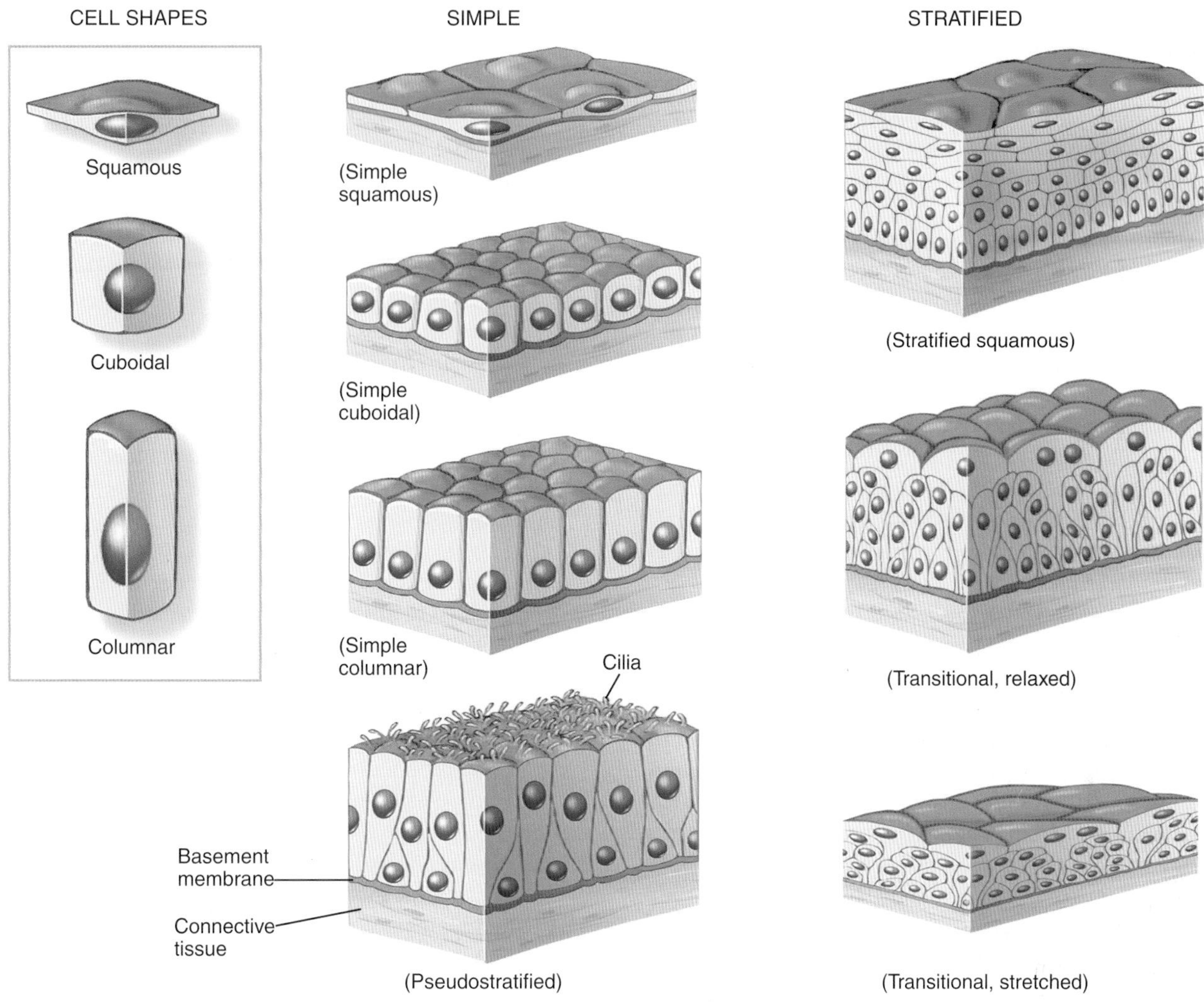


**Fig. 2.7** Classification of epithelia according to morphologic shape and number of cell layers. (From Patton KT. *Anatomy and Physiology*. 9th ed. St. Louis: Elsevier; 2016.)

b. Dentin
c. Cementum

C. Types of connective tissues—differ in composition of cell products and proportions of products present
1. Dense connective tissue—consists predominantly of heavy, tightly packed collagen fibers; main function is to resist tension; this dense collagenous connective tissue is present in the gingiva
2. Loose connective tissue—collagen and reticulin fibers extending in all directions; the main function is to provide biologic support and fill the spaces between organs and tissues

### *Connective Tissue Components*

A. Cells
1. Types of cells normally present
 a. Fibroblasts—produce the fibrous matrix and ground substance of connective tissue
 b. Macrophages—capable of digestive activity
 c. Mast cells—contain vesicles filled with heparin and histamine
 d. Mesenchymal cells—primitive cells with the capability of differentiating into various connective tissue cells; they play a key role in the replacement of connective tissue lost as a result of injury or disease
2. Cells that are normally in the bloodstream but move in and out of the blood vessels into surrounding connective tissue when needed (wandering cells)
 a. Monocytes
 b. Polymorphonuclear leukocytes (PMNs)
 c. Lymphocytes
 d. Plasma cells

B. Fibrous matrix
1. Matrix of connective tissue composed of some or all of the following fibers:
 a. Collagen fibers—consist of three long polypeptide chains coiled in a left-handed helix to form a tropocollagen unit, which is assembled in a "quarter-stagger" model outside of the cell; fibers are highly resistant to tension and are part of the anchoring mechanism by which the connective tissue attaches the basement membrane (see Fig. 2.20B); the most abundant fibers found in connective tissue
 b. Reticulin fibers—comparable with collagen fibers in their protein composition; usually found in the border areas between connective tissue and other tissues

c. Elastic fibers—consist of long fibrous proteins that differ in composition from collagen; are the branching fibers responsible for recoiling tissues when they are stretched
d. Oxytalan fibers—resemble elastic fibers in morphology and chemical composition; are believed to be immature elastic fibers

C. Ground substance
1. Amorphous substance that consists of many large, highly organized carbohydrate chains attached to long protein cores (e.g., proteoglycans)
2. Molecular structure and composition are responsible for the ground substance's resistance to compression, or compressive loading, from any direction

### *Types (Cartilage and Bone)*

**Cartilage.**

A. Cartilage and bone are sister tissues, both highly specialized forms of connective tissue, whose intercellular substances have assumed particular properties that allow them to perform support functions
1. Flexible tissue that is specialized to resist compression; has a gel-like matrix in which the ground substance predominates over the intercellular matrix
2. Relatively avascular tissue
3. In humans, most of the embryonic skeleton is preformed as hyaline cartilage that is eventually replaced by bone (during endochondral ossification); depending on the location and loading pattern imposed on the cartilage, it may specialize to form fibrous or elastic cartilage
4. All mature cartilage is surrounded by the perichondrium, a fibrous connective tissue, which serves a biomechanical function; it acts as an attachment site for muscles and tendons

B. Cartilage, as with all types of connective tissue, has three components:
1. Cells—chondroblasts and chondrocytes
2. Fibrous matrix—type II collagen fibers and, in some cases, elastic fibers
3. Ground substance—proteoglycans, which have a protein core with side chains of chondroitin sulfate and keratan sulfate (glycosaminoglycans); because of the chemical nature and organization of proteoglycans, the ground substance can readily bind and hold water, which allows the tissue to assume a gelatinous nature that can resist compression and also permit some degree of diffusion through the matrix

C. Types
1. Hyaline cartilage
   a. Found in the adult human
      (1) Covering articular surfaces of movable long bones
      (2) Forms the skeletal support parts of:
         (a) Trachea
         (b) Larynx
         (c) External ear
         (d) Nasal septum
         (e) Ends of ribs
   b. Most abundant type of cartilage; forms the embryonic skeleton in humans; is best suited to resist compression; appears as a homogeneous, translucent tissue because its intercellular matrix dominates its collagenous fibers; the major type of fiber in collagen
2. Fibrous cartilage (fibrocartilage)
   a. Has a very sparse amount of intercellular substance dominated by collagen fibers, which are in such proportion that they are visible through a light microscope and are seen running between the chondrocytic cells in the cartilage
   b. Resembles tendons except for the presence of the chondrocytes enclosed in lacunae
   c. Usually found in areas that are subjected to both compression and tension, as in:
      (1) Intervertebral disc
      (2) Temporomandibular joint of older adults
      (3) Pubic symphysis
3. Elastic cartilage
   a. In areas that are in need of elastic recoil, hyaline cartilage becomes highly specialized, and elastic fibers are added to its intercellular matrix, as in:
      (1) External ear
      (2) Epiglottis
   b. Elastic fibers are highly branched and form a delicate fibrous matrix, often obscuring the intercellular substance; fibers can be seen only through a light microscope when stained with a specific elastic stain

**Bone.**

A. A specialized vascular connective tissue composed of a mineralized organic matrix; the inorganic component of bone is hydroxyapatite:

$$Ca_{10}(PO_4)_6(OH)_2$$

B. Two main functions:
1. Provides skeletal support and protection of soft tissues
2. Acts as a reservoir for calcium and phosphorus ions; when these two ions drop below a critical level in the blood (100 mg of calcium per 100 mL of blood, and 600 mg of phosphorus per/100 mL of blood), they can be withdrawn from the bone

C. Characteristic of all bones
1. Compact bone—dense bone that appears as a continuous solid mass
2. Trabecular (cancellous or spongy) bone—composed of a central medullary cavity filled with either red or yellow marrow and with intervening spicules of bone (trabeculae); these trabeculae act to reinforce bone by increasing in number with increased function

D. Bone morphology
1. Bone-forming cells (osteoblasts) are produced from undifferentiated mesenchymal cells of the periosteum, the endosteum, and the periodontal ligament (PDL)
   a. The periosteum is the connective tissue that covers the outer aspects of bone
   b. The endosteum is a more delicate connective tissue lining the inner aspects of bone, the trabeculae, and Volkmann's canals (canals of the bone containing blood vessels)

c. The PDL is specialized periosteum because it covers the outer aspects of the alveolar bone; it is also capable of forming bone and of forming cells that produce cementum (cementoblasts)
2. Osteoblasts become incorporated into bone during their formation; they occupy a space called a *lacuna* (plural, *lacunae*)
3. Lacunae are connected to each other by means of a system of canals named *canaliculi*; these canals house the cytoplasmic extension of the osteocytes and provide a means for the transport of vascular components
4. Both compact and trabecular mature bones are formed in layers, or *lamellae.* Lamellae are found in three distinct types of arrangements present in all mature human bones (Fig. 2.8):
   a. Concentric, or haversian system, bone makes up the bulk of compact bone; it consists of lamellae arranged in concentric circles around a blood vessel (haversian canal) to form an osteon. An osteon, which consists of this concentrically arranged bone and haversian canal, is the basic metabolic unit of bone
   b. Interstitial lamellae fill the space between the concentric circles of the haversian system bone
   c. Lamellar bone is not arranged in concentric circles and is found on the surfaces of most bones. This bone is further defined by its location. When found on the outer aspects or the circumference of the bone underneath the periosteum, it is referred to as *circumferential,* or *(sub)periosteal, bone*; when found on the surfaces of trabeculae or the inner aspect of compact bone, it is referred to as *(sub)endosteal bone*

E. Bone tissue
1. Bone, as with all connective tissues, has three main components:
   a. Cells
      (1) Osteoblasts—bone-forming cells
      (2) Osteoclasts—bone-resorbing cells
      (3) Osteocytes—osteoblasts that are embedded in the lacunae of bone matrix and that maintain bone tissue
   b. Fibrous matrix—collagen fibers (type I), which are the dominant component of bone matrix
   c. Ground substance—proteoglycans containing chondroitin sulfates and seeded with the mineral salt hydroxyapatite
2. Bone is formed by osteoblasts developed in one of two ways:
   a. Intramembranous ossification—mesenchymal cells move closer together (condensation), differentiate into osteoblasts, and begin to deposit bone matrix; this is how the maxilla and the mandible are formed
   b. Endochondral ossification—future bone is preformed in a cartilage model that is eventually resorbed and replaced by new bone formed by osteoblasts (Fig. 2.9)
      (1) Cartilage must undergo two important changes before being resorbed and replaced by new bone:
         (a) Chondrocytic hypertrophy
         (b) Calcification of the cartilage model

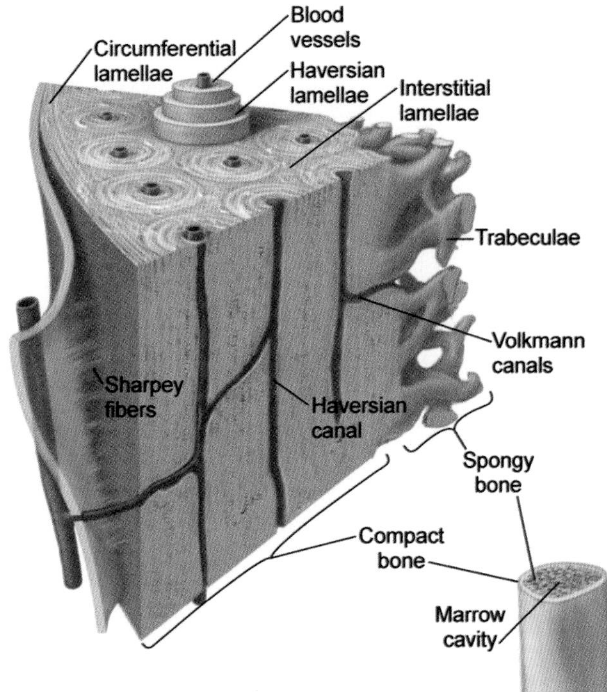


**Fig. 2.8** Microscopic morphology of bone tissue. Haversian system bone is composed of lamellae arranged in concentric circles around a canal. Interstitial bone fills the space between the concentric circles. Circumferential lamellar bone is found on the outer aspects of compact bone; endosteal lamellar bone covers the inner aspect of compact bone. Spongy bone is composed of trabeculae and marrow cavity. (From Pollard TD, Earnshaw WC. *Cell Biology*. Philadelphia: Saunders; 2002.)

      (2) Endochondral ossification is the process by which all long bones in the human body are formed
         (a) Bone growth in length—occurs in the cartilaginous epiphyseal growth plate
         (b) Bone growth in diameter—occurs in the cellular layer of the fibrous covering of connective tissue periosteum, which produces a periosteal bone collar on the outer bone surface

F. Structure of long bones (macroscopic)
1. The typical long bone is composed of:
   a. Diaphysis (shaft)—thick compact bone forming a hollow cylinder with a central marrow cavity; this is the primary center of ossification in a long bone
   b. Epiphyses (ends)—spongy bone covered by a thin layer of compact bone; these are the secondary growth centers
   c. Metaphysis—transitional region between the epiphyses and the diaphysis, where the cartilage growth plate is located
   d. All articular surfaces of long bones are covered by articular cartilage
2. While active, the epiphyseal growth plate usually has four zones, proceeding from first to last:
   a. Primary spongiosa with resorption
   b. Hypertrophy and provisional calcification
   c. Proliferation
   d. Resting zone (see Fig. 2.9)

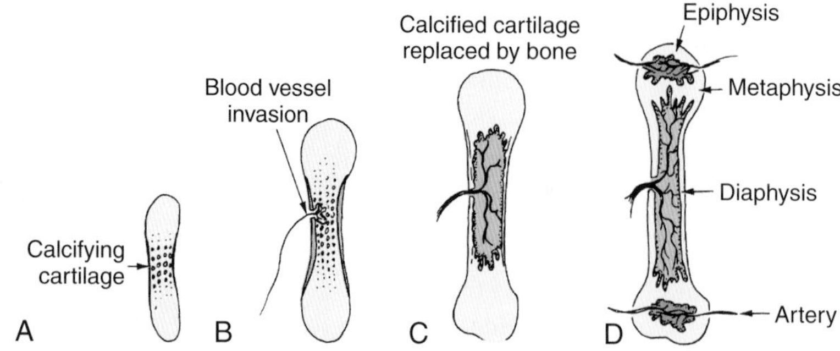


**Fig. 2.9** Stages of endochondral bone formation in long-bone growth. (A) Original hyaline cartilage is calcified in the center of the diaphysis. (B) Blood vessel invades the center of the shaft. (C) The marrow space appears in the center of the shaft, and bone forms around the diaphysis. (D) Bone formation continues in the shaft, and secondary ossification sites appear in the heads (epiphyses) of the bones. A disc of cartilage remains between bone forming in the head and the shaft (epiphyseal line). (From Chiego D. *Essentials of Oral Histology and Embryology, a Clinical Approach*. 4th ed. St. Louis: Elsevier; 2014.)

## Blood and Lymph

A. Vascular system
   1. Develops embryonically from mesenchymal cells that come together and form delicate tubular structures composed of endothelial cells
   2. Consists of the heart, blood vessels, and lymphatics
      a. Is a closed system that runs from the heart to the organs of the body and back to the heart
      b. Between the heart and the organs, the blood vessels branch progressively into finer and finer vessels and finally enter the organs
         (1) Here a delicate network of capillaries forms, called the *capillary bed*—the most essential part of the vascular system
         (2) Exchanges of gases and substances occur in this capillary bed
      c. Blood is then carried back to the heart via larger vessels, the veins
   3. Functions
      a. Carries nutrients, oxygen, and hormones to all parts of the body
      b. Carries metabolic waste products to the kidneys
      c. Transports inflammatory cells and antibodies
      d. Maintains a constant body temperature

B. Lymph vessels empty into filtering organs (nodes) and generally flow toward larger lymph vessels, the thoracic duct, and the right lymphatic duct; lymph enters the venous branches of the circulatory system

### *Blood Vessels*

A. Arteries—the largest of the blood vessels; walls are composed of:
   1. A thick layer of smooth muscle cells
   2. Elastic tissue—the largest amount is found in the large arteries close to the heart

B. Veins—usually accompany arteries but carry blood in the opposite direction
   1. Walls are composed of:
      a. A layer of endothelial cells
      b. A connective tissue layer
      c. Occasionally a few smooth muscle cells
   2. Veins contain about 70% of total blood volume of the body at any given time

C. Capillaries—the simplest of the blood vessels in the structure
   1. Walls consist of a simple layer of endothelial cells and a basal lamina
   2. Usually, the diameter of a capillary lumen is so small that only one blood cell at a time can pass through it
   3. Capillaries form a barrier between blood and tissues
   4. Transport of substances occurs at the capillary level through:
      a. Pores in the endothelial wall of the capillary
      b. Openings between adjacent endothelial cells
      c. Pinocytotic vesicles formed by the wall of the capillary

### *Microvasculature*

A. Composed of the smallest arteries and veins located in the capillary bed
   1. At the end of the arterioles is a preferential channel that has several side branches entering the capillary bed
   2. Blood passes through the capillary bed from the arterial side to the venous side

B. Selective openings and closings of the capillary bed occur in the microvasculature to ensure regulation of the amount of blood throughout the body at any given time

### *Blood Components*

A. Cells
   1. Red blood cells—erythrocytes; most numerous
   2. White blood cells—leukocytes (granular and nongranular)
   3. Platelets—cell fragments of a specific cell type found in red bone marrow; have no nuclei

B. Plasma—liquid portion of blood

**Functions of Blood Cells.**

A. Red blood cells (erythrocytes) contain hemoglobin, which carries oxygen from lungs to tissues

B. White blood cells (leukocytes) function chiefly to fight infection, to scavenge foreign invaders, and to repair injured tissue
   1. Granular leukocytes
      a. Polymorphonuclear neutrophils (PMNs)—first line of defense against bacterial invasion

b. Eosinophils—involvement in allergic reactions
c. Basophils—antigen involvement
2. Nongranular leukocytes
a. Monocytes—can become macrophages in connective tissue
b. Lymphocytes—produce antibodies
C. Platelets—promote blood clotting

**Lymphatic System.**

A. Made up of a series of vessels that carry excess tissue fluid from the capillaries to filtering organs such as lymph nodes on the return to the bloodstream
B. Lymph nodes are found along the lymphatic pathway
1. Consist of masses of lymph tissue that serve as a filtering system for the body
2. The tonsils and the spleen are both filtering organs for the body
3. Swollen and palpable lymph nodes may indicate that an infection is present somewhere in the body
C. The function of lymph is to protect and maintain the internal fluid environment of the body

## Nerve Tissue

A. Main functions of the nervous system
1. Directs and maintains the complex internal environment of the body
2. Integrates and interprets incoming stimuli and directs appropriate responses at a conscious or unconscious level
B. The nervous system can be classified as follows:
1. Central nervous system (CNS)
2. Peripheral nervous system (PNS)
3. Autonomic nervous system (ANS)
C. Afferent nerves transmit impulses (sensations) from the periphery to the CNS (sensory input); efferent nerves transmit impulses (commands) from the CNS to muscles and other organs (motor output) (Fig. 2.10)
D. Divisions of the nervous system
1. CNS
a. Includes the brain and the spinal cord
b. Main functions:
(1) Receives incoming information at a conscious or unconscious level (sensory)
(2) Integrates outgoing responses (motor) that are transmitted to various parts of the brain and the spinal cord
2. PNS
a. Composed of 31 pairs of spinal nerves and 12 pairs of cranial nerves
b. All nerves transmit information to and from the CNS
c. Contains both sensory and motor nerves (neurons)
3. ANS (Fig. 2.11)
a. Controls, regulates, and coordinates visceral activities (digestion, body temperature, blood pressure, and glandular secretions) at an unconscious level
b. Is further subdivided into:
(1) Sympathetic division—acts to regulate and mobilize activities during emergency or stress (flight activities); activities that require high outputs of energy produce an accelerated heart rate and increase in blood pressure
(2) Parasympathetic division—works in the opposite manner of the sympathetic division; stimulates activities that restore or conserve energy (e.g., decreased heart rate, constricted pupils, contraction of ciliary muscle)
(3) These two divisions are seen as acting reciprocally rather than antagonistically

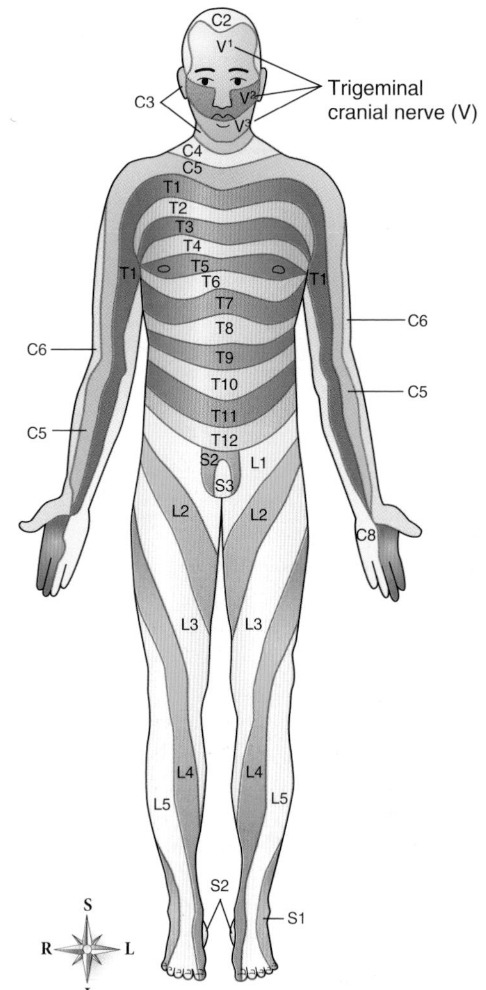


**Fig. 2.10** Cross-section of a spinal cord showing pathways used to transmit nerve impulses from the periphery to the central nervous system. (From Patton KT. *Anatomy and Physiology*. 9th ed. St. Louis: Elsevier; 2016.)

### *Structural Components*

A. Neurons (Fig. 2.12)
1. Structural components of nerve tissue
2. Receive and transmit information
3. Highly specialized cells consisting of:
a. Cell body—contains the nucleus and organelles; located in the ganglia in the CNS and the PNS
b. One or more cytoplasmic extensions
(1) Dendrites—conduct impulses toward the cell body

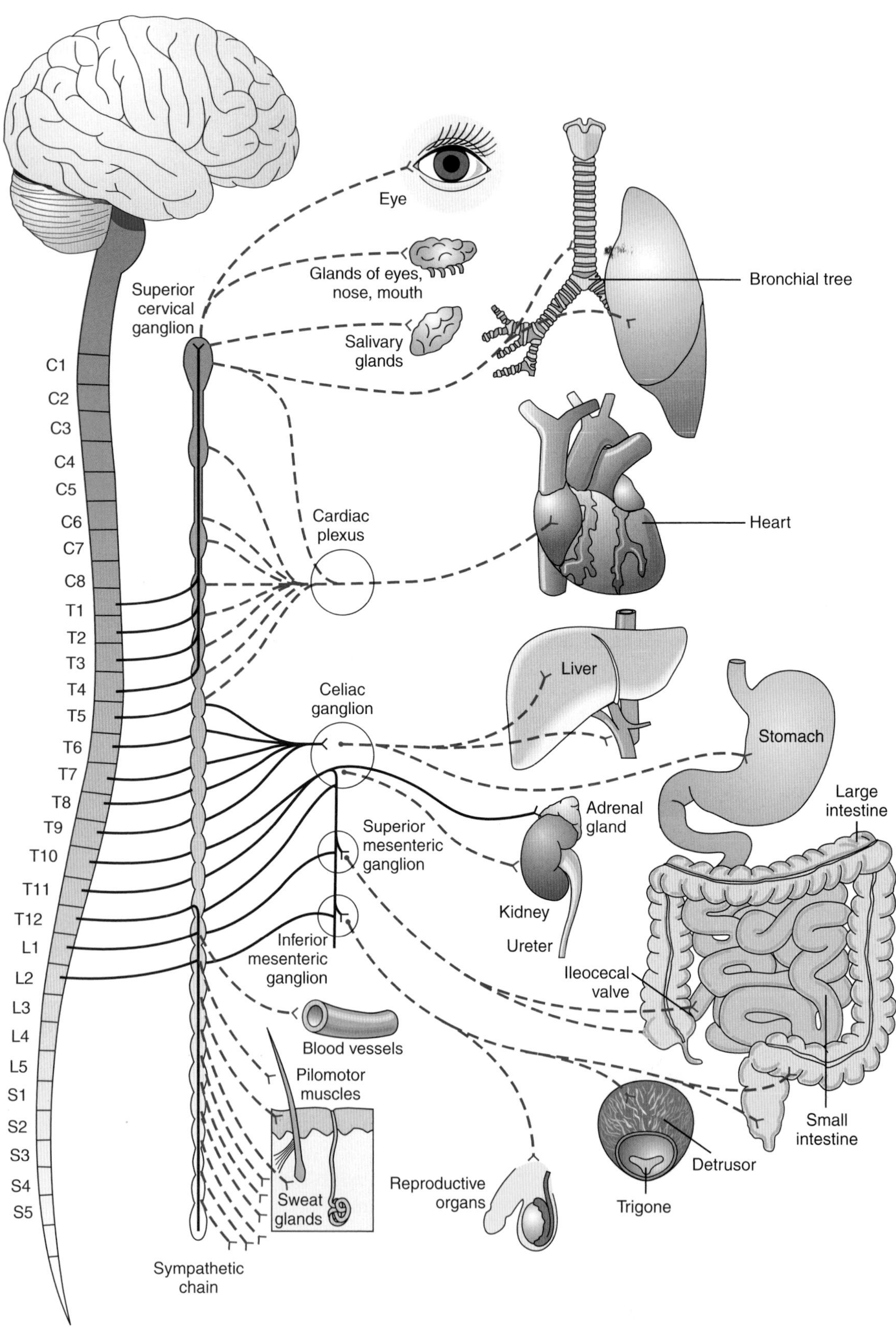


**Fig. 2.11** Distribution of sympathetic nerves. (From Copstead LC, Banasik JL. *Pathophysiology.* 5th ed. St. Louis: Elsevier; 2014.)

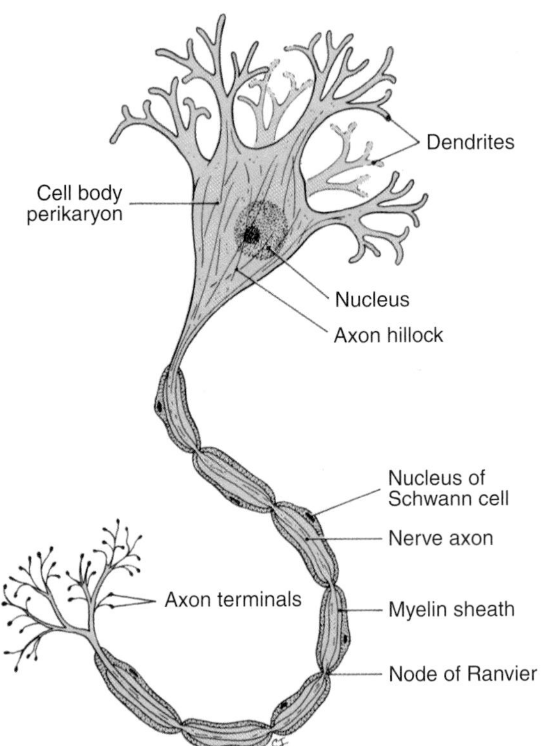


**Fig. 2.12** Neuron with its cell body, axon, dendrites, and synaptic relationships with the muscle tissue and another neuron. (From Chiego D. *Essentials of Oral Histology and Embryology, a Clinical Approach.* 4th ed. St. Louis: Elsevier; 2014.)

(2) Axons—conduct impulses away from the cell body

4. Classified according to the number of cell processes (Fig. 2.13):
   a. Multipolar neurons—located in the CNS and autonomic ganglia; usually, one process is the axon and the other processes are the dendrites
   b. Unipolar neurons—have a short cell process that leaves the cell body and divides into two long branches; one branch goes to the CNS, and the other goes to the PNS (sensory neurons)
5. Interneurons—lie within the CNS; receive and link sensory and motor impulses to bring about appropriate responses in the body

B. Glial cells—provide structural support and nourishment for the neurons; Schwann cells in the PNS and satellite cells in the ganglia

***Definitions***

A. *Synapse*—an area that occurs between two neurons or between a neuron and its effector (muscle or gland); found between the cell surfaces are:
   1. Synaptic cleft—intercellular space separating a presynaptic and postsynaptic membrane
   2. Presynaptic membrane—situated before the synapse
   3. Postsynaptic membrane—situated after the synapse

B. *Neurotransmitters*—chemicals released from the neuron as electrical impulses travel along the axon and reach the terminal end

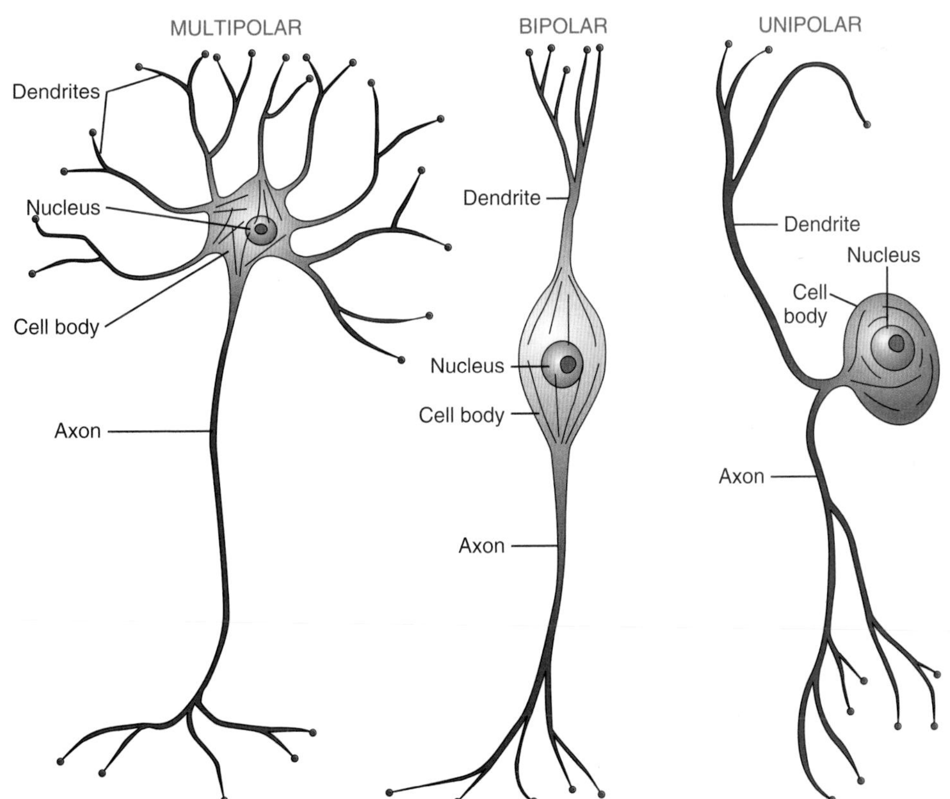


**Fig. 2.13** Classification of neurons based on the location of the cell body and the relative length and number of dendrites and axons. (From Copstead LC, Banasik JL. *Pathophysiology.* 5th ed. St. Louis: Elsevier; 2014.)

1. Neurotransmitters increase the permeability of the cell membranes; impulses are relayed to the effector; impulses can be excitatory or inhibitory
2. Two-membrane junctions
3. Types of neurotransmitters
   a. Acetylcholine—secreted by cholinergic fibers
   b. Norepinephrine—secreted by adrenergic fibers

C. *Myelin sheath*—fatty layer surrounding the axon of the nerve
   1. Myelinated—contains a fatty sheath
   2. Unmyelinated—contains no fatty sheath

D. *Neurilemma*—continuous sheath that encloses the segmented myelin sheath of some nerves

E. *Neuroglia*—extremely soft tissue that supports the nervous tissue of the brain and the spinal cord

F. *Free nerve endings*—end portions of afferent (sensory) axons no longer covered by a supportive Schwann cell; found in:
   1. Dental pulp
   2. Oral epithelium

G. *Encapsulated nerve endings*—composed of several portions of afferent axons surrounded by a capsule of several Schwann cells without a myelin sheath and some connective tissue; they are associated with:
   1. Touch perception (Meissner's corpuscles) found in the lamina propria of the oral mucosa
   2. PDL

***Cranial Nerves.*** See the section titled "The Nervous System" in Chapter 3.

A. Twelve pairs of cranial nerves originate from the brain
   1. Cranial nerves transmit information to the brain from the special sensory receptors and regulate the functions of:
      a. Smell
      b. Sight
      c. Hearing
      d. Taste
   2. Cranial nerves bring impulses from the CNS to the voluntary muscles of:
      a. Eyes
      b. Mouth (masticatory muscles)
      c. Face (facial expression)
      d. Tongue (swallowing and speech)
      e. Larynx

B. In oral health care, a local anesthetic agent is injected into a sensory peripheral nerve; it diffuses through the nerve fibers and blocks the transmission of impulses to the brain in an area of several teeth or in a localized area of soft tissue (see the section "Pain" in Chapter 18).

### Muscle Tissue

A. Composed mainly of cells called *muscle fibers,* which have differentiated from the embryonic mesenchyme and have become highly specialized in contracting (shortening)

B. Contracting ability of muscle fibers is a result of large amounts of actin and myosin, which are intracellular, contractile protein filaments

C. The three muscle tissue types are:
   1. Skeletal (striated) muscle
      a. Under conscious control; referred to as *voluntary muscle*
      b. Has rapid, short, strong contractions; requires a great deal of energy
      c. Innervated by motor nerves
      d. Skeletal muscles of the head region:
         (1) Muscles of mastication
         (2) Muscles of facial expression
      e. Muscle attachments are possible because of the connective tissues surrounding the muscle, bone, or cartilage; connecting tissues of the muscle run directly into the periosteum, cover the bone or perichondrium, cover the cartilage or perimysium, or cover the muscle. The exact nature of the attachment depends on the site and function of the muscle. The intermediate structures may be:
         (1) Tendons
         (2) Ligaments
         (3) Aponeuroses
      f. Muscles that change the shape of the tongue by their contractions are attached on both sides to the lamina propria of the oral mucosa of the tongue
   2. Smooth muscle
      a. Under the control of the ANS and not under conscious control
      b. Contractions are slow and can be maintained over a long period without the use of much energy
   3. Cardiac muscle
      a. Has some of both skeletal (striated) and smooth muscle characteristics
      b. Is involuntary; has fast, powerful contractions
      c. Purkinje fibers—specialized cells present in heart muscle that act like nerves to conduct messages through the heart
      d. Bundle of His—a band of specialized cardiac muscle fibers

***Muscle Contraction***

A. Muscle can be stimulated to contract by one nerve or by many nerves

B. Each striated muscle contains bundles of highly organized contractile proteins called *myofibrils*; each myofibril consists of regularly arranged protein filaments: actin and myosin (Fig. 2.14)

C. Protein filaments are attached to a Z band; the section of a myofibril between two Z bands is called a *sarcomere,* which is the contractile unit

D. As a muscle unit contracts, actin and myosin filaments slide past each other, shorten the length of the individual sarcomere (sliding mechanism), and cause total shortening of the muscle fiber

## GENERAL EMBRYOLOGY

A. All human development begins by fertilization, the union of a female germ cell (ovum) and a male germ cell (sperm)

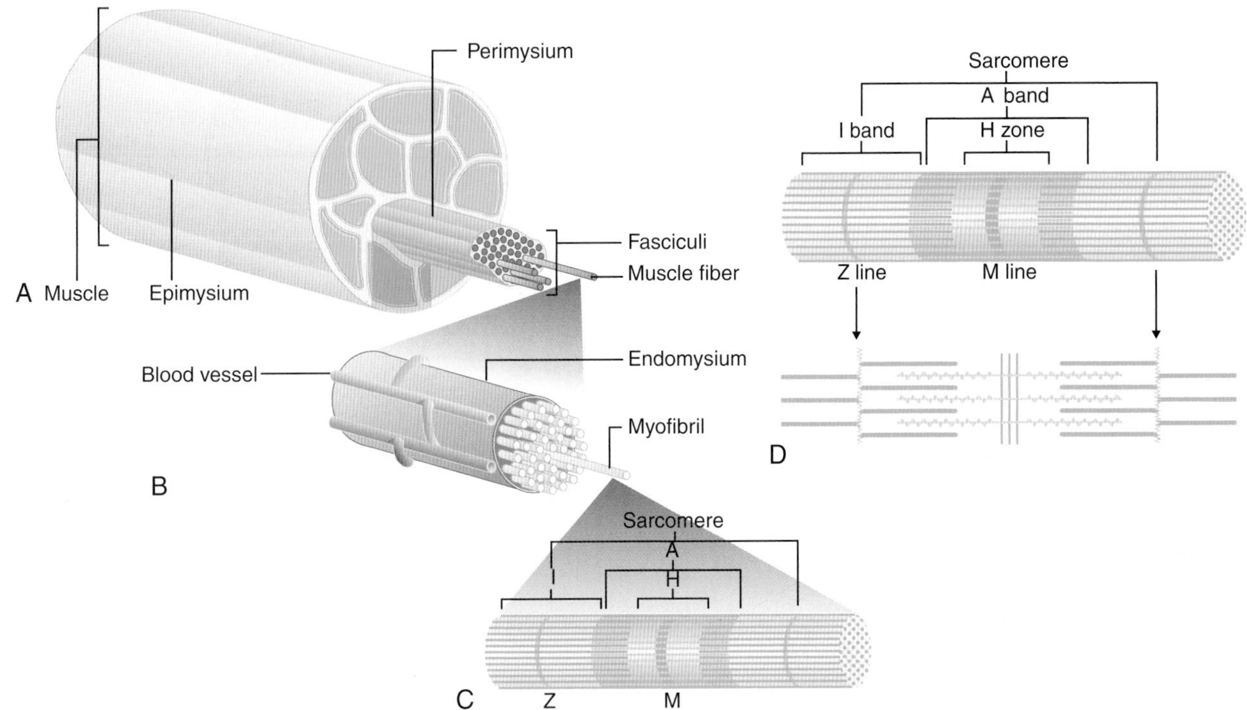


**Fig. 2.14** Muscle fiber. (A) The epimysium runs continuously with the endomysium and the perimysium. (B) The arrangement of fasciculi varies among muscles. (C) The banding pattern apparent on microscopic inspection of a muscle cell results from the organized structure of the proteins (myofibrils) of the contractile apparatus. (D) Thick and thin filaments are organized into contractile units called sarcomeres. (From Copstead LC, Banasik JL. *Pathophysiology*. 5th ed. St. Louis: Elsevier; 2014.)

B. Each germ cell contains 23 chromosomes (haploid number); during the process of fertilization, the number of chromosomes is restored to 46 (diploid number)
C. The developing organism, called the zygote, goes through a series of mitotic divisions
   1. Morula—16 to 32 cells, appearance resembles that of a mulberry
   2. Blastocele—a central cavity with an embryonic pole
   3. Blastocyst—thin-walled hollow ball of cells that attaches to and embeds in the uterine wall
      a. Two distinct layers become visible:
         (1) Epiblast (ectoderm) layer
         (2) Hypoblast (endoderm) layer
      b. These two layers constitute the embryonic disc, which will give rise to the future embryo
D. Three distinct periods in human development:
   1. Period of the ovum (1st week)—fertilized ovum develops an embryonic disc
   2. Embryonic period (2nd week to 8th week)—most of the organs and organ systems develop
      a. A period of differentiation
      b. At the end of this period, a recognizable individual has developed
      c. Most congenital malformations occur during this time
   3. Fetal period (3rd month to 9th month)—growth of existing structures takes place
E. Development of some facial and oral structures is dependent on a group of cells (neural crest cells) derived from the ectoderm as the neural tube is forming; these cells migrate cephalad and interact with the cephalic ectoderm and mesoderm to result in the development of:
   1. Facial skeleton—Meckel's cartilage
   2. Neck skeleton—hyoid bone
   3. Connective tissue components
   4. Tooth development
F. Neural crest cells migrate into each of the branchial arches and surround the existing mesoderm; in each arch, the following components develop:
   1. Cartilage rod (skeleton of each arch)—first branchial arch, Meckel's cartilage
   2. Muscular component—second branchial arch, facial musculature
   3. Vasculature component
   4. Nerve component—first branchial arch, trigeminal nerve
G. On the internal aspect of the branchial arches are corresponding pharyngeal pouches that give rise to:
   1. External auditory meatus
   2. Pharyngotympanic tube
   3. Palatine tonsils
   4. Parathyroid glands

## Facial Development

A. Initiation of the development of the oral cavity occurs in the 3rd prenatal week (embryonic period) and is complete in the 12th week
B. The future facial region is located among the bulging forebrain, the frontal nasal process, and the developing heart

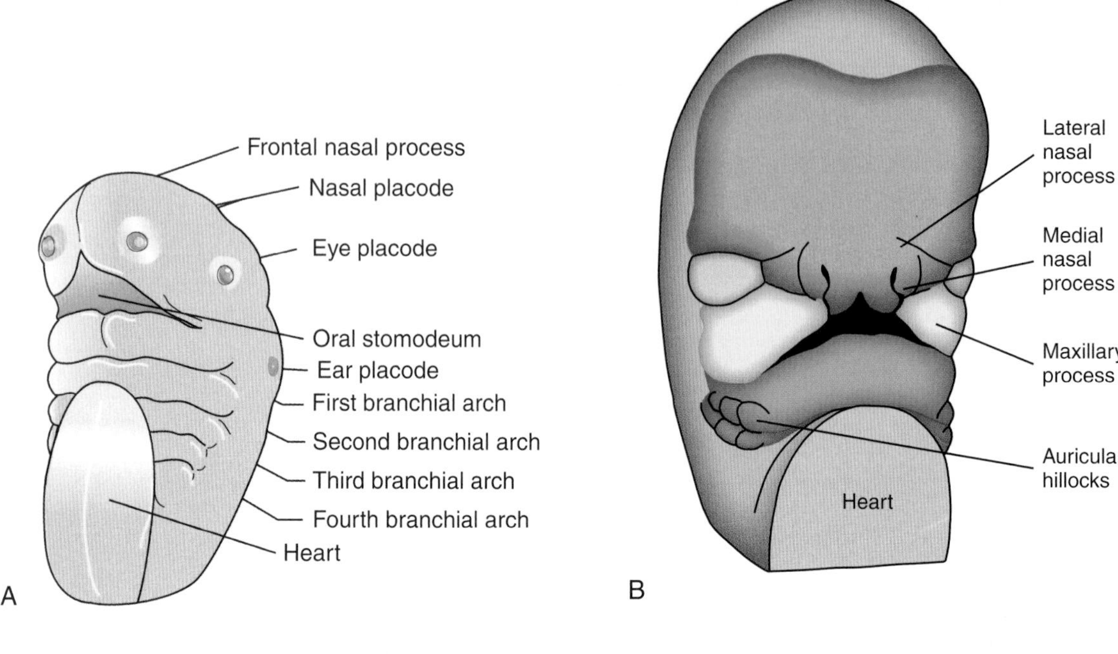


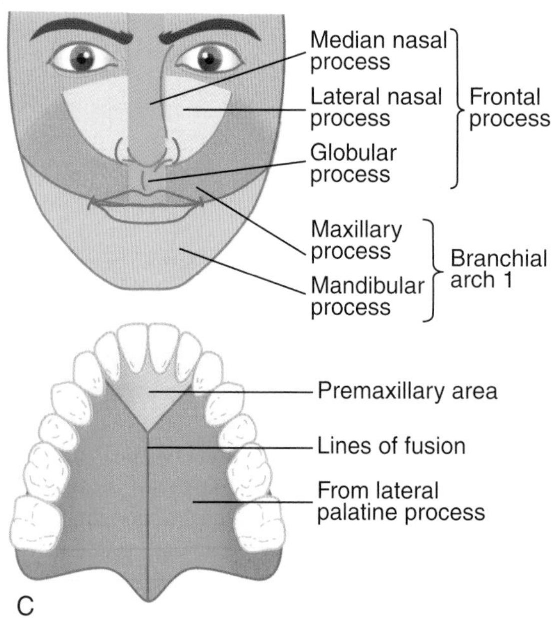


**Fig. 2.15** Facial development. (A) and (B) Facial development begins with the outgrowth of branchial arches. Note the relationship of the oral stomodeum to the heart and the developing face. Nasal pits develop from the frontal nasal process and grow to become nostrils. The nasal pits separate the frontal nasal process into the medial nasal process and the right and left lateral nasal processes. (C) Note the developmental processes and the lines of fusion on the adult face illustration. ((B) from Chiego D. *Essentials of Oral Histology and Embryology, a Clinical Approach*. 4th ed. St. Louis: Elsevier; 2014.)

C. At the beginning of the 4th week, five facial swellings, called branchial arches, appear on the embryo
   1. Located between the first branchial arch and the frontal process (forebrain) is the oral stomodeum (primitive oral cavity) (Fig. 2.15); the stomodeum is the first sign of facial development
   2. The stomodeal ectoderm invaginates until it comes in contact with the primitive foregut; the stomodeum and the foregut are initially separated by the buccopharyngeal membrane, which is composed of the ectoderm and the endoderm. It is located in the region that will eventually house the palatine tonsils
   3. Rathke's pouch—a small invagination in the roof of the stomodeum; deepens into the brain and forms the anterior lobe of the pituitary gland
   4. The maxilla and the mandible develop from the first branchial arch
   5. The second to fifth branchial arches are involved in development of the neck

D. On the lower aspect of the frontal process, nasal pits (nostrils) arise from nasal placodes (see Fig. 2.15B) and separate the lower frontal process into:
   1. Medial nasal process (area between the nasal pits); this gives rise to:
      a. The center of the nose and the nasal septum
      b. The globular process that develops into:
         (1) The center of the upper lip (philtrum)
         (2) The primary palate (premaxilla)—the anterior portion of the palate
   2. Lateral nasal processes (area to the right and left of the nasal pits) that form the sides of the nose
E. Maxillary processes arise from the superolateral border of the first branchial arch; they grow:
   1. Downward to merge with the mandibular processes and form the closure at the corner of the mouth
   2. Medially to form the sides of the upper lip, which unite with the globular process (forms the center of the lip)
   3. Inward to form the lateral palatine processes that fuse together with the primary palate (premaxilla) to form the palate
F. The lower face is formed by the bilateral swellings (mandibular processes) of the mandibular arch
G. Several facial or oral processes merge or fuse together during development; incomplete merging or fusing can result in cleft formation—cleft lip or cleft palate
   1. A cleft lip occurs more often on the left side, more frequently in males, and at the end of the second month in utero
   2. A cleft palate occurs more often in females
   3. Cleft lips and cleft palates can occur as isolated defects, meaning a cleft lip can occur without a cleft palate; most cleft palates occur in combination with a cleft lip

## Palatal Development

A. The globular process develops as medial nasal processes grow downward and gives rise to:
   1. The philtrum of the upper lip
   2. The primary palate (premaxillary process), which carries the incisor tooth buds
B. During the sixth week of embryonic life, two lateral palatine processes (palatal "shelves") develop from each side of the maxilla and lie vertically on each side of the tongue (these palatal shelves form the secondary palate)
C. During the 7th week of embryonic life, the developing tongue drops down, and the vertical lateral palatine processes flip up, assume a horizontal position, and fuse with the primary palate
D. Where the two palatal processes (shelves) fuse in the midline, trapped epithelium between the two processes may result in epithelial remnants, which may produce cysts
E. The right and left lateral palatine processes (palatal shelves) fuse with each other at the midline; anteriorly, they fuse with the primary palate in an area between the right and left laterals and the right and left canines
   1. A cleft palate occurs at the end of the 3rd month in utero
   2. Failure of fusion can occur at any of these lines of fusion
   3. A cleft in the alveolar ridge could occur unilaterally (on one side) or bilaterally (on both sides); this cleft occurs between the lateral and the canine, so the lateral incisor is the tooth most often missing or malformed
   4. The right and left lateral palatal processes can fail to fuse with each other at the midline, and the oral cavity would be open to the nasal cavity

## Tongue Development

During the 4th week of embryonic life, the tongue develops from several swellings arising on the internal aspect of branchial arches 1 to 4 (pouches); these swellings eventually merge and form the body and root of the tongue.

A. Branchial arch 1—two lateral swellings and one medial swelling (tuberculum impar) merge to form the body of the tongue
B. Branchial arches 2, 3, and part of 4—copula merge to form the base of the tongue
C. Branchial arch 4—site where the epiglottis is formed
D. Thyroid gland—develops from an invagination of ectoderm in the area of the foramen cecum of the tongue; the thyroid gland eventually migrates down to its position in the neck; thyroid tissue that remains entrapped in the tissue of the tongue may result in a developmental abnormality known as *lingual thyroid nodule*

# ORAL HISTOLOGY

## Tooth Development

A. Begins in the 7th week of embryonic life with the 20 primary teeth; continues until the late teens with sequential exfoliation of the primary dentition and development and eruption of the secondary dentition—the 32 permanent teeth
B. Tissues of the tooth
   1. Each tooth consists of four tissues (Fig. 2.16):

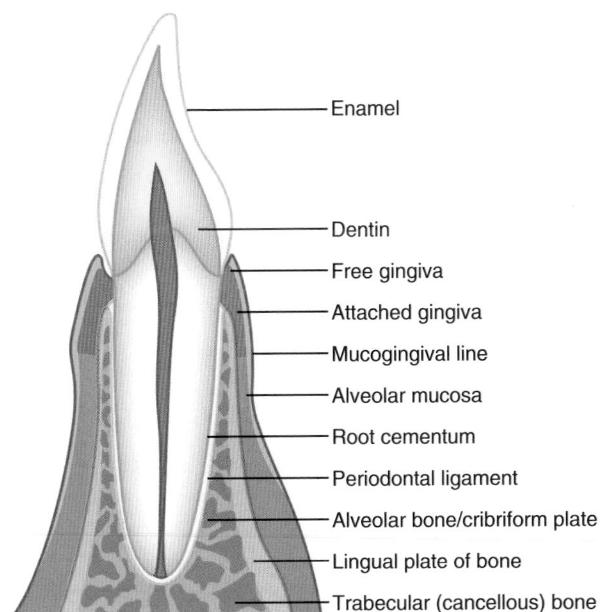


**Fig. 2.16** Four tissues of the tooth: enamel, cementum, dentin, and pulp. The periodontal ligament and alveolar bone are supporting tissues; junctional epithelium is the area where the enamel or cementum of the tooth and the epithelium of the gingival tissue form an attachment.

a. Enamel—calcified
b. Cementum—calcified
c. Dentin—calcified
d. Pulp—uncalcified
2. All tissues of the tooth are specialized forms of connective tissue, except enamel
3. Each tooth is the product of two tissues that interact during tooth development:
a. Mesenchyme (ectomesenchyme)—derived from neural crest cells
b. Epithelium—oral epithelium derived from the ectoderm

C. Involves two major events:
1. Morphodifferentiation—shaping of the tooth
2. Cytodifferentiation—cells differentiating into specific tissue-forming cells:
a. Ameloblasts—enamel-forming cells
b. Cementoblasts—cementum-forming cells
c. Odontoblasts—dentin-forming cells
d. Fibroblasts—pulp-forming cells (also capable of differentiating into a chondroblast, collagenoblast, or osteoblast)

## Morphodifferentiation

A. Oral epithelium and underlying ectomesenchyme are responsible for shaping the tooth

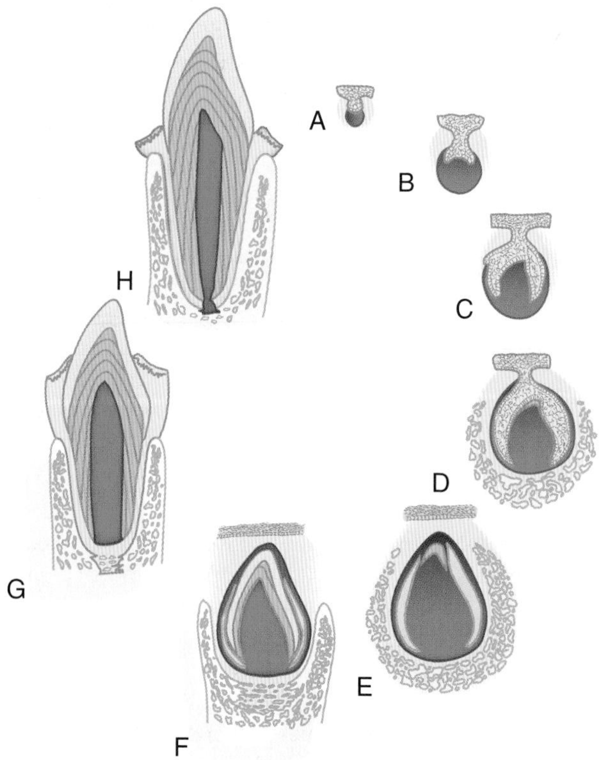


**Fig. 2.17** Sequential stages of tooth development. (A) Bud stage. (B) Cap stage. (C) Bell stage. (D) Dentinogenesis. (E) Amelogenesis. (F) Appositional dentin and enamel. (G) Eruption and root development. (H) Functional stage. (From Chiego D. *Essentials of Oral Histology and Embryology, a Clinical Approach.* 4th ed. St. Louis: Elsevier; 2014.)

1. Both primary and permanent tooth germs go through the same stages of development
2. The oral epithelium grows down into the underlying ectomesenchyme; small areas of condensed mesenchyme form future tooth germs

B. Stages (Fig. 2.17)
1. Bud stage—condensed areas of ectomesenchymal cells that are continuous with the oral epithelium; connection between the two is referred to as the *dental lamina*
2. Cap stage—future shape of the tooth becomes evident; cells specialize to form the enamel organ
3. Bell stage—final stage of morphodifferentiation; in the latter part of this stage, cytodifferentiation begins in the enamel organ
4. Dentinogenesis—origin or initial stages of dentin formation
5. Amelogenesis—differentiated cells begin initial enamel formation
6. Apposition stage—formation of dental tissue matrix; this matrix will then undergo maturation or calcification
7. Eruption and root development
8. Functional stage—the tooth is fully erupted in the mouth

## Cytodifferentiation

A. Stages of cytodifferentiation and morphodifferentiation overlap; both epithelial and mesenchymal components of the tooth germ become organized
1. Epithelial components become the enamel organ, which is organized into four distinct cell layers (Fig. 2.18):
a. Outer enamel epithelium (OEE)—outlines the shape of the future developing enamel organ on the outer surface; composed of small cuboidal cells, one cell layer thick
b. Inner enamel epithelium (IEE)—innermost layer of the enamel organ on the concave side of the developing tooth germ; this will become the future enamel-producing cells, the ameloblasts; composed of cuboidal-type cells, one cell layer thick
c. Stratum intermedium (STI)—flat, supporting, squamous-type cells, two to three cell layers thick, lying on top of the inner enamel epithelial cells
d. Stellate reticulum (STR)—mechanically and nutritionally supporting cells that fill the bulk of the developing enamel organ; are star shaped with large amounts of intercellular space between them
2. Mesenchymal components become subdivided into:
a. Dental sac (follicle)—surrounds the developing tooth germ and provides cells that will form the PDL, which in turn will produce the cementum and the alveolar bone proper
b. Dental papilla—condensed ectomesenchyme located on the concave side of the enamel organ; peripheral cells facing the IEE will differentiate into odontoblasts (dentin-forming cells)
c. The center of the dental papilla will become the dental pulp

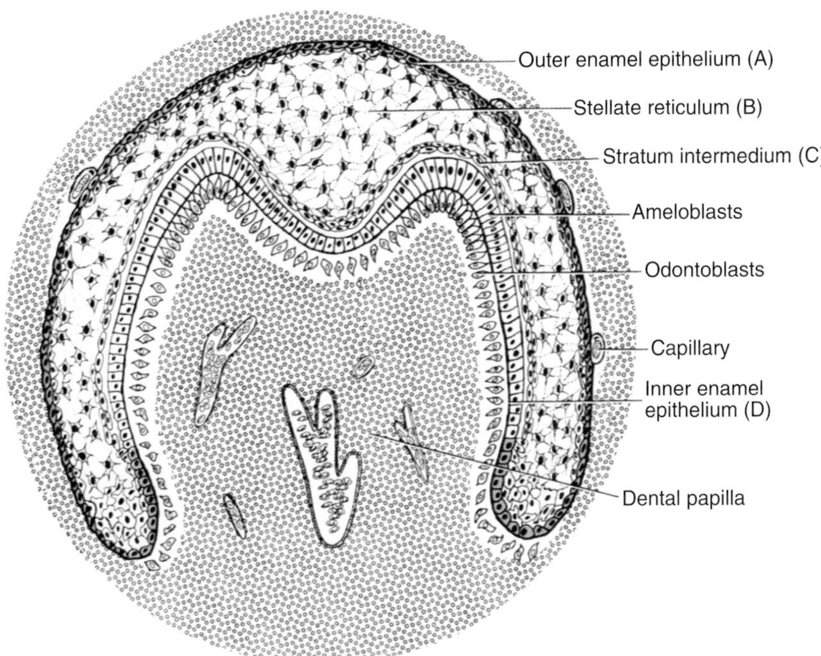


**Fig. 2.18** The four distinct layers of the enamel organ. (A) Outer enamel epithelium. (B) Stellate reticulum. (C) Stratum intermedium. (D) Inner enamel epithelium. (Modified from Chiego D. *Essentials of Oral Histology and Embryology, a Clinical Approach.* 4th ed. St. Louis: Elsevier; 2014.)

B. Tooth development depends on a series of sequential cellular interactions between the epithelial and mesenchymal components of the tooth germ
   1. First interaction—between the oral epithelium and the mesenchyme; the ectomesenchyme instructs the epithelium to grow down into the ectomesenchyme and shape the tooth
   2. Second interaction—signal given by cells of the IEE (preameloblasts) to the mesenchymal cells on the periphery of the dental papilla to differentiate into odontoblasts and begin the deposition of dentin
   3. Third interaction—as soon as odontoblasts begin to deposit dentin, preameloblasts become true secreting ameloblasts and begin the deposition of enamel
   4. Fourth interaction—occurs with the development of root dentin and cementum

## Dentin and Enamel Formation

A. Both enamel-forming and dentin-forming cells are polarized, tall, columnar, secreting cells; just before ameloblasts and odontoblasts begin to deposit enamel and dentin, organelles, especially the mitochondria, increase in number; organelles move to the basal nonsecretory end of the cell; both cells require tremendous amounts of energy for the production of their calcified tissues

B. All dentin and enamel formation begins at the dento-enamel junction (DEJ) of the cup or the incisal edge of the tooth and continues in an apical direction

C. The permanent tooth germ grows off the primary (deciduous) tooth germ by an epithelial attachment similar to dental lamina, called *successional lamina*; this applies to all the developing permanent teeth except the first, second, and third molars; these develop from the dental lamina, which continues to grow back in oral arches

D. Dentin formation
   1. Odontoblasts produce collagen fibers that unravel to produce a fibrous connective tissue matrix (fibrillar matrix) of predominantly collagen fibers with a rich proteoglycan ground substance; dentinal tissue is calcified by the deposition of the crystals of the calcium salt hydroxyapatite into the matrix
   2. Each odontoblast has a long cell extension, the odontoblastic process, left behind in the calcified dentin and enclosed in a dentinal tubule (Fig. 2.19)
   3. Dentin remains a vital tissue throughout the life of the tooth; in a vital tooth, cells continue to produce dentin when needed

E. Enamel formation
   1. Ameloblasts produce an enamel matrix with protein components called *amelogenins* and *enamelins*; the matrix is calcified immediately by the deposition of the crystals of the calcium salt hydroxyapatite
   2. Ameloblasts deposit enamel; each ameloblast has a secretory process called *Tomes' process*; Tomes' process has a six-sided pyramidal shape and is responsible for prism-shaped microscopic patterns of enamel rods; unlike the odontoblastic process, Tomes' process is not left behind embedded in the calcified tissue (see Fig. 2.19)
   3. When the tooth emerges into the oral cavity, the enamel has no vital cells associated with the tissue; enamel is not a true tissue like other dental tissues and is incapable of tissue growth or repair; once formed, the mineral substance cannot be physiologically withdrawn from the tooth

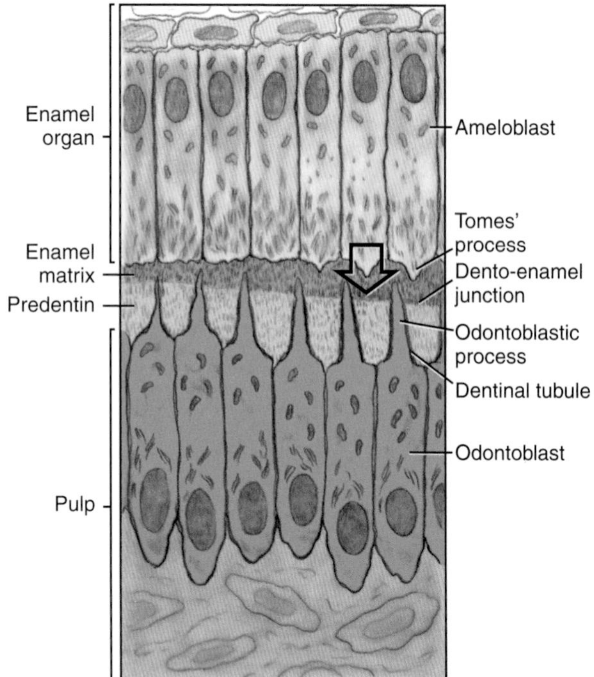


**Fig. 2.19** Odontoblasts and ameloblasts with their cell extensions. Tall, secretory odontoblast with its cell extension (odontoblastic extension). Tall, secretory ameloblast with its cell extension (Tomes' process). (From Fehrenbach MJ, Popowics. *Dental Embryology, Histology, and Anatomy*. 4th ed. St. Louis: Saunders; 2016.)

4. A final product of the ameloblasts is the primary enamel cuticle, a calcified coating on the enamel surface
5. Secondary cuticle—a noncalcified coating; a product of the reduced enamel organ
6. Nasmyth's membrane consists of the primary enamel cuticle and the secondary enamel cuticle; this membrane on the newly erupted tooth can easily pick up extrinsic stain

F. Dento-gingival junction formation
1. After the enamel formation is complete, remains of the enamel organ (OEE, IEE, STI, and STR) come together to form the reduced enamel epithelium (REE)
2. REE—plays an important role in the formation of the dento-gingival junction as the tooth emerges into the oral cavity

G. Cementum formation
1. Formation of root dentin and cementum follows after the formation of the crown of the tooth is complete
2. *Hertwig's root sheath* is formed by the joining of the OEE and the IEE; the sheath continues to grow down, shapes the root of the tooth and the formation of root dentin, and is followed by differentiation of cells from the dental sac; these cells produce:
   a. Cementum
   b. PDL
   c. Alveolar bone proper

## Soft Tissue of the Oral Cavity

### Oral Mucosa

A. Oral epithelium (Fig. 2.20)

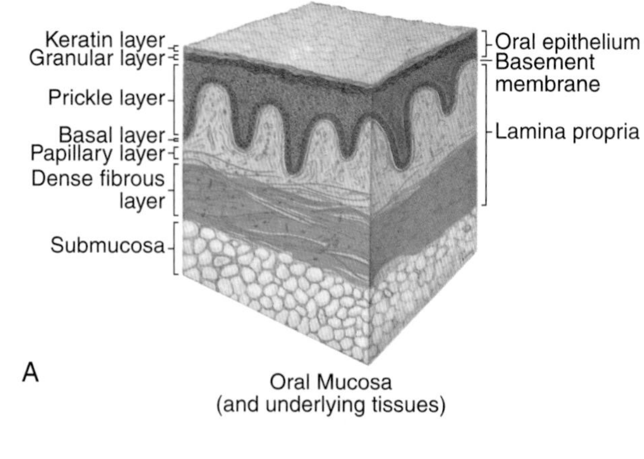


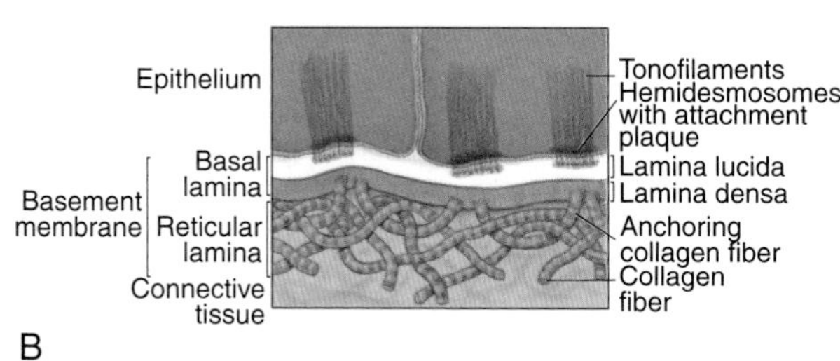


**Fig. 2.20** Basic structure of the oral epithelium. (A) Two basic tissues comprise the oral mucosa: the oral epithelium and connective tissue. Connective tissue is composed of a papillary layer and a reticular layer. A submucosal layer may or may not be present, depending on the location of the oral mucosa. Note the arrangement of rete ridges (or pegs) and connective tissue papillae. (B) Basal lamina interface between oral epithelium and connective tissue. Note the hemidesmosomes with attachment plaque between epithelial cells and the basal lamina. (From Fehrenbach MJ, Popowics. *Dental Embryology, Histology, and Anatomy*. 4th ed. St. Louis: Saunders; 2016.)

1. Covered by a layer of the stratified squamous epithelium that:
   a. Acts as a mechanical barrier
   b. Protects the underlying tissues
2. Three types of stratified squamous epithelia are found in the oral cavity:
   a. Orthokeratinized
      (1) Effective as a mechanical protector and barrier against fluids
      (2) Least common of the three types
      (3) Layers
         (a) Basal cell layer—deepest layer
         (b) Prickle cell layer (stratum spinosium)
         (c) Granular layer—contains the keratohyaline granules, the precursor to keratin
         (d) Keratinized layer (stratum corneum)—contains degenerative cells with no nuclei or organelles; cells are filled with keratin, become hard (cornified), and are eventually lost from the surface epithelium
   b. Nonkeratinized
      (1) Functions as a selective barrier; acts as a cushion and as protection against mechanical stress and wear
      (2) Layers

(a) Basal cell layer
(b) Prickle cell layer
(c) Outer surface of nonkeratinized cells (squamae); no distinctly recognizable layer above the prickle cell layer; superficial cells in the outermost layer undergo a gradual increase in size; look empty but are filled with fluid sacs; cells act as a cushion and are firmly attached to each other

c. Parakeratinized
(1) Intermediate form of the epithelium located between the orthokeratinized and nonkeratinized oral mucosa
(2) Layers
(a) Basal cell layer
(b) Prickle cell layer
(c) Keratinized layer—no distinct granular layer present; gradually becomes filled with keratin; nuclei and other cell organelles remain until the cell becomes cornified, and then they are eventually lost

3. The stratified squamous epithelium is constantly renewed by mitosis at the basal cell layer; turnover time ranges from 5 to 16 days

B. Connective tissue—referred to as *lamina propria*
1. Subdivided into two layers:
a. Papillary layer—directly under the epithelial layer; tattoo dye is injected into this portion of tissue
b. Reticular layer—dense fibrous layer located under the papillary layer; wrinkles in the skin occur because of degradation of the reticular layer
2. Forms a mechanical support system and carries
a. Blood vessels
b. Nerves

C. Submucosa
1. Layer of loosely organized connective tissue
2. Present only in areas that require a high degree of compressibility and flexibility (e.g., cheeks, soft palate)
3. When present, submucosa is located between the lamina propria and areas of muscle tissue

D. Interface
1. Area of interdigitation between the oral epithelium and connective tissue
2. Epithelial extensions into connective tissue (lamina propria) are called *ridges* or *rete pegs* (see Fig. 2.20A)
3. Connective tissue extensions into overlying epithelium are called *connective tissue papillae*
4. Corrugated arrangement
a. Increases the surface area between the two tissues
b. Increases the strength of the junction between the two tissues
c. Decreases the distance between the blood supply and the epithelium, which does not have its own blood supply; blood vessels are carried to the epithelium in connective tissue through connective tissue papillae
d. This rete peg arrangement is found in healthy attached gingiva, the stippling of which is caused by this arrangement; healthy sulcular epithelium does not have rete pegs

E. Basement membrane (see Fig. 2.20B)
1. Located between oral epithelium and connective tissue
2. Noncellular
3. Produced partly by epithelial cells and connective tissue cells
4. Composed of two layers:
a. The basal lamina is primarily the product of epithelial cells and can be further divided into two layers:
(1) The clear layer adjacent to the epithelium is the lamina lucida
(2) The denser layer closer to the connective tissue is the lamina densa and is about 20 to 70 nm thick; it contains some type IV collagen fibers that are produced by the connective tissue
b. Reticular lamina is found below the basal lamina and is much thicker than the basal layer; it contains collagen fiber produced by connective tissue cells and plays a role in anchoring the basal lamina to the underlying connective tissue
5. Epithelial cells form hemidesmosome attachments to the basal lamina (see Fig. 2.20)

F. Clinical changes in the oral mucosa
1. Inflammation, friction, heat, and chronic irritation produce changes in the degree of keratinization
a. Inflammation causes a reduction in keratinization
b. Friction, heat, and chronic irritation cause an increase in keratinization
c. Increased keratinization causes tissue appearance to be lighter or whitish; in areas of the mouth that have minor salivary glands, such as the soft palate, increased keratin may obstruct the gland openings, producing the appearance of red dots on hyperkeratinized tissue (nicotine stomatitis)
2. The appearance of the oral mucosa changes in response to pathologic, dermatologic, systemic, allergic, and localized factors

## Classifications of Mucosa

A. Masticatory—gingiva, hard palate (orthokeratinized epithelial covering)
1. Histologic structure
a. Keratinized stratified squamous epithelium; rete pegs—projections into the underlying connective tissue
b. No submucosa; no salivary glands
c. Fibrous connective tissue; gingival fibers
2. Clinical appearance
a. Coral pink; influenced by vascularity, the thickness and degree of keratinization of the epithelium, and the presence of pigment cells
b. Texture—stippled, the result of the rete peg arrangement
c. Consistency—firm, caused by the fibrous content (mostly collagen) of the underlying connective tissue

B. Lining—lips, cheeks, floor of mouth, ventral surface (underside) of tongue, soft palate, alveolar mucosa (nonkeratinized epithelial covering)

1. The floor of the mouth is the thinnest part of the nonkeratinized squamous epithelial lining mucosa (100 μm)
2. Connective tissue of the lining mucosa has more elastic fiber than that of the masticatory mucosa; fluid disperses readily in this area, making it an ideal site for local anesthetic injections

***Specialized Mucosa of the Tongue***

A. Specialized covering found only on the top of the tongue; covered with lingual papillae
B. Epithelial layer—stratified squamous epithelium that varies in thickness and degree of keratinization
C. Taste buds are epithelial organs of special sense (taste); most taste buds are found on lingual papillae; isolated buds may be found on the soft palate and on the walls of the pharynx
D. Connective tissue papillae form specialized lingual papillae
   1. Fungiform papillae—located on the dorsal aspect of the tongue; mushroom shaped; a single taste bud may be present on the top surface
   2. Filiform papillae—most abundant of papillae; found covering the entire top surface of the tongue; have no taste buds; elongated in cases of "hairy" tongue
   3. Circumvallate papillae—large papillae located in a V-shaped groove at the base of the tongue; encircled by a deep groove; mushroom shaped; taste buds are located on their sides; small salivary glands (Ebner's glands) empty into surrounding grooves of taste buds
   4. Foliate papillae—located along the sides of the tongue, near the base; taste buds may be located on only one of the sides
E. No submucosa is present

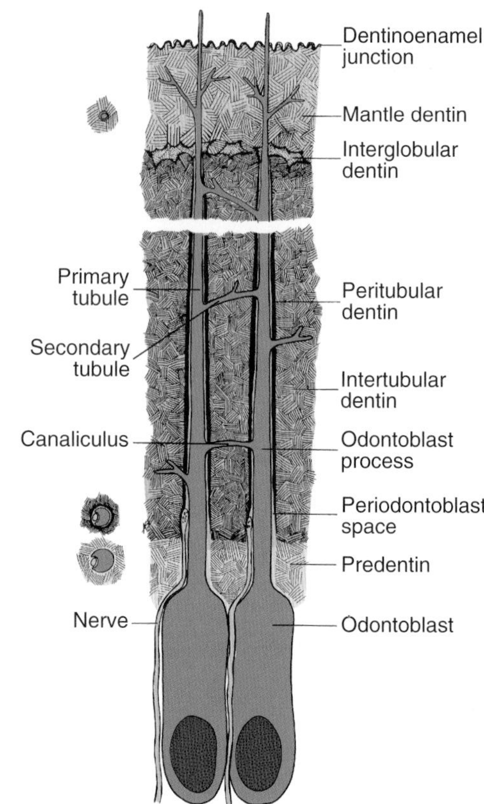


**Fig. 2.21** Odontoblastic process with its cell process enclosed in dentinal tubule. (From Chiego D. *Essentials of Oral Histology and Embryology, a Clinical Approach.* 4th ed. St. Louis: Elsevier; 2014.)

## Tissues of the Tooth

### Dentin

A. Mature dentin composition
   1. Chemical composition
      a. Organic matter, 18%
      b. Inorganic matter, 70%
      c. Water, 12%
   2. Tissue composition
      a. Cells—odontoblasts
      b. Fibrous material—collagen fibers (type I)
      c. Ground substance—proteoglycans and glycoproteins
   3. Calcification—deposition of crystals of the calcium salt hydroxyapatite in the dentin, fibrous matrix, and ground substance
B. Process of dentogenesis
   1. Dentin begins to form in the late bell stage of the developing tooth germ (see Fig. 2.17)
   2. Newly differentiated odontoblasts deposit the dentin matrix; odontoblastic processes become surrounded by predentin (a newly deposited, uncalcified dentin matrix); predentin becomes calcified as cells deposit more dentin; predentin is adjacent to the pulp in young teeth
   3. Each cell process in mature calcified dentin is enclosed in a dentinal tubule (Fig. 2.21)
      a. Dentinal tubules can run from the DEJ to the periphery of the dental pulp, where cell bodies of odontoblasts are located
      b. Tubules follow a primary S-shaped curve (pathway) and secondary S-shaped curves along the length of the tubules
         (1) Primary S-shaped curves are caused by the movement of odontoblasts from a wider area to a narrower area, which produces crowding of the odontoblasts; because of the S-shaped–curved movement, odontoblasts adjust to the new crowding while moving back toward the dental pulp
         (2) Secondary S-shaped curves are seen along the length of the dentinal tubule as small waves in the tubules, about 4 μm apart; may possibly be reflecting changes in the movement of the odontoblasts during night and day
      c. Tubules tend to have more branching at their terminal ends in the crown of the tooth than in root dentin; root dentin has more lateral branching, with fewer primary S-shaped curves
      d. Higher tubular density in peripheral dentin makes teeth particularly sensitive when exposed, almost as sensitive as the dentin near the pulp
      e. The diameter of tubules changes during the process of dentin formation; the widest dentinal tubules are found in children and are about 4 μm wide
   4. The first layer of dentin immediately adjacent to the DEJ is called *mantle dentin*; the remainder of the deposited dentin is called *circumpulpal dentin* (around the pulp)

a. Mantle dentin
(1) The layer of dentin that is about 10 to 30 μm thick
(2) Differs from circumpulpal dentin because in addition to collagen fibers normally found in dentin, it contains a second group of thicker and heavier collagen fibers
(a) These fibers are deposited perpendicular to the DEJ
(b) These heavier collagen fibers are referred to as *Korff's fibers*
(3) Mantle dentin is less calcified than is circumpulpal dentin
b. Circumpulpal dentin
(1) Contains finer collagen fibers than does mantle dentin
(2) Fibers are deposited parallel to the DEJ
5. Dentin that forms immediately around the odontoblastic process is called *peritubular dentin*
a. Forms a sheath around each odontoblastic process about 1 μm thick
b. Consists of a matrix of delicate collagen fibers
c. Is highly calcified
d. Is the first dentin to be decalcified by bacterial enzymes when exposed to caries
6. The remainder of dentin is called *intertubular dentin*
a. Consists of large, coarse collagen fibers
b. The matrix is less calcified than that of peritubular dentin
c. Produced first by the odontoblast; then the odontoblast produces its peritubular dentin
7. Once dentin is deposited, it does not undergo any remodeling
C. Types
1. Primary dentin—refers to dentin deposited before completion of the apical foramen
2. Secondary dentin—refers to dentin formed after completion of the apical foramen; tends to be more calcified than primary dentin; forms at a slower rate
3. Reactive (reparative) dentin—forms rapidly in localized areas where dental tubules have been exposed to external traumas such as:
a. Dental caries
b. Attrition or bruxism (enamel has been mechanically worn away)
c. Thermal extremes
4. Sclerotic dentin—forms when the dentinal fibers have degenerated and the tubules become filled with calcium salts
5. Dead tracts—dentinal tubules that remain unfilled after dentinal fiber degeneration
6. Interglobular dentin—small areas of unmineralized dentin near the DEJ
7. Tomes' granular layer—small unmineralized areas of dentin beneath the cementum (may play a role in root sensitivity)
D. Sensory conduction
1. Nerves associated with dentin are located in the dental pulp, but it is believed that they monitor the changes in the environment of odontoblasts, which allows for the perception of pain
2. When dentinal tubules become exposed to the outside environment, a direct contact is made with the dental pulp; fluid in open, exposed tubules begins to evaporate, and the movement of fluid caused by evaporation may stimulate the nerves closest to odontoblasts to produce pain (dentinal hypersensitivity) (see the section "Control of Dentinal Hypersensitivity" in Chapter 16)

## Pulp Tissue

A. Structure
1. Most centrally located tissue in the tooth
2. Loose connective tissue
3. Cells
a. Fibroblasts—undifferentiated mesenchymal cells
b. Histiocytes—found along blood vessels; sometimes referred to as *macrophages* when filled with ingested materials
c. Lymphocytes—when present, tend to be near the odontoblastic layer
d. Cells present in diseased pulp include monocytes, polymorphonuclear leukocytes, eosinophils, and plasma cells
e. No fat cells are present
4. Structural arrangement
a. The outer periphery of the pulp gives rise to the odontoblastic cell layer
b. The layer subjacent to the odontoblastic layer is called the *cell-free zone,* or the *zone of Weil*
c. Next to the cell-free zone is a relatively cell-rich zone
d. The core of the pulp is centrally located
B. Functions
1. Nutritive functions—very rich blood supply that forms a capillary plexus surrounding odontoblasts
2. Formative function—peripheral layer of pulp cells gives rise to odontoblasts
3. Sensory function—naked nerve fibers travel as free nerve endings and make contact with odontoblasts
4. Protective function—the pulp can respond to stimuli that occur outside the tooth; response may trigger the formation of reactive dentin
C. Blood supply and nerves
1. Blood vessels enter the pulp through the apical foramen; one or more small arterioles form a rich capillary plexus under the odontoblastic layer; exchange of nutrients occurs across the capillary wall
2. Two types of nerve fibers enter the pulp:
a. Autonomic nerve fibers—only the sympathetic autonomic nerve fibers are present; they regulate blood flow in the vessels
b. Afferent nerve fibers—come from the second and third branches of the trigeminal nerve; they lose their myelin sheath and terminate as free nerve endings in close association with odontoblasts; it is thought that the presence of free nerve endings is responsible for the perception of pain by the dental pulp

D. Pulp changes
   1. Changes resulting from aging
      a. As the tooth ages, the amount of collagen fibers increases and the number of reticulin fibers decreases; in addition, the ground substance loses considerable water
      b. The pulp becomes less cellular and more fibrous
      c. The size of the pulp decreases because of the continued deposition of dentin
   2. Small calcified bodies, called *denticles*, may be present
      a. The three types of denticles are:
         (1) True denticles—form during tooth development in the root; have dentinal tubules in their structure; odontoblasts are present on the periphery
         (2) False denticles—form when the components of the pulp start to degenerate; calcify and grow into irregular calcified bodies; dentinal tubules are not usually present
         (3) Diffuse calcifications—occur in diseased pulp in many locations; are likely to grow and cause problems
      b. Both true and false denticles may be loose in the dental pulp, attached to the dentin wall, or embedded in the dentin tissue
      c. Calcified structures in the pulp appear radiopaque on radiographs

## Comparison of Pulp and Dentin

A. Dentin and the dental pulp are closely related functionally and developmentally; both are products of the dental papilla (derived from neural crest cells)
B. Two major differences exist between these tissues:
   1. The pulp is a loose, noncalcified connective tissue; dentin is a highly specialized, calcified connective tissue
   2. The pulp is a very vascular tissue; dentin is avascular
C. Dentin and the pulp form the bulk of the fully developed tooth
D. During tooth development, the peripheral cells of the dental papilla differentiate into odontoblasts and form dentin, while the core of the dental papilla becomes the pulp

## Enamel

A. Composition
   1. Most highly calcified of all the dental tissues
   2. Composed mainly of inorganic calcium salt and hydroxyapatite, with a small amount of protein material and water in the matrix
      a. Inorganic component, 95%
      b. Organic component, 1%
      c. Water, 4%
B. Process of amelogenesis
   1. Enamel formation, as with dentin formation, begins in the late bell stage of tooth development
   2. Shortly after the deposition of dentin, the inner enamel epithelial cells of the enamel organ become secretory ameloblasts
      a. Ameloblasts begin to deposit the enamel matrix, which is mineralized almost immediately
      b. Ameloblasts have tall columnar cell bodies that appear hexagonal in cross section
      c. The secretory process of the ameloblast is the shovel-shaped Tomes' process discussed earlier; the shape of the process is closely related to the form of the structural units that make up the fully developed enamel tissue
   3. Ameloblasts pass through two main stages while depositing enamel:
      a. Secretory stage—ameloblasts deposit the enamel matrix, which contains both organic and inorganic components
      b. Resorbing stage—ameloblasts remove most of the water and organic components from the matrix
   4. Enamel maturation begins before the completion of enamel formation
      a. First, very thin and needle-like hydroxyapatite crystals are deposited in the matrix
      b. During the process of enamel maturation, the crystals increase in all dimensions, which is made possible by the continual removal of water and organic components from the matrix
      c. The hydroxyapatite crystals in enamel are four times larger than those in bone, dentin, and cementum
C. Enamel rods—structural units of enamel
   1. Enamel is composed of tightly packed masses of hydroxyapatite crystals called *enamel rods,* or *prisms*
   2. Rod formation is related to the shape of the Tomes' process and the orientation of crystals as they are deposited by ameloblasts
   3. The prisms are rod-shaped structures that run from the DEJ to the outer edge of the enamel surface
   4. They are stacked in interlocking rows, one on top of the other; the stacking arrangement causes the rods to appear as keyhole-shaped prisms when viewed in cross section, with the top of the keyhole facing the occlusal or incisal edge of the tooth and the tail facing the cervical portion; four ameloblasts contribute to form one keyhole (Fig. 2.22)
   5. The average width of an enamel rod is approximately 4 μm; the rods are narrower near the DEJ and wider near the outer surface of the enamel
   6. The crystals in the head region of the rod are oriented with their long axis parallel to the long axis of the rod; in the tail region, crystals are perpendicular to the long axis of the rod
   7. Adjacent rods are separated from each other by rod sheaths approximately 0.1 to 2.0 μm wide; they can be observed in the head region of the rods but are not as clearly defined in the tail region; and they are produced by an abrupt change in the angulation (orientation) of the crystals as they are deposited by the moving ameloblast (Fig. 2.23)
   8. Rodless enamel may be found near the DEJ and the outer surface of the enamel

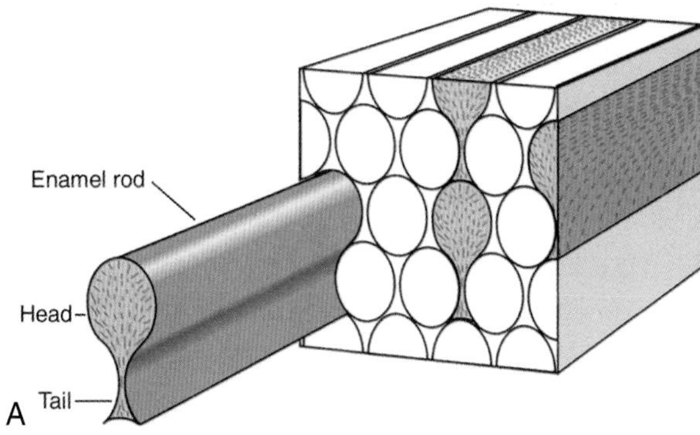


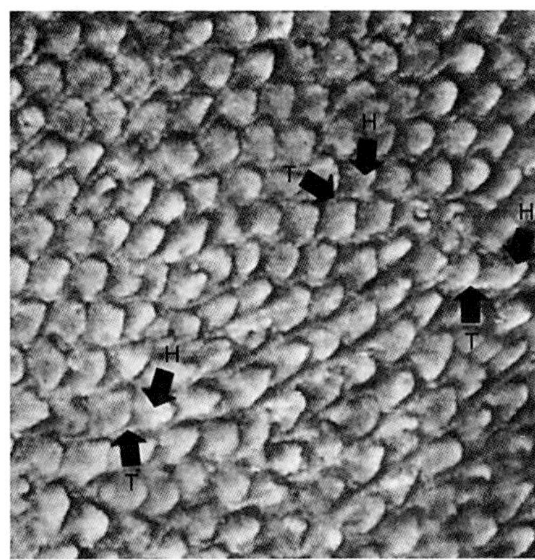


**Fig. 2.22** Enamel rod, the basic unit of enamel. (A) Relationship of the rod to enamel. (B) Scanning electron micrograph of enamel showing head *(H)* and tail *(T)*. ((B) from Fehrenbach MJ, Popowics. *Dental Embryology, Histology, and Anatomy*. 4th ed. St. Louis: Saunders; 2016.)

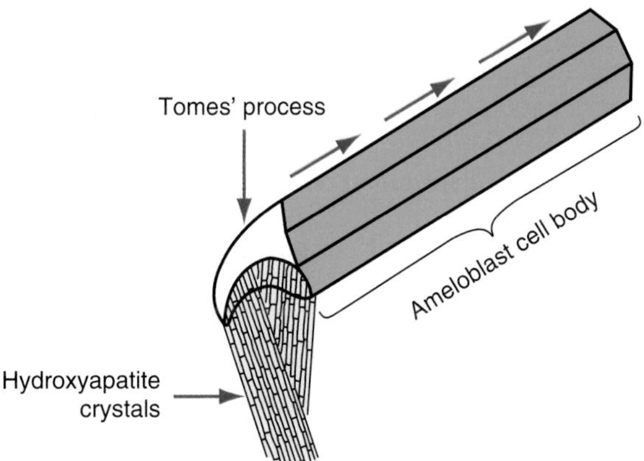


**Fig. 2.23** Ameloblast depositing hydroxyapatite crystals from the Tomes' process. Note the angular change in the orientation of crystals being deposited, which accounts for the rod sheath around the head of the rod. (Modified from Dr. Marlene Klyvert, Columbia University, School of Dental and Oral Surgery, New York.)

9. The rods are perpendicular to the outer surface of the enamel; near the cervix of the tooth, they tend to be oriented apically; toward the inner third of the enamel, groups of rods curve but then straighten out to form right angles with the enamel surface

D. Microscopic structures
   1. Bands of Hunter-Schreger—alternating light and dark bands; perpendicular to the DEJ; manifest as a result of enamel rod curvature
   2. Stripes of Retzius—narrow brown lines that extend diagonally from enamel rods; on the tooth surface, they end in shallow furrows known as *perikymata*
   3. Enamel lamellae—cracks that occur during enamel crystallization
   4. Enamel tufts—hypomineralized inner ends of some enamel rods; located in the DEJ area
   5. Enamel spindles—terminal portions of dentinal fibers that extend across the DEJ into the enamel

E. Clinical importance
   1. Dental procedures performed on enamel
      a. Application of fluoride—because enamel is semipermeable, fluoride ions are attracted to the hydroxyapatite crystals; fluoride also changes hydroxyapatite into fluorapatite; the tooth becomes more resistant to acids produced by bacteria
      b. Acid etching of enamel—the structure of enamel (rods and rod sheaths) allows acid to penetrate it for a limited distance (30 μm), and the acid attacks the mineral at the periphery of the sheaths; the acid thus creates a rough enamel surface, which helps bonding materials adhere more readily; the acid may attack the rod core and produce the same effect
      c. Cavity preparations—all rods are supported by dentin; margins will fail if enamel is left unsupported
   2. Tetracycline stains
      a. Appear clinically as dark bands through enamel, especially near the cervix of the tooth where enamel is thin
      b. Caused by the administration of tetracycline (antibiotic) during the formation of teeth
      c. Tetracycline binds chemically to organic and inorganic components of bone and dentin
      d. The resulting darkened area shows through enamel, making the fully developed tooth appear unattractive
      e. Stains are difficult to bleach out; affected teeth may need crowns or veneers, but only for aesthetic purposes
   3. Pits and fissures in enamel
      a. Are often present in less calcified areas
      b. Form where ameloblasts become crowded between adjacent areas (cusps), resulting in incomplete maturation of enamel
      c. Place teeth at increased risk for dental caries
      d. Require the application of dental sealants to prevent caries and arrest incipient caries

## Cementum

A. General properties and functions
   1. Calcified connective tissue that covers the roots of teeth; in conjunction with the alveolar bone proper and the PDL, forms the attachment apparatus of the teeth, allowing the teeth to become suspended in the jaw
   2. Derived from the dental sac (dental follicle)

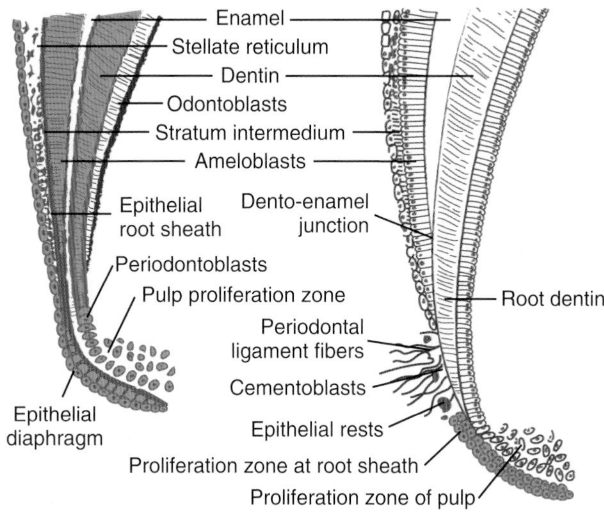


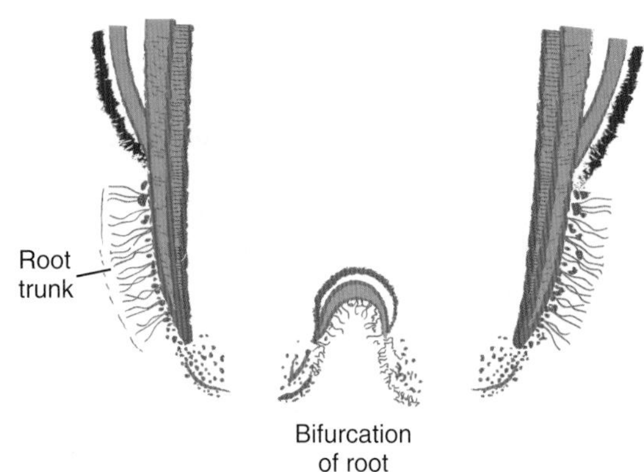


**Fig. 2.24** Relationship of the epithelial root sheath to the forming root and the formation of cementum.

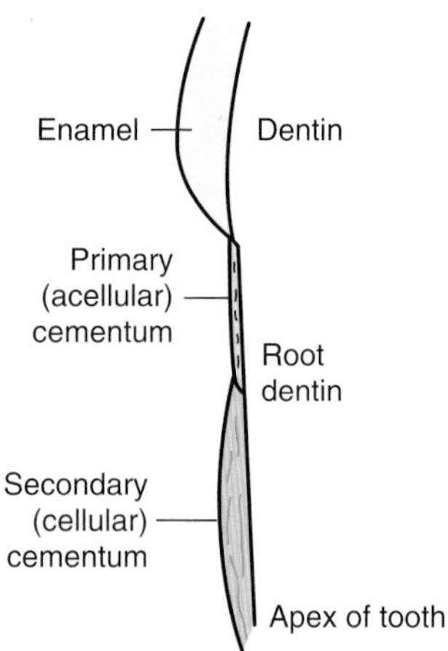


**Fig. 2.25** Relationship of the primary acellular cementum to the secondary (cellular) cementum, or root of tooth. Note the thickness of the cellular cementum near the tooth apex.

3. Resembles bone in structure and composition; major differences are:
   a. Bone is a vascularized tissue
   b. Cementum is avascular
4. Least mineralized of the calcified tissues of the tooth

B. Mature cementum composition
1. Chemical composition
   a. Organic components, 23%
   b. Inorganic components, 65%
   c. Water, 12%
2. Tissue composition
   a. Cells—cementoblasts, cementocytes
   b. Fibrous matrix—collagen fibers (type I); dominant component of the tissue, 90%
   c. Ground substance—proteoglycans

C. Process of cementogenesis (Fig. 2.24)
1. After crown formation is complete, the epithelial root sheath (Hertwig's root sheath) begins to grow down
   a. Shapes the root of the tooth
   b. Induces the formation of root dentin
2. After the first root dentin is deposited, the root sheath breaks down; cells from the dental sac migrate onto the newly deposited dentin and differentiate into cementoblasts

D. Mature cementum (fibrous matrix)
1. Very little cementum is deposited on the developing root until the tooth reaches functional occlusion (only approximately two-thirds of the root has been formed when the tooth erupts)
2. Cores of fibers remain uncalcified in the calcified cementum; referred to as *Sharpey's fibers*

E. Cellular and acellular cementum (Fig. 2.25)
1. Acellular cementum (primary cementum)
   a. Cervical half of the tooth is covered with a thin layer of cementum, approximately 10 μm thick
   b. Does not contain any embedded cementocytes (cementoblasts) in lacunae
   c. Forms at a slower rate than does cellular cementum
   d. Does not increase during the life of the tooth
   e. Appears to be involved more in maintenance than in the production of the tissue
   f. Contains less inorganic matrix than does cellular cementum
   g. Better calcified than cellular cementum
2. Cellular cementum (secondary cementum)
   a. Apical portion of the tooth is covered with cellular cementum, reaching a thickness of 100 to 150 μm
   b. Contains cementocytes trapped in the lacunae of the tissue
   c. Deposited throughout the life of the tooth
   d. Deposited at intervals (pauses), producing arrest lines—highly calcified lines similar to those seen in bone tissue

F. Abnormalities
1. Reversal lines
   a. May be present in cementum as in bone tissue
   b. Reflect resorption of tissue (remodeling)
   c. Resorption of cementum does not occur as frequently as in bone tissue; when it does occur, it is usually associated with:
      (1) Extreme orthodontic movement of the teeth
      (2) Trauma to teeth
2. Cementicles

a. Small, abnormal calcified bodies occasionally found in the PDL
b. Result of cellular debris (i.e., degenerating remnants of the epithelial root sheath)
c. May be found:
   (1) Attached to the cementum surface
   (2) Free in the PDL
   (3) Embedded in the cementum of the root
3. Hypercementosis
   a. Local abnormal thickening of parts of the cementum
   b. Usually found in the apical region, occurring on one or all of the teeth
   c. May be seen in cases of:
      (1) Chronic inflammation of the tooth
      (2) Loss of an antagonist tooth (no opposing tooth in the jaw)
      (3) Additional eruption; compensatory cementosis takes place
      (4) Tooth becoming fused with the surrounding alveolar bone proper

### Cemento-Enamel Junction

A. Three types of cemento-enamel relationships can occur during the development of the tooth:
   1. Cementum meets enamel edge to edge—occurs in approximately 76% of all teeth
   2. Cementum overlaps a small part of enamel—occurs in approximately 14% of all teeth
   3. Cementum is ditched with no exposed dentin—occurs in approximately 10% of all teeth
B. Cemento-enamel relationships occur when root-cementum development begins; this is related to the timing of the disruption (breakdown) of the epithelial root sheath and allows the cells from the dental sac to differentiate and begin depositing cementum
C. Differentiation of root dental papillae into odontoblasts is mediated by a cell-to-matrix type of inductive interaction (between the basal lamina of Hertwig's root sheath and the undifferentiated root dental papilla)
D. Differentiation of dental sac cells into cementoblasts is mediated by a cell-substrate type of inductive interaction between sac cells and newly deposited dentin
E. Practicing dental hygienists should use caution during instrumentation in areas where cementum is thin or absent; conservation of tooth structure is recommended
F. Recession of gingiva and loss of clinical attachment may also leave exposed cementum or dentin, creating root sensitivity and increased risk of root caries

## Supporting Tissues

### Alveolar Bone

A. The part of the bony maxilla and mandible, the alveolar process, in which teeth are suspended in alveoli (bony sockets)
B. Existence or presence of alveolar bone is totally dependent on the presence of dental roots; when teeth do not develop and erupt, alveolar bone does not develop; when teeth are extracted, alveolar bone is resorbed
C. Formed during the development and eruption of teeth; developing teeth, primary or permanent, are located in bony crypts in the bone of the maxilla or of the mandible
D. Has the same biophysical and chemical properties as other bone tissue in the body; has the same basic components as other connective tissue
   1. Cells—osteoblasts, osteocytes, osteoclasts
   2. Fibrous matrix—collagen fibers are the dominant component; calcified by deposition of the calcium salt hydroxyapatite into the matrix
   3. Ground substance—proteoglycans
E. Gross anatomy of a mature bone socket (Fig. 2.26)
   1. Each tooth is suspended in its own alveolus (socket), with each alveolus having the same structure and anatomy
      a. Outer cortical (compact lamellar) plate of bone—faces the cheek and lips (buccal)
      b. Inner cortical (compact lamellar) plate of bone—faces the tongue and palate (lingual)
      c. Spongiosa—cancellous bone sandwiched between the cortical plates of bone
   2. Alveolar bone proper—the part of the alveolus directly facing the root of the tooth; follows the general outline of the root; sometimes referred to as the *cribriform plate,* or lamina dura
      a. Cribriform plate
         (1) Contains numerous small openings; allows blood vessels and nerves in the PDL and bone to communicate
         (2) Consists of two layers of bone:
            (a) Compact lamellar bone
            (b) Layer of bundle bone into which the periodontal fibers insert themselves; the cores of the fibers remain uncalcified in the calcified tissues of bone or cementum, called Sharpey's fibers
      b. *Lamina dura* is purely a radiographic term based on this area appearing more radiopaque on radiographs; it is not more calcified than the rest of the bone socket; rather, the opacity is caused by the two-dimensional view of the compact bone in the area
      c. Alveolar bone proper that forms sockets around multiple-rooted teeth consists of the cribriform plates of both the roots and some spongy bone, called *inter-radicular alveolar bone*
      d. The alveolar bone proper between teeth consists of the cribriform plates of both the teeth and some spongy bone, called *interdental alveolar bone*
      e. Spongiosa is composed of small trabeculae of bone with large, narrow spaces between the trabeculae
   3. The alveolar bone proper (cribriform plate) is the only essential part of the bone socket; spongiosa and outer and inner cortical plates of bone are not always present; spongiosa may be absent, and outer and inner cortical plates may be fused together

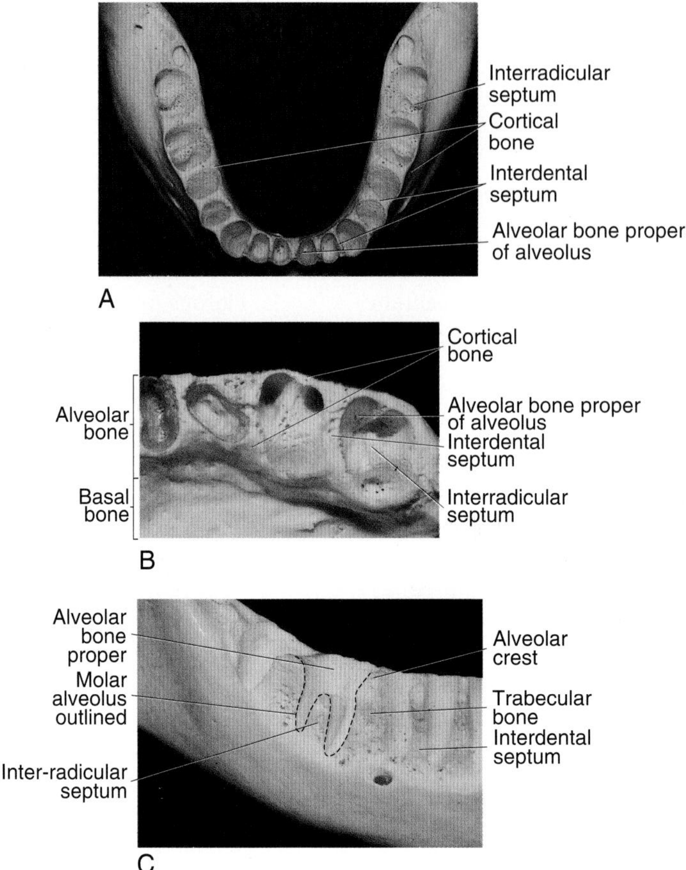


**Fig. 2.26** Components of alveolar bone. (A) Mandibular arch of the skull with teeth removed. (B) Portion of the maxilla of a skull with teeth removed. (C) Cross-section of mandible with teeth removed. (From Fehrenbach MJ, Popowics. *Dental Embryology, Histology, and Anatomy.* 4th ed. St. Louis: Saunders; 2016.)

4. Trabeculae of the spongiosa reflect functional forces or loading patterns imposed on teeth; the pattern changes when the forces are altered; two principal directions of the trabeculae are parallel and perpendicular to the direction of the imposed forces; trabecular bone orientation can be observed on radiographs; the number of trabeculae increases with increased function
5. Orthodontic movement of teeth always causes remodeling of the alveolar bone proper to accommodate movement of teeth; it affects the insertion of PDL fibers in the bundle bone but is a localized type of resorption; when the bundle bone is redeposited, fibers become firmly attached again; with pressure, bone is resorbed; when tension is applied, bone formation occurs
6. Radiographs of teeth may be used to show the height or slope (or both) of the interdental bone septum, which may reflect periodontal disease or other disease; the crest of the alveolar bone is usually between 0.75 and 1.49 mm from the cemento-enamel junction
7. The periosteum is a dense connective tissue layer on the outer portion of bone and is active in bone formation
8. The endosteum lines the inner aspects (medullary cavity) of bone

F. Alveolar bone is constantly remodeled by means of resorption and formation; this makes it the least stable of periodontal tissues
   1. Alveolar bone is affected by function, age-related and disease-related changes, hormones, and other systemic and host factors
   2. Remodeling affects the height, contour, and density of alveolar bone

## Periodontal Ligament

A. A specialized form of connective tissue derived from the dental sac that contributes to the attachment of teeth
B. Consists of groups of fiber bundles called *gingival fibers* and principal fiber bundles; areas of loose connective tissue, blood vessels, and nerves are present between principal fiber bundles; areas of loose connective tissue are called *interstitial spaces*
C. Tissue components
   1. Fibroblasts of the PDL are responsible for the production of the fibrous matrix and the ground substance; they are continually engaged in synthetic activities, rebuilding and producing new fibers to be incorporated into existing fibers, which are constantly being remodeled; PDL has a very fast turnover rate

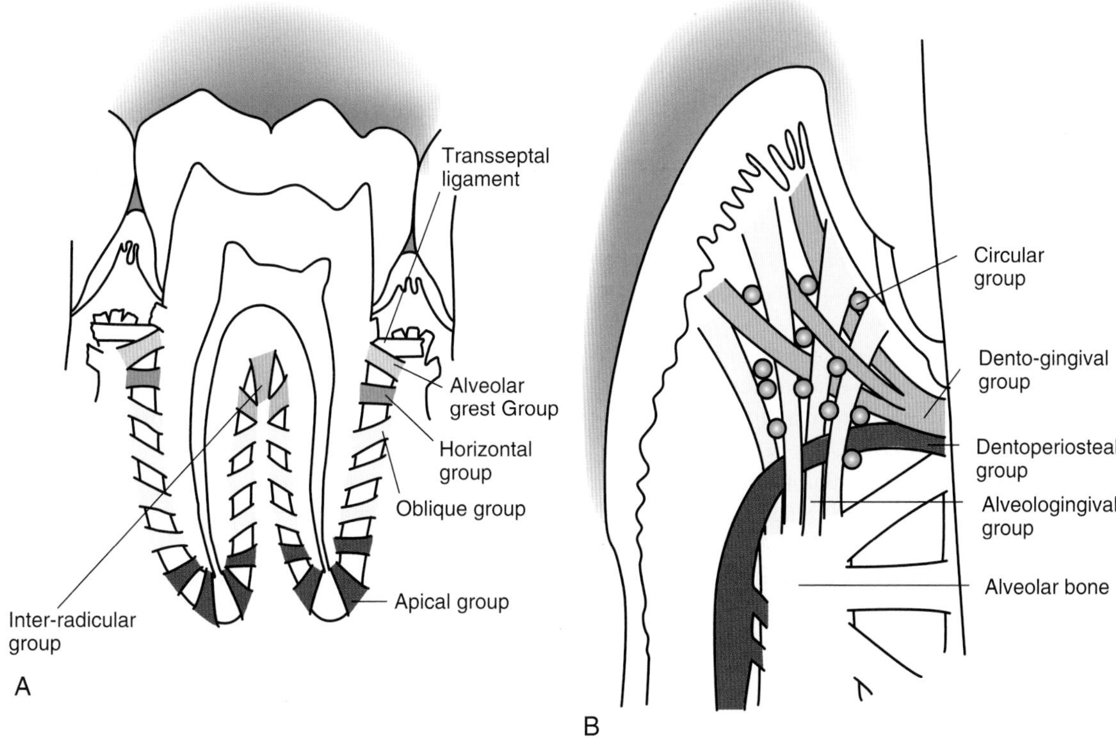


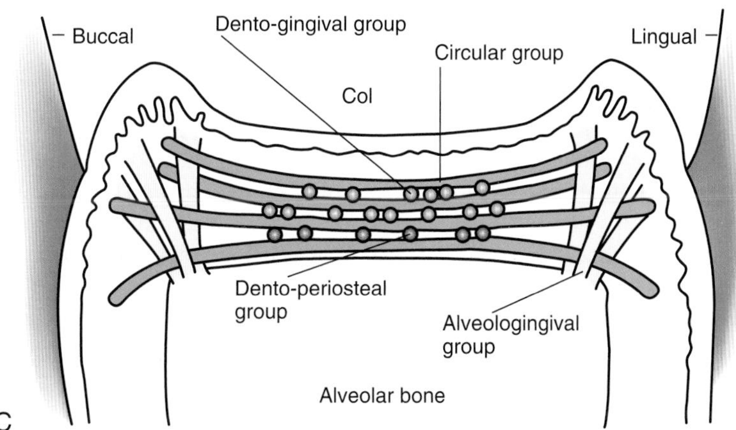


**Fig. 2.27** Connective tissue fibers. (A) Principal fiber groups of the periodontal ligament. (B) Gingival fiber groups. (C) Gingival ligament fibers in the col area. (Modified from Nanci A. *Ten Cate's Oral Histology: Development, Structure, and Function.* 8th ed. St. Louis: Elsevier; 2013.)

2. Ground substance—proteoglycans
3. The fibrous matrix is the dominant component of the PDL
   a. The fibers are collagen and oxytalan, with a few elastic fibers associated with blood vessels
   b. The fibers are arranged in dense bundles inserted into the alveolar bone proper and cementum
   c. The fibers are arranged into two groups:
      (1) Gingival fiber groups (Fig. 2.27B)
         (a) Dento-gingival fibers—extend from the cervical cementum to the free gingiva and from the cervical cementum to the lamina propria of the gingiva, over the alveolar crest
         (b) Dento-periosteal fibers—extend from cervical cementum over the alveolar crest to the periosteum of the cortical plates of bone
         (c) Trans-septal fibers—extend from the cementum of the tooth to the adjacent tooth, over the alveolar crest
         (d) Circular fibers—extend horizontally around the most cervical part of the root and insert into the cementum and lamina propria of the gingiva and the alveolar crest
      (2) Principal fiber groups (see Fig. 2.27A)
         (a) Alveolar crest fibers—extend from cervical cementum and insert themselves into the alveolar crest

(b) Horizontal fibers—extend at right angles to the long axis of the root of the tooth in a horizontal plane from alveolar bone to cementum; found in the cervical third of the root
(c) Oblique fibers—slant occlusally from cementum to alveolar bone; most abundant of the fiber bundles; start at the apical two-thirds of the root
(d) Apical fibers—radiate from apical cementum into alveolar bone
(e) Interradicular fibers (seen only in multiple-rooted teeth)—extend from the cementum in the furcation area of the tooth to the interradicular alveolar bone

d. Sharpey's fibers—the terminal portion of a PDL fiber that is embedded in bone and cementum
e. Fiber groups are oriented to give the tooth optimal resistance to all types of functional loading patterns
(1) Circular fibers resist rotational movements of the tooth (see Fig. 2.27C)
(2) Alveolar crest and apical fibers resist pull of the tooth from its socket
(3) Trans-septal fibers connect all teeth and maintain the integrity of the dental arches
f. Elastic fibers in the PDL do not contribute to the support of the tooth; the role of the oxytalan fibers is not clear

D. Blood vessels
1. The blood supply of the PDL is very rich and highly developed, more than in any other connective tissue; blood vessels are found in the interstitial spaces of the ligament
2. Each tooth, with its PDL and alveolar bone, has a common blood supply; a small artery branches off the main artery that supplies the jaw and enters the following:
a. Apical foramen of the tooth, which supplies the pulp of the tooth
b. PDL, which supplies the areas all around the tooth
c. Alveolar bone of the tooth
3. Once blood vessels enter the pulp chambers, they are isolated from surrounding tissues, but vessels supplying the PDL and alveolar bone are richly interconnected through openings in the cribriform plate

E. Nerves
1. The PDL contains two types of nerves:
a. Autonomic—sympathetic fibers that travel with blood vessels; these regulate blood flow to the tissues
b. Afferent sensory fibers—mostly myelinated nerves from the branches of the second and third divisions of the trigeminal nerve (fifth cranial nerve)
2. Two types of nerve endings are found in the PDL:
a. Free, unmyelinated nerve endings—responsible for pain sensation
b. Encapsulated nerve endings—responsible for registering pressure changes

F. The width of the PDL varies with the functional forces placed on the tooth and at different levels of the root (apex and cervix)
1. The width is greater in young adults (0.21 mm) than in older adults (0.15 mm)
2. The width is greater near the cervical and apical areas than in the middle of the root
3. Minimal movement (rotations) of any tooth occurs around the axis in the middle of the root; greatest movement occurs near the apex and the cervix, accounting for the difference in the width of the PDL along the root
4. The width is related to the amount of function and cellularity; an actively functioning tooth has a slightly wider PDL and more cellularity than does a nonfunctioning tooth

G. Abnormalities
1. Cementicles
2. Epithelial rests (cell rests of Malassez)
a. Remnants of the epithelium from the root sheath that did not disintegrate; formed from a cluster of epithelial cells surrounded by a basement membrane
b. In most cases, these rests are harmless, but they have the potential to become cystic
3. Untreated periodontal disease can result in damage to the supporting apparatus of the tooth and eventual loss of the tooth

## Dento-Gingival Junction

A. The area on the tooth where enamel and the epithelium form a junction; with aging, the junction is displaced more apically between cementum and the epithelium
B. First established as the tooth emerges into the oral cavity (Fig. 2.28)
1. Developing tooth is covered with REE, consisting of:
a. A layer of outer enamel epithelial cells
b. Remnants of the STI cell layers
c. STR
d. Postsecretory ameloblasts
2. Basal cells of oral epithelium covering the emerging tooth and outer layer of cells of the REE begin to proliferate and soon grow together to form one continuous unit; as the tooth emerges through the combined epithelia, it forms the initial dento-gingival junction on the enamel of the tooth
C. Dento-junctional epithelium
1. Gingival epithelium that faces the tooth
2. Composed of nonkeratinized stratified squamous epithelium without rete pegs and divided into:
a. Sulcular epithelium
(1) Found occlusally at the same height as the free gingiva
(2) The sulcus forms a shallow pocket around the tooth, about 0.5 mm deep
(3) In the disease state, the sulcus deepens and exhibits rete pegs and ulcerations

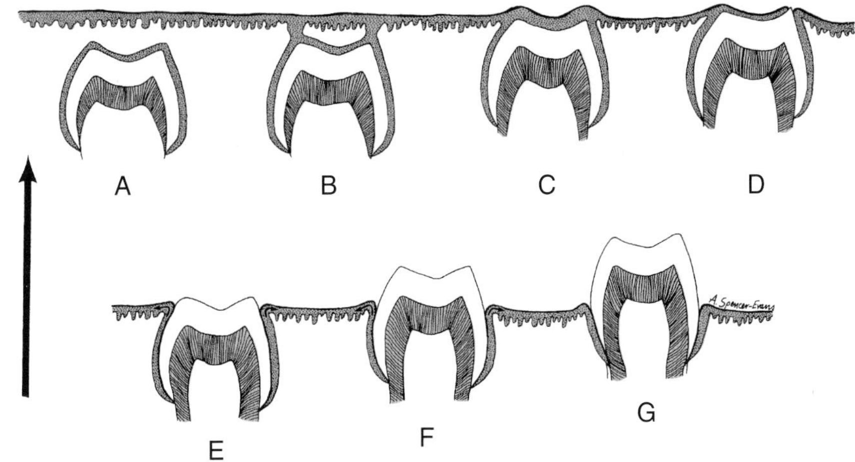


**Fig. 2.28** Tooth emerging into the oral cavity. Note that the reduced enamel epithelium covering the tooth joins the oral epithelium. The reduced enamel epithelium will form the initial junctional epithelium. (A) Crown penetrating bone and connective tissue. (B) Contact of crown with oral epithelium. (C) Fusion of epithelia. (D) Thinning of the epithelium. (E) Rupture of the epithelium. (F) Crown emergence. (G) Occlusal contact. (From Chiego D. *Essentials of Oral Histology and Embryology, a Clinical Approach*. 4th ed. St. Louis: Elsevier; 2014.)

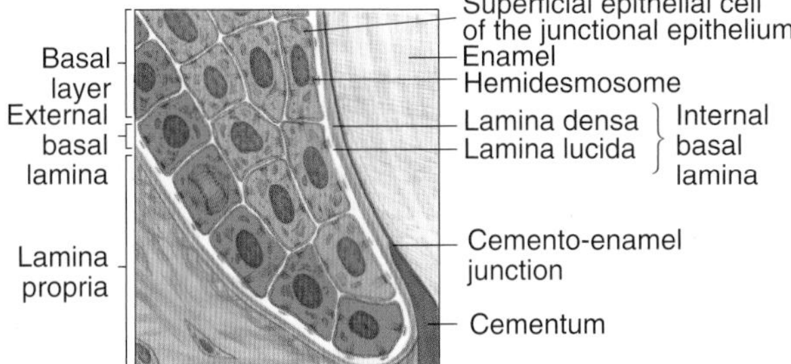


**Fig. 2.29** The epithelial attachment is the part of the junctional epithelium that attaches the junctional epithelium to the tooth surface. Note that the outer external basal lamina is continuous with the inner basal lamina, and between them are the cells of the junctional epithelium. (From Fehrenbach MJ, Popowics. *Dental Embryology, Histology, and Anatomy*. 4th ed. St. Louis: Saunders; 2016.)

b. Junctional epithelium (see Figs. 2.28 and 2.29)
   (1) Begins at the base of the sulcus
   (2) Firmly attached to the tooth, enamel, cementum, or all by hemidesmosomes
   (3) Located between two basal laminae
      (a) One basal lamina faces the enamel surface
      (b) The second basal lamina faces the connective tissue of the gingiva
      (c) Basal laminae are continuous at the base of the junctional epithelium (Fig. 2.29)

3. A membrane called the *primary cuticle* intervenes between the basal lamina of the junctional epithelium and the tooth surface
   a. The primary cuticle is formed during the late stages of eruption of the tooth
   b. The composition of the cuticle is not known, but the cuticle thickens with aging
4. The newly erupted tooth is covered with a thin, delicate membrane (Nasmyth's membrane)
   a. Will float off the tooth surface if placed in a 10% solution of hydrochloric acid
   b. Contains some cells of the REE and the dental cuticle
5. In the area of the dento-gingival junction, the junctional epithelium has the capacity to repair itself
6. The site of the dento-gingival junction is easily invaded by microorganisms and is the area where periodontal disease often begins

For a review of the histology, see the listings in the Website Information and Resources table.

Answers and rationales to chapter review questions are available on this text's accompanying Evolve site. See inside front cover for details.

## WEBSITE INFORMATION AND RESOURCES

| Source | Website Address | Description |
|---|---|---|
| University of Kentucky | http://www.uky.edu/~brmacp/oralhist/html/ohtoc.htm | Oral Histology Digital Lab & Atlas |
| Coursera, University of Pennsylvania | https://www.coursera.org/lecture/dental-medicine-penn/lecture-1-embryology-of-the-tooth-cavity-and-tooth-eruption-10min-dmqKX | Embryology of the oral cavity and tooth eruption |
| University of North Carolina at Chapel Hill | https://syllabus.med.unc.edu/courseware/embryo_images/ | Images and text on normal and abnormal human embryology |

# CHAPTER 2 REVIEW QUESTIONS

## CASE A PEDIATRIC

**Synopsis of the Patient**

| | |
|---|---|
| Age | 5 |
| Gender | Female |
| Height | 42″ |
| Weight | 40 lbs |
| Vital Signs | BP 90/60, pulse rate 85, respirations 10 |
| Chief Concern | Mother concerned about dark spots on teeth. Child complains of dental pain when eating candy. |
| Social History | Entering kindergarten, plays soccer |
| Current Medications | Rescue inhaler |
| Medical History | Diagnosis of asthma |
| Dental History | First dental appointment |
| Extraoral and Intraoral Findings | Extraoral – normal<br>Intraoral – several carious lesions on primary dentition 6-year molars are partially erupted |
| Gingival Examination | Red tissue at gingival margins |
| Dentition | 20 primary teeth |
| Radiographic Findings | Interproximal carious lesions |
| Deposits | Moderate biofilm |

***Use Case A Pediatric to answer Questions 1 to 12.***

1. The tissue(s) that have nerve innervation are:
   a. Dentin
   b. Pulp and dentin
   c. Pulp and periodontal ligament
   d. Cementum
   d. All of the above
2. The free unmyelinated nerve endings of the pulp can sense:
   a. Hot
   b. Cold
   c. Pressure
   d. Pain
   e. All of the above
3. Nonsuccedaneous permanent molars develop from buds that grow from:
   a. A successional dental lamina.
   b. Primary tooth buds.
   c. The posterior part of palatal shelves.
   d. Extension of the primary second molar's dental lamina.
4. What is the angled part of the ameloblast that secretes the enamel matrix?
   a. Inner enamel epithelium
   b. Repolarized preameloblasts
   c. Tomes' process
   d. Disintegrating basement membrane
5. The pink labial mucosa or buccal mucosa meets the redder ______ at the mucobuccal fold.
   a. Marginal gingiva
   b. Attached gingiva
   c. Alveolar mucosa
6. The outer cells of the dental papilla are induced to differentiate during tooth development into:
   a. Pulp tissue
   b. Preameloblasts
   c. Odontoblasts
   d. Cementoblast
7. Which stage of tooth formation occurs for the primary dentition during the 11th and 12th week of prenatal development?
   a. Bell Stage
   b. Initiation Stage
   c. Cap Stage
   d. Bud Stage
8. What is connective tissue derived from during prenatal development?
   a. Ectoderm
   b. Endoderm
   c. Neural crest cells
   d. Mesoderm
9. Enamel ______form the crystalline structural unit of enamel.
   a. Tubules
   b. Granules
   c. Rods
   d. Cuticles
10. The patient's mother was informed the multiple carious lesions caries on her maxillary molars had progressed into the dentin. Caries in the dentin of the tooth progresses through the
    a. Interglobular dentin
    b. Dentinal tubule
    c. Secondary dentin
    d. Predentin
11. Enamel hypocalcification is a type of enamel dysplasia that involves:
    a. an increased number of ameloblasts
    b. reduction in the quantity of enamel matrix
    c. grooves and pitting on the enamel surface
    d. interference in the metabolic processes of ameloblasts
12. During the 4th week of embryonic life, the tongue develops from several swellings arising on the internal aspect of branchial arches 1–4 (pouches). Which swellings form the body of the tongue?
    a. **Branchial arch 1**
    b. Branchial arches 2, 3, and part of 4
    c. Branchial arch 4
    d. Thyroid gland

## CASE B ADOLESCENT

**Synopsis of the Patient**

| | |
|---|---|
| Age | 10 |
| Gender | Male |
| Height | 55 in″ |
| Weight | 70 l bs |
| Vital Signs | BP 110/60, pulse rate 80, respirations 14 |
| Chief Concern | Mother concerned about crooked teeth |
| Social History | Patient is entering grade 5. He plays a reed instrument in a marching band |

## CASE B ADOLESCENT—CONT'D

**Synopsis of the Patient**

| | |
|---|---|
| Current Medications | None |
| Medical History | Patient is up to date with vaccinations |
| Dental History | Patient had repaired cleft lip/palate |
| Extraoral and Intraoral Findings | All normal |
| Gingival Examination | Coral pink, stippled attached gingiva |
| Dentition | Mixed dentition out of alignment |
| Radiographic Findings | Normal eruption pattern |
| Deposits | Light supragingival calculus on lower lingual anterior teeth |

***Use Case B Adolescent to answer Questions 13 to 25.***

13. What histologic structure(s) comprise(s) healthy attached gingiva?
    a. Circular fibers
    b. Rete pegs
    c. Connective tissue papilla
    d. Fibroblasts
    e. All of the above
14. What type of epithelium comprises attached gingiva?
    a. Keratinized stratified squamous epithelium
    b. Nonkeratinized stratified squamous epithelium
    c. Keratinized simple squamous epithelium
    d. Pseudostratified columnar epithelium
    e. Nonkeratinized simple squamous epithelium
15. A cleft lip occurs when the maxillary process fails to fuse with which *one* of the following embryonic processes?
    a. Palatine process
    b. Globular process (medial nasal process)
    c. Lateral nasal process
    d. Mandibular process
    e. Opposing maxillary process
16. Embryonically, the mandible is derived from the:
    a. Stomodeum
    b. First branchial arch
    c. Frontal process
    d. Second branchial arch
    e. Third branchial arch
17. The anterior portion, or body, of the tongue develops from the:
    a. Second branchial arch
    b. Maxillary process
    c. Mandibular process
    d. Globular process (medial nasal process)
    e. Rathke's pouch
18. Which of the following orofacial structures is located in the midline of the face or neck?
    a. Philtrum
    b. Submandibular salivary gland
    c. Naris and ala
    d. Parotid salivary gland
19. Continuous replacement of cells is characteristic of which type of epithelium?
    a. Simple squamous
    b. Stratified squamous
    c. Pseudo-stratified columnar
    d. Stratified transitional
20. When a cleft of the alveolar process is present, it occurs between the
    a. First and second premolars
    b. Central incisors
    c. Lateral incisor and canine
    d. Canine and first premolar
21. The overlapping period between the primary and permanent dentition is considered the period of:
    a. Primary
    b. Secondary
    c. Tertiary
    d. Mixed
22. During the cell cycle, interphase involves the cells engaging in:
    a. Chromatin removal
    b. Organelle replication
    c. Centromere reduction
    d. Substance destruction
23. Meckel's cartilage is derived from neural crest cells which migrate cephalad and interact with cephalic ectoderm and mesoderm to result in the development of:
    a. Facial skeleton
    b. Neck Skeleton
    c. Connective tissue components
    d. Tooth development
24. Each germ cell contains ____ chromosomes (haploid number); during the process of fertilization, the number is restored to ____ chromosomes (diploid).
    a. 22, 45
    b. 21, 44
    c. 20, 43
    d. 23, 46
25. Each tooth is the product of two tissues that interact during tooth development:
    a. Epithelium, ectomesenchyme
    b. Endoderm, epithelium
    c. Ectomesenchyme, endoderm
    d. Mesenchyme, ectoderm

## CASE C ADULT

**Synopsis of the Patient**

| | |
|---|---|
| Age | 30 |
| Gender | Female |
| Height | 5ft 4 in |
| Weight | 120 lbs |
| Vital Signs | BP 110/60, pulse rate 70, respirations 12 |
| Chief Concern | Gingival recession |
| Social History | Teacher, mother of 2 |
| Current Medications | Birth control pills |
| Medical History | Gravida para two |
| Dental History | Regular dental treatment, history of periodontal treatment |
| Extraoral and Intraoral Findings | Extraoral and intraoral – no significant findings |
| Gingival Examination | Localized gingival recession on mandibular premolar areas with no attached gingiva present |
| Dentition | History of orthodontic treatment |
| Radiographic Findings | Normal |
| Deposits | Light subgingival interproximal calculus |
| Periodontal Charting | Pocket depth between 4–6 mm, moderate bleeding on probing |

*Use Case C Adult to answer Questions 26–35.*

26. A connective tissue graft from the hard palate area was recommended for the gingival recession. What type of epithelial tissue is in this area?
   a. Nonkeratinized simple squamous epithelium
   b. Keratinized simple squamous epithelium
   c. Orthokeratinized stratified squamous epithelium
   d. Pseudostratified columnar epithelium
   e. Nonkeratinized stratified squamous epithelium
27. A graft procedure would include a surgical flap in the epithelial tissue of the palate and harvesting the underlying connective tissue. The connective tissue would be placed in the recipient site. What type of connective tissue is usually found underlying the gingiva?
   a. Loose connective tissue
   b. Dense connective tissue
   c. Mixed connective tissue
   d. Cannot be determined
28. All of the following tissues have little or no keratinization, *except one*. Which one is this *exception?*
   a. Attached gingiva
   b. Sulcular epithelium
   c. Alveolar mucosa
   d. Soft palate
29. Which of the following is *not* a component of the periodontium?
   a. Gingiva
   b. Crown
   c. Periodontal ligament
   d. Alveolar bone
30. Which of the following is *not* a histological component of the gingival connective tissue?
   a. Enamel
   b. Lymphatic tissues
   c. Collagen fibers
   d. Blood cells
31. Which tissue surrounds the tooth and creates a cuff of gingiva extending coronally approximately 1.5 mm from the CEJ?
   a. Periodontal ligament
   b. Free gingiva
   c. Attached gingiva
   d. Oral mucosa
32. What are the clinical observations noted during an examination of the gingiva indicating gingival health?
   a. Loosely attached gingiva
   b. Firm attached gingiva
   c. Purple-colored gingiva
   d. Inflamed gingiva
33. What relationship does tooth size have on the interdental papilla?
   a. The smaller the tooth the larger the papilla
   b. The larger the tooth the smaller the papilla
   c. The larger the tooth the larger the papilla
   d. Tooth size does not relate to papilla size
34. The inner and outer surfaces of alveolar bone are made up of ________________.
   a. Spongy bone
   b. Cortical plates
   c. Cementum
   d. Oblique fibers
35. The wall of the tooth socket is lined by what type of bone?
   a. Trabecular
   b. Dentin
   c. Lamina Dura
   d. Cancellous
36. The tooth is attached to the underlying bone through which of the following?
   a. Periodontal fibers
   b. Attached gingiva
   c. Cementum
   d. Interradicular bone
37. Which tooth appears in the permanent dentition but not in the primary?
   a. Molars
   b. Lateral Incisors
   c. Central Incisors
   d. Premolars
38. Which one of the tooth components has an equivalent hardness to bone?
   a. Cementum
   b. Enamel
   c. Dentin
   d. Dentin Tubules

## CASE D GERIATRIC

**Synopsis of the Patient**

| | |
|---|---|
| Age | 76 |
| Gender | Male |
| Height | 67″ |
| Weight | 200 lbs |
| Vital Signs | BP 130/85, pulse rate 80, respirations 14 |
| Chief Concern | Maintain oral health |
| Social History | Enjoying retired life |
| Current Medications | Statin, NSAIDS, inhaler |
| Medical History | Elevated cholesterol, osteoarthritis in back, asthma, sleep apnea |
| Dental History | Sporadic recall visits |
| Extraoral and Intraoral Findings | Palpable left submandibular lymph node, bilateral mandibular tori |
| Gingival Examination | Generalized gingival recession with exposed cementum |
| Dentition | Moderate restorative restorations |
| Radiographic Findings | Generalized horizontal bone loss |
| Deposits | Moderate subgingival interproximal deposits |
| Periodontal Charting | Bleeding on probing, mucogingival defects in lower molars, pockets depths range from 4–7 mm. |

*Use Case D Geriatric to answer Questions 39–50.*

39. What attachment mechanism attaches the cells in the basal layer of stratified squamous epithelium?
   a. Desmosome
   b. Hemidesmosome
   c. Gap
   d. Tight
40. Which of the following are characteristics of bundle bone?
   a. Covered by endosteum

b. Adjacent to periodontal ligament and adjacent to fatty marrow
c. Adjacent to fatty marrow and covered by endosteum
d. Contains Sharpey's fibers and is adjacent to periodontal ligament

41. What type of cells are found in Howship's lacunae?
a. Osteocytes
b. Osteoclasts
c. Cementocytes
d. Cementoblasts

42. What is the name of the space occupied by the body of the cementocyte?
a. Lamellae
b. Lacuna
c. Canaliculi
d. Centicle

43. Cementum differs from bone in that cementum:
a. Contains cells
b. Has no blood vessels
c. Is 50% inorganic and 50%organic
d. Resorbs more readily

44. What is the name for the outer, less-calcified layer of cementum?
a. Cellular cementum
b. Acellular cementum
c. Cementoid
d. Cementicles

45. What name is given to the remnants of Hertwig's epithelial root sheath found in the periodontal ligament of a functioning tooth?
a. Enamel pearls
b. Denticles
c. Rests of Malassez
d. Cementicles

46. The crystalline formation of mature bone consists of *mainly* which of the following?
a. Calcium hydroxyapatite
b. Osteoid
c. Osteocytes
d. Canaliculi

47. What tissue component of the periodontal ligament is responsible for the production of the fibrous matrix and ground substance?
a. Osteoblast
b. Cementoblast
c. Odontoblast
d. Fibroblast

48. Which portion of the tooth germ is the primary source of the periodontal ligament?
a. Dental follicle
b. Herwig's epithelial root sheath
c. Stratum intermedium
d. Central cells of dental papilla

49. The upper deep cervical nodes primarily drain all except:
a. Tonsils
b. Base of the tongue
c. Third molars
d. Soft palate

50. Pulp changes result from aging. Changes result from:
a. Increased collagen fibers
b. True denticles
c. False denticles
d. Diffuse calcification

## SUGGESTED READINGS

Fehrenbach MJ. *Popowics. Dental Embryology, Histology, and Anatomy*. 4th ed. St. Louis: Saunders; 2016.

Chiego D. *Essentials of Oral Histology and Embryology, a Clinical Approach*. 4th ed. St. Louis: Elsevier; 2014.

Finkelstein M. Oral histology image index. The University of Iowa. <http://www.healthcare.uiowa.edu/anatomy/dental/oralhist/OHMAC/index.html> Accessed July 14, 2019.

Galil, KA. Anatomy and histology quizzes, University of Western Ontario Department of Anatomy and Cell Biology. http://clinicalcases.drgalil.ca/. Accessed July 14, 2019.

Ibsen OAC, Phelan JA. *Oral Pathology for the Dental Hygienist*. 6th ed. St. Louis: Saunders; 2014.

# 3

# Anatomy and Physiology

*Alison F. Doubleday*

Anatomy and physiology are subjects that focus on the structure, organization, and function of the human body. Dental hygienists use knowledge of anatomy and physiology most often during patient assessment, treatment, and evaluation; during oral radiographic and pathologic examinations; and for the administration of local anesthetic agents. This knowledge also allows a dental hygienist to determine whether patients are functioning within normal limits, deviating from the normal, or presenting with structures that are ectopic. Moreover, this knowledge enables dental hygienists to link systemic and oral disease. This chapter covers basic concepts: definitions of terms, cell structure and function, and body systems, including the skeletal, muscular, nervous, circulatory, lymphatic, digestive, endocrine, urinary, and reproductive systems.

## BASIC CONCEPTS

### Anatomy

A. Study of the structure of an organism and the relationships of its parts; derived from the Greek word meaning "the act of cutting up"
B. Branches of anatomy
   1. Gross anatomy—study of structures that can be identified with the naked eye (see Chapter 4)
   2. Microscopic anatomy—study of cells (cytology) and tissues (histology) (see Chapter 2)
   3. Developmental anatomy (embryology)—study of human growth and development (see Chapter 2)

### Physiology

Study of body functions—how the body parts work

### Levels of Organization

See Fig. 3.1.

The intricate human body is organized in a hierarchical order from simple to complex. The levels of organization discussed below culminate in the total organism, the human body.

A. Chemical level—organization of chemical structure separates living and nonliving material; atoms, molecules, and macromolecules result in living matter
B. Organelle level—organelles are structures made of molecules and organized to perform specific functions; organelles reside within a cell and allow the cell to perform vital functions; types include:
   1. Endoplasmic reticulum
   2. Golgi apparatus
   3. Mitochondria
   4. Peroxisomes
   5. Proteasomes
C. Cellular level—cells comprise the basic structural and functional units of an organism; the smallest living units in the human body; in general, cells are characterized by:
   1. Nucleus surrounded by cytoplasm within a limiting membrane
   2. Differentiated capabilities to perform unique functions
D. Tissue level—groups of cells and materials surrounding them that work together to perform a particular function
   1. Four major tissue types:
      a. Epithelial tissue
      b. Connective tissue
      c. Muscle tissue
      d. Nervous tissue
E. Organ level—different types of tissues join together to form body structures
   1. Each organ has a unique size, shape, appearance, and placement in the body (e.g., stomach, heart, liver, lungs, brain)
F. System level—related organs that contribute to a common function (e.g., digestive system breaks down and absorbs molecules in food; organs include the mouth, salivary glands, pharynx, esophagus, stomach, liver, gallbladder, pancreas, small intestine, and large intestine)
G. Organism level—all the systems of the body working together to make up an organism

### Anatomic Nomenclature

Basic terms are needed to communicate regions and directions of the body. We describe the location of an anatomical structure in the human body in relation to other structures. The anatomic position provides a reference point for all other terms (see the section on "Anatomic Nomenclature" in Chapter 4).

A. Anatomic position—erect body position with arms at the sides and palms facing forward
B. Plane or section—imaginary flat surfaces that pass through the body (Fig. 3.2)

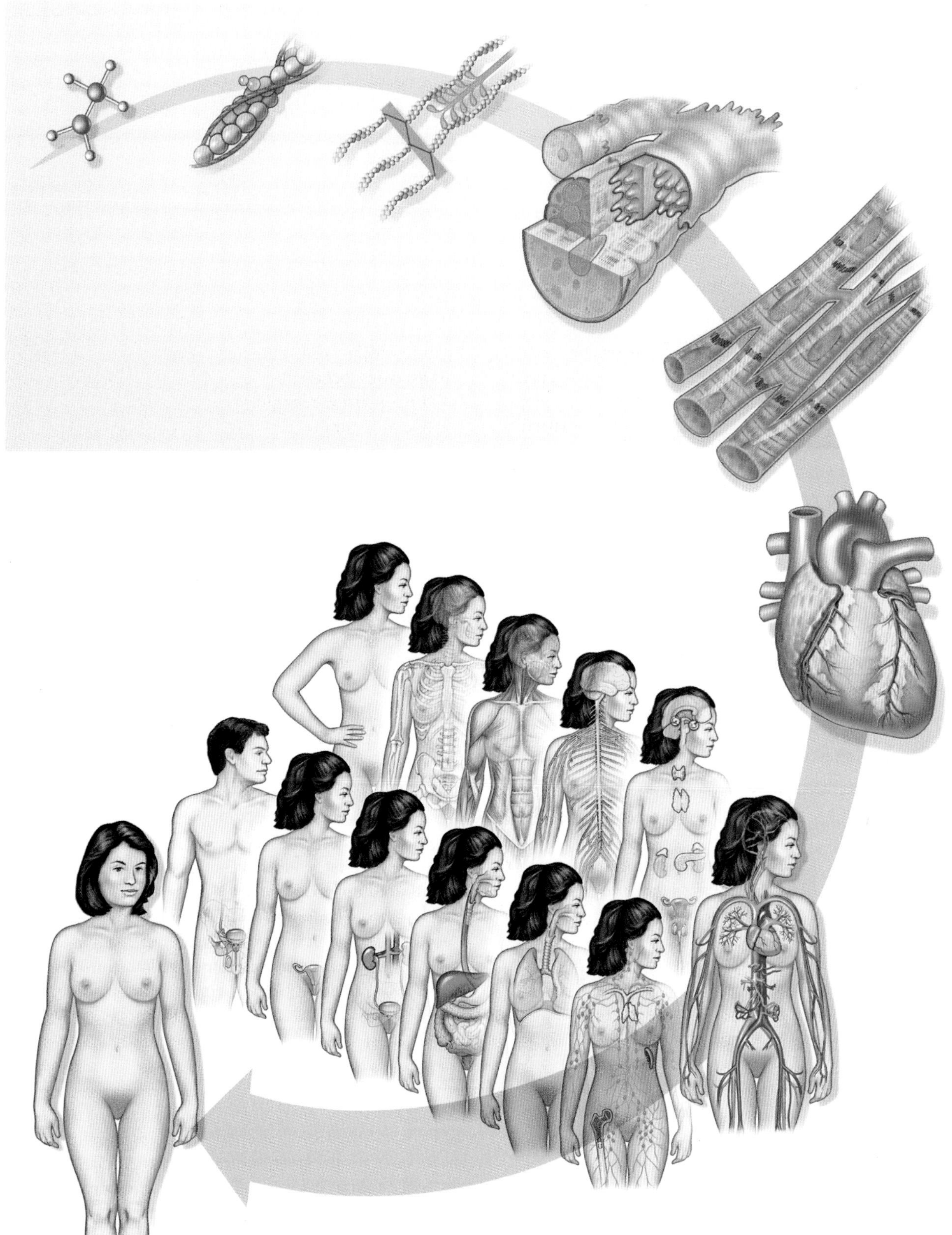

**Fig 3.1** Levels of organization. (From Patton KT, Thibodeau GA, Douglas MM: *Essentials of anatomy and physiology,* St Louis, 2012, Mosby)

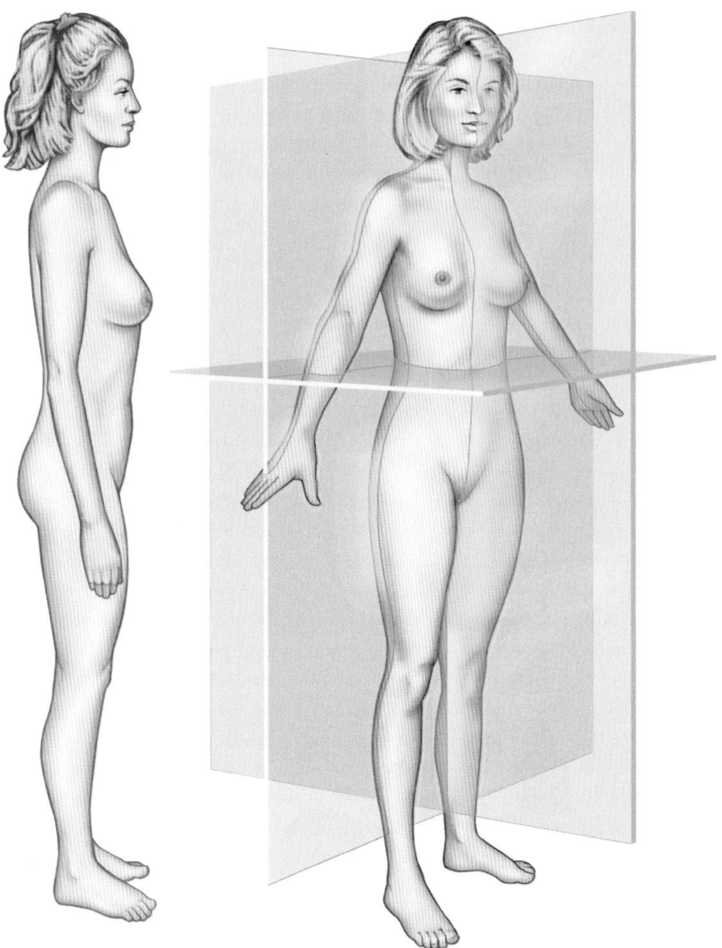

**Fig 3.2** Directions and planes of the body. (Patton KT, Thibodeau GA, Douglas MM: *Essentials of anatomy and physiology,* St Louis, 2012, Mosby.)

1. Sagittal plane—vertical plane dividing the body into right and left sides; midsagittal plane bisects the body at the exact midline
2. Frontal plane—divides the body or organ into anterior and posterior portions (may also be called the *coronal plane*)
3. Transverse plane—divides the body or organ into superior and inferior portions (may also be called *cross-sectional,* or *horizontal, plane*)

## Body Cavities

The human body contains two major cavities, the dorsal cavity and the ventral cavity. These two cavities are then sectioned into smaller cavities that contain internal organs. The dorsal body cavities are in the back part of the body. The ventral body cavities are on the front side of the trunk (Fig. 3.3 and Table 3.1).

A. Dorsal cavity
   1. Cranial cavity—formed by the cranial bones of the skull; contains the brain
   2. Vertebral cavity—formed by the vertebrae; contains the spinal cord

B. Ventral cavity
   1. Thoracic (chest) cavity comprises the upper portion
      a. Pericardial cavity—contains the heart
      b. Pleural cavities (2)—contain the lungs
      c. Mediastinum—soft tissue partition between pleural cavities; allows for passage of several thoracic organs; includes the heart, esophagus, trachea, and several large blood vessels and lymphatic structures
   2. Abdominopelvic cavity
      a. Upper (abdominal) cavity contains part of the esophagus, the stomach, spleen, liver, gallbladder, small intestine, and most of the large intestine
      b. Lower (pelvic) cavity contains the bladder, sigmoid colon, rectum, and reproductive organs

# CELLS

All living creatures or organisms are made up of one or more cells. Cells in a multicellular organism have the ability to regenerate to sustain life. As structural and functional units of the body, cells develop characteristics and functionality, resulting in a large variety of cells in the body. See Fig. 3.4.

## Cellular Structure

(See the section in Chapter 2: General Histology)

See Fig. 3.4.

A. Plasma or cell membrane
   1. Surrounds and contains the cytoplasm of a cell; composed of proteins and lipids

2. Selective permeability characteristics
   a. Protects cell from external environment
   b. Permits the entrance and exit of selected substrates
   c. Membrane proteins have several functions—channels and transporters are integral proteins that help specific solutes across the membrane; receptors serve as cellular recognition sites; some membrane proteins are enzymes
3. Basic framework—lipid bilayer; two layers of phospholipids, cholesterol, and glycolipids

B. Cytoplasm—all cellular contents between the plasma membrane and the nucleus; includes:
   1. Cytosol—fluid portion of cytoplasm; site of many chemical reactions for the cell's existence
   2. Cytoskeleton—network of several kinds of protein filaments that extend throughout the cytoplasm; structural framework for the cell; facilitates movement
   3. Organelles—specialized cellular structures, each with characteristic features and specific functions

C. Ribosomes
   1. Free ribosomes—not attached to other organelles; synthesize proteins used inside the cell
   2. Bound ribosomes—attached to the endoplasmic reticulum (ER); form rough ER; synthesize proteins destined for use in the plasma membrane or for export from the cell

D. Endoplasmic reticulum—network of membranes that form flattened sacs called *cisterns*; arranged in parallel rows within the cytoplasm of a cell; contains enzymes involved in a variety of metabolic activities
   1. Rough ER (granular)
      a. Contains ribosomes
      b. Site of protein synthesis

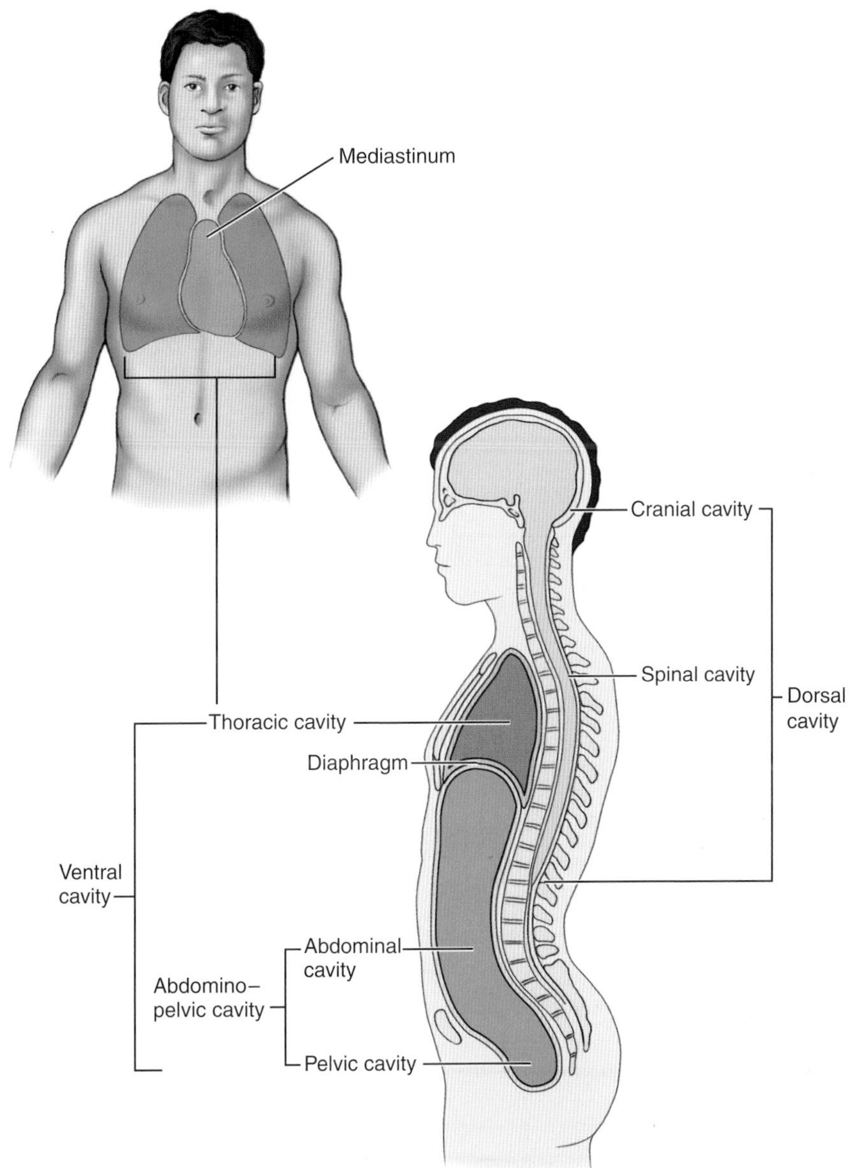


**Fig 3.3** Major body cavities. (Patton KT, Thibodeau GA: *Mosby's handbook of anatomy and physiology*, ed 2, St Louis, 2014, Mosby.)

**TABLE 3.1 Organs in the Ventral Body Cavities**

| Areas | Organ |
|---|---|
| **Thoracic** | |
| Right pleural cavity | Right lung |
| Mediastinum | Heart |
| | Trachea |
| | Right and left bronchi |
| | Esophagus |
| | Thymus gland |
| | Aortic arch and thoracic aorta |
| | Venae cavae |
| | Various lymph nodes and nerves |
| | Thoracic duct |
| Left pleural cavity | Left lung |
| **Abdominopelvic Cavity** | |
| Abdominal cavity | Liver |
| | Gallbladder |
| | Stomach |
| | Pancreas |
| | Intestines |
| | Spleen |
| | Kidneys |
| | Ureters |
| Pelvic cavity | Urinary bladder |
| | Female reproductive organs |
| | Uterus |
| | Uterine tubes |
| | Ovaries |
| | Male reproductive organs |
| | Prostate gland |
| | Seminal vesicles |
| | Part of vas deferens |
| | Part of large intestine (sigmoid colon and rectum) |

2. Smooth ER (agranular)
   a. No ribosomes present
   b. Synthesizes certain lipids and carbohydrates
   c. Contains enzymes that release glucose into the bloodstream and inactivate or detoxify a variety of drugs and potentially harmful substances, including alcohol, pesticides, and carcinogens

E. Golgi complex
   1. Stack of 3 to 20 flattened membranous sacs (cisterns)
   2. Within the cisterns, proteins are modified, sorted, and packaged into vesicles for transport to different destinations

F. Lysosomes
   1. Membrane-enclosed vesicles that form in the Golgi complex
   2. Contain digestive enzymes
   3. Function is the digestion of worn-out organelles (autophagy) and self (autolysis)

G. Mitochondria
   1. Ellipsoid bodies that consist of two membranes containing enzyme complexes in a particular array (e.g., tricarboxylic acid cycle enzymes)
   2. Function as the "powerhouse of the cell" by transforming the chemical energy bond of nutrients into the high-energy phosphate bonds of adenosine triphosphate
   3. A single cell may contain 50 to 2500 of these organelles, depending on the cell's energy needs

H. Nucleus
   1. Consists of a double nuclear membrane, nuclear pores (control the movement of substances into and out of nucleus), nucleoli (produce ribosomes), and deoxyribonucleic acid (DNA)

I. Peroxisomes
   1. Function to eliminate toxic substances from intercellular fluid

J. Proteasomes
   1. Remove abnormal and misfolded proteins
   2. Destroy specific normal proteins that are no longer needed

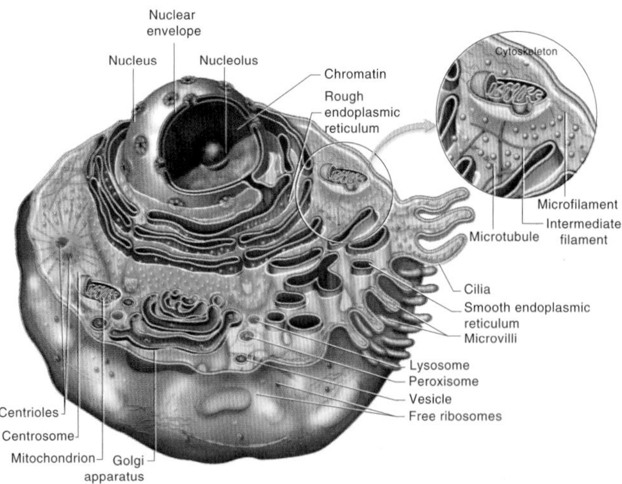


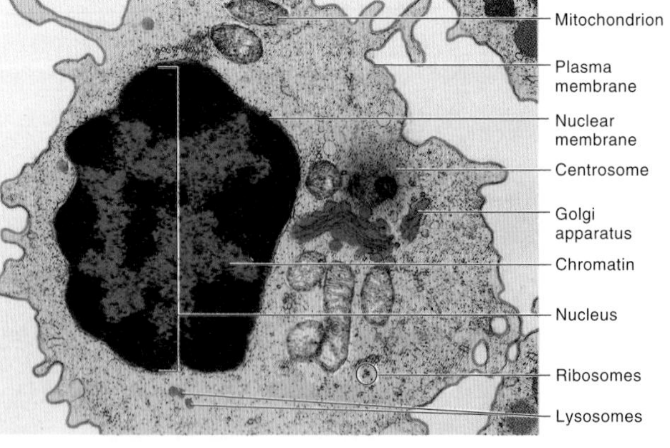


**Fig 3.4** Typical, or composite, cell. A, Artist's interpretation of cell structure. B, Color-enhanced electron micrograph of a cell. Both show the many mitochondria, known as the "power plants of the cell." Note also the innumerable dots bordering the endoplasmic reticulum. These are ribosomes, the cell's "protein factories." (From Patton KT, Thibodeau GA: *Anthony's textbook of anatomy and physiology,* ed 20, St Louis, 2013, Elsevier.)

## MOVEMENT OF SUBSTANCES THROUGH CELL MEMBRANES

See Tables 3.2 and 3.3.

A. Passive transport processes—do not require energy expenditure of the cell membrane
   1. Diffusion—a passive process
      a. Molecules move across the membranes
      b. Molecules move from an area of high concentration to an area of low concentration (down a concentration gradient)
      c. Eventually a state of equilibrium is reached
      d. Membrane channels—pores in cell membranes through which specific ions or small water-soluble molecules can pass
   2. Simple diffusion—substances diffuse across a membrane in one of two ways: lipid-soluble substances diffuse through the lipid bilayer, ions diffuse through pores
   3. Osmosis
      a. Diffusion of water through a selectively permeable membrane (limits diffusion of at least some solute particles); results in gain of volume on one side of the membrane and loss of volume on the other side of the membrane
      b. A solution containing solute particles that cannot pass through a membrane exerts osmotic pressure on the membrane
      c. Potential osmotic pressure—maximum pressure that could develop in a solution when it is separated from pure water by a selectively permeable membrane; knowledge of potential osmotic pressure allows the prediction of the direction of osmosis and resulting change of pressure
         (1) Isotonic—when two fluids have the same potential osmotic pressure
         (2) Hypertonic (higher pressure)—cells placed in solutions that are hypertonic to intracellular fluid shrivel as water flows out of cells by osmosis faster than it enters
         (3) Hypotonic (lower pressure)—a solution that has a lower concentration of solutes than the cytosol inside the cell; water molecules enter the cells by osmosis faster than they leave and the cells swell.
   4. Facilitated diffusion (carrier-mediated passive transport)
      a. Movement of molecules made more efficient by the action of specific transport mechanisms in the plasma membrane; facilitated by channel proteins or carrier proteins
      b. Transports substances down a concentration gradient
      c. Substances moved by facilitated diffusion include glucose, fructose, galactose, urea, and some vitamins
   5. Filtration
      a. Passage of water and permeable solutes through a membrane by the force of hydrostatic pressure (the

**TABLE 3.2 Passive Transport Processes**

| Process | Description | | Examples |
|---|---|---|---|
| Simple diffusion | | Movement of particles through the phospholipid bilayer or through channels from an area of high concentration to an area of low concentration—that is, down the concentration gradient | Movement of carbon dioxide out of all cells; movement of sodium ions into nerve cells as they conduct an impulse |
| Channel-mediated passive transport (facilitated diffusion) | | Diffusion of particles through a membrane by means of channel structures in the membrane (particles move down their concentration gradient) | Diffusion of sodium ions into nerve cells during a nerve impulse |
| Osmosis | | Diffusion of water through a selectively permeable membrane in the presence of at least one impermanent solute | Diffusion of water molecules into and out of cells to correct imbalances in water concentration |
| Carrier-mediated passive transport (facilitated diffusion) | | Diffusion of particles through a membrane by means of carrier structures in the membrane (particles move down their concentration gradient) | Movement of glucose molecules into most cells |

Art from Patton KT, Thibodeau GA, Douglas MM: *Essentials of anatomy and physiology,* St Louis, 2012, Mosby.

pressure exerted by a fluid on the walls of the structure containing the fluid); occurs most often in capillaries
   b. Small molecules travel down a hydrostatic pressure gradient and through a sheet of cells

B. Active transport processes—require the expenditure of metabolic energy by the cell
   1. Active transport
      a. Process that moves substances against a concentration gradient (from an area of low concentration to an area of high concentration)
      b. Opposite of diffusion
      c. Substances moved by "pumps," for example, calcium pumps and sodium-potassium pumps
   2. Endocytosis and exocytosis—allow substances to enter or leave the interior of a cell without actually moving through its plasma membrane
      a. Endocytosis—process by which the plasma membrane "traps" some extracellular material and brings it into the cell in a vesicle; the two basic types are:
         (1) Phagocytosis (cell eating)—large particles are engulfed by the plasma membrane and enter the cell in vesicles; vesicles fuse with lysosomes, where particles are digested
         (2) Pinocytosis (cell drinking)—the plasma membrane folds inward, forming a pinocytic vesicle containing a droplet of extracellular fluid; the vesicle detaches from the plasma membrane and enters the cytosol
      b. Exocytosis—process by which large molecules, notably proteins, can leave the cell, even though they are too large to move through the plasma membrane; large molecules are enclosed in membranous vesicles and then pulled to the plasma membrane by the cytoskeleton, where the contents are released
         (1) Provides a way for new material to be added to the plasma membrane

## Cell Metabolism

A. Metabolism—chemical reactions in a cell
   1. Catabolism—breaking of large molecules into smaller ones; usually releases energy
   2. Anabolism—building of large molecules from smaller ones; usually consumes energy

B. Role of enzymes
   1. Enzymes—chemical catalysts, reducing activation energy needed for a reaction
   2. Regulate cell metabolism
   3. Chemical structure of enzymes
      a. Proteins of a complex shape
      b. Active site—where the enzyme molecule fits the substrate molecule; lock-and-key model

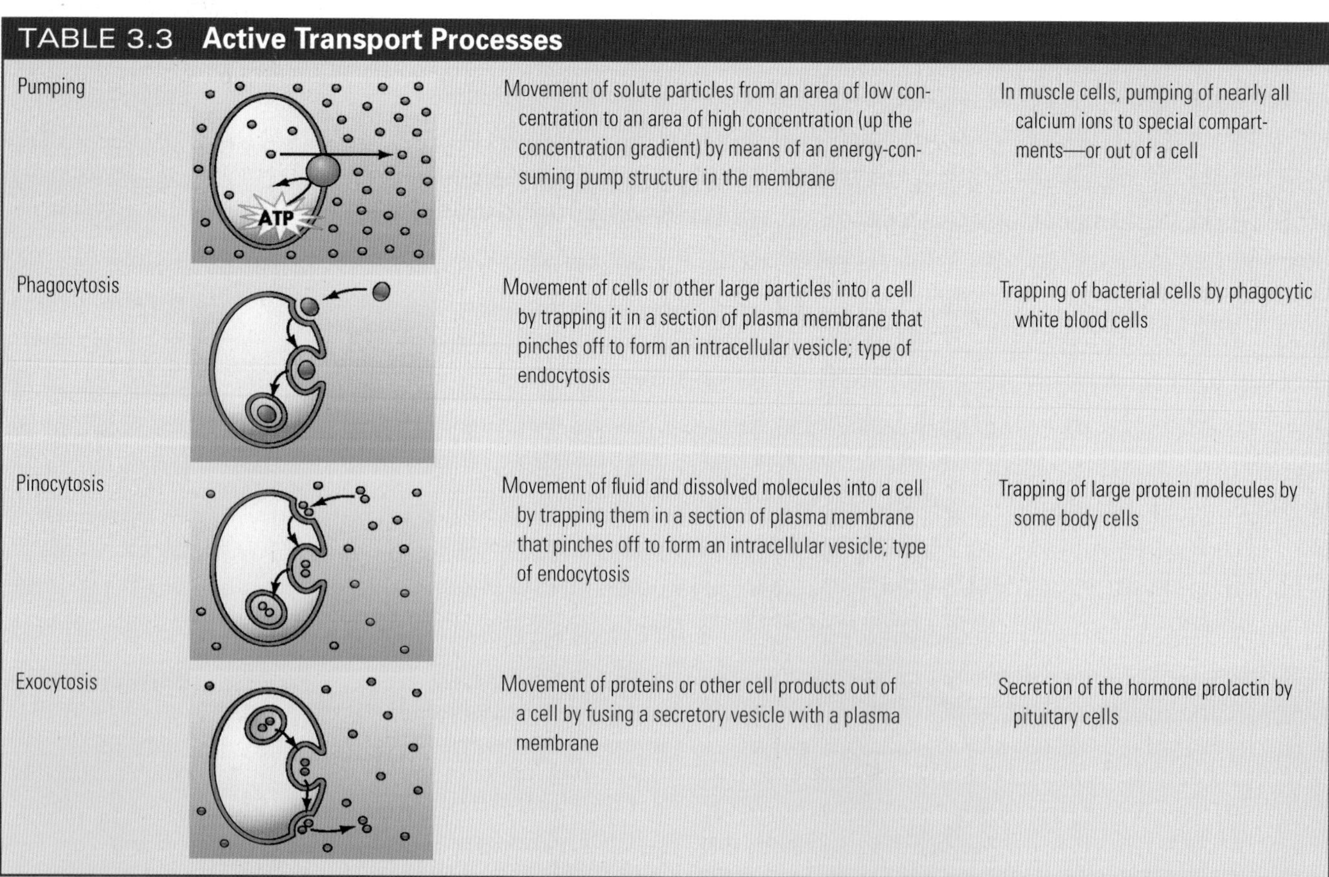

**TABLE 3.3 Active Transport Processes**

| Process | | Description | Example |
|---|---|---|---|
| Pumping | ATP | Movement of solute particles from an area of low concentration to an area of high concentration (up the concentration gradient) by means of an energy-consuming pump structure in the membrane | In muscle cells, pumping of nearly all calcium ions to special compartments—or out of a cell |
| Phagocytosis | | Movement of cells or other large particles into a cell by trapping it in a section of plasma membrane that pinches off to form an intracellular vesicle; type of endocytosis | Trapping of bacterial cells by phagocytic white blood cells |
| Pinocytosis | | Movement of fluid and dissolved molecules into a cell by trapping them in a section of plasma membrane that pinches off to form an intracellular vesicle; type of endocytosis | Trapping of large protein molecules by some body cells |
| Exocytosis | | Movement of proteins or other cell products out of a cell by fusing a secretory vesicle with a plasma membrane | Secretion of the hormone prolactin by pituitary cells |

Art from Patton KT, Thibodeau GA, Douglas MM: *Essentials of anatomy and physiology*, St Louis, 2012, Mosby.

4. Enzyme nomenclature
   a. Enzymes usually have an "-ase" suffix; the first part of the word often signifies the substrate or the type of reaction
   b. Oxidation-reduction enzymes—known as *oxidases, hydrogenases,* and *dehydrogenases*; energy release depends on these enzymes
   c. Hydrolyzing enzymes—Hydrolases are hydrolytic enzymes, biochemical catalysts that use water to **cleave** chemical bonds, usually dividing a large molecule into two smaller molecules.

Read more: http://www.chemistryexplained.com/Ge-Hy/Hydrolase.html#ixzz5mtsP7FmD

   d. Phosphorylating enzymes—phosphorylases or phosphatases; add or remove phosphate groups
   e. Carboxylases and decarboxylases—add or remove carbon dioxide
   f. Mutases or isomerases—rearrange atoms within a molecule
   g. Hydrases—add water to a molecule without splitting it
5. Functions of enzymes
   a. Regulate cell functions by regulating metabolic pathways; specific in their actions
   b. Chemical and physical agents called *allosteric effectors* alter enzyme action by changing the shape of the enzyme molecule, for example:
      (1) Temperature
      (2) Hydrogen ion ($H^+$) concentration (pH)
      (3) Ionizing radiation
      (4) Cofactors
      (5) End products of certain metabolic pathways
   c. Most catalyze chemical reactions in both directions
   d. Continually being destroyed and replaced
   e. Many are first synthesized as inactive proenzymes

C. Catabolism—breakdown of larger molecules to smaller molecules.
1. Energy is needed to function and is obtained from the foods we eat; the most efficient way for cells to harvest energy stored in food is through *cellular respiration,* a catabolic pathway for the production of adenosine triphosphate (ATP), a high-energy molecule expended by working cells
2. Cellular respiration is what cells do to break up sugars into a form that the cell can use as energy
3. There are three main stages of cellular respiration: glycolysis, the citric acid cycle, and electron transport
   a. Glycolysis
      (1) The cellular degradation of the simple sugar glucose to yield pyruvic acid, with ATP as an energy source
      (2) Pathway in which glucose is broken apart into two pyruvic acid molecules to yield a small amount of energy (which is transferred to ATP and nicotinamide adenine dinucleotide [NADH])
      (3) Includes many chemical steps (reactions that follow one another), each regulated by specific enzymes
      (4) Can occur aerobically or anaerobically, depending on whether oxygen is available
      (5) Occurs within the cytosol (outside the mitochondria)
   b. Citric acid cycle (Krebs cycle)
      (1) Pyruvic acid (from glycolysis) is converted into acetyl coenzyme A (CoA) and enters the citric acid cycle after losing carbon dioxide ($CO_2$) and transferring some energy to NADH
      (2) A cyclic sequence of reactions that occurs inside the inner chamber of a mitochondrion; the acetyl splits from the CoA and is broken down, yielding $CO_2$ and energy (in the form of energized electrons), which is transferred to ATP, NADH, and flavin adenine dinucleotide (FADH2)
   c. The electron transport system (ETS)
      (1) Energized electrons are carried by NADH and FADH2 from glycolysis and the citric acid cycle to electron acceptors embedded in the cristae of the mitochondrion
      (2) As electrons are shuttled along a chain of electron-accepting molecules in the cristae, their energy is used to pump accompanying protons ($H^+$) into the space between mitochondrial membranes
      (3) Protons flow back into the inner chamber through carrier molecules in the cristae; their energy of movement is transferred to ATP
      (4) Low-energy electrons coming off the ETS bind to oxygen and rejoin their protons, forming water ($H_2O$)

D. Anabolism—the opposite of catabolism; involves making larger molecules out of smaller molecules
1. Anabolism allows the body to grow new cells and maintain all the tissues
2. Protein synthesis is an example of a central anabolic pathway as biologic cells generate new proteins (protein synthesis pathway is outlined below)
3. DNA (see the section on "Genetics" in Chapter 7)
   a. A double-helix polymer (composed of nucleotides); functions to transfer the information encoded in genes, which directs protein synthesis
   b. Gene—a segment of a DNA molecule that consists of approximately 1000 pairs of nucleotides; contains the code for synthesizing one polypeptide
4. Transcription
   a. Messenger ribonucleic acid (mRNA) forms along a segment of one strand of DNA
   b. Noncoding introns are removed, and the remaining exons are spliced together to form the final edited version of the mRNA copy of the DNA segment
5. Translation
   a. After leaving the nucleus and being processed, mRNA associates with a ribosome in the cytoplasm
   b. Transfer ribonucleic acid (tRNA) molecules bring specific amino acids to the mRNA at the ribosome;

the type of amino acid is determined by the fit of a specific tRNA's anticodon with an mRNA's codon
    c. As amino acids are brought into place, peptide bonds join them, eventually producing an entire polypeptide chain
6. Processing—enzymes in the ER and Golgi apparatus link polypeptides into whole protein molecules or process them in other ways

### Cell Growth and Reproduction

A. Cell growth and reproduction of cells are the most fundamental of all functions in a living being; together they constitute the life cycle of the cell
    1. Cell growth—depends on the use of the genetic information in DNA to make structural and functional proteins for cell survival
    2. Cell reproduction—ensures that genetic information is passed from one generation to the next
B. Cell growth
    1. Production of cytoplasm—more cell material is made, including growth and replication of organelles and plasma membrane; a largely anabolic process
    2. DNA replication
        a. Replication of the genome prepares the cell for reproduction; mechanics similar to RNA synthesis
        b. DNA replication
            (1) DNA strand uncoils, and strands come apart
            (2) Along each separate strand, a complementary strand forms
            (3) The two new strands are called *chromatids* (attached pairs); their point of attachment is called a *centromere*
    3. Growth phase of the cell's life cycle—subdivided into the first phase (G1), the DNA synthesis phase (S), and the second growth phase (G2)
C. Cell reproduction
    1. Mitosis—process of organizing and distributing nuclear DNA during cell division; cells reproduce by splitting themselves into two smaller daughter cells (see the section on "Cell Replication" and Fig. 2.6 in Chapter 2)
    2. Meiosis—germ cell division; produces gametes (sperm and oocytes), the cells needed to form the next generation of sexually reproducing organisms
D. Regulating the cell's life cycle
    1. Cyclin-dependent kinases (CDKs)—activating enzymes that drive the cell through the phases of its life cycle
    2. Cyclins—regulatory proteins that control the CDKs and "shift" them to start the next phase; important in cancer pathways

## TISSUES

Cells that have a similar structure and function make up a tissue. Tissues working together configure, connect, and hold together organs. The study of tissues is referred to as histology (see the sections on "Concepts Relating to Dental Tissues," "Basic Tissues," "Epithelial Tissue," "Connective Tissue," "Blood and Lymph," "Nerve Tissue," and "Muscle Tissue" in Chapter 2).

### Body Membranes

A. Thin tissue layers that cover organ surfaces, line body cavities or organs, or divide spaces or organs
B. Epithelial membranes are the most common
    1. Cutaneous membranes (skin)
        a. Primary organ of the integumentary system
        b. One of the most important organs
        c. Comprises approximately 16% of body weight
    2. Serous membranes – typically two layers
        a. Parietal membranes—line closed body cavities
        b. Visceral membranes—cover visceral organs
        c. Examples:
            (1) Pleura—covers the lung and lines the thoracic cavity
            (2) Pericardium—covers the heart and lines the fibrous pericardium
            (3) Peritoneum—covers the abdominal viscera and lines the abdominal cavity
    3. Mucous membranes (see the section on "Soft Tissue of the Oral Cavity" and Fig. 2.21 in Chapter 2)
        a. Line and protect orifices that open to the exterior of the body, for example, anus, vagina, and oral cavity
        b. Line ducts and passageways of respiratory and digestive tracts
C. Connective tissue membranes
    1. Have smooth and slick synovial membranes to reduce friction between opposing surfaces in a movable joint; contain no epithelial components
    2. Synovial membranes—line bursae and the spaces between the bones in joints; secrete synovial fluid

## SYSTEMS OF THE BODY AND THEIR COMPONENTS

### The Integumentary System

The integumentary system is made up the skin, hair, nails, and glands that provide a protective barrier for the internal environment of the body from the external physical and biologic world.

A. Functions—regulation of body temperature, protection, sensation, excretion, immunity, synthesis of vitamin D
B. Parts
    1. Epidermis—thin outer portion composed of keratinized stratified squamous epithelium
        a. Components include keratin, melanin, Langerhans cells, Merkel cells
        b. Four layers:
            (1) Stratum basale
            (2) Stratum spinosum
            (3) Stratum lucidum
            (4) Stratum corneum
    2. Dermis—deeper, thicker, dense connective tissue
        a. Components include collagen and elastic fibers that give skin its extensivity and elasticity; dermal

papillae that produce fingerprints and facilitate gripping objects; corpuscles of touch (Meissner's corpuscles); and nerve endings that are sensitive to touch

C. Skin color—from melanin, carotene, and hemoglobin pigments

D. Accessory structures—hair, skin glands, and nails
   1. Hair—threads of fused, dead keratinized cells that have a protective function
      a. Consist of a shaft above the surface, a root that penetrates the dermis and subcutaneous layer, and a hair follicle
   2. Sebaceous glands—usually connected to hair follicles; absent in palms and soles of feet; produce sebum, which moistens hair and waterproofs skin
   3. Sudoriferous glands—produce perspiration; carry waste to the skin's surface; assist in maintaining body temperature
   4. Nails—hard keratinized epidermal cells covering terminal portions of fingers and toes; the principal parts are body, free edge, root, lunula, cuticle, and matrix

## Tissues and Membranes of the Body

A. Epithelial tissues
   1. Form membranes that contain and protect the internal fluid environment
   2. Absorb nutrients
   3. Secrete products that regulate functions involved in homeostasis

B. Connective tissues
   1. Hold organs and systems together
   2. Form structures that support the body and permit movement

C. Muscle tissues—work with connective tissues to permit movement

D. Nervous tissues—work with glandular epithelial tissue to regulate body function

## The Skeletal System

The skeletal system contributes about 20% of body weight. It comprises the bones and cartilages, as well as ligaments, and tendons related to the bones. Bones are rigid living organisms that furnish the framework of the body while protecting soft body parts. In addition to providing sites for muscle attachment, the skeletal system enables bones and muscle to work together for movement. It also contributes to blood cell formation and storage of inorganic ions (calcium salts, sodium, magnesium, potassium, and carbonate) (Fig. 3.5; see the section on "Connective Tissue" in Chapter 2).

A. Functions of the skeletal system
   1. Provides rigid support system
   2. Provides protection; for example, cranial bones protect the brain
   3. Serves as a source and a reservoir for calcium; involved in the formation of blood cells (hemopoiesis)
   4. Basis of attachment of muscles; allows movement

B. Types of bones
   1. Classified by shape
      a. Long bones
      b. Short bones
      c. Flat bones
      d. Irregular bones
   2. Sutural bones—found between the sutures of certain cranial bones

C. Parts of a long bone
   1. Diaphysis—shaft
   2. Epiphyses—ends
   3. Metaphysis – narrow portion between the shaft and end; contains the growth plate
   4. Articular cartilage—layer of hyaline cartilage that covers the articular surfaces of epiphyses; cushions jolts and blows to bone
   5. Periosteum—fibrous membrane that surrounds bone; contains cells that form bone, blood vessels; serves as point of attachment for ligaments and tendons
   6. Medullary (marrow) cavity
      a. Hollow space within the diaphysis
      b. Filled with marrow in adult
   7. Endosteum—epithelial membrane that lines the medullary cavity

D. Bone tissue
   1. Most distinctive form of connective tissue
   2. Extracellular components are hard and calcified
   3. Rigidity allows its supportive and protective functions
   4. Tensile strength nearly equal to cast iron at less than one-third the weight
   5. Bone matrix composition
      a. Inorganic salts
         (1) Hydroxyapatite—highly specialized chemical crystals of calcium and phosphate contribute to the hardness of bone
         (2) Slender needle-like crystals oriented to resist stress and mechanical deformation
         (3) Magnesium and sodium are also present
      b. Organic matrix
         (1) Ground substance—composite of collagenous fibers and an amorphous mixture of protein and polysaccharides; secreted by connective tissue cells
         (2) Adds to the overall strength and resilience of bone

### Microscopic Structure of Bone

See the section on "Bone" in Chapter 2.

A. Compact bones' microstructure
   1. Osteons, or haversian systems—cylinder-shaped structural units (living bone cells are located in these units); constitute the structural framework of compact bone; surround canals that run lengthwise through bone and are connected by transverse Volkmann's canals; permit the delivery of nutrients and removal of waste products
   2. Four types of structures make up each osteon:
      a. Lamellae—concentric, cylinder-shaped layers of calcified matrix
      b. Lacunae—small spaces containing tissue fluid; bone cells (osteoblasts) are located within lacunae between the hard layers of the lamellae

c. Canaliculi—ultra-small canals radiating in all directions from the lacunae and connecting them to each other and to the haversian canal; contain cell processes of osteoblasts
d. Haversian canal—extends lengthwise through the center of each osteon; contains blood vessels and lymphatic vessels

B. Cancellous (spongy) bone
1. No osteons in cancellous bone; instead, it has bony spicules called trabeculae
2. Nutrients are delivered and waste products removed by diffusion through tiny canaliculi
3. Bony spicules are arranged along the lines of stress, enhancing the bone's strength

C. Blood supply
1. Bone cells are metabolically active and need a blood supply, which comes from the bone marrow in the internal medullary cavity of cancellous bone
2. Blood vessels, lymphatic vessels, and nerves from the periosteum penetrate cortical bone by way of Volkmann's canals; connect with vessels in the haversian canals

D. Types of bone cells
1. Osteoblasts—bone-forming cells found in all bone surfaces; synthesize and secrete osteoid, an important component of ground substance; collagen fibrils line up in the osteoid and serve as a framework for the deposition of calcium and phosphate
2. Osteoclasts—giant multinucleate cells that contain powerful lysosomal enzymes that destroy bone matrix (resorption); contain large numbers of mitochondria and lysosomes
3. Osteocytes—mature bone cells; maintain metabolism such as exchange of nutrients and wastes with the blood

## Bone Marrow

A. Myeloid tissue—specialized type of soft, diffuse connective tissue found in the medullary cavities of long bones and in

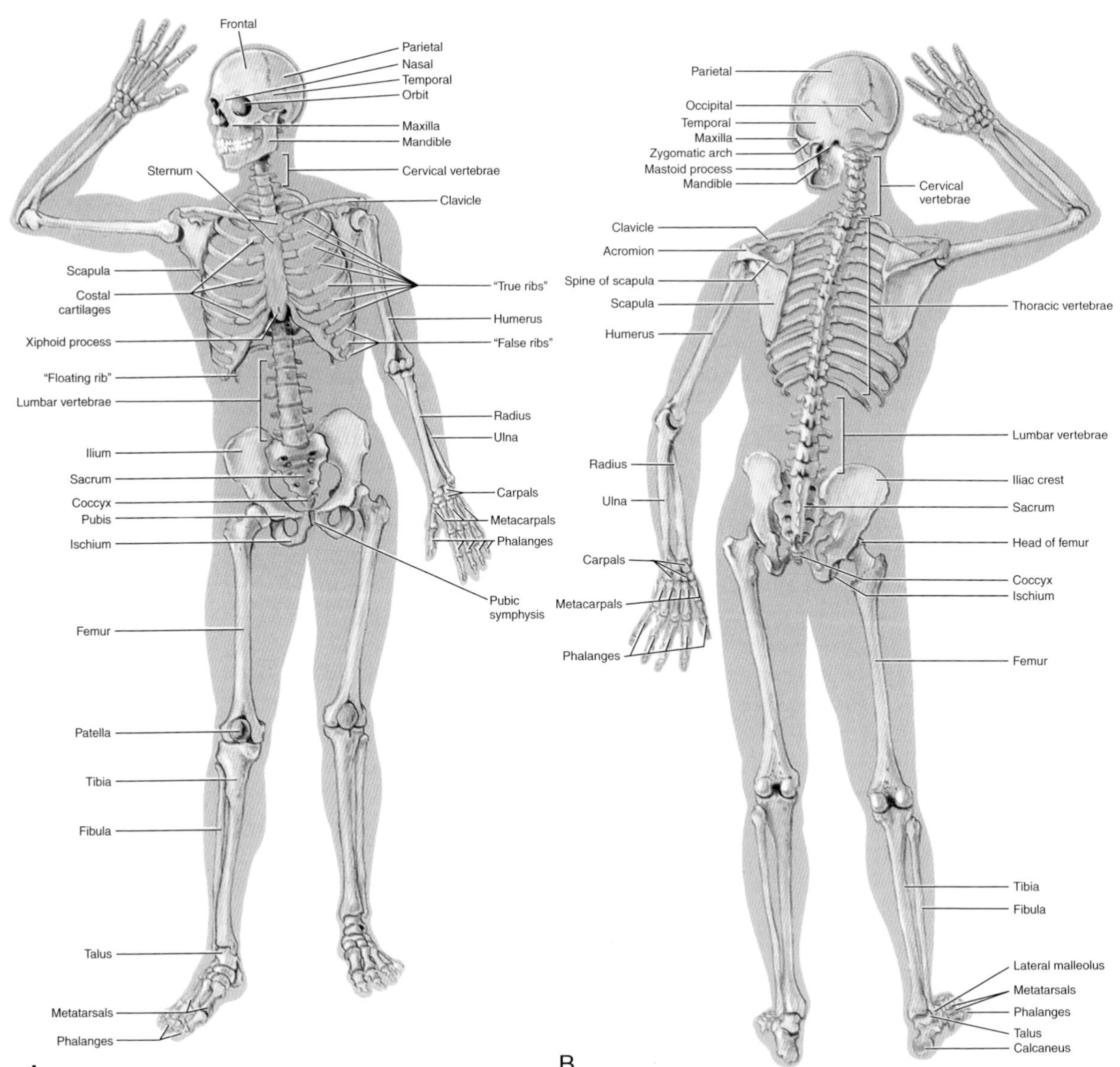


**Fig 3.5** Skeleton. **A**, Anterior view. **B**, Posterior view. (From Solomon EP: *Introduction to human anatomy and physiology*, ed 2, St Louis, 2008, Saunders.)

the spaces of spongy bone; site for the production of blood cells

B. Two types of marrow occur during a person's lifetime:
   1. Red marrow
      a. Found in virtually all bones in an infant or child's body; in an adult, red marrow found in ribs, bodies of the vertebrae, humerus, pelvis, and femur
      b. Produces red blood cells
   2. Yellow marrow
      a. As an individual ages, red marrow is replaced by yellow marrow
      b. Marrow cells become saturated with fat and are no longer active in blood cell production
      c. Yellow marrow can revert to red marrow during times of decreased blood supply, for example, anemia, exposure to radiation, and certain diseases

### Regulation of Blood Calcium Levels

A. The skeletal system serves as a reservoir for approximately 98% of body calcium reserves
   1. Helps maintain the constancy of blood calcium
      a. Calcium is mobilized in and out of blood during bone remodeling
      b. During bone formation, osteoblasts remove calcium from blood and lower circulating levels
      c. During breakdown of bone, osteoclasts release calcium into blood and increase circulating levels
   2. Homeostasis of calcium ion concentration essential for:
      a. Bone formation, remodeling, and repair
      b. Blood clotting
      c. Transmission of nerve impulses
      d. Maintenance of skeletal and cardiac muscle contraction

### Divisions of the Skeleton

A. Axial skeleton—made up of 80 bones of the head, neck, and torso
B. Appendicular skeleton—made up of 126 bones that form the appendages to the axial skeleton; the upper and lower extremities

#### *Axial Skeleton*

A. Skull (see Chapter 4)
B. Vertebral column (Fig. 3.6)
   1. Consists of 24 vertebrae plus the sacrum and the coccyx
   2. Segments of the vertebral column
      a. Cervical vertebrae (7), C1-C6 have openings in their transverse processes for passage of the vertebral artery.
      b. Thoracic vertebrae (12), T1 to T12 are stronger than cervical vertebrae; have facets for articulating with the ribs
      c. Lumbar vertebrae (5), L1 to L5 are the largest and strongest vertebrae; well adapted for the attachment of large back muscles
      d. Sacrum (5 fused vertebrae)—provides strong foundation for pelvic girdle
      e. Coccyx (4 or 5 fused vertebrae)—articulates with the sacrum
   3. Characteristics of vertebrae
      a. All vertebrae, except the first, have a flat, rounded body anteriorly and centrally, a spinous process posteriorly, and two transverse processes laterally
      b. All vertebrae except the sacrum and the coccyx have a vertebral foramen
      c. The first cervical vertebra, the atlas, supports the head
      d. The second cervical vertebra, the axis, has an upward projection (dens) to allow the rotation of the head
   4. The vertebral column as a whole articulates with the head, ribs, and iliac bones
   5. Individual vertebrae articulate with each other in joints between their bodies and between their articular processes
C. Sternum
   1. Dagger-shaped bone in the middle of the anterior chest wall made up of three parts:
      a. Manubrium—upper handle part
      b. Body—middle blade part
      c. Xiphoid process—blunt cartilaginous lower tip; ossifies during adult life; may be damaged during improper administration of chest compressions during CPR
   2. The manubrium articulates with the clavicle and the first and second ribs
   3. Ribs join the body of the sternum, either directly or indirectly, by means of costal cartilages
D. Ribs
   1. Twelve pairs of ribs form the sides of the thoracic cavity
   2. Each rib articulates with the body and the transverse process of its corresponding thoracic vertebra
   3. From its vertebral attachment, each rib curves outward and then forward and downward
   4. Rib attachment to the sternum:
      a. Ribs 1 to 8 join a costal cartilage that attaches it to the sternum
      b. The costal cartilage of ribs 8 to 10 indirectly joins the cartilage of the rib above to the sternum (false ribs)
      c. Ribs 11 and 12 are floating ribs because they are not attached to the sternum

#### *Appendicular Skeleton*

A. Upper extremity (Fig. 3.7)
   1. Consists of the bones of the shoulder girdle, arm, forearm, wrist, and hand
   2. Shoulder girdle
      a. Made up of the scapula and the clavicle
      b. The clavicle forms the only bony joint with the trunk (sternoclavicular joint)
      c. At its distal end, the clavicle articulates with the acromion process of the scapula
   3. Humerus (Fig. 3.8)
      a. Longest bone of the upper limb
      b. Articulates proximally with the glenoid fossa of the scapula and distally with the radius and the ulna
   4. Ulna (Fig. 3.9)
      a. Long bone found on the medial, little finger (pinky) side of the forearm

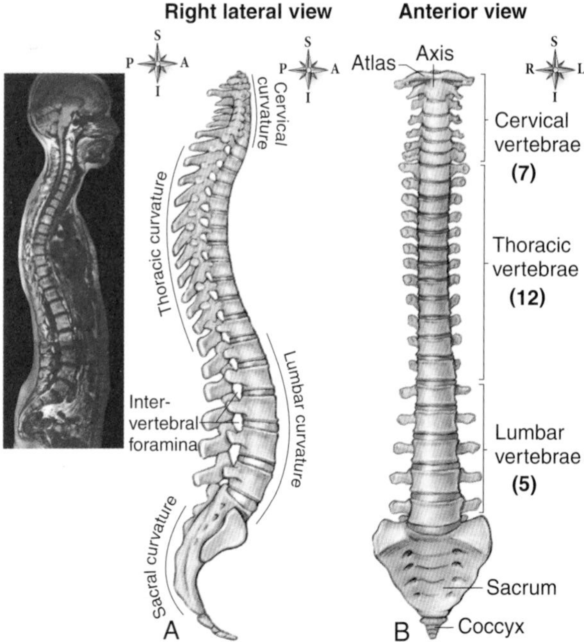


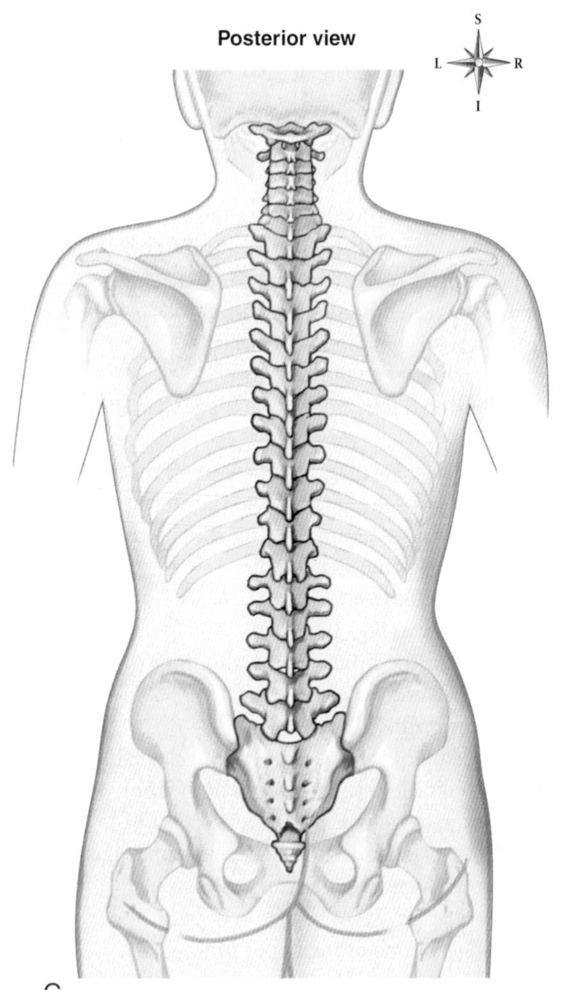


**Fig 3.6** The vertebral column. A, Right lateral view of the vertebral column, demonstrating the curvatures of the spine. B, Anterior view of the vertebral column, indicating number of vertebral types present. C, Posterior view of the vertebral column. (From Patton KT, Thibodeau GA: *Anthony's textbook of anatomy and physiology*, ed 20, St Louis, 2013, Elsevier.)

   b. Articulates proximally with the humerus and the radius and distally with a fibrocartilaginous disc
5. Radius (Fig. 3.9)
   a. Long bone found on the lateral, thumb side of the forearm
   b. Articulates proximally with the capitulum of the humerus and the radial notch of the ulna; articulates distally with the scaphoid and lunate carpals of the wrist
6. Carpal bones (Fig. 3.10)
   a. Eight small bones that form the wrist; bound closely and firmly by ligaments; arranged in two transverse rows:
      (1) Top row made up of the pisiform, the triquetrum, the lunate, and the scaphoid
      (2) Bottom row made up of the hamate, the capitate, the trapezoid, and the trapezium
   b. Joints between the radius and carpals allow wrist and hand movements
   c. Carpal tunnel—concavity formed by the pisiform and the hamate (on the ulnar side) and the scaphoid and the trapezium (on the radial side), through which the median nerve passes; narrowing or inflammation of the carpal tunnel gives rise to carpal tunnel syndrome
7. Metacarpal bones
   a. Form the framework of the hand
   b. The thumb metacarpal forms the most freely movable joint with the carpals (carpometacarpal joint)
   c. The heads of the metacarpals (knuckles) articulate with the phalanges (metacarpophalangeal joint)
8. Phalanges—bones of the fingers; articulate with metacarpals and with each other (interphalangeal joints)

B. Lower extremity
1. Consists of the bones of the hip, thigh, leg, ankle, and foot
2. The pelvic girdle is made up of the sacrum and the two coxal (hip) bones bound tightly by strong ligaments
   a. A stable circular base that supports the trunk and attaches the lower extremities to the axial skeleton
   b. Each coxal bone is made up of three fused parts:
      (1) Ilium—largest and uppermost part
      (2) Ischium—strongest and lowermost, posterior part
      (3) Pubis—anterior and inferior part
3. Femur—longest and heaviest bone in the body (Fig. 3.11)
4. Patella—kneecap; small triangular bone in front of the joint between the femur and the tibia
5. Tibia
   a. Larger bone of the leg; bears the weight of the body
   b. Articulates proximally with the femur to form the knee joint
   c. Articulates distally with the fibula and the talus of the ankle
6. Fibula
   a. Smaller, more laterally and deeply placed of the two shin bones
   b. Articulates with the tibia

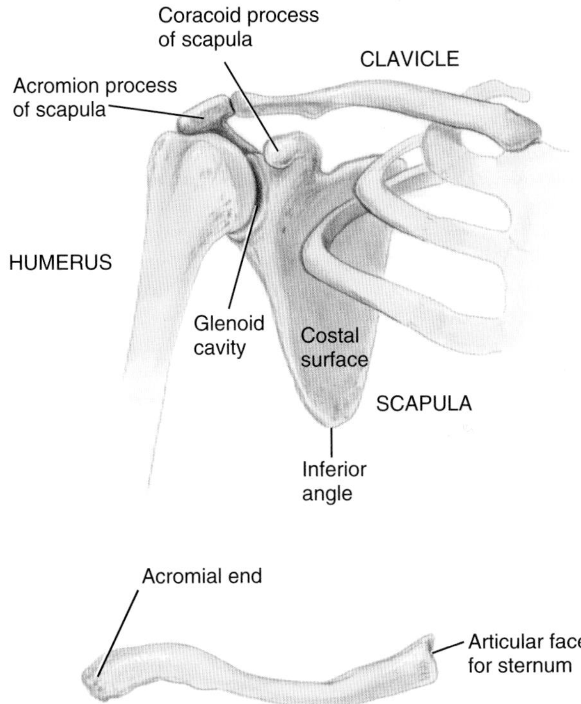


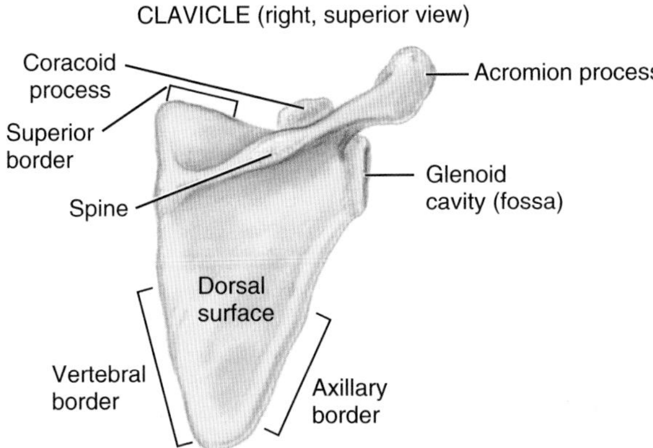


**Fig 3.7** Right scapula and clavicle. (From Applegate E: *The anatomy and physiology learning system,* ed 2, St Louis, 2011, Saunders.)

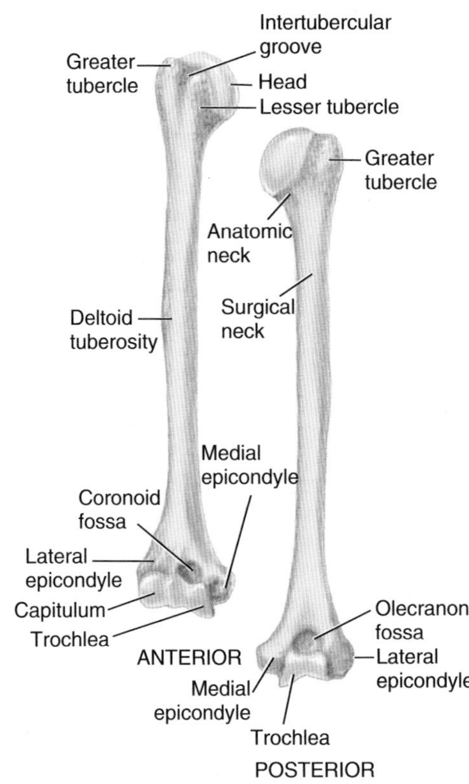


**Fig 3.8** Humerus (upper arm). (Modified from Applegate E: *The anatomy and physiology learning system,* ed 4, St Louis, 2011, Saunders.)

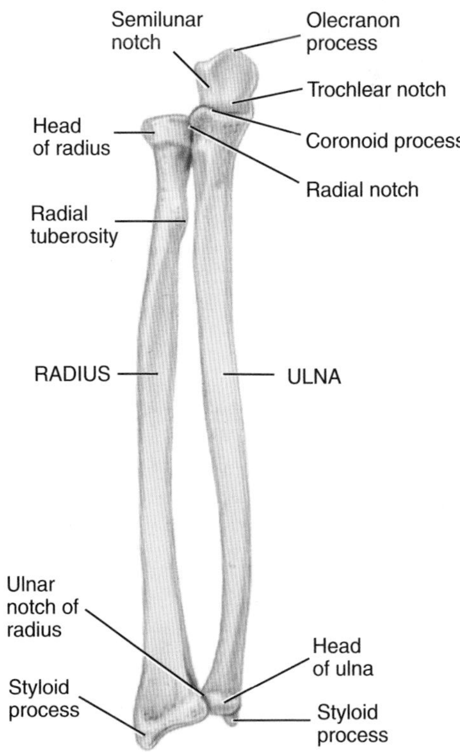


**Fig 3.9** Radius and ulna (lower arm). (Modified from Applegate E: *The anatomy and physiology learning system,* ed 4, St Louis, 2011, Saunders.)

7. Foot (Figs 3.12 and 3.13)
   a. The structure is similar to that of the hand, with adaptations for supporting weight
   b. Foot bones are held together to form spring arches
      (1) Tarsus (ankle)—contains seven bones: calcaneus (heel bone), talus (ankle bone), cuneiforms, cuboid, and navicular

## Joints

A. Classification of joints
   1. Structural—based on the presence or absence of synovial cavity and type of connecting tissue; classified as fibrous, cartilaginous, or synovial
   2. Functional—based on the degree of movement permitted; joints may be synarthroses (immovable), amphiarthroses (slightly movable), or diarthroses (freely movable)

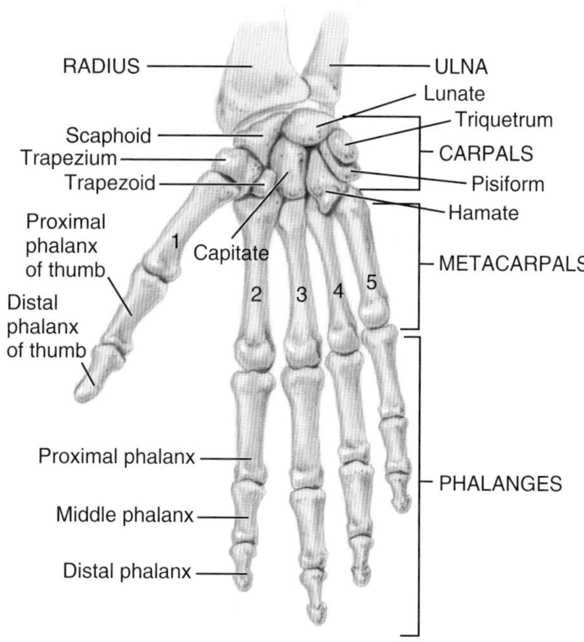


**Fig 3.10** Bones of the hand and wrist. (From Patton KT, Thibodeau GA, Douglas MM: *Essentials of anatomy and physiology,* St Louis, 2012, Mosby.)

B. Fibrous joints (Fig. 3.14)
  1. Bones held together closely by fibrous connective tissue
     a. Syndesmoses—joints in which ligaments connect two bones, for example, the joint between the radius and ulna
     b. Sutures—found only in the skull; tooth-like projections from adjacent bones interlock with each other
     c. Gomphoses—a joint in which one bone articulates within a cavity or socket of another bone; found between the root of the tooth and the alveolar process of the mandible or the maxilla

C. Cartilaginous joints (Fig. 3.15)
  1. Bones held together by hyaline cartilage or fibrocartilage; allow little motion
     a. Synchondroses—hyaline cartilage present between articulating bones
     b. Symphysis—joints in which a pad or disc of fibrocartilage connects two bones

D. Synovial joints
  1. Structures of synovial joints (Fig. 3.16)
     a. Joint capsule—sleeve-like casing around the ends of bones, which binds them together
     b. Synovial membrane—membrane lining the joint capsule; secretes synovial fluid
     c. Articular cartilage—hyaline cartilage covering the articular surfaces of the joint cavity
     d. Menisci (articular discs)—pads of fibrocartilage located between articulating bones
     e. Bursae—sac-like body cavities; reduce friction in joints
     f. Ligaments—strong cords of dense white fibrous tissue; hold the bones of a synovial joint more firmly together (temporomandibular joint [TMJ] has three ligaments)
  2. Types of synovial joints

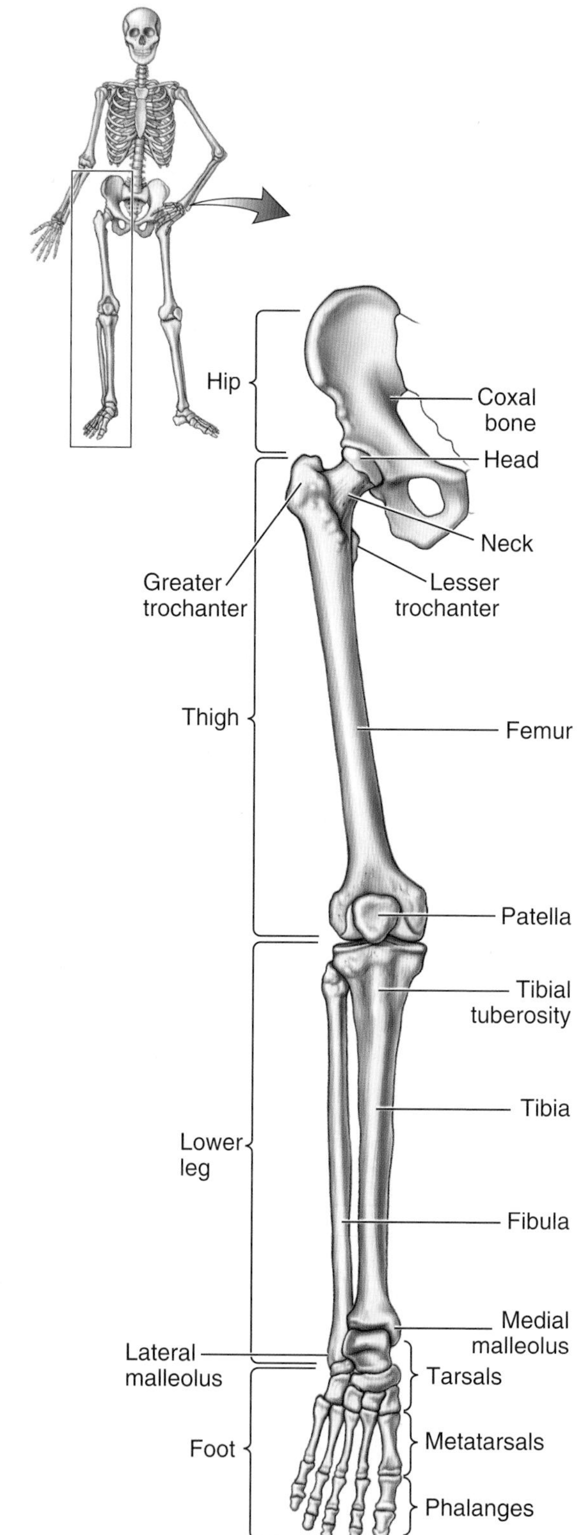


**Fig 3.11** Bones of the thigh and leg. (Modified from Herlihy B: *The human body in health and illness,* ed 5, St Louis, 2015, Elsevier.)

     a. Uniaxial joints—permit movement around only one axis and in only one plane
        (1) Hinge joints—the articulating ends of bones form a hinge-shaped unity that allows only flexion and extension

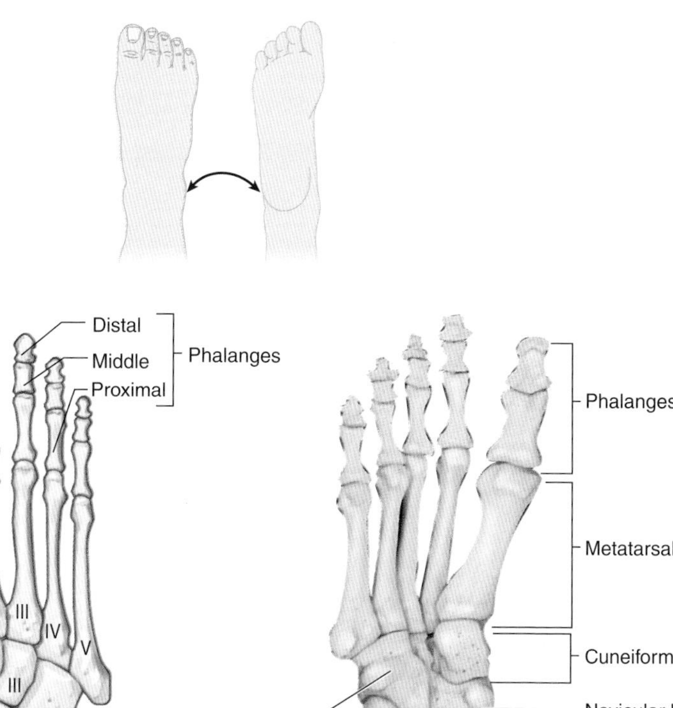


**Fig 3.12** The foot. **A,** Bones on the right foot viewed from above. Tarsal bones consist of cuneiforms, navicular, talus, cuboid, and calcaneus. **B,** Posterior aspect of the right ankle skeleton and inferior aspect of the right foot skeleton. (From Patton KT, Thibodeau GA: *Anthony's textbook of anatomy and physiology,* ed 20, St Louis, 2013, Elsevier.)

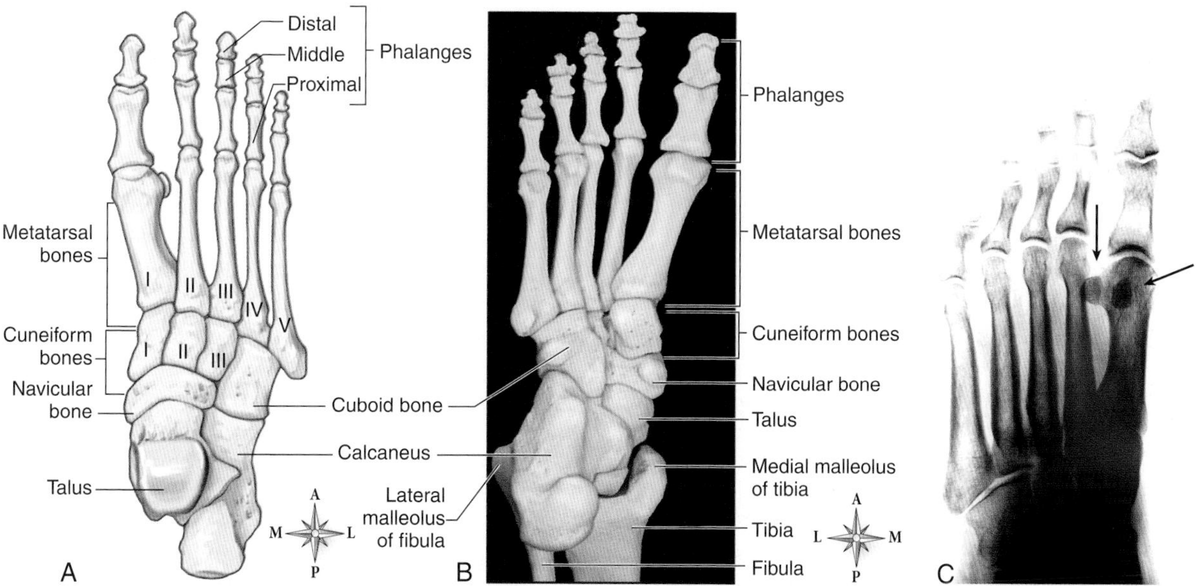


**Fig 3.13** Arches of the foot **A,** Right foot; the medial longitudinal arch is formed by the calcaneus, talus, navicular, cuneiform bones, and the first three metatarsal bones. **B,** Left foot; the lateral longitudinal arch is formed by the calcaneus, the cuboid bone, and the fourth and fifth metatarsal bones. **C,** X-ray film of the left foot showing prominent sesamoid bones near the distal end (head) of the first metatarsal bone of the great toe. (From Solomon EP: *Introduction to human anatomy and physiology,* ed 2, St Louis, 2008, Saunders.)

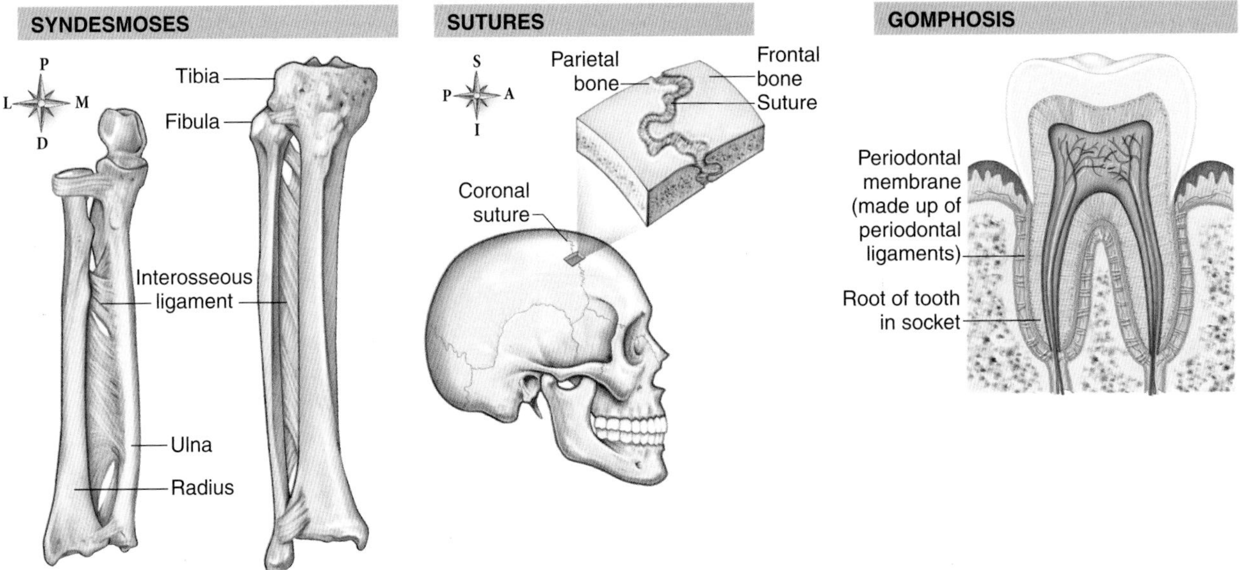


**Fig 3.14** Fibrous joints. (From Patton KT, Thibodeau GA: *Anthony's textbook of anatomy and physiology,* ed 20, St Louis, 2013, Elsevier.)

(2) Pivot joints—a projection of one bone articulates with a ring or notch of another bone

b. Biaxial joints—permit movements around two perpendicular axes in two perpendicular planes

c. Saddle joints—the articulating ends of bones are reciprocally concave-convex; one bone resembles a miniature saddle and the other bone will fit into this depression like a rider in the saddle, for example, the carpometacarpal joint of the thumb

d. Condyloid (ellipsoidal) joints—a bony projection that fits into an elliptical socket

e. Multi-axial joints—permit movements around three or more axes in three or more planes

(1) Ball-and-socket (spheroid) joints—most movable joints; the ball-shaped head of one bone fits into a concave depression, for example, shoulder

(2) Gliding joints—relatively flat articulating surfaces that allow limited gliding movements along various axes, for example, the joints between the carpals

## Muscular System

The muscular system makes up about 40% of body weight and comprises more than 600 muscles. The muscular system acts together with the skeletal system to provide form, contours, and movement. The three types of muscle are cardiac, smooth, and skeletal.

### Anatomy of the Muscular System

See Fig. 3.17.

A. Muscle tissue has five key functions:
  1. Producing body movements
  2. Stabilizing body positions
  3. Regulating organ volume
  4. Moving substances within the body
  5. Producing heat

B. Characteristics
  1. Excitability—ability of muscle fibers (and neurons) to respond to a stimulus and convert it into an action potential
  2. Contractibility—ability to contract (shorten and thicken)
  3. Extensibility—ability to be stretched
  4. Elasticity—ability to return to original shape after contraction or extension

C. Types
  1. Skeletal muscle—mostly attached to bones; striated and voluntary
  2. Cardiac muscle—forms most of the walls of the heart; striated and involuntary
  3. Smooth muscle—located in viscera; participates in internal processes; involuntary

### Skeletal Muscle Structure

See Fig. 3.18.

A. Connective tissue components (may become a tendon or an aponeurosis)
  1. Endomysium—delicate connective tissue membrane that covers specialized skeletal muscle fibers
  2. Perimysium—tough connective tissue binding muscle fascicles together
  3. Epimysium—coarse sheath covering the muscle as a whole

B. Size, shape, and fiber arrangement
  1. Size—ranging from extremely small to large masses
  2. Shape—variety of shapes, such as broad, narrow, long, tapering, short, blunt, triangular, quadrilateral, or irregular, and as flat sheets or bulky masses
  3. Arrangement of muscle fibers—variety of arrangements; the direction of fibers is significant because of its relationship to function

C. Attachment of muscle
  1. Origin—point of attachment that does not move when the muscle contracts

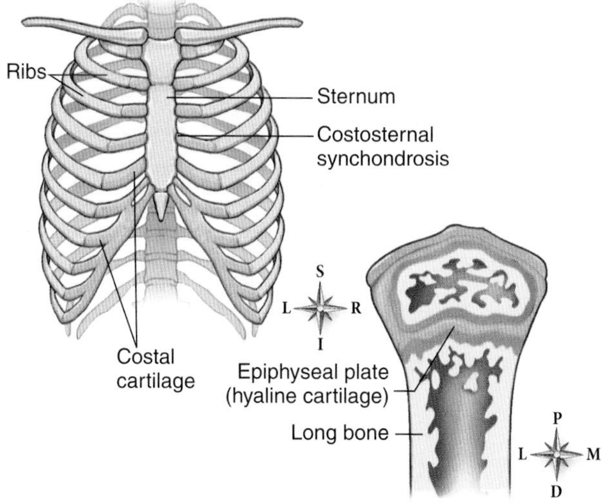


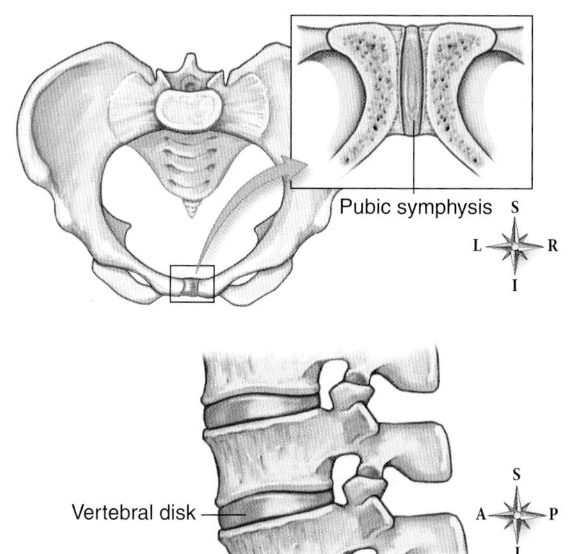


Fig 3.15 Cartilaginous joints. (From Patton KT and Thibodeau GA: *Anthony's textbook of anatomy and physiology,* ed 20, St Louis, 2013, Elsevier.)

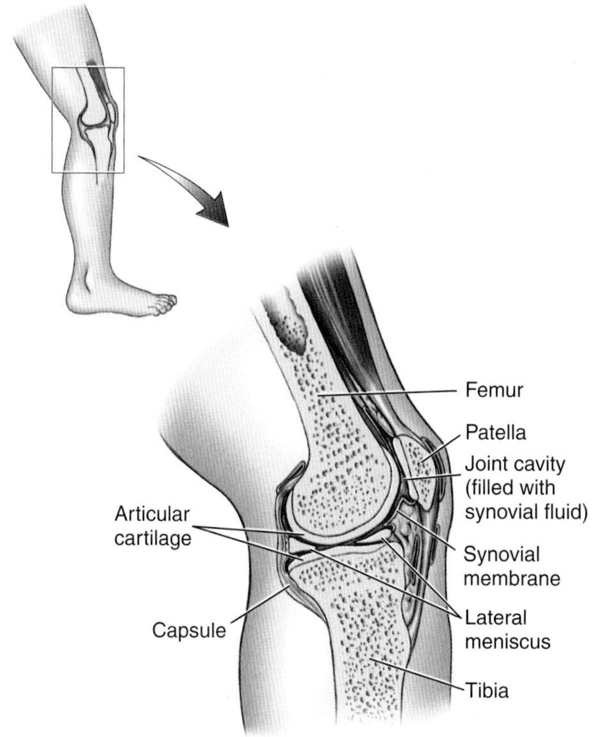


Fig 3.16 Structure of synovial joints. (From Herlihy B: *The human body in health and illness,* ed 5, St Louis, 2015, Elsevier.)

2. Insertion—point of attachment that moves when the muscle contracts

D. Muscle actions
   1. Most movements produced by the coordinated actions of several muscles; some muscles in the group contract while others relax
      a. Prime mover (agonist)—muscles that directly perform a specific movement
      b. Antagonist—when contracting, directly oppose prime movers; relax while the agonist is contracting to produce movement; provide precision and control during contraction of prime movers
      c. Synergists—contract at the same time as prime movers do; facilitate prime mover actions to produce a more efficient movement
      d. Fixator muscles—stabilize joints

E. Lever systems—bones serve as levers, and joints serve as fulcrums; the muscle applies a pulling force on a bone lever at the point of the muscle's attachment to the bone, causing the insertion bone to move about its joint fulcrum

***Head and Neck Muscles.*** See the section on "The Muscular System" and Fig. 4.4 in Chapter 4.

A. Muscles of facial expression—unique in that at least one point of attachment is to the deep layers of the skin over the face or neck
B. Muscles of mastication—responsible for chewing movements
C. Muscles that move the head—paired muscles on either side of the neck that are responsible for head movements

***Trunk Muscles***

A. Muscles of the thorax—critical in respiration
B. Muscles of the abdominal wall—arranged in three layers, with fibers in each layer running in different directions to increase strength
C. Muscles of the pelvic floor—support structures in the pelvic cavity

***Upper Limb Muscles***

A. Muscles acting on the shoulder girdle—muscles that attach the upper extremity to the torso; located anteriorly (chest) or posteriorly (back and neck); allow extensive movement
B. Muscles that move the arm—most originate on the trunk; the shoulder is a synovial joint allowing extensive movement in every plane of motion
C. Muscles that move the forearm—found proximal to the elbow and attached to the ulna and radius
D. Muscles that move the wrist, hand, and fingers—located on the anterior or posterior surfaces of the forearm and

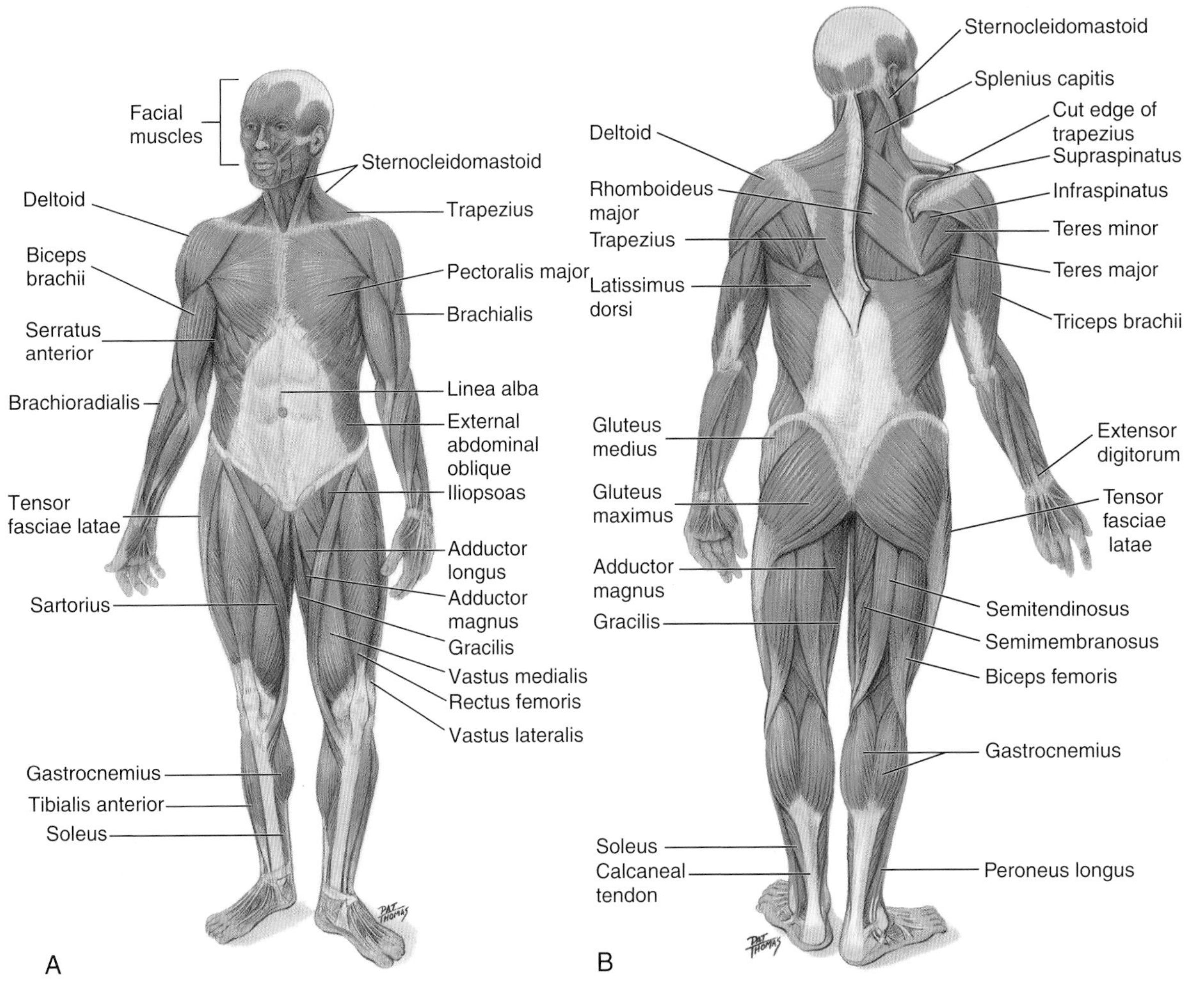


**Fig 3.17** General overview of the body musculature. **A**, Anterior view. **B**, Posterior view. (Modified from Applegate E: *The anatomy and physiology learning system*, ed 4, St Louis, 2011, Saunders.)

attaching to carpals, metacarpals or phalanges. Muscles that abduct and adduct the fingers are located within the deep palm and attach the metacarpals to phalanges.

***Lower Limb Muscles***

A. The pelvic girdle and the lower extremity function in locomotion and maintenance of stability
B. Muscles that move the thigh and the leg
C. Muscles that move the ankle and the foot
   1. Extrinsic foot muscles—located in the leg; exert their actions by pulling on tendons that insert on bones in the ankle and foot; responsible for dorsiflexion, plantarflexion, inversion, and eversion
   2. Intrinsic foot muscles—located within the foot; responsible for flexion, extension, abduction, and adduction of the toes

***Posture***

A. Maintaining body posture is an important function of muscles
B. Good posture—body alignment that favors function and requires the least muscular work to maintain, keeping the body's center of gravity over its base
C. How posture is maintained:
   1. Muscles exert a continual pull on bones in the opposite direction from gravity
   2. Structures other than muscle and bone have a role in maintaining posture
      a. The nervous system—responsible for the existence of muscle tone and for the regulation and coordination of the amount of pull exerted by individual muscles
      b. Respiratory, digestive, excretory, and endocrine systems all contribute to maintain posture

***Function of Skeletal Muscle***

A. Overview of muscle cells
   1. Muscle cells are called *fibers* because of their thread-like shape
   2. Sarcolemma—plasma membrane of muscle fibers
   3. Sarcoplasmic reticulum
      a. A network of tubules and sacs found within muscle fibers
      b. The membrane of the sarcoplasmic reticulum continually pumps calcium ions from the sarcoplasm and stores the ions within sacs
   4. Muscle fibers contain many mitochondria and several nuclei
   5. Myofibrils—numerous fine fibers packed close together in the sarcoplasm

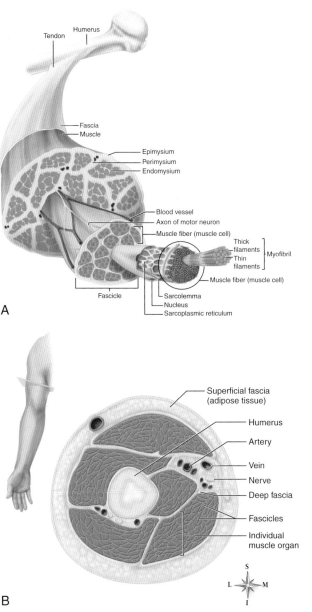

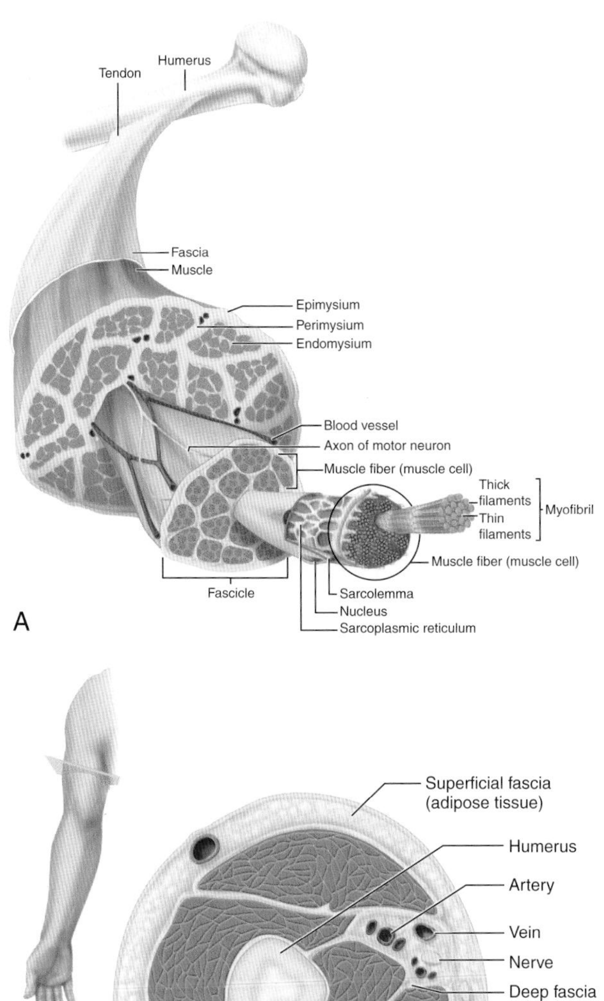


**Fig 3.18** Structure of a muscle organ **A**, Cross section of a muscle, demonstrating the components of this organ, as well as connective tissue coverings of each part. Myofibrils form a myofiber (muscle cell), each myofiber is surrounded by endoysium, many myofibers form a fascicle, surrounded by perimysium, and many fascicles form a muscle, surrounded by epimysium. **B**, A cross section through the right upper limb. (From Patton KT, Thibodeau GA: *Anthony's textbook of anatomy and physiology,* ed 20, St Louis, 2013, Elsevier.)

6. Sarcomere
   a. The segment of myofibril between two successive Z lines
   b. Each myofibril consists of many sarcomeres
   c. The contractile unit of muscle fibers
7. Striated muscle
   a. Dark stripes are called *A bands*; the light H zone runs across the midsection of each dark A band
   b. Light stripes are called *I bands*; the dark Z line extends across the center of each light I band
8. T tubules
   a. Transverse tubules that extend across the sarcoplasm at right angles to the long axis of the muscle fiber
   b. Formed by the inward extension of the sarcolemma
   c. The membrane has ion pumps that continually transport calcium ions inward from the sarcoplasm
   d. Allow electrical impulses traveling along the sarcolemma to move deeper into the cell
9. Triad
   a. Triplet of tubules; a T-tubule is sandwiched between two sacs of the sarcoplasmic reticulum; allows an electrical impulse traveling along a T-tubule to stimulate the membranes of adjacent sacs of the sarcoplasmic reticulum

B. Myofilaments
1. Each myofibril contains thousands of thick and thin myofilaments
2. Four different types of protein molecules make up myofilaments:
   a. Myosin
      (1) Makes up almost all the thick filament
      (2) Myosin "heads" are chemically attracted to actin molecules; known as *cross-bridges* when attached to actin
   b. Actin—globular protein that forms two fibrous strands twisted around each other to form the bulk of the thin filament
   c. Tropomyosin—protein that blocks the active sites on actin molecules
   d. Troponin—protein that holds tropomyosin molecules in place
3. Thin filaments attached to both Z lines of a sarcomere and extend partway toward the center
4. Thick myosin filaments are not attached to Z lines

C. Mechanism of contraction
1. Excitation and contraction
   a. A skeletal muscle fiber remains at rest until stimulated by a motor neuron
   b. Neuromuscular junction—motor neurons connect to the sarcolemma at the motor endplate
   c. Neuromuscular junction—synapse where neurotransmitter molecules transmit signals
   d. Acetylcholine—neurotransmitter released into the synaptic cleft, which diffuses across the gap, stimulates receptors, and initiates an impulse in the sarcolemma
   e. A nerve impulse travels over the sarcolemma and inward along T-tubules to trigger the release of calcium ions
   f. Calcium binds to troponin, causing the tropomyosin to shift and expose the active sites on actin
   g. Sliding filament theory
      (1) When active sites on actin are exposed, myosin heads bind to them
      (2) Myosin heads bend, pulling the thin filaments past them
      (3) Each head releases itself, binds to the next active site, and pulls again

(4) The entire myofibril becomes shortened

2. Relaxation
   a. Immediately after calcium ions are released, the sarcoplasmic reticulum begins actively pumping them back into sacs
   b. Calcium ions are removed from troponin molecules, ending the contraction
3. Energy sources for muscle contraction
   a. Hydrolysis of ATP yields the energy required for muscular contraction
   b. ATP binds to the myosin head to perform the work of pulling the thin filament during contraction
   c. Muscle fibers continually synthesize ATP from the breakdown of creatine phosphate
   d. Catabolism by muscle fibers requires glucose and oxygen
   e. At rest, excess oxygen ($O_2$) in the sarcoplasm is stored by myoglobin
      (1) Red fibers—muscle fibers with high levels of myoglobin
      (2) White fibers—muscle fibers with minimal myoglobin
   f. Aerobic respiration occurs when adequate $O_2$ is available
   g. Anaerobic respiration occurs when low levels of $O_2$ are available and results in the formation of lactic acid
   h. Skeletal muscle contraction produces excess heat that can be used to maintain body temperature

### *Function of Skeletal Muscle Organs*

A. Motor unit
   1. Motor unit—comprised of the motor neuron and the muscle fibers to which it is attached
   2. Motor units can consist of only a few or numerous muscle fibers
   3. Generally, with a smaller number of fibers in a motor unit, more precise movements are possible; the larger the number of fibers in a motor unit, the more powerful is the contraction

B. Twitch contraction
   1. A quick jerk of a muscle that is produced as a result of a single, brief threshold stimulus (generally occurs only in experimental situations)
   2. Three phases:
      a. Latent phase—the nerve impulse travels to the sarcoplasmic reticulum to trigger the release of calcium
      b. Contraction phase—calcium binds to troponin, and the sliding of filaments occurs
      c. Relaxation phase—the sliding of filaments ceases

C. Treppe—the "staircase phenomenon"
   1. Gradual, step-like increase in the strength of a contraction; observed in a series of twitch contractions that occur 1 second apart
   2. Eventually, the muscle responds with less forceful contractions, and the relaxation phase becomes shorter
   3. If the relaxation phase disappears completely, a contracture (abnormal shortening of muscle tissue that can cause disability) occurs

D. Tetanus—smooth, sustained contractions
   1. Multiple-wave summation—multiple twitch waves are added together to sustain muscle tension for a longer time
   2. Incomplete tetanus—very short periods of relaxation occur between peaks of tension
   3. Complete tetanus—twitch waves fuse into a single, sustained peak

E. Muscle tone
   1. Tonic contraction—continual, partial contraction of a muscle
   2. At any one time, a small number of muscle fibers within a muscle contract, producing tightness of muscle tone
   3. Muscles with less tone than normal are *flaccid*
   4. Muscles with more tone than normal are *spastic*
   5. Muscle tone is maintained by negative feedback mechanisms

F. Principle of graded strength
   1. Skeletal muscles contract with varying degrees of strength at different times
   2. Factors that contribute to the phenomenon of graded strength:
      a. Metabolic condition of individual fibers
      b. Number of muscle fibers contracting simultaneously; the greater the number of fibers contracting, the stronger the contraction
      c. Number of motor units recruited
      d. Intensity and frequency of stimulation
   3. Length-tension relationship
      a. The maximal strength that a muscle can develop bears a direct relationship to the initial length of its fibers
      b. A shortened muscle's sarcomeres are compressed; therefore the muscle cannot develop much tension
      c. An overstretched muscle cannot develop much tension because the thick myofilaments are too far from the thin myofilaments
      d. The strongest maximal contraction is possible only when the skeletal muscle has been stretched to its optimal length
   4. Stretch reflex
      a. The load imposed on a muscle influences the strength of a skeletal contraction
      b. The body tries to maintain a consistency of muscle length in response to increased load
      c. Maintains a relatively constant length as the load is increased up to a maximum sustainable level

G. Isotonic and isometric contractions
   1. Isotonic contraction
      a. Contraction in which the tone or tension within a muscle remains the same as the length of the muscle changes
         (1) Concentric—the muscle shortens as it contracts
         (2) Eccentric—the muscle lengthens as it contracts
      b. *Isotonic* means "same tension"
      c. All the energy of contraction is used to pull on the thin myofilaments and thereby change the length of a fiber's sarcomeres
   2. Isometric contraction

a. Contraction in which muscle length remains the same while muscle tension increases
b. *Isometric* means "same length"
3. Body movements occur as a result of both types of contractions

***Function of Cardiac and Smooth Muscle Tissue***

A. Cardiac muscle (also known as *striated involuntary muscle*)
1. Found only in the heart; forms bulk of the walls of each chamber
2. Contracts rhythmically and continuously to maintain a constant blood flow
3. Resembles skeletal muscle but has specialized features related to its role in continuous pumping of blood
a. Each cardiac muscle contains parallel myofibrils
b. Cardiac muscle fibers form strong, electrically coupled junctions (intercalated discs) with other fibers; individual cells also exhibit branching
c. Syncytium—continuous, electrically coupled mass; important for coordinating muscle contractions
d. Cardiac muscle fibers form a continuous, contractile band around the heart chambers and conduct a single impulse across a virtually continuous sarcolemma
e. T-tubules are larger and form dyads with a rather sparse sarcoplasmic reticulum
f. Cardiac muscle sustains each impulse longer than does skeletal muscle; therefore, impulses cannot come rapidly enough to produce tetanus
g. Cardiac muscle does not run low on ATP and does not experience fatigue
h. Cardiac muscle is self-stimulating

B. Smooth muscle
1. Smooth muscle is composed of small, tapered cells with single nuclei
2. T-tubules are absent; only a loosely organized sarcoplasmic reticulum is present
3. Calcium comes from outside the cell and binds to calmodulin instead of troponin to trigger a contraction
4. No striations are present because both the thick and the thin myofilaments have an arrangement different from that in skeletal or cardiac muscle fibers; myofilaments are not organized into sarcomeres
5. Two types of smooth muscle tissue:
a. Visceral muscle (single unit)
(1) Gap junctions join smooth muscle fibers into large, continuous sheets
(2) Most common type; forms a muscular layer in the walls of hollow structures such as the digestive, urinary, and reproductive tracts
(3) Exhibits autorhythmicity, which produces peristalsis
b. Multi-unit
(1) Does not act as a single unit; is composed of many independent cell units
(2) Each fiber responds only to input from nerves

## The Nervous System

The nervous system is primarily composed of the brain, the spinal cord, nerves, and ganglia. Along with the endocrine system, the nervous system regulates and maintains homeostasis. It allows the human body to communicate, integrate, and regulate body functions vital for living. Subdivisions of the nervous system aid in the understanding of structure, direction of information flow, and motor output or motor function (see the section on "Nerve Tissue" in Chapter 2).

A. Two main subsystems (Fig. 3.19):
1. The central nervous system (CNS)—consists of the brain and the spinal cord
2. The peripheral nervous system (PNS)—includes all nervous tissue outside the CNS; contains the nerves to and from the body wall

B. Other divisions of the nervous system
1. Direction of information flow
a. *Afferent* consists of incoming sensory pathways
b. *Efferent* consists of outgoing motor pathways
2. Control of effectors
a. The somatic nervous system (SNS) carries information to the somatic effectors (skeletal muscle)
b. The autonomic nervous system (ANS) carries information to the autonomic effectors (e.g., cardiac and smooth muscle, glands, adipose tissue)

C. Functions
1. Sensory—detection of different types of stimuli both inside and outside the body
a. Afferent or sensory neurons—carry information from the PNS to the CNS
2. Integrative—processing of sensory information by analyzing and storing some of it and by making decisions regarding appropriate responses; interneurons carry out this function
3. Motor—responses to integrative decisions
a. Efferent or motor neurons carry information from the CNS to the PNS

D. The central nervous system
1. Brain—housed within the skull; contains about 100 billion neurons
2. Spinal cord—contains about 100 million neurons; is connected directly to the brain and is protected by the vertebral column
3. Source of thoughts, emotions, memories; source of most nerve impulses that stimulate muscles to contract and glands to secrete
4. Communication to and from CNS accomplished by:
a. Cranial nerves
b. Spinal nerves
c. Ganglia—small clusters of neuronal cell bodies that relay signals traveling along cranial and spinal nerves
d. Enteric plexuses—in the walls of the organs of the gastrointestinal (GI) tract; help regulate the digestive system

E. The peripheral nervous system
1. Subdivisions
a. The somatic nervous system

(1) Sensory neurons—convey information to the CNS from the somatic receptors in the head, body wall, and limbs and also from the receptors for the special senses of vision, hearing, taste, and smell
(2) Motor neurons—conduct impulses from the CNS to skeletal muscles only; motor responses are voluntary

b. The autonomic nervous system (ANS)
(1) Sympathetic division (thoracolumbar) involves motor (efferent) nerves from the ANS; initiates the "flight or fight" response.
(2) Parasympathetic division (craniosacral) involves motor (efferent) nerves from the ANS: stimulates "resting and digesting" responses.

c. The enteric nervous system
(1) "Brain of the GI system"
(2) Enteric motor neurons govern the contraction of GI tract smooth muscle, secretions of the GI tract organs (e.g., acid secretions by stomach), and activity of GI tract endocrine cells

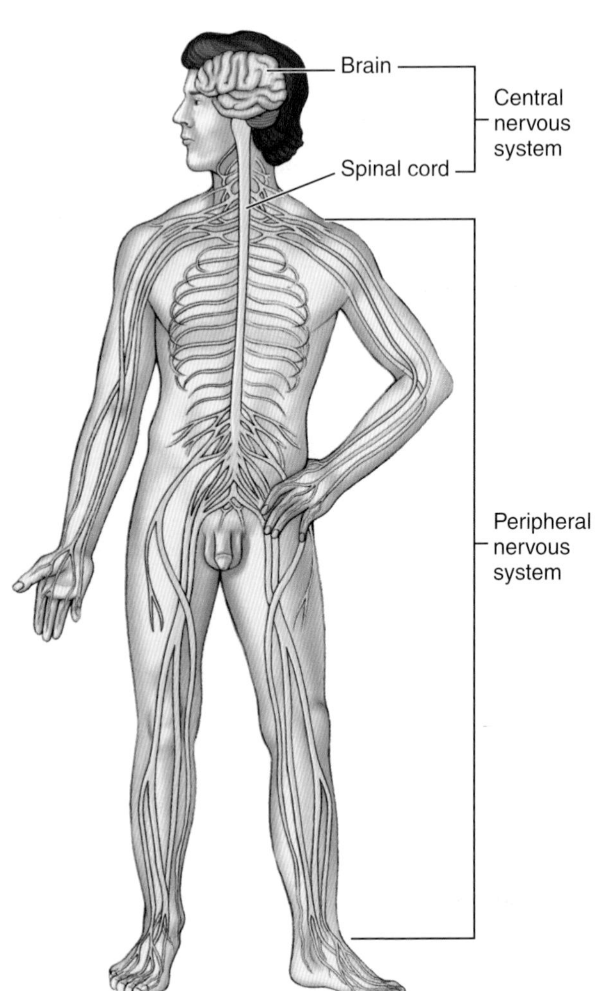


**Fig 3.19** The nervous system. (From Herlihy B: *The human body in health and illness,* ed 5, St Louis, 2015, Elsevier.)

### Cellular Organization

***Nervous System Structure.*** See Fig. 3.20 and the section on "Nerve Tissue" and Figs 2.12 and 2.13 in Chapter 2.

A. Each neuron (nerve cell) consists of a cell body containing a nucleus
B. Dendrite—sends impulses toward the cell body or to a muscle or gland
C. Axon—conducts nerve impulses away from the cell body
D. Neuroglia—specialized tissue cells that support neurons, attach neurons to blood vessels, produce the myelin sheath around the axons of the CNS, carry out phagocytosis, and retain the ability to undergo mitosis
E. Myelin—fatty substance around axons; provides insulation and increases the speed of nerve conduction; deposited by Schwann cells in layers in the PNS
   1. Neurilemma—outermost layer of the Schwann cell
   2. Nodes of Ranvier—located between myelin segments; unmyelinated
   3. Oligodendrocytes—processes from one cell assist in myelination of multiple CNS axons
F. White matter consists of aggregations of myelinated processes from many neurons
G. Gray matter contains the neurons, dendrites, and axon terminals of unmyelinated axons and neuroglia; forms an H-shaped inner core in the spinal cord that is surrounded by white matter; a superficial shell of gray matter covers the cerebrum and the cerebellum
H. The nervous system exhibits plasticity—the capability to change on the basis of experiences; limited ability to regenerate
I. Axons and dendrites that are associated with a neurilemma in the PNS may undergo repair if the cell body is intact, Schwann cells are functional, and scar tissue does not form too rapidly

***Action Potentials.*** See the section on "Characteristics and Physiology of Pain" in Chapter 18.

A. Neurons communicate by means of nerve action potentials (impulses)
B. Generation of action is dependent on:
   1. The presence of special types of ion channels and the existence of a resting membrane potential
   2. Membrane potential—a difference in electrical charge across the plasma membrane; a cell that has a membrane potential is said to be *polarized*
   3. A nerve impulse results from the concentration of two ions on the inside and outside of the nerve
   4. Resting membrane potential—the outside surface of plasma membrane has a positive charge; the inside surface has a negative charge; the resting membrane in neurons is ≈ 70 millivolts (mV)
   5. During an action potential, voltage-gated sodium ($Na^+$) and potassium ($K^+$) channels open in sequence; opening of voltage-gated $Na^+$ channels results in depolarization, followed by the loss and reversal of membrane polarization (from − 70 mV to + 30 mV); then, the opening of voltage-gated $K^+$ channels allows repolarization, the recovery of the resting membrane potential

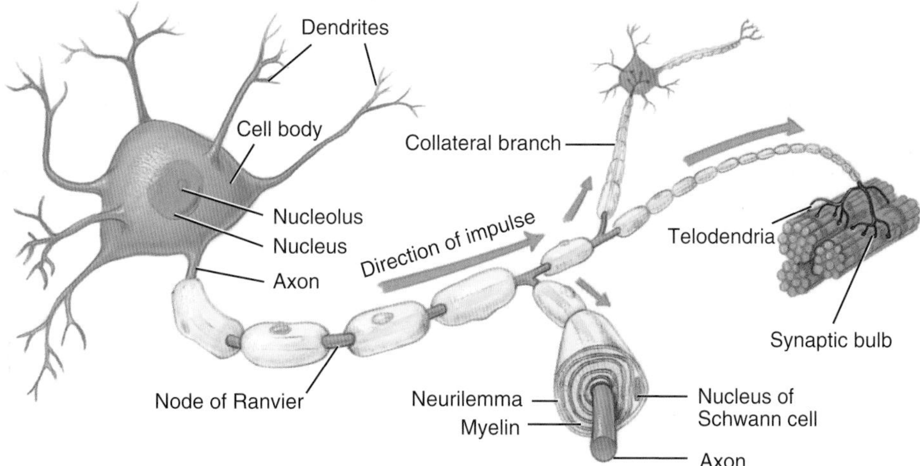


**Fig 3.20** Structure of a typical neuron. (From Applegate E: *The anatomy and physiology learning system*, ed 4, St Louis, 2011, Saunders.)

6. According to the "all-or-none" principle, if a stimulus is strong enough to generate an action potential, the impulse generated is of a constant size; a stronger stimulus does not generate a larger impulse
7. During the absolute refractory period, another impulse cannot be generated; during the relative refractory period, an impulse can be triggered only by a supra-threshold stimulus
8. Nerve impulse conduction that occurs as a step-by-step process along an unmyelinated axon is called *continuous conduction*; in *salutatory conduction,* a nerve impulse "leaps" from one node of Ranvier to the next along a myelinated axon
9. Axons with larger diameters conduct impulses faster than those with smaller diameters; myelinated axons conduct impulses faster than unmyelinated axons

#### *Synaptic Transmission*

A. Neurons communicate with each other and with effectors at synapses in a series of events known as *synaptic transmission*
B. Two types of synapses:
   1. Electrical synapses—gap junctions allow ions to flow from one cell to another
   2. Chemical synapses—neurotransmitter is released from a presynaptic neuron into the synaptic cleft and then binds to receptors on the postsynaptic plasma membrane
C. Types of neurotransmitters
   1. Excitatory neurotransmitter—depolarizes the membrane of the postsynaptic neuron to bring the membrane potential closer to threshold
   2. Inhibitory neurotransmitter—hyperpolarizes the membrane of the postsynaptic neuron
D. The postsynaptic neuron integrates excitatory and inhibitory signals in a process called *summation* and then responds accordingly
E. The neurotransmitter is removed from the synaptic cleft in three ways: diffusion, enzymatic degradation, and reuptake by neurons or neuroglial cells
F. Important neurotransmitters include acetylcholine, gamma-aminobutyric acid (GABA), glycine, norepinephrine, epinephrine, dopamine, serotonin, neuropeptides, and nitric oxide

### Spinal Cord

See Fig. 3.21

A. Location—in the vertebral canal; extends from the foramen magnum of the occipital bone of the skull to the superior border of the second lumbar vertebrae in the vertebral column; approximately 40 to 45 cm (16 to 18 inches)
B. Meninges—three layers of connective tissue coverings that extend around the spinal cord and the brain
   1. Dura mater—outermost of three layers
   2. Arachnoid—middle layer composed of collagen and elastic fibers
   3. Pia mater—inner layer composed of collagen and elastic fibers that adhere to the surface of the spinal cord and brain; contains numerous blood vessels
C. Spinal cord does not run the entire length of the vertebral column; nerves called *cauda equina* arise from the lowest portion of a cord and angle down the vertebral canal
D. Functions
   1. White matter tracts in the spinal cord are pathways for nerve impulse conduction; sensory impulses flow from the periphery to the brain, and motor impulses flow from the brain to the periphery
   2. Gray matter receives and integrates incoming and outgoing information
   3. Spinal reflexes—fast automatic responses to sensory impulses that enter the spinal cord via spinal nerves
   4. Reflex arc—pathway followed by nerve impulses that produce a reflex
      a. Somatic reflex—reflex involving involuntary contraction of skeletal muscles (e.g., knee-jerk reflex)
      b. Withdrawal reflex—causes immediate withdrawal of a limb from a source of injury before awareness of pain
      c. Autonomic reflex—reflexes involving smooth muscle, cardiac muscle, and glands (e.g., swallowing, urinating)

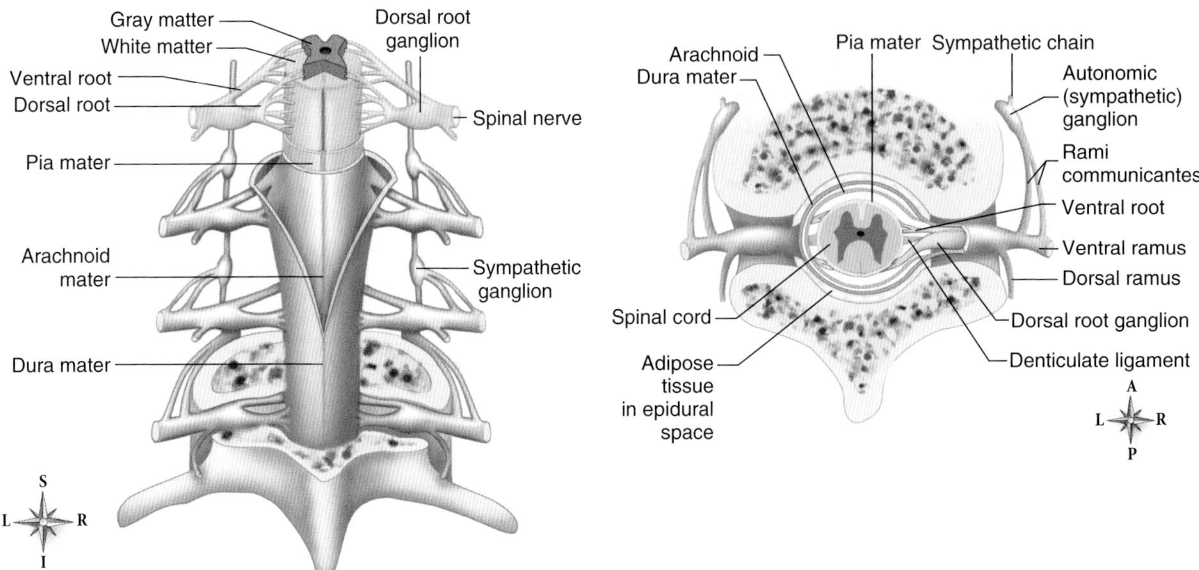


**Fig 3.21** Coverings of the spinal cord. (From Patton KT, Thibodeau GA: *Anthony's textbook of anatomy and physiology*, ed 20, St Louis, 2013, Elsevier.)

E. Spinal nerves
 1. Thirty-one pairs of spinal nerves; each has a dorsal (afferent) root and a ventral (efferent) root
 2. Named and numbered according to the region and level of the vertebral column from which they emerge
 3. Emerge from the spinal cord to form plexuses along the cord, except in the thoracic region
  a. The cervical plexus (C1 to C4) innervates muscles, skin, posterior head, neck, upper shoulders, and diaphragm
  b. Brachial plexus (C5 to T1) nerves supply upper limbs, neck, and muscles
   (1) Radial nerve—posterolateral side of the arm, forearm and posterior hand (afferent) and posterior muscles of arm and forearm (efferent)
   (2) Median nerve—anterolateral side of forearm (afferent) and hand, most muscles of forearm and thumb (efferent)
   (3) Ulnar nerve—anteromedial side of the forearm and hand (afferent), muscles of the deep palm and pinky finger (efferent)
  c. T2 to T12 comprise the intercostal nerves; do not form a plexus
  d. Lumbosacral plexus—includes L1 to S4
   (1) Lumbar portion—first four lumbar nerves contribute to the femoral nerve; supplies abdominal wall, external genitals, and part of lower limbs
   (2) Sacral portion—sacral nerves, the last lumbar nerve, and the coccygeal nerve supply the pelvis and legs; contribute to the sciatic nerve (longest nerve in the body)

## Brain

See Fig. 3.22.

A. Principal parts—brain stem (consists of the medulla oblongata, pons, and midbrain), diencephalon (consists of the thalamus and hypothalamus), cerebrum, and cerebellum
B. Supplied with oxygen and nutrients by the cerebral arterial circle, or circle of Willis
 1. Any interruption of the oxygen supply may permanently damage or kill brain cells
 2. Glucose deficiency may produce dizziness, convulsions, and unconsciousness
C. The blood-brain barrier (BBB) limits the passage of certain materials from the blood into the brain
D. The brain is protected by cranial bones, meninges, and the cerebrospinal fluid
 1. Cranial meninges are continuous with the spinal meninges (dura mater, arachnoid, and pia mater)
 2. Cerebrospinal fluid (CSF)—formed in the choroid plexuses; circulates continually through the subarachnoid space, ventricles, and central canal; protects the brain and spinal cord by serving as a shock absorber; delivers nutritive substances from the blood and removes wastes
E. Medulla oblongata (also called *medulla*)—is continuous with the upper part of the spinal cord
 1. Contains regions for regulating heart rate, diameter of blood vessels, respiratory rate, swallowing, coughing, vomiting, sneezing, and hiccupping
 2. The vestibulocochlear, accessory, vagus, and hypoglossal nerves originate at the medulla
F. Pons—connects the spinal cord to the brain; links parts of the brain to one another; relays impulses related to voluntary skeletal movements from the cerebral cortex to the cerebellum
 1. Contains two regions that control respiration
 2. The trigeminal, abducens, facial, and vestibular branches of the vestibulocochlear nerves originate at the pons

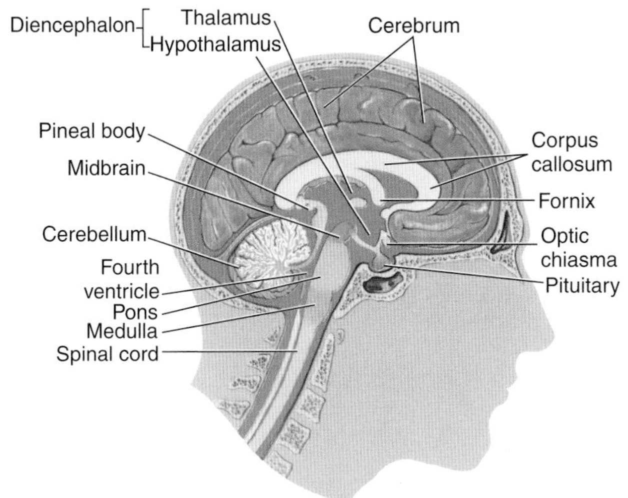


**Fig 3.22** Divisions of the brain. (From Solomon EP: *Introduction to human anatomy and physiology,* ed 2, St Louis, 2008, Saunders.)

G. Midbrain—conveys motor impulses from the cerebrum to the cerebellum and the spinal cord, and transmits sensory impulses from the spinal cord to the thalamus
H. Reticular formation—net-like arrangement of gray and white matter extending throughout the brain stem; alerts the cerebral cortex to incoming sensory signals; helps regulate muscle tone
I. Diencephalon—consists of the thalamus and the hypothalamus
   1. Thalamus—contains nuclei that serve as relay stations for sensory impulses to the cerebral cortex; provides crude recognition of pain, temperature, touch, pressure, and vibration
   2. Hypothalamus—located below the thalamus; controls and integrates the ANS and pituitary gland; functions in rage and aggression; controls body temperature; regulates food and fluid intake; maintains consciousness and sleep patterns
J. The reticular activating system—functions in arousal (awakening from deep sleep) and consciousness (wakefulness)
K. Cerebrum—largest part of the brain; the cortex contains convolutions, fissures, and sulci
   1. Cerebral lobes—frontal, parietal, temporal, and occipital
   2. White matter under the cerebral cortex consists of myelinated axons extending in three principal directions
   3. Sensory areas receive and interpret sensory impulses; motor areas govern muscular movement
   4. Contains tissues associated with emotional and intellectual processes
   5. Generates brain waves measurable by electroencephalogram (EEG), which may be used to diagnose epilepsy, infections, and tumors
L. Basal ganglia—paired masses of gray matter in the cerebral hemispheres that control muscle movements
M. The limbic system—found in cerebral hemispheres and the diencephalon; functions in the emotional aspects of behavior and memory
N. Hemispheres of the brain
   1. Left hemisphere—receives sensory signals from and controls the right side of the body; more important for language, numerical and scientific skills, and reasoning
   2. Right hemisphere—receives sensory signals from and controls the left side of the body; more important for musical and other artistic awareness, spatial and pattern perception, recognition of faces, emotional content of language, and generating mental images of sight, sound, touch, taste, and smell
O. Cerebellum—occupies the inferior and posterior aspects of the cranial cavity; consists of two hemispheres with a cerebellar cortex of gray matter and an interior of white matter tracts; attaches to the brain stem by three pairs of cerebellar peduncles; coordinates skeletal muscles and maintains normal muscle tone and body equilibrium

## Cranial Nerves

See the section on "The Nervous System" in Chapter 4.

A. Twelve pairs of cranial nerves originate from the brain
B. As with spinal nerves, cranial nerves are part of the PNS

## The Autonomic Nervous System

A. Regulates smooth muscle, cardiac muscle, and certain glands; usually operates without conscious control by the centers in the brain, in particular by the hypothalamus
B. Two principal divisions—sympathetic and parasympathetic; most organs have dual innervation; in general, nerve impulses from one division stimulate excitation, and impulses from the other division cause inhibition
   1. Sympathetic (thoracolumbar division)—sympathetic ganglia are classified as sympathetic trunk ganglia (lateral to the vertebral column)—provide sympathetic innervation to structures in skin and organs above the diaphragm; and prevertebral ganglia (anterior to the vertebral column)—provide sympathetic innervation to structures below the diaphragm.
   2. Parasympathetic—parasympathetic ganglia are called *terminal ganglia*; located near or within visceral effectors; there is no parasympathetic innervation in the limbs.
   3. Neurons of preganglionic autonomic neurons are myelinated; those of postganglionic autonomic neurons are unmyelinated
C. Functions
   1. Cholinergic neurons release acetylcholine (ACh); adrenergic neurons release norepinephrine (NE)
   2. Activation of the sympathetic division causes widespread responses; the "fight-or-flight" response
   3. Activation of the parasympathetic division produces more restricted responses that typically are concerned with "rest-and-digest" activities

## Special Senses

A. Sensation—conscious or subconscious awareness of external and internal conditions of the body; for a sensation to occur, three conditions must be satisfied:
   1. A stimulus, or change in environment, capable of activating certain sensory neurons must occur

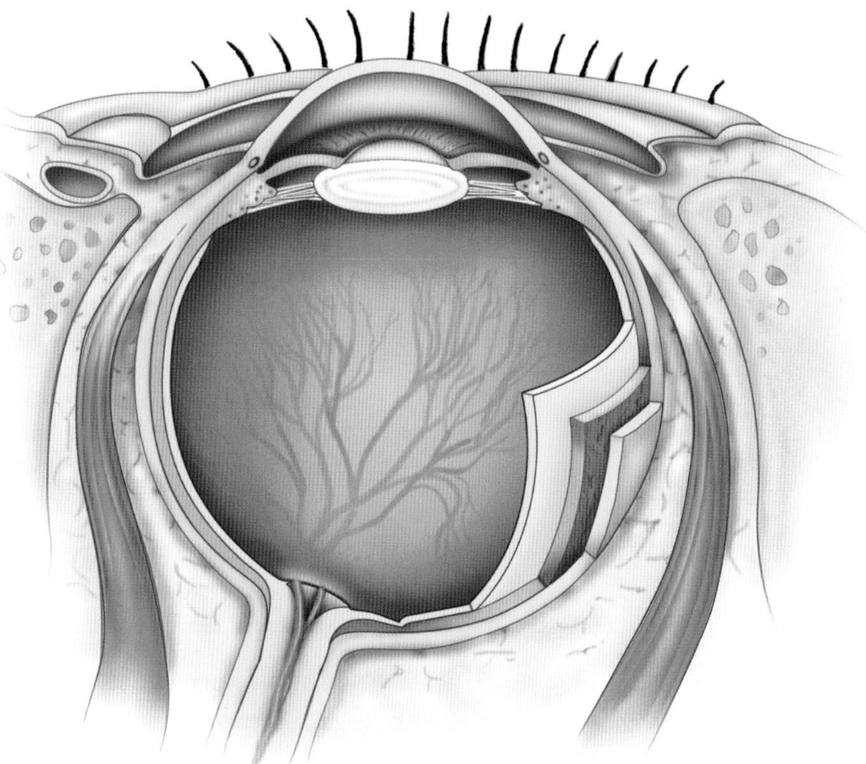

**Fig 3.23** Horizontal cross section of the eye. (From Patton KT, Thibodeau GA, Douglas MM: *Essentials of anatomy and physiology,* St Louis, 2012, Mosby.)

2. A sensory receptor must convert the stimulus to nerve impulses
3. The nerve impulses must be conducted along a neural pathway from the sensory receptor to the brain

B. Components of the eye (Fig. 3.23)
1. Conjunctiva—thin mucous membrane that covers the front of the eye and lines the eyelid
2. Lacrimal glands—located bilaterally on the outer borders of the orbital cavity; secrete about 1 milliliter (mL) of fluid per day; contain lysozyme to destroy bacteria
3. Nasolacrimal duct—carries fluid away from the eye and towards the nasal cavity
4. Iris—the colored part of the eye that is a circular diaphragm; regulates the amount of light that enters the pupil
5. Pupil—where light enters the eye
6. Lens—biconvex disc; avascular
7. Sclera—white covering on the anterior aspect of the eye; posterior to the cornea
8. Vitreous body—colloid inside the posterior chamber of the eyeball; maintains the shape
9. Optic disc—located on the posterior surface of the eyeball; contains no rods or cones, only optic nerves
10. Retina—contains cones in its center (fovea) and rods on the outer periphery; process of forming an image on the retina is similar to a camera producing a picture:
    a. Light rays are bent as they enter the eye
    b. The lens adjusts to the amount of light
    c. Light rays are converged on the fovea
    d. Rays cause changes in the chemistry of rods and cones
    e. Optic nerve sends impulses to the occipital lobes of the brain

C. Hearing and equilibrium (Fig. 3.24)
1. The external ear consists of an ear flap
2. The middle ear is separated from the external ear by the tympanic membrane (eardrum); contains the ossicles (malleus, incus, and stapes) and the eustachian tube (to equalize pressure)
3. The inner ear contains the vestibule, the cochlea, and semicircular canals
    a. Cranial nerve VIII innervates this structure
    b. Small hair cells detect various frequencies and pitches; impulses are sent to the temporal lobes of the brain
    c. Semicircular canals maintain equilibrium

D. Tongue
1. Cranial nerve VII provides special sensory fibers for taste to the anterior two-thirds of the tongue, including fungiform and foliate papillae; umami taste sensation and sensations of sweet, sour and salty tastes are detected sensations of sweet, sour, and salty tastes are detected
2. Cranial nerve IX provides special sensations of taste to the posterior one-third of the tongue's circumvallate papillae; the bitter taste is detected there
3. Food must be in solution in the mouth before taste buds can transfer the information to the brain
4. Most taste sensations are made up of various combinations of the four basic tastes

E. Olfactory sense
1. Stimulates hairs (cilia) that are sensitive to slight odors

2. On each side of the nose, bundles of slender, unmyelinated axons of olfactory receptors extend through holes in the cribriform plate of the ethmoid bone
3. These bundles of axons form cranial nerve I, the olfactory nerve; they terminate in the brain in olfactory bulbs, which are located inferior to the frontal lobes of the cerebrum
4. Within the olfactory bulbs, the axon terminals of olfactory receptors synapse with the dendrites and cell bodies of the next neurons in the olfactory pathway
5. The axons of the neurons extending from the olfactory bulb form the olfactory tract
6. The olfactory tract projects into the primary olfactory area in the temporal lobe, where the conscious awareness of smell begins

F. Tactile sensation (Table 3.4)
1. Meissner's corpuscles—receptors that control the sensation of touch
2. Pacinian corpuscles—receptors that control the sensation of pressure
3. Ruffini's corpuscles—receptors that control the sensation of heat
4. Krause's end bulbs—receptors that control the sensation of cold
5. Nociceptors—sensory receptors for pain; during tissue irritation or injury, release of chemicals such as prostaglandins stimulates nociceptors

G. Proprioceptive sensations—inform consciously and subconsciously; sense the degree of muscle contraction, amount of tension present in tendons, position of joints, and orientation of head and equilibrium

## The Endocrine System

A. The endocrine system is a collection of glands, each of which secretes different types of hormones that regulate metabolism, growth and development, tissue function, sexual function, reproduction, sleep, mood, and other processes

B. Communication, integration, and control of body processes is accomplished by secreting cells that send hormone molecules through the blood to specific target cells contained in target tissues or target organs
1. Works in conjunction with the nervous system to achieve and maintain homeostasis
2. The neuroendocrine system—interaction of the endocrine and nervous systems to perform similar functions

C. Endocrine glands—"ductless glands"; many are made of glandular epithelium whose cells manufacture and secrete hormones; a few endocrine glands are made of neurosecretory tissue; widely scattered throughout the body

### Hormones

A. Function of hormones—regulate most cells to stimulate a physiologic activity; work more slowly and last longer than neurotransmitters; carried to almost every point in the body

B. Classification of hormones
1. Classification by general function
   a. Tropic hormones—target other endocrine glands and stimulate their growth and secretion
   b. Sex hormones—target reproductive tissues
   c. Anabolic hormones—stimulate anabolism in target cells
2. Classification by chemical structure
   a. Steroid hormones
      (1) Synthesized from cholesterol
      (2) Lipid soluble; can easily pass through plasma membrane of target cells

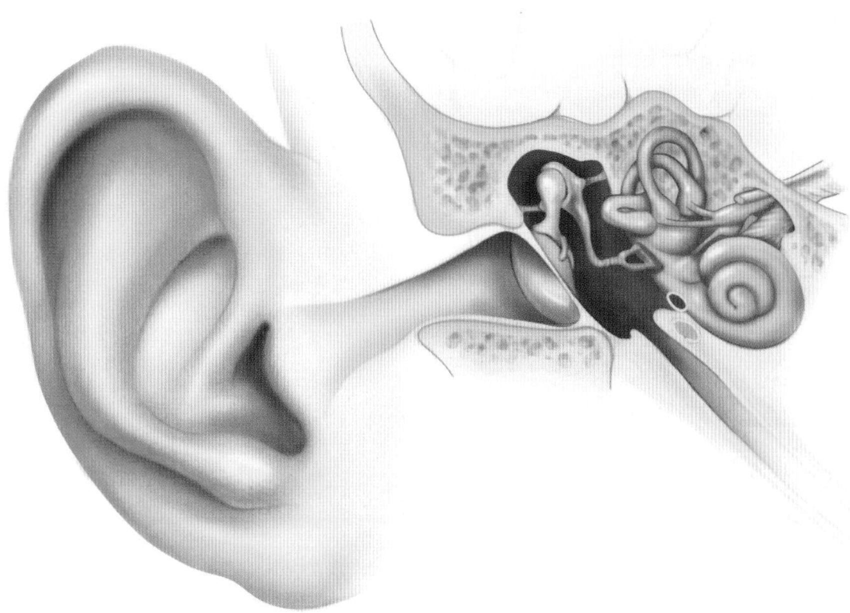

**Fig 3.24** The ear. (From Patton KT, Thibodeau GA, Douglas MM: *Essentials of anatomy and physiology,* St Louis, 2012, Mosby.)

**TABLE 3.4 Classification of Somatic Sensory Receptors**

| By Structure | By Location and Type | By Activation Stimulus | By Sensation or Function |
|---|---|---|---|
| **Free Nerve Endings** | | | |
| Nociceptors | Both exteroceptors and visceroceptors—most body tissues | Almost any noxious stimulus; temperature change; mechanical | Pain; temperature; itch; tickle; stretching |
| Merkel discs | Exteroceptors | Light pressure; mechanical | Discriminative touch |
| Root hair plexuses | Exteroceptors | Hair movement; mechanical | Sense of "deflection" hair movement |
| **Encapsulated Nerve Endings** | | | |
| ***Touch and Pressure Receptors*** | | | |
| Meissner's corpuscle | Exteroceptors; epidermis, hairless skin | Light pressure, mechanical | Discriminative touch; low-frequency vibration |
| Krause's corpuscle | Mucous membranes | Mechanical; thermal | Touch; low-frequency vibration |
| Ruffini's corpuscle | Dermis of skin, exteroceptors | Mechanical; thermal | Crude and persistent touch |
| Pacinian corpuscle | Dermis of skin, joint capsules | Deep pressure, mechanical | Deep pressure; high-frequency vibration; stretch |
| ***Stretch Receptors*** | | | |
| Muscle spindles | Skeletal muscle | Stretch, mechanical | Sense of muscle length |
| Golgi tendon receptors | Musculotendinous junction | Force of contraction and tendon stretch, mechanical | Sense of muscle tension |

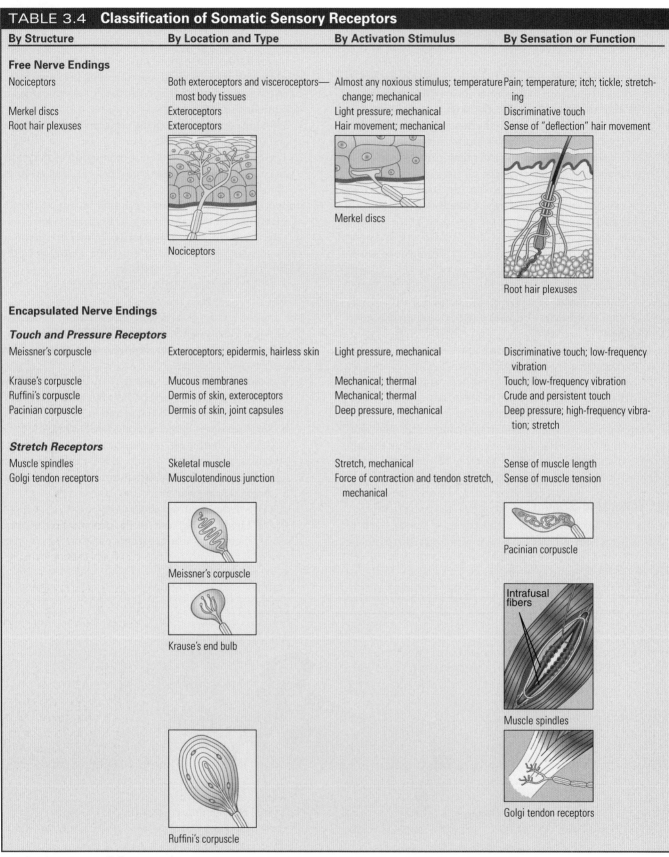

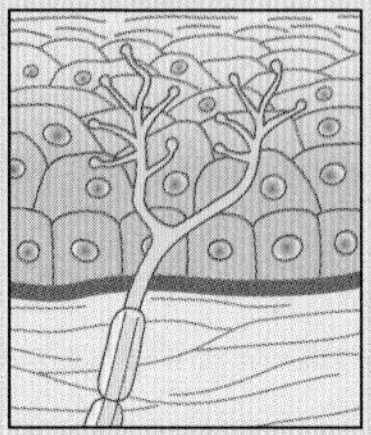

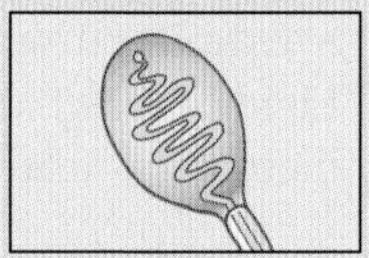

Nociceptors

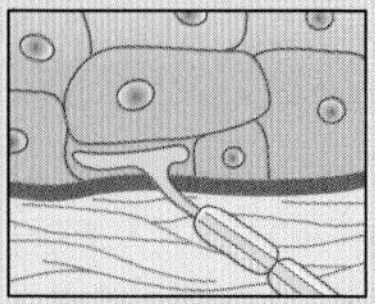

Merkel discs

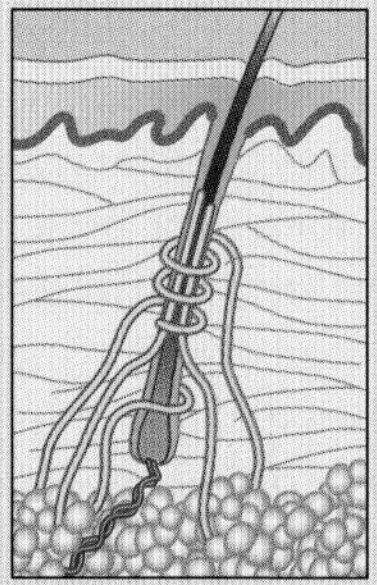

Root hair plexuses

Meissner's corpuscle

Pacinian corpuscle

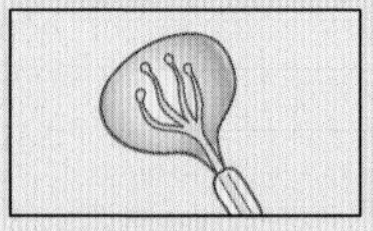

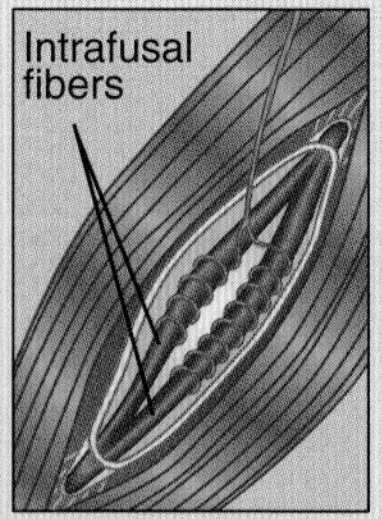

Krause's end bulb

Intrafusal fibers

Muscle spindles

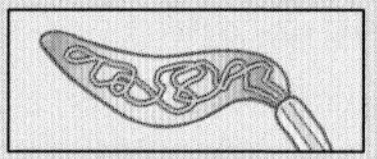

Golgi tendon receptors

Ruffini's corpuscle

Modified from Patton KT, Thibodeau GA: *Anthony's textbook of anatomy and physiology,* ed 20, St Louis, 2013, Elsevier.

(3) Examples include cortisol, aldosterone, estrogen, progesterone, and testosterone
b. Nonsteroid hormones—synthesized primarily from amino acids
c. Protein hormones—long, folded chains of amino acids (e.g., insulin, parathyroid hormone)
d. Glycoprotein hormones—protein hormones with carbohydrate groups attached to the amino acid chain
e. Peptide hormones—smaller than protein hormones; short chain of amino acids (e.g., oxytocin, antidiuretic hormone)
f. Amino acid derivative hormones—each is derived from a single amino acid molecule
(1) Amine hormones—synthesized by modifying a single molecule of tyrosine; produced by neurosecretory cells and by neurons (e.g., epinephrine, norepinephrine)
(2) Amino acid derivatives produced by the thyroid gland; synthesized by adding iodine to tyrosine

C. Mechanism of action
1. General principles
a. Hormones signal a cell by binding to the specific receptors of a target cell in a "lock-and-key" arrangement
b. Different hormone-receptor interactions produce different regulatory changes within the target cell through chemical reactions
c. Combined hormone actions
(1) Synergism—combinations of hormones acting together have a greater effect on a target cell than the sum of the effects that each would have if acting alone
(2) Permissiveness—when a small amount of one hormone allows a second one to have its full effects on a target cell
(3) Antagonism—one hormone produces the opposite effects of another hormone; used to fine-tune the activity of target cells with great accuracy
d. Endocrine glands produce more hormone molecules than needed; unused hormones are quickly excreted by the kidneys or broken down by metabolic processes
2. Mechanism of steroid hormone action
a. Steroid hormones are lipid soluble, and their receptors are normally found within the target cell
b. After a steroid hormone molecule has diffused into the target cell, it binds to a receptor molecule to form a hormone-receptor complex
c. Mobile receptor hypothesis—the hormone passes into the nucleus, where it binds to a mobile receptor and activates a certain gene sequence to begin transcription of mRNA; newly formed mRNA molecules move into the cytosol, associate with ribosomes, and begin synthesizing protein molecules that produce the effects of the hormone
d. The amount of steroid hormone present determines the magnitude of the target cell's response
e. Because transcription and protein synthesis take time, responses to steroid hormones are often slow
3. Mechanisms of nonsteroid hormone action
a. Second messenger mechanism—also known as the *fixed-membrane-receptor hypothesis*
(1) A nonsteroid hormone molecule acts as a "first messenger" and delivers its chemical message to receptors that are fixed in the plasma membrane of the target cell
(2) The message is then passed by way of a G-protein into the cell where a "second messenger" triggers the appropriate cellular response
(3) The second messenger mechanism produces target cell effects that differ from steroid hormone effects in several important ways:
(a) The effects of the hormone are amplified by a cascade of reactions
(b) The second messenger mechanisms include inositol trisphosphate ($IP_3$), guanosine monophosphate (GMP), and calcium calmodulin
(c) The second messenger mechanism operates much more quickly than the steroid mechanism
b. Nuclear receptor mechanism—small iodinated amino acids ($T_4$ and $T_3$) enter the target cell and bind to receptors associated with a DNA molecule in the nucleus; this binding triggers transcription of mRNA and synthesis of new enzymes

D. Regulation of hormone secretion
1. Usually part of a negative feedback loop called an *endocrine reflex*; the simplest regulatory mechanism is when an endocrine gland is sensitive to the physiologic changes produced by its target cells
2. Regulated by a hormone produced by another gland
3. May be influenced by the input of the nervous system; this fact emphasizes the close functional relationship between the two systems

## Prostaglandins

A. Function of prostaglandins
1. Unique group of lipid molecules (20-carbon fatty acid with 5-carbon ring); serve important, widespread integrative functions, but do not meet the usual definition of a hormone; tend to integrate activities of neighboring cells
2. Called *tissue hormones* because the secretion is produced in a tissue and diffuses only a short distance to other cells within the same tissue

B. Structural classes of prostaglandins
1. Prostaglandin A (PGA)—intra-arterial infusion resulting in an immediate drop in blood pressure accompanied by an increase in regional blood flow to several areas
2. Prostaglandin E (PGE)—regulation of red blood cell deformability and platelet aggregation; regulation of hydrochloric acid secretion in the GI tract

3. Prostaglandin F (PGF)—causes uterine contractions; affects intestinal motility; required for normal peristalsis

## Pituitary Gland

A. The function of pituitary gland is divided by two separate glands:
   1. The anterior pituitary gland: secretory cells produce growth hormone, prolactin, and a number of tropic hormones
   2. The posterior pituitary gland: serves as a storage site for antidiuretic hormone and oxytocin
B. Structure of the pituitary gland
   1. Also known as *hypophysis*, the "master gland"
   2. Size: 1.2 to 1.5 cm
   3. Located on the ventral surface of the brain within the skull
   4. Infundibulum—stem-like stalk that connects the pituitary to the hypothalamus
   5. Composed of two separate glands, the adenohypophysis (anterior pituitary gland) and the neurohypophysis (posterior pituitary gland)
C. Adenohypophysis (anterior pituitary)
   1. Divided into two parts:
      a. Pars anterior—forms the major portion of the adenohypophysis
      b. Pars intermedia
   2. Tissue is composed of irregular clumps of secretory cells supported by fine connective tissue fibers and surrounded by a rich vascular network
   3. Three types of cells can be identified by their stain affinity:
      a. Chromophobes—do not stain
      b. Acidophils—stain with acidic stains
      c. Basophils—stain with basic stains
   4. Five functional types of secretory cells:
      a. Somatotrophs—secrete GH
      b. Corticotrophs—secrete ACTH
      c. Thyrotrophs—secrete TSH
      d. Lactotrophs—secrete prolactin
      e. Gonadotrophs—secrete LH and FSH
D. Hormones secreted by the adenohypophysis
   1. Growth hormone (GH); also known as *somatotropin* (STH)
      a. Promotes growth of bone, muscle, and other tissues by accelerating amino acid transport into the cells
      b. Stimulates fat metabolism by mobilizing lipids from storage in adipose cells and speeding up the catabolism of lipids after they have entered another cell
      c. Shifts cell chemistry away from glucose catabolism and toward lipid catabolism as an energy source; this leads to increased blood glucose levels
      d. Functions as an insulin antagonist; vital to maintaining the homeostasis of blood glucose levels
   2. Prolactin (PRL); also known as *lactogenic hormone*
      a. Produced by acidophils in the pars anterior
      b. Promotes breast development during pregnancy in anticipation of milk secretion; stimulates lactation after delivery
   3. Tropic hormones—have a stimulating effect on other endocrine glands; four principal tropic hormones are produced and secreted by the basophils of the pars anterior:
      a. Thyroid-stimulating hormone (TSH), or thyrotropin—promotes and maintains the growth and development of the thyroid; causes the thyroid to secrete its hormones
      b. Adrenocorticotropic hormone (ACTH), or adrenocorticotropin—promotes and maintains normal growth and development of the cortex of the adrenal gland; stimulates the adrenal cortex to secrete some of its hormones
      c. Follicle-stimulating hormone (FSH)—stimulates primary graafian follicles to grow toward maturity in females; also stimulates follicle cells to secrete estrogens; in males, stimulates the development of the seminiferous tubules of the testes and maintains spermatogenesis
      d. Luteinizing hormone (LH)—stimulates the formation and activity of the corpus luteum of the ovary in females; the corpus luteum secretes progesterone and estrogens when stimulated by LH; LH also supports FSH in stimulating the maturation of follicles; in males, LH stimulates the interstitial cells in the testes to develop and secrete testosterone
      e. FSH and LH are called *gonadotropins* because they stimulate the growth and maintenance of the gonads
   4. Control of secretion in the adenohypophysis
      a. The hypothalamus secretes releasing hormones into the blood, which are then carried to the hypophyseal portal system; through negative feedback, the hypothalamus adjusts the secretions of the adenohypophysis, which then adjusts the secretions of the target glands, which in turn adjust the activity of their target tissues
      b. The hypophyseal portal system carries blood from the hypothalamus directly to the adenohypophysis, where the target cells of the releasing hormones are located; releasing hormones influence the secretion of hormones by acidophils and basophils
      c. Under stress, hypothalamus translates nerve impulses into hormone secretions by endocrine glands, creating a neuroendocrine link
E. Neurohypophysis (posterior pituitary)
   1. Serves as storage and release site for antidiuretic hormone (ADH, vasopressin) and oxytocin (OT), which are synthesized in the hypothalamus
   2. ADH and OT are released into blood; controlled by nervous stimulation
   3. Antidiuretic hormone
      a. Prevents the formation of a large volume of urine, thereby helping the body conserve water
      b. Causes the tubules in the kidney to resorb water from urine
      c. Dehydration triggers the release of ADH
   4. Oxytocin—has two actions:
      a. Causes the release of milk from the lactating breast; regulated by the positive feedback mechanism; PRL cooperates with OT

b. Stimulates the contractions of uterine muscles during childbirth; regulated by positive feedback mechanism

### Pineal Gland

A. Function of pineal glands
   1. A member of the nervous system because it receives visual stimuli; also a member of the endocrine system because it secretes hormones
   2. Supports the body's biologic clock
      a. Principal pineal secretion is melatonin
B. Structure of pineal glands
   1. Tiny, pinecone-shaped structure located on the dorsal aspect of the brain's diencephalon

### Thyroid Gland

See the section on "Glands of the Head and Neck Region" and Fig. 4.8 in Chapter 4.

A. Function of the thyroid gland
   1. Increases metabolic rate and essential for growth and development; crucial for brain development in children
   2. Influences body temperature
B. Structure of the thyroid gland
   1. Two large lateral lobes and a narrow connecting isthmus; located in the neck, on the anterior and lateral surfaces of the trachea, just below the larynx
   2. A thin, worm-like projection of thyroid tissue, often extends upward from the isthmus
   3. The weight of the thyroid in an adult is approximately 30 grams (g)
   4. Composed of follicles
      a. Small hollow spheres
      b. Filled with thyroid colloid that contains thyroglobulins
C. Thyroid hormone
   1. Two different hormones:
      a. Triiodothyronine ($T_3$)—contains three iodine atoms; considered to be the principal thyroid hormone; $T_3$ binds efficiently to the nuclear receptors in target cells
      b. Tetraiodothyronine ($T_4$), or thyroxine—contains four iodine atoms; approximately 20 times more abundant than $T_3$; its major importance is its role as a precursor to $T_3$
   2. The thyroid gland stores considerable amounts of a preliminary form of its hormones before secreting them
   3. Before being stored in the colloid of follicles, $T_3$ and $T_4$ are attached to globulin molecules to form thyroglobin complexes
   4. On release, $T_3$ and $T_4$ detach from globulin and enter the bloodstream
   5. Once in the blood, $T_3$ and $T_4$ attach to plasma globulins and travel as a hormone-globulin complex
   6. $T_3$ detaches from plasma globulin as it nears the target cells; $T_4$ also detaches, but to a lesser extent
   7. Thyroid hormone—helps regulate the metabolic rate of all cells, cell growth, and tissue differentiation; it is said to have a "general" target
D. Calcitonin
   1. Produced by the thyroid gland in the parafollicular cells
   2. Influences the processing of calcium by bone cells by decreasing blood calcium levels and promoting the conservation of the hard bone matrix
   3. Parathyroid hormone acts as antagonist to calcitonin to maintain calcium homeostasis

### Parathyroid Glands

A. Function of the parathyroid glands
   1. Control calcium in the blood by stimulating bone breakdown, increasing calcium absorption in the digestive tract, and decreasing loss of calcium in the urine
B. Structure of the parathyroid glands
   1. Four or five parathyroid glands are embedded in the posterior surface of the thyroid's lateral lobes
   2. Tiny, rounded bodies within thyroid tissue formed by compact, irregular rows of cells
C. Parathyroid hormone (PTH, parathormone)
   1. An antagonist to calcitonin; acts to maintain calcium homeostasis
   2. Acts on bone and the kidneys
      a. Causes more bone to be dissolved, yielding calcium and phosphate, which enter the bloodstream
      b. Causes phosphate to be secreted by the kidney cells into urine to be excreted
      c. Increases the intestinal absorption of calcium by stimulating the kidney to produce active vitamin D

### Adrenal Glands

A. Function of the adrenal glands
   1. Work with the hypothalamus and pituitary gland to stimulate and produce hormones that influence metabolism, body characteristics, ability to cope with physical and emotional stress, and aids in the regulation of sodium and potassium levels
B. Structure of the adrenal glands
   1. Located on top of the kidneys like caps
   2. Made up of two portions:
      a. Adrenal cortex—the outer part of the gland; produces hormones that are vital to life, such as cortisol, which regulates metabolism and the body's response to stress, and aldosterone, which helps regulate blood pressure
      b. Adrenal medulla—produces nonessential hormones, such as adrenaline, which helps the body react to stress
C. Adrenal cortex
   1. All cortical hormones are steroids; known as *corticosteroids*
   2. Composed of three distinct layers of secreting cells:
      a. Zona glomerulosa—outermost layer, directly under the outer connective tissue capsule of the adrenal gland; secretes mineralocorticoids
      b. Zona fasciculata—middle layer; secretes glucocorticoids
      c. Zona reticularis—inner layer; secretes small amounts of glucocorticoids and gonadocorticoids
   3. Mineralocorticoids—important role in regulating sodium levels

a. Aldosterone
   (1) The only physiologically important mineralocorticoid; its primary function is to maintain sodium homeostasis in blood by increasing sodium resorption in the kidneys
   (2) Increases water retention; promotes the loss of potassium and hydrogen ions
   (3) Secretion is controlled by the renin-angiotensin mechanism and by blood potassium concentration
b. Glucocorticoids
   (1) Secreted by the zona fasciculata
   (2) Examples include cortisol, cortisone, and corticosterone
   (3) Affect every body cell
   (4) Are protein mobilizing, gluconeogenic, and hyperglycemia inducing
   (5) Tend to cause a shift from carbohydrate catabolism to lipid catabolism
   (6) Essential for maintaining normal blood pressure by helping norepinephrine and epinephrine to have their full effect; cause vasoconstriction
   (7) High blood concentration causes eosinopenia and marked atrophy of lymphatic tissues
   (8) Act with epinephrine to bring about normal recovery from injury produced by inflammatory agents
   (9) Secretion increases in response to stress
   (10) Except during stress response, secretion is mainly controlled by a negative feedback mechanism involving ACTH from the adenohypophysis

4. Gonadocorticoids—sex hormones (androgens) released from the adrenal cortex

D. Adrenal medulla
   1. Neurosecretory tissue—composed of neurons specialized to secrete their products into blood
   2. Secretes epinephrine and norepinephrine, part of the class of nonsteroid hormones called *catecholamines*; both hormones bind to the receptors of sympathetic effectors to prolong and enhance the effects of sympathetic stimulation by the ANS

## Pancreatic Islets

A. Function of pancreatic islets
   1. From the liver, increases breakdown of glycogen to increase blood glucose levels
   2. Decreases blood glucose by influencing uptake and use of the body's cells
B. Structure of the pancreatic islets
   1. Elongated gland; its head lies in the duodenum; extends horizontally behind the stomach and touches the spleen
   2. Composed of endocrine and exocrine tissues
      a. Islets of Langerhans—endocrine portion; each islet contains four primary types of endocrine glands joined by gap junctions:
         (1) Alpha cells ($\alpha$-cells)—secrete glucagon
         (2) Beta cells ($\beta$-cells)—secrete insulin; account for up to 75% of all pancreatic islet cells
         (3) Delta cells ($\delta$-cells)—secrete somatostatin
         (4) Pancreatic polypeptide cells (F- or PP-cells)—secrete pancreatic polypeptides
      b. Acini—exocrine portion; secretes a serous fluid containing digestive enzymes into the ducts draining into the small intestine
C. Pancreatic hormones—work as a team to maintain the homeostasis of food molecules
   1. Glucagon—produced by $\alpha$-cells; tends to increase blood glucose levels; stimulates gluconeogenesis in liver cells
   2. Insulin—produced by $\beta$-cells; lowers the blood concentration of glucose and fatty acids; promotes their metabolism by tissue cells
   3. Somatostatin—produced by $\delta$-cells; primary role is regulating the other endocrine cells of pancreatic islets
   4. Pancreatic polypeptide—produced by F-cells (PP-cells); influences the digestion and distribution of food molecules to some degree

## Gonads

A. Testes
   1. Paired organs within the scrotum in a male
   2. Composed of seminiferous tubules and a scattering of interstitial cells
   3. Testosterone—produced by interstitial cells; responsible for the growth and maintenance of male sexual characteristics; secretion is mainly regulated by gonadotropin levels in blood
B. Ovaries
   1. Primary sex organs in a female
   2. Set of paired glands in the pelvis that produce several types of sex hormones
      a. Estrogens—steroid hormones secreted by ovarian follicles; promote development and maintenance of female sexual characteristics
      b. Progesterone—secreted by the corpus luteum; maintains the lining of the uterus necessary for successful pregnancy
      c. Ovarian hormone secretion depends on the changing levels of FSH and LH from the adenohypophysis

## Placenta

A. Tissues that form on the lining of the uterus as a connection between the circulatory systems of the mother and the developing fetus
B. Serves as a temporary endocrine gland; produces human chorionic gonadotropin, estrogens, and progesterone

## Thymus Gland

A. Function of thymus gland
   1. Important for immune system development and function
B. Structure of thymus gland
   1. Located in the mediastinum just beneath the sternum
   2. Large in children, begins to atrophy at puberty, and is a vestige of fat and fibrous tissue by old age
   3. Considered to be primarily a lymphatic organ

4. Thymosin—isolated from thymus tissue; stimulates development of T cells

### Gastric and Intestinal Mucosa

A. The mucous lining of the GI tract contains cells that produce both endocrine and exocrine secretions
B. GI hormones such as gastrin, secretin, and cholecystokinin-pancreozymin (CCK) play regulatory roles in coordinating the secretory and motor activities involved in the digestive process
C. Ghrelin—a hormone secreted by endocrine cells in the gastric mucosa; stimulates the hypothalamus to boost appetite; slows metabolism and fat burning; may be a contributor to obesity

### Heart

A. Has a secondary endocrine role; hormone-producing cells produce the hormone atrial natriuretic peptide (ANP)
B. ANP opposes increases in blood volume or blood pressure; also an antagonist to ADH and aldosterone

## The Cardiovascular System

The purpose of the cardiovascular system is to transport oxygen to all the tissues in the body and remove, from these same tissues, metabolic waste products. The cardiovascular system consists of three interrelated components: blood, the heart, and blood vessels.

A. Blood—a vital liquid that has three general functions:
    1. Transportation—transports oxygen from the lungs to the cells throughout the body and carbon dioxide from the cells to the lungs; carries nutrients from the GI tract to body cells, heat and waste products away from cells, and hormones from endocrine glands to other body cells
    2. Regulation—helps regulate the pH of body fluids; helps adjust body temperature; blood osmotic pressure also influences the water content of cells
    3. Protection—blood clots in response to injury to protect against excessive blood loss; white blood cells protect against disease through phagocytosis and by producing antibodies; blood contains interferons, which also help protect against disease
B. Characteristics of blood
    1. Viscosity greater than that of water; temperature of 38°C (100.4°F); pH ranges between 7.35 and 7.45
    2. Blood constitutes about 8% of body weight in an adult
C. Components of blood (Fig. 3.25)
    1. Consists of 55% plasma; 45% formed elements that include red blood cells (RBCs, erythrocytes), white blood cells (WBCs, leukocytes), and platelets
    2. Hematocrit—the percentage of RBCs in whole blood
    3. Plasma contains 91% water, 7% proteins, and 2% solutes
    4. Principal solutes include proteins (albumins, globulins, fibrinogen), nutrients, hormones, respiratory gases, electrolytes, and waste products
    5. Hemopoiesis—the formation of blood cells from pluripotent stem cells; in the adult occurs in red bone marrow
    6. Red blood cells—biconcave discs without a nucleus that contain hemoglobin
        a. Hemoglobin transports oxygen
        b. RBCs live for about 120 days; in terms of a normal blood count, a healthy male has about 4.7 to 6.1 million/mm$^3$ RBCs; a healthy female has about 4.2 to 5.4 million/mm$^3$ RBCs
        c. After phagocytosis of aged RBCs by macrophages, hemoglobin is recycled
        d. Erythropoiesis—RBC formation occurring in adult red bone marrow; stimulated by hypoxia, which stimulates the release of erythropoietin by the kidneys
    7. White blood cells—nucleated cells with two principal groups:
        a. Granular leukocytes (neutrophils, eosinophils, basophils)
        b. Agranular leukocytes (lymphocytes and monocytes)
        c. Function—to combat inflammation and infection; neutrophils and monocytes do so by phagocytosis
        d. Eosinophils combat the effects of histamine in allergic reactions and increase with allergies and parasites
        e. Basophils develop into mast cells that liberate heparin, histamine, and serotonin in allergic reactions that intensify the inflammatory response
        f. B cells (lymphocytes)—effective against bacteria and other toxins
        g. T cells (lymphocytes)—effective against viruses, fungi, and cancer cells
        h. WBCs usually live for only a few hours or a few days
        i. Normal blood contains 5000 to 10,000 WBCs/mm$^3$
    8. Platelets—disc-shaped cell fragments without nuclei
        a. Formed from megakaryocytes; take part in hemostasis by forming a platelet plug
        b. Normal blood contains 150,000 to 450,000 platelets/mm$^3$
D. Hemostasis—stoppage of bleeding
    1. Three mechanisms:
        a. Vascular spasm—when a blood vessel is damaged, the smooth muscle in its walls contracts immediately
        b. Platelet plug—when platelets come into contact with parts of a damaged blood vessel, their characteristics change drastically, and they come together to form a plug that helps fill the gap in the injured vessel
        c. Blood clotting—a series of reactions
            (1) Prothrombinase is formed
            (2) Conversion of prothrombin into thrombin
            (3) Conversion of soluble fibrinogen into insoluble fibrin
    2. Clot—a network of insoluble protein fibers (fibrin), in which formed elements of blood are trapped
    3. Normal coagulation requires vitamin K and also involves clot retraction and fibrinolysis
    4. Anticoagulants prevent clotting
    5. Thrombosis—clotting in an unbroken blood vessel; a thrombus that moves from its site of origin is called an *embolus*
E. Blood groups
    1. Surfaces of RBCs contain a genetically determined assortment of glycolipids and glycoproteins called *isoantigens*

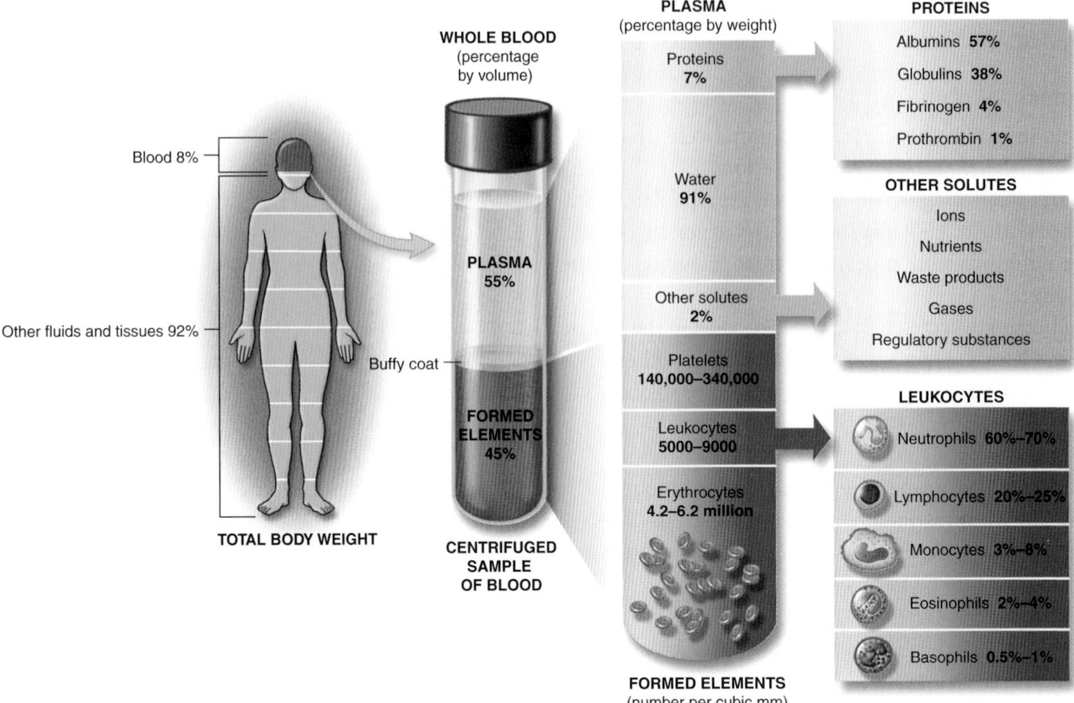


**Fig 3.25** Composition of whole blood. (From Patton KT, Thibodeau GA: *Anthony's textbook of anatomy and physiology*, ed 20, St Louis, 2013, Elsevier.)

   a. Based on the presence or absence of various isoantigens, blood is categorized into different blood groups
   b. Within a blood group, two or more different blood types may be present
2. ABO blood group system—based on isoantigens A and B
   a. Type A—red cells display only antigen A
   b. Type B—red cells display only antigen B
   c. Type AB—red cells display both antigens A and B
   d. Type O—red cells display neither antigen A nor B

F. Heart
1. Located in the space between the lungs, behind the sternum, in the thoracic cavity known as the *mediastinum*; size of a human fist; apex of the heart points down and to the left
2. Consists of four chambers: two atria and two ventricles (Fig. 3.26)
   a. Blood from superior and inferior venae cavae fills the right atrium and passes into the right ventricle through the tricuspid valve (three flaps)
   b. From the right ventricle, the unoxygenated blood is sent to the lungs by passing through the pulmonary semilunar valve and the pulmonary artery
   c. Oxygenated blood is sent from the lungs to the left atrium through the pulmonary veins
   d. From the left atrium, blood flows through the mitral valve (two flaps) into the left ventricle
   e. Blood enters the circulation by passing through the left (aortic) semilunar valve into the aorta
3. The heart walls consist of three layers:
   a. Visceral pericardium or epicardium—outermost connective tissue covering
   b. Myocardium—intermediate, muscular layer
   c. Endocardium—smooth, endothelial-like internal lining
   d. All valves and chambers are lined by the endothelium
4. The valves of the heart are unique
   a. Atrioventricular (AV) valves—tough, fibrous tissue; remain open except at maximal ventricular filling; held in place by chordae tendineae at the edge of the valves; chordae tendinae are anchored to papillary muscles in the inferior ventricular walls (one papillary muscle per valve cusp).
      (1) Tricuspid AV valve—present in the right side of the heart; formed by three flaps
      (2) Bicuspid AV valve (mitral valve)—present in the left side of the heart; formed by two parts
   b. Semilunar (SL) valves—pressure exerted by ejection of blood during ventricular contraction opens them, and pressure in response to gravitation forces closes them; remain closed until ventricles contract
      (1) Pulmonary SL valve—emerges from the right ventricle
      (2) Aortic SL valve—emerges from the left ventricle
5. Heart rate averages 70 to 72 beats per minute; the heart cannot contract without nerve impulses; nerves regulate heart rate
   a. Sinoatrial (SA) node—specialized cardiac muscle cells located in the walls of the right atrium near the superior vena cava; the heartbeat begins there
      (1) From there, the action current spreads out and passes to the fibrous layer of the tricuspid valve
      (2) The current goes through the AV node at the upper end of the interventricular septum
      (3) Modified cardiac muscle within the interventricular septum (the AV bundle) divides into right and left bundle branches that head toward each ventricle

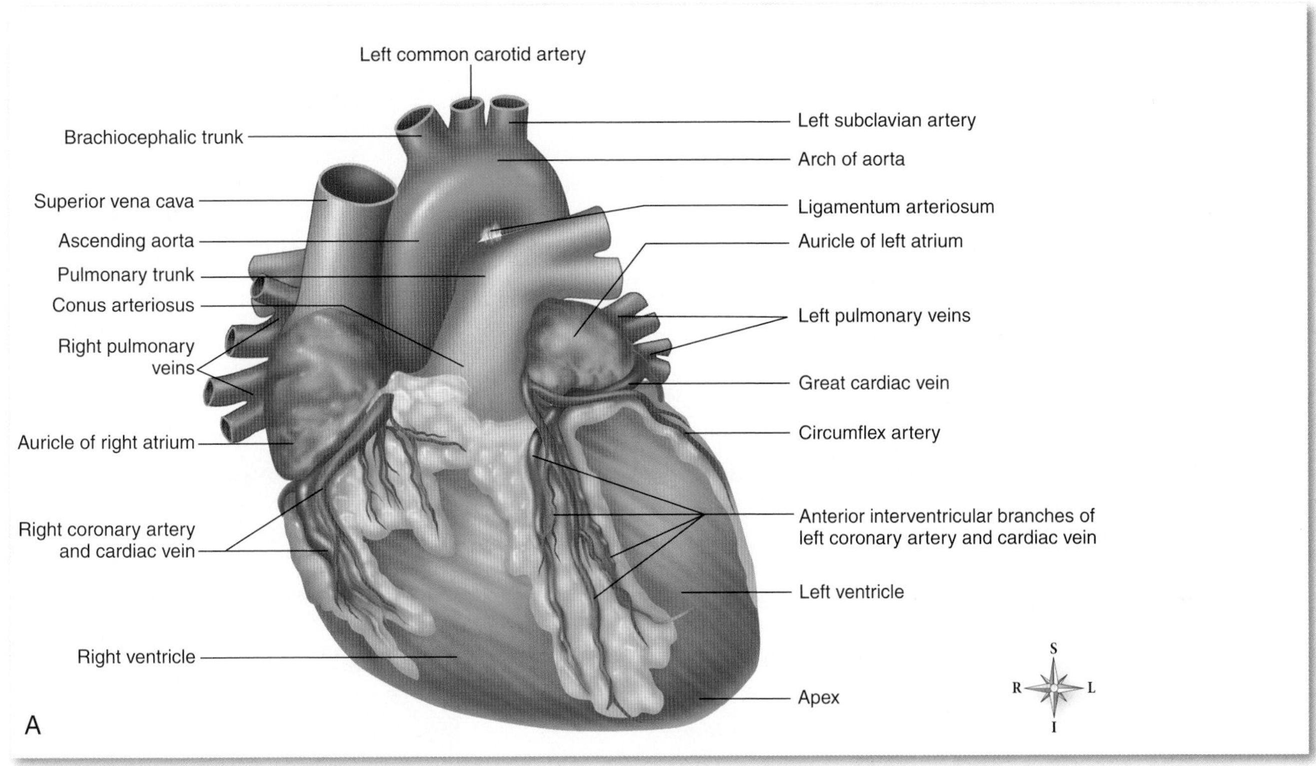


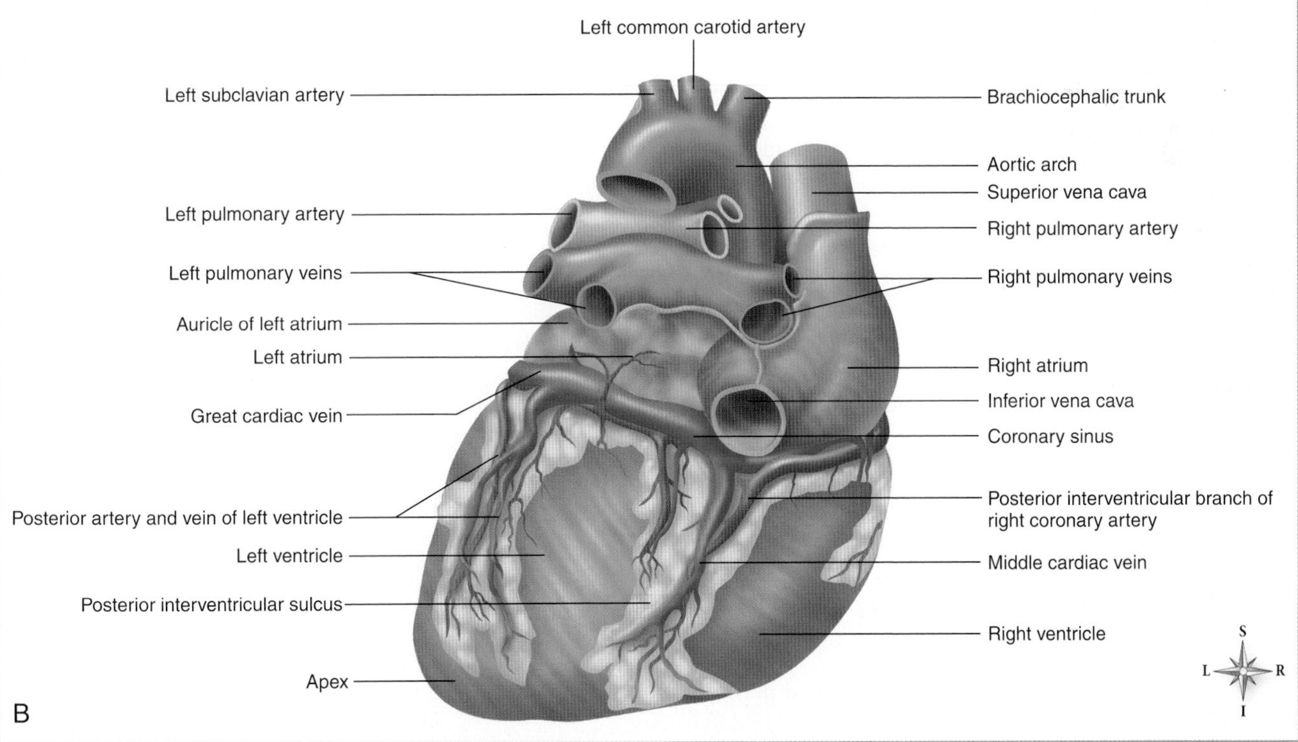


**Fig 3.26** The heart and great vessels **A**, Anterior view of the heart and great vessels. **B**, Posterior view of the heart and great vessels. (From Patton KT, Thibodeau GA, Douglas MM: *Essentials of anatomy and physiology,* St Louis, 2012, Mosby.)

(4) Along the AV bundle and bundle branches, fibers pass out into the cardiac muscle (Purkinje fibers)

b. The action current consists of an impulse starting at the SA node, spreads to the atria, passes to the AV node, is picked up and sent down through the AV bundle, then to the right and left bundle branches, and then through all the cardiac fibers from Purkinje fibers; muscle contracts after the impulse spreads over the heart
   (1) Purkinje fibers are specialized cardiac muscle cells, provide for uniform contraction
   (2) If the SA node is blocked, the AV node can initiate heartbeat but at a slower rate; if AV node is blocked, ventricles will set up their own rhythm

6. Cardiac cycle—includes all the events associated with one heartbeat (Fig. 3.27)
   a. In a normal cardiac cycle, the two atria contract while the two ventricles relax; then, while the two ventricles contract, the two atria relax
      (1) Systole—phase of contraction
      (2) Diastole—phase of relaxation
   b. Three phases of cardiac cycle (each cycle lasts about 0.8 second):
      (1) Relaxation period—begins at the end of a cardiac cycle; ventricles start to relax, and all four chambers are in diastole; repolarization of ventricular muscle fibers initiates relaxation; as ventricles relax, pressure within them drops; when ventricular pressure drops below atrial pressure, AV valves open, and ventricular filling begins
      (2) Contraction (atrial systole)—an action potential from the SA node causes atrial depolarization; atria contract and force the last 25% of blood into ventricles; AV valves are still open, and SL valves are closed
      (3) Contraction (ventricular systole)—maximal ventricular filling and ventricular contraction pushes blood against AV valves, forcing them to shut; pressure inside chambers rises when left ventricular pressure surpasses aortic pressure; right ventricular pressure rises above the pressure in the pulmonary trunk; both SL valves open, and ejection of blood from the heart begins; ejection continues until ventricles start to relax; ventricular pressure drops, SL valves close, and another relaxation period begins
   c. Heart sounds
      (1) First sound—AV valves close
      (2) Second sound—SL valves close
   d. Cardiac output—volume of blood ejected per minute from the left ventricle into the aorta; determined by:
      (1) Stroke volume (SV)—amount of blood ejected by the left ventricle during each contraction or beat; in a resting adult, stroke volume averages 70 mL, and heart rate is about 75 beats/min
      (2) Number of heartbeats per minute

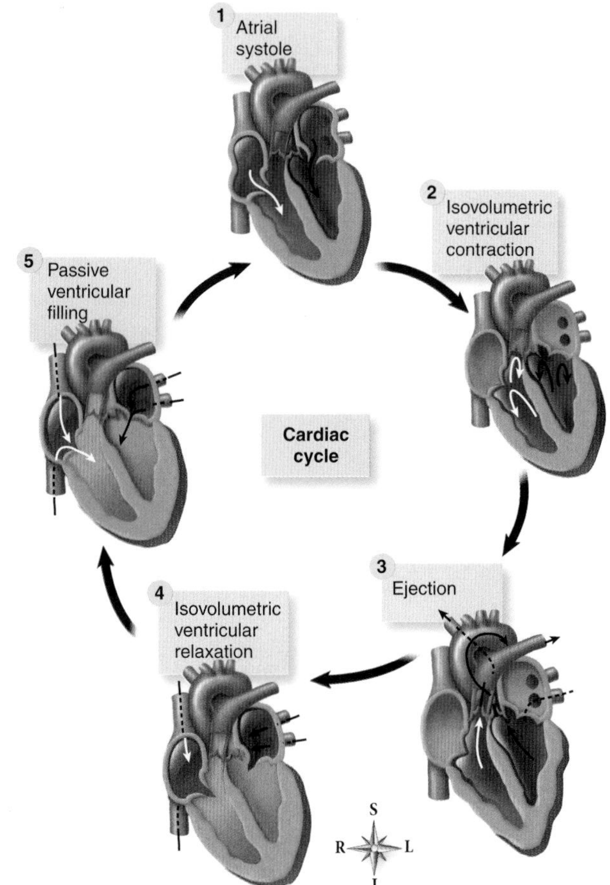


**Fig 3.27** The cardiac cycle. (From Patton KT, Thibodeau GA: *Anthony's textbook of anatomy and physiology,* ed 20, St Louis, 2013, Elsevier.)

      (3) Regulation of stroke volume depends on three factors:
         (a) Starling's law—the more the heart is stretched as it fills during diastole, the greater the force of contraction during systole
         (b) The forcefulness of the contraction of individual ventricular muscle fibers
         (c) The pressure required to eject blood from the ventricles
      (4) Regulation of heart rate—adjustments of heart rate are important in the short-term control of cardiac output and blood pressure; for example, during exercise, cardiac output rises to supply working tissues with increased amounts of oxygen and nutrients
         (a) The most important factors are the autonomic nervous system and the hormones epinephrine and norepinephrine released by adrenal glands
         (b) The regulation of the nervous system originates in the cardiovascular center in the medulla oblongata
         (c) Sympathetic impulses increase heart rate and force of contraction; parasympathetic impulses decrease heart rate

(d) Sensory receptors help adjust heart rate; for example, baroreceptors (neurons sensitive to blood pressure) are strategically located in the arch of the aorta and carotid arteries; if an increase in blood pressure occurs, baroreceptors send nerve impulses along the sensory neurons that are part of the glossopharyngeal and vagus nerves to the cardiovascular center; the center responds, and the result is a decrease in heart rate that lowers cardiac output, thus lowering blood pressure; if a decrease in blood pressure occurs, baroreceptors decrease firing so that sympathetic innervation can stimulate heart rate.

(5) Chemical regulation of heart rate
 (a) Epinephrine and norepinephrine enhance the heart's pumping effectiveness by increasing both heart rate and contraction force
 (b) Thyroid hormones also increase heart rate; a sign of hyperthyroidism is tachycardia
 (c) Ions—elevated blood levels of $K^+$ or $Na^+$ decrease heart rate and contraction force

## The Circulatory System

The circulatory system contributes to the homeostasis of other body systems by transporting and distributing blood throughout the body to deliver oxygen, nutrients, and hormones and to carry away wastes.

A. Types of blood vessels
 1. Arteries—carry blood away from the heart to body tissues; walls have three layers of tissue surrounding a hollow space called the *lumen*
  a. Inner layer composed of endothelium
  b. Middle layer composed of smooth muscle and elastic tissue
  c. Outer layer composed mainly of elastic and collagen fibers
  d. Vasoconstriction—increase in sympathetic stimulation stimulates smooth muscle to contract, squeezing the vessel wall and narrowing the lumen
  e. Vasodilation—sympathetic stimulation is inhibited/decreases; smooth muscle fibers relax
 2. Arteriole—very small artery that delivers blood to capillaries
 3. Capillaries—microscopic vessels that connect arterioles to venules; present near almost every body cell; permit the exchange of nutrients and wastes between the body's cells and blood; the number of capillaries varies with the metabolic activity they serve
  a. Because capillaries are so numerous, blood flows more slowly through them than through larger blood vessels
  b. Slow flow aids the prime mission of the entire cardiovascular system—to keep blood flowing through capillaries so that capillary exchange (movement of substances into and out of capillaries) can occur
  c. Methods of capillary exchange
   (1) Diffusion
   (2) Bulk flow (filtration and resorption)—capillary blood pressure "pushes" fluid out of capillaries into interstitial fluid (filtration); blood colloid osmotic pressure "pulls" fluid into capillaries from interstitial fluid (resorption)
 4. Venules—small vessels that emerge from capillaries and merge to form veins; they receive blood from capillaries and empty blood into veins, which return blood to the heart
 5. Venous return—volume of blood flowing back to the heart occurs because of the pumping action of the heart, aided by skeletal muscle contractions (skeletal muscle pump) and breathing (respiratory pump).
 6. Hormonal regulation of blood pressure—several hormones regulate blood pressure and blood flow by altering cardiac output, changing vascular resistance, or adjusting the total blood volume
  a. Renin-angiotensin-aldosterone (RAA) system—when blood volume or blood flow to the kidneys decreases, certain cells in the kidneys secrete renin into the bloodstream
   (1) Renin and angiotensin together produce the hormone angiotensin II, which raises blood pressure by causing vasoconstriction
   (2) Angiotensin II also stimulates the secretion of aldosterone, which increases resorption of sodium ions ($Na^+$) and water by the kidneys; water resorption increases the total blood volume, which in turn increases blood pressure
  b. Epinephrine and norepinephrine—in response to sympathetic stimulation, the adrenal medulla releases these hormones, which in turn increase cardiac output by increasing the rate and force of heart contractions; also cause vasoconstriction of arterioles

B. Blood pressure—pressure exerted by blood on the walls of a blood vessel; generated by the contraction of ventricles (see the sections on "Health History Evaluation" in Chapter 15 and "Vital Signs" in Chapter 21)
 1. Blood pressure is highest in the aorta and in the large systemic arteries; it drops progressively as distance from the left ventricle increases
 2. An increase in blood volume increases blood pressure; a decrease in blood volume decreases blood pressure
 3. Vascular resistance—the opposition to blood flow because of friction between blood and the walls of blood vessels; depends on the size of the blood vessel lumen (smaller lumen = higher resistance), blood viscosity (increased viscosity = higher resistance), and total length of the blood vessel (increased length = higher resistance)
 4. Neural regulation—the nervous system regulates blood pressure through negative feedback loops that occur as two types of reflexes, baroreceptor and chemoreceptor
  a. Baroreceptors—neurons sensitive to pressure; send impulses to the cardiovascular center to regulate blood pressure

b. Chemoreceptors—neurons sensitive to concentrations of $O_2$, $CO_2$, and hydrogen ions ($H^+$); chemoreceptors detect changes in the blood levels of $O_2$, $CO_2$, and $H^+$ and in the veins in skin and abdominal organs
c. Antidiuretic hormone—produced by the hypothalamus and released from the pituitary gland in response to dehydration or decreased blood volume; also causes vasoconstriction
d. Atrial natriuretic peptide—released by cells in the atria of the heart; lowers blood pressure by causing vasodilation and by promoting loss of salt and water in urine, which reduces blood volume

5. *Autoregulation* refers to local adjustments of blood flow in response to physical and chemical changes in a tissue

C. Assessing circulation through pulse and blood pressure (see the section on "Health History Evaluation".
1. Pulse—alternative expansion and elastic recoil of an artery with each heartbeat
2. Blood pressure—pressure exerted by blood on the walls of an artery when the left ventricle undergoes systole and then diastole
3. Shock—failure of the cardiovascular system to circulate blood adequately or to deliver adequate amounts of $O_2$ and nutrients to meet the metabolic needs of cells

D. Circulatory route
1. Systemic circulation—takes oxygenated blood from the left ventricle through the aorta to all parts of the body and returns deoxygenated blood to the right atrium
   a. Parts of the aorta include the ascending aorta, the arch of the aorta, and the descending aorta; each part gives off arteries that branch to supply the whole body
   b. Blood leaving the aorta and traveling through systemic arteries has a bright-red color; as it moves through the capillaries, it loses some of its $O_2$ and takes on $CO_2$ so that the blood in systemic veins has a dark-red color
2. Pulmonary circulation—takes deoxygenated blood from the right ventricle to the air sacs of the lungs and returns oxygenated blood from the air sacs to the left atrium; allows blood to be oxygenated for systemic circulation; deoxygenated blood is returned to the heart through systemic veins; all veins of systemic circulation flow into the superior vena cava, inferior vena cava, or coronary sinus, which empty into the right atrium
3. Hepatic portal circulation—collects deoxygenated blood from the veins of the GI tract and spleen and directs it into the hepatic portal vein of the liver; allows the liver to extract, modify, and detoxify harmful substances in blood; the liver also receives oxygenated blood from the hepatic artery

## The Lymphatic and Immune System

The primary purpose of the lymphatic and immune system is to aid in the body's resistance against disease. Primary functions include absorption of fats from the digestive system, transportation of fats and surplus interstitial fluid, and a defense system against attacking microorganisms and disease.

A. Components (Fig. 3.28)
1. Lymph
2. Lymphatic vessels
3. Structures and organs that contain lymphatic tissue (specialized reticular tissue containing large numbers of lymphocytes)
4. Red bone marrow

B. Function
1. Drains tissue spaces of excess interstitial fluid
2. Transports dietary lipids (triglycerides, cholesterol, and lipid-soluble vitamins A, D, E, K) from the GI tract to blood
3. With the help of macrophages, protects the body from foreign invasion by microbes and cancer cells
4. The major difference between the interstitial fluid and lymph is location; when fluid bathes tissue cells, it is called *interstitial fluid,* or *intercellular fluid*; when it flows through lymphatic vessels, it is called *lymph*

C. Lymphatic vessels and lymph circulation
1. Lymphatic vessels—begin as lymphatic capillaries in tissue spaces between cells; have thinner walls and more valves than veins
2. Lymphatic capillaries—merge to form larger vessels, called *lymphatic vessels,* which ultimately converge into the thoracic duct or the right lymphatic duct
3. Lymph flows from the interstitial spaces, to lymphatic capillaries, to lymphatic vessels, to lymph trunks, to the thoracic duct or right lymphatic duct, and to the subclavian veins, as a result of skeletal muscle contractions, respiratory movements, and the valves in the lymphatic vessels
   a. The milking action of skeletal muscle contractions compresses lymphatic vessels and forces lymph toward subclavian veins (skeletal muscle pump)
   b. Lymphatic vessels contain valves that ensure the one-way movement of lymph; lymph flow is also maintained by pressure changes that occur during inhalation (respiratory pump); lymph flows from the abdominal region, where the pressure is higher, toward the thoracic region, where it is lower; when the pressures reverse during exhalation, valves prevent the backflow of lymph
   c. Edema—accumulation of the interstitial fluid in tissue spaces that may be caused by an obstruction such as an infected lymph node, blockage of lymphatic vessels, injury, or inflammation (see the section on "Inflammation" in Chapter 7).

D. Lymphatic organs and tissues)
1. Primary lymphatic organs (red bone marrow)—sites where stem cells divide and mature into B cells and T cells
2. Secondary lymphatic organs and tissues—lymph nodes, spleen, and lymphatic nodules; sites where most immune responses occur
3. Thymus—a two-lobed organ located posterior to the sternum and medial to the lungs
   a. Site of T cell maturation

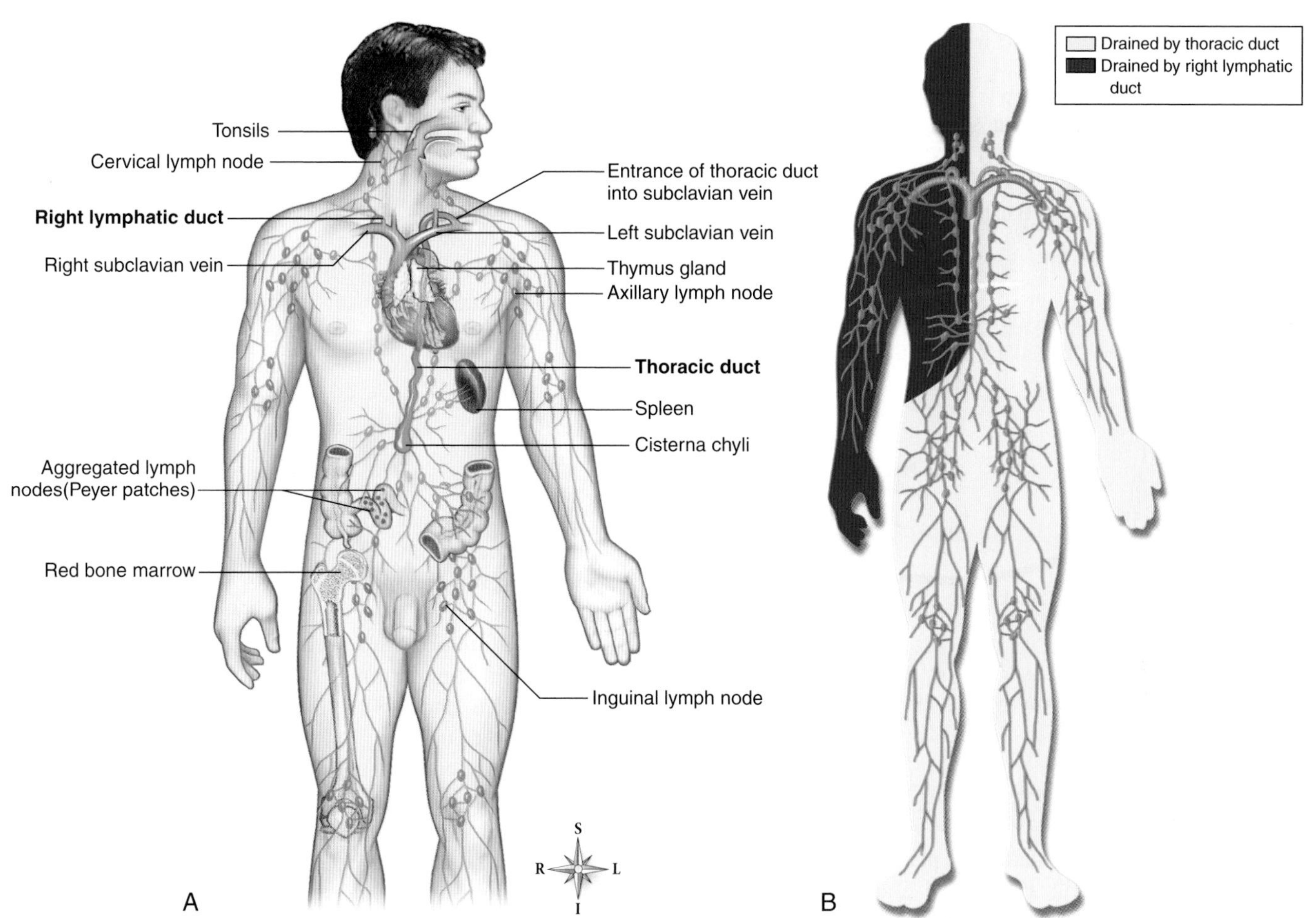


**Fig 3.28** Components of the lymphatic system. **A**, Major components of the lymphatic system. **B**, Anatomic regions drained by the right lymphatic duct (dark purple) and by the thoracic duct (yellow). (From Patton KT, Thibodeau GA, Douglas MM: *Essentials of anatomy and physiology*, St Louis, 2012, Mosby.)

b. Produces hormones
c. Large in infants; after puberty, much of thymic tissue is replaced by fat and connective tissue; the gland continues to function throughout life

4. Lymph nodes—approximately 600 bean-shaped organs located along lymphatic vessels; scattered throughout the body, both in superficial and deep locations; usually occur in groups (see the section on "Blood and Lymph" in Chapter 2; "The Lymphatic System" and "Extraoral and Intraoral Assessment" in Chapter 15)
   a. Contain B cells that develop into plasma cells, which secrete antibodies, T cells, and macrophages
   b. Function as filters of lymphatic fluid

## The Immune System

The immune system comprises a wide variety of body reactions or responses to fight the invasion of pathogens. This is accomplished by detecting pathogens and differentiating them from the body's own healthy tissue. The defense mechanisms are categorized as either nonspecific or specific immunity, providing mechanical and chemical barriers, inflammatory responses, phagocytosis, antibodies, and many other means to protect the body (Fig. 3.29; see the section on "Disease Barriers," and Figs. 9.2 in Chapter 9).

A. Nonspecific (innate) immunity—mechanisms that provide general defense by acting against anything recognized as "not self" or foreign
B. Specific (adaptive) immunity—mechanisms that recognize specific threatening agents

### *Nonspecific Immunity*

A. Species resistance—genetic characteristics of an organism or species that defend against pathogens
B. First line of defense—mechanical and chemical barriers, for example, skin, mucous membranes, sebum, mucus, enzymes, and hydrochloric acid in the stomach
C. Second line of defense—inflammation (see Fig. 3.29; see the sections on "Inflammation," "Acute Inflammation," and "Chronic Inflammation" in Chapter 7)
   1. Inflammatory response—tissue damage elicits responses to counteract injury and promote normalcy
   2. Phagocytosis—ingestion and destruction of microorganisms or other small particles by phagocytes, for example, neutrophils, macrophages, histiocytes in connective tissue, microglia in the nervous system, and Kupffer cells in the liver

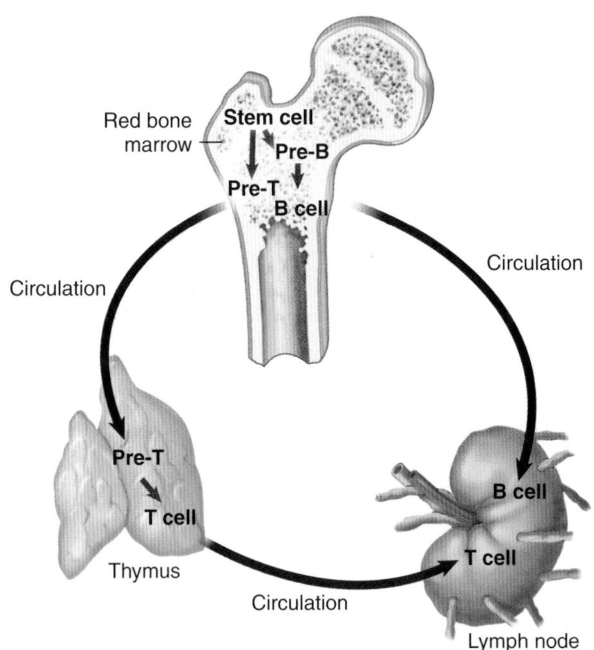


**Fig 3.29** Lines of defense. (From Patton KT, Thibodeau GA: *Anthony's textbook of anatomy and physiology*, ed 20, St Louis, 2013, Elsevier.)

D. Third line of defense—natural killer cells (lymphocytes that kill tumor cells and cells infected by viruses); method of killing cells: lysing cells by damaging plasma membranes
   1. Interferon—protein synthesized and released into the circulation by certain cells if invaded by viruses
   2. Complement—group of enzymes lyse cells when activated by either specific or nonspecific mechanisms

***Specific Immunity***

A. Specific immunity—part of the third line of defense consisting of lymphocytes; lymphocytes are densest where they develop in bone marrow, thymus gland, lymph nodes, and spleen; lymphocytes flow through the bloodstream, become distributed in tissues, and return to the bloodstream in a continuous recirculation; lymphocytes are named by the CD protein surface markers that the cells carry, for example, CD4 and CD cells (called the CD system)
B. Two classes of lymphocytes—B lymphocytes (B cells) and T lymphocytes (T cells)
   1. B cells—produce antibodies that attack pathogens (antibody-mediated immunity)
   2. T cells—attack pathogens more directly (cell-mediated immunity)

**B Cells and Antibody-Mediated Immunity.** See the section on "Disease Barriers" in Chapter 9.

A. B cells develop in two stages:
   1. Pre-B cells develop by a few months of age
   2. The second stage occurs in lymph nodes and the spleen—activation of B cell when it binds to a specific antigen
   3. B cells serve as ancestors to antibody-secreting plasma cells
B. Antibodies—proteins (immunoglobulins) secreted by activated B cell; resist disease first by recognizing foreign abnormal substances
C. Antibody molecule—consists of two heavy and two light polypeptide chains; each molecule has two antigen-binding sites and two complement-binding sites; produces antibody-mediated immunity (humoral immunity) within plasma
D. Classes of immunoglobulin (Ig)
   1. IgM—inactive B cells synthesize and insert themselves into their own plasma membranes; predominant class produced after initial contact with an antigen
   2. IgG—makes up 75% of antibodies in blood; predominant antibody of the secondary antibody response
   3. IgA—major class of antibody in external secretions of the mucous membranes, saliva, and tears
   4. IgE—role in immediate hypersensitivity reactions and parasitic infections
   5. IgD—small amount in blood; precise function unknown; thought to activate B cells
E. Complement—component of blood plasma consisting of several protein compounds; serves to kill foreign cells by cytolysis; causes vasodilation and enhances phagocytosis and other functions; complement protein 3 activated without antigen stimulation; produces full complement effect by binding to bacteria or viruses in presence of properdin
F. Clonal selection theory
   1. The human body contains many diverse clones of cells, each committed by its genes to synthesize a different antibody
   2. When an antigen enters the body, it selects the clone whose cells are synthesizing its antibody and stimulates them to proliferate and create more antibodies
   3. The clones selected by antigens consist of lymphocytes and are selected by the shape of antigen receptors on the lymphocyte's plasma membrane

**T Cells and Cell-Mediated Immunity.** See the section on "Disease Barriers" and Fig. 9.2 in Chapter 9.

A. T cells—lymphocytes that go through the thymus gland before migrating to the lymph nodes and spleen; function to produce cell-mediated immunity and regulate specific immunity in general
   1. Pre-T cells develop into thymocytes while in the thymus
   2. Thymocytes stream into blood and are carried to the T-dependent zones in the spleen and lymph nodes
B. T cells display antigen receptors on their surface membranes; the T cell is activated when an antigen (presented by a macrophage) binds to its receptors, causing it to divide repeatedly to form a clone of identical sensitized T cells
   1. Sensitized T cells go to the site where the antigen entered, bind to antigens, and release cytokines (lymphokines)
C. Killer T cells—release lymphotoxin to kill cells
D. Helper T cells—regulate the function of B cells
E. Suppressor T cells—suppress B cell differentiation into plasma cells

## The Respiratory System

In order to maintain life, the body needs oxygen for metabolic processes. The respiratory system, working with the cardiovascular system, provides oxygen and removal of waste products. Air is filtered and warmed by the respiratory system while providing a mechanism for vocal communication. It aids in homeostasis of circulation, metabolism, electrolyte and water balance, and acidity of the blood.

A. The respiratory system functions as an air distributor and gas exchanger that supplies $O_2$ and removes $CO_2$ from cells, and warms, filters, and humidifies air (Fig. 3.30)
   1. Alveoli serve as gas exchangers; all other parts of the respiratory system serve as air distributors
   2. Respiratory organs influence speech, homeostasis of body pH, and olfaction
B. Divided into two parts:
   1. Upper respiratory tract—organs located outside of the thorax and consist of the nose, nasopharynx, oropharynx, laryngopharynx, and larynx
   2. Lower respiratory tract—organs located within the thorax and consist of the trachea, bronchial tree, and lungs
C. Accessory structures—oral cavity, rib cage and associated muscles, sternum, and diaphragm

## Upper Respiratory Tract

See the section on "Osteology" in Chapter 4.

A. Nose—passageway for air traveling to and from the lungs; filters air, aids speech, and makes the sense of smell possible
   1. The external portion of the nose consists of a bony and cartilaginous frame covered by skin containing sebaceous glands; two nasal bones meet and are surrounded by frontal bone to form the roof; the floor of the nose is bound by the maxilla
   2. The internal nose (nasal cavity) lies over the roof of the mouth, separated by the palatine bones
      a. Cribriform plate—separates the roof of the nose from the anterior cranial cavity
      b. Septum—separates the nasal cavity into right and left cavities; consists of four structures: the perpendicular plate of the ethmoid bone, the vomer bone, the vomeronasal cartilages, and the septal nasal cartilage
   3. Each nasal cavity is divided into three passageways: superior, middle, and inferior meatus
   4. Anterior nares—external openings to nasal cavities, open into the vestibule
   5. Nasal mucosa—a mucous membrane over which air passes; contains a rich blood supply
      a. Olfactory epithelium—specialized membrane containing many olfactory nerve cells and a rich lymphatic plexus
   6. Paranasal sinuses (see the section on "Paranasal Sinuses" in Chapter 4)
B. Pharynx (throat) (see the section on "Clinical Oral Structures" and Table 5.1 in Chapter 5)
C. Larynx
   1. Located between the root of the tongue and the upper end of the trachea; functions as part of the airway to the lungs and produces the voice
   2. Consists of cartilages attached to each other by muscle; lined by a ciliated mucous membrane that forms two pairs of folds:
      a. Vestibular (false) vocal folds
      b. True vocal cords
   3. The framework of the larynx is formed by nine cartilages:
      a. Single laryngeal cartilages—the three largest cartilages: the thyroid cartilage, the epiglottis, and the cricoid cartilages
      b. Paired laryngeal cartilages—three pairs of smaller cartilages: the arytenoid, corniculate, and cuneiform cartilages
   4. Muscles of the larynx
      a. Intrinsic muscles both insert and originate within the larynx
      b. Extrinsic muscles insert in the larynx but originate on another structure

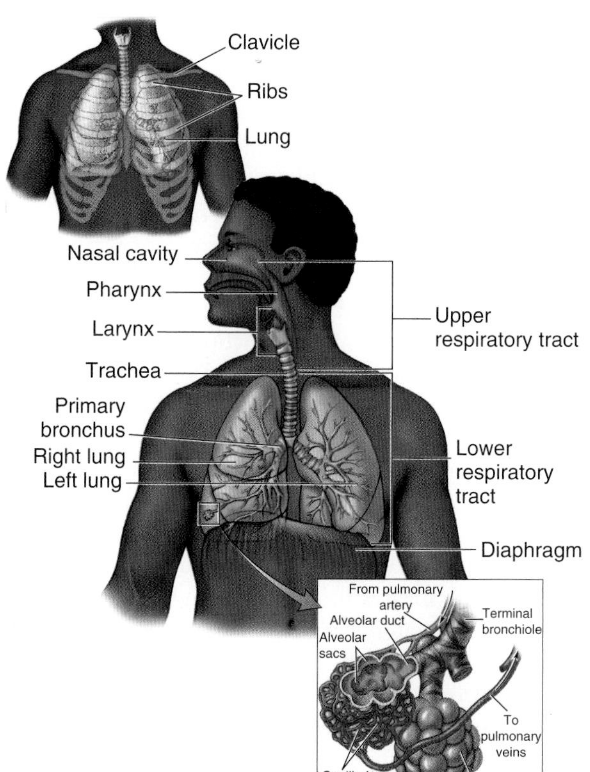


**Fig 3.30** Structural plan of the respiratory system. (From Herlihy B: *The human body in health and illness*, ed 5, St Louis, 2015, Elsevier.)

## Lower Respiratory Tract

A. Trachea (windpipe)—extends from the larynx to the primary bronchi; furnishes part of the open airway to the lungs; obstruction causes death
B. Bronchi and alveoli
   1. The lower end of the trachea divides into two primary bronchi (one at the right and one at the left), which continue into each lung and then divide into secondary bronchi (one per lung lobe); these branch into tertiary bronchi (one per bronchopulmonary segment) that branch into bronchioles, which then divide into respiratory bronchioles and then alveolar ducts

2. Alveoli—the primary gas exchange structures
   a. Respiratory membrane—the barrier between which gases are exchanged by alveolar air and blood; consists of the alveolar epithelium, the capillary endothelium, and their joined basement membranes
   b. Surfactant—a component of the fluid coating the respiratory membrane that reduces surface tension

C. Lungs
1. Cone-shaped organs extending from the diaphragm to above the clavicles; function in air distribution and gas exchange
   a. Hilum—indentation on lung's medial surface, where primary bronchi and pulmonary blood vessels enter and exit the lung
   b. Base—the inferior surface of the lung; rests on the diaphragm
   c. Costal surface—area in contact with the ribs
   d. Left lung—divided into two lobes (superior and inferior)
   e. Right lung—divided into three lobes (superior, middle, and inferior)
   f. Lobes—further divided into functional units called *bronchopulmonary segments*
      (1) Ten segments in the right lung
      (2) Eight or nine segments in the left lung

D. Thorax
1. Part of the body between the neck and the abdomen; encased by the ribs, sternum (anteriorly) and vertebral column (posteriorly) and containing the heart and lungs
2. Functions to bring about inspiration and expiration

## Respiratory Physiology

The respiratory system includes pulmonary ventilation, gas exchange in the lungs and tissues, transport of gases by blood, and regulation of respiration.

A. Pulmonary ventilation (breathing)
1. Mechanism
   a. Establishes two gas pressure gradients: in one gradient, the pressure within the alveoli of the lungs is lower than atmospheric pressure to produce inspiration; in the other, the pressure in the alveoli of the lungs is higher than atmospheric pressure to produce expiration
   b. Pressure gradients—established by changes in the size of the thoracic cavity through the contraction and relaxation of muscles
   c. Boyle's law—the volume of gas varies inversely with pressure at a constant temperature (expansion of the thorax results in decreased intrapleural pressure, leading to a decreased alveolar pressure and causing air to move into the lungs)
2. Two components of respiration:
   a. Inspiration—contraction of the diaphragm produces inspiration; as the diaphragm contracts, the thoracic cavity enlarges; the ability of pulmonary tissues to stretch, which makes inspiration possible, is termed *compliance*
   b. Expiration—a passive process that begins when the inspiratory muscles are relaxed, decreasing the size of the thorax and increasing intrapleural pressure from about – 6 mm Hg to a preinspiration level of – 4 mm Hg
      (1) The pressure between the parietal and visceral pleurae is always less than atmospheric pressure
      (2) Elastic recoil—tendency of pulmonary tissues to return to a smaller size after having been stretched passively during expiration
3. Pulmonary volumes—amount of air moved in and out and air remaining; important for normal exchange of $O_2$ and $CO_2$ to take place
   a. Spirometer—instrument used to measure the volume of air
   b. Tidal volume (TV, $V_T$)—amount of air inhaled and exhaled during a normal breath
   c. Expiratory reserve volume (ERV)—largest volume of additional air that can be forcibly exhaled after normal exhalation (normal ERV is 1.0 to 1.2 liters [L])
   d. Inspiratory reserve volume (IRV)—amount of air that can be forcibly inhaled after normal inspiration (normal IRV is 3.3 L)
   e. Residual volume—amount of air that cannot be forcibly exhaled because it remains in the airways (1.2 L)
   f. Pulmonary capacity—the sum of two or more pulmonary volumes
   g. Vital capacity—the sum of IRV + TV + ERV; depends on many factors, including the size of the thoracic cavity and posture
   h. Minimal volume—the minimal amount of air needed in the lung to prevent collapse (atelectasis)
   i. Functional residual capacity—the sum of ERV + RV; amount of air at the end of passive expiration
   j. Total lung capacity—sum of all four lung volumes; the total amount of air a lung can hold
   k. Anatomic dead space—air in passageways that does not participate in gas exchange
   l. Physiologic dead space—anatomic dead space plus the volume of any nonfunctioning alveoli (as in pulmonary disease)
   m. Alveolar ventilation— exchange of gas between alveoli and external environment; volume of inspired air that reaches the alveoli per unit of time; alveoli must be properly ventilated for adequate gas exchange

B. Pulmonary gas exchange
1. Once alveolar ventilation has occurred and the alveolar spaces are filled with air, the second stage of respiration takes place: pulmonary gas exchange occurs in the lungs between the alveoli and the blood; also referred to as "external respiration" because it involves the respiratory processes that have contact with the external environment
2. Gas exchange in the lungs takes place between alveolar air and blood flowing through lung capillaries
   a. Four factors determine the amount of $O_2$ that diffuses into blood:

(1) $O_2$ pressure gradient between alveolar air and blood
(2) Total functional surface area of the respiratory membrane
(3) Respiratory minute volume
(4) Alveolar ventilation

b. Structural facts that facilitate $O_2$ diffusion from alveolar air to blood
(1) The walls of alveoli and capillaries form only a very thin barrier for gases to cross
(2) Alveolar and capillary surfaces are large
(3) Blood is distributed through capillaries in a thin layer so that each red blood cell comes close to alveolar air

C. How blood transports gases
1. $O_2$ and $CO_2$ are transported as solutes and as parts of the molecules of certain chemical compounds
2. Transport of $O_2$
a. Hemoglobin—made up of four polypeptide chains (two α-chains, two β-chains), each with an iron-containing heme group; $CO_2$ can bind to amino acids in the chains, and $O_2$ can bind to iron in the heme groups
b. Oxygenated blood contains about 0.3 mL of dissolved $O_2$ per 100 mL of blood
c. Hemoglobin increases the $O_2$-carrying capacity of blood
d. $O_2$ travels in two forms: as dissolved $O_2$ in plasma ($PO_2$) and associated with hemoglobin (oxyhemoglobin)
(1) Increasing blood $PO_2$ accelerates the association of hemoglobin with $O_2$
(2) Oxyhemoglobin carries the majority of the total $O_2$ transported by blood
3. Transport of $CO_2$
a. A small amount of $CO_2$ dissolves in plasma and is transported as a solute (10%)
b. Less than one-fourth of blood $CO_2$ combines with $NH_2$ (amine) groups of hemoglobin and other proteins to form carbaminohemoglobin (20%)
c. The association of $CO_2$ with hemoglobin is accelerated by an increase in blood $PO_2$
d. More than two-thirds of the $CO_2$ in plasma is bicarbonate ions ($HCO_3$-, 70%)

D. Systemic gas exchange
1. Gas exchange in tissues takes place between arterial blood flowing through tissue capillaries and cells
a. $O_2$ diffuses out of arterial blood because the $O_2$ pressure gradient favors its outward diffusion
b. As dissolved $O_2$ diffuses out of arterial blood, blood $PO_2$ decreases, which accelerates oxyhemoglobin dissociation to release more $O_2$ to plasma for diffusion to cells
2. $CO_2$ exchange between tissues and blood occurs in the opposite direction from $O_2$ exchange
a. Bohr effect—increased $PO_2$ decreases the affinity between $O_2$ and hemoglobin
b. Haldane effect—increased $CO_2$ loading is caused by a decrease in $PO_2$

E. Regulation of respiration
1. Respiratory control centers—main integrators that are located in the brain stem and control the nerves that affect inspiratory and expiratory muscles
a. Medullary rhythmicity center—generates the basic rhythm of the respiratory cycle
(1) Consists of two interconnected control centers:
(a) Inspiratory center, which stimulates inspiration
(b) Expiratory center, which stimulates expiration
b. The basic breathing rhythm can be altered by different inputs to the medullary rhythmicity center
(1) Input from the apneustic center in the pons stimulates the inspiratory center to increase the length and depth of inspiration
(2) Pneumotaxic center in the pons—inhibits the apneustic center and the inspiratory center to prevent overinflation of the lungs
2. Factors that influence breathing—sensors from the nervous system provide feedback to the medullary rhythmicity center
a. Changes in the partial pressure of oxygen ($Po_2$) and carbon dioxide ($Pco_2$) and the pH of arterial blood influence the medullary rhythmicity area
(1) $Pco_2$ acts on the chemoreceptors in the medulla; an increase in $Pco_2$ results in faster breathing; a decrease results in slower breathing
(2) A decrease in blood pH stimulates the chemoreceptors in the carotid and aortic bodies
(3) Arterial blood $Po_2$ presumably has little influence if it stays above a certain level
b. Arterial blood pressure controls breathing through the respiratory pressor reflex mechanism
c. Hering-Breuer reflexes control respirations by regulating the depth of respirations and the volume of tidal air
d. The cerebral cortex influences breathing by increasing or decreasing the rate and strength of respirations

## The Digestive System

The digestive system is vital in preparing nutrients to be absorbed and utilized by body cells. The chemical and physical alteration of nutrients to aid in absorption is called *digestion*. The digestive system includes the digestive tract and other accessory organs (Fig. 3.31).

A. System of organs that breaks down food into molecules small enough for cells to use; the two groups are:
1. Gastrointestinal tract—continuous tube that extends from the mouth to the anus; organs include the mouth, pharynx, esophagus, stomach, and small and large intestines
2. Accessory digestive organs—teeth, tongue, salivary glands, liver, gallbladder, and pancreas; teeth and tongue only accessory organs that come into direct contact with food

B. Functions
1. Ingestion—taking foods and liquids into mouth
2. Secretion—cells within the walls of the GI tract and accessory organs secrete a total of about 7L of water, acid, buffers, and enzymes into the lumen of the tract

3. Mixing and propulsion—alternating contraction and relaxation of smooth muscle in the walls of the GI tract mix food and secretions and propel them toward the anus; motility is the ability of the GI tract to mix and move material along its length
4. Digestion—mechanical and chemical processes break down ingested food into small molecules
5. Absorption—entrance of ingested and secreted fluids, ions, and small molecules that are products of digestion into the epithelial cells lining the lumen of the GI tract; absorbed substances pass into blood or lymph and circulate to cells throughout the body
6. Defecation—wastes, indigestible substances, microorganisms, and digested materials that were not absorbed leave the body through the anus; the eliminated material is called feces

C. Organs
1. Mouth
   a. Formed by cheeks, palates, lips, and tongue, which aid mechanical digestion
   b. Fauces—opening from the mouth to the throat
   c. Tongue—composed of skeletal muscle covered with mucous membrane and forms the floor of the oral cavity; superior and lateral surfaces covered with papillae, some of which contain taste buds
   d. Salivary glands empty via ducts into the oral cavity; three pairs of salivary glands: parotid, submandibular, and sublingual glands; secrete saliva that lubricates food and starts the chemical digestion of carbohydrates (salivary amylase begins the digestion of starches in the mouth); salivation is entirely under the control of the nervous system
   e. Teeth—see the sections on “Dental Terminology” and “Dental Anatomy” in Chapter 5.
   f. Mastication—food is chewed, mixed with saliva, and shaped into a bolus
2. Pharynx
   a. Food that is swallowed passes from the mouth into the oropharynx
   b. From the oropharynx, food passes into the laryngopharynx
3. Esophagus
   a. Muscular tube that connects the pharynx to the stomach
   b. Swallowing—moves the bolus from the mouth to the esophagus, which passes the food bolus into the

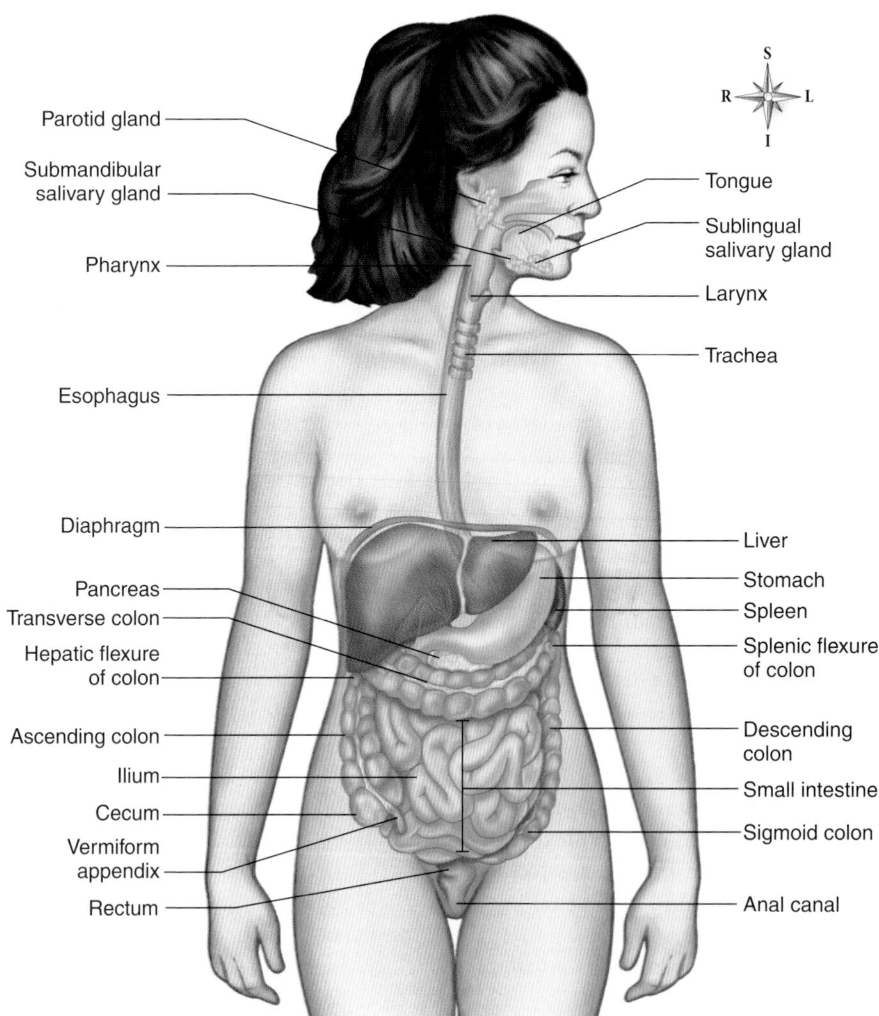


**Fig 3.31** Location of digestive organs. (From Patton KT, Thibodeau GA, Douglas MM: *Essentials of anatomy and physiology,* St Louis, 2012, Mosby.)

stomach by peristalsis; consists of a voluntary stage, a pharyngeal stage (involuntary), and an esophageal stage (involuntary)

4. Stomach
   a. Is attached to the esophagus and ends at the pyloric sphincter
   b. Anatomic subdivisions: cardia, fundus, body, and pylorus
   c. Adaptations for digestion include rugae; glands that produce mucus, hydrochloric acid, a protein-digesting enzyme (pepsin), intrinsic factor, and gastrin; and a three-layered muscularis for efficient mechanical movement
   d. Mechanical digestion consists of mixing waves; chemical digestion consists of conversion of proteins into peptides by pepsin; mixing waves and gastric secretions reduce food to chyme
   e. Gastric secretion and motility are regulated by neural and hormonal mechanisms; parasympathetic impulses and gastrin cause the secretion of gastric juices; food in the small intestine, secretin, and cholecystokinin inhibit gastric secretion
   f. Gastric emptying
      (1) Stimulated in response to stretching; gastrin released in response to the presence of certain foods
      (2) Inhibited by reflex action and hormones (secretin and cholecystokinin)
   g. Impermeable to most substances; the stomach can absorb water, certain ions, some drugs, and alcohol
5. Pancreas
   a. Connected to the duodenum by the pancreatic duct
   b. Pancreatic islets (islets of Langerhans)—secrete hormones; endocrine portion of the pancreas
   c. Acinar cells—secrete pancreatic juice; exocrine portion of the pancreas
   d. Pancreatic juice—contains enzymes that digest starch, glycogen, and dextrins (pancreatic amylase); proteins (trypsin, chymotrypsin, and carboxypeptidase); triglycerides (pancreatic lipase); and nucleic acids (nucleases)
6. Liver and gallbladder
   a. Liver—has left and right lobes; produces bile, detoxifies chemicals, metabolizes products of digestion and drugs, stores lipid soluble vitamins (A,D,E,K),
   b. Gallbladder—a sac located in a depression under the liver; stores and concentrates bile

D. Layers of the GI tract
   1. Basic arrangement from deep to superficial: mucosa, submucosa, muscularis, and serosa/adventitia
   2. The mucosa contains extensive patches of lymphatic tissue

## The Urinary System

The function of the urinary system is not only to produce urine, but also to balance the composition of blood plasma. The primary organs of the urinary system are the kidneys, which control the homeostasis of water, electrolytes, and pH in body fluids. The accessory organs that aid in the excretion of waste are the ureters, urinary bladder, and urethra.

A. Kidneys—principal organs of the urinary system; accessory organs are ureters, urinary bladder, and urethra
B. Regulates content of blood plasma to maintain the "dynamic constancy," or homeostasis, of the internal fluid environment within normal limits
C. Anatomy of the urinary system—structure
   1. Kidneys (Fig. 3.32)
      a. Shape, size, and location
         (1) Roughly oval, with a medial indentation; each kidney approximately 11 × 7 × 3 cm
         (2) The left kidney is often larger than the right; the right kidney is located slightly lower than the left because of the presence of the liver on the right side of the body.
         (3) The kidneys are located in the retroperitoneal position; lie on either side of the vertebral column between T12 and L3
         (4) Superior poles of both kidneys extend above the level of the twelfth rib and the lower edge of the thoracic parietal pleura
         (5) The renal fascia anchors the kidneys to surrounding structures; heavy cushion of fat surrounds each kidney
      b. Internal structures of the kidney
         (1) Cortex and medulla
         (2) Renal pyramids: constitute much of the medullary tissue
         (3) Renal columns: where cortical tissue dips into the medulla between the pyramids
         (4) Calyx: cup-like structure at each renal papilla that collects urine; the structures join together to form the renal pelvis
         (5) Renal pelvis: narrows as it exits the kidney to become the ureter
      c. Kidneys are highly vascular

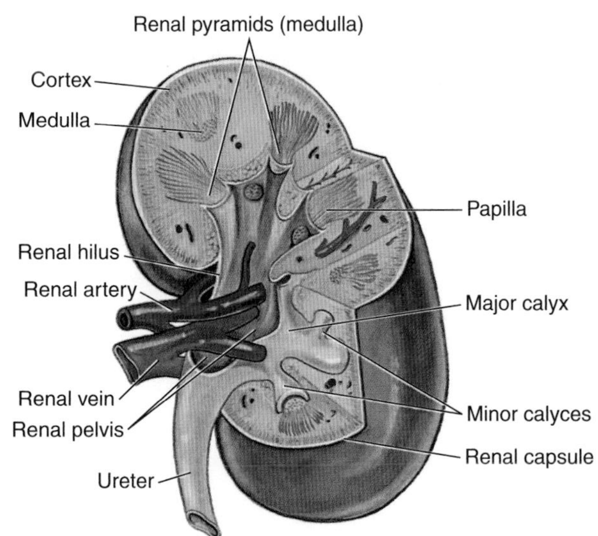


**Fig 3.32** Internal structure of the kidney. (From Solomon EP: *Introduction to human anatomy and physiology*, ed 2, St Louis, 2008, Saunders.)

2. Renal artery: a large branch of the abdominal aorta; brings blood into each kidney (Fig. 3.33)
3. Interlobar arteries—the renal artery branches between the pyramids of the medulla; interlobar arteries extend toward the cortex, arch over the bases of the pyramids, and form arcuate arteries; from arcuate arteries, interlobular arteries penetrate the cortex and lead towards the afferent arteriole and glomerular capillaries.
4. Juxtaglomerular apparatus—located where the afferent arteriole brushes past the distal tubule; important for the maintenance of blood flow homeostasis by reflexively secreting renin when blood pressure in the afferent arteriole drops
5. Ureter—tube running from each kidney to the urinary bladder; composed of three layers: mucous membrane lining, muscular middle layer, and fibrous outer layer
6. Urinary bladder (Fig. 3.34)
   a. Collapsible, bag-like structure located behind the symphysis pubis; made mostly of smooth muscle tissue; lining forms rugae; can distend considerably
   b. Functions
      (1) Reservoir for urine before it is voided
      (2) Expels urine from the body with the aid of the urethra
   c. Mechanism for voiding
      (1) Voluntary relaxation of external sphincter muscle
      (2) Reflexive contraction of regions of the detrusor muscle
      (3) Urine forced out of bladder through the urethra
7. Urethra
   a. Small mucous membrane–lined tube; extends from the trigone to the exterior of the body
   b. In the female, lies posterior to the symphysis pubis and anterior to the vagina; approximately 3 cm long
   c. In the male, after leaving the bladder, passes through the prostate gland, where it is joined by two ejaculatory ducts; from the prostate, it extends to the base of the penis and then through the center of the penis and ends as the urinary meatus; approximately 20 cm long; the male urethra is part of the urinary system as well as the reproductive system

D. Microscopic structure of the nephron
   1. Nephrons—microscopic functional units; make up the bulk of the kidney; those located in the renal cortex are called *cortical nephrons*; those near the junction of the cortical and medullary layers are called *juxtamedullary nephrons*; each nephron is made up of various structures
      a. Renal corpuscle
      b. Bowman's capsule—cup-shaped mouth of the nephron
         (1) Formed by parietal and visceral layers, with a space between them
         (2) Pedicles (cellular foot processes) in the visceral layer are packed closely together to form filtration slits; slit diaphragm prevents filtration slits from enlarging under pressure
         (3) Glomerulus—network of fine capillaries in Bowman's capsule; together called *renal corpuscle*; located in the cortex of the kidney

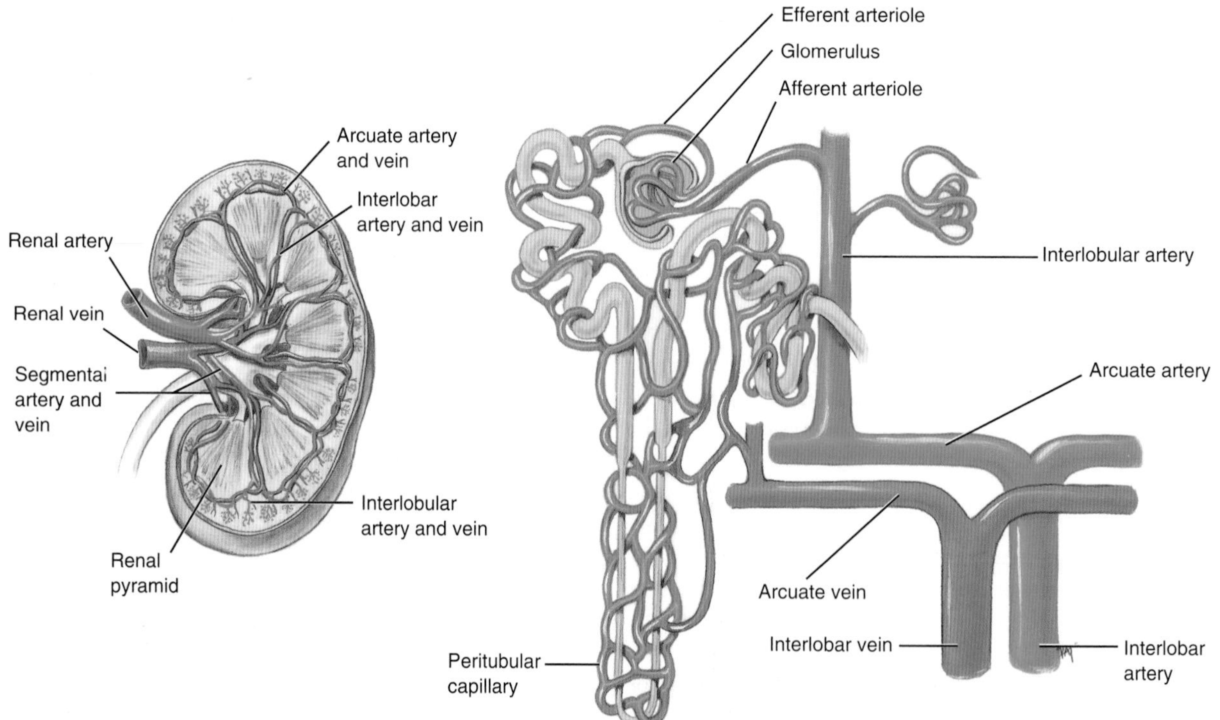


**Fig 3.33** Circulation of blood through the kidney. (Modified from Applegate E: *The anatomy and physiology learning system*, ed 4, St Louis, 2011, Saunders.)

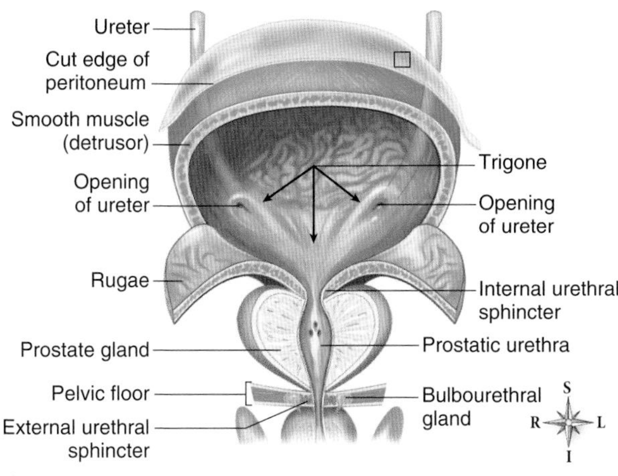


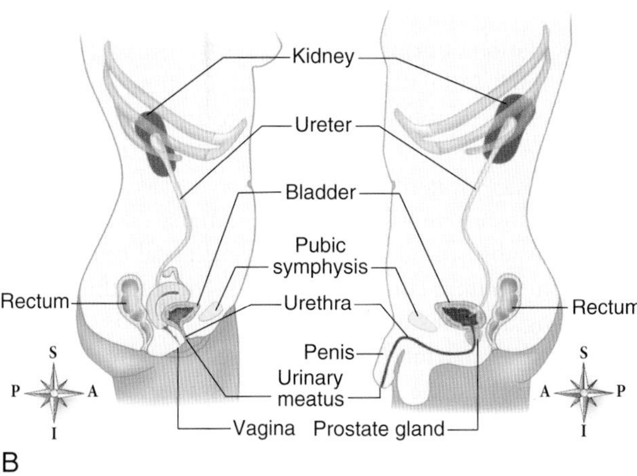


**Fig 3.34** Structure and location of the urinary bladder. **A**, Frontal view of a dissected urinary bladder (male) in a fully distended position. **B**, Sagittal view of the female urinary system *(left)* and male urinary system *(right)*, each showing a partially distended bladder. (From Patton KT, Thibodeau GA: *Anthony's textbook of anatomy and physiology*, ed 20, St Louis, 2013, Elsevier.)

(4) The basement membrane lies between the glomerulus and Bowman's capsule

(5) Glomerular-capsular membrane—formed by the glomerular endothelium, the basement membrane, and the visceral layer of Bowman's capsule; function is filtration

c. Proximal tubule—first part of the renal tubule nearest to Bowman's capsule; follows a winding, convoluted course; also known as *proximal convoluted tubule*

d. Loop of Henle
   (1) Renal tubule segment just beyond proximal tubule
   (2) Consists of a thin descending limb, a sharp turn, and a thick ascending limb
   (3) Juxtamedullary nephron—a nephron with a loop of Henle that dips far into the medulla
   (4) Cortical nephron—a nephron with a loop of Henle that does not dip into the medulla but remains almost entirely within the cortex; constitutes about 85% of the total number of nephrons

e. Distal tubule—convoluted tubule beyond the loop of Henle; also known as *distal convoluted tubule*

f. Collecting duct
   (1) Straight tubule joined by the distal tubules of several nephrons
   (2) Joins larger ducts; larger collecting ducts of one renal pyramid converge to form one tube that opens at a renal papilla into a calyx

E. Physiology of the urinary system—the kidneys are important organs with many functions in the body, including producing hormones, absorbing minerals, and filtering blood and producing urine

1. Functions of the kidneys
   a. Waste excretion—the kidneys filter out toxins, excess salts, and urea, a nitrogen-based waste created by cell metabolism
      (1) While filtering waste, kidneys measure out chemicals (e.g., sodium, phosphorus, potassium) and release these back to the blood to return to the body; in this way, kidneys regulate the body's level of these substances
      (2) Urea is synthesized in the liver and transported through the blood to the kidneys for removal
   b. Water level balance—kidneys are key in the production of urine
      (1) The kidneys react to changes in the body's water level throughout the day
      (2) As water intake decreases, the kidneys adjust accordingly and leave water in the body instead of helping to excrete it
   c. Blood pressure regulation—the kidneys need constant pressure to filter the blood
      (1) When it drops too low, the kidneys increase the blood pressure
      (2) One way is by producing a blood vessel–constricting protein (angiotensin) that also signals the body to retain sodium and water
      (3) Both constriction and retention help restore normal blood pressure
   d. Red blood cell regulation—when the kidneys do not receive enough oxygen, they send out a "distress call" in the form of *erythropoietin*, a hormone that stimulates the bone marrow to produce more oxygen-carrying RBCs
   e. Acid regulation—as cells metabolize, they produce acids
      (1) Foods eaten can either increase the acid in the body or neutralize it
      (2) To function properly, the body needs to keep a healthy balance of these chemicals, as is done by the kidneys
   f. Nephron—basic functional unit; forms urine through:
      (1) Filtration—movement of water and protein-free solutes from the plasma in the glomerulus into the capsular space of Bowman's capsule
      (2) Tubular resorption—movement of molecules out of the tubule and into peritubular blood

(3) Tubular secretion—movement of molecules out of peritubular blood and into the tubule for excretion

2. Filtration—first step in blood processing that occurs in the renal corpuscles
   a. From the blood in glomerular capillaries, about 180 L of water and solutes filter into Bowman's capsule each day; takes place through the glomerular-capsular membrane
   b. Occurs because of the existence of a pressure gradient (hydrostatic or oncotic pressure)
   c. Occurs rapidly because of the increased number of fenestrations
   d. Glomerular hydrostatic pressure and filtration are related to systemic blood pressure
3. Tubular reabsorption—second step in urine formation; results from passive and active transport mechanisms from all parts of the renal tubules; major portion of resorption occurs in proximal tubules
   a. Tubular reabsorption in the proximal tubule—most water and solutes are recovered by blood, leaving only a small volume of tubule fluid to move on to the loop of Henle
      (1) Sodium—actively transported out of the tubule fluid and into blood
      (2) Glucose and amino acids—passively transported out of the tubule fluid by means of the sodium co-transport mechanism
      (3) Chloride, phosphate, and bicarbonate ions passively move into blood because of an imbalance of electrical charge
      (4) Water—movement of sodium and chloride into blood causes an osmotic imbalance, moving water passively into blood
      (5) Urea—approximately one-half of urea passively moves out of the tubule; the remaining urea moves on to the loop of Henle
   b. Reabsorption in the loop of Henle
      (1) Water is reabsorbed from the tubule fluid, and urea is picked up from the interstitial fluid in the descending limb
      (2) Sodium and chloride are resorbed from the filtrate in the ascending limb, where the reabsorption of salt dilutes the tubule fluid and creates and maintains a high osmotic pressure of the medulla's interstitial fluid
4. Reabsorption in the distal tubules and collecting ducts
   a. The distal tubule resorbs sodium by active transport, but in smaller amounts than in the proximal tubule
   b. ADH—secreted by the posterior pituitary gland; targets the cells of distal tubules and collecting ducts to make them more permeable to water
   c. With the reabsorption of water in the collecting duct, urea concentration of the tubule fluid increases, causing urea to diffuse out of the collecting duct into the medullary interstitial fluid
   d. Urea participates in a countercurrent multiplier mechanism that, along with countercurrent mechanisms of the loop of Henle and the vasa recta, maintains the high osmotic pressure needed to form concentrated urine and avoid dehydration
5. Tubular secretion
   a. Tubular secretion—movement of substances out of blood and into the tubular fluid
   b. The descending limb of the loop of Henle secretes urea by diffusion
   c. Distal and collecting tubules secrete potassium, hydrogen, and ammonium ions
   d. Aldosterone—hormone that targets the cells of distal and collecting tubules; causes increased activity of sodium-potassium pumps
   e. Secretion of hydrogen ions increases with increased $H^+$ concentration in blood
6. Regulation of urine volume
   a. ADH influences water reabsorption; as water is resorbed, the total volume of urine is reduced by the amount of water removed by the tubules; ADH reduces water loss
   b. Aldosterone—secreted by the adrenal cortex; increases the absorption of sodium by the distal tubule, raising the sodium concentration of blood and thus promoting the reabsorption of water
   c. Atrial natriuretic peptide—secreted by specialized atrial muscle fibers; promotes the loss of sodium through urine; opposes aldosterone, causing the kidneys to resorb less water and thereby produce more urine
   d. Tubuloglomerular feedback mechanism—maintains constant glomerular filtration rate (GFR) by regulating resistance in afferent arterioles; protects kidney GFR function from rapid blood pressure variations; dependent on macula densa cells and the juxtaglomerular apparatus; may influence the renin-angiotensin mechanism
   e. Myogenic mechanism—rapid and effective regulation of GFR through changes in the contraction and relaxation of afferent arteriole smooth muscle
   f. Related to the total amount of solutes other than sodium excreted in urine; generally, the more solutes present, the higher the volume of urine
7. Urine composition—approximately 95% water with several substances dissolved in it, for example:
   a. Nitrogenous wastes—result of protein metabolism; for example, urea, uric acid, ammonia, and creatinine
   b. Electrolytes—mainly the ions sodium, potassium, ammonium, chloride, bicarbonate, phosphate, and sulfate; amounts and types of minerals vary with diet and other factors
   c. Toxins—during disease, bacterial poisons leave the body in urine
   d. Pigments—especially urochromes
   e. Hormones—high hormone levels may spill into the filtrate

f. Abnormal constituents such as blood, glucose, albumin, casts, or calculi

## The Reproductive System

The primary function of the reproductive system is to produce offspring. Other systems in the endocrine system function to maintain homeostasis, whereas the reproductive system is vital for survival of the species. The primary reproductive organs are the gonads (ovaries and testes), producing gametes (egg or sperm) and hormones. All other organs in the reproductive system are considered secondary and function to nurture and transport the gametes and developing offspring.

### Male

A. Testes
   1. Two ovoid bodies that lie in the scrotum and are suspended in the inguinal region by the spermatic cord
   2. Sperm—formed and stored in the seminiferous tubules of the testes
   3. Testosterone—produced in the testes
   4. The epididymis is adjacent to the testes in the scrotum
      a. Acts as a storage reservoir for sperm along with the seminiferous tubules
      b. Sperm may live for as long as 1 month in both the epididymis and the seminiferous tubules
   5. If the testes fail to descend during infancy, the condition is referred to as cryptorchidism

B. Vas deferens
   1. Conducts sperm from the epididymis to the urethra
   2. Acts as a storage site for sperm

C. Urethra
   1. Passageway for semen from the vas deferens through the penis
   2. Passage for urine from the bladder through the penis
   3. Ends at the urinary meatus, which is the opening in the glans penis through which urine and semen are excreted

D. Seminal vesicles
   1. Membranous pouches located posterior to the bladder
   2. Produce a secretion that contains fructose, amino acids, and mucus
   3. Secrete mucoid material into the upper end of the vas deferens

E. Prostate gland
   1. Located inferior to the bladder
   2. Secretes an alkaline fluid to activate sperm
   3. Secretes its milky fluid into the vas deferens

F. Bulbourethral glands (Cowper's glands)
   1. Located inferior to the prostate gland
   2. Secrete a mucous secretion into the urethra before ejaculation to aid in lubrication

G. Penis
   1. Organ of copulation; divided into the shaft and the glans penis
      a. Glans penis—most sensitive portion of the penis
      b. The foreskin covers the glans penis (removed by circumcision)
   2. Erectile tissue (corpus cavernosum) surrounds the penile urethra; causes erection when engorged with blood

H. Sperm
   1. Spermatozoa formed in the testes
   2. Contains head, neck, body, and tail
      a. The head contains the genetic material of the male
      b. The tail provides motility through flagellar movement
      c. Sperm move through the female genital tract to seek the ovum at a velocity of approximately 1 to 4 mm per minute
   3. Spermatogenesis
      a. After a spermatogonium has been divided by mitosis for the last time, it increases in size and forms a primary spermatocyte
      b. The primary spermatocyte is divided by meiosis to form the secondary spermatocyte, with a haploid number of chromosomes
      c. Division of the secondary spermatocytes results in the formation of spermatoids
      d. Spermatoids are transformed into motile cells called *spermatozoa*

I. Physiology of ejaculation
   1. Erection—stiffening of a flaccid penis
   2. Rhythmic peristalsis in the genital ducts during orgasm causes semen to be propelled through the epididymis, vas deferens, seminal ducts, and urethra
   3. Semen—a thick, whitish fluid of high viscosity
      a. Between 2.5 and 5 mL are secreted at ejaculation
      b. Each milliliter contains 10 million to 150 million sperm
      c. Sperm usually move at about 3 mm per minute

J. Hormonal influences
   1. Hormones are essential to the mechanism of reproduction and to the development and maintenance of secondary sex characteristics
   2. The anterior pituitary gland secretes FSH and LH, which cause the growth and function of testes at puberty
   3. Secondary sex characteristics in the male (appear during adolescence)
      a. Deepening of voice; widening of the musculature of the chest and shoulders
      b. Growth of facial and body hair

### Female

A. Pelvis
   1. Wider and shallower than the male's pelvis
   2. Shaped like a funnel with a wide mouth
   3. Divided into true and false pelvis by the inlet, or brim; the sacral promontory and ileopectineal lines are dividing points between true and false pelvis
   4. Forms part of the birth canal
   5. The perineum, vagina, muscles, and ligaments form the soft structures of the pelvis
      a. Retain pelvic organs in place
      b. During labor, the direct presenting part of the infant is forward

B. Ovaries
   1. Flat, oval-shaped bodies about 2.5 cm long

2. Supported in the pelvis by the broad ligament, ovarian ligament, and suspensory ligament
3. Three types of follicles in the ovaries:
   a. Primordial follicles contain a primary oocyte
      (1) Present at birth
      (2) Follicles complete their first maturation under the influence of FSH
   b. Growing follicles—contain a mature ovum and spaces that contain fluid
   c. Mature follicles—bulge from the surface of the ovary

C. Fallopian tubes (oviducts)
1. Lie in the folds of the broad ligaments
2. Fimbriae (finger-like projections) located at the ovarian ends; the isthmus portion is connected to the uterus
3. Important events occurring in the fallopian tube are fertilization of the ovum by a spermatozoon, segmentation, and formation of the blastocyst

D. Uterus
1. Hollow, pear-shaped organ with thick muscular walls; located behind the bladder and in front of the rectum
2. Divided into three parts:
   a. Fundus—rounded upper part
   b. Body—narrows from the fundus
   c. Cervix—tapering projection; projects into the vagina
3. Muscular layers
   a. Endometrium—one layer of ciliated columnar cells except for the lower one-third of the cervical canal where it changes to stratified squamous epithelium; contains glands and a good blood supply
   b. Myometrium—contains smooth muscle and large blood vessels
   c. Exometrium—contains the pelvic peritoneum
4. Serves as the womb for a developing fetus

E. External genitalia
1. Vagina—female organ of copulation
   a. Passageway for menstrual flow
   b. Connects the uterus to the external surface (vaginal orifice)
   c. Serves as the birth canal
2. Mons pubis—rounded eminence in front of the pubic symphysis
3. Labia majora—two longitudinal folds; protect the inner vulva; homologue of the scrotum in the male.
4. Labia minora—two smaller inner folds; protect the clitoris
5. Clitoris
   a. Contains erectile tissue; homologue of the penis in the male
   b. Increases in size with sexual stimulation

F. The perineum contains the structures found between the pubic symphysis and the coccyx

G. Mammary glands
1. Composed of compound alveolar glands
2. Secrete milk to the nipples under the influence of lactogenic hormone from the pituitary gland
3. Pigmented circular region (areolae surround the nipple)
4. Active glandular growth occurs during pregnancy to prepare mammary glands to produce milk (lactation)

H. Hormonal cycle
1. Begins at puberty and ends at menopause
2. FSH—secreted by the anterior pituitary gland; activates the primary graafian follicle; maturing follicle produces estrogen; causes the endometrium to become engorged with blood and prepares it to receive the fertilized ovum
3. Both hormones (FSH and estrogen) allow the ovum to mature
4. The mature ovum is released into the fallopian tube by a ruptured graafian follicle; LH assists ovulation; the follicle forms the corpus luteum and secretes progesterone
5. Increased progestogen levels reduce FSH and increase LH; cause the corpus luteum to secrete progesterone
   a. Stimulate the uterus to store glycogen and increase the uterine blood supply
   b. The corpus luteum begins to involute as a result of lowered FSH levels
6. Menstrual cycle lasts 21 to 35 days
   a. Menstruation begins if the ovum is not fertilized
   b. If fertilization occurs, the placenta will secrete chorionic gonadotropin to maintain the corpus luteum; estrogens and progesterone continue to be secreted to maintain the rich vascular supply in the endometrium for the developing embryo

## CHAPTER 3 REVIEW QUESTIONS

Answers and rationales to chapter review questions are available on this text's accompanying Evolve site. See inside front cover for details.

**1.** A sagittal MRI would visualize the body bisected into:
**a.** Anterior and posterior portions
**b.** Superior and inferior portions
**c.** Right and left portions
**d.** None of the above

**2.** Which cellular organelle synthesizes lipids and carbohydrates?
**a.** Golgi complex
**b.** Rough endoplasmic reticulum
**c.** Lysosomes
**d.** Smooth endoplasmic reticulum

**3.** A solution that has a lower concentration of solutes than the cytosol inside the cell is said to be:
**a.** Isotonic
**b.** Hypertonic
**c.** Hypotonic
**d.** Stable

**4.** Which active transport process allows large molecules to leave the cell after being enclosed in membranous vesicles?
**a.** Active transport pump

b. Endocytosis
c. Exocytosis
d. Phagocytosis

5. Pyruvic acid is converted into acetyl coenzyme A (CoA) during which stage of cellular respiration?
a. Glycolysis
b. Citric acid cycle
c. Electron transport
d. Protein synthesis

6. A dental hygienist created a treatment plan and divided his patient's oral cavity at the transverse plane. He plans to debride two quadrants per appointment (UR, upper right; UL, upper left; LR, lower right; LL, lower left). Which quadrants will be treated at each scheduled appointment?
a. Appointment one: UR and LR; Appointment two: UL and LL
b. Appointment one: LR and LL; Appointment two: UR and UL
c. Appointment one: UR and LL; Appointment two: UL and LR
d. Appointment one: all anterior teeth; Appointment two: all posterior teeth

7. What type of enzyme functions to rearrange atoms within a molecule?
a. Oxidation-reduction enzymes
b. Mutases (isomerases)
c. Hydrases
d. Phosphorylating enzymes

8. Which membrane covers the outer surface of organs?
a. Visceral serous membranes
b. Mucous membranes
c. Cutaneous membranes
d. Parietal serous membranes

9. Which of the following is NOT a function of the integument?
a. Regulation of body temperature
b. Immunity
c. Synthesis of vitamin D
d. Storage of vitamin A

10. Which portion of a long bone contains the growth plate?
a. Diaphysis
b. Epiphysis
c. Metaphysis
d. Medullary cavity

11. Parathyroid hormone can result in increased blood calcium by stimulating these cells:
a. Osteoblasts
b. Osteocytes
c. Osteoclasts
d. Chondrocytes

## CASE A

Stacey, a RDH, has not maintained good ergonomics during her 20-year professional career as a dental hygienist and has been recently diagnosed with carpal tunnel syndrome. Stacey is experiencing some paresthesia along the anterolateral forearm and hand and muscle weakness in her right thumb.

***Use Case A to answer questions 12 to 16.***

12. Injury to which nerve has likely led to Stacey's symptoms of paresthesia and weakness in her thumb?
a. Femoral nerve
b. Median nerve
c. Radial nerve
d. Ulnar nerve

13. The carpometacarpal joint of the thumb can be categorized as which type of joint?
a. Ball and socket
b. Condyloid
c. Gliding
d. Saddle

14. Which long bone is located in the forearm, on the same side of the body as the thumb?
a. Humerus
b. Radius
c. Scapula
d. Ulna

15. One muscle that is affected in this case is called flexor pollicis longus, which directly performs the action of thumb flexion. For this function, this muscle is an example of what muscle action group?
a. Antagonist
b. Fixator
c. Agonist
d. Synergist

16. Which neurotransmitter will stimulate contraction of skeletal muscle?
a. Acetylcholine
b. Gamma-aminobutyric acid (GABA)
c. Dopamine
d. Nitric oxide

17. All of the following may result from a disorder in calcium ion concentration EXCEPT:
a. Faster transmission of nerve impulses
b. Skeletal muscle weakness
c. Abnormal bleeding
d. Osteoporosis

18. Where do muscles that move the shoulder joint typically originate?
a. In the forearm
b. In the palm
c. On the trunk
d. On the carpals

19. Binding of calcium to the regulatory domain of which protein induces a conformational change which causes the active sites on actin to be exposed?
a. Tropomyosin
b. Myosin
c. Troponin
d. Meromyosin

20. During which phase of muscle contraction is the sarcoplasmic reticulum triggered to release calcium?
a. Latent phase
b. Contraction phase
c. Relaxation phase
d. Tetanus

21. Which type of muscle contraction is an example of an isometric contraction?
    a. Biceps curl
    b. Pushing against a wall
    c. Sitting in a chair
    d. Walking down the stairs
22. ALL of the following characterize cardiac muscle EXCEPT:
    a. T-tubules from dyads in the sarcoplasmic reticulum
    b. Contains parallel myofibrils
    c. Calcium binds to calmodulin to stimulate contraction
    d. Operates as a continuous, electrically coupled mass
23. A demyelination disorder that primarily impacts peripheral nerves would target which cells?
    a. Schwann cell
    b. Oligodendrocyte
    c. Astrocytes
    d. Neuron
24. During the relative refractory period, what can trigger an action potential?
    a. An action potential is not possible during this period
    b. A supra threshold stimulus
    c. A continuous stimulus
    d. A sub threshold stimulus
25. A subdural hematoma would occur between which two structures?
    a. Dura mater and arachnoid
    b. Dura mater and pia
    c. Arachnoid and pia
    d. Pia and the spinal cord
26. A lesion in the medulla would impact which cranial nerve?
    a. CN III
    b. CN IV
    c. CN VII
    d. CN XII
27. The area of the brain is responsible for coordinating and regulating skeletal muscle movement and equilibrium:
    a. Diencephalon
    b. Cerebellum
    c. Pons
    d. Medulla
28. Lesions to the prevertebral ganglia would interfere with the function of which organ?
    a. Stomach
    b. Heart
    c. Lungs
    d. Eye
29. An upper respiratory infection can spread via the eustachian tube from the nasopharynx to which anatomical space?
    a. Middle ear
    b. Inner ear
    c. External ear
    d. Middle cranial fossa
30. Cranial nerve VII is injured during an inferior alveolar nerve block that penetrates too deeply into the parotid gland. What would you expect to see as a consequence of this?
    a. Loss of somatic sensation on the posterior tongue
    b. Difficulty maintaining balance when walking
    c. Loss of taste sensation of the anterior tongue
    d. Loss of movement of facial muscles
31. A patient with acute pancreatitis is likely to have problems with:
    a. Digestion of proteins
    b. Digestion of fats
    c. Digestion of carbohydrates
    d. All of the above
32. All the following describe a steroid hormone EXCEPT:
    a. Can pass easily through plasma membranes
    b. Synthesized from amino acids
    c. Response time to steroid hormones is slow
    d. Must bind to a receptor
33. All of the following organs are targeted by tropic hormones produced in the hypothalamus EXCEPT:
    a. Ovaries
    b. Thyroid gland
    c. Pancreas
    d. Adrenal cortex
34. When palpating the thyroid gland on a patient, where would you expect to find the isthmus of the thyroid gland in a healthy individual?
    a. Between the hyoid bone and the thyroid cartilage
    b. Directly beneath the manubrium of the sternum
    c. Between the mandible and the hyoid bone
    d. Inferior to the cricoid cartilage
35. What is a major function of natural killer (NK) cells?
    a. Target virus-infected cells and tumor cells
    b. Phagocytize gram negative bacteria
    c. Secrete antibodies
    d. Help activate B cells
36. What is the corresponding effect on pressure in the alveolar and interpleural spaces as the volume of the thoracic cavity increases during inspiration?
    a. Alveolar pressure and intrapleural pressure both decrease
    b. Alveolar pressure and intrapleural pressure both increase
    c. Alveolar pressure and intrapleural pressure both equal atmospheric pressure
    d. Alveolar pressure increases but intrapleural pressure decreases
37. Metabolic alkalosis typically results in respiratory acidosis. The compensatory mechanism is hypoventilation.
    a. Both statements are TRUE
    b. Both statements are FALSE
    c. The first statement is TRUE; the second statement is FALSE
    d. The first statement is FALSE; the second statement is TRUE

## CASE B

Sharon is a 34-year-old woman who presents at the dental office for an initial dental exam and prophylaxis. Sharon suffers from severe asthma. In addition to her albuterol inhaler, her physician has prescribed prednisone, an oral corticosteroid, to combat airway inflammation resulting from asthma attacks. Sharon's current blood pressure is 130/85, pulse is 72 beats per minute, and respiration 16 breaths per minute. Further questioning reveals that the patient frequently experiences xerostomia after using her inhaler.

*Use Case B to answer questions 38 to 43.*

38. In the human body, where are naturally occurring corticosteroids produced?
    a. Adrenal cortex
    b. Adrenal medulla
    c. Anterior pituitary
    d. Posterior pituitary
39. Input from what structure stimulates the medullary inspiratory center to increase the length and depth of respiration?
    a. Medullary expiratory center
    b. Apneustic center
    c. Pneumotaxic center
    d. Respiratory pressor reflex
40. Sharon is having a hard time expelling air from her lungs during expiration. Which term refers to the total amount of air left in the airways after a normal, passive expiration?
    a. Vital capacity
    b. Total lung capacity
    c. Functional residual capacity
    d. Tidal volume
41. What is a direct physiological effect of an increase in partial pressure of carbon dioxide ($Pco_2$) in the arterial blood?
    a. Breathing rate increases (becomes faster)
    b. Heart rate decreases (becomes slower)
    c. Arterial chemoreceptors are inhibited
    d. Arterial baroreceptors increase firing
42. Which term refers to gas exchange between blood and the alveoli?
    a. Alveolar ventilation
    b. External respiration
    c. Internal respiration
    d. Perfusion
43. Which of the following BEST describes this patient's blood pressure?
    a. Blood pressure rate is considered prehypertensive, and she should be encouraged to see a physician
    b. Blood pressure rate is considered high, and she should be encouraged to see a physician
    c. Blood pressure rate is considered too high, and she should not receive dental treatment until seen by a physician
    d. Blood pressure is within normal limits

## CASE C

A 68-year-old man with a history of mild aortic stenosis presents for a dental hygiene appointment. He is on anticoagulant therapy and has a resting heart rate of 80 bpm. When reviewing his health history, the patient reveals that he often experiences fatigue and can also have chest pain and lightheadedness, on occasion.

*Use Case C to answer questions 44 to 49.*

44. If the aortic semilunar valve does not open properly, there is a decrease in the volume of blood that is ejected through the aorta. This has the most immediate consequences for which heart chamber?
    a. Right atrium
    b. Right ventricle
    c. Left atrium
    d. Left ventricle
45. When listening to the patient's heart with a stethoscope what does the second heart sound indicate?
    a. Opening of AV valves
    b. Closure of AV valves
    c. Opening of semilunar valves
    d. Closure of semilunar valves
46. The use of an anticoagulant would lead to which of the following:
    a. Increased aggregation of platelets
    b. Increased vitamin K synthesis
    c. Decreased fibrin formation
    d. Decreased red blood cell formation
47. Decreased blood volume leaving the aorta leads to reduced blood pressure in the vessels of the head and neck. Decreased blood pressure increases baroreceptor firing.
    a. Both statements are TRUE
    b. Both statements are FALSE
    c. The first statement is TRUE; the second statement is FALSE
    d. The first statement is FALSE; the second statement is TRUE
48. What specific prostaglandin regulates platelet aggregation?
    a. Prostaglandin A (PGA)
    b. Prostaglandin D (PGD)
    c. Prostaglandin E (PGE)
    d. Prostaglandin F (PGF)
49. Which class of immunoglobulin is the predominant antibody in external secretions of the mucous membranes?
    a. IgM
    b. IgG
    c. IgA
    d. IgE

## CASE D

After working as a dental hygienist for 35 years, Shirley's neck and shoulder pain has become nearly unbearable. She used to have better posture in the clinic, but as she's gotten older, she's noticed that her shoulders curve forward more and she slumps when she's working at the computer and driving. A recent visit to her physician revealed that she has herniated discs in her cervical and lumbar spine.

*Use Case D to answer questions 50 to 54*

50. Which system is involved in maintaining posture?
    a. Muscular system
    b. Nervous system
    c. Respiratory system
    d. All of the above are involved in maintaining posture*
51. What receptor initiates the sensation of pain?
    a. Meissner's corpuscles
    b. Nociceptors
    c. Ruffini's corpuscles
    d. Krause's end bulbs
52. A herniated disc in the cervical region may affect innervation to muscles of the upper limb. A herniated disc in the region of the L1-L2 part of the spinal cord may affect the femoral nerve.
    a. Both statements are TRUE

b. Both statements are FALSE
c. The first statement is TRUE; the second statement is FALSE
d. The first statement is FALSE; the second statement is TRUE

53. Which vertebrae have openings in their transverse processes for passage of the vertebral artery?
   a. Cervical vertebrae
   b. Thoracic vertebrae
   c. Lumbar vertebrae
   d. Sacral vertebrae
54. Which reflex arc involves involuntary contraction of skeletal muscle?
   a. Autonomic reflex
   b. Withdrawal reflex
   c. Somatic reflex
   d. Stretch reflex
55. What would the expected prothrombin time (PT) look like for a patient with poor liver function?
   a. Lower than normal
   b. Normal
   c. Higher than normal
   d. It would not be possible to obtain PT
56. Which of the following will stimulate secretion of gastric juice in the stomach?
   a. Cholecystokinin
   b. Presence of food in the duodenum
   c. Secretin
   d. Gastrin
57. Which of the following will result in increased urine production?
   a. ADH (antidiuretic hormone)
   b. Aldosterone
   c. ANP (atrial natriuretic peptide)
   d. All of the above result in increased urine production.
58. Glucose reabsorption occurs in which part of the nephron?
   a. Proximal convoluted tubule
   b. Loop of Henle
   c. Distal convoluted tubule
   d. Collecting ducts
59. Which structure is a reservoir for sperm and site of sperm maturation?
   a. Testis
   b. Epididymis
   c. Vas deferens
   d. Prostate gland
60. Hepatocytes in the liver are responsible for metabolism of drugs. The hepatic portal circulation bypasses the liver and brings blood directly to the inferior vena cava.
   a. Both statements are TRUE
   b. Both statements are FALSE
   c. The first statement is TRUE; the second statement is FALSE
   d. The first statement is FALSE; the second statement is TRUE

## SUGGESTED READINGS

Colbert BJ, Ankney JJ, Lee KT. *Anatomy & Physiology for Health Professions: An Interactive Journey*. ed 4. Pearson; 2019.

Patton KT, Thibodeau GA. *Structure and Function of the Body*. ed 16. Mosby; 2019.

Patton KT, Thibodeau GA, Swisher L. *Study Guide for Structure and Function of the Body*. ed 16. Mosby; 2019.

4

# Head and Neck Anatomy and Physiology

*Kim T. Isringhausen*

For the dental hygienist, knowledge of the skeletal, muscular, circulatory, endocrine, and nervous systems within the head and neck is essential for patient assessment and evaluation; radiologic examination and interpretation; identification of sources of infection and pathways of spread; and patient referral for abnormal findings. An understanding of the nervous system will facilitate treatment planning and safe and effective delivery of local anesthesia by the dental hygienist.

## ANATOMIC NOMENCLATURE

A. All references to body structures are made assuming the body is in anatomic position; *anatomic position* is the erect position of the body, feet together, with head, eyes, and palms facing forward (Fig. 4.1) (see the section on "Anatomical Nomenclature" in Chapter 3)
B. Planes—sections of the body divided by imaginary lines; the body may be sectioned in one of three planes: (see Fig. 4.1)
   1. Sagittal plane—a vertical plane that passes through the body from front to back; divides the body into right and left sections
      a. Median or midsagittal plane—a sagittal plane passing through the midline of the body from front to back; divides the body into equal right and left halves
   2. Frontal or coronal plane—a vertical plane passing through the body from one side to the other; divides the body into front (anterior) and back (posterior)
   3. Transverse or horizontal plane—a horizontal plane dividing the body into upper (superior) and lower (inferior) parts
C. Directional terms—used to describe the location of one body structure in relation to another
   1. Anterior or ventral—structures toward or at the front of the body; in front
   2. Posterior or dorsal—structures toward or at the back of the body; behind
   3. Tongue surfaces—the ventral surface of the tongue is the bottom surface, toward the belly; and the dorsal surface of the tongue is the top surface, toward the back when the tongue is upright in the mouth with the tip of the tongue touching the palate
   4. Medial—structures toward or at midline of the body; inner side (e.g., eyes)
   5. Lateral—structures away from the midline of the body; outer side (e.g., ears)
   6. Contralateral—structures on opposite sides of the body
   7. Superficial—structures located toward the body surface
   8. Deep—structures located away from the body surface
   9. Proximal—closer to the point of attachment of a limb to the body trunk; closer to the shoulder or hip (e.g., the elbow is proximal to the wrist)
   10. Distal—farther from the point of attachment of a limb to the body trunk; farther from the shoulder or hip (e.g., the ankle is distal to the knee)
   11. Superior or cranial—structures toward the head; upper
   12. Inferior or caudal—structures away from the head; lower
   13. Apex—the narrow end or tip of a conical structure

## OSTEOLOGY

A. Definition—the study of bones (see the section on "Skeletal System" in Chapter 3)
B. Classification—bones are classified on the basis of shape (each shape has a distinct function), pattern of development (membranous, cartilaginous, or mixed), region (axial or appendicular), and structure (arrangement of material, compact or spongy)
C. Function—bone supports organs and structures; protects the soft tissues and organs of the body; enables movement by providing attachments for muscles and ligaments; and is involved in mineral storage and blood cell formation
D. Histology of bone (see the section on "Connective Tissue" in Chapter 2)
   1. Intramembranous ossification—one of two processes resulting in bone formation, no cartilage is present; begins as a fibrous membrane of collagen and blood vessels; osteoblasts form a sponge-like network of bony processes (e.g., flat bones of the skull)
      a. Osteoblasts—bone-forming cells, deposit calcium for remodeling
      b. Osteoclasts—bone resorbing cells, break down bone by freeing calcium to initiate bone remodeling
      c. Osteocytes—mature bone cell embedded in bone matrix; maintain bone; most abundant cells

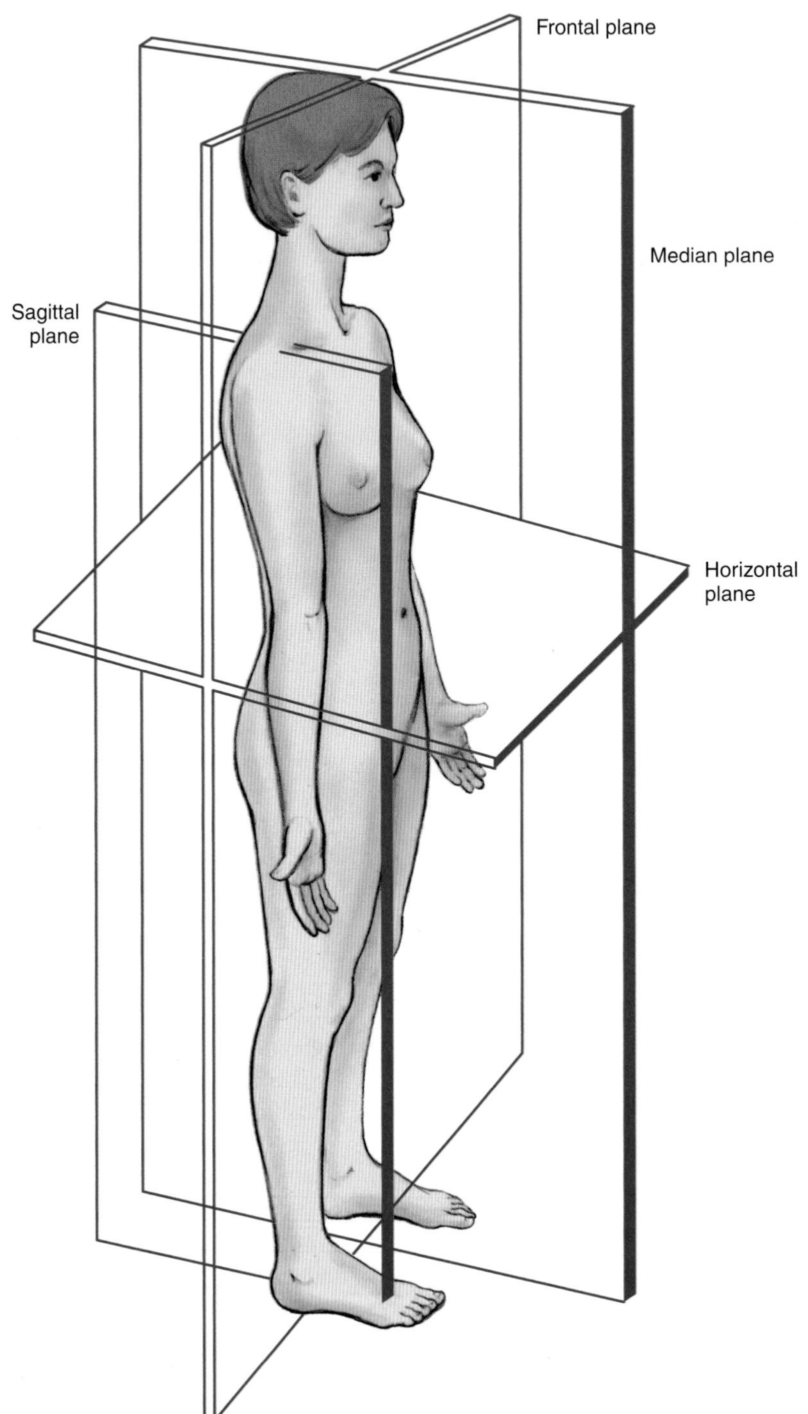


**Fig. 4.1** Body in anatomic position with median, sagittal, horizontal, and frontal planes noted. (From Fehrenbach M, Herring S. *Illustrated Anatomy of the Head and Neck*. 5th ed. St. Louis: Elsevier; 2017.)

2. Endochondral ossification— one of two processes resulting in bone formation; cartilage is present as a precursor; cartilage is gradually replaced by bone produced by osteoblasts (e.g., long bones)
3. Cartilage—noncalcified, avascular, pliable connective tissue; three types of cartilage:
   a. Hyaline cartilage—most abundant, precursor to bone, facilitates smooth movement at joints
   b. Fibrocartilage—strongest, contains collagen fibers in its matrix, provides rigidity (e.g., intervertebral discs)
   c. Elastic cartilage—contains elastic fibers in its matrix; provides support and defines shape (e.g., external ear)

E. Descriptive terminology
   1. Bony prominences—an area where bone is immediately below the skin surface; usually landmarks for the attachment of muscles, ligaments, and tendons; *process* is a general term used to describe any prominence on the bony surface
      a. Condyle—a rounded articular process; forms joints
      b. Tuberosity—a large, rough, rounded process on the surface of bone for the attachment of connective tissue

c. Tubercle or eminence—a small, rough, rounded process on the surface of bone for the attachment of connective tissue
d. Arch—a bridge-like bony structure
e. Cornu (plural, cornua)—a horn-like prominence
f. Crest—a raised, prominent border or ridge; attachment for connective tissue, usually muscle
g. Spine—a sharp, slender projection; higher than a crest; often a site for muscle attachment
2. Bony depressions—on the surface of bones; provide for the passage of blood vessels and other soft tissue
a. Notch—an indentation at the edge of the bone; an articulatory surface
b. Sulcus (plural, sulci)—a channel-like, shallow depression or groove that usually accommodates a blood vessel, nerve, or tendon
c. Fossa (plural, fossae)—a deeper depression on a bone surface, basin-like; can be an area for muscle attachment or articulating bone
d. Sinus—a cavity within a bone
3. Bony openings—occur primarily where blood vessels and nerves pass into or through the bone
a. Foramen (plural, foramina)—a short, window-like opening in a bone; round hole (e.g., incisive foramen)
b. Canal—a longer, tube-like opening in a bone (e.g., mandibular canal)
c. Meatus—a type of canal or channel within the bone (e.g., internal acoustic meatus)
d. Fissure—a narrow, slit-like opening between adjacent parts of bones forming a passageway for blood vessels and nerves (e.g., superior orbital fissure)
4. Skeletal articulations—connections between bones that may be movable or immovable
a. Joints—articulation classified by the amount of movement allowed (e.g., immovable, slightly movable, free); the temporomandibular joint (TMJ) is the only movable joint in the skull
b. Sutures—fibrous joints found on the skull where bones are held together, immovable

## Axial Skeleton: Skull

Bones of the head are grouped into two categories—cranial bones and facial bones.

A. Cranial bones, or neurocranium (eight bones)—bones that surround the brain; four singular bones, two paired bones
1. Frontal bone (single bone) (Fig. 4.2)
a. Forms the forehead and the top portion of the orbits
b. Contains the frontal sinuses
c. Supraorbital ridges form the roof of the orbits
d. Articulates with many of the cranial and facial bones; articulation with the parietal bones forms the coronal suture
e. Landmarks include the supraorbital notch, the zygomatic process of the frontal bone, and the lacrimal fossa, which contains the tear-producing lacrimal gland
2. Parietal bones (paired bones) (see Fig. 4.2)
a. Constitute a large part of the vault and sides of the cranium
b. Articulate with each other at the sagittal suture and with various bones to form the coronal, lambdoidal, and squamosal sutures of the skull
3. Temporal bones (paired bones) (see Fig. 4.2)
a. Form the lateral walls of the skull
b. Articulate on each side of the skull with the zygomatic and parietal bones, the sphenoid and occipital bones, and the mandible
c. Divided into three portions:
(1) Squamous portion—largest portion; forms the zygomatic process of the temporal bone, which is a portion of the zygomatic arch; the zygomatic process contains the articular (mandibular) fossa and articular eminence, which articulate with the mandible; this area also forms the cranial portion of the TMJ
(2) Tympanic portion—forms most of the external acoustic meatus; it is separated from the petrous portion by the petrotympanic fissure, through which the chorda tympani nerve emerges
(3) Petrous portion—located inferiorly; contains the mastoid process that serves as an attachment for the sternocleidomastoid muscle; other landmarks include the styloid process, stylomastoid foramen, jugular notch, and internal acoustic meatus (exit for the facial nerve)
4. Occipital bone (single bone) (see Fig. 4.2)
a. Forms the posterior portion of the skull
b. Articulates with the parietal bones to form the lambdoidal suture and temporal and sphenoid bones
c. Foramen magnum is formed completely by occipital bone
d. Jugular notches on both the occipital and the temporal bones form the jugular foramen (Fig. 4.3)
e. Occipital condyles on each side form a movable articulation with the first cervical vertebrae (atlas)
f. Occipital bone has paired hypoglossal canals that are openings for cranial nerve (CN) XII (see Fig. 4.3)
5. Sphenoid bone (single bone) (see Figs 4.2 and 4.3)
a. Articulates with the frontal, parietal, ethmoid, temporal, zygomatic, maxillary, palatine, vomer, and occipital bones
b. Body of the sphenoid bone contains the sphenoid sinuses and the sella turcica, the seat of the pituitary gland, which supplies numerous hormones to the body
c. Three paired processes: lesser wing of the sphenoid bone, greater wing of the sphenoid bone, and the pterygoid processes
d. Lesser sphenoid wings—anterior process
(1) Forms the top of the superior orbital fissure
(2) Optic foramen—entrance point of CN II
e. Greater sphenoid wings—lateral projections in the temporal area
(1) Forms the inferior border of the superior orbital fissure

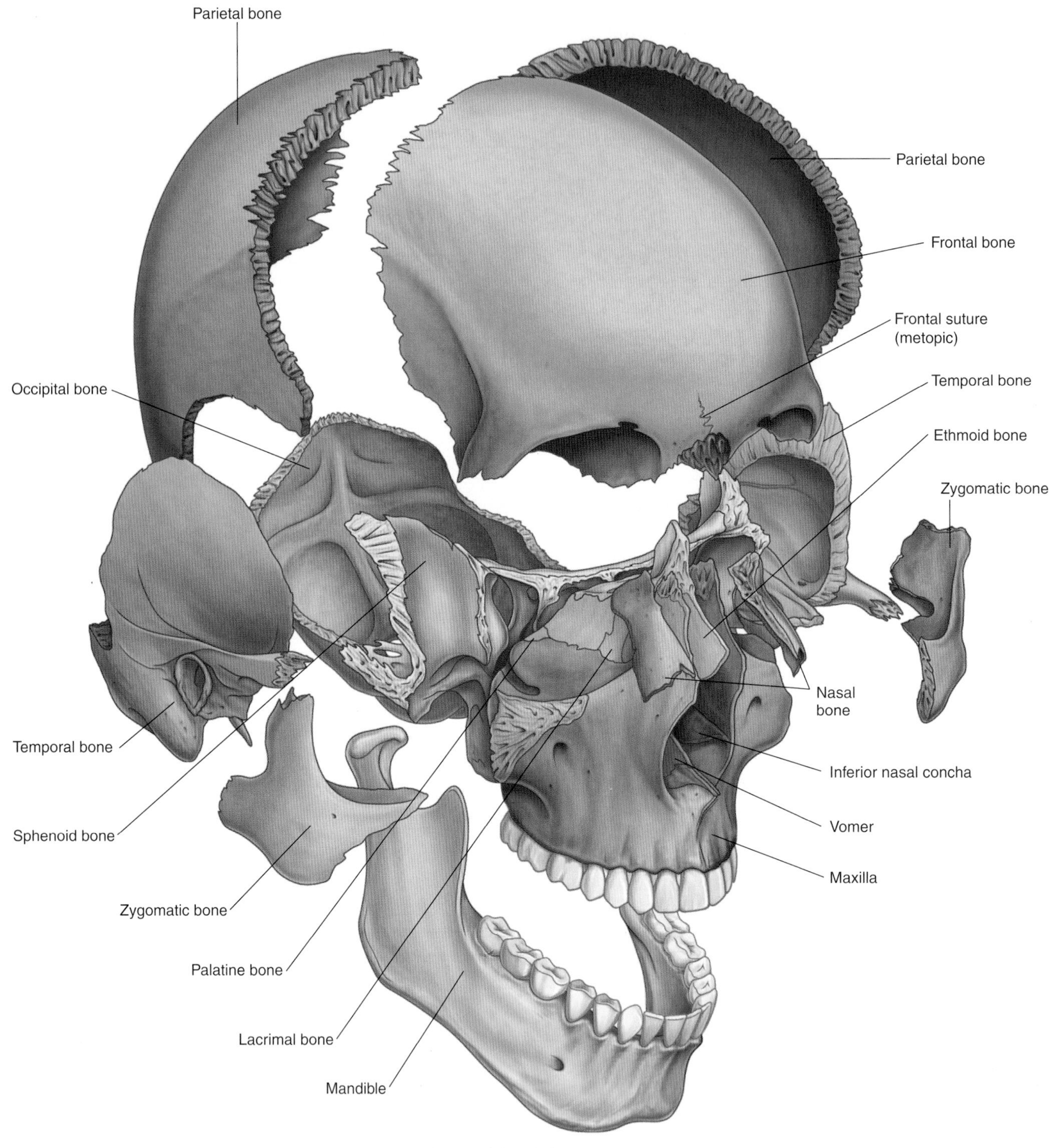


**Fig. 4.2** Bones of the skull, exploded view. (From Brand RW, Isselhard DE. *Anatomy of Orofacial Structures*. 8th ed. St. Louis: Elsevier; 2019.)

(2) Infratemporal crest—union of the temporal and infratemporal surfaces
(3) Foramen rotundum—maxillary division of CN V (see Fig. 4.3)
(4) Foramen ovale—mandibular division of CN V (see Fig. 4.3)
(5) Foramen spinosum—opening that gives passage to the middle meningeal artery (see Fig. 4.3)
(6) Superior orbital fissure—a cleft between the lesser and greater wings; transmits CNs III, IV, and VI and the ophthalmic division of CN V (see Fig. 4.3)

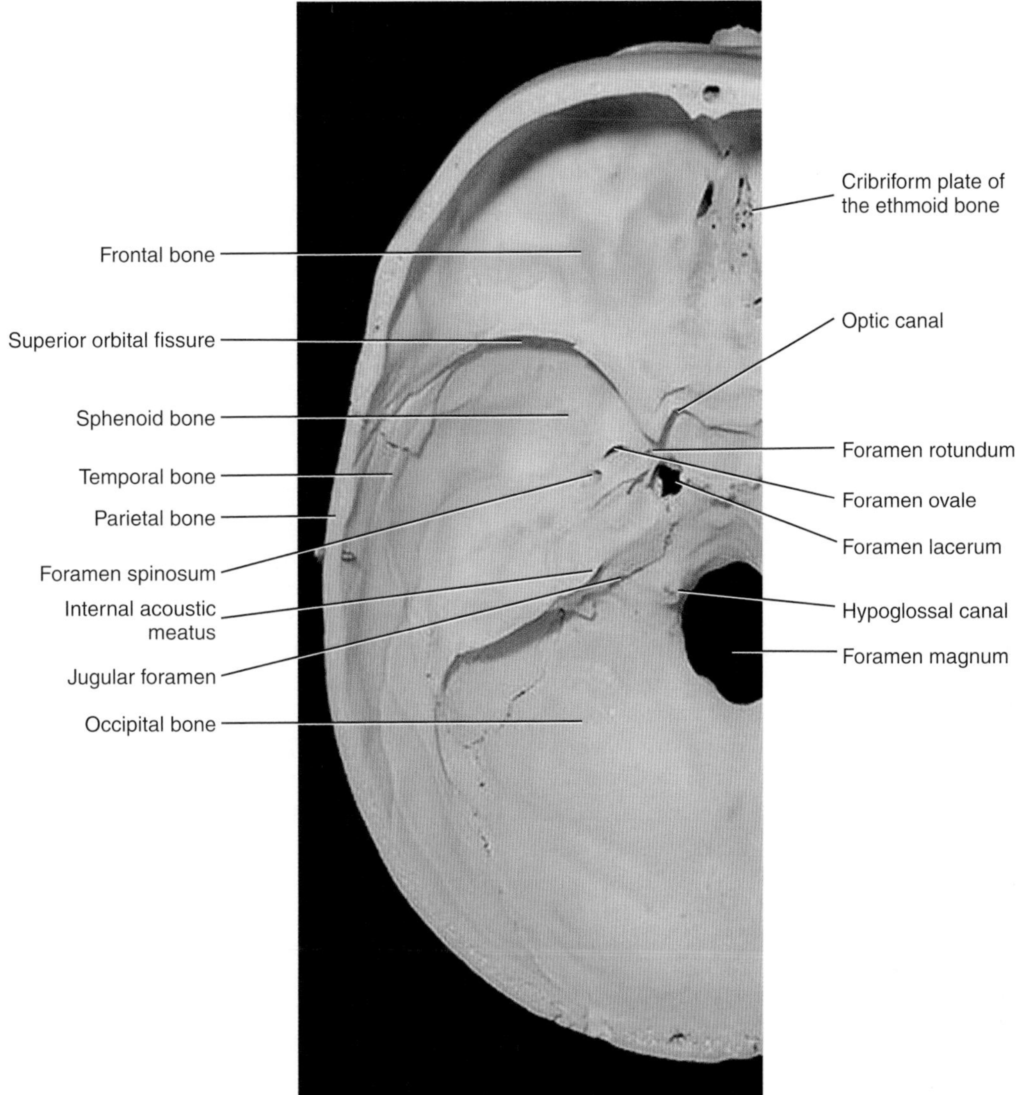


**Fig. 4.3** Superior view of the internal surface of the skull with its foramina and associated structures. (From Fehrenbach M, Herring S. *Illustrated Anatomy of the Head and Neck*. 5th ed. St. Louis: Elsevier; 2017.)

f. Pterygoid process—long process projecting downward from the junction of the body and greater wing of the sphenoid bone; formed by two plates
   (1) Medial and lateral pterygoid plates—attachment points for pterygoid muscles
   (2) Pterygoid fossa—formed by divergence of the medial and lateral pterygoid plates
   (3) Hamulus—inferior termination of the medial pterygoid plate; also provides attachment for a tendon of the soft palate

6. Ethmoid bone (single bone) (see Fig. 4.2)
   a. Single midline bone of the skull, anterior to the sphenoid
   b. Articulates with the sphenoid, frontal, lacrimal, and maxillary bones; joins the vomer inferoposteriorly
   c. Contains ethmoid sinuses
   d. Cribriform plate—horizontal plate with numerous openings for passage of olfactory nerves (see Fig. 4.3)
   e. Crista galli—midline process of the ethmoid bone that serves as an attachment for the dura mater (meninges) of the brain
   f. Perpendicular plate—projects downward from the crista galli, assists in forming the nasal septum
   g. Superior and middle nasal conchae—located laterally in the nasal cavity; part of ethmoidal labyrinth; protect olfactory bulb and buffer sinuses

B. Facial bones, or viscerocranium (14 bones)— surround the face; two singular bones, six paired bones
   1. Inferior nasal conchae (paired bones) (see Fig. 4.2)
      a. Arise from the maxilla horizontally into the nasal cavity
      b. Responsible for airflow direction, humidification, and heating and filtering of inhaled air
   2. Nasal bones (paired bones) (see Fig. 4.2)
      a. Form the bridge of the nose, articulating with each other
      b. Articulate with the maxillae, and the frontal and ethmoid bones

3. Lacrimal bones (paired bones) (see Fig. 4.2)
   a. Thin bones that form part of the medial wall of the orbit of the eye
   b. The nasolacrimal duct is located at the junction of the lacrimal and maxillary bones
   c. Fluid (tears) from the lacrimal gland is drained through this duct into the inferior nasal meatus
4. Zygomatic bones (paired bones) (see Fig. 4.2)
   a. Zygomatic arch (cheekbone)—composed of the temporal process of the zygomatic bone and the zygomatic process of the temporal bone
   b. Three processes are named for the bones with which the zygomatic bones articulate: frontal process, maxillary process, and temporal process
5. Maxillae (paired bones)—fused; each has a body and four processes (see Fig. 4.2)
   a. The body contains the maxillary sinus and forms the lower and medial rims of the orbits and the borders of the nasal cavity; other landmarks are:
      (1) Infraorbital (IO) foramen—originates as the inferior orbital fissure and becomes the IO canal that carries the IO nerve, the inferior ophthalmic vein, and the IO artery; it is a landmark for the administration of local anesthesia (IO nerve block) to achieve facial/pulpal anesthesia to the maxillary premolars, canines, and incisors
      (2) Canine fossa—inferior to the IO foramen and distal to the roots of the maxillary canines
   b. The frontal process articulates with the frontal bone, forming the medial orbital rim with the lacrimal bone
   c. The alveolar process (see the section on “Supporting Tissues” in Chapter 2)
      (1) Less dense bone containing the roots of the maxillary teeth; thinner facially; less dense than mandibular alveolar process, making infiltration of local anesthesia more successful; may resorb completely in edentulous arch
      (2) Sockets (alveoli) for maxillary teeth
      (3) Canine eminence—a protuberance over the root of the maxillary canine
      (4) Maxillary tuberosity— a soft tissue depression distal to the last maxillary molar; contains foramina for the passage of the posterior superior alveolar (PSA) nerve; it is a landmark for the administration of local anesthesia (PSA nerve block) to achieve buccal/pulpal anesthesia for the maxillary molar teeth
   d. Zygomatic process
      (1) Articulates with the zygomatic bone
      (2) Completes the IO rim
   e. Palatine processes
      (1) Articulate with each other to form the anterior, major portion of the hard palate and the median palatine suture
      (2) Contains the incisive foramen, a landmark for the administration of local anesthesia (nasopalatine [NP] nerve block) to the lingual of maxillary canines and incisors
6. Palatine bones (paired bones)
   a. The horizontal plates of the palatine bones articulate with each other to form the posterior portion of the hard palate
   b. Articulate with the maxillary and sphenoid bones
   c. The vertical plates form part of the lateral walls of the nasal cavity and a small part of the orbital apex
   d. Contain the greater palatine (GP) foramen, located at the apex of the maxillary second or third molar, a landmark for the administration of local anesthetic agent (GP nerve block) to palatal soft tissues distal to the canine
7. Vomer (single bone)
   a. Located in the midsagittal line; forms the posterior portion of the nasal septum
8. Mandible (single bone) (see Fig. 4.2)
   a. Largest, strongest, and only movable facial bone; articulates with the temporal bones on both sides
   b. Body—curved, horizontal portion with two surfaces and two borders; landmarks include:
      (1) Mental protuberance—the chin
      (2) Symphysis—midline, faint ridge formed by fusion
      (3) Alveolar process of the mandible—contains roots of mandibular teeth; less dense around mandibular incisors than posterior molars, allowing for improved infiltration of local anesthetic to anterior teeth; may resorb completely in edentulous arch
      (4) Sockets (alveoli)—for mandibular teeth
      (5) Mental foramen—located bilaterally on the external surface, below and between the first and second premolars; the landmark for the administration of local anesthesia (mental nerve block) to facial periodontium of mandibular premolars and incisors; also important landmark on radiographs, not to be confused with periapical or other lesions
      (6) Genial tubercles—near the midline on the internal surface, provide points of muscle attachment
      (7) Retromolar triangle—distal to the last mandibular molar
      (8) Sublingual and submandibular fossae—shallow depressions on the internal surface, these fossae contain their corresponding salivary glands (Fig. 4.4)
   c. Ramus—extends vertically and backward from the body of the mandible
      (1) External oblique line—a crest on the external surface where the ramus joins the body of the mandible
      (2) Mandibular foramen—located bilaterally on the internal surface; forms the opening of the mandibular canal and the exit for blood vessels and the inferior alveolar (IA) nerve; the landmark for the administration of local anesthesia (IA nerve block) to the lingual periodontium and pulp of mandibular teeth, and the facial periodontium of mandibular anterior and premolar teeth (see Fig. 4.4)
      (3) Condyle—articulates with temporal bone, forming the movable part of the TMJ

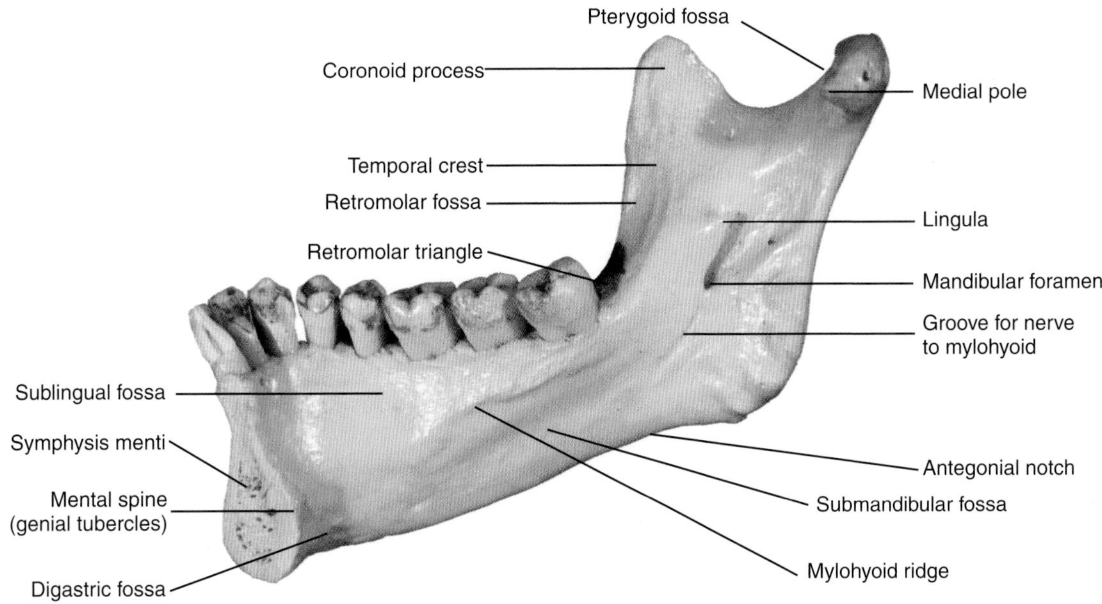


**Fig. 4.4** Medial view of the mandible. (From Brand RW, Isselhard DE, Erdman K. *Anatomy of Orofacial Structures: A Comprehensive Approach*. 8th ed. St. Louis: Elsevier, Inc.; 2019.)

(4) Lingula—a sharp bony spine overlapping the mandibular foramen, giving attachment to the sphenomandibular ligament
(5) Coronoid process—the superior margin, which forms the anterior border of the ramus and provides points of muscle attachment
(6) Coronoid notch—greatest concavity on the anterior border of the ramus; landmark for determining height of injection for the IA nerve block
(7) Mandibular notch—concave area between the condyle and the coronoid process

C. Neck bones
1. Hyoid bone—U-shaped bone suspended in the neck; located superior and anterior to the thyroid cartilage; paired projections are the greater and lesser cornua for the attachment for many muscles and ligaments of the tongue and throat
2. Atlas—first cervical vertebra; its lateral masses articulate superiorly with the occipital condyles of the skull and inferiorly with the axis
3. Axis—second cervical vertebra; along with the atlas, the axis provides attachment points for many muscles responsible for the movement of the head

## PARANASAL SINUSES

A. Air-filled, mucus-lined cavities in the bones of the skull that function to lighten the weight of the skull and act as sound resonators; the four paired sinuses are:
1. Frontal sinuses—frontal bone above the nasal cavity; drain into the middle nasal meatus
2. Sphenoid sinuses—body of sphenoid bone; drain into the superior nasal meatus
3. Ethmoid sinuses—small compartments in ethmoid bone: anterior and middle compartments drain into the middle meatus; posterior compartment drains into the superior meatus of the nasal cavity
4. Maxillary sinuses—largest, pyramid shaped, drain into the middle meatus; infection and diseases of these sinuses can cause complications of the maxillary posterior teeth

## THE MUSCULAR SYSTEM

A. Descriptive terminology (see the section on "Muscle Tissue" in Chapter 2)
1. Muscle tissue, one of the four classifications of body tissue, consists of specialized fibers for contraction; three types of muscle tissue are skeletal (voluntary), cardiac (involuntary), and smooth (involuntary); muscles in the head and neck region are skeletal muscles
2. Movement—muscles are under neural control to shorten or contract; contraction is the action of the muscle fibers
3. Origin—origin of a muscle is bone; less movable structure (e.g., sternocleidomastoid muscle originates on the clavicle and sternum)
4. Insertion—the structure muscle attaches to and tends to be moved by the contraction of the muscle (e.g., tendon); more movable structure; during muscle contraction the insertion moves toward the origin (e.g., sternocleidomastoid muscle inserts on the mastoid process of the temporal bone; when contracted, the head bends to the side)

B. Muscles of facial expression—most facial muscles are superficial, paired muscles originating in bone and inserting into skin; responsible for functions related to speech, emotional expression, and mastication; innervated by the seventh cranial, or facial, nerve; damage to this nerve results in facial paralysis (Fig. 4.5)

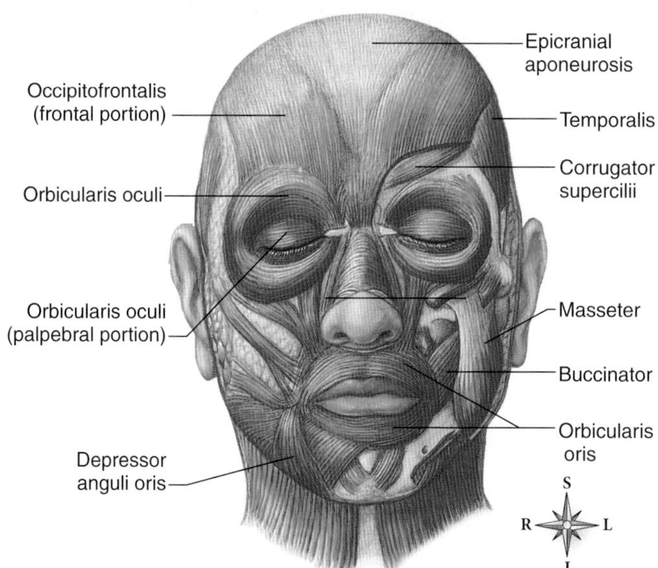


**Fig. 4.5** Muscles of facial expression. (From Patton K. Anatomy & Physiology. 10th ed. St. Louis: Elsevier, Inc.; 2019.)

1. Epicranial muscle—scalp region; composed of two bellies, the frontal and occipital, which are connected by the epicranial aponeurosis; raise the eyebrows and scalp when a person shows surprise
2. Orbicularis oculi muscle—surrounds the eye; closes the eyelid
3. Corrugator supercilii muscle—superior to the orbicularis; wrinkles the forehead when a person frowns
4. Orbicularis oris muscle—encircles the mouth; closes lips
5. Buccinator muscle—anterior part of the cheek; functions to pull the mouth laterally, thereby shortening the cheek, and as an aid in keeping food on the chewing surfaces of the teeth
6. Risorius muscle—mouth region; widens mouth when a person smiles broadly
7. Levator labii superioris muscle—upper lip; raises the upper lip
8. Levator labii superioris alaeque nasi muscle—upper lip; raises the upper lip and dilates the nose, as in sneering
9. Zygomaticus minor muscle—upper lip; raises the upper lip
10. Zygomaticus major muscle—angle of the upper lip; pulls the angle of the upper lip laterally, creating the appearance of a smile
11. Levator anguli oris muscle—angle of the mouth; elevates the angle of the mouth, as in smiling
12. Depressor anguli oris muscle—angle of the mouth; depresses the angle of the mouth, as when frowning
13. Depressor labii inferioris muscle—lower lip; lowers the lower lip to expose lower mandibular incisors
14. Mentalis muscle—chin area; raises the chin, narrows the vestibule near mandibular incisors
15. Platysma muscle—neck region; originates in the clavicle fascia and inserts in the region of the mandible and facial muscles of the mouth; pulls down the corners of the mouth, raises the skin of the neck

C. Muscles of mastication—four paired muscles, all inserting on the mandible; innervated by the mandibular division of the fifth cranial, or trigeminal, nerve; they are responsible for movement of the jaw: depression, elevation, protrusion, retraction, and lateral deviation (Table 4.1)
   1. Masseter muscle—most superficial, largest, and strongest of the four muscles
      a. Originates on the zygomatic arch; originates from two heads, one superficial and one deep, and inserts on the lateral surface of the angle of the mandible
      b. Action—elevates the mandible, raising the lower jaw during closing
   2. Temporalis muscle
      a. Originates from a fan-like attachment on the temporal fossa; inserts on the coronoid process of the mandible
      b. Action—when the entire muscle contracts, it elevates the mandible, raising the jaw; contraction of only the posterior portion causes retraction of the mandible
   3. Medial (internal) pterygoid muscle (Fig. 4.6)
      a. Originates from two heads: the superficial head arises from the maxillary tuberosity; the deep head from the medial surface of the pterygoid plate of the sphenoid bone; inserts on the medial surface of the angle of the mandible
      b. Action—elevates the mandible, raising the lower jaw
   4. Lateral (external) pterygoid muscle; lies within the infratemporal fossa (see Fig. 4.6)
      a. Originates from two heads: the superior head originates from the infratemporal crest of the greater

**TABLE 4.1 Muscles of Mastication**

| Muscle | Origin | Insertion | Action |
|---|---|---|---|
| Masseter | Inferior border of zygomatic arch | Lateral surface angle of mandible | Elevates mandible |
| Temporalis | Temporal fossa | Coronoid process of mandible | Elevates mandible, retracts mandible |
| Medial Pterygoid | Lateral pterygoid plate and fossa, and maxillary tuberosity | Medial surface angle of mandible | Elevates the mandible |
| Lateral Pterygoid | Infratemporal crest and lateral pterygoid plate | Anterior border of TMJ and neck of mandibular condyle | Protrudes and depresses mandible, lateral excursion |

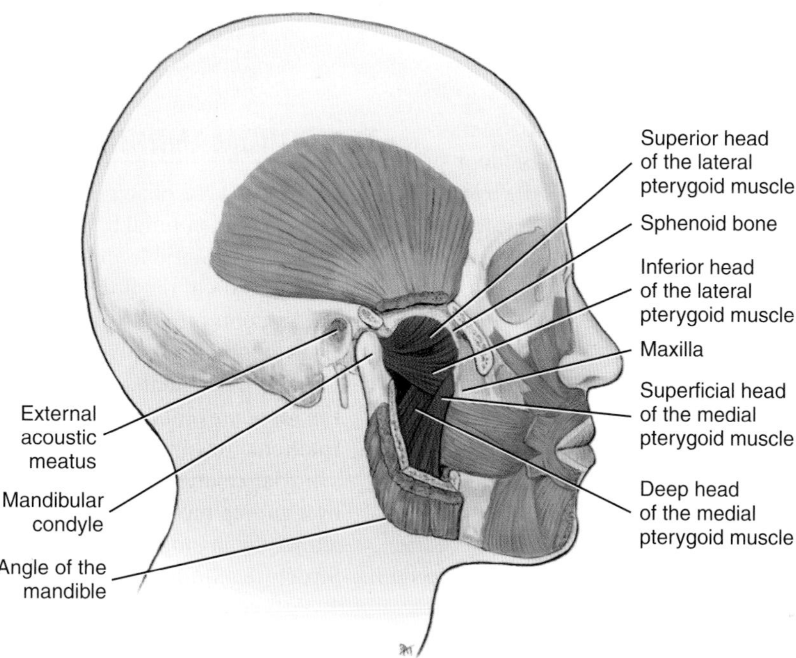


**Fig. 4.6** Origin and insertion of both the medial pterygoid muscle and lateral pterygoid muscle with both heads of each muscle highlighted. Note that the inferior part of temporalis muscle, zygomatic arch, and most of the mandibular ramus have been removed. (From Fehrenbach M, Herring S. *Illustrated Anatomy of the Head and Neck*. 5th ed. St. Louis: Elsevier; 2017.)

wing of the sphenoid bone; the inferior head originates from the lateral surface of the pterygoid plate of the sphenoid bone; both heads run horizontally to insert on the anterior neck of the mandibular condyle, and the anterior border of the TMJ

b. Action—both heads working together protrude the mandible, which occurs during opening; when only one side is contracted, the jaw shifts to the opposite side, causing lateral deviation of the mandible; lateral pterygoid is the only muscle of mastication that depresses the mandible

D. Cervical muscles—superficial, paired, large, easily palpated muscles

1. Sternocleidomastoid muscle—large, well-defined muscle; important landmark for palpating lymph nodes
   a. Originates from the clavicle and sternum; inserts on the mastoid processes of the temporal bone
   b. Action—contraction of one side makes the head bend to the same side, turning the face to the opposite side; contraction of both muscles causes the head to flex forward
   c. Innervated by CN XI (accessory nerve)
2. Trapezius muscle—broad, superficial muscles covering lateral and posterior surfaces of the neck
   a. Originates from the occipital bone and the cervical and thoracic vertebrae; inserts on the clavicle and the scapula
   b. Action—lifts the clavicle and scapula, as when shrugging shoulders
   c. Innervated by CN XI (accessory nerve) and third and fourth cervical nerves

E. Hyoid muscles—all are attached to the hyoid bone; usually grouped as suprahyoid or infrahyoid muscles, depending on their relationship to the hyoid; aid in mastication and swallowing

1. Suprahyoid muscle group—located superior to the hyoid; act to raise the hyoid and the larynx during swallowing and depress the mandible during mastication
   a. Digastric muscle
      (1) Two separate bellies—anterior belly originates from the intermediate tendon on the hyoid bone and inserts near the symphysis of the mandible; posterior belly originates from the mastoid notch and inserts on the intermediate tendon of the hyoid; form the submandibular triangles and submental triangle
      (2) Action—pulls the jaw back; anteriorly innervated by the mylohyoid nerve and posteriorly by the posterior digastric nerve
   b. Mylohyoid muscle
      (1) Originates from the inner surface of the mandible; unites with counterpart to form the floor of the mouth, and inserts on the body of the hyoid
      (2) Action—depresses mandible, helps elevate the tongue; innervated by the mylohyoid nerve, a division of CN V (trigeminal nerve)
   c. Stylohyoid muscle
      (1) Originates from the styloid process; inserts on the body of the hyoid; innervated by the stylohyoid branch of the seventh cranial, or facial, nerve
   d. Geniohyoid muscle
      (1) Originates from the genial tubercles on the mandible; inserts into the body of the hyoid
      (2) Innervated by CN XII (hypoglossal nerve)
2. Infrahyoid muscle group—act to depress the hyoid bone; all muscles in the group innervated by the second and third cervical nerves
   a. Sternothyroid muscle
      (1) Originates on the sternum; inserts on the thyroid cartilage
      (2) Depresses the thyroid cartilage and the larynx (but not the hyoid)
   b. Sternohyoid muscle
      (1) Originates on the sternum; inserts on the body of the hyoid
   c. Omohyoid muscle
      (1) Two separate bellies—inferior belly originates from the scapula and attaches to the tendon of the superior belly, which is the origin of the superior belly that inserts on the body of the hyoid
   d. Thyrohyoid muscle
      (1) Originates on the thyroid cartilage; inserts on the body and greater cornu of the hyoid
      (2) Raises the thyroid cartilage and larynx in addition to depressing the hyoid

F. Muscles of the tongue—all are innervated by CN XII (hypoglossal nerve); aid in speech, mastication, and swallowing; grouped into intrinsic and extrinsic muscles
1. Intrinsic tongue muscles
   a. Located entirely within the tongue; include the superior longitudinal, transverse, vertical, and inferior longitudinal muscles; considered by some to be one muscle; act together to change the shape of the tongue
2. Extrinsic tongue muscles
   a. All insert inside the tongue but originate elsewhere; their names indicate their origin; these muscles move the tongue
      (1) Genioglossus muscle—acts in the protrusion of the tongue, helps prevent airway obstruction; originates from the genial tubercles
      (2) Styloglossus muscle—acts in the retraction of the tongue; originates from the styloid process of the temporal bone
      (3) Hyoglossus muscle—depresses the tongue; originates on areas of the hyoid bone

## TEMPOROMANDIBULAR JOINT (TMJ)

A. Description—a bilateral articulation between the articular fossa of the temporal bones (immovable) and condylar process of the mandible (movable); innervated by the mandibular division of the fifth cranial, or trigeminal, nerve; blood supply comes from the external carotid artery
B. Type of joint—a synovial joint by structure
C. Type of movement—orientation of mandibular condyle in the fossa prevents complete opening (depression); first is a rotational or hinge movement of the condyles in the lower synovial cavities to partially open the mandible, followed by a gliding movement in the upper synovial cavities which allows the mandible to open fully
D. Structure of joint (Fig. 4.7)
   1. Articular (joint) capsule—completely surrounds the TMJ
   2. Articular (joint) disc—a fibrous disc that divides the synovial cavity of the TMJ into superior and inferior synovial cavities; both cavities are filled with synovial fluid secreted by the articular capsule; perforation or displacement can cause TMJ problems

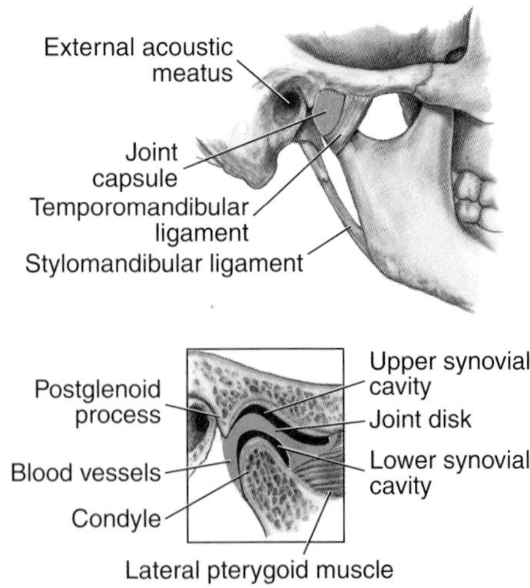


**Fig. 4.7** View of the temporomandibular joint depicting upper and lower synovial cavities and the joint disk. (From Avery JK, Chiego DJ. *Essentials of Oral Histology and Embryology: A Clinical Approach.* 5th ed. St. Louis: Mosby; 2018.)

3. TMJ ligament—located laterally on each joint, extending from the zygomatic arch to the posterior neck of the condyle; prevents posterior and inferior displacement of the mandible
4. Sphenomandibular ligament—located medially; extends from the spine of the sphenoid to the lingula of the mandible; the IA nerve is located in the space between the mandibular ramus and the sphenomandibular ligament, making it an important landmark for the administration of the IA nerve block
5. Stylomandibular ligament—located medially; runs from the styloid process of the temporal bone to the angle of the mandible; also assists in stabilizing the jaw; separates the submandibular salivary and parotid glands

## THE CIRCULATORY SYSTEM

A. Classification and function
   1. Blood is classified as connective tissue and consists of two main components, plasma and formed elements (blood cells and platelets)
   2. Three main functions of blood: (see the section on "Blood and Lymph" in Chapter 2)
      a. Transportation—transports gases (oxygen [$O_2$] and carbon dioxide [$CO_2$]), nutrients, waste products of metabolism, hormones, and heat to the skin for maintenance of body temperature
      b. Regulation—sustains the pH of the body; maintains fluid balance
      c. Protection—defends the body against infections and blood loss
B. Four components of blood (see the section on "Blood and Lymph" in Chapter 2)
   1. Plasma—liquid portion of blood; consists of 90% water, the remaining mixture comprises proteins, glucose, hormones, and electrolytes; makes up more than half the total volume of blood
   2. Erythrocytes—red blood cells (RBCs) lack nuclei and have a biconcave shape; produce hemoglobin, which functions to transport $O_2$ from the lungs to body tissues in exchange for $CO_2$; then delivered to the lungs
   3. Leukocytes—white blood cells (WBCs); much less numerous than RBCs; protect the body against infections
      a. Granulocytes—contain granules in their cytoplasm
         (1) Neutrophils are the first to respond to bacterial invasion; fight infection by the digesting bacteria (phagocytosis) and releasing enzymes that destroy bacteria; make up the majority of leukocytes
         (2) Eosinophils function in the destruction of allergens and release enzymes that destroy parasites
         (3) Basophils secrete histamine and heparin in allergic reactions, intensifying inflammatory reactions
      b. Agranulocytes—lack granules in their cytoplasm
         (1) Lymphocytes produce antibodies and provide immune response; second most abundant leukocyte
         (2) Monocytes reach sites of infection after neutrophils and can phagocytize more microbes than neutrophils; clean up cellular debris after an infection
   4. Platelets—thrombocytes; cell fragments that participate in blood clotting
C. Vascular system
   1. Arteries carry blood, typically oxygenated, away from the heart to arterioles and capillaries, which supply blood directly to the tissue
   2. Venules (smaller veins that drain capillaries) and veins carry blood, typically deoxygenated, to the heart
   3. Arteries supply blood to all structures in their surrounding vicinity, and veins drain blood from all their regional structures
D. Descriptive terminology
   1. Anastomosis—connection between vessels by channels
   2. Arteriole—smaller artery that connects with a capillary
   3. Capillary—smaller blood vessel branching off an arteriole to supply blood directly to tissue
   4. Plexus—a congregation of multiple veins
   5. Venous sinus—blood-filled space between two layers of tissue
E. Arterial blood supply to the head and neck
   1. Common carotid and subclavian arteries supply the head and neck; pathways from the aorta to the head and neck differ on the right and left sides:
      a. Right side of the body—the right common carotid and right subclavian arteries arise from the brachiocephalic artery
      b. Left side of the body—the left common carotid and left subclavian arteries ascend directly from the aorta
      c. The subclavian artery terminates in the upper arm extremity
   2. Each common carotid artery ends by dividing into the internal carotid and external carotid arteries (Fig. 4.8)
      a. Internal carotid artery—enters the skull to the brain area
      b. External carotid artery—supplies the principal areas of the oral cavity and face
      c. Carotid sinus—just before the common carotid artery bifurcates; a swelling; most reliable arterial pulse in the body
   3. Anterior branches of the external carotid artery (see Fig. 4.8)
      a. Lingual artery—runs above the hyoid bone; supplies the floor of the mouth, the tongue, and the suprahyoid muscles; gives rise to the sublingual artery, which supplies the mylohyoid muscle, sublingual salivary gland, and mucous membranes of the floor of the mouth

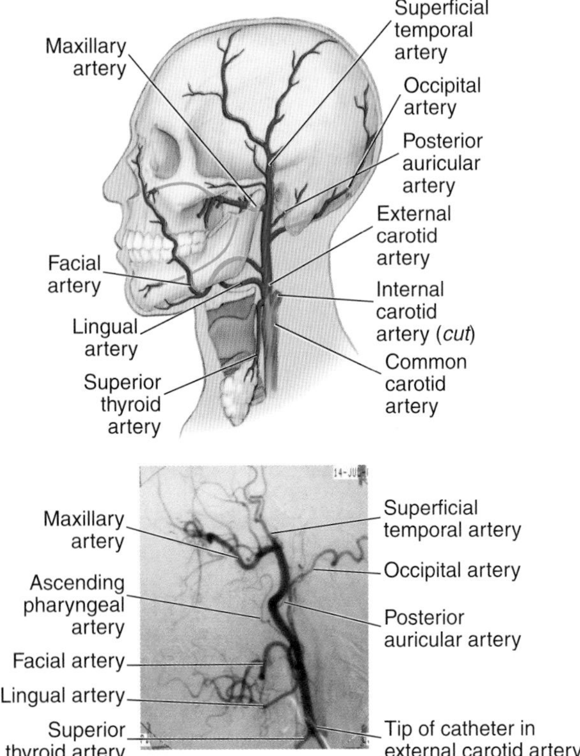


**Fig. 4.8** Carotid vasculature. Note the arteries branching from the external carotid artery. (From Reynolds PA, Abrahams PH. *McMinn's Interactive Clinical Anatomy: Head and Neck.* 2nd ed. London: Mosby Ltd; 2001.)

b. Facial artery—complicated path that runs over the submandibular gland, crossing the lower border of the mandible laterally, anterosuperiorly near the angle of the mouth and alongside the nose, terminating near the eye; supplies the muscles of the face in the oral, buccal, nasal, IO, and orbital regions; branches from the facial artery are:
   (1) Ascending palatine artery—supplies the soft palate, palatine muscles, and palatine tonsils
   (2) Submental artery—supplies the submandibular lymph nodes, the submandibular salivary gland, and mylohyoid and digastric muscles
   (3) Inferior labial artery—supplies lower lip muscles of facial expression
   (4) Superior labial artery—supplies the upper lip tissues

4. Medial branch of the external carotid artery (see Fig. 4.8)
   a. Ascending pharyngeal artery—supplies the pharyngeal walls, where they form an anastomosis with the ascending palatine artery; supplies the soft palate and meninges of the brain
5. Posterior branch of the external carotid artery (see Fig. 4.8)
   a. Occipital artery—supplies the suprahyoid and sternocleidomastoid muscles as well as the scalp and meningeal tissue of this region
   b. Posterior auricular artery—supplies the inner ear and mastoid air cells
6. Terminal branches of the external carotid artery (see Fig. 4.8)
   a. Superficial temporal artery—gives rise to smaller arteries supplying the temporalis muscle, the parotid salivary gland duct, and the scalp in the frontal and parietal regions
   b. Maxillary artery—three parts:
      (1) The first diverges from the external carotid artery near the neck of the condyle in the parotid gland; the second runs between the mandible and the sphenomandibular ligament anteriorly and through the infratemporal fossa superiorly; within the infratemporal fossa, this part of the maxillary artery gives off many branches:
         (a) IA artery—enters the mandibular canal by way of the mandibular foramen, along with the IA nerve; supplies the mandibular teeth and the floor of the mouth and diverges into three branches
         (b) Mylohyoid artery—travels in mylohyoid groove; supplies the mylohyoid muscle and the floor of the mouth
         (c) Mental artery—exits the mandibular canal by the mental foramen; supplies the chin region; forms an anastomosis with the inferior labial artery
         (d) Incisive artery—remains in the mandibular canal, dividing into branches that supply the teeth, periodontium, and gingiva of the anterior mandibular region
      (2) The second part of the maxillary artery also has muscle branches:
         (a) Deep temporal artery—supplies the temporalis muscle
         (b) Pterygoid artery—supplies the lateral and medial pterygoid muscles
         (c) Masseteric artery—supplies the masseter muscle
         (d) Buccal artery—supplies the buccinator muscle and buccal region
      (3) After traversing the infratemporal fossa, the maxillary artery enters the pterygopalatine fossa as the third part:
         (a) PSA artery—exits the infratemporal fossa and descends into the maxillary tuberosity; supplies the maxillary posterior teeth and periodontium and maxillary sinus
         (b) IO artery—branches off the maxillary artery in the pterygopalatine fossa; travels through the inferior orbital fissure, enters the IO canal, giving off branches to the orbit, and then branches off as the anterior superior alveolar (ASA) artery; it travels through the IO foramen, exiting on the face
         (c) ASA artery—travels down the maxillary sinus to supply the anterior maxillary teeth and the periodontium; forms an anastomosis with the PSA artery

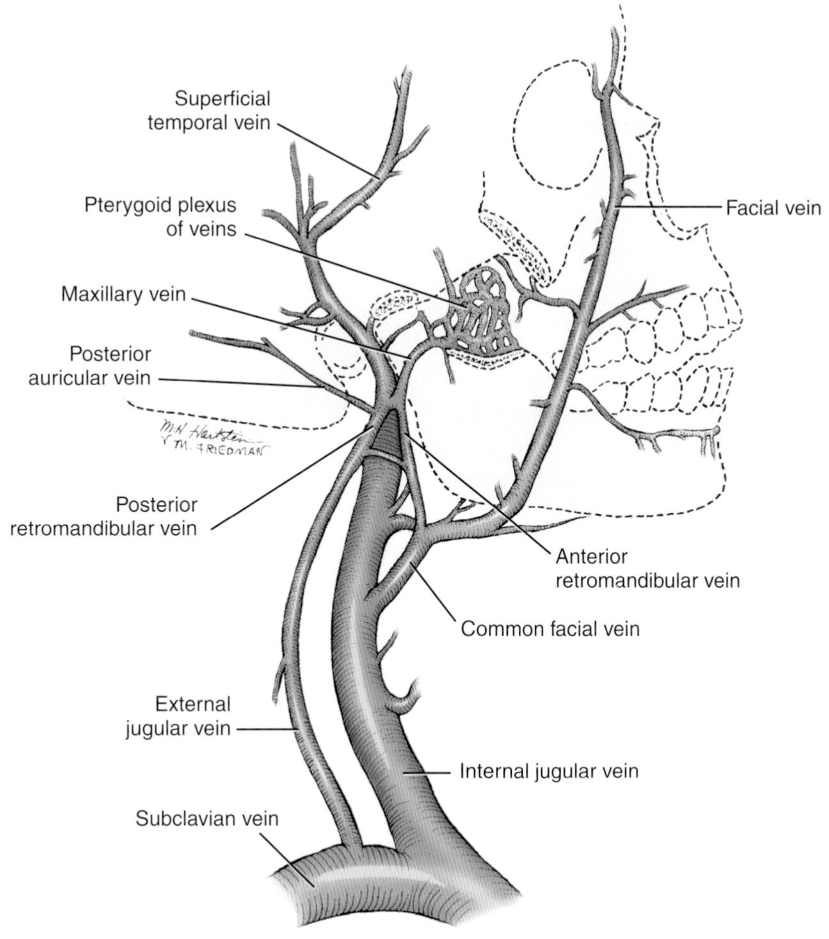




**Fig. 4.9** General drainage areas of the internal and external jugular veins. The retromandibular vein connects the internal and external jugular veins and distributes blood between them. (From Brand RW, Isselhard DE. *Anatomy of Orofacial Structures*. 8th ed. St. Louis: Elsevier; 2019.)

(d) GP and lesser palatine arteries—travel to the palate through the pterygopalatine canal and the greater and lesser foramina, supplying the hard and soft palates

F. Venous drainage of the head and neck (Fig. 4.9)
1. Generalizations—the venous system originates as small venules, which become larger veins in the neck region that carry blood back to the heart; veins anastomose freely with one another; veins lack one-way valves, which would prevent backflow, they are easily involved in the spread of infections
2. Internal and external jugular veins
   a. Internal jugular vein—drains the brain and most tissue of the head and neck
   b. External jugular vein—drains a small portion of extracranial tissue
3. Facial vein—drains into the internal jugular vein
   a. Drains the veins from the tissues of the frontal region and orbit of the eye; communicates with the cavernous venous sinus, which may become fatally infected through spread of dental infection
   b. Drains the veins of the lower lip, chin, and submandibular region
   c. Variations of the facial vein drain the tongue and floor of the mouth; sometimes drain indirectly into the facial vein or directly into the internal jugular vein
4. Retromandibular vein—formed by the superficial temporal and maxillary veins
   a. Posterior division—drains the temporal, maxillary, and posterior auricular areas and joins the external jugular vein
   b. Anterior division—joins the facial vein
5. Maxillary vein—originates in the infratemporal fossa; drains the pterygoid plexus, which drains the veins from the area served by the maxillary artery, such as the middle meninges, oral cavity, nose, and palate
6. Pterygoid plexus of veins—collection of vessels that form anastomoses with the facial and retromandibular veins located in the infratemporal fossa
   a. Drains portions of the face into the maxillary vein
   b. Drains the meninges of the brain
   c. Surrounds and protects the maxillary artery
   d. Can be pierced during the administration of a local anesthetic agent

e. Can be involved in the spread of dental infections during improper administration of local anesthetic agent
7. External and internal jugular veins on both sides of the neck merge with the subclavian veins to form the brachiocephalic veins, which then drain into the superior vena cava, directly to the heart

## THE LYMPHATIC SYSTEM

A. Function—part of the circulatory system; primary function is to help fight disease through ridding the body of toxins.
B. Descriptive terminology (see the section on "Blood and Lymph" in Chapter 2)
1. Lymph—tissue fluid that drains into lymphatic vessels from surrounding regions
2. Lymphatic vessels—a system of structures paralleling blood vessels that transport fluid (lymph) away from tissues; only carries fluid one direction, away
3. Lymph nodes—oval shaped organs of lymphatic system clustered along connecting lymphatic vessels; contain lymphocytes that filter toxins from lymph; not visible or palpable during extraoral examination in a healthy patient
4. Lymphadenopathy—an increase in size or consistency of lymphoid tissue; allows lymph node to be visualized and palpated; can indicate infection or disease
5. Tonsils—masses of lymphoid tissue located in the oral cavity and pharynx, remove toxins
C. Superficial cervical lymph nodes (Fig. 4.10)
1. Submental nodes
a. Located beneath the chin near the midline
b. Drain the chin, lower lip, floor of the mouth, mandibular incisors, and the apex of the tongue
c. Empty into the submandibular nodes or superior deep cervical nodes
2. Submandibular nodes
a. Located along the inferior border of the mandible superficial to the submandibular gland
b. Drain the cheek, upper, lip, anterior portion of the hard palate, the body of the tongue, and all teeth except maxillary third molars and mandibular incisors
c. Empty into the superior deep cervical nodes
D. Deep cervical lymph nodes
1. Superior deep cervical nodes
a. Located deep beneath the sternocleidomastoid muscle, 2 inches (5 cm) below the ear
b. Primary nodes for the drainage of the posterior nasal cavity, posterior hard palate, base of tongue, and maxillary third molars
c. The jugulodigastric lymph node in this area is easily palpable in clients with tonsillar lymphadenopathy
d. Empty into the inferior deep cervical nodes or directly into the jugular trunk

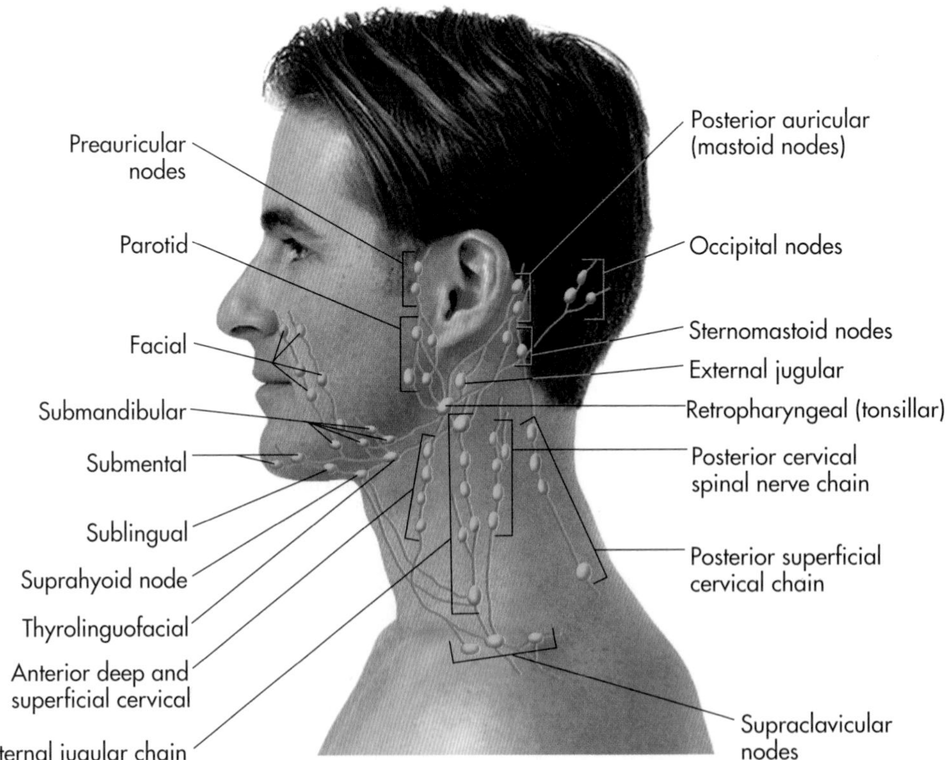


**Fig. 4.10** The lymphatic drainage system of the head and neck. If the group of nodes is often referred to by another name, the second name appears in parentheses. (From Ball JW, et al. *Seidel's Guide to Physical Examination*. 9th ed. St. Louis: Elsevier; 2019.)

2. Inferior deep cervical nodes
    a. Continuation of the superior deep cervical nodes, two inches above the clavicle
    b. Primary nodes for the drainage of the posterior part of the scalp and neck as well as part of the arm
    c. The inferior deep cervical node also communicate with the axillary lymph nodes, which can become involved in breast cancer
    d. Empty into the jugular trunk

E. Superficial lymph nodes of the head (see Fig. 4.10)
  1. Occipital nodes
      a. Located in the occipital region on the posterior head; drain the occipital portion of the scalp
      b. Empty into the deep cervical nodes
  2. Three groups of nodes drain the external ear and lacrimal gland; all empty into the deep cervical nodes:
      a. Retroauricular nodes—located posterior to the ear; also drain adjacent region
      b. Anterior auricular nodes—located anterior to the ear; also drain adjacent region
      c. Superficial parotid nodes—located on the surface of the parotid gland; also drain adjacent region
  3. Facial nodes
      a. Located along the facial vein; subgroups include buccal and mandibular; all drain the skin where they are located
      b. Infections from teeth may cause lymphadenopathy, described as being "firm like a pea"
      c. Drain into submandibular nodes, which empty into deep cervical nodes

F. Deep lymph nodes of the head—all located too deep for palpation; include deep parotid and retropharyngeal nodes (see Fig. 4.10)

G. Tonsils—not located along lymphatic vessels; drain into the superior deep cervical nodes
  1. Palatine tonsils—located between the anterior and posterior pillars, commonly referred to as "tonsils"
  2. Lingual tonsils—located on the dorsal surface of the base of the tongue
  3. Pharyngeal tonsils—located on the midline of the posterior wall of the nasopharynx, commonly referred to as "adenoids," enlarged in children
  4. Tubal tonsils—located in the nasopharynx, posterior to the openings of the auditory tube

## GLANDS OF THE HEAD AND NECK REGION

A. General definition—a *gland* is an organ that secretes chemical substances for use in normal body functioning; two main types of glands (see the section on "Glandular Tissue" in Chapter 2):
  1. Exocrine glands—have ducts; empty directly to a body location where secretions will be used (e.g., salivary glands)
  2. Endocrine glands—have no ducts; empty directly into the circulatory system, which transports secretions to the region to be used (e.g., thyroid gland)

B. Exocrine glands of the head
  1. Major salivary glands—paired glands, have named ducts
      a. Parotid salivary gland—located on the surface of the masseter muscle behind the ramus of the mandible, anterior and inferior to the ear; has a superficial and deep lobe and is the largest salivary gland, but produces only 25% of the total salivary volume, mainly serous; the associated duct is the parotid, or Stensen duct; the duct pierces the buccinator muscle and opens opposite the second maxillary molar; the parotid papilla marks the opening of the duct
      b. Submandibular salivary gland—located medially underneath the angle of the mandible; the second largest salivary gland, providing 60% to 65% of the total salivary volume, mixed serous and mucous; the associated duct is the submandibular, or Wharton duct; the duct opens at the sublingual caruncle on the floor of the mouth; the submandibular gland is the most common salivary gland involved in salivary stone formation
      c. Sublingual salivary gland—located in the sublingual fossa, anterior to the submandibular gland; the smallest, most diffuse salivary gland, providing 10% of the total salivary volume, mixed serous and mucous; associated ducts are located along the sublingual fold, combine to form the sublingual or Bartholin duct
  2. Minor salivary glands—smaller and more numerous than major salivary glands
      a. Numerous small glands—located in oral cavity tissues such as the soft palate; buccal, labial, and lingual mucosa; and the floor of the mouth; most secrete mainly mucous fluid
      b. Von Ebner glands—located in the circumvallate lingual papillae of the dorsal surface of the tongue; only minor salivary gland that secretes serous fluid only
  3. Lacrimal glands—located in the lacrimal fossa of the frontal bone; secrete lacrimal fluid, or tears; the associated duct is the nasolacrimal duct, at the junction of the lacrimal and maxillary bones

C. Endocrine glands of the neck region
  1. Thyroid gland—located below the hyoid bone; consists of two lobes connected by an isthmus; largest of the endocrine glands; secretes the hormone thyroxine, which regulates body metabolism; in a healthy patient, the thyroid gland moves with the thyroid cartilage when swallowing (Fig. 4.11)
  2. Parathyroid glands—located behind or within the thyroid gland; secrete parathyroid hormone, which regulates calcium metabolism and phosphorus uptake; not visible or palpable during examination
  3. Thymus gland—located inferior to the thyroid in the upper part of the chest; secretes thymosin, which assists in the maturation of T cell lymphocytes, which play a role in the immune system of the body; shrinks after puberty

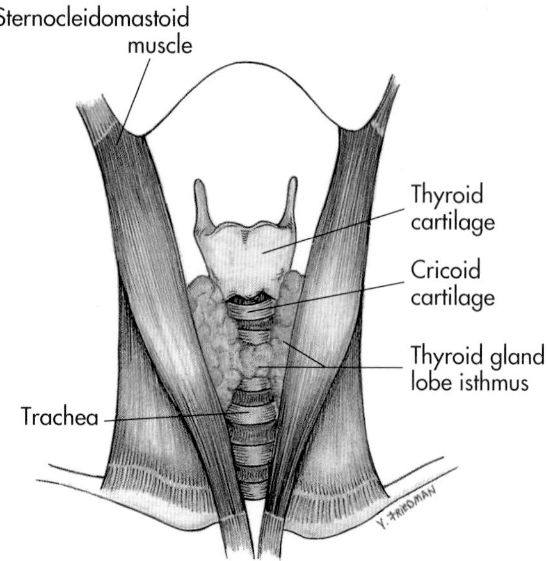


**Fig. 4.11** Anatomic position of the thyroid gland. (From Potter PA, et al. *Fundamentals of Nursing*. 9th ed. St. Louis: Elsevier; 2017.)

## THE NERVOUS SYSTEM

A. Classification and function—a complex network of nerves and cells that coordinates voluntary and involuntary actions through transmission of information from one location to another; the nervous system controls all body functions essential to life

B. Descriptive terminology (see the section on "Nerve Tissue" in Chapter 2 and the section on "Nervous System" in Chapter 3)
   1. Neuron—a nerve cell that is the basic building block of the nervous system, specialized to transmit information; contains a nucleus, which holds genetic information; dendrites, which conduct impulses to the cell body; and axons, which conduct impulses away from the cell body
   2. Nerve—a collection of neurons in the peripheral nervous system (PNS)
   3. Synapse— connection that allows the transmission of nerve impulses between two neurons or between a neuron and an effector organ
   4. Ganglion—a group of nerve cell bodies in the PNS
   5. Afferent, or sensory, neurons carry nerve impulses toward the central nervous system (CNS) away from a body structure (e.g., information sent to the brain for analysis or action)
   6. Efferent, or motor, neurons carry nerve impulses away from the CNS toward a body structure (e.g., information sent to a muscle for activation)

C. The nervous system—two major divisions:
   1. CNS—comprises the brain and spinal cord
   2. PNS—composed of nerves outside the CNS, such as sensory neurons carrying impulses to the CNS and motor neurons carrying messages from the CNS
      a. Autonomic nervous system (ANS)—responsible for control of body functions not consciously directed, such as respiratory rate, heart rate, and salivation; functions performed involuntarily and reflexively; two subdivisions of the ANS:
         (1) Sympathetic nervous system—prepares the body for stressful situations (e.g., increases heart rate, dilates airways); known as the "fight-or-flight" response; also slows body processes that are less important in emergencies, such as digestion (salivation) and urination
         (2) Parasympathetic nervous system—controls the body in ordinary situations (e.g., slows heart rate, decreases blood pressure); known as the "rest and digest" system; it generally conserves and restores body functions

D. CNs (12 pairs)—part of the PNS; designated with Roman numerals, for example, CNs V, VI, and VII; provide afferent (sensory), efferent (motor), or mixed impulses (Table 4.2)
   1. CN I (olfactory nerve)—afferent; carries smell from the nasal mucosa to the brain; exits the skull through the cribriform plate of the ethmoid bone
   2. CN II (optic nerve)—afferent; carries visual impulses from retina to the brain; exits the skull through the optic canal of the sphenoid bone
   3. CN III (oculomotor nerve)—efferent; innervates muscles of the eye for movement; exits the skull through the superior orbital fissure of the sphenoid bone
   4. CN IV (trochlear nerve)—efferent; supplies only one eye muscle which depresses and abducts the eye; exits the skull through the superior orbital fissure of the sphenoid bone
   5. CN V (trigeminal nerve)— largest CN, both efferent and afferent; efferent component for the muscles of mastication and some cranial muscles; afferent component for the teeth, tongue, oral cavity, and most of the skin of the face and head; knowledge of CN V is critical for the successful administration of a local anesthetic agent (Tables 4.3 and 4.4; see Tables 18.3 and 18.5 in Chapter 18, Management of Pain and Anxiety)
   6. Three divisions or branches of the trigeminal nerve:
      a. Ophthalmic nerve, first division, or $V_1$—afferent nerve; carries information to the brain via the superior orbital fissure of the sphenoid bone; divides into three major branches:
         (1) Frontal nerve—a large branch which courses superiorly in the orbit; innervates skin of upper eyelids, forehead, scalp, and frontal sinus
         (2) Lacrimal nerve—small branch that passes laterally through the orbit; innervates lacrimal gland and adjacent skin, and conjunctiva
         (3) Nasociliary nerve—most complex branch with numerous small branches; innervates eye, skin of nose, and frontal, ethmoid, and sphenoid sinuses
      b. Maxillary nerve, second division, or $V_2$—afferent nerves exits the skull through the foramen rotundum of the sphenoid bone to supply the maxillae and related skin, maxillary sinuses, nasal cavity, palate, and nasopharynx (Figs. 4.12 and 4.13) (see the section on "Trigeminal Nerve, maxillary nerve, second division ($V_2$) in Chapter 18)

TABLE 4.2 **Cranial Nerves**

| Number | Nerve | Exit | Modality | Basic Function |
|---|---|---|---|---|
| I | Olfactory | Cribriform plate | Sensory | Smell |
| II | Optic | Optic canal | Sensory | Vision |
| III | Oculomotor | Superior orbital fissure | Motor | Eye movement: supply to several muscles |
| IV | Trochlear | Superior orbital fissure | Motor | Eye movement: supply to one muscle only |
| V | Trigeminal | | Mixed | |
| | • Ophthalmic | Superior orbital fissure | Sensory | Sensation to orbit and anterior portion of the scalp |
| | • Maxillary | Foramen rotundum | Sensory | Sensation to nasal and oral cavities, maxillary teeth, and surrounding soft tissues |
| | • Mandibular | Foramen ovale | Mixed | Sensation to mandibular teeth and surrounding soft tissues, tongue, floor of the mouth<br>Motor supply to muscles of mastication |
| VI | Abducens | Superior orbital fissure | Motor | Eye movement: supply to one muscle only |
| VII | Facial | Internal acoustic meatus<br>Stylomastoid foramen | Mixed | Muscles of facial expression, taste to anterior tongue, submandibular and sublingual glands |
| VIII | Vestibulocochlear | Internal acoustic meatus | Sensory | Hearing, equilibrium, balance |
| IX | Glossopharyngeal | Jugular foramen | Mixed | Pharynx, taste to posterior tongue, parotid gland |
| X | Vagus | Jugular foramen | Mixed | Muscles of larynx, pharynx, and palate |
| XI | Accessory | Juglar foramen | Motor | Muscles in the neck (two) |
| XII | Hypoglossal | Hypoglossal canal | Motor | Muscles of the tongue |

TABLE 4.3 **Summary of Maxillary Injection Sites for Local Anesthetic Agent Administration**

| Landmark and Nerve | Injection | Teeth or Tissue Anesthetized |
|---|---|---|
| Maxillary tuberosity/posterosuperior alveolar nerve of the maxillary branch of trigeminal nerve (second division, $V_2$) | Posterosuperior alveolar (PSA) | Maxillary first,[a] second, and third molars and related buccal tissues |
| Apex of second premolar/middle superior alveolar nerve of $V_2$ (not present in all people) | Middle superior alveolar (MSA) | Maxillary first and second premolars; mesiobuccal root of maxillary first molar and buccal tissues |
| Apex of maxillary canine/anterosuperior alveolar nerve of $V_2$ | Anterosuperior alveolar (ASA) | Maxillary premolars, canines, and incisors and associated buccal tissues |
| Greater palatine foramen/greater palatine nerve of $V_2$ | Greater palatine (GP) | Palatal roots of maxillary molars and premolars and related lingual tissues |
| Incisive foramen/nasopalatine nerve of $V_2$ | Nasopalatine (NP) | Anterior portion of palate or lingual aspects of anterior maxillary teeth |
| Infraorbital foramen/infraorbital nerve of $V_2$ | Infraorbital (IO) | Facial aspects of anterior maxillary teeth and buccal aspects of the premolars |

[a]In some cases, the mesiobuccal root is not innervated by the PSA nerve, but by the MSA nerve.

TABLE 4.4 **Summary of Mandibular Injection Sites for Local Anesthetic Agent Administration**

| Landmark and nerve | Injection | Teeth or Tissue Anesthetized |
|---|---|---|
| Mandibular foramen/inferior alveolar nerve of the mandibular branch of the trigeminal nerve (third division, $V_3$) | Inferior alveolar (IA) | Mandibular teeth to midline; buccal mucoperiosteum; mucous membrane anterior to mandibular first molar; anterior two-thirds of tongue and floor of oral cavity; lingual soft tissues |
| Mental foramen/inferior alveolar nerve; mental and incisive nerve branches of $V_3$ | Mental block (MB) or incisive block (IB) | IB: mandibular premolars, canines, and incisors; lower lip and skin of chin; buccal mucous membrane anterior to the mental foramen<br>MB: buccal mucous membranes anterior to mental foramen to midline; skin of lower lip and chin |
| Buccal tissue distal and buccal to the most distal molar/buccal nerve of $V_3$ | Buccal block (LB) | Buccal periodontium and gingiva of mandibular molars |

(1) Zygomatic nerve—merger of two smaller nerves emerging from the lateral wall of the orbit that serve the skin of the cheek and the temple

(2) IO (inferior alveolar) nerve—formed from the merger of nerve branches from the upper lip, medial portion of the cheek, lower eyelid, and side of the nose; passes into the IO foramen of the maxilla, which is the landmark for anesthetic injection of the IO nerve block; gives off two important branches that supply the maxillary teeth:

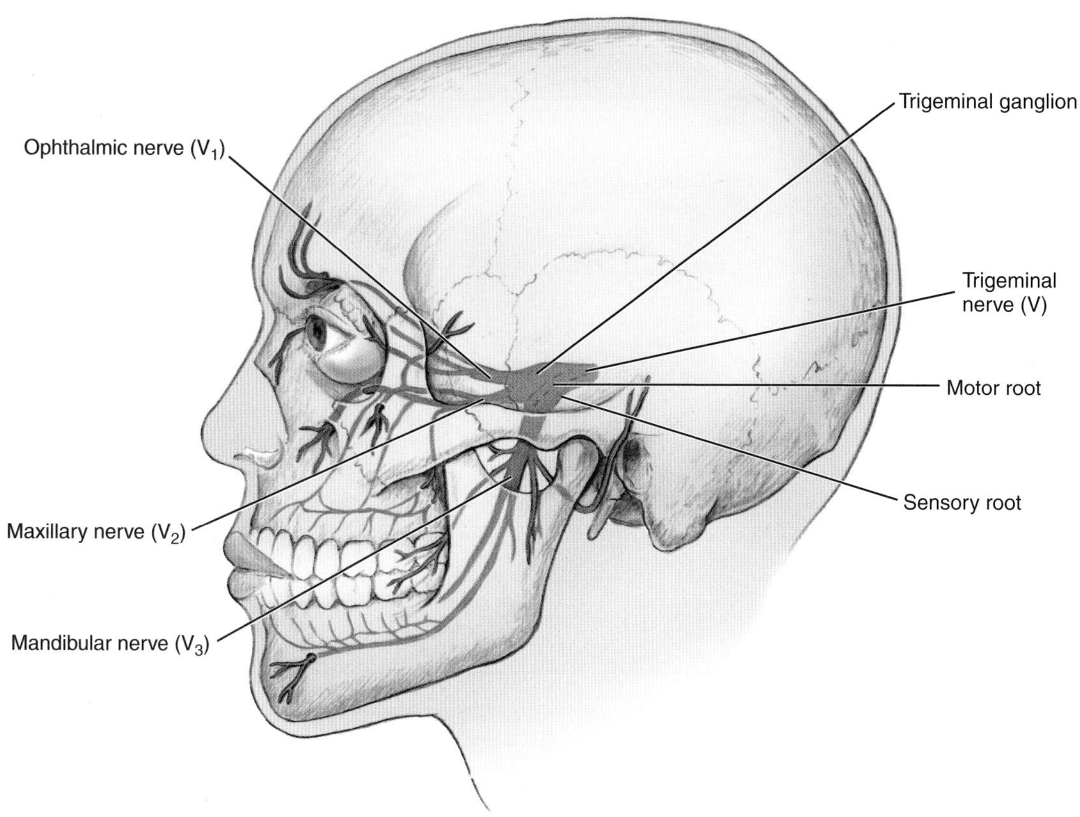


**Fig. 4.12** Pathway of the maxillary nerve or second division of the trigeminal nerve is highlighted; note the innervation coverage for the maxillary nerve (see inset). (From Fehrenbach M, Herring S. *Illustrated Anatomy of the Head and Neck*. 5th ed. St. Louis: Elsevier; 2017.)

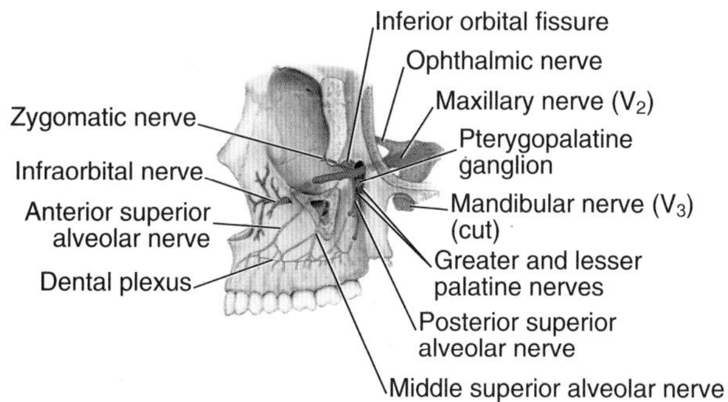


**Fig. 4.13** Lateral view of the skull with part of lateral wall of orbit removed; the branches of the maxillary nerve are highlighted. (From Fehrenbach M, Herring S. *Illustrated Anatomy of the Head and Neck*. 5th ed. St. Louis: Elsevier; 2017.)

(3) ASA nerve—carries sensations from the dental branches in the pulp tissue of maxillary central incisors, lateral incisors, and canines and their associated tissues; forms a nerve network with interdental branches, which is the landmark for anesthetic injection of the ASA nerve block

(4) Middle superior alveolar (MSA) nerve—carries sensations from the dental branches in the pulp tissue of the maxillary premolar teeth and mesial buccal root of the maxillary first molar, the associated periodontium, and buccal gingiva; forms a nerve network that is the landmark for anesthetic injection of the MSA nerve block; about 30% of the time, the MSA is not present in patients. In this case, the area is innervated by the ASA primarily and PSA nerves

(5) PSA nerve—carries sensations from the dental branches in the pulp tissue of the maxillary molars (except mesial buccal root of the maxillary first molar), periodontium, buccal gingiva, and the maxillary sinus; internal branches of the PSA nerve exit from several PSA foramina on the maxillary tuberosity, these foramina are landmarks for anesthetic injection of the PSA nerve block

(6) GP nerve, anterior nerve—carries sensations from the hard palate and posterior lingual gingiva; enters the greater palatine foramen near the maxillary second or third molar, which is the landmark for anesthetic injection of the GP block

(7) Lesser palatine nerve, posterior nerve—carries sensations from the soft palate and palatine tonsil; enters the lesser palatine foramen where it joins the GP nerve within the pterygopalatine canal

(8) NP nerve—carries sensations from the anterior hard palate and lingual gingiva of maxillary anterior teeth and canine teeth; enters the incisive canal through the incisive foramen, which is the landmark for anesthetic injection of the NP block

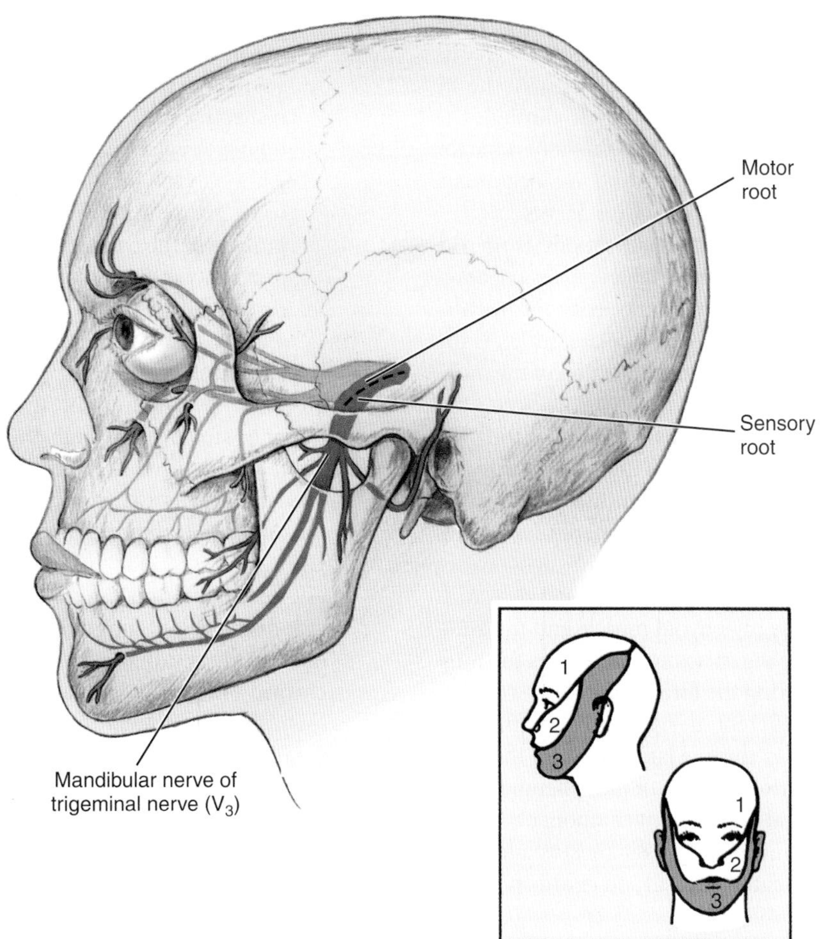


**Fig. 4.14** Pathway of the mandibular nerve or third division of the trigeminal nerve is highlighted; note the innervation coverage for the mandibular nerve (see inset). (From Fehrenbach M, Herring S. *Illustrated Anatomy of the Head and Neck*. 5th ed. St. Louis: Elsevier; 2017.)

c. Mandibular nerve, third division, or $V_3$—the only division containing both afferent and efferent types; largest of the trigeminal branches; exits the skull through the foramen ovale on the sphenoid bone and divides into anterior and posterior divisions (Figs. 4.14 and 4.15) (see the section on "Trigeminal Nerve, mandibular nerve, third division ($V_3$) and Table 18.4 in Chapter 18)
   (1) Long buccal nerve—(anterior)carries sensations from the cheek, buccal mucosa, and buccal gingiva of mandibular posterior teeth; the nerve crosses in front of the anterior border of the ramus between the two heads of the lateral pterygoid muscle, which is the landmark for anesthetic injection of the buccal nerve block
   (2) Muscular branches—(anterior) efferent nerves supplying the four muscles of mastication, deep temporal nerves, masseteric nerve, and lateral pterygoid nerve
   (3) Auriculotemporal nerve—(posterior) carries sensations from the ear and temporal skin, parotid gland, and TMJ
   (4) Lingual nerve—(posterior) carries sensations from the floor of the mouth, the lingual mandibular gingiva, and the anterior two-thirds of the tongue; it communicates with CN VII (facial nerve) supplying parasympathetic fibers to the submandibular and sublingual salivary glands; because of its location in the floor of the mouth, it is often anesthetized when an IA nerve block is administered

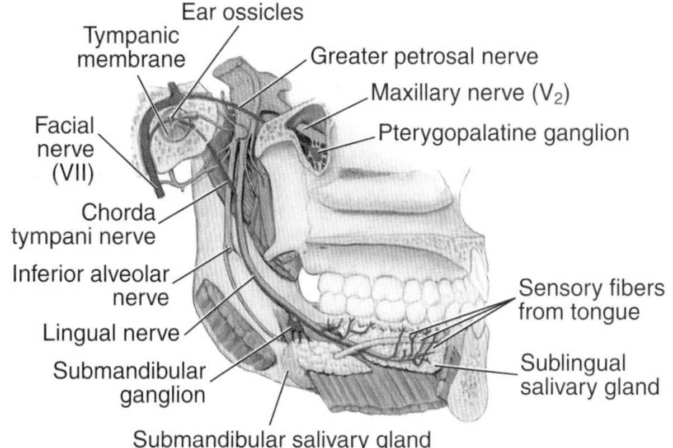


**Fig. 4.15** Medial view of the mandible with the motor and sensory branches of the mandibular nerve or third division highlighted. (From Fehrenbach M, Herring S. *Illustrated Anatomy of the Head and Neck*. 5th ed. St. Louis: Elsevier; 2017.)

(5) IA nerve—(posterior) carries sensations from mandibular teeth and buccal gingiva; it travels through the mandibular canal, along with the IA artery and vein; exits the mandible through the mandibular foramen, which is the landmark for anesthetic injection of the IA nerve block; it is a merger of the mental and incisive nerves

(a) Mental nerve—carries sensations from the chin, lower lip, and the labial mucosa of anterior teeth and premolars; exits the mental foramen between the premolars, which is the landmark for anesthetic injection of the mental nerve block

(b) Incisive nerve—carries sensations from the dental branches of the pulp tissue of the mandibular anterior teeth; merges with the mental nerve to form the IA nerve and travels through the mandibular canal

(6) Mylohyoid nerve—a small efferent nerve branch that supplies the mylohyoid muscle and the anterior belly of the digastric muscle; it joins the inferior nerve entering the foramen ovale

7. CN VI (abducens)—efferent nerve; supplies only one eye muscle which moves the eye laterally; exits the skull through the superior orbital fissure of the sphenoid bone
8. CN VII (facial)—efferent and afferent components, leaves the brain through the internal acoustic meatus and gives off two branches, the greater petrosal and chorda tympani (see Fig. 4.15)
   a. Greater petrosal nerve—efferent nerve; fibers are carried through the pterygopalatine ganglion to the lacrimal gland, nasal cavity, and minor salivary glands of the hard and soft palate; the afferent nerve fibers also carry taste sensations from the palate
   b. Chorda tympani nerve—parasympathetic efferent nerve supplying submandibular and sublingual salivary glands; has an afferent component carrying taste sensations for the body of the tongue
   c. Facial nerve continues anteriorly, passing through the parotid gland, and separates into efferent branches supplying the muscles of facial expression in their respective areas; temporal, zygomatic, buccal, mandibular, and cervical branches
   d. Although the facial nerve passes into the parotid salivary gland, it does not innervate the gland; disease process in the parotid gland may be painful due to the proximity of the facial nerve
   e. Knowledge of the facial nerve is important for avoidance of complications in the administration of local anesthesia
9. CN VIII (vestibulocochlear nerve)—afferent nerve for hearing, supplied through the cochlear nerve, and balance, supplied by the vestibular nerve in the semicircular canals; exits the brain through the internal acoustic meatus of the temporal bone
10. CN IX (glossopharyngeal nerve)—afferent and efferent nerve; afferent innervation provides taste to posterior one-third of tongue, general sensation to posterior one-third of tongue, pharynx, tonsillar regions and carotid sinus; the efferent innervation controls swallowing; exits the cranial cavity through the jugular foramen
11. CN X (vagus nerve)—mixture of afferent and efferent nerves; the larger efferent component supplies the muscles of the soft palate, pharynx, larynx, and parasympathetic fibers to the organs in the thoracic and abdominal cavities; the smaller afferent component conveys to skin around the ear and taste sensation of the epiglottis; exits the skull through the jugular foramen
12. CN XI (accessory nerve)—efferent nerve; impulses to the trapezius and sternocleidomastoid muscles; exits the skull through the jugular foramen
13. CN XII (hypoglossal nerve)—efferent nerve; innervates all muscles of the tongue; exits the skull through the hypoglossal canal of the occipital bone

## WEBSITE INFORMATION AND RESOURCES

| Source | Web Address | Description |
|---|---|---|
| Innerbody | https://www.innerbody.com/ | Interactive learning tool featuring over 300 high-resolution 3D CAD views of over 1500 objects in the body, covering all 13 major anatomical systems |
| TeachMeAnatomy | https://teachmeanatomy.info/ | Containing over 700 vibrant, full-color images, TeachMeAnatomy is a comprehensive anatomy encyclopedia presented in a visually appealing, easy-to-read format |

## CHAPTER 4 REVIEW QUESTIONS

Answers and rationales to chapter review questions are available on this text's accompanying Evolve site. See inside front cover for details.

1. The term used to describe structures located toward the surface of the body is:
   **a.** Superficial
   **b.** Proximal
   **c.** Distal
   **d.** Deep
   **e.** Anterior
2. The term that describes a window-like opening in the bone is:
   **a.** Canal
   **b.** Meatus
   **c.** Foramen
   **d.** Fissure
3. Each of the following bones are cranial bones EXCEPT one. Which is the EXCEPTION?

a. Occipital bone
b. Sphenoid bone
c. Ethmoid bone
d. Frontal bone
e. Zygomatic bone

4. The horizontal plates of the palatine bones articulate with each other to form the posterior portion of the hard palate. An important landmark for the administration of local anesthesia found here is:
   a. Incisive foramen
   b. Greater palatine foramen
   c. Infraorbital foramen
   d. Mental foramen
5. The sphenoid bone is important to dental professionals because it has processes that serve as part of the attachment for two of the four pairs of the muscles of mastication. The sphenoid bone also has formina that are the passageway for important nerves and blood vessels of the head and neck.
   a. Both statements are TRUE
   b. Both statements are FALSE
   c. The first statement is TRUE; the second statement is FALSE
   d. The first statement is FALSE; the second statement is TRUE
6. The paired hypoglossal canals that are openings for cranial nerve XII (hypoglossal nerve) are formed by which of the following bones?
   a. Sphenoid bone
   b. Occipital bone
   c. Maxilla
   d. Mandible
7. Cranial Nerve VII, or the facial nerve, exits the skull through the:
   a. External acoustic meatus
   b. Superior orbital fissure
   c. Internal acoustic meatus
   d. Cribriform plate
8. All of the following features are located on the temporal bone EXCEPT one. Which is the EXCEPTION?
   a. Pterygoid process
   b. Mastoid process
   c. External acoustic meatus
   d. Jugular notch
9. The maxillary tuberosity is a landmark for the administration of local anesthesia to which of the following?
   a. Lesser palatine nerve
   b. Infraorbital nerve
   c. Nasopalatine nerve
   d. Posterior superior alveolar nerve
10. Which of the following landmarks is used to locate the hyoid bone?
    a. Thyroid cartilage
    b. First cervical vertebra
    c. Second cervical vertebra
    d. Lingula
11. All of the following paranasal sinuses drain into the middle meatus of the nasal cavity EXCEPT one. Which one is the EXCEPTION?
    a. Posterior ethmoidal sinuses
    b. Anterior ethmoidal sinuses
    c. Frontal sinuses
    d. Maxillary sinuses
12. The origin of muscle is a fixed attachment. The insertion of muscle is a less moveable structure.
    a. Both statements are TRUE
    b. Both statements are FALSE
    c. The first statement is TRUE; the second statement is FALSE
    d. The first statement is FALSE; the second statement is TRUE
13. Difficulty in accessing the lower anterior teeth during instrumentation is caused by contraction of which of the following muscles?
    a. Mentalis muscle
    b. Zygomaticus major muscle
    c. Depressor anguli oris muscle
    d. Levator anguli oris muscle
14. The muscle of facial expression that assists the muscles of mastication during chewing is the
    a. Risorius muscle
    b. Mentalis muscle
    c. Buccinator muscle
    d. Orbicularis oris muscle
15. Each of the following is a muscle of mastication EXCEPT one. Which one is the EXCEPTION?
    a. Masseter muscle
    b. Buccinator muscle
    c. Temporalis muscle
    d. Lateral pterygoid muscle
16. Contraction of both sternocleidomastoid muscles causes which of the following?
    a. Face and front of the neck to rotate to the opposite side
    b. Neck skin to be raised
    c. Head and neck to be bent to the same side
    d. Head to flex at the neck
17. Which of the following muscles originates partially from the maxillary tuberosity?
    a. Masseter muscle
    b. Medial pterygoid muscle
    c. Lateral pterygoid muscle
    d. Temporalis muscle
18. The only muscle of mastication that depresses the mandible or opens the mouth is which of the following?
    a. Masseter muscle
    b. Medial pterygoid muscle
    c. Lateral pterygoid muscle
    d. Temporalis muscle
19. All the following are suprahyoid muscles EXEPT one. Which one is the EXCEPTION?
    a. Geniohyoid muscle
    b. Stylohyoid muscle
    c. Thyrohyoid muscle
    d. Digastric muscle
20. Deviation of the mandible to one side during protrusion is caused by which of the following?
    a. Contraction of both lateral pterygoid muscles
    b. Contraction of the temporalis muscle
    c. Contraction of the masseter muscle
    d. Contraction of one lateral pterygoid muscle
21. The muscles of facial expression are innervated by

a. Cranial Nerve VII, facial nerve
b. Cranial Nerve XI, accessory nerve
c. Cranial Nerve X, vagus nerve
d. Cranial Nerve $V_3$, trigeminal nerve, mandibular division

22. The intrinsic muscles of the tongue originate and insert inside the tongue while the extrinsic muscles originate elsewhere and insert inside the tongue. Both extrinsic and intrinsic muscles are innervated by the hypoglossal nerve.
    a. Both statements are TRUE
    b. Both statements are FALSE
    c. The first statement is TRUE; the second statement is FALSE
    d. The first statement is FALSE; the second statement is TRUE
23. Which one of the following structures prevents posterior and inferior displacement of the mandible?
    a. Sphenomandibular ligament
    b. Temporomandibular joint ligament
    c. Articular disc
    d. Stylomandibular ligament
24. The posterior superior alveolar artery supplies blood to
    a. The mandibular teeth and floor of the mouth
    b. The hard and soft palate
    c. Maxillary posterior teeth and periodontium, and maxillary sinus
    d. Maxillary anterior teeth and periodontium
25. All of the following are branches of the facial artery EXCEPT one. Which one is the EXCEPTION?
    a. Ascending palatine artery
    b. Inferior labial artery
    c. Submental artery
    d. Lingual artery
26. Which of the following veins is formed by the merger of the maxillary vein and the superficial temporal vein?
    a. Facial vein
    b. Internal jugular vein
    c. Retromandibular vein
    d. Brachiocephalic vein
27. The pterygoid plexus of veins is of clinical importance for all of the following reasons EXCEPT one. Which one is the EXCEPTION?
    a. Connections with the cavernous sinus could cause an infection of dental origin to spread to the cranial cavity
    b. Connections of the plexus drain into the superior vena cava, directly to the heart
    c. Connections with the facial vein could allow an infection on the surface of the face to reach the plexus and spread to more internal structures
    d. Trauma to the plexus such as puncture during the administration of local anesthesia could result in a hematoma
28. During an extraoral examination of a patient, the dental hygienist notes lymphadenopathy beneath the chin near the midline. Which one of the following lymph nodes is involved?
    a. Retroauricular nodes
    b. Inferior deep cervical nodes
    c. Submandibular nodes
    d. Submental nodes
29. All of the following are endocrine glands EXCEPT one. Which one is the EXCEPTION?
    a. Parotid gland
    b. Thyroid gland
    c. Parathyroid gland
    d. Thymus gland
30. The parotid salivary glands empty through the
    a. Sublingual fold
    b. Stensen duct
    c. Wharton duct
    d. Sublingual caruncle
31. An exocrine gland is a gland having a duct associated with it that allows secretions to be emptied directly into the location where the secretion is to be used. An endocrine gland is a ductless gland, with secretion being poured directly into the blood.
    a. Both statements are TRUE
    b. Both statements are FALSE
    c. The first statement is TRUE; the second statement is FALSE
    d. The first statement is FALSE; the second statement is TRUE
32. The minor salivary gland associated the circumvallate lingual papillae are:
    a. Parotid salivary glands
    b. Submandibular salivary glands
    c. Sublingual salivary glands
    d. Ebner's salivary glands
33. A sensory nerve that carries information from the body to the brain or spinal cord is called:
    a. Efferent nerve
    b. Nerve
    c. Afferent nerve
    d. Neuron
34. Which one of the following cranial nerves is the largest?
    a. Fifth cranial nerve
    b. Ninth cranial nerve
    c. Eighth cranial nerve
    d. Twelfth cranial nerve
35. All of the following cranial nerves supply innervation for eye movement EXCEPT one. Which one is the EXCEPTION?
    a. Cranial Nerve I
    b. Cranial Nerve III
    c. Cranial Nerve IV
    d. Cranial Nerve VI
36. The three divisions or branches of the trigeminal nerve are:
    a. Frontal nerve, lacrimal nerve, nasociliary nerve
    b. Zygomatic nerve, infraorbital nerve, inferior alveolar nerve
    c. Ophthalmic nerve, maxillary nerve, mandibular nerve
    d. Long buccal nerve, auriculotemporal nerve, lingual nerve
37. The muscles of mastication are supplied by the trigeminal nerve. The muscles of facial expression are supplied by the facial nerve.
    a. Both statements are TRUE
    b. Both statements are FALSE

c. The first statement is TRUE; the second statement is FALSE
d. The first statement is FALSE; the second statement is TRUE

38. All of the following cranial nerves serve only head and neck structures EXCEPT one. Which one is the EXCEPTION?
a. Vagus nerve
b. Glossopharyngeal nerve
c. Vestibulocochlear nerve
d. Accessory nerve

39. The infraorbital nerve innervates which of the following?
a. Lacrimal gland and adjacent skin, and conjunctiva
b. Skin of the lower eyelid, medial portion of the cheek, side of the nose, upper lip
c. Skin of the cheek and the temple
d. Skin of the upper eyelid, forehead, scalp, and frontal sinus

40. Which one of the following nerves innervates the parotid salivary gland?
a. Vagus nerve CN X
b. Facial nerve CN VII
c. Hypoglossal nerve CN XII
d. Glossopharyngeal nerve CN IX

41. The sensation of taste on the anterior one-third of the tongue is supplied by the
a. Facial nerve
b. Glossopharyngeal nerve
c. Hypoglossal nerve
d. Accessory nerve

42. The only division of the trigeminal nerve that contains both afferent and efferent components
a. Ophthalmic nerve
b. Mandibular nerve
c. Maxillary nerve
d. Facial nerve

## CASE A

A 56-year-old female presents for scaling and root planing. Review of the medical history reveals a prescription for oral bisphosphonate for treatment of osteoporosis. The patient reports taking calcium and vitamin D; no other medications are noted, and no allergies reported other than seasonal allergies. Vitals signs are normal. Extraoral examination findings include lymphadenopathy located approximately 2 inches below the ear and bilateral crepitus of the temporomandibular joint (TMJ) upon opening of the jaw. Intraoral examination findings are within normal limits except patient notes a loss of taste on the back of her tongue. Due to the patient's history of bisphosphonate usage, the dental hygienist has planned quadrant scaling and root planing, starting with the maxillary right, in order to evaluate the reaction of the bone and tissue before treating the entire mouth.

***Use Case A to answer questions 43 to 50.***

43. Bisphosphonates disturb the process of bone resorption and remodeling. Which of the following cells is responsible for the majority of bone resorption in the remodeling process?
a. Osteocyte
b. Osteoblast
c. Osteoclast
d. Monocyte

44. While performing the extraoral examination, the dental hygienist noted lymphadenopathy along the neck approximately 2 inches below the ear. Given the location, which of the following lymph nodes are involved?
a. Inferior deep cervical nodes
b. Anterior auricular nodes
c. Occipital nodes
d. Superior deep cervical nodes

45. In order to examine the temporomandibular joint (TMJ), the dental hygienist asks the patient to open and close her mouth slowly. All of the following muscles of mastication are responsible for elevation of the mandible EXCEPT one. Which one is the EXCEPTION?
a. Lateral pterygoid
b. Temporalis
c. Medial pterygoid
d. Masseter

46. The dental hygienist should explain to the patient that crepitus of the TMJ can occur when the articular disc becomes displaced which affects the normal movement of the TMJ. Which of the following describes the movement of the TMJ?
a. Hinge movement followed by gliding movement
b. Hinge movement only
c. Gliding movement only
d. Gliding movement followed by hinge movement

47. Which one of the following cranial nerves is responsible for the patient's loss of taste on the back of the tongue?
a. Trigeminal nerve
b. Glossopharyngeal nerve
c. Vestibulocochlear nerve
d. Hypoglossal nerve

48. The dental hygienist plans to perform scaling and root planing on the maxillary right quadrant. In order to achieve anesthesia of the maxillary first molar, the hygienist may need to target which of the following two nerves?
a. Middle superior alveolar nerve and posterior superior alveolar nerve
b. Posterior superior alveolar nerve and anterior superior alveolar nerve
c. Middle superior alveolar nerve and anterior superior alveolar nerve
d. Infraorbital nerve and posterior superior alveolar nerve

49. After administering local anesthesia to the maxillary right quadrant, the dental hygienist notices that the patient is experiencing sensitivity of the lingual tissues. In order to keep the patient comfortable, the hygienist should also anesthetize which one of the following nerves?
a. Middle superior alveolar nerve
b. Lesser palatine nerve
c. Greater palatine nerve
d. Lingual nerve

50. Due to the patient's seasonal allergies, which one of the following sinuses could become infected and cause discomfort and complications with the maxillary posterior teeth?
a. Maxillary
b. Ethmoid
c. Sphenoid
d. Frontal

5

# Clinical Oral Structures, Dental Anatomy, and Root Morphology

*Miranda A. Drake*

The practice of dental hygiene is based on oral anatomy, a fundamental dental science. A thorough knowledge of oral anatomy provides the basis for assessing, diagnosing, planning, implementing, and evaluating patients during the dental hygiene process of care. Oral anatomy provides the basis for nonsurgical periodontal therapy, pit-and-fissure sealant placement, and patient education. The dental hygienist also uses oral anatomy to assess the relationship of teeth, both within and between the arches. These factors influence evidence-based decision making, care plans, professional recommendations, and referral to other health care practitioners.

## CLINICAL ORAL STRUCTURES

The dental hygienist must be proficient in performing a clinical examination of the head and neck both extraorally and intraorally to detect variations of normal and abnormal conditions that may be indicators of overall health. Abnormal conditions can be recognized if the appearance of normal oral structures is known (Figs. 5.1 to 5.8 and Table 5.1). Oral structures are identified according to their specific locations and functions. Generally, oral structures appear in shades of pink and may be pigmented in dark-complexioned individuals. In the oral cavity, the presence of melanin pigmentation is random, scattered, and unpredictable. The dental hygienist must be able to communicate the clinical examination findings professionally (Figs. 5.9 to 5.16 and Table 5.2).

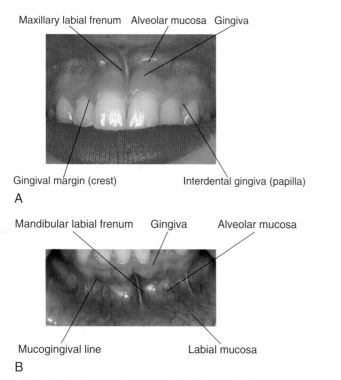

Maxillary labial frenum
Alveolar mucosa
Gingiva
Gingival margin (crest)
Interdental gingiva (papilla)
A
Mandibular labial frenum
Gingiva
Alveolar mucosa
Mucogingival line
Labial mucosa
B

**Fig 5.1** Labial and oral mucosa. (A) Maxillary. (B) Mandibular.

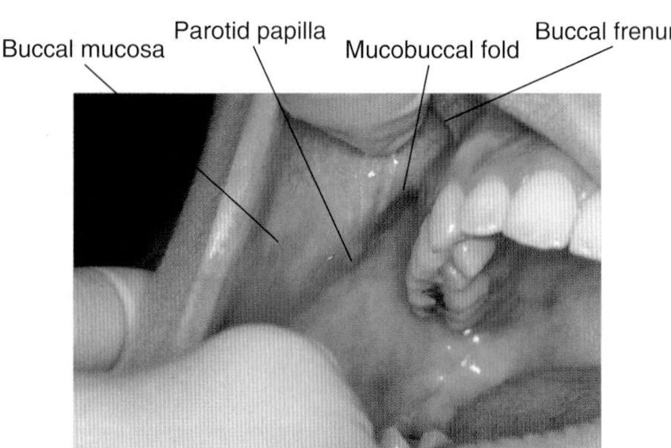


**Fig 5.2** Buccal mucosa.

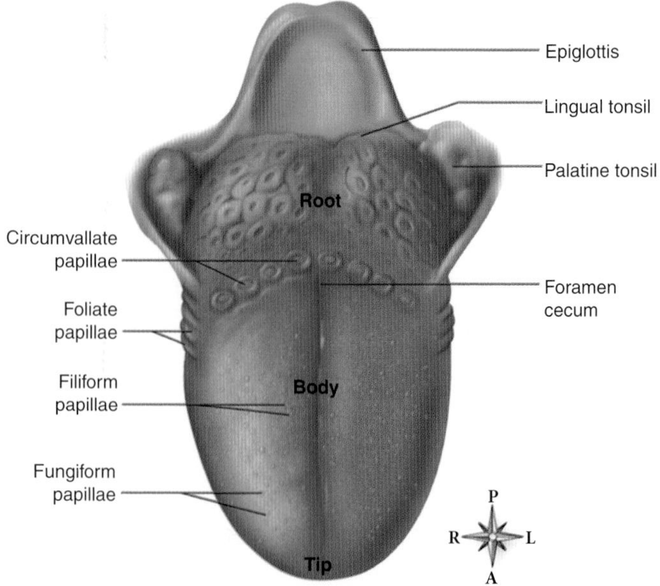


**Fig 5.3** Dorsum of the tongue. (From: Patton K. Anatomy and Physiology. 10th ed. St. Louis: Elsevier; 2018.)

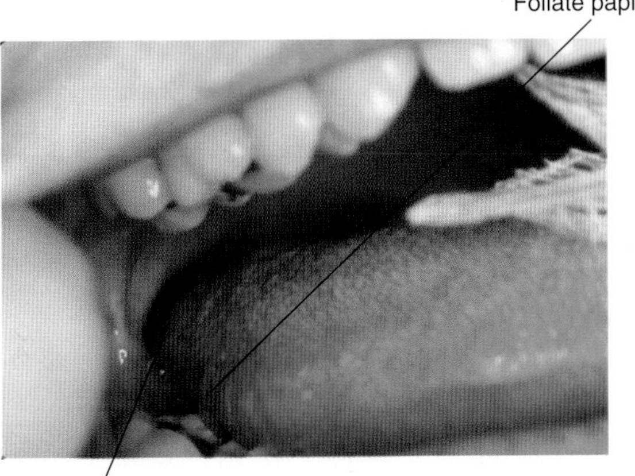

**Fig 5.4** Lateral surface of the tongue.

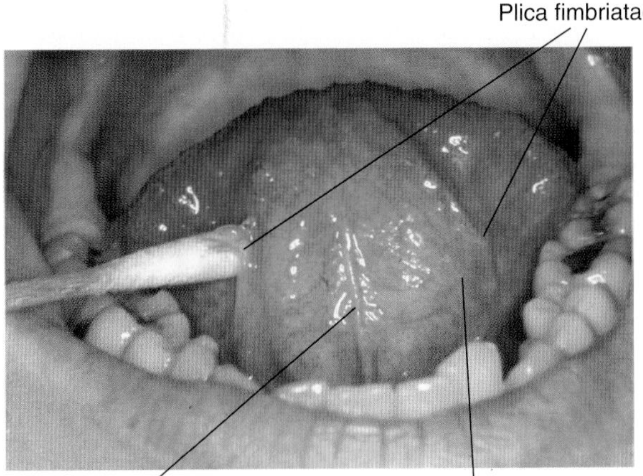

**Fig 5.5** Ventral surface of the tongue.

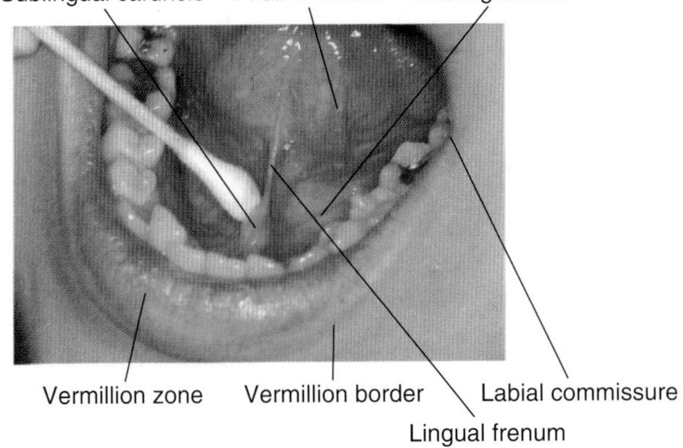

**Fig 5.6** Ventral surface of the tongue and the floor of the mouth.

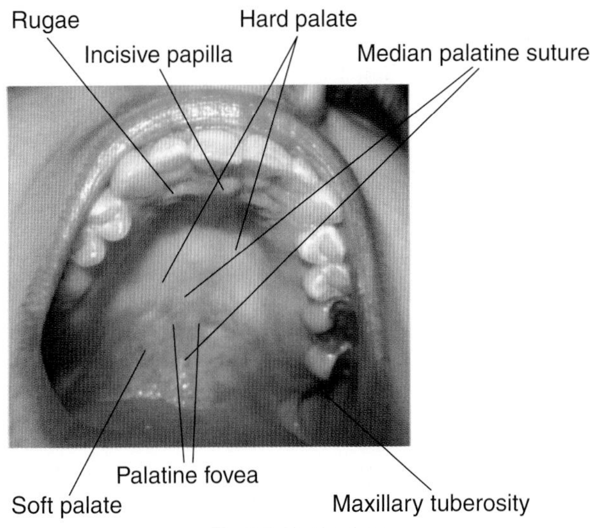

**Fig 5.7** Hard palate.

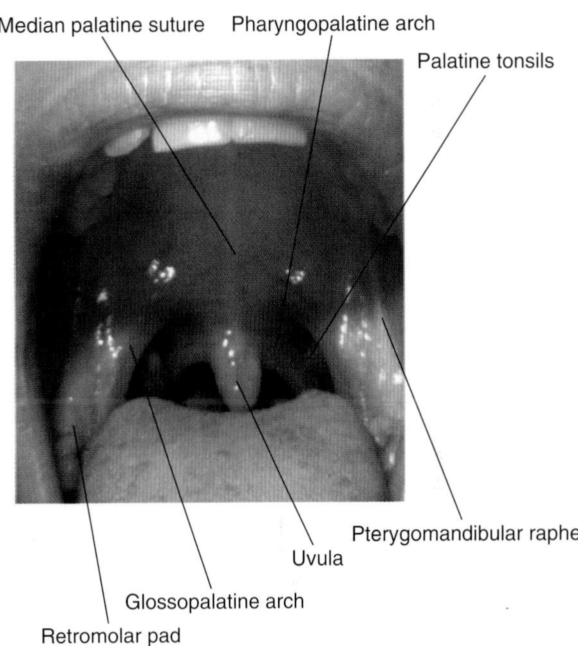

**Fig 5.8** Soft palate and oropharynx.

## DENTAL ANATOMY

A. Permanent dentition (Table 5.3)
   1. Humans are diphyodonts, with two sets of teeth in a lifetime—a primary/deciduous dentition and a permanent dentition; span three dentition periods: primary, mixed/transitional, and permanent
   2. The permanent dentition consists of 32 teeth if all are present; arranged in four quadrants: maxillary right, maxillary left, mandibular left, and mandibular right (quadrants 1–4)
   3. When naming teeth use this order: set, arch, side, type, class (e.g., permanent mandibular right second molar)

B. Classes of teeth: incisors, canines, premolars, and molars; each quadrant (from the midline) has two incisors (central and lateral), one canine, two premolars (first and second), and three molars (first, second, and third); incisors and canines are anterior teeth; premolars and molars are posterior teeth
   1. Anatomic features of anterior teeth
      a. Incisors—two in each quadrant; function in cutting
         (1) Incisal ridge—found on incisors; newly erupted incisors have *mamelons*: three rounded elevations on the incisal ridge, delineating the three facial developmental lobes, which are usually worn away with normal function after eruption

## TABLE 5.1 Oral Structures.

| Structure | Clinical Description | Clinical Consideration |
|---|---|---|
| **Lips, Cheeks, and Oral Mucosa (see Figs. 5.1 and 5.2)** | | |
| Philtrum | Midline vertical depression of the skin between the nose and upper lip | Common location for cleft lip |
| Vermillion zone/ border | Transitional area between the skin of the face and the oral mucosa of lips; medium pink in light-skinned individuals, and pigmented with melanin in dark-skinned individuals | Junction between vermillion zone and skin of face is a frequent site of herpetic lesions<br>The lower lip is a frequent site of oral cancer<br>Fordyce's granules or spots (small white spots of ectopic sebaceous material) may be present |
| Labial commissure | Junction of upper and lower lips at the corner of the mouth | Frequent site of chafing, herpetic lesions, and cracking (angular cheilitis); avoid pulling with instrument handle |
| Vestibule | Space between the teeth (alveolar processes) and the lips and cheeks | Frequent site of aphthous ulcers |
| Labial mucosa | Mucosal lining of the inner lip next to the anterior teeth; vascular; small elevations are external manifestation of numerous labial salivary glands | Frequent site of mucoceles, mucus-retention cysts, aphthous ulcers, and scars |
| Labial frenum (plural, frena) (maxillary and mandibular) | Fold of tissue at the midline (maxillary and mandibular) between the inner surface of the lip and the alveolar mucosa; attaches the lips to the mucosal tissue between central incisors | Maxillary fold is sometimes overdeveloped, which results in a space between the central incisors, (diastema); frequently has an extra flap of tissue<br>If overextended onto the attached gingiva, mandibular fold may cause recession |
| Buccal mucosa | Mucous membrane lining of the inner cheek next to the posterior teeth | Frequent site of linea alba, cheek bites, and Fordyce's granules |
| Parotid papilla | Flap of tissue on the cheek opposite the maxillary first and second molars; contains the opening of Stensen duct, which carries saliva from the parotid gland | Large amounts of mainly serous saliva come from this duct; the opening can often be seen as a dark spot |
| Buccal frena (muscle attachments) | Folds of epithelium between the cheek and attached gingivae (maxillary and mandibular) in the premolar area | Overextension may cause gingival recession<br>Movement of the frena aids in guiding food during mastication |
| Mucobuccal fold | Fold between the alveolar and buccal or labial mucosa | The height of the mucobuccal fold is a penetration site for injection techniques |
| Alveolar mucosa | Thin movable mucosal lining covering alveolar bone; between the attached gingiva and the mucobuccal fold on the facial aspect of maxillary and mandibular arches and between the attached gingiva and the floor of the mouth on the lingual aspect of the mandibular arch | Very thin and fragile epithelium; frequent site of apthous ulcers |
| Gingiva | Keratinized mucosa that surrounds teeth and alveolar bone. Attached gingiva: part attached to the alveolar bone<br>Free gingiva: part that surrounds the necks of the teeth | Ideally, except for a narrow band around the necks of teeth, it is firmly attached to teeth and bone |
| Mucogingival line or junction | A visible line where the pink, keratinized, attached gingiva meets the more vascular, nonkeratinized, looser alveolar mucosa | Found on maxillary facial and mandibular facial and lingual areas |
| Gingival margin or crest | The most coronal edge of keratinized gingiva | Can change positionally because of inflammation, recession, and attachment loss |
| **Tongue (see Figs. 5.3 to 5.6)** | | |
| The tongue is a flat, muscular organ of speech, taste, mastication, and swallowing; the lateral border and undersurface are frequent sites of oral cancer; dorsum is the top surface covered by papillae (projections for taste); ventral is the underside of the tongue. | | |
| Median sulcus | Midline depression on the dorsum of the tongue | Presence and depth vary.<br>Additional deep depressions are called *fissures* (a fissured tongue) |
| Lingual tonsils | Mass of lymphoid tissue on the base of the tongue, posterior to circumvallate papillae | Difficult to observe; extend and move the tongue to the right and left to examine |
| Fungiform papillae | Large, round, mushroom-shaped, red to dark-brown elevations scattered over the anterior third of the dorsum of the tongue (tip) | In dark-skinned individuals, these papillae may contain melanin pigmentation<br>Function in taste sensations of sweet, sour, and salty |
| Filiform papillae | Fringe-like, fine, keratinized projections concentrated in the middle third of the dorsum of the tongue | Readily collect plaque and stain<br>Tongue with moving patches devoid of these papillae is called a *geographic tongue* |
| Circumvallate papillae | From 8 to 12 large papillae arranged in an inverted V-shaped row posterior to filiform papillae | Function in the taste sensation of bitter<br>Ducts of von Ebner salivary glands open around these papillae and secrete serous saliva |
| Foliate papillae | Vertical ridges on the lateral borders of the tongue | Function in the taste sensation of sour<br>May be a site of precancerous or cancerous findings (white or red areas, ulcers, masses, pigmentations) |

**TABLE 5.1 Oral Structures.—cont'd**

| Structure | Clinical Description | Clinical Consideration |
|---|---|---|
| Lingual frenum | Thin fold of epithelium attaching the undersurface of the tongue to the floor of the mouth | A short frenum limits movement (ankyloglossia, tongue-tied) and makes exposing radiographs and taking impressions difficult; if located too close to the mandibular central incisors, cause periodontal issues |
| Sublingual folds (plica sublingualis) | Two ridges of tissue on the floor of the mouth arranged in a V-shaped direction, from the lingual frenum to the base of the tongue | Contains Wharton duct from the submandibular (also called *submaxillary*) salivary gland, Bartholin duct, and the openings of the sublingual salivary glands<br>Limited amounts of mixed saliva secreted there |
| Sublingual caruncle | Round elevation of the floor of the mouth on either side of the lingual frenum; contains the openings for both the submandibular and the sublingual salivary glands | Wharton duct carries large amounts of saliva from the submandibular salivary gland |
| Lingual veins | Blue line on the undersurface of the tongue on either side of the lingual frenum | With age, these veins become more prominent in size and color; varicosities may be present |
| Plica fimbriata | Delicate, fringe-like projections of the mucous membranes on the undersurface of the tongue, lateral to the lingual vein | May be dark colored, with more melanin pigmentation |
| **Palate (see Figs. 5.7 and 5.8)** | | |
| Hard palate: the anterior two-thirds of the roof of the mouth; soft palate: the posterior third of the roof of the mouth; a frequent site of oral cancer | | |
| Incisive papilla | Midline, elevated pad of tissue lingual to the maxillary central incisors | Often burned or traumatized when eating<br>Protects the nasopalatine nerve, which enters through the underlying incisive foramen<br>The palatal mucosa immediately lateral to the papilla is needle insertion site for nasopalatine nerve block anesthesia |
| Rugae | Firm, irregular ridges of masticatory mucosa on anterior half of the hard palate branching off of the palatine raphe (see later) | If prominent, rugae may be burned or traumatized more easily<br>Functions include tactile sensation of food and aiding sounds in speech |
| Palatine fovea | Small dimple on either side of the midline at the junction of the hard and soft palates | Touching area posterior to this may initiate the gag reflex<br>Site for the greater palatine nerve block |
| Palatal salivary duct openings | Small, dark spots scattered on the hard and soft palates | Represent the duct openings of minor palatal salivary glands |
| Palatine raphe | Hard, linear elevated ridge of tissue along the midline of the hard palate; external manifestation of the palatine suture, which joins the right and left maxillary and palatine bones | Excess bone (tori) or a deep depression may be present there<br>Site of hyperkeratinization or associated nicotine stomatitis |
| Maxillary tuberosity | Protuberance of alveolar bone distal to the last maxillary molar | Erupting third molar may be present there |
| **Tonsillar Region (see Fig. 5.8)** | | |
| Retromolar area | Triangular area of bone and pad of movable tissue distal to the last mandibular molar | An erupting third molar may be present, and a flap of tissue (operculum) is often associated with infection in this area |
| Pterygomandibular raphe | Fold of tissue from the retromolar area to an area near the maxillary tuberosity; separates the soft palate from the cheek; lies medial to the posterior border of the ramus of the mandible | Covers a ligament from the mandible to sphenoid bone<br>Used as a guide for needle insertion for inferior alveolar nerve block |
| Anterior or glossopalatine arch | Thin fold of epithelium extending laterally and inferiorly from both sides (two pillars) of the soft palate to the base of the tongue | Marks the entry into the pharynx; the anterior boundary of the tonsillar recess |
| Posterior or pharyngopalatine arch | Thin fold of epithelium (two pillars) that is more posterior and narrower than the anterior arch | Marks the posterior boundary of the palatine tonsillar recess |
| Tonsillar recess | Recessed area between the anterior and posterior arches | May or may not contain palatine tonsils |
| Palatine tonsils | Globules of lymphoid tissue in the tonsillar recess | Vary greatly in size<br>Not visible if removed or atrophied, or may be so large that the fauces is very narrow |
| Uvula | Fleshy tissue suspended from the midline of the posterior border of the soft palate | Closes the opening to the nasopharynx when swallowing<br>Varies in size and shape |
| Pharyngeal tonsils | Globules of lymphoid tissue on the oropharyngeal wall | Nontechnical term is *adenoids*; appear as globules of reddish orange tissue<br>Mucosal secretions from the sinuses may be seen here |
| Fauces or faucial isthmus | Isthmus (narrowing) of the space from the oral cavity into the pharynx; posterior border of the oral cavity | |

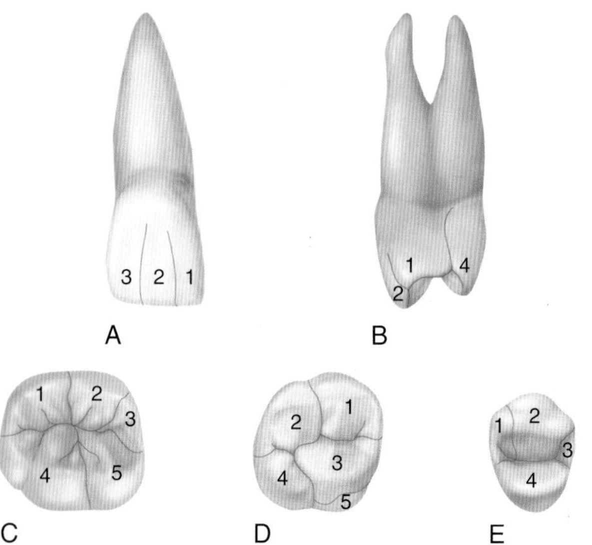

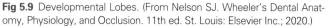

**Fig 5.9** Developmental Lobes. (From Nelson SJ. Wheeler's Dental Anatomy, Physiology, and Occlusion. 11th ed. St. Louis: Elsevier Inc.; 2020.)

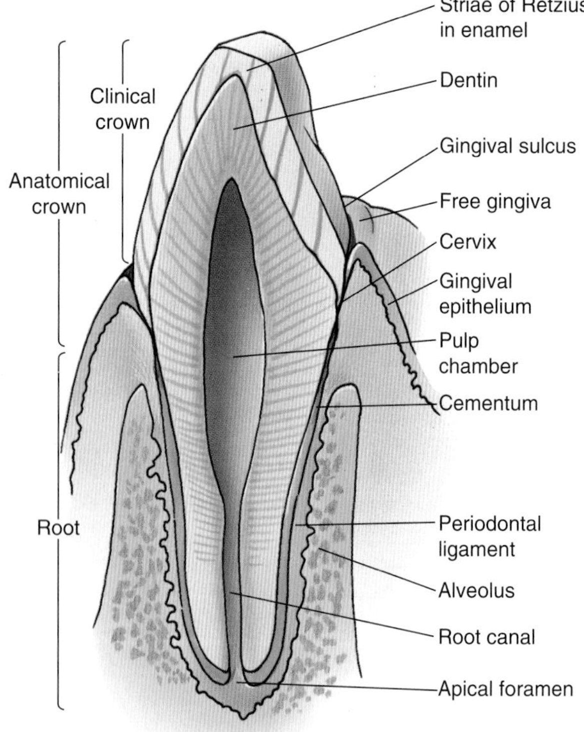

**Fig. 5.10** Clinical and anatomical crown. (From Gartner LP. Textbook of Histology. 5th ed. St. Louis: Elsevier Inc.; 2021.)

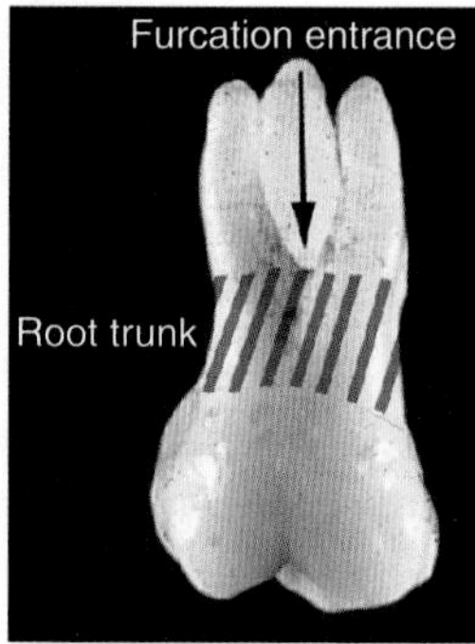

**Fig. 5.11** Furcation. (LA Bergstrom-Bryan, BSDH, RDH, MEd, Marquette University School of Dentistry and former Department of Dental Hygiene.)

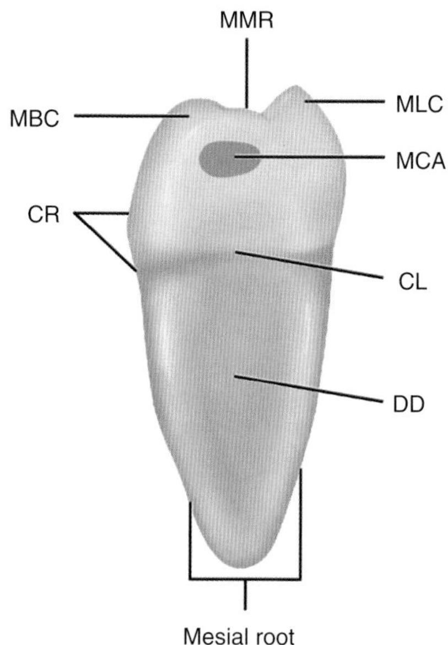

**Fig. 5.12** Mandibular right first molar, mesial aspect. *CL,* cervical line; *CR,* cervical ridge; *DD,* developmental depression; *MBC,* mesiobuccal cusp; *MCA,* mesial contact area; *MLC,* mesiolingual cusp; *MMR,* Mesial marginal ridge. (From: Nelson. Wheeler's Dental Anatomy, Physiology, and Occlusion, 10th edition).

(2) Incisal angles—formed by the proximal surfaces and the incisal ridge; central incisor angles are sharper and more acute than lateral incisor angles, and mesioincisal angles are sharper than distoincisal angles
(3) Maxillary lateral incisors vary the most in size and shape and may be congenitally missing or anomalous, as in the case of a peg lateral (smaller and more pointed)

b. Canines—one in each quadrant; only teeth with one cusp; function in grasping and tearing
   (1) Considered the cornerstone of the dentition because of the long, large root, which is externally manifested by the canine eminence of maxillary alveolar bone
   (2) Have a prominent lingual ridge between two fossae; lingual anatomy is more prominent on maxillary canines

2. Anatomic features of posterior teeth
   a. Premolars—two in each quadrant; first and second premolars; function in cracking/chopping
      (1) Generally have two cusps; the mandibular second premolar also typically has a three-cusped type
      (2) Have one root, except maxillary first premolars, which have two roots 60% of the time
      (3) Replace (succeed) primary molars when exfoliated
      (4) First premolars are frequently extracted for orthodontic reasons

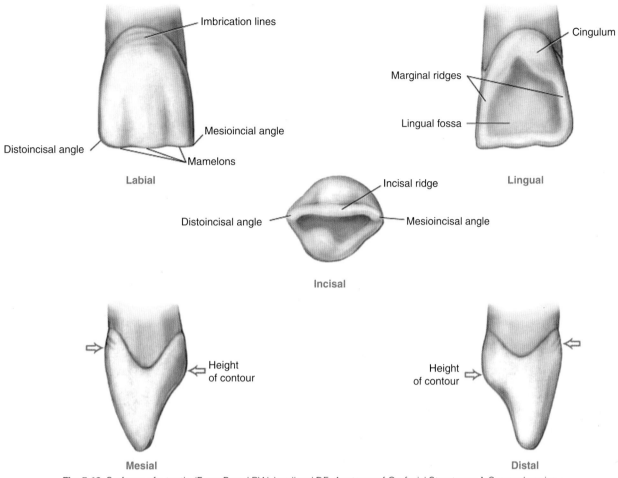

Fig. 5.13 Surfaces of a tooth. (From Brand RW, Isselhard DE. Anatomy of Orofacial Structures: A Comprehensive Approach. 8th ed. St. Louis: Elsevier Inc.; 2019.)

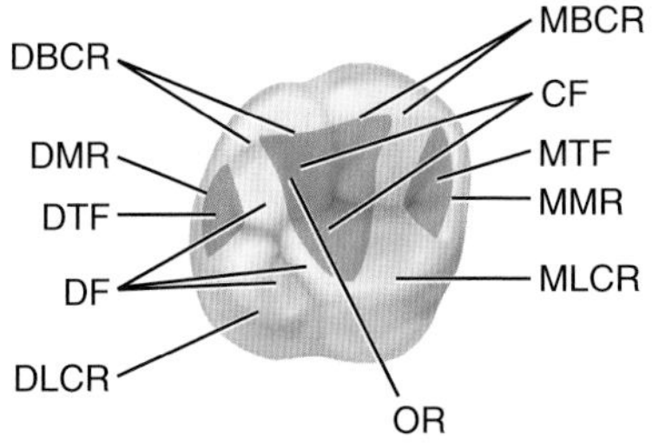


Fig. 5.14 Occlusal anatomy. (From Nelson SJ: Wheeler's Dental Anatomy, Physiology, and Occlusion, ed. 11, St. Louis, 2020, Elsevier Inc.)

b. Molars—three in each quadrant; named first, second, and third molars; function in grinding
   (1) Largest crown in the dentition both mesiodistally and faciolingually; shorter cervico-occlusally
   (2) Only teeth that do not replace primary teeth (nonsuccedaneous); erupt posterior to primary molars
   (3) The mandibular first molar is the first permanent tooth to erupt
   (4) Multicusped, with each having a distinct cusp-and-groove pattern
   (5) Maxillary molars have three roots; mandibular molars have two roots
   (6) The presence, size, and shape of third molars vary greatly, roots commonly fused

C. Tooth-numbering systems (Fig. 5.17)
   1. Universal Numbering System—Arabic numerals 1 to 32 to specify permanent teeth, beginning with the maxillary right third molar and ending with the mandibular right third molar.
   2. International Numbering System—a two-digit code: the first digit—1 to 4—designates the quadrant location; the second digit—1 to 8—designates the tooth, starting from the midline, from the central incisor to the third molar (e.g., 1-1 is the maxillary right central incisor)
   3. Palmer/Zsigmondy System—uses quadrant symbols with the tooth number, teeth are numbered 1–8 from the midline

D. General characteristics of tooth form (Fig. 5.18)
   1. Crest of curvature (crest of convexity) or height of contour (HOC)—the greatest curvature on each axial surface; four on each tooth
   2. All proximal surfaces narrow mesiodistally from the HOC to the cemento-enamel junctions (CEJ)
   3. The proximal crest (HOC) convergence provides spacing for the interproximal gingiva and bone
   4. Contact area—ideally formed by the proximal HOC area, which functions to stabilize adjacent teeth and protect the interproximal gingiva

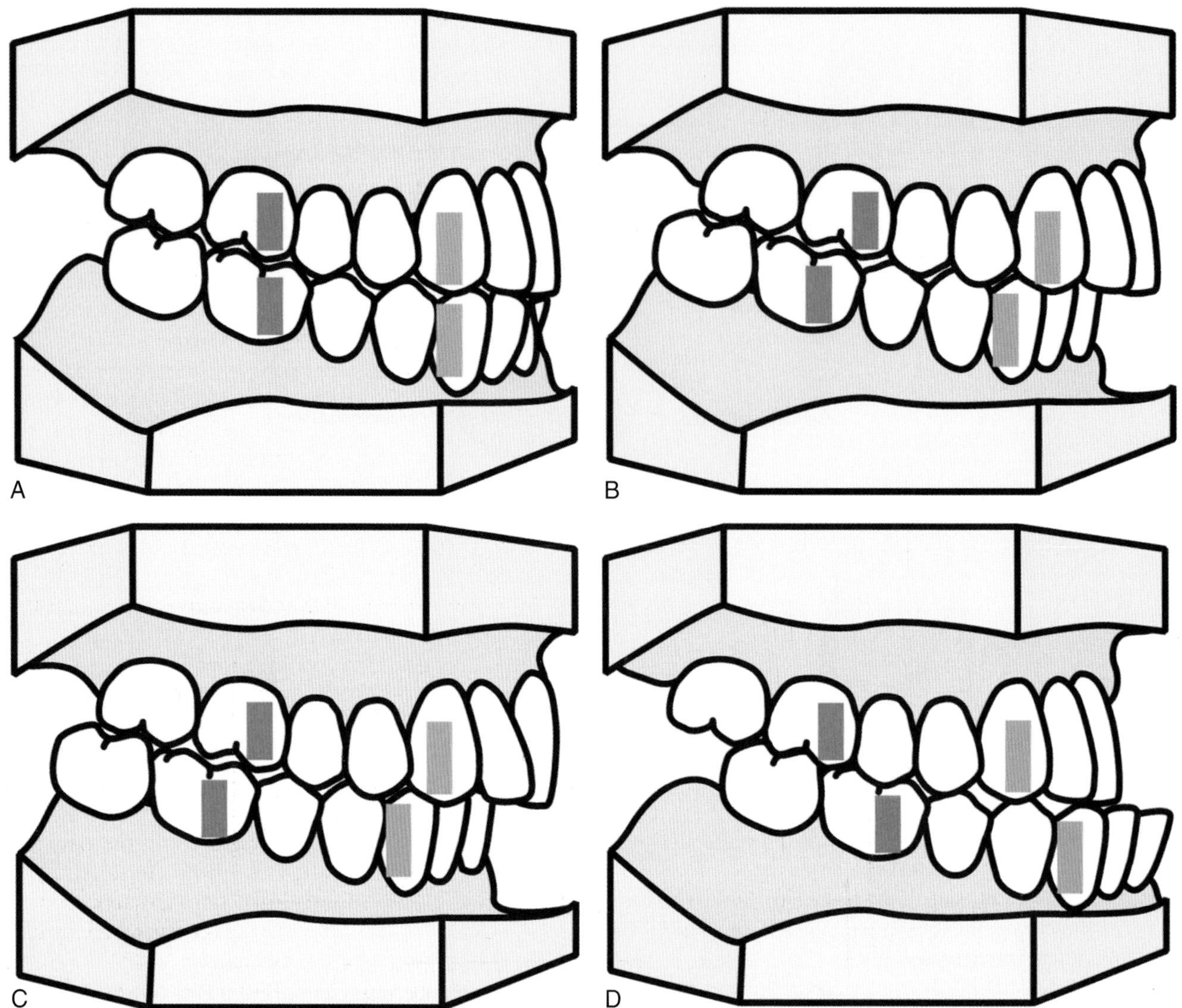


**Fig. 5.15** Malocclusion classified using Angle's system. (A) Angle's class I occlusion. (B) Angle's class II malocclusion (division 1). (C) Angle's class II malocclusion (division 2). (D) Angle's class III malocclusion. (From Nelson SJ: Wheeler's Dental Anatomy, Physiology, and Occlusion, ed 11, St. Louis, 2020, Elsevier Inc.)

5. Proximal crests (HOC) gradually move from the incisal third on incisors to the middle third on molars; as a general rule, the mesial crest is more incisal-occlusal than the distal crest
6. Facial and lingual crests (HOC) are generally in the cervical third on anterior teeth, with the lingual HOC more in the middle third on premolars and molars; mandibular posteriors, especially molars, have their lingual HOC more toward the occlusal third
7. Mesial cusp ridges are shorter than distal cusp ridges (except the maxillary first premolar); mesial outlines are straighter than distal outlines
8. All facial and lingual surfaces converge toward the apex and toward the incisal-occlusal surface from the crests of curvature
   a. This convergence facilitates mastication
   b. These contours deflect food away from the gingiva and facilitate the function of teeth
9. CEJs
   a. The CEJ on the proximal surface curves toward the incisal-occlusal; more prominent on anterior teeth than on posterior teeth; curves more on the mesial surface than on the distal surface
   b. Maxillary CEJs curve more than mandibular
10. Crown and root inclination—from a proximal view, the long axes of the crown and the root are in line, except for the mandibular posterior teeth crowns, which tilt lingually to the long axes of the root; this lingual inclination enables the intercuspal relationship of posterior teeth and the distribution of forces along their long axes
11. Proximal surfaces converge toward the lingual; this is most prominent on maxillary incisors and canines
   a. Lingual embrasures are larger than facial embrasures
   b. The two exceptions are the mandibular second premolar, three-cusp type, and the maxillary first molar, because of its large distolingual cusp (Table 5.3)

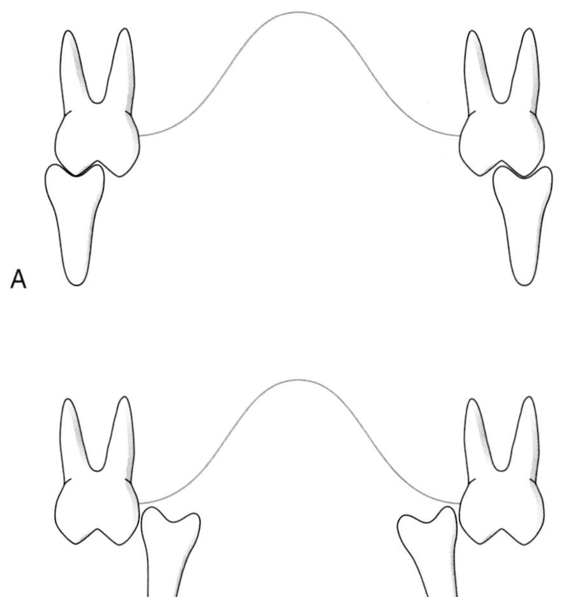


**Fig. 5.16** **A**, Bilateral buccal crossbite, **B**, Bilateral lingual crossbite. (From Heasman P: Master Dentistry: Volume 2: Restorative Dentistry, Paediatric Dentistry and Orthodontics, ed. 3, 2013, Churchill Livingstone.)

D. General characteristics of roots
   1. Root anatomy varies in size, shape, and number
   2. Teeth have 1 to 3 roots; some roots may divide in the apical third
      a. One root—incisors, canines, maxillary second premolars, mandibular premolars
      b. Two roots—maxillary first premolars (buccal and lingual) and mandibular molars (mesial and distal)
      c. Three roots—maxillary molars (mesiobuccal, distobuccal, and lingual)
   3. Teeth with 2 to 3 roots have a root trunk with depressions that deepen until the trunk divides at the furcation
      a. The more cervical the furcation, the more stable the tooth because of the divergence of roots with interradicular bone; first molars have the shortest root trunk
      b. Furcation involvement—loss of attachment of tissue and bone exists
      c. Furcations closer to the CEJ are more likely to become involved in periodontal disease, but are more accessible
      d. Individual roots are basically cone-shaped, widest at the CEJ and converge (taper) to the apex; more root surface area is present in the cervical third than apical third
      e. A cervical cross section of a tooth with one root shows three basic shapes (Fig. 5.19; see Table 5.3), which may be slightly altered by the presence of root concavities
         (1) Triangular—maxillary incisors; have narrower mesiodistal dimension on the lingual surface
         (2) Ovoid (egg shaped)—canines and some mandibular premolars
         (3) Elliptical (oblong)—maxillary premolars, mandibular incisors, and some mandibular premolars
      g. A cervical cross section of molars follows the form of the crown, with depressions on most axial surfaces
      h. From a facial or lingual view, roots often have distal flexion; more reliably on posterior teeth
      i. Second-molar and third-molar roots are more likely to be closer together or fused, and distally inclined

E. Clinical considerations of permanent tooth form—as a general rule, proximal surfaces of most teeth are more accessible from the lingual approach because of the convergence (tapering) of lingual teeth surfaces producing larger lingual embrasures
   1. Incisors
      a. Maxillary lingual anatomy is more prominent than mandibular lingual anatomy; however, plaque, calculus, and stain readily collect on mandibular lingual surfaces
      b. Repeated instrumentation on the narrow roots of mandibular incisors makes them subject to loss of structure, resulting in unsupported cervical enamel
      c. Deep fossae and narrow dimensions of roots are difficult for instrumentation
      d. Pits on maxillary lateral incisors more subject to caries
   2. Canines
      a. Crown length, bulk, and long roots make these teeth very stable
      b. Prominent distal crown and root depression
   3. Premolars
      a. Distinctive pit-and-groove patterns facilitate the identification of premolars
      b. Proximal root concavities, especially the mesial of the maxillary first premolar, make subgingival instrumentation difficult on the proximal surfaces
      c. Lingual inclination of mandibular premolar crowns makes instrumentation difficult
      d. Self-care more difficult with root depressions and lingual inclination
   4. Molars
      a. Complex pit-and-groove patterns make molars susceptible to dental caries; sealants should be placed shortly after eruption
      b. Lingual inclination of mandibular molar crowns makes self-care and instrumentation difficult
      c. Maxillary molar furcations better accessed from the lingual approach because of locations
      d. Furcation involvement challenging for access; requires more time and possible surgical intervention

F. Primary/deciduous dentition
   1. The primary (deciduous) dentition consists of 20 teeth (5 per quadrant): 8 incisors, 4 canines, and 8 molars
   2. Numbering systems (Fig. 5.20)
      a. The Universal Numbering System uses capital letters: A through T for primary teeth, beginning with the maxillary right second primary molar and ending with the mandibular right second primary molar
      b. The International System uses a two-digit code: the first digit—5 to 8—designates the quadrant in the dentition, clockwise from the upper-right

**TABLE 5.2 Dental Terminology.**

| Terminology | Description |
|---|---|
| **Parts of a tooth (see Figs. 5.9 to 5.12)** | |
| Developmental lobe | Developmental centers; anterior teeth are formed by four lobes; posterior teeth are formed by four to five lobes |
| Anatomic crown | Part of the tooth covered by enamel |
| Clinical crown | Portion of the tooth that is visible in the oral cavity; determined by the location of the gingival margin |
| Note: the anatomic and clinical crown are the same when the marginal gingiva is at the cemento-enamel junction (CEJ) | |
| Root | Part of the tooth covered by cementum; can be single-root or multirooted |
| Apex/apices | Rounded end of the root |
| Periapex/periapical | Area around the apex |
| Root trunk | Area from the CEJ to the furcation |
| Foramen/foramina | Opening at the apex through which blood vessels and nerves enter |
| Furcation | Area of a multirooted tooth when the root divides |
| Root concavity/depression | Concave, vertical depression on the root; named by location (mesial, distal, lingual); can be narrow or broad, shallow or deep |
| Enamel | Hardest calcified tissue covering the dentin in the crown of the tooth; 96% mineralized (inorganic); thinnest at the CEJ |
| Dentin | Hard calcified tissue surrounding the pulp and underlying enamel and cementum; makes up the bulk of the tooth; 70% mineralized (inorganic) |
| Cementum | Bone-like calcified tissue covering the dentin on the root of the tooth; 65% mineralized (inorganic) |
| Pulp | Innermost, noncalcified tissue containing blood vessels, lymph, and nerves |
| Pulp chamber | Portion of the pulp in the crown of the tooth |
| Pulp canal | Portion of the pulp in the root of the tooth |
| Pulp cavity | The pulp chamber and the pulp canal; space containing the pulp |
| Pulp horns | Pointed, crown-ward extensions of the pulp chamber; generally one horn per cusp on posterior teeth and one to three horns per cusp on anterior teeth |
| **Junction of tooth tissues** | |
| CEJ | Junction of cementum and enamel; also known as cervical line |
| Dento-enamel junction (DEJ) | Junction of dentin and enamel |
| Cemento-dentin junction (CDJ) | Junction of cementum and dentin |
| **Tooth surfaces (see Fig. 5.13)** | |
| Facial | Surface toward the face<br>Labial: toward the lips; facial surfaces of anterior teeth<br>Buccal: toward the cheeks; facial surfaces of posterior teeth |
| Lingual | Surface toward the tongue; may also be called palatal for maxillary teeth |
| Proximal | Surface toward the adjacent tooth |
| Mesial | Proximal surface toward the midline |
| Distal | Proximal surface farthest away from the midline |
| Incisal | Surface of an anterior tooth that is toward the opposite arch; the biting surface |
| Occlusal | Surface of a posterior tooth that is toward the opposite arch; the biting surface |
| Embrasure | The interproximal space between teeth; functions in deflecting food and reducing the forces placed on the periodontium during mastication |
| **Features of incisal/occlusal surfaces (see Figs. 5.14)** | |
| Cusp | Large, rounded, elevated area of enamel found on posterior teeth; usually named for its location |
| Ridge | Rounded, linear elevation of enamel |
| Marginal ridge | Forms the mesial and distal borders of the lingual surface of anterior teeth and the occlusal proximal surfaces of posterior teeth |
| Triangular ridge | Ridges on posterior teeth from the tip of the cusp to the central groove |
| Oblique ridge | Two triangular ridges meeting in an oblique line; a characteristic of some maxillary molars |
| Transverse ridge | Two triangular ridges meeting in a faciolingual line (often on two-cusped premolars) |
| Groove | Narrow linear depression |
| Developmental groove/depression | Groove or line that indicates the primary anatomic divisions (cusps, developmental lobes) of a crown |
| Supplemental groove | A less distinct groove that branches from a developmental groove |
| Fossa/fossae | A depression on anterior teeth between marginal ridges on the lingual surfaces, and on occlusal surfaces of posterior teeth |
| Fissure | Narrow crevice within a groove where fusion is incomplete |

**TABLE 5.2 Dental Terminology.—cont'd**

| Terminology | Description |
|---|---|
| Pit | A sharp, pointed depression generally located at the junction of developmental grooves (fissures) or at their termination; narrow or wide; pits in primary teeth are not as deep as those in permanent teeth |
| Cingulum/cingula | Large, rounded elevation of enamel on the linguocervical third of anterior teeth (the lingual developmental lobe) |
| **Miscellaneous terminology** | |
| Line angle | The junction of two tooth surfaces; each tooth has eight line angles |
| Point angle | The junction of three tooth surfaces; each tooth has four point angles |
| Fused roots | No division of furcations |
| Supernumary roots | Extra roots |
| Dilaceration | Unusual bending or root curvature |
| Hypercementosis | Deposition of extra cementum |
| Enamel pearls | Spherical enamel formed on cementum, usually near a furcation |
| Cervical enamel projections | CEJ curves more apically near a furcation; a linear projection of enamel towards the apex |
| Bifurcational ridge | Ridge of cementum between mesial and distal roots on mandibular molars |
| Overjet (horizontal overlap) | The characteristic of maxillary teeth to overlap mandibular teeth in a horizontal direction; the maxillary arch is slightly larger; it functions to protect the narrow edge of incisors and to provide for an intercusping relationship of posterior teeth |
| Overbite (vertical overlap) | The characteristic of the anterior maxillary teeth to overlap the anterior mandibular teeth in a vertical direction normally; facilitating the scissors-like cutting function of incisors |
| Intercuspation | The characteristic of posterior teeth to intermesh in a faciolingual direction; mandibular facial cusps and maxillary lingual cusps are centric cusps (supporting cusps) that contact interocclusally in the opposing arch |
| Interdigitation | The characteristic of each tooth to articulate with two opposing teeth (except for mandibular central incisors and maxillary last molars); a mandibular tooth occludes with its counterpart in the upper arch and the one mesial to it; a maxillary tooth occludes with its counterpart in the mandibular arch and the one distal to it |
| Guiding cusps | Maxillary facial and mandibular lingual cusps that help to protect the teeth and tissues |
| **Angle's classifications (see Fig. 5.16)** | |
| Class I (orthognathic profile) | Normal molar relationships (mesiobuccal groove of the mandibular first permanent molar aligns with the mesiobuccal cusp of the maxillary first permanent molar) with alterations in other characteristics of the occlusion, such as versions, crossbites, excessive overjets, or overbites |
| Class II (retrognathic profile: Division 1 | Distal relationship of the mesiobuccal groove of the mandibular first permanent molar to the mesiobuccal cusp of the maxillary first permanent molar; protruded anterior maxillary teeth |
| Class II division 2 | Distal relationship of the mesiobuccal groove of the mandibular first permanent molar to the mesiobuccal cusp of the maxillary first permanent molar; one or more retruded anterior maxillary teeth |
| Class III (prognathic profile) | A mesial relationship of the mesiobuccal groove of the mandibular first permanent molar to the mesiobuccal cusp of the maxillary first permanent molar |
| **Disturbances in interarch alignment (see Fig. 5.17)** | |
| Excessive overbite | The incisal edges of maxillary incisors extend to the cervical third of mandibular incisors |
| Excessive overjet | Horizontal overlap of maxillary teeth to mandibular teeth by more than 3 mm |
| End-to-end relationships | Edge-to-edge bite; anterior teeth meet at their incisal edges with no overjet or overbite; cusp-to-cusp bite in which posterior teeth meet cusp to cusp with no intercuspation |
| Open bite | No incisal or occlusal contact between maxillary and mandibular teeth; teeth cannot be brought together, a space is created, may be caused by tongue thrust or thumb sucking |
| Crossbites | Altered normal faciolingual relationship between maxillary teeth and mandibular teeth; for anterior teeth, mandibular teeth are facial rather than lingual to maxillary teeth; for posterior teeth, normal intercuspation is not observed; numerous alterations are possible and result in maxillary or mandibular, buccal or lingual, or partial or total crossbites |

quadrant; the second digit—1 to 5—designates the tooth, from the central incisor to the second primary molar

c. Palmer/Zsigmondy System—uses quadrant symbols with the tooth letter, teeth are lettered A–E from the midline

3. Set traits—the anatomy of primary teeth is similar to that of permanent teeth, except:
   a. Primary teeth are smaller in size than their permanent counterparts; primary molars are wider than the premolars *(leeway space)*
   b. Primary teeth are whiter than permanent teeth
   c. The crowns of primary teeth are shorter cervico-incisally/occlusally, with pronounced labial and lingual cervical ridges
   d. Occlusal tables of primary teeth narrower faciolingually (smaller intercuspal width), and the cuspal anatomy is not as pronounced as in permanent teeth (smaller intercuspal depth)
   e. Enamel thickness is more consistent and thinner: 0.5 to 1 mm thick, compared with that of permanent teeth, 2.5 mm

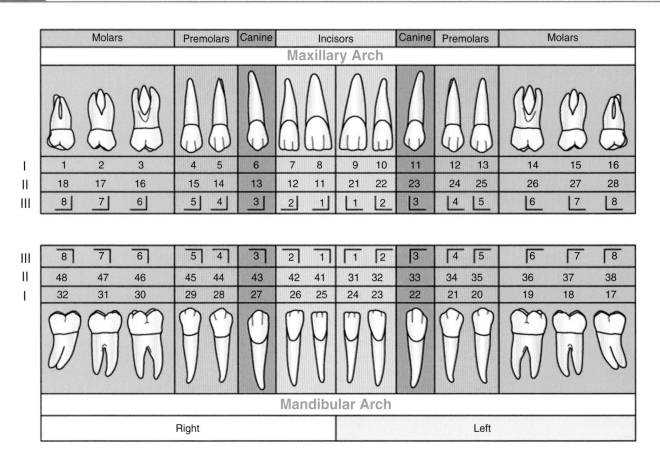

| | Molars | | | Premolars | | Canine | Incisors | | | | Canine | Premolars | | Molars | | |
|---|---|---|---|---|---|---|---|---|---|---|---|---|---|---|---|---|
| | Maxillary Arch | | | | | | | | | | | | | | | |
| I | 1 | 2 | 3 | 4 | 5 | 6 | 7 | 8 | 9 | 10 | 11 | 12 | 13 | 14 | 15 | 16 |
| II | 18 | 17 | 16 | 15 | 14 | 13 | 12 | 11 | 21 | 22 | 23 | 24 | 25 | 26 | 27 | 28 |
| III | 8⌋ | 7⌋ | 6⌋ | 5⌋ | 4⌋ | 3⌋ | 2⌋ | 1⌋ | ⌊1 | ⌊2 | ⌊3 | ⌊4 | ⌊5 | ⌊6 | ⌊7 | ⌊8 |
| III | 8⌉ | 7⌉ | 6⌉ | 5⌉ | 4⌉ | 3⌉ | 2⌉ | 1⌉ | ⌈1 | ⌈2 | ⌈3 | ⌈4 | ⌈5 | ⌈6 | ⌈7 | ⌈8 |
| II | 48 | 47 | 46 | 45 | 44 | 43 | 42 | 41 | 31 | 32 | 33 | 34 | 35 | 36 | 37 | 38 |
| I | 32 | 31 | 30 | 29 | 28 | 27 | 26 | 25 | 24 | 23 | 22 | 21 | 20 | 19 | 18 | 17 |
| | Mandibular Arch | | | | | | | | | | | | | | | |
| | Right | | | | | | | | Left | | | | | | | |

I Universal Numbering System
II International Numbering System
III Palmer Notation Method

**Fig. 5.17** Permanent dentition. (From: Fehrenbach MJ, Herring SW. *Illustrated Anatomy of the Head and Neck*. 4th ed. St. Louis: Saunders/Elsevier; 2012.)

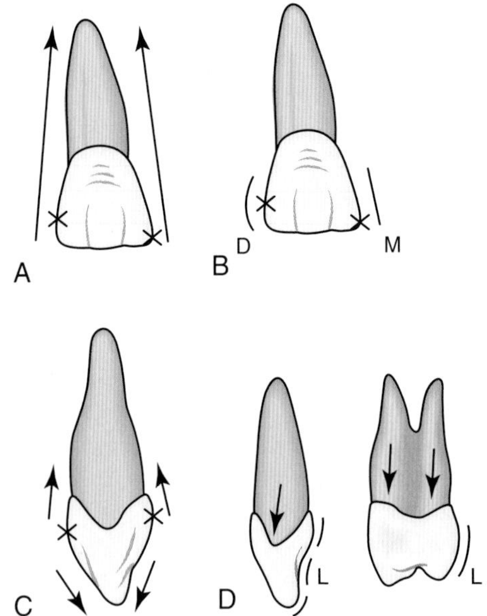


**Fig. 5.18** (A–D) General characteristics of permanent tooth form. A: shows tapering towards the apex B: mesial usually more straight, distal move convex C: from proximal perspective tapers towards incisal edge and tapers towards apex D: CEJ more curvature in anteriors compared to posteriors, anteriors lingual side concave, whereas posteriors lingual side more convex. (From Heasman P. Master Dentistry: Volume 2: Restorative Dentistry, Paediatric Dentistry and Orthodontics. 3rd ed. Churchill Livingstone; 2013.)

f. Pulp chambers (relative to the size of the tooth) are larger, and pulp horns extend more occlusally than in permanent teeth; the amount of dentin is proportionately less

g. Roots are slender and longer than in permanent teeth, approximately twice the length of the crown (larger root-crown ratio)

h. Molar root trunks are shorter (furcations closer to the CEJ); roots are more divergent to accommodate the developing premolar crown

i. Primary teeth have fewer anomalies and variations in tooth form

5. Class traits—anatomy of primary teeth
   a. Incisors—resemble the outline of their permanent counterparts, except no mamelons on the incisal ridge and no pits on the lingual surface
   b. Canines—resemble the outlines of their permanent counterparts; maxillary canine has a sharp cusp, wide and short; mesial cusp ridge is longer than the distal cusp ridge
   c. Molars
      (1) First primary molars—do not resemble any other teeth

## TABLE 5.3 Characteristics of the Crowns and Roots of Permanent Teeth.

| Maxillary | Crown | Root(s) | Visual Characteristics |
|---|---|---|---|
| Central incisor | Largest of incisors<br>The mesiodistal is greater than the faciolingual width<br>Distinct lingual anatomy; broad cingulum with tubercles<br>The lingual surface (mesiodistal) is smaller than the facial surface because of proximal surface convergence | One root, conical in shape<br>Proximal root concavities uncommon<br>Prominent incisal curvature of proximal cemento-enamel junctions<br>Smallest root-crown ratio<br>Cervical cross section is "rounded triangular" in shape with a flat mesial surface | 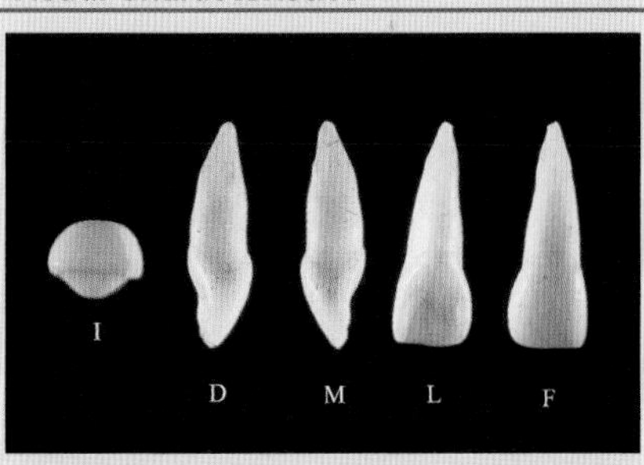 Tooth #8 |
| Lateral incisor | Similar to central but smaller, more slender; rounded incisal angles<br>Cingulum is narrow, and a lingual pit is common | One root, conical in shape<br>The root is longer and more rounded than the central incisor<br>The root is 1⅓ times the length of the crown; may have a narrow lingual or palato–radicular groove extending from the crown to the root | 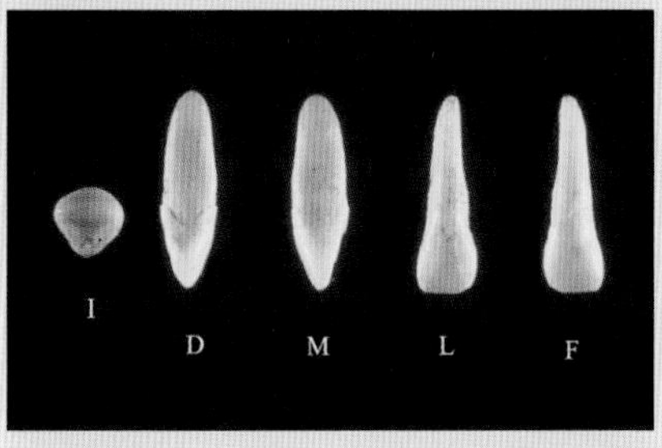 Tooth #7 |
| Canine | Single cusp formed by cusp ridges, facial and lingual ridges; one-third the length of the crown<br>Lingual anatomy is distinct: large cingulum; lingual ridge between two lingual fossae; rarely has pits | One long root, conical in shape<br>Proximal root concavities; distal crown and root depression more significant<br>Bulbous distal height of contour (HOC) may hinder access to the mesial surface of the first premolar.<br>Cervical cross section is ovoid in shape<br>The root is 1½ times the length of the crown | 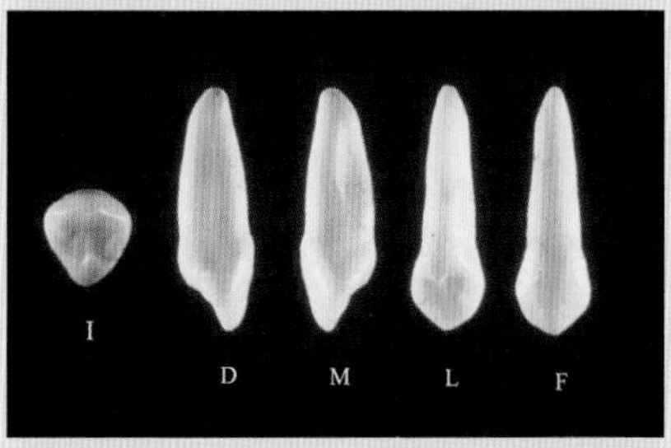 Tooth #6 |
| First premolar | Two cusps, facial longer and wider mesiodistally than the lingual; pentagonal shape from the occlusal with sharper angles on the facial cusp<br>Occlusal: long central developmental groove; mesial and distal pits<br>Mesial marginal ridge groove interrupts the mesial marginal ridge | Two roots (40% have one root); one facial, one lingual<br>Bifurcated in the apical to middle thirds; mesial and distal furcation entrances<br>Prominent mesial concavity begins on the crown cervical to the mesial contact; extends apically to the furcation | 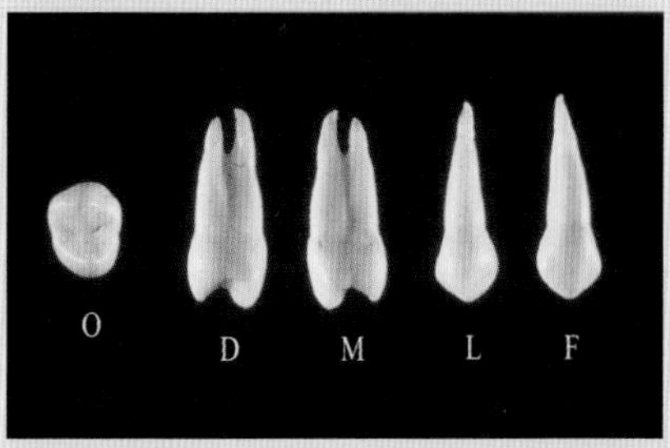 Tooth #4 |
| Second premolar | Two cusps of more equal length and width<br>Occlusal outline is more rounded.<br>Short central developmental groove; supplemental grooves<br>No mesial crown concavity or groove | One root<br>Proximal root concavities common; mesial root concavity not as pronounced as the first premolar<br>Elliptical in cross section; broad proximally<br>The root is 1¾ times the length of the crown. | 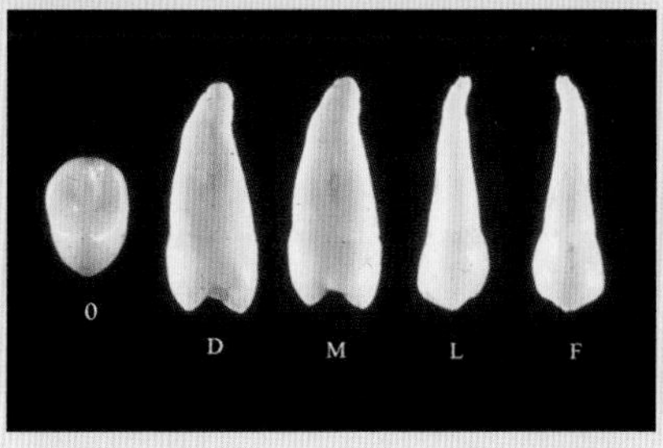 |

Continued

**TABLE 5.3 Characteristics of the Crowns and Roots of Permanent Teeth.—cont'd**

| Maxillary | Crown | Root(s) | Visual Characteristics |
|---|---|---|---|
| | | | Tooth #5 |
| First molar | Largest tooth faciolingually<br>Rhomboidal occlusal view outline<br>Oblique ridge from mesiolingual to distobuccal cusp<br>Four cusps and one minor cusp on the mesiolingual cusp *(cusp of Carabelli)*<br>An occlusal lingual groove ends with a pit on the lingual surface<br>Pits on occlusal, in mesial, central, and distal fossae<br>Lingual surface wider than facial surface due to large distolingual cusp (exception) | Three roots: mesiofacial, distofacial, and lingual; lingual root the longest<br>Furcations on mesial, facial, and distal surfaces<br>Root concavities: palatal surface of lingual root, mesial surface of mesiofacial root, and furcal surfaces (furcal concavities)<br>Mesiofacial and distofacial root apices curve toward each other; resembles a pliers handle<br>Furcations begin gradually before the entrance, which is generally located near the junction of the cervical and middle third of the root; the mesial furcation is located more toward the lingual surface (mesiofacial root is broad in the faciolingual dimension)<br>Root is 1¾ times the length of the crown | 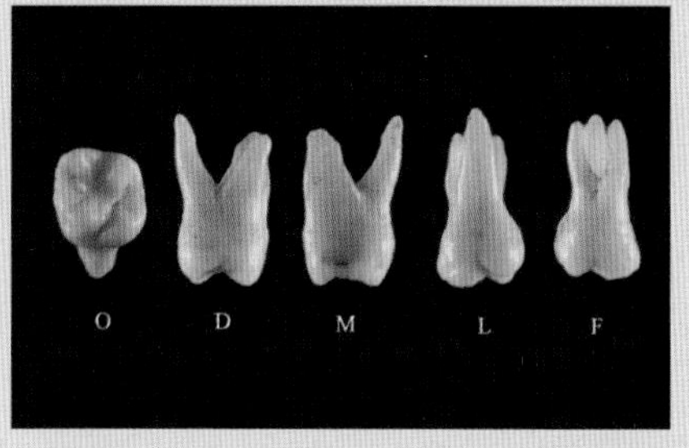 Tooth #3 |
| Second molar | Resembles the first molar, but is smaller; more rhomboidal from occlusal view<br>Four cusps; distolingual cusp is smaller (lingual surface is narrower in the mesiodistal dimension) and sometimes absent<br>Pits in mesial, central, and distal fossae | Three roots: mesiofacial, distofacial, and lingual<br>Roots are closer together; more distally oriented; less interradicular bone<br>Longer root trunk<br>The root is 1¾ times the length of the crown | 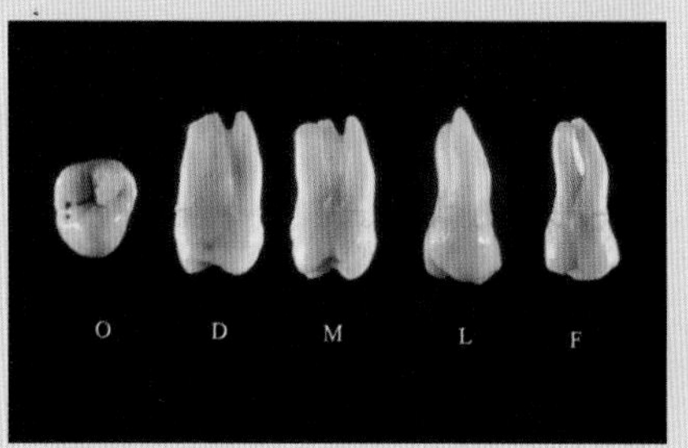 Tooth #2 |
| Third molar | Resembles the second molar, but varies frequently | May have three roots; varies frequently<br>Roots frequently fused | |
| **Mandibular** | **Crown** | **Root(s)** | **Visual Characteristics** |
| Central and lateral incisors | Central incisor is the smallest tooth; symmetrical<br>Lateral incisor is slightly larger; asymmetrical<br>Sharp incisal angles<br>Contact areas near the incisal ridge<br>Lingual surface is concave, less distinct lingual anatomy<br>Lateral crown has a distal twist; incisal ridge is more lingually located on the distal, but cingulum is displaced toward the distal<br>More prominent distal concavity on lateral incisor | One root, wider faciolingually than mesiodistally<br>Proximal root concavities are likely<br>Cervical cross section, elliptical in shape<br>The root is 1½ times the length of the crown | 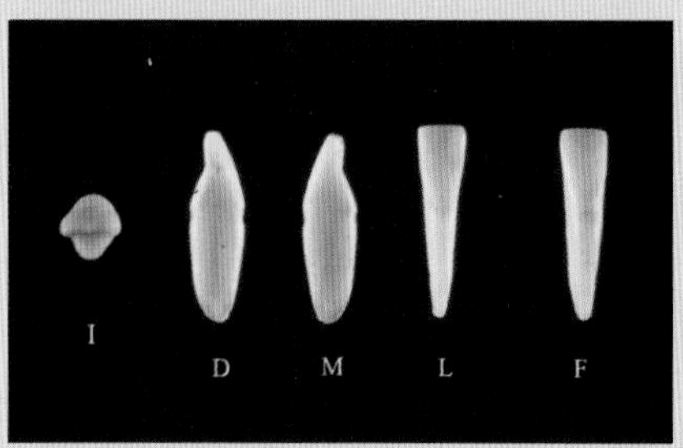 Tooth #25 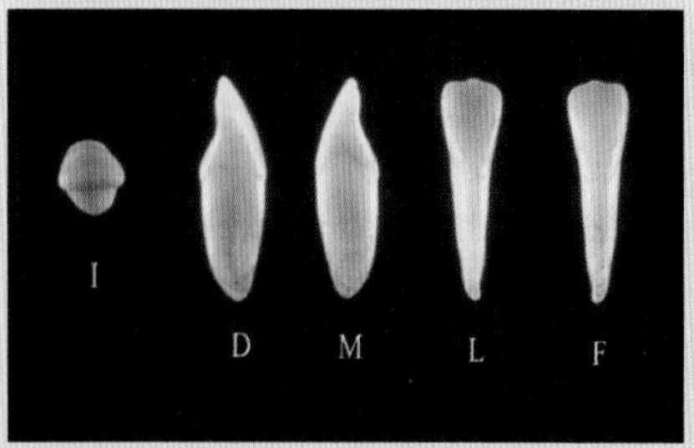<br>Tooth #26 |

## TABLE 5.3 Characteristics of the Crowns and Roots of Permanent Teeth.—cont'd

| Mandibular | Crown | Root(s) | Visual Characteristics |
|---|---|---|---|
| Canine | Cusp ridges and tip occupy ¼ to ⅕ of crown length<br>Lingual anatomy same as that of the maxillary canine, not as prominent<br>Mesial surfaces of the crown and the root are in a straight line; mesial proximal crests (HOC) more incisal than the maxillary canine | One root, conical in shape<br>Proximal root concavities are present<br>In cervical cross section, ovoid in shape, small lingual surface<br>Occasionally is bifurcated into a facial and lingual root in apical third<br>The root is 1½ times the length of the crown | 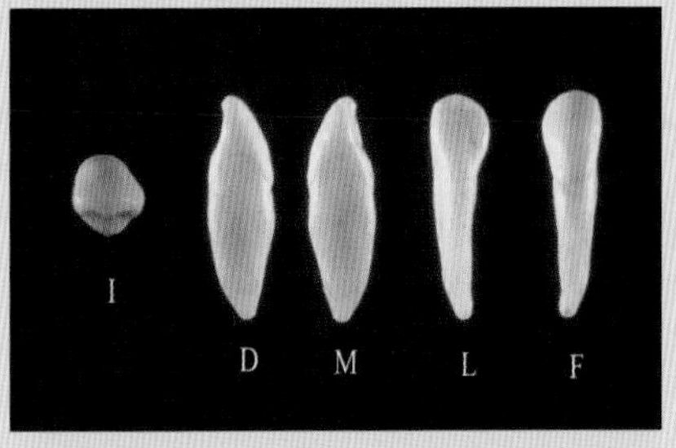 Tooth #27 |
| First premolar | Two cusps: large facial with small, nonfunctional lingual<br>Prominent transverse ridge, two pits, and a mesiolingual groove<br>Crowns of all mandibular posterior teeth are inclined lingually | One root, conical in shape<br>In cervical cross section, may be ovoid or elliptical in shape<br>May have a mesiolingual proximal root concavity<br>The root is 1⅔ times the length of the crown | 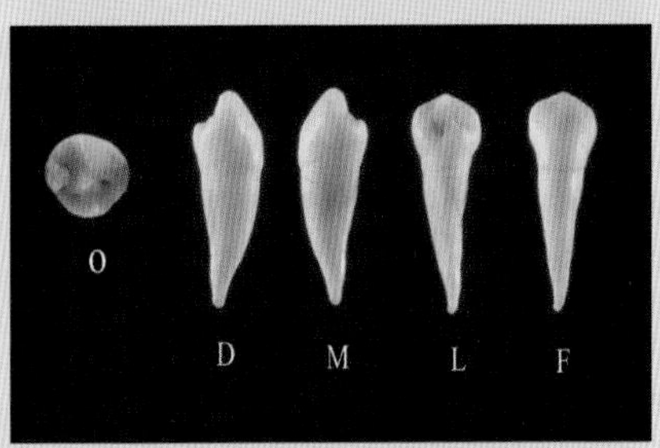 Tooth #28 |
| Second premolar | Bicuspidate (2) or tricuspidate (3) forms<br>Two-cusped form: H-shaped or U-shaped groove pattern<br>Three-cusped form: Y-shaped groove pattern with large facial cusp and smaller mesiolingual and distolingual cusps | One root, conical in shape<br>In cervical cross section, may be ovoid or elliptical in shape<br>The root is 1⅔ times the length of the crown<br>No significant root concavities | 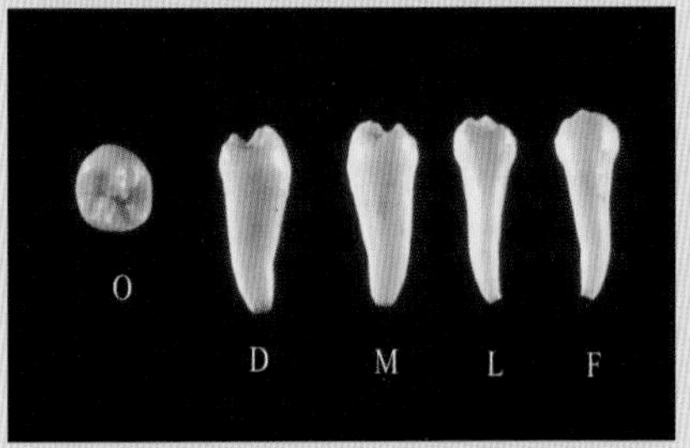 Tooth #29 |
| First molar | Largest tooth mesiodistally<br>Five cusps: mesiofacial, distofacial, distal, mesiolingual, and distolingual; Y-shaped occlusal groove pattern; extends onto facial surface and forms two facial grooves with a mesiofacial pit<br>Occlusal pits in mesial, central, and distal fossae | Two roots, mesial is wider faciolingually and longer then the distal root.<br>Furcations on facial and lingual surfaces; concavity before the furcation on facial surface begins just apical to cemento-enamel junction<br>Short root trunk; larger interradicular area<br>Major proximal concavity and two root canals on the mesial root<br>Cervical enamel projections may occur<br>The root is 1¾ times the length of the crown | 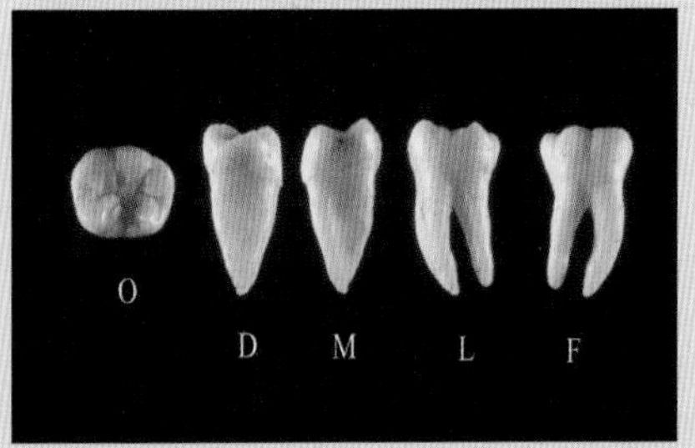 Tooth #30 |
| 3<br>Second molar | Similar to the first molar<br>Four cusps: two facial and two lingual; "+"-shaped occlusal groove pattern; extends onto facial surface to form one groove and pit<br>Occlusal pits in mesial, central, and distal fossae | Two roots, mesial and distal<br>Roots are more likely to be closer together with a longer root trunk<br>Mesial root concavity is not as prominent<br>Roots are 1¾ times the length of the crown | 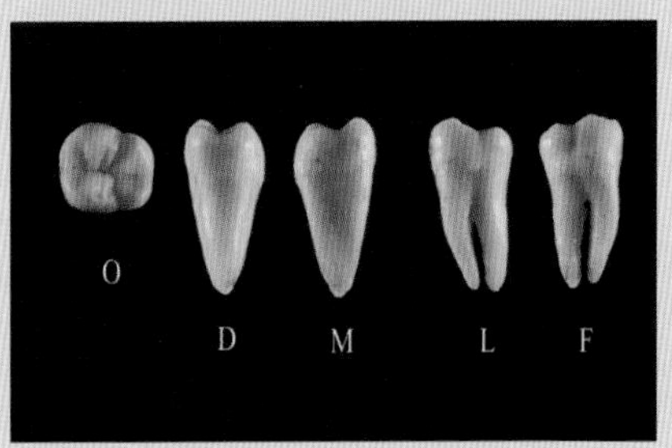 Tooth #31 |
| Third molar | Similar to the second molar<br>Varies greatly in form | Usually two roots<br>Roots are short, frequently fused, and angled to the distal | |

(2) Have the same number and position of roots as that of permanent molars
(3) The CEJ on the mesial half of the buccal surface curves apically around a very prominent cervical ridge
(4) The maxillary first primary molar has an H-shaped central groove pattern and usually has three to four cusps; the mesial cusps are the largest; a prominent cervical ridge is present
(5) The mandibular first primary molar has four cusps; the mesial cusps are larger, and the mesiolingual cusp is long, pointed, and angled toward the occlusal surface

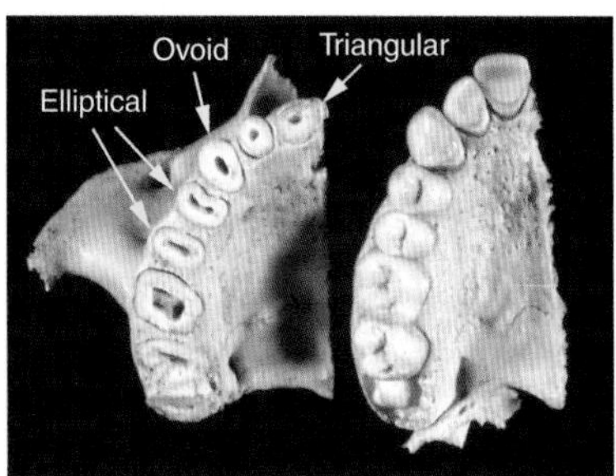


**Fig. 5.19** Root shapes as seen in cervical cross section: elliptical, ovoid, and triangular.

(6) Second primary molars are larger than the first primary molars and resemble the form of the first permanent molar (isomorphic)

## ERUPTION

A. General comments
1. *Eruption* frequently is defined as "the emergence of the tooth through the gingiva"
2. Also defined as the movements a tooth makes to attain and maintain a relationship with the teeth in the same and opposing arches; follows distinct stages:
   a. Beginning of hard tissue formation
   b. Enamel (crown) completion, after which actual tooth movement begins
   c. Eruption; approximately 50% of the root is formed when eruption begins
   d. Root completion
3. Ages at which eruption occurs are given in classic eruption tables
4. Sequential pattern (order) is more predictable than age of eruption
5. As a generalization, the mandibular tooth of a class (e.g., incisor, canine) emerges before the maxillary tooth of the

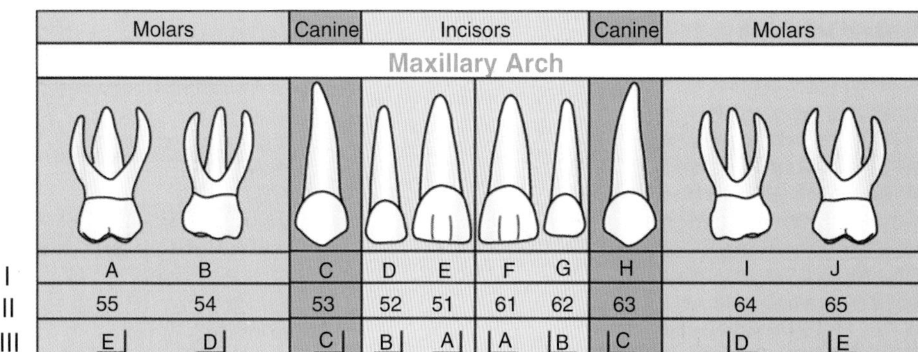


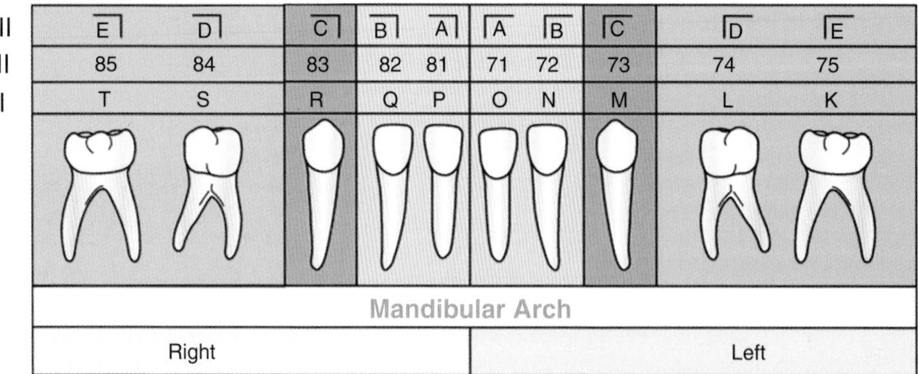


I Universal Numbering System

II International Numbering System

III Palmer Notation Method

**Fig. 5.20** Primary dentition. (From: Fehrenbach MJ, Herring SW. Illustrated anatomy of the head and neck. ed. 4. St. Louis. 2012. Saunders/Elsevier.)

same type, and the first before the second (e.g., the central incisor emerges before the lateral incisor)

B. Primary dentition development and eruption
   1. A guide for the emergence of primary teeth into the oral cavity is provided in the following table:

| | Mandibular | Maxillary |
|---|---|---|
| Central incisor | 6 months | 7 ½ months |
| Lateral incisor | 7 months | 9 months |
| Canine | 16 months | 18 months |
| First molar | 12 months | 14 months |
| Second molar | 20 months | 24 months |

   2. The order of eruption for primary tooth development is: central incisor, lateral incisor, first molar, canine, and second molar
   3. Hard tissue formation begins in utero between 4 and 6 months
   4. Crowns are completed between 1.5 and 10 months of age
   5. Roots are completed between 1.5 and 3 years of age, 6 to 18 months after eruption
   6. By 3 years of age, all primary teeth are erupted, and permanent teeth (except the third molars) are in some stage of development
   7. Root resorption of a primary tooth is triggered by the pressure exerted by the developing permanent tooth; followed by primary tooth exfoliation in sequential patterns

C. Mixed/transitional dentition—period with both primary/deciduous and permanent teeth present; begins with the eruption of the first permanent tooth (often the mandibular first molar) and ends with the exfoliation of the last primary tooth
   1. Mixed/transitional dentition occurs between 6 and 12 years of age
   2. Characteristics
      a. Edentulous areas
      b. Perception of disproportionately sized teeth
      c. Varying clinical crown heights
      d. Crowding
      e. Enlarged and edematous gingiva
      f. Enamel color variations between dentitions

D. Permanent dentition development and eruption
   1. Succedaneous teeth replace primary teeth: incisors, canines, and premolars; nonsuccedaneous teeth are the permanent molars
   2. Permanent tooth formation begins between birth and 3 years of age (except for the third molars)
   3. The crowns of permanent teeth are completed between 4 and 8 years of age, at approximately one-half the age of eruption
   4. The order of eruption in permanent tooth development follows:

| Mandibular | Maxillary |
|---|---|
| First molar | First molar |
| Central incisor | Central incisor |
| Lateral incisor | Lateral incisor |
| Canine | First premolar |
| First premolar | Second premolar |
| Second premolar | Canine |
| Second molar | Second molar |
| Third molar | Third molar |

   5. A guide for the emergence of permanent teeth into the oral cavity follows:

| | Mandibular | Maxillary |
|---|---|---|
| First molar[a] | 6–7 years | 6–7 years |
| Central incisor | 6–7 years | 7–8 years |
| Lateral incisor | 7–8 years | 8–9 years |
| Canine | 9–10 years | 11–12 years |
| First premolar | 10–12 years | 10–11 years |
| Second premolar | 11–12 years | 10–12 years |
| Second molar | 11–13 years | 12–13 years |
| Third molar | 17–21 years | 17–21 years |

[a]First permanent tooth to erupt.

   6. Roots of permanent teeth are completed between 10 and 16 years of age, 2 to 3 years after eruption

## INTRAARCH AND INTERARCH RELATIONSHIPS

Each tooth has a relationship with adjacent teeth in the same and opposing arches. These relationships are influenced by size and shape of the maxilla, the mandible, the teeth themselves, spacing, and a variety of external factors, such as oral habits and dental disease.

A. Intraarch relationship—the alignment of the teeth within an arch
   1. Position of teeth in the jaw
      a. Interproximal contacts—in an ideal alignment, teeth contact at their proximal crests of curvature (HOC); a continuous arch form is observed from an occlusal view
         (1) Anterior teeth contacts are in the middle of the faciolingual dimension
         (2) Posterior teeth contacts are facial of center in a faciolingual dimension
         (3) Some permanent dentitions have normal alignment with no contact
         (4) Primary dentitions often have developmental spacing in the anterior area; some have *primate spaces* between the primary maxillary lateral incisor and the canine and between the primary mandibular canine and the first molar (Fig. 5.21)
      b. Axial positioning—relationship of the long axis of individual teeth to an imaginary horizontal or median plane (mesiodistally and faciolingually); ideally, each tooth "sits" at an angle that best withstands the forces placed on it (Fig. 5.22)
         (1) Most teeth are inclined facially, with the incisors having the greatest inclination
         (2) The mandibular posterior teeth tip lingually toward the median plane

c. Curves of the occlusal plane (a line connecting the cusp tips of canines, premolars, and molars)
   (1) Curve of Spee—from the buccal aspect in centric occlusion, the cusp tips of posterior teeth curve anteroposteriorly; for mandibular teeth, the curve is concave, and for maxillary teeth, it is convex
   (2) Curve of Wilson—mediolateral curve connecting cusp tips of posterior mandibular teeth on opposite sides of the mouth (side to side); for mandibular teeth, the curve is concave because of their lingual tilt, and for maxillary molars, it is convex
   (3) The matching curve is termed the *compensating curve*

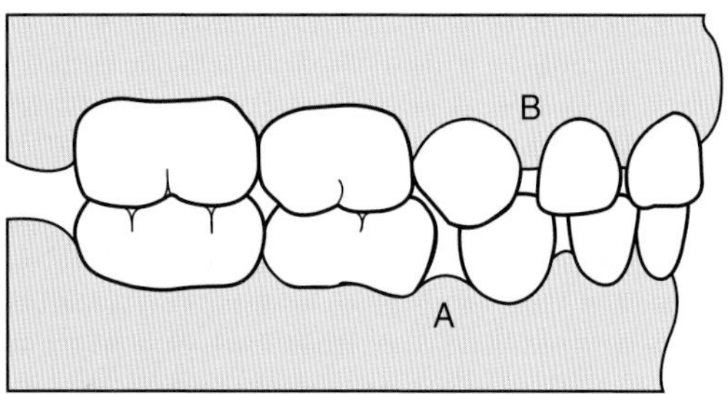


**Fig. 5.21** Primary teeth showing primate spaces. A, Mandibular primate space between the canine and the first molar. B, Maxillary primate space between the lateral incisor and the canine. (Modified from Wilkins E. *Clinical Practice of the Dental Hygienist.* 10th ed. Philadelphia: Lippincott, Williams & Wilkins; 2008.)

2. Disturbances in intraarch alignment
   a. Open contacts—sites where an interproximal space exists because proximal crests (HOC) do not meet; from developmental disturbances, missing teeth, oral habits, dental disease, or overdeveloped frena
   b. Positional variations, or versions—misplaced positioning of teeth from developmental disturbances, crowding, oral habits, dental caries, or periodontal disease; named for their positions: facioversion (facial of normal alignment), linguoversion, mesioversion, distoversion, supraversion (supraerupted), infraversion (undererupted), and torsiversion (rotated); interproximal contacts are often not normal

B. Interarch relationships—alignment between arches; can be viewed from a stationary (fixed) perspective and a dynamic (movable) perspective
   1. Stationary relationships
      a. Centric relationship—the most retruded position of the mandible, as in swallowing; muscles contract fully, not usually resulting in maximum tooth contact

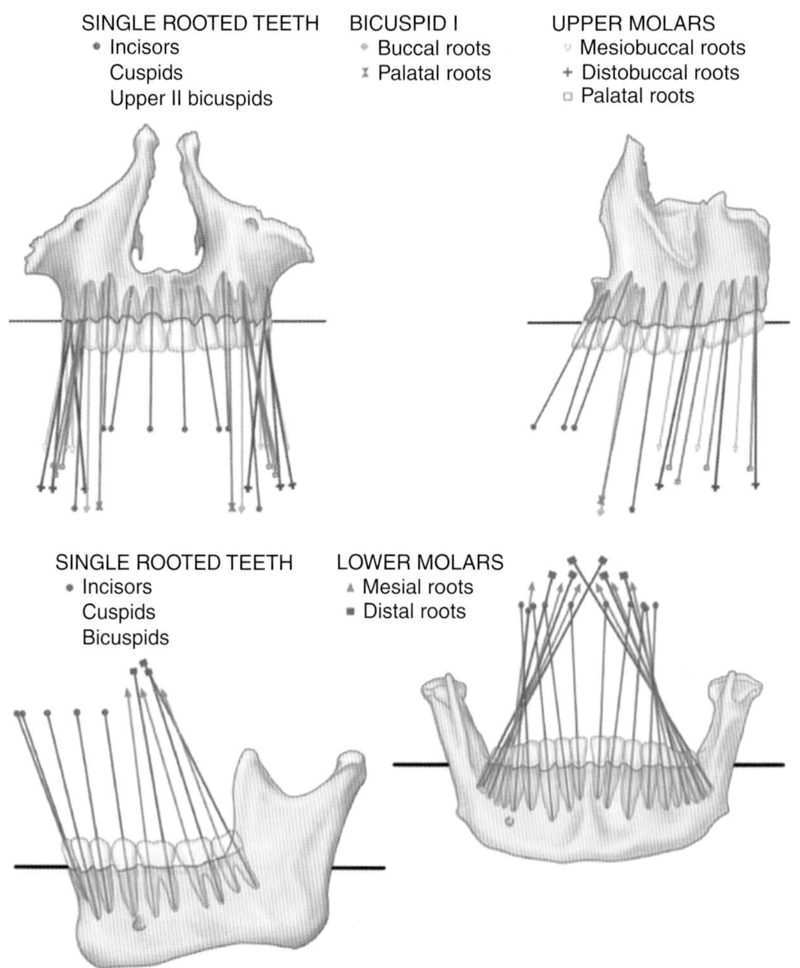


**Fig. 5.22** Tooth positioning in relation to the horizontal plane. (From: Nelson S. Wheeler's Dental Anatomy, Physiology, and Occlusion. 10th ed. Elsevier: St. Louis, Missouri: p.285:2015)

b. Centric occlusion—habitual occlusion where maximum tooth contact between arches (intercuspation) occurs (*note*: a normal physiologic rest position of the mandible during nonfunction)
c. Angle's classification of occlusion—using the first permanent molars, Edward H. Angle classified these relationships (Fig. 5.15; see Table 5.2)
   (1) Canines may also be used to classify occlusion when a molar is missing
   (2) Class I canine relationship: cusp tip of the maxillary canine is facial to and between the mandibular canine and the first premolar
   (3) Class II canine relationship: maxillary canine is mesial to normal position
   (4) Class III canine relationship: maxillary canine is distal to normal position
d. Occlusion in a primary dentition is assessed by the relationship of the distal terminus (surface) of second primary molars in centric occlusion; three relationships are possible: a flush terminal plane, a distal step, or a mesial step
e. Mixed dentition represents a transitional stage of occlusal development; the initial contact of permanent first molars usually begins at age 7, and by 12 years of age, the final occlusion of the first molars is established
   (1) Distal-step primary dentitions always lead to a class II permanent molar occlusion
   (2) Exaggerated mesial-step primary dentitions lead to a class III permanent molar occlusion
   (3) Development of occlusion from a flush terminus or a mild mesial-step primary dentition is variable but frequently leads to a class I first permanent molar relationship

2. Dynamic interarch relationships are a result of functional mandibular movements that start and end with centric occlusion during mastication
   a. Mandibular movements involve complex neuromuscular functions
      (1) Depression (opening)
      (2) Elevation (closing)
      (3) Protrusion (thrusting forward)
      (4) Retrusion (bringing back)
      (5) Lateral movements right and left; one side is always the working, or chewing, side; the opposite side is the nonworking, or balancing, side; ideally, these alternate during chewing
   b. Mandibular movements from centric occlusion are guided by maxillary teeth
      (1) Protrusion is guided by incisors; called *incisal guidance*
      (2) Lateral movements are guided by the canines on the working side in young, unworn dentitions (canine-protected occlusion); lateral movements may be guided by incisors and posterior teeth in worn dentitions
   c. As mandibular movements commence from a centric occlusion, posterior teeth should disengage in protrusion; on the balancing side, posterior teeth should disengage in lateral movement
   d. If tooth contact occurs where teeth should be disengaged, occlusal interferences or premature contacts exist

## SUMMARY OF TOOTH DIMENSIONS

A. Crowns
   1. From 7 to 11 mm cervico-incisally
   2. Anterior teeth are longer cervico-incisally (2 to 3 mm longer) than posterior teeth in both arches
   3. Smallest crown mesiodistally is the mandibular central incisor
   4. Maxillary first molar is the widest tooth faciolingually; mandibular first molar is the widest tooth mesiodistally
B. Roots
   1. From 12 to 17 mm in length
   2. Incisor roots are shortest
   3. Longest root is the maxillary canine
C. Ratio of root length to crown length is smaller in anterior teeth (root-to-crown ratio)
   1. Smallest ratio is the maxillary central incisor, where the root is only slightly longer
   2. Molars have a greater root-crown ratio because of short crowns cervico-occlusally
   3. Largest ratio is the mandibular first molar, where the root is 1.83 times longer

## WEBSITE INFORMATION AND RESOURCES

| Source | Website Address | Description |
|---|---|---|
| National Institute of Dental and Craniofacial Research | http://www.nidcr.nih.gov | Information and links related to awareness of craniofacial development and disorders; publications aimed at client/patient education are available. |
| Dental Hygiene Education Net | www.dhed.net | Links to both professional dental and dental hygiene organizations as well as numerous healthcare resource centers. |
| | | Dental anatomy information for professionals and patients is available, as well as resources such as journals and research sites for and by dental hygienists. |
| Medscape from WebMD | https://www.medscape.com | Numerous topics concerning oral health, including the oral examination, diseases of the oral cavity, and links to the Centers for Disease Control and Prevention (CDC) and other resources. |
| Medline Plus | https://www.nlm.nih.gov/medlineplus/ | Current health information, including a medical encyclopedia; a service of the US National Library of Medicine and the National Institutes of Health. |

## CHAPTER 5 REVIEW QUESTIONS

Answers and rationales to review questions are available on this text's accompanying Evolve site. See inside front cover for details.

### CASE A

**Permanent Dentition**

A 29-year-old male presents for an initial dental hygiene appointment. The patient has no significant medical history. The patient brushes once a day. It has been 4 years since he has been to a dentist because he did not have dental insurance. He presents today with a chief concern about his front teeth breaking and would like a cleaning. He also notes that he thinks his teeth are getting yellower and is interested in whitening. During dietary counseling the clinician noted the patient drinks Mountain Dew all day.

***Use Case A and Figs. 5.23, 5.24, and 5.25 to answer questions 1 to 10.***

1. After reviewing Fig. 5.23, what term would you use to describe this wear?
   - **a.** Abfraction
   - **b.** Abrasion
   - **c.** Attrition
   - **d.** Erosion
2. Using the Universal Numbering System what tooth numbers are wearing in Fig. 5.23?
   - **a.** 8, 9
   - **b.** 24, 25
   - **c.** 2.1, 1.1
   - **d.** 1.1, 3.1
3. What in the patient's history could be contributing to his condition?
   - **a.** Not being to the dentist in 4 years
   - **b.** Drinking Mountain Dew
   - **c.** Not having dental insurance
   - **d.** Brushing his teeth

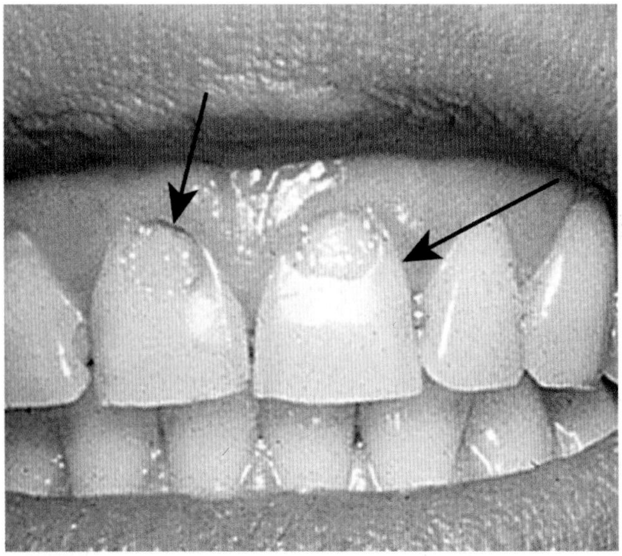

**Fig. 5.23** (From: Darby M, Walsh M. Dental Hygiene Theory and Practice. 4th ed. Elsevier: St. Louis, Missouri: p.259:2015.)

4. Using Fig. 5.24, what would you call the enamel projections seen on the maxillary molars?
   - **a.** Enamel pearl
   - **b.** Enamel projection
   - **c.** Hypercementosis
   - **d.** Dens in dente
5. What is the structure called on the hard palate that is firm and has irregular ridges branching off the palatine raphe?
   - **a.** Palatine fovea
   - **b.** Rugae
   - **c.** Incisive papilla
   - **d.** Maxillary tuberosity
6. What tooth tissue is seen in Fig. 5.23 that is yellow in color?
   - **a.** Enamel
   - **b.** Dentin
   - **c.** Cementum
   - **d.** Pulp
7. What is wear called on cusps of posterior teeth?

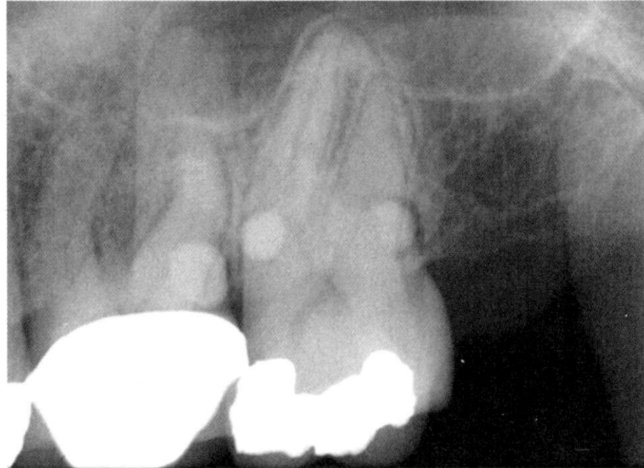

**Fig. 5.24** (From: Mallya S, Lam E. White and Pharaoh's Oral Radiology: Principles and Interpretation. 8th ed. Elsevier: St. Louis, Missouri:2018. Mosby.)

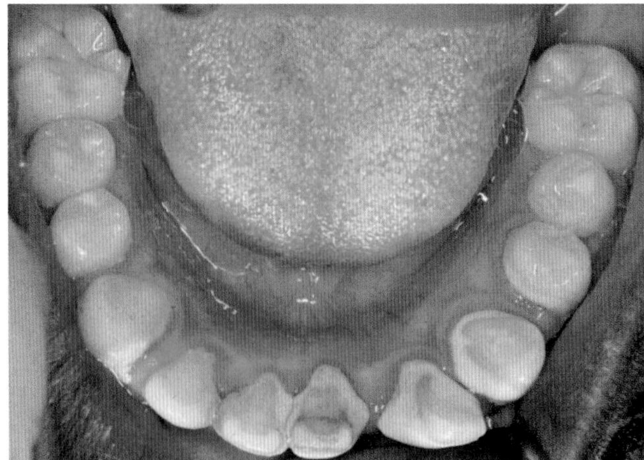

**Fig. 5.25** (From: Darby, Walsh: Dental hygiene theory and practice, ed 4, St. Louis, 2015 Saunders.)

a. Wear facets
b. Grooves
c. Pits
d. Decalcification

8. Looking at Fig. 5.25, what gingiva is edematous?
a. Gingival margin
b. Attached gingiva
c. Interdental papilla
d. a. and c.

9. Looking at Fig. 5.23, which tooth/teeth looks suspicious on the mesial surface using the International Numbering System?
a. 1.2
b. 1.3
c. 2.3
d. b. and c.

10. What would you call a tooth that is malpositionally rotated?
a. Torsiversion
b. Extrusion
c. Infraocclusion
d. Linguoversion

## CASE B

**Mixed dentition**

A 12-year-old female presents to your clinic for an initial hygiene appointment. Her medical history is significant for congenital syphilis.

***Use Case B and Figs. 5.27 and 5.28 to answer questions 11 to 15.***

11. After the clinical exam notching of the maxillary incisors is seen, what are these incisors called?
a. Hutchinson's incisors
b. Mulberry incisors
c. Peg incisors
d. Macrodontia incisors

12. What other anatomy anomalies can be caused due to congential syphilis?
a. Microdontia
b. Fusion
c. Mulberry molars
d. Dens in dente

13. Using the Universal Number System, which teeth are showing notching of the incisors?
a. O and P
b. 24 and 25
c. E and F
d. 8 and 9

14. What surface of the incisors is affected by the notching (Hutchinson's incisors)?
a. Marginal ridge
b. Facial ridge
c. Lingual ridge
d. Incisal ridge

15. A small fold of soft tissue located on each side of the frenulum linguae in the floor of the mouth is called:
a. Sublingual folds
b. Labial folds
c. Vermillion folds
d. Foliate folds

16. Which trait would distinguish a premolar from a canine?
a. Set trait
b. Type trait
c. Class trait
d. Arch trait

17. Another term for cervical line would be?
a. Gingival crest
b. Line angle
c. Cemento-dentinal junction
d. Cemento-enamel junction

18. In which quadrant is tooth #4.3 located?
a. Maxillary right
b. Maxillary left
c. Mandibular right
d. Mandibular left

19. What is formed by the junction of the distal and occlusal surfaces of a posterior tooth?
a. An incisal edge
b. A point angle
c. A cusp tip
d. A line angle

20. For mandibular incisors, on which surface is a root depression usually more distinct?
a. Facial
b. Lingual
c. Mesial
d. Distal

21. Which tooth has the longest root in the oral cavity?
a. Maxillary canine
b. Mandibular canine
c. Maxillary first premolar
d. Mandibular first premolar

22. Which premolar develops from five lobes?
a. Maxillary first premolar
b. Maxillary second premolar
c. Mandibular first premolar
d. Mandibular second premolar

23. Which premolar usually has a deep, mesial depression on the crown and the root?
a. Maxillary first premolar
b. Maxillary second premolar
c. Mandibular first premolar
d. Mandibular second premolar

24. Which term is used to describe an extra rounded projection on a tooth usually found on the cingulae of anterior teeth or occlusal surface of posterior teeth?
a. Enamel pearl
b. Mammelon
c. Tubercle
d. Exostosis

25. What class of teeth is present in the permanent dentition that is NOT present in the primary dentition?
a. Incisors

b. Canines
c. Premolars
d. Molars

26. Which tooth tissue is the most calcified?
a. Pulp
b. Cementum
c. Dentin
d. Enamel

27. Which permanent tooth erupts into the space previously held by the primary second molar?
a. First molar
b. Second molar
c. First premolar
d. Second premolar

28. How many pulp horns does tooth #13 have?
a. 1
b. 2
c. 3
d. 4

29. Which anterior tooth may have a bifurcated root?
a. Maxillary canine
b. Mandibular canine
c. Maxillary central incisor
d. Maxillary lateral incisor

30. Which tooth has a mesial marginal ridge groove?
a. Maxillary first premolar
b. Maxillary second premolar
c. Mandibular first premolar
d. Mandibular second premolar

31. Which molar usually has the roots closest together?
a. First premolar
b. First molar
c. Second molar
d. Third molar

32. Name the roots of the maxillary first molar.
a. Mesial and distal
b. Facial and lingual
c. Mesiobuccal, distobuccal, and buccal
d. Mesiobuccal, distobuccal, and lingual

33. Where is a cervical enamel projection normally found?
a. Near any furcation
b. Near the incisal edge
c. Near the apex
d. Near the occlusal surface

34. Which term is used to describe the amount of vertical overlap of maxillary teeth?
a. Crossbite
b. Overjet
c. Overbite
d. Supraversion

35. Which is usually the first permanent tooth to erupt in the oral cavity?
a. Mandibular central incisors
b. Maxillary central incisors
c. Maxillary first molars
d. Mandibular first molars

36. What statement is TRUE of teeth that are dilacerated?

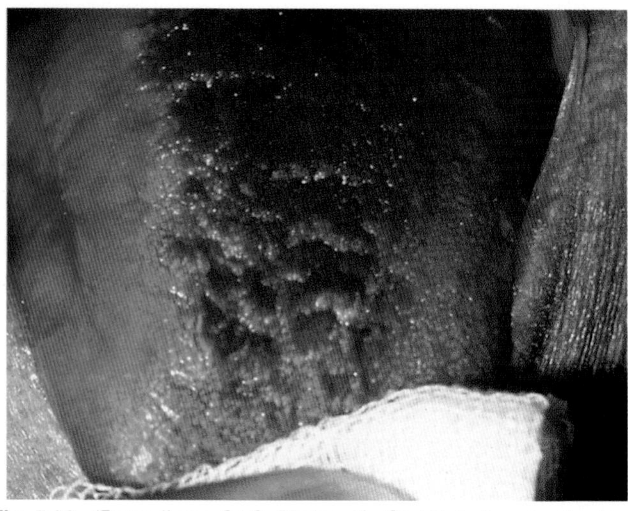

Fig. 5.26 (From: Ibsen OAC, Phelan JA. Oral Pathology for the Dental Hygienist: with General Pathology Introductions. 7th ed. St. Louis: Saunders/Elsevier; 2018.)

a. The root and/or crown may be unusually bent
b. The root is unusually short
c. The marginal ridges are very prominent
d. There is a deep crevice in the cingulum

37. The anterior teeth in Fig. 5.29 exhibits:
a. Perikymata
b. Fluorosis
c. Attrition
d. Mamelons

38. What type of papillae is involved with the condition seen in Fig. 5.26?
a. Fungiform
b. Circumvallate
c. Foliate
d. Filiform

39. Which of the following is the correct assessment of the following patient's tongue? (Fig. 5.26)
a. Hairy
b. Fissured
c. Coated
d. Ulcerated

40. When there is a space between the maxillary central incisors, what is the space called?
a. Open bite
b. Fremitus
c. Centric relation
d. Diastema

41. What is seen on the incisal edge of the picture (Fig. 5.27)?
a. Recession
b. Abrasion
c. Attrition
d. Abfraction

42. What is seen in the radiograph (Fig. 5.28) on tooth #7?
a. Peg lateral
b. Dens in dente
c. Supernumerary tooth
d. Bifurcated root

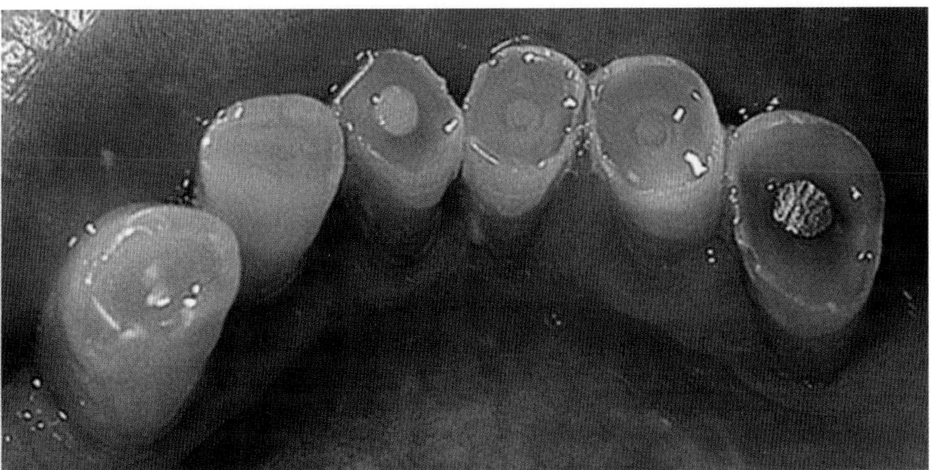
**Fig. 5.27** (From: Darby, Walsh: Dental hygiene theory and practice, ed 4, St. Louis, 2015 Saunders.)

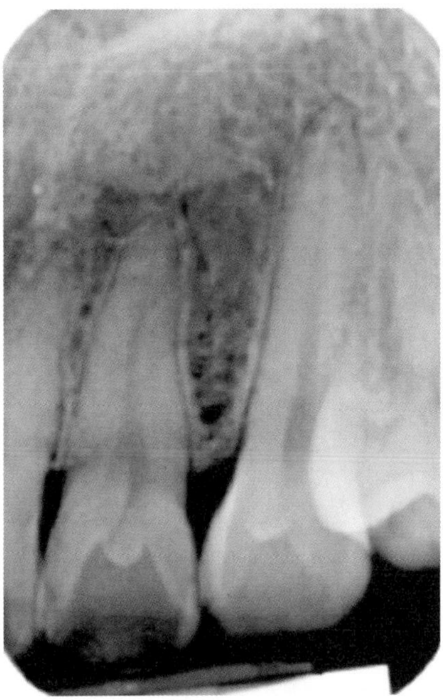
**Fig. 5.28** (From: Nelson S. Wheeler's Dental Anatomy, Physiology, and Occlusion. 10th ed. Elsevier: St. Louis, Missouri. p.234:2015.)

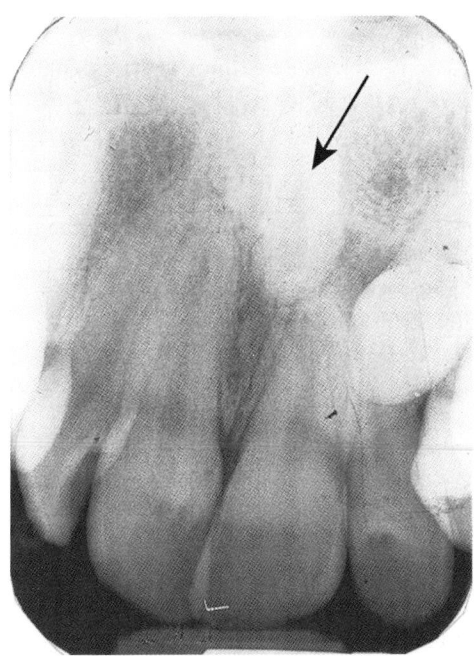
**Fig. 5.29** (From: Darby M, Walsh M. Dental Hygiene Theory and Practice. 4th ed. Elsevier: St. Louis, Missouri: p.1065:2015.)

43. What is the term for the extra tooth in Fig. 5.29 pointed out by the arrow?
    a. Mesiodens
    b. Macrodontia
    c. Microdontia
    d. Anodontia
44. What is another name for the corner of the mouth?
    a. Philtrum
    b. Buccal mucosa
    c. Commissure
    d. Frenum
45. What tonsillar tissue hangs from the soft palate and closes the nasopharynx when swallowing?
    a. Palatine tonsils
    b. Uvula
    c. Pterygomandibular raphe
    d. Pharyngeal tonsils
46. The mesiobuccal cusp of the maxillary first molar meets up with the buccal groove of the mandibular first molar. What type of occlusion relationship is this?
    a. Class I
    b. Class II Division I
    c. Class II Division II
    d. Class III
47. What papilla on the tongue function in taste of bitter?
    a. Fungiform
    b. Filiform
    c. Foliate
    d. Circumvallate
48. What structure on the buccal mucosa carries saliva from the parotid gland?

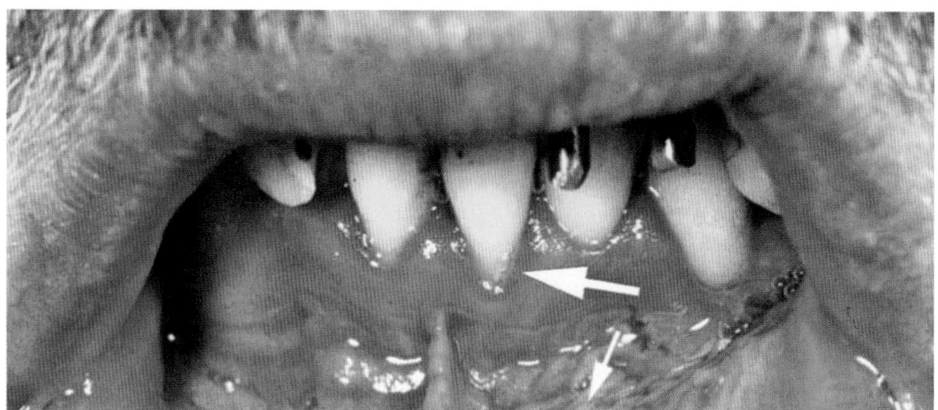

Fig. 5.30 (From: Darby, Walsh: Dental hygiene theory and practice, ed 4, St. Louis, 2015 Saunders.)

   a. Parotid papilla
   b. Stenson's duct
   c. Wharton's duct
   d. a. and b.
49. What is a possible cause of the recession seen in Fig. 5.30?
   a. Labial frenum attachment
   b. Chewing tobacco
   c. Toothbrushing
   d. All of the above
50. What terminology would you use to describe the location of tooth #24 seen in Fig. 5.31?
   a. Torsiversion
   b. Infraocclusion
   c. Labioversion
   d. Linguoversion

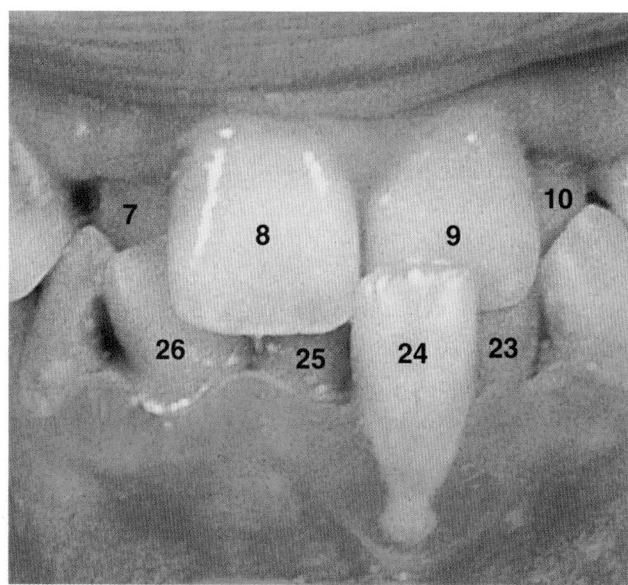


Fig. 5.31 (From: Wolters Kluwer. Woelfel's Dental Anatomy. 8th ed. Philadelphia: Scheid, RC. Weiss G. p.253:2012.)

## SUGGESTED READINGS

Bath-Balogh M, Fehrenbach MF. *Illustrated Dental Embryology, Histology, and Anatomy*. 4th ed. St Louis: Saunders; 2015.

Bryan L. Root morphology and instrumentation implications. In: Darby ML, Walsh MM, eds. *Dental Hygiene: Theory and Practice*. 4th ed. Philadelphia: Saunders; 2015.

Darby W, Walsh M. *Dental hygiene Theory and Practice*. 4th ed. St. Louis: Saunders; 2015.

Ibsen OAC, Phelan JA. *Oral Pathology for the Dental Hygienist: With General Pathology Introductions*. 7th ed. St. Louis: Saunders/Elsevier; 2018.

Mallya S, Lam E. *White and Pharaoh's Oral Radiology: Principles and Interpretation*. 8th ed. St. Louis: Missouri, Mosby; 2018.

Nelson S. *Wheeler's Dental Anatomy, Physiology, and Occlusion*. 10th ed. Philadelphia: Saunders; 2014.

Norton N. *Netter's Head and Neck Anatomy for Dentistry*. 3rd ed. Philadelphia: Saunders; 2016.

Patton K. *Anatomy and Physiology*. 10th ed. St. Louis: Elsevier; 2018.

Scheid RC, Weiss G. *Woelfel's Dental Anatomy*. 9th ed. Baltimore: Wolters Kluwer, Lippincott, Williams & Wilkins; 2017.

Wilkins E. *Clinical Practice of the Dental Hygienist*. 12th ed. Philadelphia: Lippincott, Williams & Wilkins; 2017.

Zwemer T, Thomas J, eds. *Mosby's Dental Dictionary*. 3rd ed. St Louis: Mosby; 2014.

6

# Oral and Maxillofacial Radiology

*Laura Jansen Howerton*

Diagnostic dental images are an important and necessary component of total patient care. Radiographic images enable the practitioner to see conditions that may otherwise go undetected. The goal of dental radiography is to obtain the highest-quality radiographic image while maintaining the lowest possible radiation exposure dose to the patient. The dental hygienist must be not only capable of producing diagnostic images but also competent in interpretation skills.

Knowledge and skill in applying this information are critical for the safe use of ionizing radiation in the oral health care setting. This chapter emphasizes basic information on radiation, film processing, digital imaging, intraoral and extraoral techniques and errors, and radiographic interpretation.

## GENERAL CONSIDERATIONS

### Discovery of X-Radiation

A. Radiation—a form of energy carried through space in the form of waves or a stream of particles
B. Radiation characteristics
  1. Bundles of energy that have neither mass nor charge
  2. Travels at the speed of light (186,000 miles per second)
  3. Electromagnetic energies exist over a wide range of magnitudes, termed the *electromagnetic spectrum* (Fig. 6.1)
  4. Interaction of radiation with biologic tissues causes change in the tissue due to ionization
  5. Electromagnetic spectrum is measured according to frequency, velocity, and wavelength
C. X-ray—a beam of energy that has the power to penetrate substances and record image shadows on receptors
D. Wilhelm Roentgen discovered the x-ray in 1895
  1. He experimented with vacuum tubes, photographic plates, and electrical currents
  2. Dr. Roentgen was awarded a Nobel Prize in physics

### Radiation Physics

A. Ion—an atom that gains or loses an electron and becomes electronically unbalanced
B. Ionization— the process by which radiant energy removes an orbital electron from an atom to yield an ion pair
C. Ionizing radiation—radiation capable of producing ions; two types:
  1. Particulate radiation
    a. Tiny particles have both mass and energy, travel in straight lines at high speeds
    b. Examples: neutrons, protons, alpha and beta particles
  2. Electromagnetic radiation
    a. Electromagnetic radiation
    b. The propagation of wave-like energy *without mass* through space
    c. Arranged in an electromagnetic spectrum and measured according to wavelength, velocity, and frequency (see Fig. 6.1)
      (1) Wavelength—distance from one crest of a wave to the crest of the next wave; the shorter the wavelength, the greater the energy and penetrating ability of the radiation
      (2) Velocity—the speed of a wave
      (3) Frequency—number of wavelength crests passing a particular point per unit of time; the shorter the wavelength, the higher the frequency
      (4) Photon and quantum—a single unit or bundle of energy
      (5) Energy—ability to do work; electromagnetic radiation is measured in electron volts (eV)
D. X-ray machine
  1. Control panel—contains on/off switch exposure button and the controls to regulate the exposure factors (milliamperage [mA], kilovoltage peak [kVp], time); modern x-ray machines have preset exposure factors for various anatomic areas of the maxilla and mandible
  2. Extension arm—suspends the x-ray tubehead and houses electrical wires
  3. X-ray tubehead—lead-lined metal casing for the x-ray tube designed to prevent excessive radiation exposure and electrical shock
    a. Protects the x-ray tube
    b. Insulating oil surrounds x-ray tube and absorbs excess heat produced during x-ray production
    c. Transformers alter voltage of incoming electricity
    d. Aluminum discs filter the longer-wavelength x-rays
    e. Lead collimator restricts the size and shape of the x-ray beam
    f. Position-indicating device (PID) aims and shapes the x-ray beam; the longer PID produces an x-ray beam less divergent, decreases radiation exposure to patient, and provides less image magnification
    g. X-ray tube is the heart of the x-ray–generating system
      (1) Cathode
        (a) Negative electrode
        (b) Consists of a tungsten wire filament and molybdenum (focusing) cup

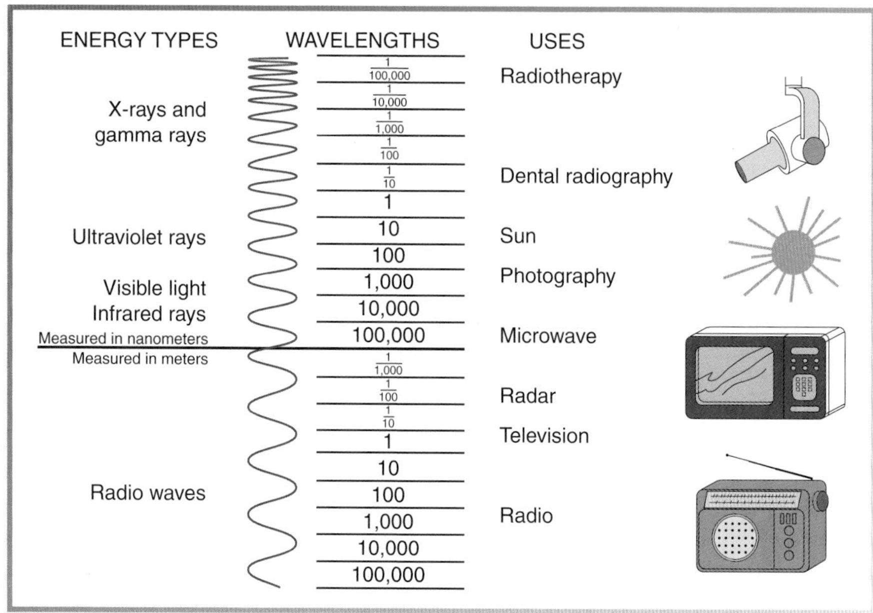


**Fig. 6.1** Electromagnetic energy spectrum. (From Iannucci JM, Howerton LJ. *Dental Radiography: Principles and Techniques.* 4th ed. St. Louis: Elsevier Saunders; 2012.)

(c) Supplies the electrons necessary to generate x-rays; mA control regulates the step-down transformer, the quantity of x-rays produced, and heating of the filament

(d) Because like charges repel, the electron beam is directed to a small area on the anode

(2) Anode

(a) Positive electrode

(b) Consists of a tungsten plate fixed to a copper arm

(c) The tungsten target serves as a focal spot and converts bombarding electrons into x-ray photons

(d) kVp regulates the step-up transformer, voltage between cathode and anode, and speed of electrons

(3) Aluminum filters are placed in the path of the x-ray beam to filter and selectively remove the low-energy, nonpenetrating x-rays from the beam

(4) A lead collimator is positioned next to the aluminum filter to restrict the size and shape of the x-ray beam

E. Production of x-radiation (Fig. 6.2)

1. Control panel is activated by the on/off switch; appropriate mA, kVp, and time selections are chosen
   a. mA—allows for warming of the cathode filament and determines the number of electrons available for x-ray production; the higher the mA setting, the hotter the filament becomes, resulting in a greater number of available electrons
   b. kVp—controls the current passing from cathode to anode; the higher the kVp setting, the greater the penetrating power and speed of acceleration of electrons from the cathode to the anode
   c. Exposure time establishes the time during which electrons are available for the bombardment of target material; the higher the time setting, the more electrons available for x-ray production
2. Exposure button is pressed
   a. The heated filament provides electrons for x-ray production by *thermionic emission,* referred to as a "boiling off" of electrons; an electron cloud surrounding the filament is formed
   b. An electrical potential difference is created whereby electrons are attracted from the negative cathode to the positive anode
   c. The directional flow of electrons is influenced by the focusing cup of the cathode; electrons are repelled away from the negatively charged focusing cup; this mechanism controls the size and shape of the electron stream
   d. Less than 1% of the kinetic energy leaving the cathode is converted into x-ray energy; more than 99% of the energy leaving the cathode is converted into heat and absorbed by the insulating oil

F. Types of x-rays produced

1. General (braking or "bremsstrahlung") radiation
   a. Produces 70% of x-ray photons by dental x-ray machines
   b. The accelerating electron passes near the nucleus of the target atom and is slowed down by the attraction of the nucleus
   c. The slowing-down process results in the transference of the kinetic energy of the electron into x-ray energy
2. Characteristic radiation
   a. Can only occur at levels of 70 kVp or higher with a tungsten target; accounts for a small portion of x-rays produced by dental x-ray machines
   b. Occurs when an electron removes an orbital electron from the target atom

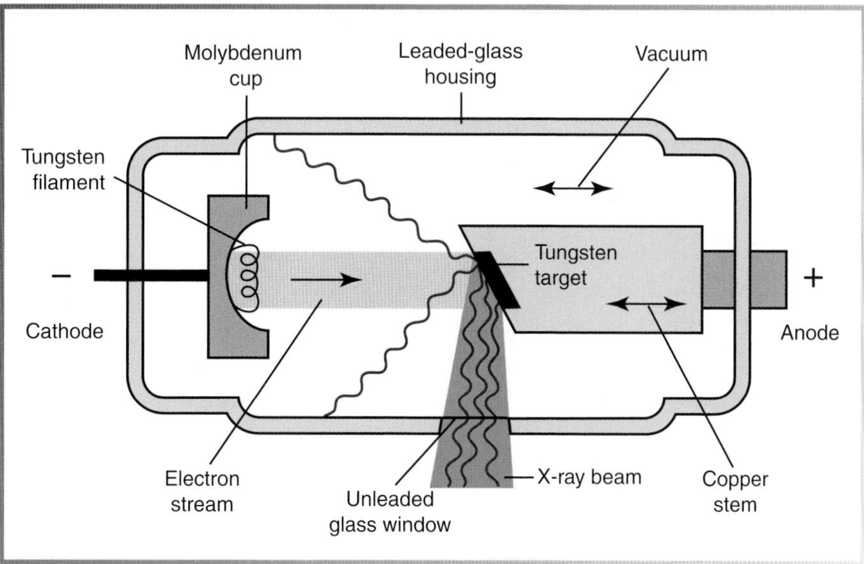


**Fig. 6.2** Diagram of x-ray tube. (From Iannucci JM, Howerton LJ. *Dental Radiography: Principles and Techniques.* 5th ed. St. Louis: Elsevier; 2017.)

c. During restabilization of the ionized atom, the movement of the outer-shell electron results in the transference of electron-binding energy into x-ray energy

G. Interactions of x-rays with matter
1. Definitions
a. Primary radiation—penetrating beam produced at the target anode; also termed *primary* or *useful beam*
b. Secondary radiation—results from the interaction of primary radiation and matter
c. Scatter radiation—one form of secondary radiation in which the direction of travel of the x-ray has been altered
2. Interactions of x-ray photons and matter; four possibilities may occur when x-rays interact with matter
a. No interaction
(1) The passing of x-ray photons through a material without any alteration of the photon or the material
(2) Photons proceed to strike the image receptor
b. Photoelectric effect
(1) Results from an incident photon colliding with a tightly bound inner-shell electron
(2) Incident photon ceases to exist; the electron is ejected as a recoil electron; ionization of the atom occurs
(3) Accounts for approximately 30% of interactions
c. Compton scatter
(1) Results from an incident photon colliding with a loosely bound outer-shell electron
(2) Incident photon gives up part of its energy in the ejection of the orbiting electron; ionization of the atom occurs
(3) Accounts for approximately 62% of interactions
d. Coherent scatter
(1) The interaction of an incident photon passing near an outer-shell electron and being scattered without energy loss
(2) Incident photon ceases to exist, and a new photon of identical energy is released from the electron; no ionization of the atom occurs
(3) Accounts for approximately 8% of interactions

## Characteristics of X-Radiation

A. Beam quality—the mean energy or penetrating ability of the x-ray beam
1. Controlled by kVp; increasing the kVp will result in a higher-energy x-ray beam with increased penetrating ability
2. Increasing the kVp will create a beam with shorter wavelength and higher frequency
3. Density—the overall darkness of an image
a. Increase kVp = increase density (darker image)
b. Decrease kVp = decrease density (lighter image)
4. Contrast—the differences between the dark and light areas on an image
a. Increase kVp = low contrast (many shades of gray visible)
b. Decrease kVp = high contrast (few shades of gray, mostly dark and light areas seen)

B. Beam quantity—the number of x-rays produced in the dental x-ray machine
1. Controlled by mA; determines the amount of electrons passing through the cathode filament
2. Increasing the mA will increase the number of x-rays produced and will also increase the temperature of the cathode filament
a. Increase mA = increased density (darker image)
b. Decrease mA = decreased density (lighter image)
c. Milliamperage does not have an effect on image contrast
3. Exposure time also has an effect on the beam quantity; an increase in exposure time results in an increase in the number of x-rays produced

C. Beam intensity—the product of the quality and quantity of x-radiation; beam intensity is affected by kVp, mA, exposure time, and distance
   1. Increase kVp = increase beam intensity
   2. Increase mA = increase beam intensity
   3. Increase exposure time = increase beam intensity
   4. Increase distance = decrease beam intensity
      a. The distance between the source of radiation and the receptor has an influence on the intensity of the x-ray beam
      b. The inverse square law is defined as "the intensity of radiation is inversely proportional to the square of the distance from the source of radiation"

$$\frac{\text{Original intensity}}{\text{New intensity}} = \frac{\text{New distance}^2}{\text{Original distance}^2}$$

         (1) As the distance between the source of radiation and an object increases, the intensity of the x-ray beam decreases
         (2) As the distance between the source of radiation and an object decreases, the intensity of the x-ray beam increases
         (3) For example, if the intensity of an x-ray beam is 400 millisieverts (mSv) at 36 inches, at 72 inches the intensity is only one-fourth as great, or 100 mSv

## RADIATION BIOLOGY AND PROTECTION

A. Radiation exposure
   1. Harmful to all living tissues; should be used cautiously
   2. Injury to cells, tissues, and organs occurs at the time of exposure but may take hours, days, or generations to manifest
   3. Two mechanisms of radiation injury are possible
      a. Radiation injury is caused by ionization
         (1) May cause a breakage in the molecule or a relocation of the atom in the molecule
         (2) Such changes may have a profound effect of structures of great importance, such as DNA
      b. Radiolysis of water
         (1) Yields free radicals that combine to form hydrogen peroxide ($H_2O_2$)
         (2) $H_2O_2$ is toxic to living tissues; its formation is an indirect, damaging effect of ionizing radiation
B. Characteristics of dose-response relationships
   1. Linear—the response is directly proportional to the dose
   2. Nonthreshold—any dose, regardless of its size, is expected to produce a response
   3. Threshold—from zero to a particular point, no response would be expected; above the threshold point, any dose will produce a response
C. Interactions of ionizing radiation with cells, tissues, and organs
   1. Stochastic effects—occur as a direct function of dose
   2. Nonstochastic effects—increase in severity with an increase in dose
   3. Genetic effects— not seen in the irradiated person but are passed to future generations
   4. Somatic effects—seen in the irradiated person but are not passed to future generations
   5. Short-term effects—associated with large amounts of radiation absorbed in a short time
   6. Long-term effects—associated with small amounts of radiation absorbed repeatedly over a long period of time
D. Sequence of radiation injury
   1. Latent period—the time between exposure to radiation and the appearance of the first observable clinical signs
   2. Period of injury—a variety of cellular injuries may occur
   3. Recovery period—not all cellular radiation injuries are permanent
   4. Cumulative effects—repeated radiation exposures can lead to problems with the health of the patient
E. Radiation effects on cells
   1. Not all cells respond to radiation in the same manner
   2. Several factors determine tissue sensitivity
      a. Mitotic activity—cells that divide frequently or undergo many divisions are more sensitive to radiation
      b. Cell differentiation—cells that are immature are more sensitive to radiation
      c. Cell metabolism—cells that have a higher metabolism are more sensitive to radiation
   3. Tissue and organ sensitivity
      a. Radiosensitive—a cell that is sensitive to radiation effects
         (1) Lymphatic (most sensitive)
         (2) Erythrocytes
         (3) Reproductive cells
      b. Radioresistant—a cell that is resistant to radiation effects
         (1) Nerve (most resistant)
         (2) Liver
         (3) Muscle
      c. Organ tissues considered critical for dental radiography are skin, thyroid gland, lens of the eyes, and bone marrow
      d. Continued low-dose exposure negatively affects the repair mechanism; overloading of the repair system by time or amount of exposure can result in somatic or genetic damage

### Radiation Measurements and Sources

A. Two systems are used to define the radiation measurements: an older system, or traditional system (found in literature dated before 1985), and a newer or metric equivalent system known as International System of Units (SI)
B. The International Commission on Radiation Units and Measurements (ICRU) has established units for the measurement of radiation[1]
   1. Radiation exposure—the measurement of ionization in air produced by x-rays
      a. Traditional unit of exposure is the roentgen (R)
      b. SI unit of exposure—defined as electrical charge per unit mass of air or coulomb per kilograms (C/kg)
      c. $1\ R = 2.58 \times 10^{-4}\ C/kg$
         $1\ C/kg = 3.88 \times 103\ R$

2. Radiation absorbed dose (rad)—the amount of radiation absorbed by a tissue
   a. Traditional unit is the rad
   b. SI unit is the gray (Gy)
   c. 1 Gy = 100 rad
3. Dose equivalent—the measure of biologic effects produced by different types of radiation
   a. Traditional unit is the roentgen-equivalent man (rem)
   b. SI unit is the sievert (Sv)
   c. 1 Sv = 100 rem

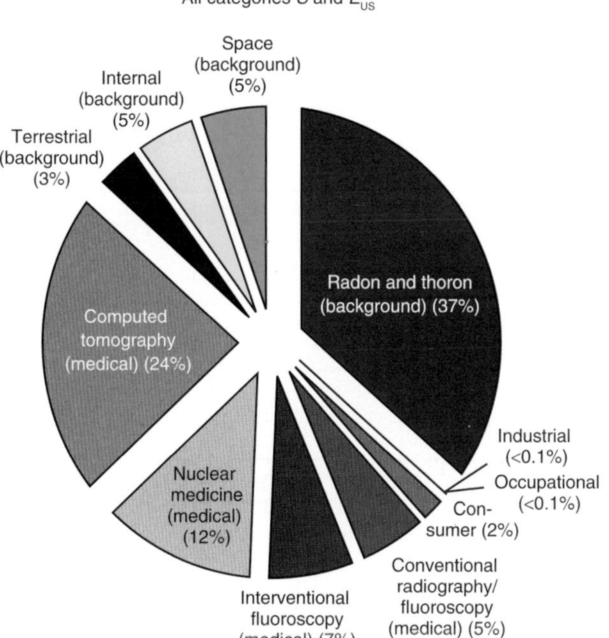


**Fig. 6.3** Annual effective dose equivalent of ionizing radiations. This chart illustrates the approximate percentage of exposure of the US population to background and artificial radiations. (From http://www.NCRPonline.org.)

C. Radiation risks and sources of radiation
1. Naturally occurring (or background) radiation constitutes 50% of the overall exposure to the United States population[2]
   a. Radon gas, the result of naturally occurring radionuclides found in soil (a *radionuclide* is an unstable atom that decays by emitting particles and energy from the nucleus to become electrically stable), accounts for 37% of the natural background radiation (Fig. 6.3)
   b. Other terrestrial sources, cosmic radiation from outer space, and internal sources constitute another 13% of natural exposure
2. Medical applications account for 48% of the overall exposure to the US population[2]
   a. Computed tomography (CT) and nuclear medicine lead medical exposures by 24% and 12%, respectively
   b. Other conventional images, including those produced with oral and maxillofacial radiography, constitute 5% of medical exposures
   c. Consumer products and industrial and occupational exposures account for the remaining 2% of total exposure to the US population
3. *Exposure* is defined as the average annual effective dose equivalent of ionizing radiation
   a. Average annual effective dose equivalent of ionizing radiation to a member of the US population is 6.2 mSv, up from 3.6 mSv in the early 1980s[2] (Fig. 6.4)
   b. Significant increase largely arising from the increased use of large-dose medical imaging technologies

## Radiation Protection

A. Before exposure
1. Proper prescribing of radiographs (Table 6.1)
   a. To limit the amount of radiation received by the patient, radiographs must be ordered on an individual basis, based on the patient need
   b. Evidence-based selection criteria is recommended[3]

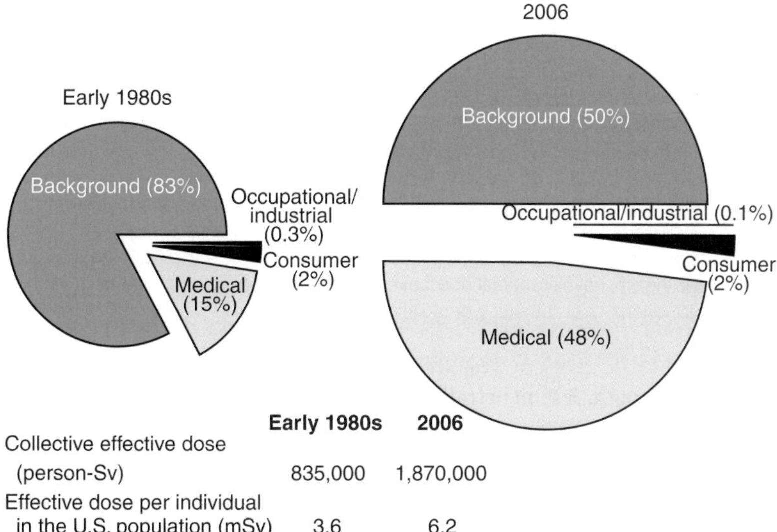


**Fig. 6.4** Comparison of effective dose equivalents. These charts illustrate the difference in approximate percentage of exposure of the US population to background and artificial radiations in the early 1980s and 2006. (From http://www.NCRPonline.org.)

**TABLE 6.1 Guidelines for Prescribing Dental Radiographs**

| TYPE OF ENCOUNTER | CHILDREN | | ADOLESCENT | | ADULT |
|---|---|---|---|---|---|
| | **Primary Dentition (before eruption of first permanent tooth)** | **Transitional Dentition (after eruption of first permanent tooth)** | **Permanent Dentition (before eruption of third molars)** | **Dentate or Partially Edentulous** | **Edentulous** |
| New patient[a] being evaluated for dental diseases and dental development | Individualized radiographic examination consisting of selected periapical views, occlusal views, or both; posterior bitewings if proximal surfaces cannot be visualized or probed<br>Patients without evidence of disease and with open proximal contacts may not require a radiographic examination at this time | Individualized radiographic examination consisting of posterior bitewings with panoramic examination or posterior bitewings and selected periapical images | Individualized radiographic examination consisting of posterior bitewings with panoramic examination or posterior bitewings and selected periapical images<br>A full-mouth intraoral radiographic examination is preferred when the patient has clinical evidence of generalized dental disease or a history of extensive dental treatment | | Individualized radiographic examination based on clinical signs and symptoms |
| Recare patient[a] with clinical caries or at increased risk for caries[b] | Posterior bitewing examination at 6- to 12-month intervals if proximal surfaces cannot be examined visually or with a probe | | | Posterior bitewing examination at 6- to 18-month intervals | Not applicable |
| Recare patient[a] with no clinical caries and not at risk for caries[b] | Posterior bitewing examination at 12- to 24-month intervals if proximal surfaces cannot be examined visually or with a probe | | Posterior bitewing examination at 18- to 36-month intervals | Posterior bitewing exam at 24- to 36-month intervals | Not applicable |
| Recare patient[a] with clinical periodontal disease | Clinical judgment as to the need for and type of radiographic images for the evaluation of periodontal disease. Imaging may consist of, but is not limited to, selected bitewing images, periapical images, or both, of areas where periodontal disease (other than nonspecific gingivitis) can be identified clinically | | | | Not applicable |
| Patient for monitoring of growth and development | Clinical judgment as to the need for and type of radiographic images for evaluation, monitoring, or both, of dentofacial growth and development | | Clinical judgment as to the need for and type of radiographic images for evaluation, monitoring, or both, of dentofacial growth and development<br>Panoramic or periapical exam to assess developing third molars | | Not usually indicated |
| Patient with other circumstances, including, but not limited to, proposed or existing implants, pathology, needs, treated periodontal disease, and caries remineralization | Clinical judgment as to the need for and type of radiographic images for evaluation, monitoring, or both, in these circumstances | | | | |

[a]Clinical situations for which radiographs may be indicated include, but are not limited to the following. *Positive historical finding:* previous periodontal or endodontic treatment, history of pain or trauma, familial history of dental anomalies, postoperative evaluation of healing, remineralization monitoring, presence of implants or evaluation for implant placement. *Positive clinical signs and symptoms:* clinical evidence of periodontal disease; large or deep restorations; deep carious lesions; malposed or clinically impacted teeth; swelling; evidence of dental or facial trauma; mobility of teeth; fistula involving sinus tract; clinically suspected sinus pathology; growth abnormalities; oral involvement in known or suspected systemic disease; positive neurologic findings in the head and neck; evidence of foreign objects; pain, dysfunction, or both, of the temporomandibular joint; facial asymmetry; abutment teeth for fixed or removable partial prosthesis; unexplained bleeding; unexplained sensitivity of teeth; unusual eruption, spacing, or migration of teeth; unusual tooth morphology, calcification, or color; unexplained absence of teeth; clinical erosion.

[b]Factors increasing the risk for caries may include, but are not limited to the following: high level of caries experience or demineralization, history of recurrent caries, high titers of cariogenic bacteria, existing restoration(s) of poor quality, poor oral hygiene, inadequate fluoride exposure, prolonged nursing (bottle or breast), high-sucrose diet, poor familial oral health, developmental or acquired enamel defects, developmental or acquired disability, xerostomia, genetic abnormality of teeth, many multisurface restorations, chemotherapy or radiation therapy, eating disorders, drug or alcohol abuse, irregular dental care.

2. Proper equipment must be used
   a. Filtration removes long-wavelength, less penetrating x-rays from the beam; dental x-ray machines operating at or below 70 kVp require 1.5-mm aluminum filtration; machines operating above 70 kVp require 2.5-mm aluminum filtration (Fig. 6.5)
   b. Collimation restricts the size and shape of the x-ray beam; federal regulations require that the x-ray beam be collimated to a diameter of no more than 2.75 inches as it reaches the skin of the patient (Fig. 6.6)
   c. The PID must be an open-ended, lead-lined cylinder; the longer the focal spot to object distance, the less divergent beam is created

B. During exposure
   1. Use of the fastest image receptor
      a. Currently, "F" speed is the fastest speed intraoral film available

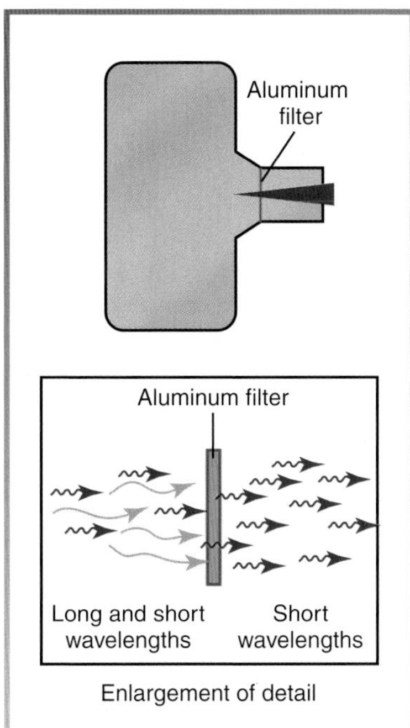


**Fig. 6.5** Aluminum discs are placed in the path of the beam to filter out the low-energy, longer-wavelength x-rays that are harmful to the patient. (From Iannucci JM, Howerton LJ. *Dental Radiography: Principles and Techniques*. 5th ed. St. Louis: Elsevier; 2017.)

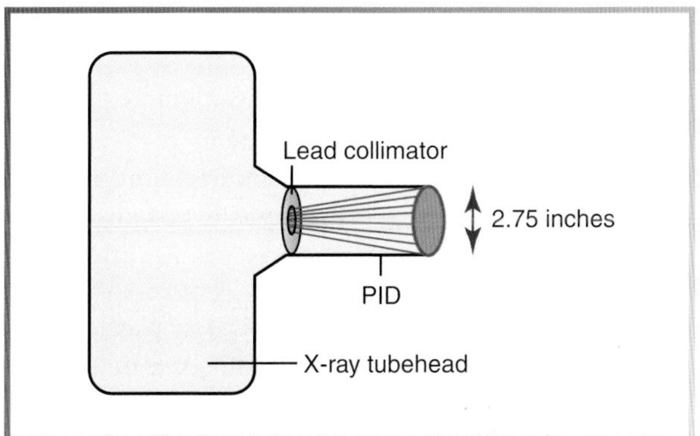


**Fig. 6.6** Federal regulations require that the diameter of a collimated x-ray beam be restricted to 2.75 inches at the patient's skin. (From Iannucci JM, Howerton LJ. *Dental Radiography: Principles and Techniques*. 5th ed. St. Louis: Elsevier; 2017.)

b. Digital imaging further reduces patient exposure and is recommended over film
2. Use of the lead apron and thyroid collar limits the amount of radiation received by the patient
3. Beam alignment devices and proper technique also reduce the chance of retakes, thereby reducing unnecessary exposure to the patient

C. After exposure
1. Correct receptor handling is necessary to produce diagnostic images
2. Proper film processing and retrieval of digital images is necessary to produce diagnostic results

D. Operator protection
1. The dental radiographer should remain behind a barrier during patient exposure

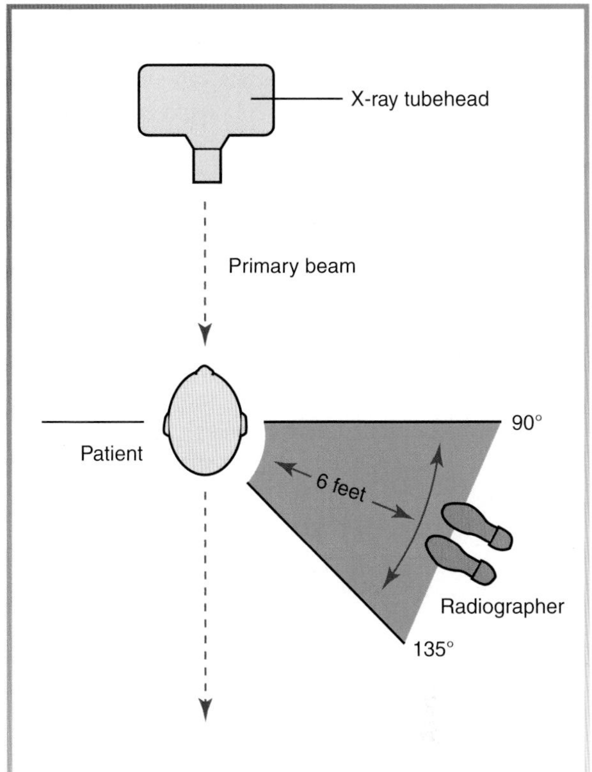


**Fig. 6.7** Operator protection guidelines suggest that the dental radiographer stand at an angle of 90 to 135 degrees to the primary beam. (From Iannucci JM, Howerton LJ. *Dental Radiography: Principles and Techniques*. 5th ed. St. Louis: Elsevier; 2017.)

2. If a structural wall or shield is not available, the radiographer should stand at least 6 feet away from the source of radiation and should be in a position at an angle of 90 to 135 degrees to the primary beam (Fig. 6.7)

E. Maximum permissible dose (MPD)—defined by the National Council on Radiation Protection and Measurements (NCRP) as the maximum dose equivalent that a body is permitted to receive within a specific period[2]
1. The current MPD for occupationally exposed persons is 50 mSv/year
2. The current MPD for nonoccupationally exposed persons is 5 mSv/year (one-tenth [1/10] the dose of the occupational radiation worker)

F. ALARA concept—individuals working with radiation should attempt to keep all radiation exposures "as low as reasonably achievable"

## DIGITAL IMAGING

A. Digital imaging is a filmless system in which a radiographic image is captured using a sensor, the image is broken down into electronic pieces and viewed and stored on a computer
1. Source of radiation—a conventional dental x-ray unit
2. Intraoral sensor—replaces the traditional dental x-ray film
3. Computer—converts the electronic signal received by the sensor; processes and stores the information

B. Methods of obtaining digital images

1. Direct digital imaging
   a. Uses an x-ray machine, intraoral sensor, and computer
   b. The sensor contains a fiberoptic cable linked to the computer as it is placed into the mouth of the patient; the sensor is rigid, and patients may complain of bulkiness
   c. Within seconds of exposure, the image appears on the computer monitor
2. Indirect digital imaging
   a. Uses an x-ray machine, intraoral sensor, and computer
   b. The sensor is a reusable imaging plate coated with phosphors (often termed *PSP plate*); this sensor is thin and flexible, similar to an intraoral film packet
   c. After exposure, the plate is scanned to convert the information into electronic files
   d. Because of the laser scanning step, this type of digital imaging is less rapid than direct digital imaging

C. Advantages of digital imaging[5]
1. Superior resolution produces images with increased diagnostic capabilities
2. Because of the sensitivity of the sensors, patients are exposed to less radiation than with traditional film
3. Increased speed of image viewing leads to increased time efficiency in the dental office
4. The images on the computer monitor can be manipulated to highlight areas of concern, which helps in patient education. Image manipulation can also increase or decrease contrast, making areas of concern more easily viewed.

D. Disadvantages of digital imaging
1. Initial expense of purchasing and setting up equipment may be costly
2. Depending on the system used, sensor size and bulkiness may be an issue
3. Infection control procedures may be difficult, especially with corded sensors
4. Learning a new computer language may be problematic for the staff

## DENTAL X-RAY FILM

A. Film composition
1. The base material (polyester) must possess the dimensional stability to withstand processing procedures and support the emulsion
2. An adhesive is applied evenly to the base to provide for uniform attachment of emulsion to the base
3. The emulsion consists of gelatin and silver halide crystals; gelatin suspends the silver halide crystals, which are sensitive to radiation and light
4. A protective layer is applied to protect the emulsion from being scratched

B. Classifications of dental x-ray film
1. *Intraoral* and *extraoral* film refer to the designated use of the film
   a. Intraoral film is placed inside the oral cavity (e.g., bitewing, periapical, or occlusal)
   b. Extraoral film is placed outside the mouth for exposure of larger areas of the head or skull (e.g., panoramic, cephalometric, skull)
2. Film speed—the amount of radiation needed to produce an image with standard density
   a. Film speed is determined by the size of silver halide crystals in the emulsion, the thickness of the emulsion, and the presence of radiosensitive dyes
   b. Speed ranges used in dental radiography are designated from "D" (slowest) to "F" (fastest)
   c. E-speed intraoral film requires only 50% of the exposure of D-speed intraoral film; F-speed film requires only 77% of the exposure of E-speed film[4]
3. Film size—various sizes are available for both intraoral and extraoral films
   a. Intraoral film
      (1) No. 0 size film—22 × 35 mm
      (2) No. 1 size film—24 × 40 mm
      (3) No. 2 size film—31 × 41 mm (standard film size)
      (4) No. 3 size film—27 × 54 mm
      (5) No. 4 size film—57 × 76 mm

C. Components of intraoral film packets
1. Light-tight, leakproof wrapping protects film from light and moisture
2. Black protective paper is used for additional protection of the film from light
3. Lead foil is inserted between the black paper and the outer wrapping on the back side of the film packet; the purpose of the lead foil is to prevent backscattered radiation from fogging the film
4. Single or double films are enclosed in the packet

D. Intensifying screens used with extraoral film only
1. Housed inside a light-tight cassette
2. Used as a component of the indirect imaging system to reduce patient exposure time to x-radiation when reviewing large anatomic areas
3. Screen construction
   a. Base material composed of polyester plastic
   b. Reflective layer is coated onto the base material; redirects light toward the film to increase film efficiency
   c. Phosphor layer composed of phosphorescent crystals; calcium tungstate emits blue light to expose the film; rare-earth crystals emit green light and respond more efficiently to reduce radiation exposure needed to produce the image
   d. Protective coating is applied to phosphor layer

E. Film storage and protection
1. Unexposed film must be stored away from heat, moisture, chemical vapors, and radiation; film should be stored in a cool, dry place
2. Film has a limited shelf life and must be used before the expiration date

### Dental X-Ray Film Processing

A. Manual film processing consists of five steps: development, rinse, fixation, rinse, drying
1. Developer solution reduces the exposed silver halide crystals into black metallic silver and softens the emulsion
   a. Reducing agent (hydroquinone and elon) reduces the exposed silver halide crystals to black metallic silver

b. Alkalizer (sodium carbonate) softens and swells the gelatin of the emulsion to allow the reducing agent to reach the silver halide crystals
c. Preservative (sodium sulfite) slows the oxidation of the solution to prolong its life span
d. Restrainer (potassium bromide) slows down the action of chemicals
2. A water bath is used to wash or rinse the film and stop the development process
3. Fixer solution removes the unexposed silver halide crystals from the emulsion and hardens the emulsion
a. Clearing or fixing agent (sodium or ammonium thiosulfate) removes the unexposed or undeveloped crystals from the emulsion
b. Acidifier (acetic acid) provides the required acidity so that the fixing solutions can work; stops the action of the developer
c. Preservative (sodium sulfite) slows the solution's oxidation to prolong its life span
d. Hardener (potassium aluminum) shrinks and hardens the emulsion
4. A water bath is used to wash the films and remove all chemicals
5. Films must be completely dried before handling for mounting or viewing
6. Total time involved for manual film processing: approximately 45 to 60 minutes

B. Equipment needed for manual film processing
1. Darkroom: to provide a completely darkened environment for film handling
2. Processing tanks: two insert tanks hold the developer and fixer solutions, while a master tank holds circulating water
3. A thermometer is needed to determine the temperature of the developer solution
a. The optimum time/temperature for manual processing is 68°F (20°C) for 5 minutes
b. Higher temperatures require shorter development time; cooler temperatures require longer development time
4. A timer, film hangers, and stirring paddles are also recommended for manual film processing

C. Automatic film processing consists of four steps: development, fixation, rinse, drying
1. Films are carried from solutions to the dryer by a roller assembly
2. Processing solutions are highly concentrated to work quickly
3. Total time involved for automatic film processing: approximately 4 to 5 minutes

D. Equipment needed for automatic film processing
1. Darkroom: to provide a completely darkened environment for film handling
a. Some processors are equipped with daylight loaders
b. Daylight loaders are light-shielded compartments that allow processing to be completed in a room with white light
2. Automatic processor is built with a housing; film feed slot; roller film transporter; compartments for developer, fixer, and water; a drying chamber; and replenisher pumps

E. Darkroom design and requirements
1. Light-tight room with a revolving light-sealed door, or door with an inside lock
2. Safelight to allow sufficient illumination without exposing or damaging the film
a. Low-wattage bulb of 7.5 or 15 watts
b. Must be placed at least 4 feet from the work surface
c. The GBX-2 filter is recommended, as it is safe to use with both intraoral and extraoral films
3. Overhead white light provides illumination for cleaning and stocking materials
4. Adequate work space and ventilation

F. Film duplication
1. Copies of original radiographs may be needed for third-party payment, a change to another oral health care practitioner, referrals to specialists, or use in litigation
2. The duplication of film requires the use of a film duplicator machine and specialized duplicating film

## FILM-PROCESSING ERRORS

A. Fogged radiographs; appear gray and lack contrast (Fig. 6.8)
1. Improper safelighting in the darkroom
2. Exposure to scatter radiation, heat, humidity, or chemical vapors
3. Contaminated processing chemicals
4. Old, expired, or damaged film

B. Dark radiographs (Fig. 6.9)
1. Temperature of developer solution too high; developer solution too concentrated
2. Excessive developing time used
3. Inaccurate timer or thermometer

C. Light radiographs (Fig. 6.10)
1. Temperature of developer solution too cool; developer solution too weak

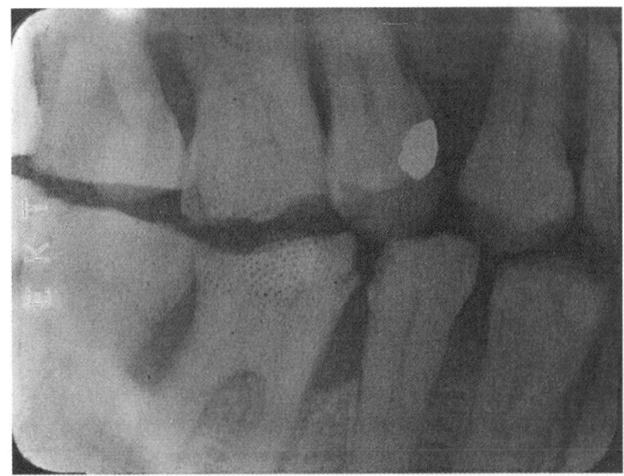

**Fig. 6.8** A fogged film appears gray and lacks detail and contrast. (From Iannucci JM, Howerton LJ. *Dental Radiography: Principles and Techniques.* 5th ed. St. Louis: Elsevier; 2017.)

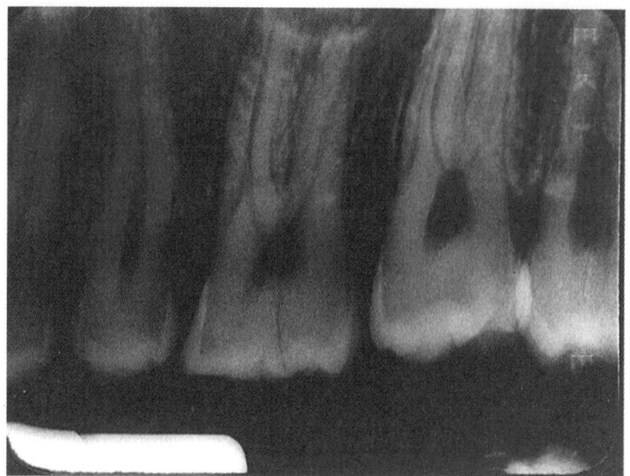

**Fig. 6.9** An overdeveloped film appears dark. (From Iannucci JM, Howerton LJ. *Dental Radiography: Principles and Techniques.* 5th ed. St. Louis: Elsevier; 2017.)

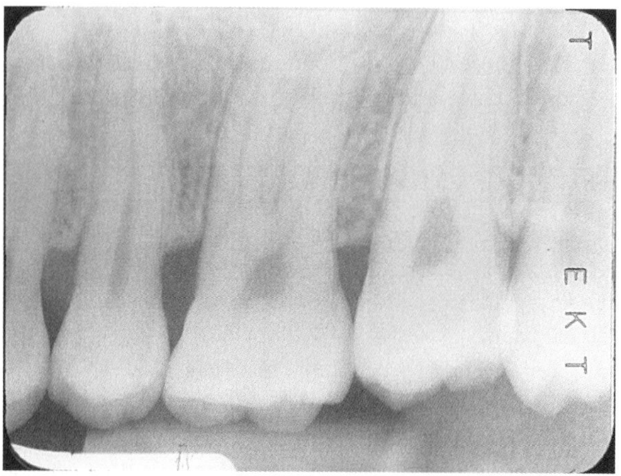

**Fig. 6.10** An underdeveloped film appears light. (From Iannucci JM, Howerton LJ. *Dental Radiography: Principles and Techniques.* 5th ed. St. Louis: Elsevier; 2017.)

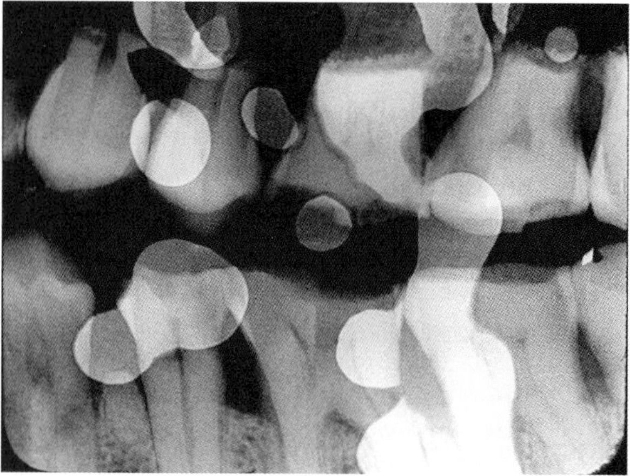

**Fig. 6.11** Fixer spots appear light or white. (From Iannucci JM, Howerton LJ. *Dental Radiography: Principles and Techniques.* 5th ed. St. Louis: Elsevier; 2017.)

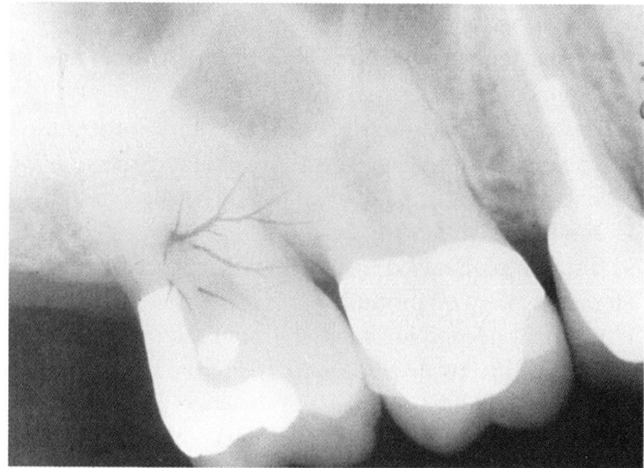

**Fig. 6.12** Static electricity appears as black branching lines. (From Iannucci JM, Howerton LJ. *Dental Radiography: Principles and Techniques.* 5th ed. St. Louis: Elsevier; 2017.)

   2. Insufficient developing time
   3. Inaccurate timer or thermometer

D. Clear (blank) radiographs
   1. Film was not exposed to radiation; most common reason for a clear radiograph
   2. Film placed in fixer solution prior to developer solution
   3. Excessive washing, which causes the removal of film emulsion

E. Completely black radiographs are caused by film exposure to white light before processing

F. Radiographs with spots (Fig. 6.11)
   1. Developer splashing on film before processing causes dark or black spots
   2. Fixer splashing on film before processing causes white or light spots
   3. Water splashing on film before processing causes light spots

G. Yellow-brown stained radiographs
   1. Insufficient fixing or washing times
   2. Processing solutions are exhausted and must be replaced or replenished

H. Dark roller lines or marks
   1. Dirty or contaminated processing chemicals cause dark lines to appear on automatically processed films
   2. Dirty or contaminated automatic processor rollers may also cause roller marks

I. Static electricity artifacts (Fig. 6.12)
   1. Caused by the rapid removal of the film from the packet or the cassette when the humidity level is very low, such as during winter months
   2. Yields black artifacts in tree-shaped streaks, smudges, or dots

## Dental X-Ray Image Characteristics

Table 6.2 summarizes the characteristics and respective influencing factors.

A. Radiolucent—refers to a portion of an image that is dark or black

B. Radiopaque—refers to a portion of an image that is light or white

C. Density—the overall darkness or blackness of an image
   1. Increase kVp, increase density

**TABLE 6.2 Radiation Characteristics and Influencing Factors**

| Characteristics | Influencing Factors | Effect of Influencing Factors | Result |
|---|---|---|---|
| Sharpness | Focal spot size | Decrease focal spot size | Increase sharpness |
| | Film composition | Decrease crystal size | Increase sharpness |
| | Movement | Decrease movement | Increase sharpness |
| Magnification | Target-receptor distance | Increase target-receptor distance | Decrease magnification |
| | Object-receptor distance | Decrease object-receptor distance | Decrease magnification |
| Distortion | Object-receptor alignment | Object and receptor parallel | Decrease distortion |
| | X-ray beam alignment | Beam perpendicular to object and receptor | Decrease distortion |

2. Increase mA, increase density
3. Increase time, increase density

D. Contrast—the difference in the degrees of darkness between adjacent areas on an image
   1. Increase kVp, low contrast (many shades of gray)
   2. Decrease kVp, high contrast (many areas of black and white)

E. Sharpness—the capability of the image receptor to reproduce the distinct outlines of an object
   1. The smaller the focal spot size, the sharper the image
   2. The smaller the silver halide crystals in the film emulsion, the sharper the image
   3. The less movement of the patient, tubehead, or receptor, the sharper the image

F. Magnification—a radiographic image that is larger than its actual size
   1. The longer the target-to-receptor distance, the less image magnification produced
   2. The shorter the tooth-to-receptor distance, the less image magnification produced

G. Distortion—a variation in the true size and shape of an object
   1. Align the tooth and receptor parallel to each other to avoid distortion
   2. Position the x-ray beam perpendicular to the tooth and receptor to avoid distortion

## QUALITY ASSURANCE

A. A quality control plan in dental radiography ensures the production of diagnostic-quality radiographs while minimizing radiation exposure through a plan of action; in addition, the means of testing and regulating x-ray equipment and procedures used to expose, process, and store radiographs are reviewed

B. Components of a quality control plan
   1. Competence of radiographer
      a. Evaluation of radiographs for self-analysis of technique
      b. Peer review of radiographs for technique analysis
      c. Continuing education courses to maintain state-of-the-art practice
   2. Equipment inspections by state and local radiation regulatory agencies
      a. Milliamperage, kilovoltage, timer accuracy
      b. Collimation and alignment of the x-ray beam
      c. Measures to avoid leakage radiation
      d. Mechanical support of the unit; may include tube drifting
      e. Penetrating quality of the beam tested by using the half-value layer (HVL); uses a material (usually aluminum) that reduces exposure by one-half when placed within path of radiation beam
   3. Quality assurance procedures for digital imaging
      a. Daily back-up of digital data on computer
      b. Periodic examination of receptors for wear and tear
      c. Monitoring of digital equipment should be completed in accordance with equipment manufacturer
   4. Quality assurance procedures for film processing
      a. Periodic evaluation of the darkroom
         (1) Checks for light leaks
         (2) Coin test for safelight evaluation involves the placement of a coin on an unwrapped, unexposed film under a safelight for 2 to 3 minutes; if the outline of the coin is present on the processed film, corrective action is necessary
   5. Creation of a reference or step-wedge radiograph to compare strengths of processing solutions; evaluates films for consistency in density and contrast
   6. Periodic cleaning, maintenance, and daily monitoring of processing equipment
      a. Clean the automatic roller assembly and manual racks to prevent debris buildup and artifacts; schedule cleaning maintenance on the basis of usage
      b. Schedule preventive maintenance for optimal equipment operation
      c. Monitor solution temperatures daily
      d. Replenish solutions in accordance with the volume of films processed

## RADIOLOGY TECHNIQUES: INTRAORAL AND EXTRAORAL

A. Adhering to shadow-casting principles produces diagnostic radiographic images
   1. Smallest focal spot possible
   2. Longest source-to-object distance possible (focal spot to tooth)
   3. Shortest object-to-receptor distance possible (tooth to receptor)
   4. Tooth and receptor should be in a parallel relationship
   5. X-ray beam should be perpendicular to the tooth and the receptor

B. Angulation of the x-ray beam
   1. Vertical angulation refers to the position of the PID in the vertical plane
      a. Positive vertical angulation indicates the PID is pointing downward
      b. Negative vertical angulation indicates the PID is pointing upward
   2. Horizontal angulation refers to the position of the PID in the horizontal plane

## Intraoral Radiographic Techniques

A. Paralleling
   1. Yields radiographic images with a minimum of image distortion
   2. Minimizes the superimposition of adjacent oral structures
   3. Application of the paralleling technique
      a. The receptor is placed parallel to the long axis of the tooth
      b. The x-ray beam is directed perpendicular to the long axis of the tooth and the receptor
      c. The x-ray beam is directed perpendicular through interproximal spaces
      d. The x-ray beam is centered over the anatomic structures and the receptor

B. Bisecting the angle
   1. Applies the rule of isometry: the accurate length of the tooth is obtained if the x-ray beam is perpendicular to the imaginary bisector of the angle formed by the plane of the receptor and the long axis of the tooth (Fig. 6.13)
   2. Allows for ease of receptor placement for certain patients with a small mouth, shallow palate, large tori, or gag reflex
   3. Application of the bisecting angle technique
      a. The receptor is placed against the teeth
      b. The x-ray beam is directed perpendicular to the imaginary bisector of the angle formed by the plane of the receptor and the long axis of the tooth
      c. The x-ray beam is directed perpendicular through the interproximal spaces
      d. The x-ray beam is centered over the anatomic structures and the receptor

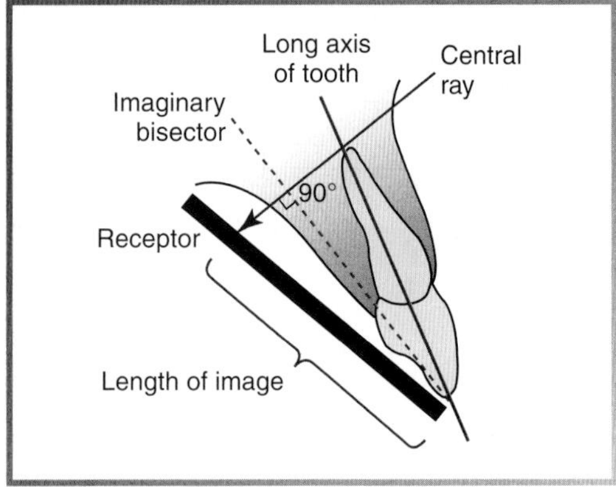


**Fig. 6.13** The image on the receptor is equal to the length of the tooth when the central ray is directed at 90 degrees to the imaginary bisector. A tooth and its image will be equal in length when two equal triangles are formed that share a common side (imaginary bisector). (From Iannucci JM, Howerton LJ. *Dental Radiography: Principles and Techniques*. 5th ed. St. Louis: Elsevier; 2017.)

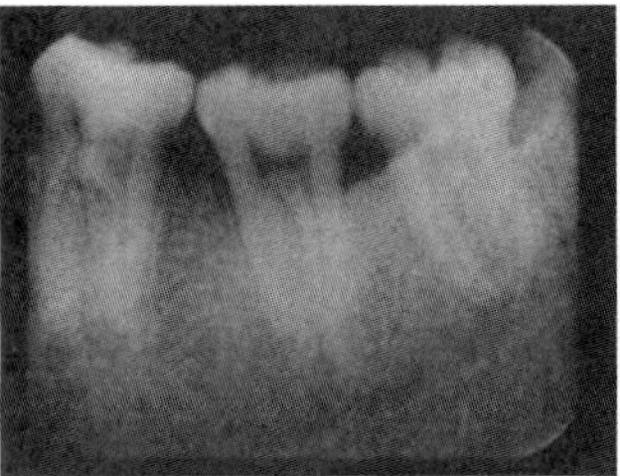

**Fig. 6.14** Periapical radiograph.

## Types of Intraoral Radiographic Examinations

A. Periapical
   1. Periapical examination demonstrates the entire tooth and surrounding bone (Fig. 6.14)
   2. Indications for periapical radiographs[3]
      a. Suspected periapical conditions
      b. Evidence of periodontal disease
      c. Injury or trauma to teeth
      d. Endodontic therapy
      e. Deep or large carious lesions
      f. Suspected impacted teeth
      g. Unusual eruption, malposition, or unexplained missing teeth
      h. Unexplained sensitivity or tooth mobility
      i. Unusual tooth morphology or color
      j. Dental implant evaluation

B. Bitewing
   1. Bitewing radiographs demonstrate the anatomic crowns of maxillary and mandibular teeth as well as the height of alveolar bone (Fig. 6.15)
   2. Indications for bitewing radiographs[3]
      a. Suspected interproximal caries
      b. Defective restorations
      c. Early periodontal disease
   3. Horizontal bitewing radiographs are considered the traditional placement; the long dimension of the receptor positioned horizontally
   4. Bitewing radiographs may also be exposed by placing the receptor with the long dimension vertically; vertical bitewing radiographs are typically prescribed for patients with periodontal disease as the vertical image increases the viewing area of alveolar bone

C. Occlusal
   1. An occlusal radiograph demonstrates a large anatomic region or the entire arch; it is usually exposed in conjunction with other intraoral radiographs (Fig. 6.16)
   2. Indications for the exposure of occlusal radiographs[6]
      a. Image margins of large pathologic conditions
      b. Localization of objects (foreign or impactions)
      c. Injury or trauma to surrounding bone structure
      d. Suspected supernumerary teeth
      e. Unexplained swelling or growth abnormality
      f. Salivary stone detection

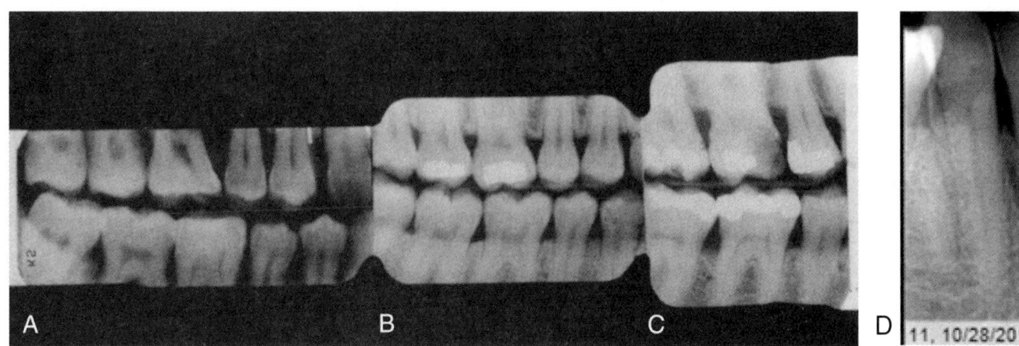
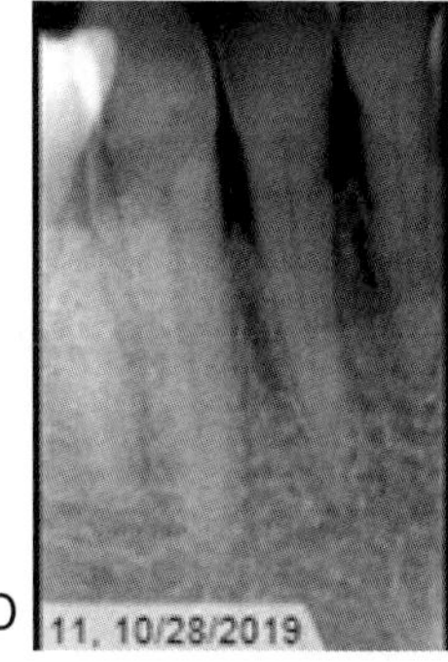
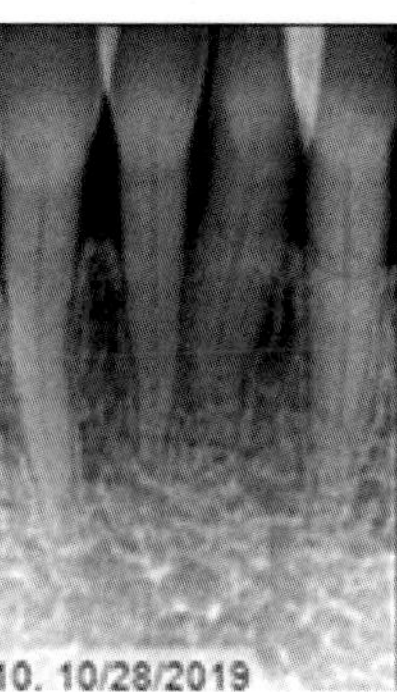

**Fig. 6.15** Bitewing radiographs. (A) Long horizontal bitewing. (B) Traditional horizontal bitewing. (C) Vertical bitewing (D) Vertical bitewings illustrating periodontal disease and bone loss.

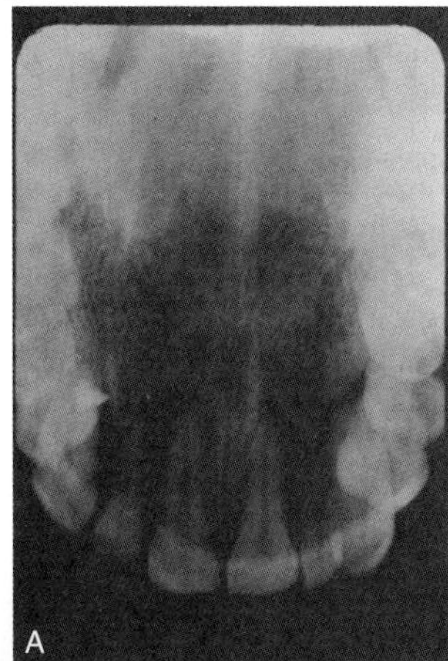
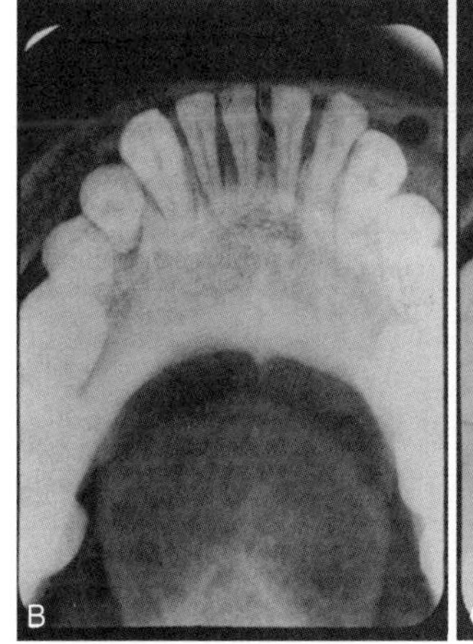
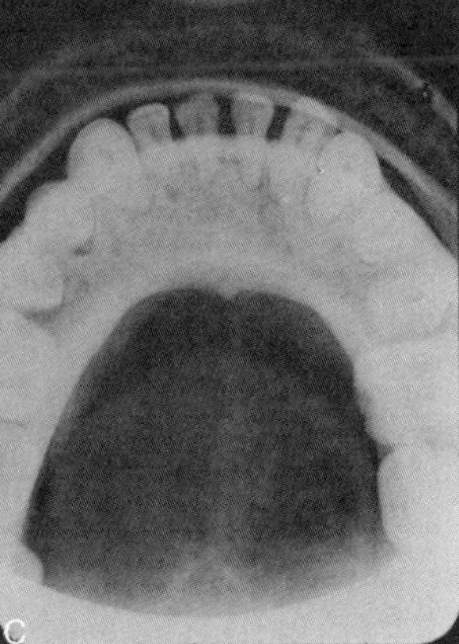

**Fig. 6.16** Occlusal radiographs. (A) Topographic maxillary occlusal radiograph. (B) Topographic mandibular occlusal radiograph. (C) Cross-sectional mandibular occlusal radiograph.

3. Occlusal radiographs may be prescribed for children, patients with limited jaw opening or those who cannot tolerate periapical receptor placement

D. Full-mouth survey (Fig. 6.17)
   1. A series of intraoral radiographs that reveal all the tooth-bearing areas of the maxilla and mandible
   2. Usually a combination of periapical and bitewing radiographs
   3. May include dentulous and edentulous areas

## Types of Extraoral Radiographic Examinations

A. The panoramic radiograph is the most common extraoral exposure (Fig. 6.18)

B. Provides an overall view of the maxilla, mandible, and surrounding structures; used to supplement intraoral images

C. Indications for the exposure of panoramic radiographs[6]
   1. Impacted teeth
   2. Eruption patterns; growth and development
   3. Assessment of trauma
   4. Examination of the extent of large lesions or pathologic conditions

D. Image production is created while the receptor and tubehead rotate around the patient
   1. The image is produced through a process termed *tomography*
   2. Tomography is a radiographic technique that permits visualization of structures in a chosen plane or layer while intentionally blurring the images above and below the selected plane
   3. The zone in which structures are most clearly demonstrated is termed the *focal trough*
      a. The size and shape of each focal trough varies, determined by the manufacturer of the panoramic machine
      b. The focal trough is designed to accommodate the average-size maxilla and mandible

E. Patient positioning is important in preparation of exposure of panoramic radiographs
   1. Follow the directions from the manufacturer for specific positioning guidelines for determining the location of the focal trough
   2. Insert the receptor into the cassette and panoramic unit
   3. Position the patient with the midsagittal plane perpendicular to the floor and the Frankfort plane parallel to the floor
   4. Instruct the patient to occlude on the bite stick or similar device and to hold still throughout the exposure
   5. Consult the manufacturer's instructions to select appropriate exposure settings
   6. Maintain pressure on the exposure button until the procedure is completed

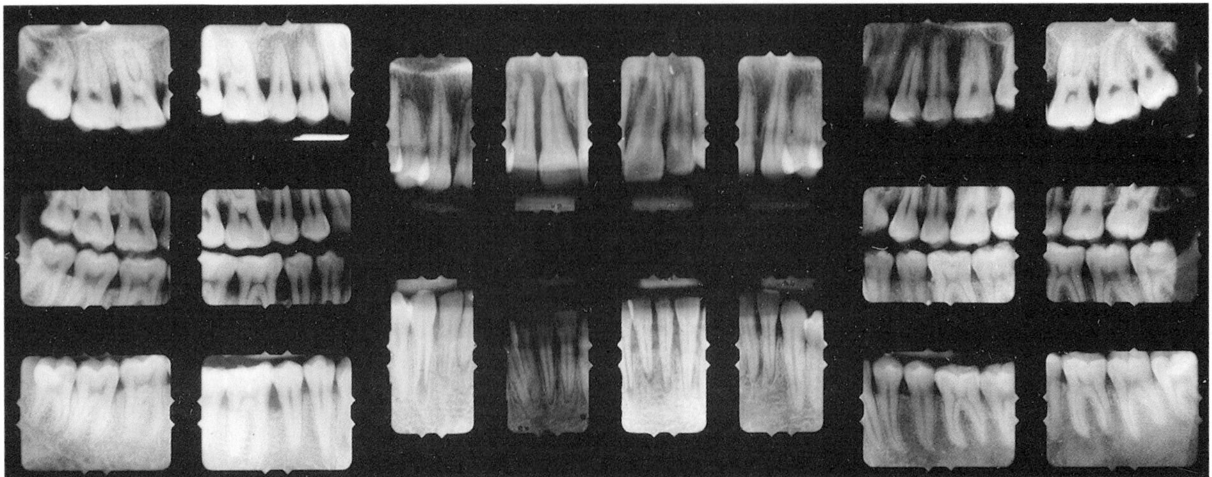

**Fig. 6.17** Full-mouth radiographic survey. (From Bird DL, Robinson DS. *Modern Dental Assisting.* 11th ed. St. Louis: Elsevier; 2015.)

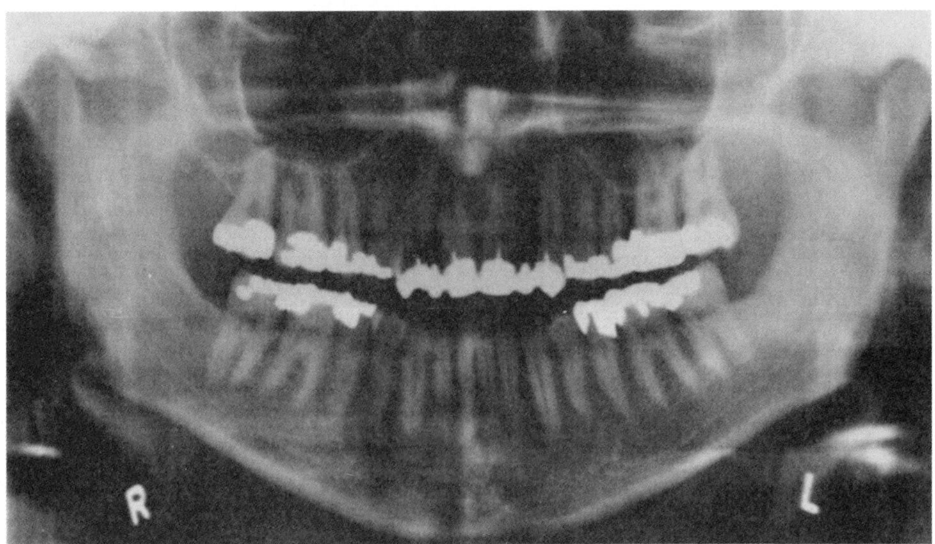


**Fig. 6.18** Panoramic radiograph.

## RADIOGRAPHIC ERRORS: INTRAORAL AND EXTRAORAL

### Intraoral Technique Errors[7]

A. Receptor placement
   1. Correct receptor placement is important for the production of diagnostic images
   2. Improper receptor placement includes not centering the receptor over the area of interest, inadequate coverage of the apical areas, and tipped occlusal/incisal edges (Fig. 6.19)

B. Vertical angulation
   1. Too much or excessive vertical angulation causes foreshortened images (Fig. 6.20)
   2. Too little or insufficient vertical angulation causes elongated images (Fig. 6.21)

C. Horizontal angulation
   1. Correct horizontal angulation directs the central ray of the beam through the interproximal regions
   2. Incorrect horizontal angulation causes overlapping of the contact areas; the adjacent teeth appear overlapped onto each other (Fig. 6.22)

D. PID alignment problems
   1. If the PID is not aligned correctly and the x-ray beam is not centered over the receptor, a partial image is seen on the resultant image
   2. A clear, unexposed area is seen on the image known as a *cone-cut* (Fig. 6.23)

E. Blurred images
   1. If the patient or tubehead is not still during exposure, blurring will appear on the image (Fig. 6.24)
   2. Instruct patients to keep all movement to a minimum during x-ray exposure

F. Reversed film
   1. If the film is placed backward in the mouth and then exposed, a light image with a herringbone (or "tire track") pattern will appear (Fig. 6.25)

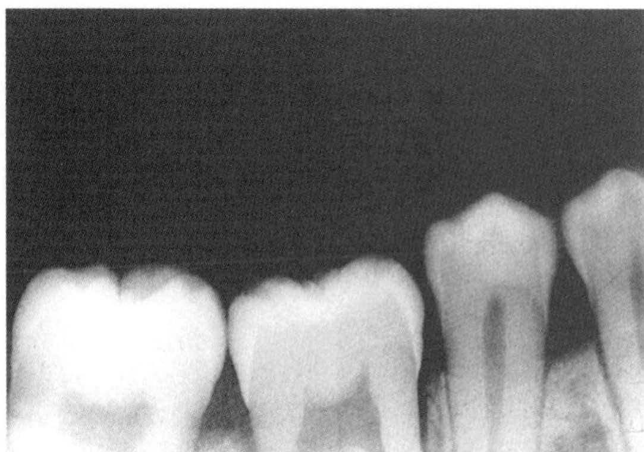

**Fig. 6.19** Improper placement; no apices are seen on this periapical image. (From Iannucci JM, Howerton LJ. *Dental Radiography: Principles and Techniques*. 5th ed. St. Louis: Elsevier; 2017.)

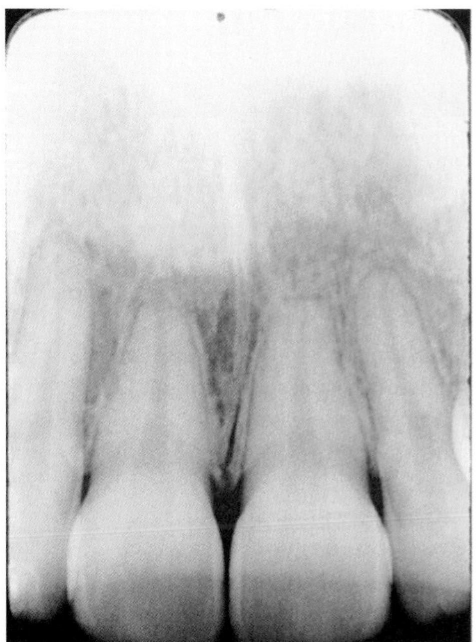

**Fig. 6.20** If the vertical angulation is too steep, the image of the tooth on the receptor is shorter than the actual tooth; the images are foreshortened. (From Iannucci JM, Howerton LJ. *Dental Radiography: Principles and Techniques*. 5th ed. St. Louis: Elsevier; 2017.)

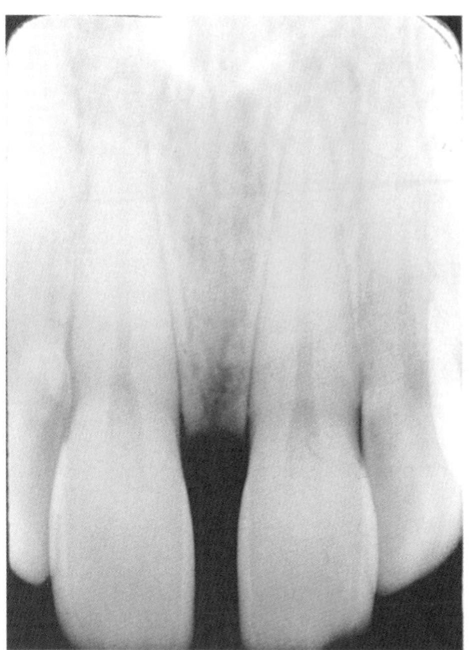

**Fig. 6.21** If the vertical angulation is too flat, the image of the tooth on the receptor is longer than the actual tooth; the images are elongated. (From Iannucci JM, Howerton LJ. *Dental Radiography: Principles and Techniques*. 5th ed. St. Louis: Elsevier; 2017.)

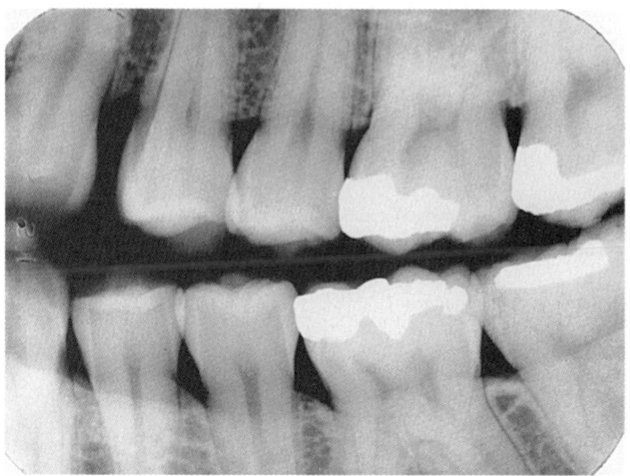

**Fig. 6.22** Nondiagnostic bitewing image with overlapped interproximal contacts. (From Iannucci JM, Howerton LJ. *Dental Radiography: Principles and Techniques*. 5th ed. St. Louis: Elsevier; 2017.)

2. Since the primary beam penetrated the lead foil inside the packet before reaching the film, the image demonstrates a lighter appearance and the herringbone pattern

## Extraoral Technique Errors[7]

A. Frankfort plane positioning errors
   1. If the chin is too low or tipped down, the mandibular incisor region will appear blurred, the condyles may not be visible, and an exaggerated smile line is seen on the image (Fig. 6.26A)
   2. If the chin is too high or tipped upward, the hard palate will be superimposed over the maxillary roots, the maxillary incisors will be blurred and magnified, and a reverse smile line is seen on the image (Fig. 6.26B)

B. Focal trough positioning errors
   1. Anterior teeth appear blurred and magnified in size if the dental arches are positioned too far back (posterior) in the focal trough (Fig. 6.27A)
   2. Anterior teeth will appear narrowed and diminished in size if the dental arches are positioned too far forward (anterior) in the focal trough (Fig. 6.27B)

C. Midsagittal plane errors
   1. If the head of the patient is not centered in the panoramic machine, the ramus and posterior teeth will be unequally magnified
   2. The side closest to the receptor will appear smaller, whereas the side farther away from the receptor will appear magnified

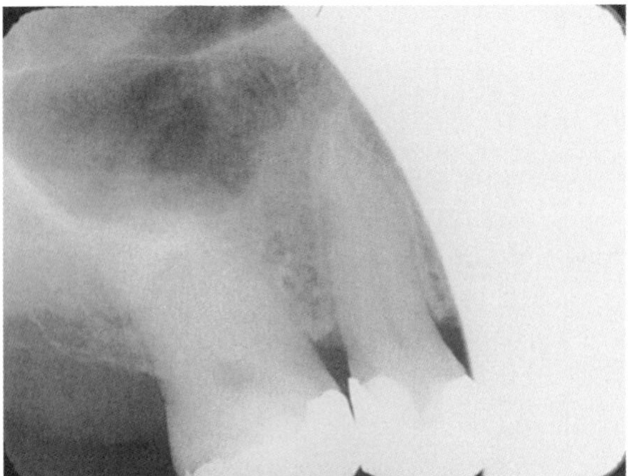

**Fig. 6.23** A cone-cut is seen as a curved unexposed (clear) area on the radiograph. (From Iannucci JM, Howerton LJ. *Dental Radiography: Principles and Techniques*. 5th ed. St. Louis: Elsevier; 2017.)

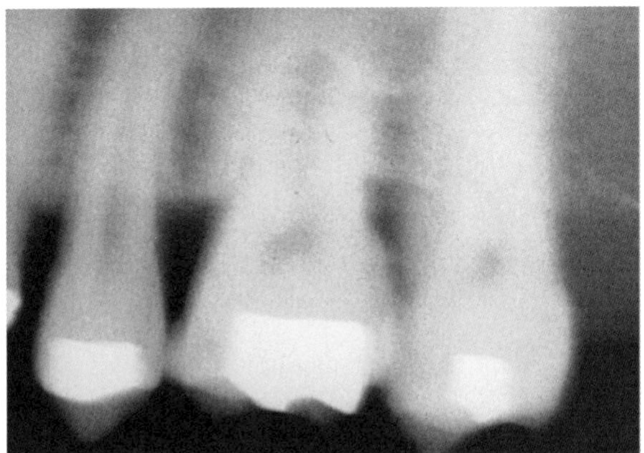

**Fig. 6.24** Movement results in a blurred image. (From Iannucci JM, Howerton LJ. *Dental Radiography: Principles and Techniques*. 5th ed. St. Louis: Elsevier; 2017.)

D. Cervical spine errors—if the patient is not standing or sitting up, the cervical spine will appear as a vertical radiopacity in the middle of the image
E. Lead apron errors—if the lead apron is placed too high on the neck of the patient, the apron will block the x-ray beam from reaching the receptor, and a radiopaque, cone-shaped artifact will obscure the mandible
F. Ghost images
   1. Any metallic object that remains in the head and neck region during panoramic radiography may cause a ghost image to appear
   2. Earrings, hearing aids, napkin chains, removable dental appliances, and hair clips are some examples of items that may cause a ghost image
   3. Ghost images are seen on the panoramic image on the opposite side of the original item, located higher than the original item, and indistinct or distorted

## FILM MOUNTING

A. Purpose—film mounting provides a systematic approach for viewing and evaluating radiographs, with placement of radiographs in a holding device according to anatomic considerations

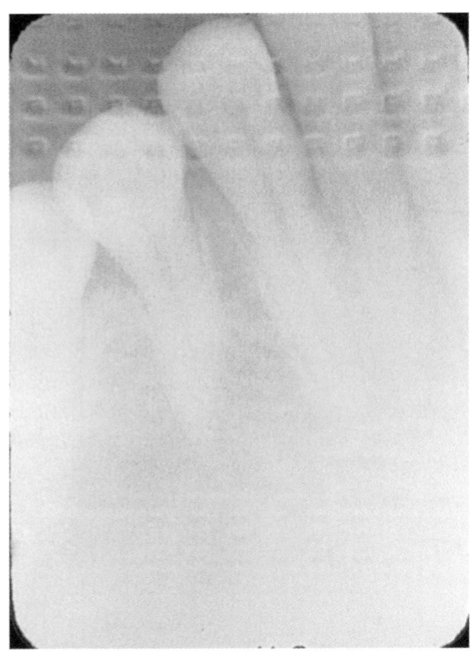

**Fig. 6.25** A reversed film causes an image that appears light with a herringbone (or tire track) pattern. (From Iannucci JM, Howerton LJ. *Dental Radiography: Principles and Techniques*. 5th ed. St. Louis: Elsevier; 2017.)

B. Mount construction—made of cardboard or plastic; available with windows for placement of radiographs in various number and size combinations (see Fig. 6.17)
C. Mounting procedures
   1. Intraoral radiographs—labial mounting; recommended by the American Dental Association (ADA)
      a. Raised portion of the embossed dot is toward the radiographer
      b. The patient's left side is the radiographer's right side
      c. The orientation is that of the radiographer facing the patient
   2. Intraoral radiographs—lingual mounting
      a. Raised portion of the embossed dot is away from the radiographer
      b. The patient's left side is the radiographer's left side
      c. The orientation is that of the radiographer behind the patient
   3. Extraoral radiographs
      a. During exposure, side(s) under examination should be identified with a metal letter (R or L) placed on the cassette
      b. A commercial film identification imprinter can be used to label after exposure but before processing

## RADIOGRAPHIC INTERPRETATION

A. Radiographic tooth anatomy (Fig. 6.28)
   1. Enamel—outermost layer of the crown; radiopaque
   2. Dentin—found beneath the enamel and surrounds the pulp cavity; less radiopaque than enamel

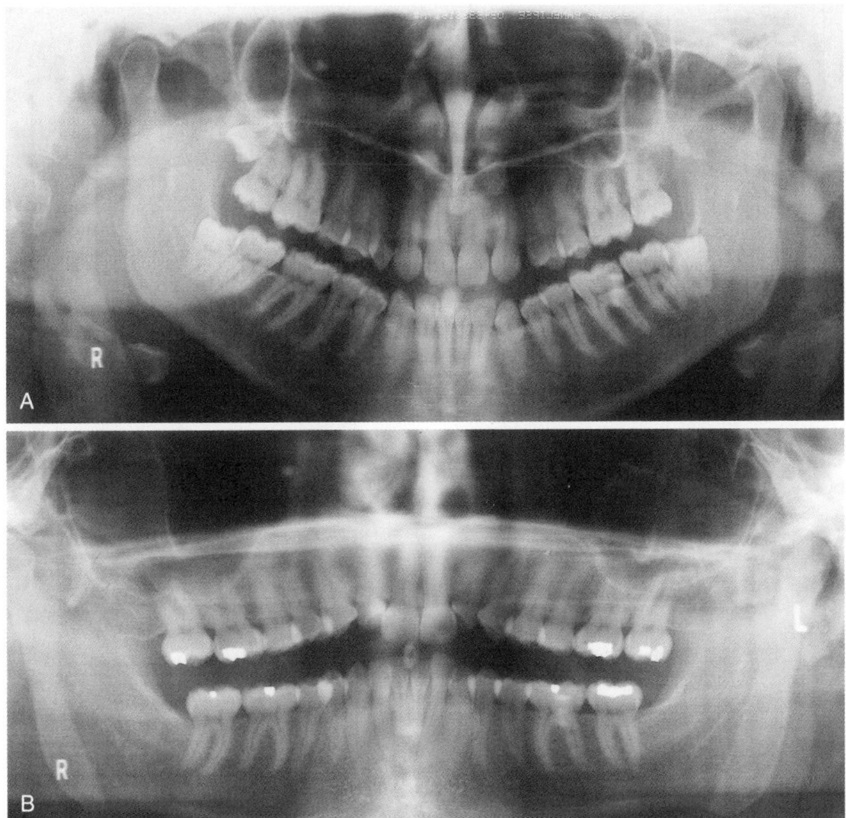


**Fig. 6.26** (A) Chin positioned too far down; the Frankfort plane is angled downward. (B) Chin positioned too far up; the Frankfort plane is angled upward.

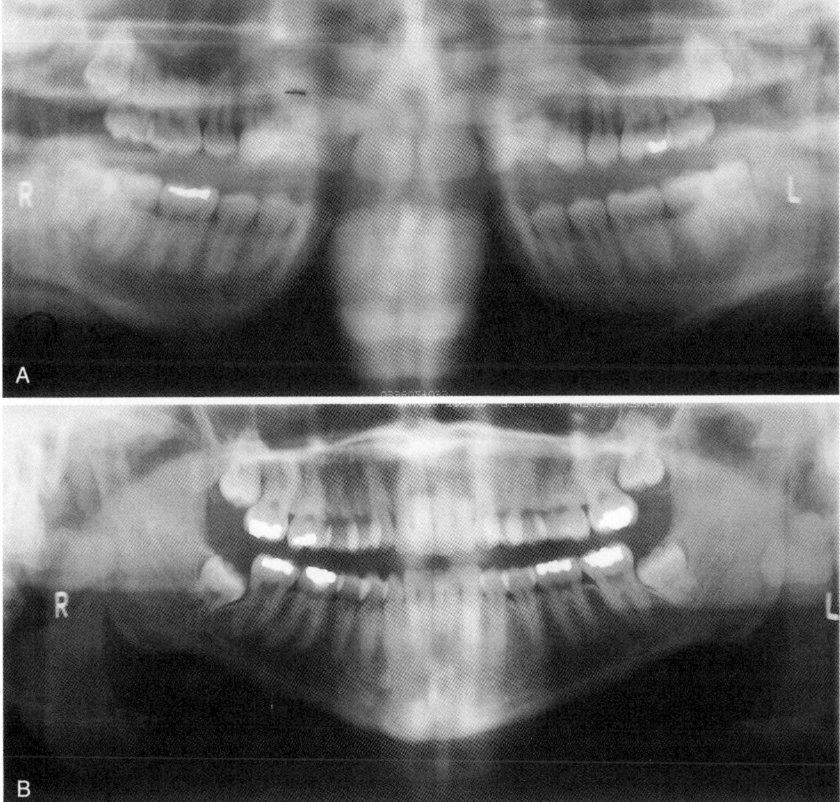


**Fig. 6.27** (A) Dental arches positioned too far posterior to the focal trough. (B) Dental arches positioned too far anterior to the focal trough.

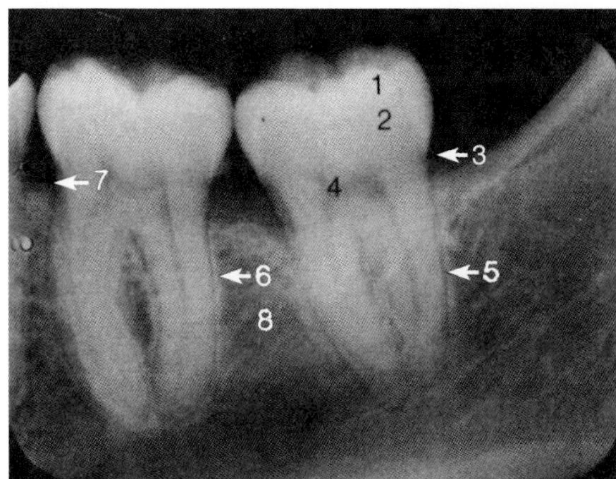

Fig. 6.28 Tooth anatomy. *1,* Enamel. *2,* Dentin. *3,* Cementum. *4,* Pulp. *5,* Periodontal ligament space. *6,* Lamina dura. *7,* Alveolar crest. *8,* Trabeculae.

3. Pulp cavity—relatively radiolucent
4. Alveolar bone—composed of cancellous and cortical bone; radiopaque
5. Lamina dura—dense radiopaque line that surrounds the root of a tooth
6. Periodontal ligament space—the space between the root of a tooth and the lamina dura; appears as a thin radiolucent line

B. Radiographic anatomic landmarks of the maxilla (Fig. 6.29)
1. Incisive foramen—a hole in bone found at the midline of the anterior portion of the hard palate; oval radiolucency located between the maxillary central incisors
2. Lateral fossa (canine fossa)—diffuse radiolucency located between the maxillary lateral incisor and the canine
3. Median palatine suture—radiolucent line extending vertically between maxillary central incisors
4. Nasal fossae (nasal cavity)—two paired radiolucent compartments seen superior to the maxillary central incisors; outlined by the floor of the nasal cavity
5. Nasal septum—vertical bony radiopaque wall that divides the nasal cavity
6. Inferior nasal conchae—curved plates of bone that extend from the lateral walls of the nasal cavity; appear as a diffuse radiopacity within the nasal cavity
7. Anterior nasal spine—V-shaped radiopacity seen at the intersection of the floor of the nasal cavity and the nasal septum
8. Inverted Y—Y-shaped radiopacity seen at the intersection of the lateral wall of the nasal cavity and the anterior portion of the maxillary sinus
9. Maxillary sinus—paired cavities of bone seen as bilateral radiolucencies that originate at the maxillary canine region and extend posteriorly; outlined by a radiopaque wall or floor
10. Nutrient canals—tiny, tube-like passageways through bone that appear as thin radiolucent lines with radiopaque borders; may be seen within the maxillary sinus
11. Zygomatic process of the maxilla—J- or U-shaped radiopacity seen superior to the maxillary posterior teeth
12. Maxillary tuberosity—rounded prominence bone seen as a radiopaque bulge in the most posterior region of the maxilla

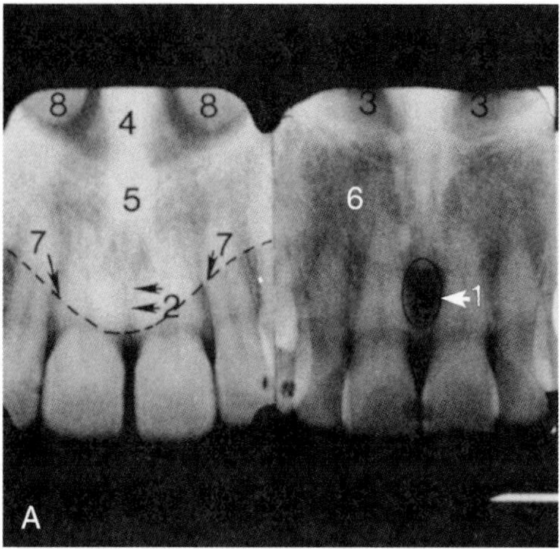


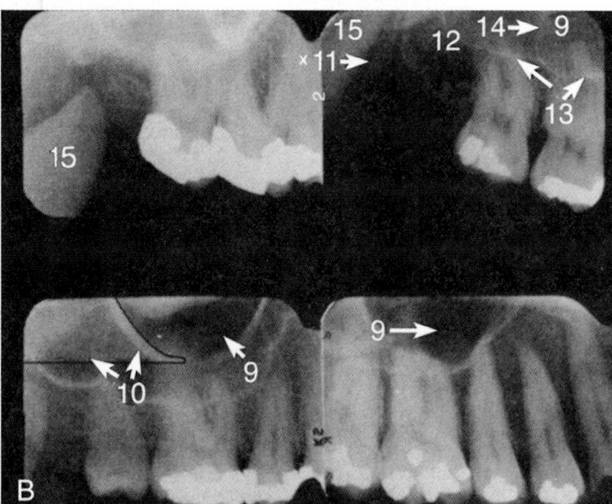

Fig. 6.29 Radiographic anatomy of the maxillary arch. (A) Maxillary anterior region. *1,* Incisive foramen. *2,* Median palatal suture. *3,* Nasal cavity (fossae). *4,* Nasal septum. *5,* Anterior nasal spine. *6,* Lateral (canine) fossa. *7,* Soft tissue outline of the nose *(dashed line)*. *8,* Inferior nasal conchae. (B) Maxillary posterior region. *9,* Maxillary sinus. *10,* Zygomatic process. *11,* Hanulus. *12,* Maxillary tuberosity. *13,* Floor of the maxillary sinus. *14,* Septa dividing the sinus. *15,* Coronoid process.

13. Hamulus—radiopaque spine located on the medial pterygoid plate seen posterior to the maxillary tuberosity
14. Lateral pterygoid plate—radiopaque extension of sphenoid bone; distinguished as separate from the maxillary tuberosity

C. Radiographic anatomic landmarks of the mandible (Fig. 6.30)
1. Genial tubercles—circular radiopaque spines located inferior to mandibular central incisors
2. Lingual foramen—tiny opening in bone found on the internal surface of the mandible; small radiolucent dot seen in the center of the genial tubercles
3. Nutrient canals—tiny, tube-like passageways through bone that appear as thin radiolucent lines with radiopaque borders; may be seen in the mandibular anterior region
4. Mental ridge—radiopaque ridge of bone that extends from the mandibular premolar region to the midline, extending upward
5. Mylohyoid ridge—radiopaque ridge of bone that extends downward and forward from the mandibular

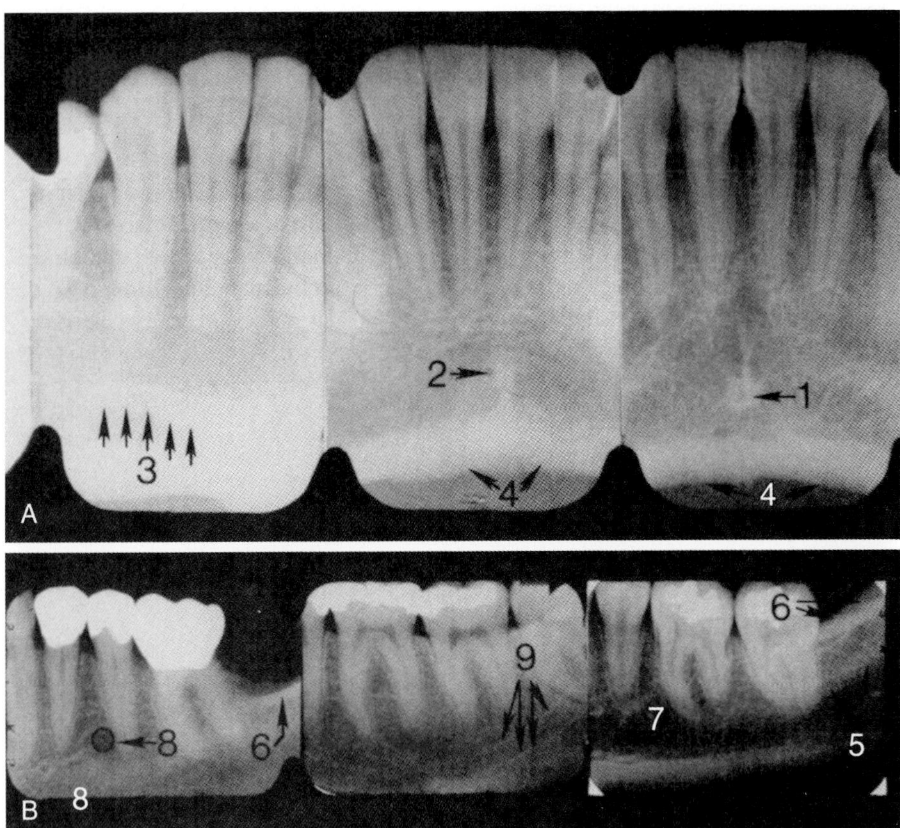

Fig. 6.30 Radiographic anatomy of the mandibular arch. (A) Mandibular anterior region. *1,* Genial tubercles. *2,* Lingual foramen. *3,* Mental ridge. *4,* Inferior border of the mandible. (B) Mandibular posterior region. *5,* Mylohyoid ridge. *6,* External oblique ridge. *7,* Submandibular fossa. *8,* Mental foramen. *9,* Mandibular canal.

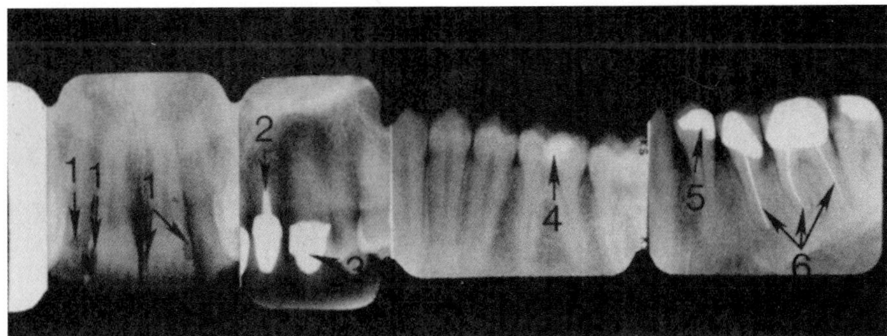

Fig. 6.31 Common restorative materials. *1,* Composite. *2,* Post-and-core restoration with a porcelain-fused-to-metal crown. *3,* Porcelain-fused-to-metal crown. *4,* Occlusal composite or temporary restoration. *5,* Amalgam. *6,* Porcelain-fused-to-metal crowns with endodontic material, silver points.

molar region; may be superimposed over the roots of the mandibular posterior teeth

6. Internal oblique ridge—radiopaque ridge of bone that extends downward and forward from the ramus; may continue as the mylohyoid ridge
7. External oblique ridge—radiopaque ridge of bone that ends at the anterior border of the ramus
8. Submandibular fossa—large radiolucent area in the posterior body of the mandible; represents the lingual depression corresponding to the location of the submandibular salivary gland
9. Mental foramen—a hole in bone found on the external surface of the mandible; seen as a round radiolucency in the area of the apical portion of the mandibular premolars
10. Mandibular canal—a tube-like passageway through bone; seen as a radiolucent horizontal canal with radiopaque borders that runs in the mandible below the apices of mandibular posterior teeth
11. Coronoid process of the mandible—a marked prominence of bone seen on the anterior portion of the mandible; this radiopacity is the only mandibular landmark to be viewed on maxillary posterior periapical images

D. Radiographic appearance of restorative materials (Fig. 6.31)
   1. Amalgam—completely radiopaque, irregular borders
   2. Gold—completely radiopaque, smooth borders

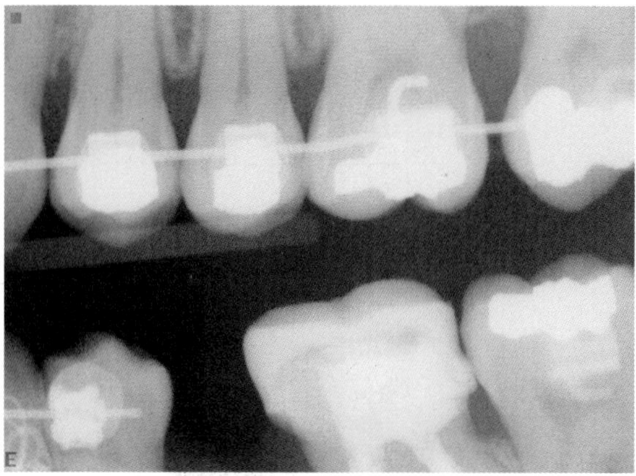

Fig. 6.32 Orthodontic appliances are easily recognized on this bitewing image.

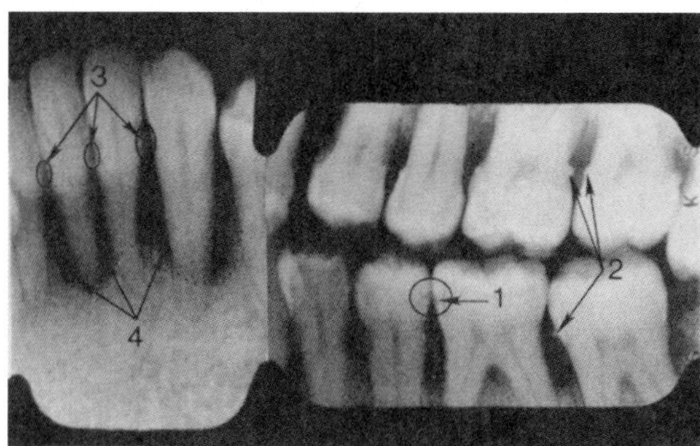


Fig. 6.35 Dental caries and bone loss. *1,* Interproximal caries. *2,* Interproximal calculus deposits. *3,* Heavy calculus deposits. *4,* Severe bone loss.

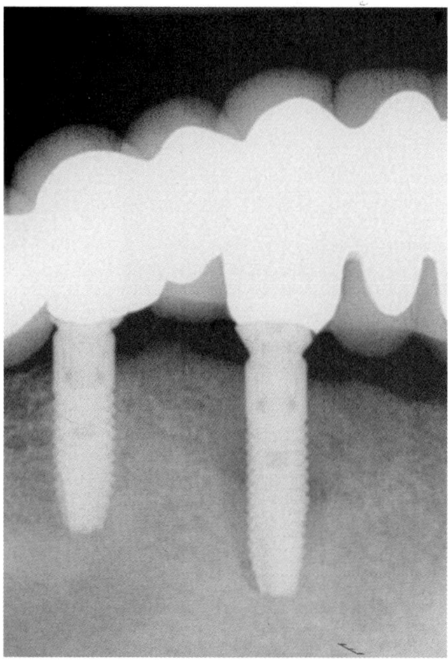

Fig. 6.33 Two dental implants support a mandibular bridge.

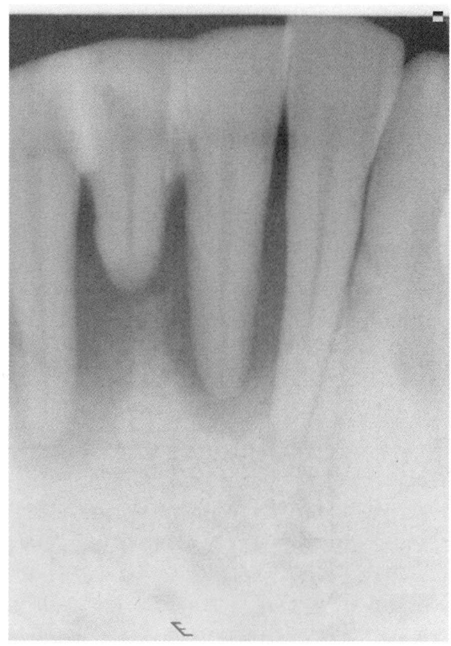

Fig. 6.36 Severe bone loss in the mandibular anterior region.

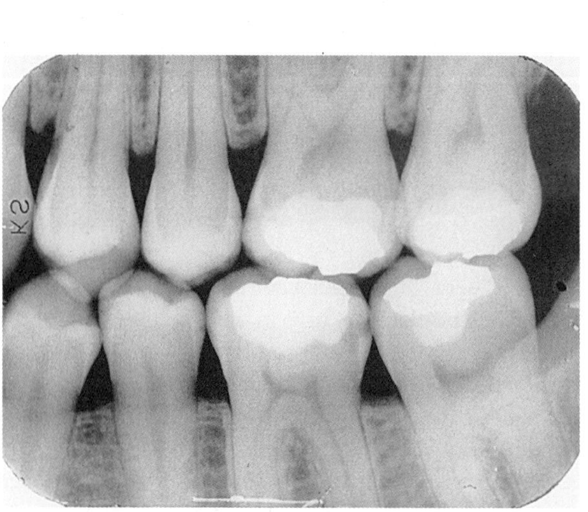

Fig. 6.34 Dental caries are evident on this bitewing image. (From Iannucci JM, Howerton LJ. *Dental Radiography: Principles and Techniques.* 5th ed. St. Louis: Elsevier; 2017.)

3. Stainless steel crown (temporary crown)—slightly radiopaque with a "see-through" component
4. Porcelain crown—slightly radiopaque; thin radiopaque line represents cement
5. Porcelain-fused-to-metal crown—metal component is completely radiopaque; porcelain component is slightly radiopaque
6. Composite—radiolucent to radiopaque
7. Endodontic materials—gutta percha is slightly radiopaque; silver points are radiopaque
8. Orthodontic appliances—radiopaque bands, brackets, and wires representing the materials (Fig. 6.32)
9. Dental implants—radiopaque metallic post positioned in bone replacing a natural tooth (Figure 6.33)

E. Radiographic appearance of dental caries[7] (Fig. 6.34)
   1. Interproximal caries—seen as a radiolucent area at or just below the contact area

2. Occlusal caries—seen as a radiolucent area in the chewing surfaces of posterior teeth
3. Buccal or lingual caries—seen as a circular radiolucency in the buccal or lingual surface of a tooth
4. Root surface caries—seen as a radiolucent area that involves only the roots of teeth; usually preceded by bone loss or gingival recession
5. Recurrent caries—a radiolucent area seen below or adjacent to an existing restoration
6. Rampant caries—radiolucent areas seen in numerous teeth

F. Radiographic appearance of periodontal disease[7] (Fig. 6.35)
   1. Bone loss
      a. Pattern—horizontal or vertical bone loss
      b. Distribution—localized or generalized bone loss
      c. Severity—slight, moderate, or severe bone loss (Fig. 6.36)
   2. The periodontitis classification system has been updated to identify stages and grades of periodontal disease; refer to the section on "Classifications of Periodontal Diseases" in Chapter 14.

| Source | Website Address | Description |
|---|---|---|
| American Academy of Oral and Maxillofacial Radiology | http://www.aaomr.org | Promotes and advances the art and science of radiology in dentistry and provides a forum for communication among its members and to the health care community and the public |
| International Commission on Radiological Protection (ICRP) | http://www.icrp.org | Provides recommendations and guidance on all aspects of protection against ionizing radiation |
| National Council on Radiation Protection and Measurements (NCRP) | http://www.ncrponline.org | Dissemination of information and recommendations on protection against radiation |
| International Commission on Radiological Units and Measurements (ICRU) | http://www.icru.org | Develops and promulgates internationally accepted recommendations on radiation-related quantities and measurement procedures and references data for the safe and efficient application of ionizing radiation |

## CHAPTER 6 REVIEW QUESTIONS

Answers and rationales to review questions are available on this text's accompanying Evolve site. See inside front cover for details.

### CASE A

An adult male patient presents to the dental office with a chief complaint of heat/cold sensitivity in his teeth, along with discontent of the appearance of the anterior crown. It has been 5 years since his last dental visit. Tooth #30 was recently avulsed due to advanced periodontal disease and trauma.

***Use Case A and the panoramic radiograph in Fig. 6.37 to answer questions 1 to 5.***

1. Which type of caries is visible on teeth #3 and #14?
   **a.** Interproximal
   **b.** Occlusal
   **c.** Buccal/lingual
   **d.** Root
2. Which type of caries is visible on tooth #29?
   **a.** No caries are visible
   **b.** Interproximal
   **c.** Occlusal
   **d.** Root

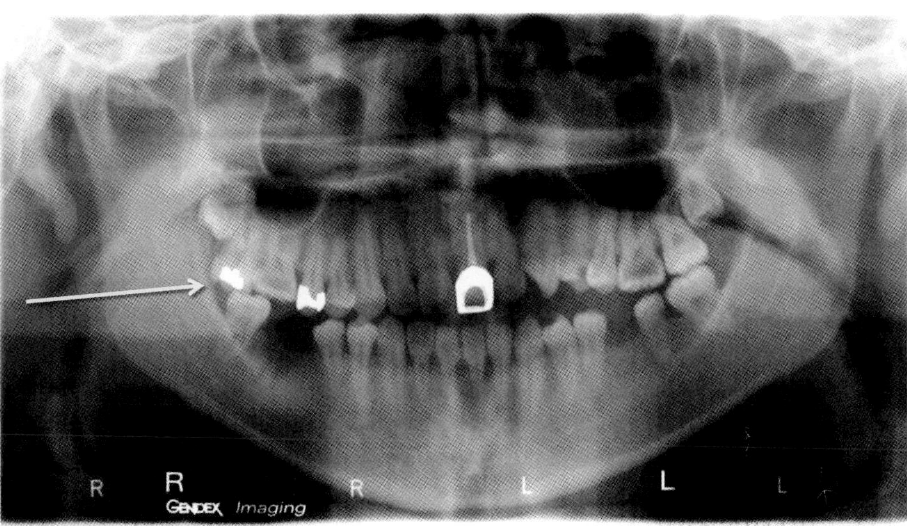


**Fig. 6.37** Panoramic view.

3. Which restorative material is seen on tooth #9?
   a. Gutta percha and metal crown
   b. Silver points and all-porcelain crown
   c. Gutta percha and composite
   d. Post-and-core restoration
4. The arrow is pointing to which radiopaque anatomic structure?
   a. External oblique ridge
   b. Mandibular canal
   c. Condensing bone
   d. Descending ramus
5. In addition to the panoramic image, which intraoral images would be most beneficial for the total care of this patient?
   a. Maxillary and mandibular occlusal images
   b. Four horizontal bitewing images
   c. Four vertical bitewing images
   d. A full-mouth series

*Use Fig. 6.38 to answer questions 6 and 7.*

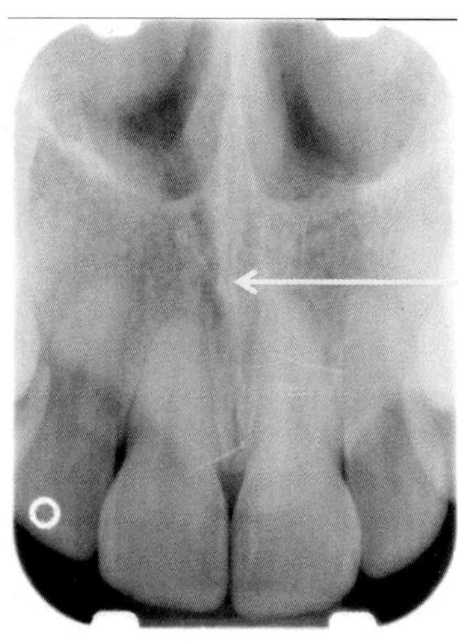

Fig. 6.38

6. All the anatomic landmarks may be viewed on this image EXCEPT:
   a. Incisive foramen
   b. Median palatal suture
   c. Maxillary torus
   d. Inferior nasal conchae
7. The yellow arrow is pointing to a V-shaped radiopacity. What is this radiographic finding?
   a. Anterior nasal spine
   b. Nasal septum
   c. Nutrient canal
   d. Root fracture

*Use Fig. 6.39 to answer questions 8 to 10.*

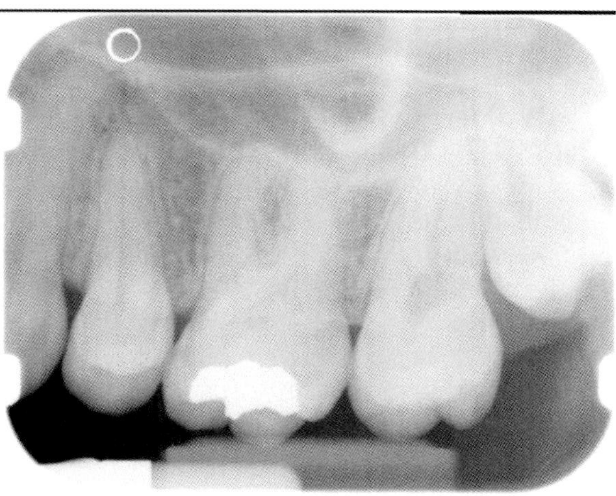

Fig. 6.39

8. Which tooth has been extracted and is not visible on this periapical image?
   a. #4
   b. #5
   c. #12
   d. #13
9. Which tooth surface demonstrates interproximal caries?
   a. Distal of maxillary premolar
   b. Mesial of maxillary first molar
   c. Distal of maxillary first molar
   d. Mesial of maxillary second molar
10. Which restorative material is present on the maxillary first molar?
    a. Amalgam
    b. Amalgam with base material
    c. Gold
    d. Composite

*Use Fig. 6.40 to answer questions 11 to 13.*

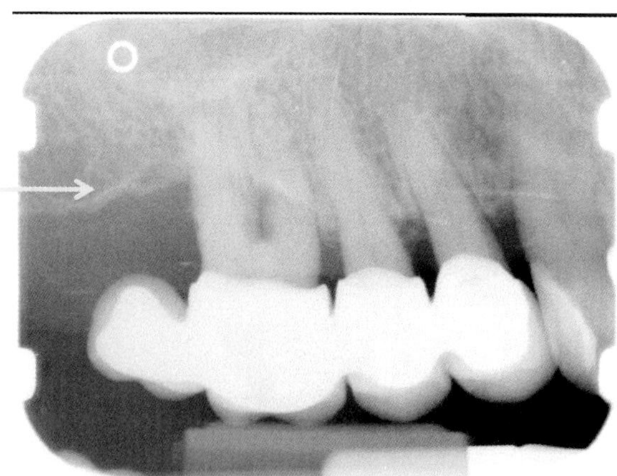

Fig. 6.40

11. Along with bone loss and calculus deposits, what other radiographic sign indicative of periodontal disease is present?
    a. Furcation involvement
    b. Cantilevered bridge
    c. Root caries
    d. Attachment loss
12. The cantilevered bridge is fabricated from what dental material?
    a. Gold
    b. Porcelain
    c. Stainless steel
    d. Porcelain-fused-to-metal
13. The yellow arrow is pointing to which radiographic finding?
    a. Zygomatic arch
    b. Zygoma
    c. Maxillary tuberosity
    d. Scratched emulsion

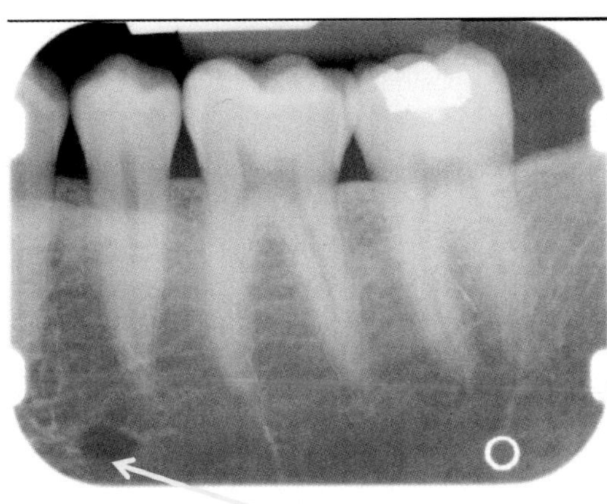

Fig. 6.41

*Use Fig. 6.41 to answer questions 14 and 15.*

14. The overlapped contact area between teeth #18 and #19 was the result of:
    a. Too much vertical angulation
    b. Too little vertical angulation
    c. Incorrect horizontal angulation
    d. Improper receptor placement
15. The yellow arrow is pointing to which radiographic finding?
    a. The identification dot
    b. Submandibular fossa
    c. Mental foramen
    d. Periapical pathology
16. Which is an appropriate condition to expose a periapical image?
    a. Pulpitis
    b. Slight bone loss
    c. Amalgam overhang
    d. Interproximal caries
17. Which would be an appropriate reason to expose an occlusal image?
    a. Mucocele
    b. Salivary stones
    c. Advanced bone loss
    d. Temporomandibular joint (TMJ) disorder
18. Which is a suitable use of a panoramic image?
    a. Diagnosis of occlusal caries
    b. Assessment of eruption patterns
    c. Evaluation of periapical pathology
    d. Measurement of periodontal bone loss
19. Which type of caries does NOT involve the enamel surface?
    a. Root
    b. Rampant
    c. Recurrent
    d. Interproximal
20. A male patient has been diagnosed with slight to moderate periodontitis. He declines the prescription of a full-mouth series due to concern with x-radiation. Which exposures would be appropriate to replace the intraoral periapical series?
    a. Maxillary and mandibular occlusal radiographs
    b. Panoramic
    c. Four vertical bitewings
    d. Four horizontal bitewings
21. Which exposure factor controls the penetrating power of the x-ray beam?
    a. Time
    b. Voltage
    c. Milliamperage
    d. Kilovoltage peak
22. Which speed of film is currently recommended by the American Dental Association (ADA) and the American Academy of Oral and Maxillofacial Radiology (AAOMR)?
    a. C
    b. D
    c. E
    d. F
23. Which error will produce a lighter radiographic image?
    a. Timer set too long
    b. Film exposed to light
    c. Fixer solution too weak
    d. Developer solution too warm
24. Your film exits the automatic processor completely clear. What is the most common reason for this appearance?
    a. Expired film
    b. Exposed to white light
    c. Not exposed to radiation
    d. Exposed backward in the mouth
25. The patient states that movement occurred during x-ray exposure. Which error will result on the image?
    a. Decreased distortion
    b. Increased sharpness
    c. Decreased sharpness
    d. Increased magnification

26. All are examples of particulate radiation EXCEPT:
   a. UV rays
   b. Neutrons
   c. Protons
   d. Alpha particles
27. The directional flow of electrons inside the x-ray tube is influenced by which component?
   a. Aluminum filters
   b. Focusing cup of the cathode
   c. Heated filament
   d. Tungsten target
28. After the exposure button is pressed, what is the approximate amount of x-ray energy produced in the x-ray tube?
   a. Less than 1%
   b. 10%
   c. 25%
   d. 50%
29. Which term describes the speed of a wave?
   a. Frequency
   b. Velocity
   c. Wavelength
   d. Quantum
30. The useful beam is also referred to as which type of radiation?
   a. Primary radiation
   b. Secondary radiation
   c. Scatter radiation
   d. General radiation
31. Free radicals are produced during the radiolysis of water that combine to form which toxin to living tissues?
   a. Cancer
   b. Lead
   c. Hydrogen peroxide
   d. Radon
32. Film speed is determined by three factors. Which is the EXCEPTION?
   a. Size of the silver halide crystals
   b. Thickness of the emulsion
   c. Volume of adhesive layer utilized
   d. Presence of radiosensitive dyes
33. Which location would be unsuitable for storing intraoral film?
   a. Inside a protected drawer near the automatic film processor
   b. On a countertop in the office kitchen, near a microwave
   c. A temperature-regulated storage closet
   d. A supply inventory area with low humidity
34. A tubehead that drifts or moves during exposure may cause which radiographic error?
   a. Magnification
   b. Distortion
   c. Streak artifact
   d. Sharpness
35. Which factor will increase the density of an image?
   a. Decrease time
   b. Increase milliamperage
   c. Align the tooth and receptor parallel to each other
   d. Use of a long position-indicating device (PID)
36. All these factors can account for a fogged film image EXCEPT:
   a. Old, expired film
   b. Exposure to overhead light
   c. Contaminated darkroom chemicals
   d. Improper safelight bulb
37. What is the most common reason for a totally clear film?
   a. Film is exposed to white light
   b. Developer solution was too warm
   c. Developer solution was too weak
   d. Film was not exposed to x-radiation
38. Clinical indications for exposure of periapical images include the following EXCEPT:
   a. Previous endodontic therapy
   b. Dental implant evaluation
   c. Suspected tooth fracture
   d. Interproximal caries
39. The rule of isometry is applied in which intraoral radiographic technique?
   a. Paralleling
   b. Bisecting angle
   c. Bitewing
   d. Occlusal
40. Proper patient positioning for panoramic exposure requires which plane parallel to the floor?
   a. Frankfort
   b. Midsagittal
   c. Coronal
   d. Frontal
41. The bisecting angle technique may be helpful in patients with which clinical finding?
   a. Large tori
   b. Large oral cavity
   c. Little to no gag reflex
   d. High vaulted palate
42. Which dental x-ray equipment item is NOT used with digital imaging?
   a. Film
   b. X-ray tubehead
   c. Lead apron
   d. Position indicating device (PID)
43. Vertical bitewing images may be prescribed for a patient with which oral finding?
   a. Occlusal caries
   b. Supernumerary teeth
   c. Periodontal disease
   d. Salivary stones
44. During panoramic exposures, which error will appear if the patient is not sitting or standing straight?
   a. Anterior teeth appear narrow
   b. Hard palate is superimposed over the maxillary roots
   c. Vertical radiopacity seen in the center of the image
   d. Ramus and posterior teeth are unequally magnified
45. Identify a radiolucent landmark of the maxilla:
   a. Mental ridge
   b. Lateral fossa
   c. Coronoid process
   d. Nasal conchae

46. Identify a radiopaque landmark of the mandible:
   a. External oblique ridge
   b. Nutrient canals
   c. Submandibular fossa
   d. Mental foramen
47. Identify the tiny opening in bone located on the internal surface of the mandible which appears as a small, radiolucent dot:
   a. Genial tubercles
   b. Incisive foramen
   c. Lingual foramen
   d. Septum
48. The zygomatic process is seen as a J-shaped radiopacity in which anatomic area?
   a. Dividing the nasal cavity
   b. Superior to the maxillary posterior teeth
   c. Inferior to the mandibular central incisors
   d. At the apical portion of the mandibular premolars

*Use Fig. 6.42 to answer questions 49 to 52.*

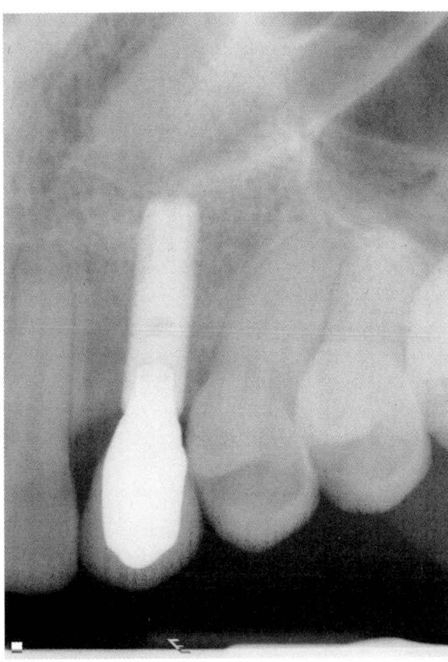

Fig. 6.42

49. Which restorative material has been used at the coronal aspect of the dental implant?
   a. Gold crown
   b. Amalgam
   c. Porcelain
   d. Porcelain-fused-to-metal crown
50. The inverted Y represents the intersection of two structures: the nasal cavity and which structure?
   a. Nasal conchae
   b. Lateral fossa
   c. Anterior nasal spine
   d. Maxillary sinus
51. Which technique error occurred in that the roots of the maxillary premolars appear shorter than their actual length?
   a. Incorrect horizontal angulation
   b. Vertical angulation too steep
   c. Vertical angulation too flat
   d. Patient movement
52. Identify the thin, radiolucent line surrounding the apex of the maxillary lateral incisor:
   a. Root fracture
   b. Lamina dura
   c. Periodontal ligament space
   d. Accessory pulp canal

*Use Fig. 6.43 to answer questions 53 to 55.*

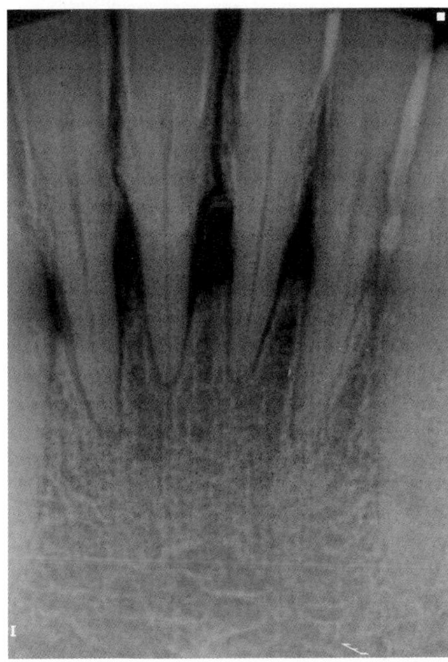

Fig. 6.43

53. Which anatomic landmark would you expect to see on this periapical image?
   a. Mental foramen
   b. Hamulus
   c. Coronoid process
   d. Genial tubercles
54. Nutrient canals appear as thin, radiolucent lines running vertically below the mandibular anterior teeth. Which additional area may nutrient canals be seen radiographically?
   a. Anterior maxilla
   b. Posterior maxilla
   c. Mandibular premolar region
   d. Mandibular molar region
55. In addition to the bone loss, what other radiographic finding is indicative of periodontal disease?
   a. Gingivitis
   b. Bleeding
   c. Calculus
   d. Mobility

*Use Fig. 6.44 to answer questions 56 to 60.*

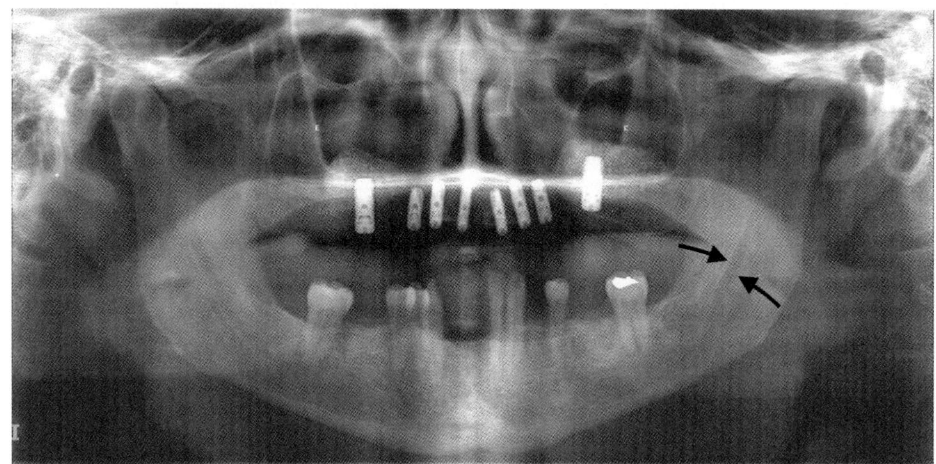

Fig. 6.44

56. Which tooth has been restored with amalgam?
    a. 17
    b. 18
    c. 30
    d. 31
57. What is the number of natural teeth present in the maxillary arch?
    a. No natural teeth are present in the maxilla
    b. Six
    c. Seven
    d. Eight
58. The mandibular anterior teeth are slightly narrowed and diminished in size. What is the appropriate step to correct this positioning error?
    a. Tell the patient to stand up as straight as possible
    b. Tip the chin downward
    c. Place the teeth slightly posterior into the focal trough
    d. Place the midsagittal plane perpendicular to the floor
59. The arrows are pointing at which radiolucent anatomic landmark?
    a. Coronoid process
    b. Internal oblique ridge
    c. Mandibular canal
    d. Mental foramen
60. The following materials would be appropriate for placing the patient correctly into the focal trough EXCEPT:
    a. Plastic bite stick
    b. Metal dental appliance
    c. Cotton roll
    d. Folded gauze square

*Use Fig. 6.45 to answer questions 61 to 65.*

61. Identify the technique error seen on this vertical bitewing image:
    a. Too steep vertical angulation
    b. Incorrect horizontal angulation
    c. Position indicating device (PID) not aligned with receptor
    d. Herringbone pattern is visible

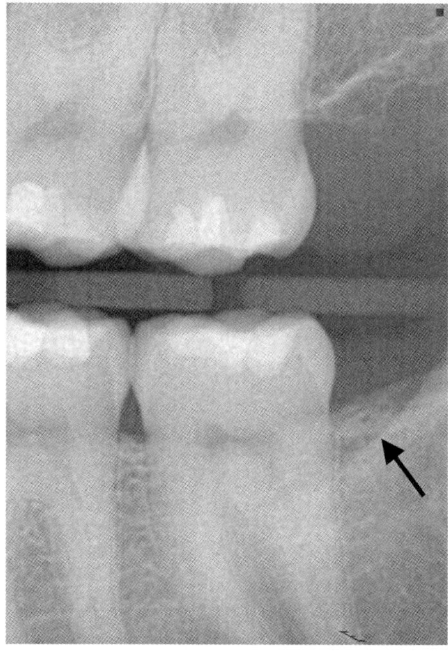

Fig. 6.45

62. What is one reason the dentist may have prescribed vertical bitewing images for this patient?
    a. Patient presented with bleeding gingiva and increased pocket depths since last visit
    b. Patient has a severe gag reflex
    c. Patient has a history of occlusal decay
    d. Patient presents with a broken amalgam on a maxillary molar
63. What is a reason for the lightness of this image?
    a. Developer solution was too warm
    b. Fixer solution was too cool
    c. Kilovoltage peak (kVp) setting was too high
    d. Exposure time setting was too low

64. Because of the lightness of this image, this film can be described as having:
   a. High density
   b. Low contrast
   c. High contrast
   d. Distortion
65. The arrow is pointing to which radiopaque landmark extending downward and forward from the ramus of the mandible?
   a. Mental ridge
   b. Internal oblique ridge
   c. Zygomatic process
   d. Median suture
66. What is the restorative material used in the occlusal surfaces of the posterior teeth?
   a. Amalgam
   b. Gold
   c. Porcelain-fused-to-metal
   d. Composite
67. What periapical film is placed in the top left corner of a full mouth series mount?
   a. Maxillary right molar
   b. Maxillary left molar
   c. Mandibular right molar
   d. Mandibular left molar
68. A quality assurance plan suggests the creation of a reference radiograph to check what x-ray equipment?
   a. Strengths of processing solutions
   b. Light leaks in the darkroom
   c. Correct wattage of the safelight
   d. Penetrating quality of the x-ray beam
69. What exposure factor has a direct effect on image contrast?
   a. Milliamperage
   b. Time
   c. Length of position indicating device (PID)
   d. Kilovoltage peak
70. Ionization occurs in which two interactions of x-ray photons and matter?
   a. No interaction and photoelectric effect
   b. Photoelectric effect and Compton scatter
   c. Photoelectric effect and coherent scatter
   d. Compton scatter and coherent scatter
71. The intensity of the x-ray beam is affected by the following EXCEPT:
   a. Distance
   b. kVp
   c. Thermionic emission
   d. mA
72. Large amounts of radiation absorbed in a short time describes which type of radiation effects?
   a. Short-term effects
   b. Somatic effects
   c. Stochastic effects
   d. Long-term effects
73. Organ tissues considered critical for dental radiography include the following EXCEPT:
   a. Skin
   b. Thyroid gland
   c. Muscle
   d. Bone marrow
74. What source produces the majority of natural background and artificial radiation exposure for the US population?
   a. Radon gas
   b. Nuclear medicine
   c. Computed medical tomography
   d. Cosmic radiation
75. Which term describes a radiopaque landmark?
   a. Process
   b. Fossa
   c. Suture
   d. Canal

## REFERENCES


1. International Commission on Radiation Units and Measurements, http://www.icru.org.
2. National Council on Radiation Protection and Measurements. *Ionizing Radiation Exposure of the Population of the United States. Report No 160.* Bethesda, MD: NCRP; 2009.
3. American Dental Association, US Food and Drug Administration. The Selection of Patients for Dental Radiographic Examinations. www.ada.org.
4. Radiation Safety in Dentistry, https://www.fdiworlddental.org/resources/policy-statements-and-resolutions/radiation-safety-in-dentistry.
5. Van der Stelt PF. Better imaging: the advantages of digital radiography. *J Am Dent Assoc.* 2008;139:7S–13S.
6. Thomson EM, Johnson ON. *Essentials of Dental Radiography for Dental Assistants and Hygienists.* 9th ed. Upper Saddle River, NJ: Pearson Education, Prentice Hall; 2012.
7. Iannucci JM, Howerton LJ. *Dental Radiography: Principles and Techniques.* 5th ed. St. Louis: Elsevier; 2017.

# 7

# General Pathology

*JoAnn R. Gurenlian, Jessica N. August*

Concepts of general pathology relate to multiple facets of dental hygiene care. Inflammatory diseases significantly affect the oral cavity, and research continues to focus on the linkages among inflammatory processes, systemic diseases, and oral diseases. Advances in genomics contribute to our understanding of the genetic basis of oral health conditions and their treatment. Individuals vary in their genetic makeup and thus responses to microbial challenges, injury, risk factors, and treatments will vary. Dental hygienists use genomic information to assess patients for periodontal and other disease risks and will use genetics in planning effective care and evaluating therapeutic outcomes in the near future.

This chapter reviews major concepts related to inflammation, wound healing, and repair; genetics; and the differential diagnostic process that enables dental hygienists to integrate the biologic basis of health and disease into patient care and acquire skills in diagnostic decision making.

## INFLAMMATION[1–3]

A. A host response to cellular injury that consists of vascular responses, migration and activation of leukocytes, and systemic reactions
B. Cellular injury may occur because of trauma, genetic defects, physical and chemical agents, tissue necrosis, foreign bodies, immune reactions, and infections
C. A protective response designed to rid the body of the initial cause of cell injury and the consequences of that injury, paving the way for a return to normal structure and function
D. Inflammatory response consists of a vascular reaction and a cellular reaction
   1. Reactions are mediated by chemical factors derived from plasma proteins or cells
   2. Reactions are produced in response to or activated by the inflammatory stimulus
E. Cardinal signs of inflammation
   1. Rubor (redness)—caused by increased vascularity
   2. Tumor (swelling)—caused by exudation of fluid; synonymous with edema or increased fluid in the interstitial space
   3. Calor (heat)—caused by a combination of increased blood flow and the release of inflammatory mediators
   4. Dolor (pain)—caused by the stretching of pain receptors and nerves by inflammatory exudates and by the release of chemical mediators
   5. Functio laesa (loss of function)—caused by a combination of the previous signs
F. Types of inflammation
   1. Acute
      a. Characterized by rapid onset and short duration
      b. Manifests with exudation of fluid and plasma proteins and emigration of leukocytes, mainly neutrophils
   2. Chronic
      a. Sustained inflammatory reaction characterized by longer duration
      b. Histologic manifestation identified by the presence of lymphocytes and macrophages, blood vessels, fibrosis, and tissue necrosis
G. Cells involved in inflammation (Fig. 7.1)
   1. Neutrophil or polymorphonuclear leukocyte (PMN)
      a. First cell to emigrate to the site of injury
      b. Primary cell involved in acute inflammation
      c. Capable of phagocytosis and contribute to repair
   2. Monocyte or macrophage
      a. Second white blood cell (WBC) to emigrate to injured tissue, where it becomes a macrophage
      b. Capable of phagocytosis; helper during the immune response
      c. Produces potent vasoconstrictive mediators (prostaglandins, leukotrienes, platelet-activating factor [PAF], and inflammatory cytokines), which maintain chronic inflammation
   3. Lymphocytes and plasma cells—involved in both chronic inflammation and immune response
   4. Eosinophils—involved in immune reactions and parasitic infections
   5. Mast cells
      a. Involved in both acute and chronic inflammatory reactions (releasing chemical mediators) and in immune responses
      b. Important in regulating vascular permeability and bronchial smooth muscle tone, especially in allergic hypersensitivity reactions

### Acute Inflammation

A. Vascular changes (Fig. 7.2)
   1. Transient vasoconstriction of arterioles caused by neurogenic reflex lasting several seconds to minutes
   2. Vasodilation
      a. First involves arterioles, then results in the opening of new capillary beds

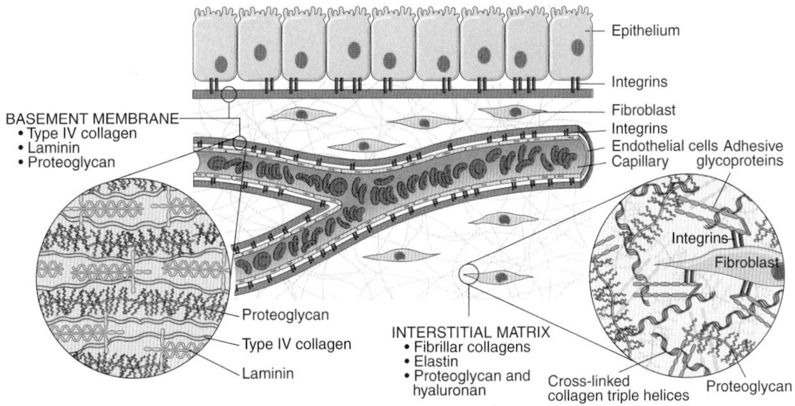


**Fig. 7.1** Components of acute and chronic inflammatory responses: circulating cells and proteins, cells of blood vessels, and cells and proteins of the extracellular matrix. (Modified from Kumar V, Abbas AK, Fausto N, Aster JC. *Robbins and Cotran Pathologic Basis of Disease*. 8th ed. Philadelphia: Saunders; 2010.)

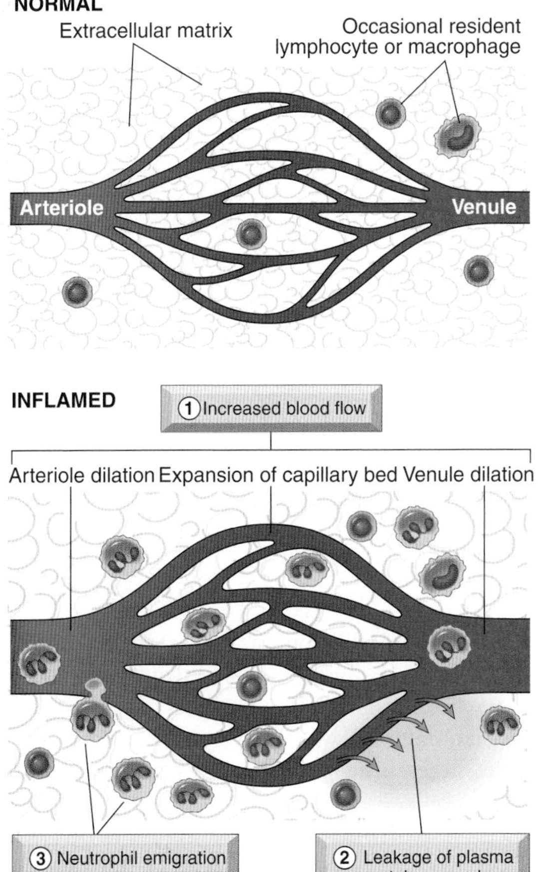


**Fig. 7.2** Major local manifestations of acute inflammation, compared with normal. (1) Vascular dilation and increased blood flow (causing erythema and warmth). (2) Extravasation and deposition of plasma fluid and proteins (edema). (3) Leukocyte emigration and accumulation at the site of injury. (Modified from Kumar V, Abbas AK, Fausto N, Aster JC. *Robbins and Cotran Pathologic Basis of Disease*. 8th ed. Philadelphia: Saunders; 2010.)

b. Results in increased blood flow, which causes heat and redness, known as *hyperemia*
c. Induced by chemical mediators such as histamine and nitric oxide (NO) on vascular smooth muscle

3. Increased permeability of microvasculature
    a. An exudate of protein-rich fluid escapes into extravascular tissue, resulting in edema
    b. Proposed mechanisms to explain the leakage of endothelium in inflammation to allow this response:
        (1) Formation of endothelial gaps in venules elicited by chemical mediators
            (a) Usually reversible
            (b) Lasts 15 to 30 minutes
        (2) Direct endothelial injury resulting in endothelial cell necrosis and detachment
            (a) Occurs in severe burns or lytic bacterial infections
            (b) Sustained for several hours
            (c) Venules, capillaries, and arterioles affected
        (3) Delayed prolonged leakage
            (a) Begins after a delay of 2 to 12 hours
            (b) Lasts for several hours or days
            (c) Involves venules and capillaries
            (d) Caused by thermal injury, radiation, and certain bacterial toxins
        (4) Leukocyte-mediated endothelial injury
        (5) Increased transcytosis across the endothelial cytoplasm
        (6) Leakage from new blood vessels until new endothelial cells mature and form intercellular junctions
4. Concentration of red blood cells (RBCs) in small vessels and increased viscosity of blood, known as *stasis*
5. Leukocytes, mainly neutrophils, accumulate along the vascular endothelium (margination); the endothelium becomes lined by leukocytes ("pavementing"); leukocytes adhere to the endothelium and, soon after, migrate through the vascular wall into interstitial tissue (*diapedesis* or emigration)
    a. Neutrophils predominate in the inflammatory infiltrate during the first 6 to 24 hours
    b. Neutrophils are replaced by monocytes in 24 to 48 hours

B. Chemotaxis
1. Chemical attraction of leukocytes to emigrate in tissues
2. Exogenous agents are bacterial products

3. Endogenous chemoattractants
   a. Components of the complement system, particularly C5a
   b. Products of the lipoxygenase pathway, such as leukotriene $B_4$ ($LTB_4$)
   c. Cytokines, such as interleukin-8 (IL-8)

C. Phagocytosis
1. Recognition and attachment
   a. Mannose receptors and scavenger receptors bind and ingest microbes
   b. Phagocytosis is greatly enhanced by *opsonins*, specific proteins such as immunoglobulin G (IgG) antibodies, fragments of the complement protein C3, and plasma lectins, which are recognized by specific receptors on leukocytes
2. Engulfment
   a. Extensions of the cytoplasm flow around the particle to be engulfed, resulting in the complete enclosure of the particle within a phagosome created by cell's plasma membrane
   b. Neutrophils and monocytes become degranulated during this process
3. Killing and degradation
   a. Eliminate infectious agents and necrotic cells
   b. After the killing, acid hydrolases degrade the microbes within phagolysosomes
   c. pH drops to between 4 and 5
4. Release of leukocyte products
   a. Include lysosomal enzymes, reactive oxygen intermediates, and products of arachidonic acids such as prostaglandins and leukotrienes
   b. These products may cause endothelial injury and tissue damage
   c. If unchecked, this leukocyte infiltrate becomes harmful and is associated with many chronic systemic diseases
   d. Also produce growth factors that aid in repair after tissue injury
5. Apoptosis—defined as programmed cell death, used by the body to eliminate old cells
   a. After phagocytosis, neutrophils undergo apoptotic cell death and are then ingested by macrophages

D. Chemical mediators (Table 7.1)
1. General principles
   a. Originate from plasma proteins or from cells
      (1) Plasma-derived mediators such as complement proteins and kinin are in precursor form and must be activated
      (2) Cell-derived mediators such as histamine, prostaglandins, and cytokines come from mast cells, platelets, neutrophils, and monocytes/macrophages
   b. Production of active mediators is triggered by microbial products or by host proteins
   c. Mediators perform their activities by binding to specific receptors on target cells, performing direct enzymatic activity, or mediating oxidative damage
   d. Once activated, most mediators are short-lived, but cause harmful effects

**TABLE 7.1 Principal Mediators of Inflammation and Their Actions**

| Mediator | Source | Action |
|---|---|---|
| Histamine | Mast cells, basophils, platelets | Vasodilation, increased vascular permeability, endothelial activation |
| Prostaglandins | Mast cells, leukocytes | Vasodilation, pain, fever |
| Leukotrienes | Mast cells, leukocytes | Increased vascular permeability, chemotaxis, leukocyte adhesion, and activation |
| Cytokines (TNF, IL-1, IL-6) | Macrophages, endothelial cells, mast cells | Local: endothelia activation (expression of adhesion molecules)<br>Systemic: fever, metabolic abnormalities, hypotension (shock) |
| Chemokines | Leukocytes, activated macrophages | Chemotaxis, leukocyte activation |
| Platelet-activating factor | Leukocytes, mast cells | Vasodilation, increased vascular permeability, leukocyte adhesion, chemotaxis, degranulation, oxidative burst |
| Complement | Plasma (produced in liver) | Leukocyte chemotaxis and activation, direct target killing (membrane attack complex) vasodilation (mast cell stimulation) |
| Kinins | Plasma (produced in liver) | Increased vascular permeability, smooth muscle contraction, vasodilation, pain |

Modified from: Kumar, V, Abbas, AK, Aster, JC. *Robbins and Cotran Pathologic Basis of Disease.* 9th ed Philadelphia: Elsevier Saunders; 2015.

2. Vasoactive amines
   a. Histamine
      (1) Found in mast cells, blood basophils, and platelets
      (2) Causes dilation of the arterioles, edema, and smooth muscle contraction; increases the permeability of venules; constricts large arteries
   b. Serotonin
      (1) Present in platelets and certain neuroendocrine cells
      (2) Causes increased permeability during immunologic reactions
3. Plasma proteins
   a. Complement system
      (1) Consists of 20 component proteins found in greatest concentration in plasma; primary function is defense against microbes
      (2) Causes increased vascular permeability, chemotaxis, and *opsonization* (the process by which certain cells are made more susceptible to phagocytosis)
      (3) C3 and C5 are the most important inflammatory mediators of the complement components
         (a) Vascular phenomenon created by C3a, C5a, and to a lesser extent, C4a; stimulate

histamine release from mast cells; called *anaphylatoxins* because they have similar effects in the reaction of anaphylaxis

(b) Leukocyte adhesion, chemotaxis, and activation occur through C5a as a chemotactic agent for neutrophils, monocytes, eosinophils, and basophils

(c) Phagocytosis enhanced by C3b, which acts as opsonin to facilitate foreign bodies being more efficiently engulfed by phagocytosis

(d) Acquired or congenital deficiencies of specific complement components or regulatory proteins result in increased susceptibility to infectious agents and a propensity for autoimmune diseases associated with circulating immune complexes (e.g., systemic lupus erythematosus, pyogenic infections, hereditary angioedema)

b. Kinin system

(1) Generates vasoactive peptides from plasma proteins called *kininogens* by the action of proteases known as *kallikreins*

(2) Bradykinin increases vascular permeability; causes the contraction of smooth muscle, dilation of blood vessels, plasma extravasation, cell migration, inflammatory cell activation, and inflammatory-mediated pain responses

(3) Is triggered by the activation of Hageman factor (factor XII of the intrinsic clotting pathway)

(4) Is short-lived; quickly inactivated by the enzyme kininase

c. Clotting system

(1) Induces the formation of thrombin, fibrinopeptides, and factor XII, which have inflammatory properties

(2) Activated by substances released during tissue destruction, such as collagen, proteinases, kallikrein, and bacterial endotoxins

(3) Prevents the spread of infection and inflammation; localizes microorganisms at the site of phagocytosis; helps clot formation to stop bleeding and for repair, chemotaxis of neutrophils, and increased permeability of vessels

4. Other mediators

a. Arachidonic acid

(1) A lipid mediator that is a short-range hormone; is formed rapidly and acts locally

(2) Produces prostaglandins, leukotrienes, and lipoxins

(a) Prostaglandins (e.g., $PGE_2$, $PGD_2$, $PGF_{2a}$, $PGI_2$) and thromboxane $A_2$ ($TXA_2$), are most important in inflammation, causing increased permeability, the chemotactic effects of other mediators, and vasodilation resulting in edema as well as pain and fever in inflammation

(b) Pathway initiating these prostaglandins occurs by two different enzymes, Cyclooxygenase-1 (COX-1) and Cyclooxygenase-2 (COX-2)

[1] COX-1 produces prostaglandins that are involved in inflammation and also maintains homeostasis, protecting the gastrointestinal mucosal lining, regulating water/electrolyte balance, stimulating platelet aggregation, and maintaining resistance to thrombosis on vascular endothelial cell surfaces

[2] COX-2 stimulates the production of prostaglandins involved in the inflammatory reactions previously noted and may play a role in normal homeostasis

(c) Leukotrienes cause intense vasoconstriction, bronchospasm, and increased vascular permeability; important in the pathogenesis of bronchial asthma

(d) Lipoxins are synthesized by platelets and neutrophils; inhibit leukocyte recruitment, neutrophil chemotaxis, and adhesion to the endothelium; may play a role in resolving inflammation

(e) Pro-resolving lipid mediators or specialized pro-resolving mediators (SPM) include lipoxins, resolvins, protectins, and maresins and are produced by resolving exudates with distinct actions for return to homeostasis; they evoke potent antiinflammatory and pro-resolving mechanisms and enhance microbial clearance; resolvins inhibit leukocyte recruitment and activation by inhibiting the production of cytokines; maresins regulate inflammation resolution, tissue regeneration, and resolve pain; aspirin may work by stimulating the production of resolvins

(f) PAF causes platelet stimulation, vasoconstriction, bronchoconstriction, vasodilation, and increased venular permeability; far more potent than histamine; increased leukocyte adhesion to endothelium; chemotaxis, degranulation, and oxidative burst; also boosts synthesis of other mediators, such as serotonin, causing changes in vascular permeability

(g) Tumor necrosis factor (TNF) and interleukin-1 (IL-1)

[1] Two major cytokines that mediate inflammation and are produced primarily by macrophages

[2] Responsible for endothelial activation, which induces the synthesis of endothelial adhesion molecules and chemical mediators, producing enzymes associated with matrix remodeling and increasing the surface thrombogenicity of endothelium

[3] Induces the systemic acute-phase responses of infection and injury, including fever, loss of appetite, release of neutrophils, corticotropin, and corticosteroids

[4] TNF—responsible for the hemodynamic effects of septic shock; regulates body mass and contributes to *cachexia* (wasting away), which is part of some infections and diseases

(h) Interleukin-6 (IL-6) is a multifunctional cytokine synthesized in response to infection and trauma by macrophages, neutrophils, keratinocytes, fibroblasts, and endothelial cells; activity in inflammation is both antiinflammatory and pro-inflammatory; also believed to have growth factor properties in the development of many types of cancers including oral cancer; may modulate the susceptibility, development, and progression of autoimmune and inflammatory diseases such as therosclerosis, rheumatoid arthritis, and myeloma; also associated with lichen planus, gingivitis and periodontal diseases, and dental granulomas

(i) Chemokines—small proteins that act as chemoattractants for leukocytes and control the normal migration of cells through various tissues

(i) NO—released from endothelial cells; causes vasodilation by relaxing vascular smooth muscle; microbicidal; a mediator of host defense against infection

(j) Lysosomal components of leukocytes

[1] Neutrophils and monocytes, contain lysosomal granules; granules contain a variety of enzymes used for phagocytosis (e.g., lysozyme, collagenase, alkaline phosphatase, elastase)

[2] These enzymes are destructive and, if unchecked, can potentiate further inflammation and tissue damage

(k) Oxygen-derived free radicals may be released from leukocytes following a phagocytic event and are potent mediators

[1] Can be damaging to the host, causing endothelial cell damage and increased vascular permeability, inactivation of antiproteases, and injury to other cell types, such as parenchymal cells and RBCs

b. Neuropeptides
   (1) Include substance P and neurokinin A
   (2) Play a role in the initiation and propagation of inflammatory response

E. Outcomes of inflammation
   1. Complete resolution
   2. Healing by connective tissue replacement
   3. Abscess
   4. Lymphadenitis
   5. Progression of tissue response to chronic inflammation

## Chronic Inflammation

A. Causes
   1. Persistent infections
   2. Prolonged exposure to potentially toxic agents
   3. Autoimmunity

B. Characteristics
   1. Infiltration with macrophages, lymphocytes, and plasma cells
   2. Tissue destruction, a hallmark of chronic inflammation
   3. Attempts at healing by connective tissue replacement and fibrosis

C. Cells involved
   1. Macrophages, lymphocytes, plasma cells, eosinophils, mast cells, and fibroblasts
   2. Produce granulomatous inflammation, characterized by focal accumulation of activated macrophages that develops an epithelioid appearance, and fibrosis
   3. Products of these cells eliminate injurious agents and help initiate repair, but are also responsible for much of the tissue injury in chronic inflammation

D. Role of lymphatics
   1. Secondary line of defense that monitors the extravascular fluids
   2. Help drain edema from the extravascular space

E. Systemic effects of inflammation—acute-phase response or the systemic inflammatory response syndrome (SIRS)
   1. Fever—produced in response to pyrogens that act by stimulating prostaglandin synthesis
   2. Acute-phase proteins, including C-reactive protein (CRP), fibrinogen, and serum amyloid A protein (SAA) increase during the inflammatory process
      a. Bind to microbial cell walls; act as opsonin and fix complement
      b. Prolonged activation causes secondary amyloidosis in chronic inflammation
      c. Elevated CRP used as a marker for increased risk of myocardial infarction in persons with coronary artery disease
   3. Leukocytosis
      a. Common feature in bacterial infections resulting in elevated to extremely high levels of different types of leukocytes, depending on the type of infection
      b. Normal count of WBCs is 4000 to 10,000/mm$^3$ in blood
      c. In an inflammatory reaction, particularly with an infection, WBC count can increase to 15,000 or 20,000 and sometimes to extremely high levels exceeding 40,000/mm$^3$
   4. Sepsis
      a. In severe bacterial infections, large quantities of cytokines, particularly TNF and IL-1, cause thrombosis and coagulation
      b. Eventually, hypoglycemia and cardiovascular failure occur, resulting in septic shock
      c. Multiple organs can be affected by inflammation and intravascular thrombosis, resulting in organ failure

F. Systemic disease affected by chronic inflammation
   1. Cardiovascular disease
   2. Cancer
   3. Diabetes mellitus
   4. Asthma
   5. Chronic obstructive pulmonary disease (COPD)
   6. Alzheimer's disease
   7. Periodontal diseases

## REGENERATION AND WOUND HEALING[1–3]

A. Definitions
   1. Regeneration—growth of cells and tissues to replace lost structures; favored when the matrix composition and architecture are unaltered
   2. Healing—a tissue response to a wound, inflammatory process, or cell necrosis in organs that cannot regenerate; involves either regeneration or scar formation (Fig. 7.3)
B. General concepts
   1. Involves a complex process that includes a number of steps
      a. A thrombus (clot) is formed at the site of injury; scab results from the drying of the exposed surfaces of the clot; forms a barrier to invading microorganisms
      b. An inflammatory response caused by the initial injury
      c. Proliferation of parenchymal and connective tissue cells
      d. Formation of new blood vessels (angiogenesis) and granulation tissue (transient, specialized tissue of repair)
      e. Synthesis of extracellular matrix (ECM) proteins and collagen deposition
      f. Tissue remodeling
      g. Wound contraction
      h. Acquisition of wound strength
   2. Repair process—a combination of regeneration and scar formation influenced by local and systemic factors that may inhibit or prolong the wound-healing process
      a. Local factors
         (1) Size, location, and type of wound
         (2) Persistent infection
         (3) Early movement
         (4) Foreign material
         (5) Ionizing radiation
      b. Systemic factors
         (1) Blood supply
         (2) Metabolic factors (e.g., diabetes)
         (3) Corticosteroids
         (4) Cytotoxic drugs
         (5) Nutritional deficiencies
   3. Generally, repair begins early in inflammation—formation of granulation tissue, which is a hallmark of healing
      a. Pink, soft, granular appearance on the surface of wounds
      b. Formation of new small blood vessels and proliferation of fibroblasts
      c. New vessels tend to leak; edematous
      d. Amount of granulation tissue that forms depends on the size of the wound and the intensity of the inflammation
C. Angiogenesis (new blood vessels formed through preexisting vessels)
   1. Occurs from the branching and extension of adjacent blood vessels and the recruitment of endothelial progenitor cells (EPCs) from bone marrow
   2. Angiogenesis from adjacent blood vessels occurs through the vasodilation and increased permeability of existing vessels, degradation of ECM, migration of endothelial cells, maturation of endothelial cells and remodeling into capillary tubes, and recruitment of periendothelial cells to support endothelial tubes and to form the mature vessel

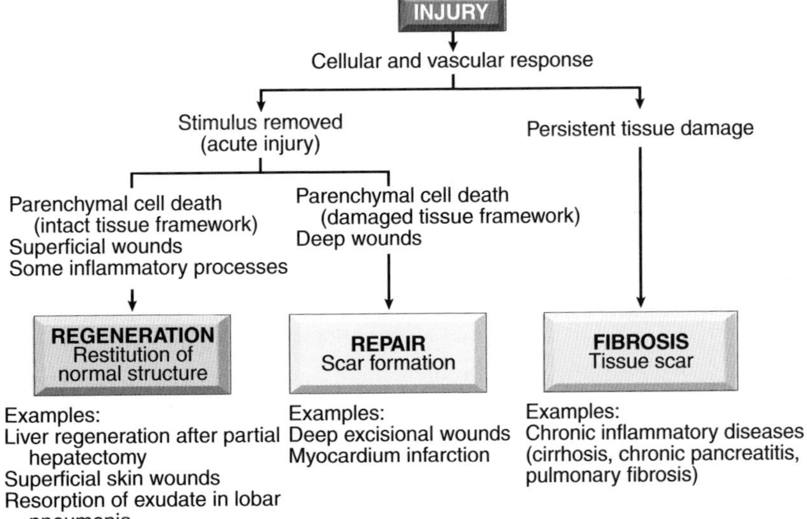


**Fig. 7.3** Repair responses after injury and inflammation. Repair after acute injury has several outcomes, including normal tissue restitution and healing with scar formation. Healing in chronic injury involves scar formation and fibrosis. (Modified from Kumar V, Abbas AK, Fausto N, Aster JC. *Robbins and Cotran Pathologic Basis of Disease*. 8th ed. Philadelphia: Saunders; 2010.)

3. Growth factors such as vascular endothelial growth factor (VEGF) support adult tissues undergoing angiogenesis
4. Directed migration of endothelial cells—controlled by ECM proteins, including integrins, matricellular proteins, and proteinases

D. Scar formation—three processes occur: emigration and proliferation of fibroblasts in the site of injury, deposition of ECM, and tissue remodeling
   1. Fibroblast emigration and proliferation
      a. Migration of fibroblasts to the site of injury and their proliferation triggered by growth factors that come from platelets, inflammatory cells, and activated endothelium
   2. ECM deposition
      a. Fibroblasts deposit increased amounts of ECM
      b. Fibrillar collagens form a major portion of connective tissue in repair sites; help develop the strength of the healing wound
      c. Fibroblasts begin forming 3 to 5 days after injury and continue for several weeks
      d. Growth factors that stimulate fibroblasts also stimulate ECM synthesis
      e. Granulation tissue is converted into a scar composed of fibroblasts, dense collagen, fragments of elastic tissue, and other ECM components; richly vascularized granulation tissue transforms into a pale, avascular scar
   3. Tissue remodeling
      a. Degradation of ECM components causes tissue remodeling; achieved through matrix metalloproteinases (MMPs)
      b. MMPs are produced by fibroblasts, macrophages, neutrophils, synovial cells, and some epithelial cells
         (1) MMP secretion is induced by certain growth factors, physical stress, and phagocytosis; inhibited by steroids and other growth factors
         (2) MMPs degrade matrix proteins at the site of injury, allowing reorganization of the tissue capable of influencing cell growth and apoptosis

E. Cutaneous wound healing (Fig. 7.4)
   1. Healing by primary intention—primary union (e.g., surgical incision and placement of sutures)
      a. Narrow incisional space fills with clotted blood, a clot forms, and a scab covers the surface of the wound; the clot stops the bleeding and acts as a scaffold for migrating cells
      b. Within 24 hours, neutrophils appear at the margins of the incision and move toward the clot
      c. In 24 to 48 hours, epithelial cells move from the wound edges and fuse in the midline beneath the scab to close the wound; a basement membrane is formed
      d. Within 3 days, neutrophils are replaced by macrophages, and granulation tissue forms
         (1) Collagen fibers begin to form in the margins of the incision
         (2) Epithelial cells proliferate and thicken the epidermal layer
      e. By day 5, the incisional space is filled with granulation tissue
         (1) Collagen fibers become more abundant and start to bridge the incision
         (2) A mature epidermal architecture with surface keratinization appears
      f. During week 2, proliferation of collagen and fibroblasts continues
         (1) The inflammatory process has largely dissipated
         (2) Blanching begins as the incisional scar forms
      g. By week 4, the scar is composed of connective tissue and an intact epidermis; the tensile strength of the wound increases
   2. Healing by secondary intention—secondary union (e.g., wounds with separated edges)
      a. Abundant granulation tissue grows in from the margin to complete the repair
      b. The inflammatory reaction is more intense because of the presence of a larger clot and more necrotic debris and exudates that must be removed from the defect
      c. Wound contraction occurs in larger surface wounds because of myofibroblasts that have the characteristics of smooth muscle cells
      d. Substantial scar formation and thinning of the epidermis occurs
   3. Healing by tertiary intention (delayed primary closure)
      a. Reserved for highly contaminated wounds
      b. Contaminated wound is initially treated with repeated debridement and either topical or systemic antibiotics to control infection
      c. Once wound is ready for closure, surgery is performed (suturing, skin graft replacement, flap)

F. Wound strength
   1. Tissues recover approximately 70% to 80% of tensile strength over a 3-month period compared with intact skin
   2. Recovery of wound strength comes from an excess of collagen synthesis over collagen degradation during the first 2 months of healing and from structural modifications of collagen fibers after collagen synthesis is complete

G. Complications of cutaneous wound healing
   1. Deficient scar formation leading to wound dehiscence or ulceration—often seen after abdominal surgery and in lower extremity wounds in patients with peripheral vascular disease, diabetes, or severe atherosclerosis
   2. Excessive scar formation
      a. Raised scar (hypertrophic scar, keloid)
      b. Scar grows beyond the boundaries of the original wound and does not regress (keloid)
   3. Contracture
      a. Exaggeration of the normal contraction process of wound healing, resulting in the deformity of the wound and surrounding tissues

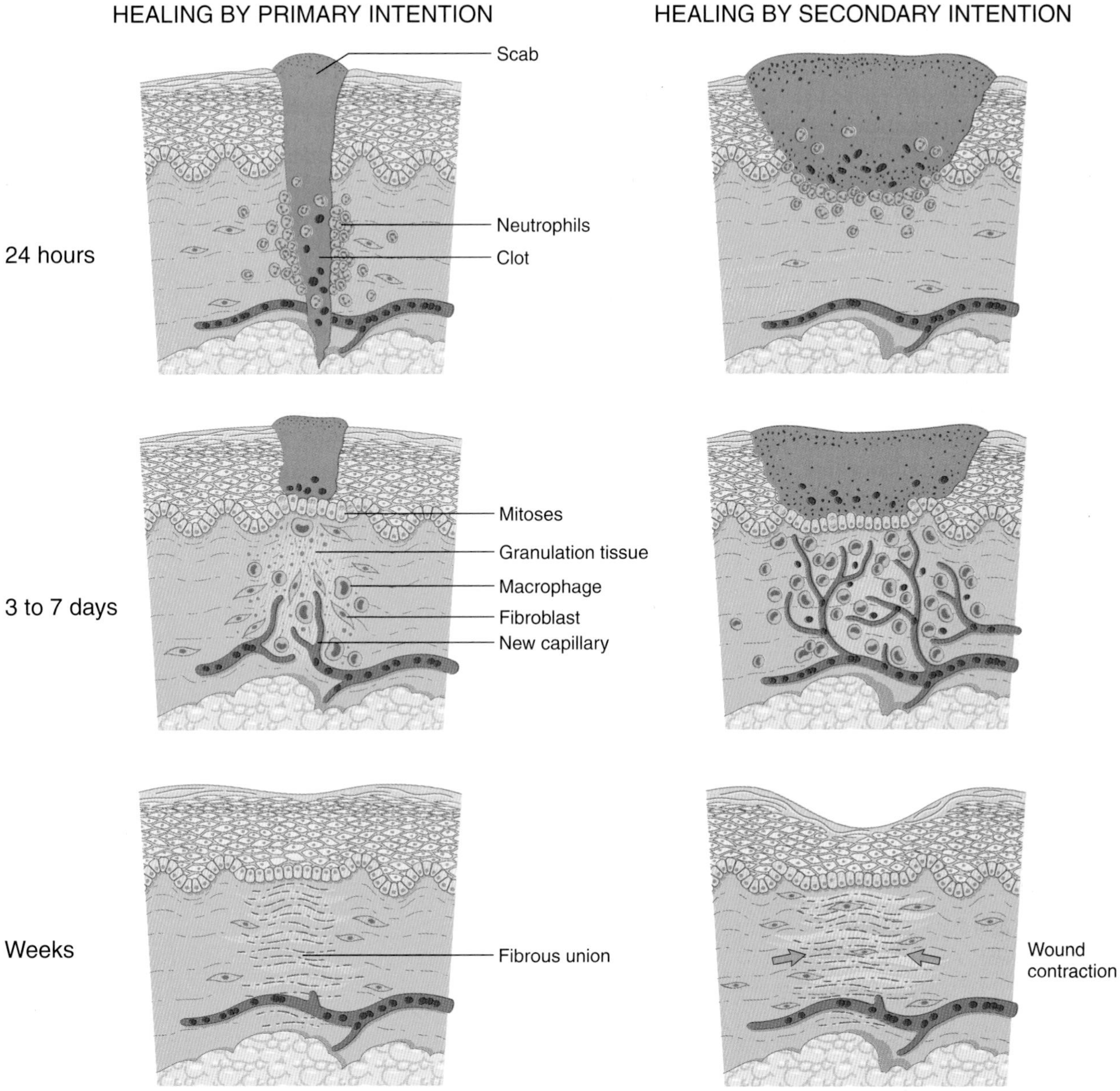

HEALING BY PRIMARY INTENTION HEALING BY SECONDARY INTENTION

Scab

24 hours

Neutrophils

Clot

3 to 7 days

Mitoses

Granulation tissue

Macrophage

Fibroblast

New capillary

Weeks

Fibrous union

Wound contraction

**Fig. 7.4** Steps in wound healing by primary intention *(left)* and secondary intention *(right)*. Note large amounts of granulation tissue and wound contraction in healing by secondary intention. (From Kumar V, Abbas AK, Aster JC. *Robbins and Cotran Pathologic Basis of Disease*, 9th ed. Philadelphia: Elsevier; 2015.)

   b. Common after serious burn injuries; can affect joint mobility
4. Blood supply
   a. Wounds of the lower extremity in person with diabetes may heal poorly or require amputation due to advanced atherosclerosis in the legs associated with peripheral vascular disease and defective angiogenesis that compromise blood supply and impede repair
   b. Varicose veins can cause edema, formation of thick (fibrin) cuffs around microvessels, ulceration, and poor healing
5. Systemic factors
   a. Coagulation defects, thrombocytopenia, and anemia impede repair
   b. Complications and/or treatments (infections, obesity, diabetes, chemotherapy, ionizing radiation) slow repair and processes

H. Fibrosis
1. Processes that occur in cutaneous scar formation because of extensive deposition of collagen; similar to the fibrosis associated with chronic inflammatory diseases (e.g., rheumatoid arthritis, cirrhosis); a major component of diseases that involve ongoing injury
2. Characterized by the persistence of initial stimuli for fibrosis or the development of immune and autoimmune reactions that sustain the synthesis and secretion of growth factors and other biologically active molecules
3. May cause permanent dysfunction

## REGENERATIVE MEDICINE[3,4]

A. Stem cells
1. Characterized by self-renewal abilities and the capacity to generate differentiated cells; stem cells from bone marrow and basal layer of epidermis provide a renewal source of epidermal and dermal cells that can form new blood vessels and epithelium and regenerate skin structures
   a. Autogenous stem cells—derived from the individual being treated
   b. Allogenous stem cells—derived from other individuals
   c. May be totipotent, multipotent, or unipotent
   d. Process of differentiation is known as *plasticity* or *transdifferentiation*
2. Stem cells are defined by common properties
   a. Ability to divide without limit, avoid senescence, and maintain genomic integrity
   b. Capacity to intermittently undergo division or to remain quiescent
   c. Ability to propagate by self-renewal and differentiation of daughter cells
   d. Absence of lineage markers
   e. In some cases, specific anatomic localization
   f. Shared presence of growth and transcription markers common to uncommitted cells
3. Types
   a. Embryonic stem cells
      (1) Pluripotent and can generate all tissue of the body
      (2) Isolated from inner cell mass of blastocytes
      (3) May be used in the future for the treatment of organs affected by diabetes, neurologic defects, myocardial infarction, and liver damage
   b. Adult stem cells or somatic stem cells
      (1) More restricted capacity to generate different cell types
      (2) Potential for adult stem cells to be reprogrammed into pluripotent cells similar to embryonic stem cells
      (3) Found in skin, lining of intestine, cornea, brain, and hematopoietic tissue (e.g., bone marrow, umbilical cord)
4. Types of adult stem cells
   a. Induced pluripotent stem cells (iPs)—adult cells that behave similar to embryonic cells
   b. Amniotic fluid–derived stem cells (AFSCs)
      (1) Isolated from the aspirates of amniocentesis during genetic screening
      (2) Capacity to differentiate into multiple lineages, such as chondrocytes, adipocytes, osteoblasts, myocytes, endothelial cells, neuron-like cells, and live cells
   c. Umbilical cord blood stem cells (UCBSCs)
      (1) Derived from the blood of the umbilical cord
      (2) Differentiate into cells that resemble liver cells, skeletal muscle, neural tissue, pancreatic cells, immune cells, and mesenchymal stem cells
   d. Bone marrow–derived stem cells (BMSCs)
      (1) Consists of both hematopoietic stem cells and stromal cells (mesenchymal stem cells) that generate bone, cartilage, other connective tissues, and fat
      (2) Most common commercially available stem cells
   e. Adipose-derived stem cells (ASCs)
      (1) Derived from lipectomy or liposuction aspirates
      (2) Differentiate into adipocytes, chondrocytes, myocytes, and neuronal and osteoblastic lineages; may provide hematopoietic support
   f. Dental stem cells
      (1) Develop from material created during the development of the nervous system and can differentiate into neural cell lines
      (2) Sources include primary teeth, permanent third molars, or extracted healthy permanent teeth and periodontal ligament
      (3) Have been transdifferentiated in the laboratory to form bone, nervous tissue, and pancreatic islet beta cells that produce insulin
      (4) Current animal studies are exploring applications to regenerate bone, cartilage, skin, nerve and brain tissues, adipose, and heart and muscle tissues
      (5) Dental application may include tooth, root, jaw, and salivary gland regeneration and cranial bone repair

## GENETICS[2]

A. General concepts
1. Almost all health-related conditions (except trauma) have a genetic component; common diseases such as cardiovascular disease, dyslipidemia, diabetes, and cancer, as well as dental caries, periodontitis, oral cancer, cleft lip, and craniofacial abnormalities, are associated with genetic factors
2. Draft sequencing of the human genome has been completed; provides information about biologic inheritance and health consequences
3. Genome—all the deoxyribonucleic acid (DNA) of a given organism
4. Genomics—the study of all the genes in the genome, their extensive DNA sequences, and their interactions
5. Gene—a segment or sequence of DNA that contains instructions for making a specific protein or proteins required by the human body; found in succession along the length of chromosomes; humans have 20,000 to 25,000 genes
6. About 99.5% of DNA sequences are shared among humans; the diversity of humans is encoded in approximately 0.5% of human DNA; this 0.5% represents 15 million base pairs
7. Chromosomes—thread-like structures in the nucleus of a cell; made of DNA and structural proteins; human cells other than egg and sperm have 46 chromosomes (23 pairs); egg and sperm cells have 23 chromosomes

8. Molecular biology has resulted in the development of recombinant DNA technology that has allowed the isolation and characterization of genes through cloning, production of human biologically active agents, study of gene therapy, and development of molecular probes to aid in disease diagnosis

B. Mutations
   1. Mutations represent permanent changes in the DNA code; they can be beneficial, neutral, or harmful
      a. Four letters of the DNA code: A = adenine, T = thymine, C = cytosine, and G = guanine; one letter can be changed, deleted, or added; entire pieces of code can be spelled backward, cut and pasted, or cut short, which can change the form and function or the end protein product in the body
      b. The impact of a mutation depends on the environment in which it is expressed
      c. Classification of mutations
         (1) Genome mutations—involve the loss or gain of whole chromosomes, resulting in monosomy or trisomy
         (2) Chromosome mutations—rearrangement of genetic material that gives rise to structural changes in the chromosome; most are incompatible with survival
         (3) Submicroscopic gene mutations—represent the vast majority of mutations associated with hereditary diseases; may result in a partial or complete deletion of a gene or may affect a single base

C. Single-gene disorders
   1. Autosomal dominant inheritance
      a. An affected person usually has one affected parent
      b. An affected person has a 50% chance of passing the trait to an offspring
      c. Both genders are equally likely to be affected, and both can transmit the condition
      d. Dominant traits are usually seen in multiple, successive generations
   2. Additional characteristics of autosomal dominant disorders
      a. Some affected persons do not have affected parents; the disorder is caused by new mutations involving either the egg or the sperm and seems to occur in the germ cells of older fathers
      b. Some inherit the mutant gene but are phenotypically normal (called *reduced* or *incomplete penetrance*)
      c. If the trait is seen in all individuals but is expressed differently among them, the phenomenon is called *variable expressivity*; combinations of these traits can be less or more severe among individuals even within the same family
      d. In many conditions, onset is delayed, and symptoms do not appear until adulthood
      e. Biochemical mechanism is either loss-of-function mutations or gain-of-function mutations; the effects of these mutations depend on the nature of the enzyme protein affected
      f. Examples of autosomal dominant disorders
         (1) Huntington's disease
         (2) Neurofibromatosis
         (3) Polycystic kidney disease
         (4) Von Willebrand disease
         (5) Marfan syndrome
         (6) Ehlers-Danlos syndrome
         (7) Osteogenesis imperfecta
         (8) Familial hypercholesterolemia
   3. Autosomal recessive inheritance
      a. Both genders equally likely to be affected
      b. Disease often found in siblings; affected individuals often have unaffected parents
      c. Offspring of the affected person are carriers of the gene mutation
      d. If a child is born to two carrier parents and is not affected, a two-thirds chance of the child being a carrier is present
      e. Carriers are usually not clinically affected
      f. Two carrier parents have a 25% chance with each conception to have an affected child
      g. Onset is frequently early in life
      h. In many cases, enzyme proteins are affected by a loss of function
      i. Examples of autosomal recessive disorders
         (1) Cystic fibrosis
         (2) Phenylketonuria
         (3) Sickle cell anemia
         (4) Thalassemias
         (5) Congenital adrenal hyperplasia
         (6) Neurogenic muscular atrophies
         (7) Spinal muscular atrophy
   4. X-linked recessive inheritance
      a. Primarily affects males
      b. Sons of carrier females have a 50% chance of receiving the gene and expressing that trait or condition
      c. Carrier females may show no disease trait or mild symptoms only
      d. No male-to-male transmission
      e. Affected males transmit the genes to all daughters but not to their sons; all daughters are carriers
      f. Uncles and cousins may also be affected
      g. Examples of X-linked recessive disorders
         (1) Duchenne muscular dystrophy
         (2) Hemophilia A and B
         (3) Chronic granulomatous disease
         (4) Glucose-6-phosphate dehydrogenase (G6PD) deficiency
         (5) Agammaglobulinemia
         (6) Diabetes insipidus
         (7) Fragile X syndrome
   5. Biochemical and molecular basis of single-gene disorders
      a. The genetic defect may lead to the formation of an abnormal protein as reduction in the output of gene product
      b. The pattern of inheritance is related to the type of protein affected by the mutation

c. The mechanisms are classified into four categories:
   (1) Enzyme defects and their consequences
   (2) Defects in membrane receptors and transport systems
   (3) Alterations in structure, function, or quality of nonenzyme proteins
   (4) Mutations resulting in unusual reactions to drugs—pharmacogenetics

6. Disorders with multifactorial inheritance
   a. Result from the combined actions of environmental influences and two or more mutant genes having additive effects
   b. The greater the number of inherited deleterious genes, the more severe the expression of the disease
   c. Risk is greater in siblings of persons having severe expressions of the disorder
   d. Frequency of concordance for identical twins is 20% to 40%
   e. Examples of disorders with multifactorial inheritance
      (1) Cleft lip, cleft palate, or both
      (2) Congenital heart disease
      (3) Coronary heart disease
      (4) Hypertension
      (5) Gout
      (6) Diabetes mellitus
      (7) Pyloric stenosis

7. Diagnosis of genetic diseases—requires examination of genetic material through cytogenetic analysis or molecular analysis
   a. Cytogenetic analysis involves *karyotyping*, an organized graphic representation of the chromosomes in a single cell
      (1) Normal human karyotypes show 23 pairs of chromosomes (22 pairs of autosomal chromosomes and one pair of sex chromosomes), numbered from larger to smaller
      (2) The 23rd pair comprises the sex chromosomes (XX = female, XY = male)
      (3) Karyotypes are described using a shorthand notation, with the total number of chromosomes listed first, followed by the sex chromosome complement, and then a description of the abnormalities in ascending numerical order
   b. Prenatal chromosome analysis should be offered to individuals at risk; can be performed on cells obtained by amniocentesis, on chorionic villus biopsy, or on umbilical cord blood
   c. Postnatal chromosome analysis can be performed on peripheral blood lymphocytes in cases of multiple congenital anomalies, unexplained mental retardation or developmental delay, suspected genetic disorders such as Turner syndrome or fragile X syndrome, infertility, or multiple spontaneous abortions
   d. Recombinant DNA technology is also used for the diagnosis of inherited diseases because it is highly sensitive; tests are not dependent on a gene product produced only in certain specialized cells
      (1) Testing performed through either direct gene diagnosis using polymerase chain reaction (PCR) analysis or indirect DNA diagnosis through linkage analysis, which involves studying several relevant family members
      (2) 0.1 μL of blood or cells scraped from the buccal mucosa is sufficient for PCR analysis
      (3) Salivary DNA-PCR used to evaluate periodontal status
         (a) MyPerioPath identifies the type and quantity of periodontopathic bacteria
         (b) MyPerioPath + MyPerioID IL-6 determines if the patient is genetically predisposed to periodontal disease by evaluating IL-6 polymorphism
         (c) MyPerioID IL-1 and MyPerioID IL-6 identify individual genetic susceptibility to periodontal disease
         (d) Celsus One is a salivary DNA test to evaluate eight gene markers related to inflammatory response related to periodontal disease, diabetes, and cardiovascular disease
   e. Identifying molecular genetic signatures for acquired diseases
      (1) Diagnosis and management of cancer
         (a) Detection of tumor-specific acquired mutations and cytogenic alterations that are hallmarks of specific tumors
         (b) Determination of clonality as an indicator of neoplastic condition
         (c) Identification of specific gene alterations that can direct therapeutic choices
         (d) Determination of treatment efficacy
         (e) Determination of Gleeve-resistant forms of chronic myeloid leukemia or gastrointestinal stromal tumors
      (2) Diagnosis and management of infectious diseases
         (a) Detection of microorganisms and specific genetic material for definitive diagnosis (i.e., human immunodeficiency virus [HIV], human papillomavirus [HPV], herpes simplex virus [HSV])
         (b) Identification of specific genetic alterations in the genomes of microbes that are associated with drug resistance
         (c) Determination of treatment efficacy (e.g., assessing viral loads in HIV and hepatitis C virus [HCV])
   f. Ribonucleic acid (RNA) analysis
      (1) Not as stable as DNA-based diagnosis, but useful for the detection and quantification of RNA viruses such as HIV and HCV
      (2) Becoming an important tool for the molecular stratification of tumors

8. Referral for genetic counseling
   a. Patients who present with evidence of suspected or diagnosed genetic disorder should be referred to a genetics center for evaluation and counseling; any genetic health condition or risk that affects one individual can affect that person's biologic and extended family
   b. Genetics professionals can be consulted through the National Society for Genetics Counselors (NSGC) website at http://www.nsgc.org
   c. Document referrals are made to a physician, a genetics professional, or both by recording:
      (1) Causes for concern
      (2) Possible diagnosis (if known)
      (3) Family history information obtained
      (4) Relevant oral examination findings, radiographs, and records
   d. Genetics consultation involves:
      (1) Confirming, diagnosing, or ruling out the genetic condition
      (2) Identifying medical management issues
      (3) Determining genetic risks
      (4) Providing psychosocial support

## DIFFERENTIAL DIAGNOSIS[5]

A. Diagnostic approaches
   1. Appearance recognition—clinical manifestations of routine oral diseases can be recognized by their characteristic appearances because no other diseases produce these lesions (e.g., dental caries, gingivitis, periodontitis)
   2. Differential diagnosis—determination of which when two or more diseases with similar signs and symptoms is the one manifested in the patient
      a. Requires a comparison of signs and symptoms and other pertinent details against the known features of all diseases that can produce the observed primary manifestation
      b. Reflects a conceptual process and a listing of pathologic conditions in the order of most likely to least likely
      c. Pathoses are ruled out on the basis of examinations, tests such as blood assays (see reference for specific examples), urinalysis, biopsy, and so on
B. Conceptual stages of the differential diagnosis process
   1. Stage 1: classification of the abnormality by primary manifestation—describe the general nature of the lesion that makes it different from normal tissue
      a. A white mucosal discoloration without loss of mucosal integrity or enlargement
      b. A dark discoloration without loss of mucosal integrity or enlargement
      c. Loss of mucosal integrity or ulceration without enlargement
      d. Enlargement of soft tissues
      e. Radiographic manifestations of a lesion originating in bone
      f. Concurrence of several dissimilar abnormalities suggestive of a syndrome
   2. Stage 2: listing of secondary features and contributing factors—objectively describe the secondary features of the lesion; reserve making judgments about the diagnosis based on information obtained
      a. Visual examination
         (1) Specific location of the lesion
         (2) Shape of the lesion and contours of tissue
         (3) Size of the lesion
         (4) Occurrence of the lesion as isolated, multifocal, or diffuse
         (5) Delineation of the borders of the abnormality from adjacent tissue
         (6) Consistency of appearance as homogeneous or heterogeneous
         (7) Surface color and texture
         (8) Alteration of adjacent structures, such as displacement of teeth
      b. Palpation
         (1) Degree of compressibility
         (2) Tenderness during compression
         (3) Alteration in color during compression
      c. Auscultation
         (1) Wheezing
         (2) Popping and clicking of the temporomandibular joint
         (3) Clicking of poorly fitting dentures
      d. Probing
         (1) Tissue defects
         (2) Exudates
      e. Aspiration
         (1) Pus
         (2) Cysts and nodules
      f. Evaluation of function
         (1) Tear production
         (2) Salivary glands
         (3) Tongue
         (4) Muscles of mastication
         (5) Neurologic function
      g. Patient awareness
         (1) Pain, discomfort, or altered function
         (2) Duration
         (3) Course as constant, healing with recurrence, or steady progression
         (4) Response to factors such as stress and certain foods
      h. Demographics
         (1) Age
         (2) Gender
         (3) Race and ethnicity
      i. Habits
         (1) Alcohol use
         (2) Tobacco use
         (3) Oral
         (4) Other (ask patient)
      j. Recent history
         (1) Injury
         (2) Infection
         (3) Surgery

k. Medical conditions
  (1) Chronic diseases
  (2) Recent acute illnesses
l. Current medical treatment
  (1) Medications
  (2) Other treatment

3. Stage 3: listing of conditions capable of causing primary manifestations
   a. Consider the variety of abnormalities that cause the condition, and compare them with the patient's abnormality
   b. Create a list of plausible diagnoses
4. Stage 4: elimination of unlikely causes
   a. Identify contradictions between the features of the lesion and the known characteristics of the diagnostic possibilities
   b. The category of the lesion determines the secondary features that are most reliable; then eliminate those conditions that appear least likely
   c. Elimination of malignant neoplasia as a possible cause is often more important than achieving a definitive diagnosis
5. Stage 5: ranking of possible causes by probability
   a. Rank the diseases that could explain the abnormality on the basis of the number of secondary features exhibited that correspond with the typical features of each possible diagnosis
6. Stage 6: Determination of a working diagnosis
   a. The condition considered the most likely cause of the lesion is referred to as the *working, tentative,* or *preliminary diagnosis* or the *clinical impression*
   b. Provides the basis for additional diagnostic testing and for the initial clinical management of the condition
   c. When all the diseases except one have been eliminated from the differential diagnosis, then that provides the definitive diagnosis
   d. Reevaluate to verify the correct diagnosis and that the patient has responded to treatment without recurrence

## WEBSITE INFORMATION AND RESOURCES

| Source | Website Address | Description |
|---|---|---|
| National Human Genome Research Institute/ Talking Genetics Glossary | https://www.genome.gov/genetics-glossary | Talking glossary of genetic terms; text-only version available |
| Centers for Disease Control and Prevention/ Office of Genomics and Disease Prevention | www.cdc.gov/genomics | Information about human genomic discoveries and how they can be used to improve health and prevent disease<br>Timely and credible information for the effective and responsible translation of genomics research into population health benefits |
| National Library of Medicine/Genetics Home Reference | http://ghr.nlm.nih.gov/ | Allows users to search for information on diseases, tutorials about basic concepts in genetics, and educational resources |
| National Institutes of Health | https://stemcells.nih.gov/ | Reviews stem cells; unique properties, types, and potential uses of human stem cells |
| International Society for Stem Cell Research | http://www.isscr.org | Provides overview of research related to stem cells; promotes professional and public education in all areas of stem cell research and application |
| Medline Plus | http://www.nlm.nih.gov/medlineplus/stemcells.html | Consumer health database that includes news, health resources, and clinical trials related to stem cells |

## CHAPTER 7 REVIEW QUESTIONS

Answers and rationales to review questions are available on this text's accompanying Evolve site. See inside front cover for details

### CASE A

Mr. Steve Perry is a new patient to your dental practice. He presents with generalized gingivitis indicated by gingival inflammation, edema, bleeding upon probing, and red fiery tissue. You also notice generalized heavy biofilm at the gingival margin. As you begin to explain your clinical findings to Mr. Perry, he explains he often feels discomfort and pain when flossing his teeth so he has discontinued his flossing routine.

***Use Case A to answer questions 1 to 4.***

**1.** What is the cause of the redness described above?
   **a.** Vasoconstriction of blood vessels
   **b.** Increased vascularity
   **c.** Stretching of pain receptors
   **d.** Exudation of fluid

**2.** What is the cause of the gingival edema?
   **a.** Vasoconstriction of blood vessels
   **b.** Increased vascularity
   **c.** Stretching of pain receptors
   **d.** Exudation of fluid

**3.** Which of the following signs of inflammation can explain the pain Mr. Perry is reporting?
   **a.** Rubor
   **b.** Calor
   **c.** Dolor
   **d.** Functio laesa

**4.** Mr. Perry's gingival tissue is reacting in response to an inflammatory stimulus. The inflammatory response has what type of reaction?
   **a.** Vascular and cellular reaction
   **b.** Vascular and regenerative reaction
   **c.** Regenerative and reparative reaction
   **d.** Cellular and regenerative reaction

## CASE B

Mrs. Evelyn Goddard presents with a periodontal abscess on the buccal mucosa adjacent to tooth #30. She noticed swelling and mild pain in this area when she woke up in the morning and called the dental office immediately for an appointment. Upon examination with the dental hygienist, the area was significantly enlarged with redness and edema. A fistula was present. When the tissue was compressed, suppuration was expressed.

***Use Case B to answer questions 5 to 10.***

**5.** The body's response to the development of an abscess most likely represents:
- **a.** Acute inflammation
- **b.** Chronic inflammation
- **c.** Regeneration
- **d.** Repair

**6.** Redness at the site of the abscess is a cardinal sign of inflammation. This sign is also referred to as:
- **a.** Dolor
- **b.** Calor
- **c.** Tumor
- **d.** Rubor

**7.** The edema present at tooth #30 is caused by which of the following?
- **a.** Increased vascularity
- **b.** Increased fluid in the interstitial space
- **c.** Release of inflammatory mediators
- **d.** Stretching of pain receptors

**8.** The suppuration present most likely represents a collection of which white blood cells?
- **a.** Lymphocytes and plasma cells
- **b.** Eosinophils and mast cells
- **c.** Neutrophils and macrophages
- **d.** Eosinophils and neutrophils

**9.** Recent evidence demonstrates that in addition to phagocytosis, neutrophils also perform which function?
- **a.** Regulate vascular permeability
- **b.** Release chemical mediators
- **c.** Regulate bronchial smooth muscle tone
- **d.** Contribute to the repair process

**10.** The dental hygienist debrides the affected abscess area and the dentist decides to prescribe an antibiotic. The tissue will heal by:
- **a.** Primary intention
- **b.** Secondary intention
- **c.** Tertiary intention
- **d.** Delayed primary closure

## CASE C

Sam Adams presents for extraction of tooth #32, which is impacted. The extraction is performed and surgery is uneventful. Sutures are placed and the patient is discharged with instructions to alternate acetaminophen and ibuprofen as needed for pain, apply ice on the outside of the mouth to reduce swelling, gently rinse the mouth with a mild antiseptic mouth rinse, consume liquid based foods/soft diet for 1–2 days, and return in one week for post-op evaluation and suture removal.

***Use Case C to answer questions 11 to 17.***

**11.** The first step in the healing process following this tooth extraction is:
- **a.** An inflammatory response
- **b.** Thrombus is formed
- **c.** Angiogenesis
- **d.** Granulation tissue forms

**12.** Because sutures were placed, healing will occur by primary intention. Epithelium will form a basement membrane under the scab within:
- **a.** 6–12 hours
- **b.** 12–24 hours
- **c.** 24–48 hours
- **d.** 48–72 hours

**13.** By day 5 in the wound healing process, granulation tissue fills the incisional space. All of the following are characteristics of granulation tissue EXCEPT one. Which one is the EXCEPTION?
- **a.** Tissue is pink and soft
- **b.** New small blood vessels appear
- **c.** New vessels are fully patent
- **d.** Amount of granulation tissue depends on the size of the wound

**14.** Tissues recover ____________ percent of tensile strength over a 3-month period of healing as compared with intact skin?
- **a.** 60–70
- **b.** 70–80
- **c.** 80–90
- **d.** 100

**15.** Local factors that could prolong the wound healing of the extraction site include all of the following EXCEPT one. Which one is the EXCEPTION?
- **a.** Size of the wound
- **b.** Foreign material
- **c.** Location of the wound
- **d.** Blood supply

**16.** Complications can occur during the wound healing process. Deficient scar formation could lead to which of the following?
- **a.** Wound dehiscence
- **b.** Keloid
- **c.** Contracture
- **d.** Fibrosis

**17.** Systemic factors that influence wound healing include all the following EXCEPT one. Which one is the EXCEPTION?
- **a.** Blood supply
- **b.** Size, location, and type of wound
- **c.** Corticosteroids
- **d.** Nutritional deficiencies

## CASE D

Mrs. Monica Salt is a female patient scheduled for periodontal maintenance. As you are reviewing her health history, Mrs. Salt tells you that she is pregnant. She is concerned about her baby being born with a cleft lip and palate because there is a family history.

*Use Case D to answer questions 18 to 21.*

**18.** Prenatal chromosome analysis should be offered to Ms. Salt for which of the following reasons?
**a.** Exposure to BPA
**b.** Clinical evidence of high palatal vault
**c.** Medical history of high triglycerides
**d.** Previous family history

**19.** The majority of mutations associated with hereditary disease are:
**a.** Genome mutations
**b.** Chromosome mutations
**c.** Submicroscopic gene mutations
**d.** Cytosine gene mutations

**20.** In this case, genetic testing for the fetus can be performed on cells obtained by ____________.
**a.** Amniocentesis
**b.** Chorionic villus biopsy
**c.** Umbilical cord blood
**d.** All of the above

**21.** Cleft lip and/or cleft palate is considered a disorder of ____________.
**a.** Single gene disorders
**b.** Multiple factorial inheritance
**c.** Autosomal dominant inheritance
**d.** Autosomal recessive inheritance

## CASE E

Mr. and Mrs. Dorchester present to the dental practice for a consult. They would like to bring their 4-year-old son to the office for comprehensive oral health care; however, he has Duchenne muscular dystrophy. They are concerned that the practice can provide care managing their son's condition as the disease progresses.

*Use Case E to answer questions 22 to 25.*

**22.** What type of genetic disease does Duchenne muscular dystrophy represent?
**a.** Autosomal dominant disorder
**b.** Autosomal recessive disorder
**c.** X-linked recessive disorder
**d.** Disorders with multifactorial inheritance

**23.** All of the following are characteristics of Duchenne muscular dystrophy EXCEPT one. Which one is the EXCEPTION?
**a.** Primarily affects males
**b.** All sons are carriers
**c.** No male-to-male transmission
**d.** Affected males transmit the genes to all daughters but not to their sons

**24.** All of the following are examples of genetic diseases similar to Duchenne muscular dystrophy EXCEPT one. Which one is the EXCEPTION?
**a.** Fragile X syndrome
**b.** Diabetes insipidus
**c.** Hemophilia A and B
**d.** Coronary heart disease

**25.** Diagnosis of Duchenne muscular dystrophy requires examination of genetic material through:
**a.** Karyotyping
**b.** Chromosome analysis
**c.** Polymerase chain reaction
**d.** All of the above

## CASE F

Janis Johnson presents to your practice with a chief complaint of a mass on the left buccal mucosa of normal tissue coloration. The lesion has been present for 2 months, is painless, but interferes occasionally with chewing activities. The patient reports that she has been known to bite the mass causing it to become ulcerated. Answer the following items as they relate to the diagnostic process.

*Use Case F to answer questions 26 to 30.*

**26.** Classify the abnormality based on the primary manifestation.
**a.** A white mucosal discoloration without loss of mucosal integrity or enlargement
**b.** A dark discoloration without loss of mucosal integrity or enlargement
**c.** Loss of mucosal integrity or ulceration without enlargement
**d.** Enlargement of soft tissues

**27.** All of the following examination procedures would be appropriate for this lesion EXCEPT one. Which one is the EXCEPTION?
**a.** Probing
**b.** Visual examination
**c.** Palpation
**d.** Evaluation of function

**28.** Alcohol use, tobacco use, oral behaviors all describe the patient's:
**a.** Demographics
**b.** Habits
**c.** Recent history
**d.** Awareness of condition

**29.** Pain, discomfort, or altered function, duration, and response to factors such as stress or certain foods all describe the patient's:
**a.** Demographics
**b.** Habits
**c.** Recent history
**d.** Awareness of condition

**30.** All of the following are terms for a working diagnosis EXCEPT one. Which one is the EXCEPTION?
**a.** Differential diagnosis
**b.** Probable diagnosis
**c.** Preliminary diagnosis
**d.** Tentative diagnosis

**31.** The white blood cells responsible for producing vasoconstrictive chemical mediators that maintain chronic inflammation are:
**a.** Eosinophils
**b.** Lymphocytes
**c.** Macrophages
**d.** Mast cells

**32.** The white blood cells responsible for assisting in immune responses and parasitic infections are:
**a.** Eosinophils
**b.** Lymphocytes
**c.** Macrophages
**d.** Mast cells

33. The chemical mediator that is responsible for causing dilation of arterioles and constricting large arteries, edema, and smooth muscle contraction is:
  a. Serotonin
  b. Bradykinin
  c. Histamine
  d. Arachidonic acid
34. Programmed cell death in phagocytosis is referred to as:
  a. Engulfment
  b. Degradation
  c. Apoptosis
  d. Chemotaxis
35. Pro-resolving mediators perform all of the following functions EXCEPT one. Which one is the EXCEPTION?
  a. Evoke potent antiinflammatory mechanisms
  b. Returns cells to homeostasis
  c. Enhance microbial clearance
  d. Induce pain
36. Which of the following chemical mediators moderates the susceptibility, development, and progression of autoimmune and inflammatory diseases?
  a. IL6
  b. TNF
  c. IL1
  d. NO
37. All of the following are possible outcomes of inflammation EXCEPT one. Which one is the EXCEPTION?
  a. Complete resolution
  b. Healing by connective tissue replacement
  c. Progression of tissue to chronic inflammation
  d. Leukopenia
38. Which systemic disease is associated with chronic inflammation?
  a. Gingivitis
  b. von Willebrand disease
  c. Anemia
  d. Caries
39. A hallmark of healing is the formation of:
  a. A scab
  b. Granulation tissue
  c. Adjacent blood vessels
  d. Endothelial growth factor
40. Extensive deposition of collagen that sustains the synthesis and secretion of growth factors during the wound healing process causing significant scar formation represents:
  a. Wound dehiscence
  b. Keloid
  c. Contracture
  d. Fibrosis
41. Poor wound healing with a compromised blood supply can lead to:
  a. COPD
  b. Rheumatoid arthritis
  c. Amputation
  d. Cirrhosis
42. Stem cells derived from other individuals refers to:
  a. Autogenous
  b. Allogenous
  c. Unipotent
  d. Totipotent
43. Characteristics of embryonic stem cells include all of the following EXCEPT one. Which one is the EXCEPTION?
  a. Pluripotent
  b. Isolated from inner cell mass of blastocytes
  c. Found in skin, lining of intestine, cornea, and brain.
  d. May be used to treat organs affected by diabetes, spinal cord injuries, heart disease, and liver damage
44. What is the most common commercially available stem cell?
  a. Umbilical cord blood stem cells
  b. Dental stem cells
  c. Adipose-derived stem cells
  d. Bone marrow–derived stem cells
45. A common property of stem cells is:
  a. Ability to have senescence
  b. Capacity to intermittently undergo division or remain quiescent
  c. Presence of lineage markers
  d. Absence of growth and transcription markers
46. Sources of dental stem cells include all of the following EXCEPT one. Which one is the EXCEPTION?
  a. Pulp chamber
  b. Periodontal ligament
  c. Third molars
  d. Primary teeth
47. How many genes do humans have?
  a. 10,000 to 15,000
  b. 15,000 to 20,000
  c. 20,000 to 25,000
  d. 25,000 to 30,000
48. The four letters of the DNA code represent:
  a. Adenine, thymus, cytosine, guanine
  b. Adenine, thymus, cytosine, guanasine
  c. Adenine, thymine, cytosine, guanasine
  d. Adenine, thymine, cytosine, guanine
49. A person has what percent chance of passing a trait to an offspring for an autosomal dominant inheritance disorder?
  a. 25%
  b. 50%
  c. 75%
  d. 100%
50. With autosomal recessive inheritance, two carrier parents have what percent chance with each conception of having an affected child?
  a. 25%
  b. 50%
  c. 75%
  d. 100%

## REFERENCES

1. Goljan EF. *Rapid Review: Pathology*. 4th ed. Philadelphia: Elsevier; 2014.
2. Kumar V, Abbas AK, Fausto N, Aster JC. *Robbins and Cotran Pathologic Basis of Disease*. 9th ed. Philadelphia: Saunders; 2015.
3. Rubin E, Resiner HM. *Principles of Rubins' Pathology*. 7th ed. Philadelphia: Wolters Kulwer; 2019.
4. Mao JJ, Giannobile WV, Helms JA, et al. Craniofacial tissue engineering by stem cells. *J Dent Res*. 2006;85(11):966–979.
5. Coleman GC, Nelson JF. *Principles of Oral Diagnosis*. St Louis: Mosby; 1993.

## SUGGESTED READINGS

Core Competencies in Genetics (n.d), https://www.jax.org/education-and-learning/clinical-and-continuing-education/ccep-non-cancer-resources/core-competencies-for-health-care-professionals. Accessed April 22, 2019.

Lee HN, Surh YJ. Therapeutic potential of resolvins in prevention and treatment of inflammatory disorders. *Biochem Pharmacol*. 2012;84(10):1340–1350.

Mariotti A. A primer on inflammation. *Compend Cont Educ Dent*. 2004;25(7 suppl 1):7–15.

Nadig RR. Stem cell therapy—hype or hope? A review. *J Conserv Dent*. 2009;12(4):131–138.

Pagana KD, Pagana TS. *Mosby's Manual of Diagnostic and Laboratory Tests*. 4th ed. Philadelphia: Mosby; 2010.

US Department of Health and Human Services. National Institutes of Health. *Stem Cell Basics*. 2015. https://stemcells.nih.gov/sites/default/files/508-Compliant-Stem-Cell%20Basics-2020.pdf. Accessed August 14, 2020.

8

# Oral Pathology

*Sandra L. Myers*

Dental hygienists perform comprehensive extraoral and intraoral examinations, identify pathologic conditions, and communicate these findings to the dentist for diagnosis, treatment, or referral. Knowledge of oral pathology is essential for the preliminary evaluation of oral lesions. The dental hygienist differentiates between normal and abnormal findings and relates significant medical, dental, and cultural histories to clinical, radiographic, and histologic findings. Although the dental hygienist is not responsible for a definitive (final) diagnosis, skill in the use of the diagnostic process is essential to establish a dental hygiene diagnosis and contribute to collaborative practice of the dental team.

## BENIGN SOFT TISSUE LESIONS

### General Characteristics

A. Etiology—varies, may be unknown
B. Age and gender—predilections associated with lesion type
C. Clinical features of benign lesions
   1. Lesions well-demarcated, may be encapsulated
   2. Slow growing, easily palpable, with sessile or pedunculated base
   3. Lack malignant features such as fixed to underlying tissues (invasion) and metastasis (spread of tumor cells to distant body sites)
D. Histologic features reflect lesion type (e.g., a lipoma is composed of fat cells)
E. Features such as slow growth and encapsulation contribute to determination of benign status
F. Benign lesions not expected to recur after complete removal

### Irritation Fibroma (Traumatic Fibroma)

A. Etiology—chronic irritation or trauma
B. Age and gender—more common in adults aged 40 to 60 years; females (2:1)
C. Location—buccal mucosa along occlusal plane; also lips, tongue, and gingiva
D. Clinical features Fig. 8.1
   1. Benign lesion of fibrous connective tissue
   2. Pink color, often same coloration as adjacent normal mucosa
   3. Round to oval shape
   4. Most often <1 cm in size
   5. Sessile or pedunculated base
   6. Exophytic
E. Histologic characteristics
   1. Surface covered with stratified squamous epithelium; may be hyperkeratinized or ulcerated (result of secondary trauma)
   2. Contains dense connective tissue with sparse blood vessels
F. Treatment—complete excision, does not recur

### Oral Squamous Papilloma

A. Etiology—due to virus; human papilloma virus (HPV) types 6 and 11
B. Age and gender—may arise at any age, but there is a 50% incidence between ages 20 and 50 years; no gender predilection
C. Location—most often seen on hard and soft palate or tongue, but can occur anywhere
D. Clinical features (Fig. 8.2A)
   1. Benign lesion of squamous epithelium
   2. Cauliflower-like appearance or cluster of finger-like projections
   3. Usually white but can also be pink; color depends on surface keratinization
   4. Well-delineated, exophytic, sessile base
   5. Most often <0.5 cm in size
E. Histologic characteristics (Fig. 8.2B)
   1. Stratified squamous epithelium covering multiple slender cores of connective tissue
   2. Variable keratinization of surface
F. Treatment and prognosis
   1. Surgical excision, includes base of lesion to prevent recurrence
   2. Does not undergo malignant transformation
   3. Does not normally recur

### Verruca Vulgaris (Common Wart)

A. Etiology—due to virus; HPV most common types HPV-2 and HPV-4 , other viral subtypes also implicated
B. Age and gender—more common in children; but lesions have also been identified in adults; no gender predilection
C. Location—common skin lesion; lips are the most common oral site; not normally observed intraorally

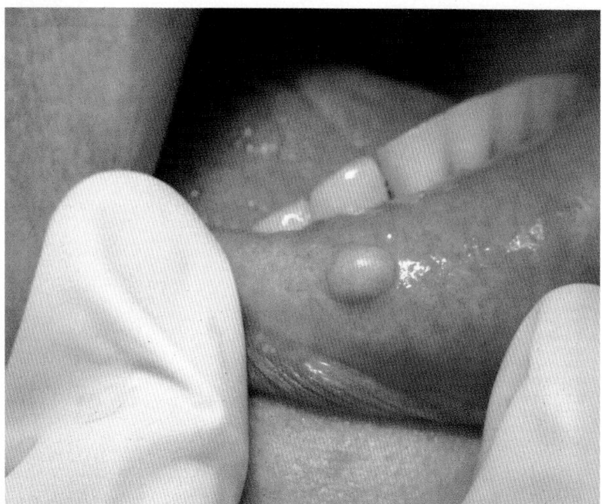

**Fig. 8.1** Fibroma with a sessile base. (From Ibsen OAC, Phelan JA. *Oral Pathology for the Dental Hygienist.* 6th ed. St. Louis: Elsevier Saunders; 2014.)

D. Clinical features (Fig. 8.3)
   1. Benign lesion of stratified squamous epithelium; rough thickened keratotic surface
   2. Sessile base, color depends on location, may be lighter or darker than surrounding skin or mucosa
   3. Self-innoculation (finger to lips) and spread to other epithelial areas can occur
E. Histologic characteristics
   1. Well circumscribed exophytic growth with marked hyperkeratotic stratified squamous epithelium
   2. Cauliflower or finger-like extensions, with central cores of connective tissue, slope inward at lesion edges
F. Treatment and prognosis
   1. Various therapies include excision, cryotherapy, electrocautery, topical agents
   2. May resolve spontaneously, but recurrence is common

## Hemangioma

A. Etiology—congenital or developmental origin; may develop as response to trauma (vascular anomaly) in adults
B. Age and gender—lesions present at birth or develop shortly thereafter; more common in females (3:1)
C. Location—most common on tongue; also found on buccal and labial mucosa, and vermilion border of lips
D. Clinical features (Fig. 8.4A)
   1. Benign proliferation of blood vessels, deep red or bluish purple in color
   2. Flat or raised, often well-circumscribed
   3. Lesions are compressible and color may blanch when pressure applied
E. Histologic characteristics (Fig. 8.4B)
   1. Capillary hemangioma—numerous small dilated blood filled capillaries lined by a single layer of endothelial cells supported by connective tissue stroma of varying density
   2. Cavernous—large, dilated endothelial lined vessels and sinuses with thin walls and filled with blood, supported by connective tissue stroma of varying density

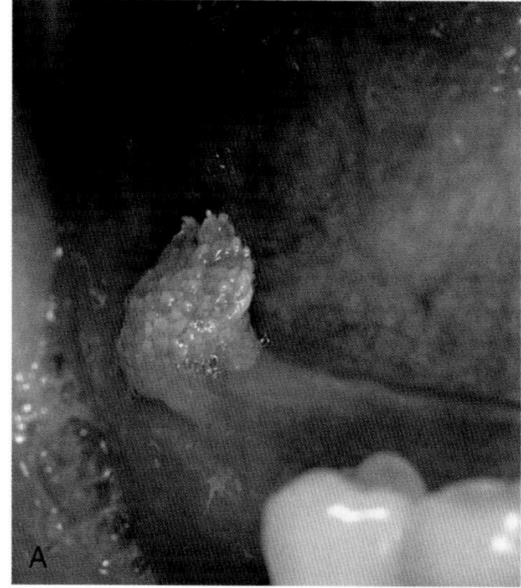



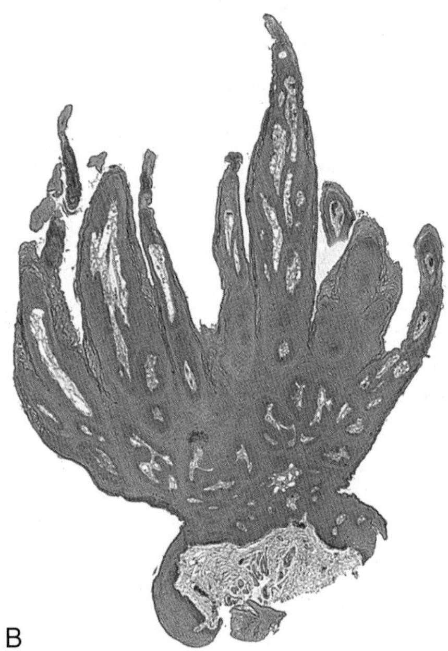



**Fig. 8.2** (A) Clinical appearance of a papilloma showing a cauliflower-like appearance and rough surface resulting from finger-like projections. (B) Microscopic appearance of a papilloma showing finger-like projections covered by a squamous epithelial layer and supported by thin cores of fibrous tissue. (From Odell E: Cawson's Essentials of Oral Pathology and Oral Medicine. 9th ed. Elsevier; 2017.)

F. Treatment
   a. Spontaneous remission may occur in some cases and intervention not necessary
   b. Surgical excision, laser procedures may be indicated for persisting lesions
   c. Sclerosing agents injected into lesions may result in resolution
G. Prognosis is good, recurrence not expected

## Lipoma

A. Etiology—unknown; rare in oral cavity
B. Age and gender—often over 40 years; no gender predilection
C. Location—most common in buccal mucosa or mucobuccal fold

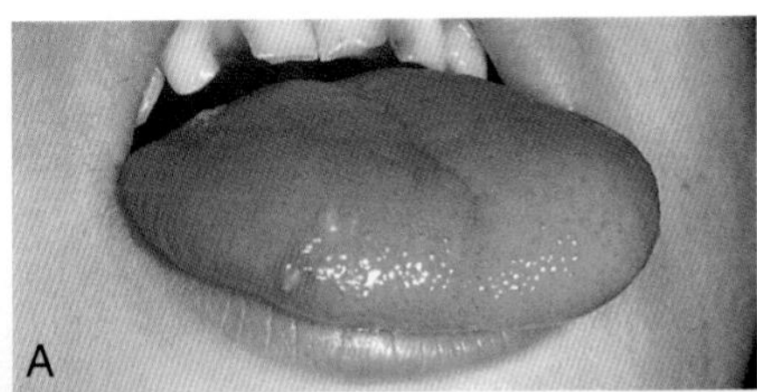

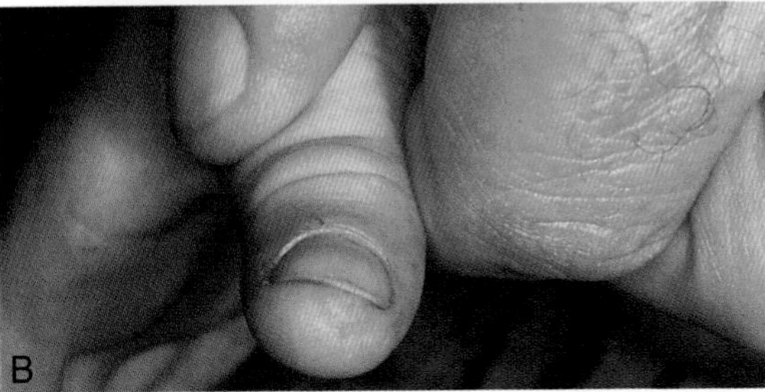

**Fig. 8.3** (A) and (B) Verruca vulgaris on the tongue of a child, with a similar lesion on the thumb. (Courtesy of Dr. Edward V. Zegarelli; from Ibsen OAC, Phelan JA. *Oral Pathology for the Dental Hygienist.* 6th ed. St. Louis: Elsevier Saunders; 2014.)

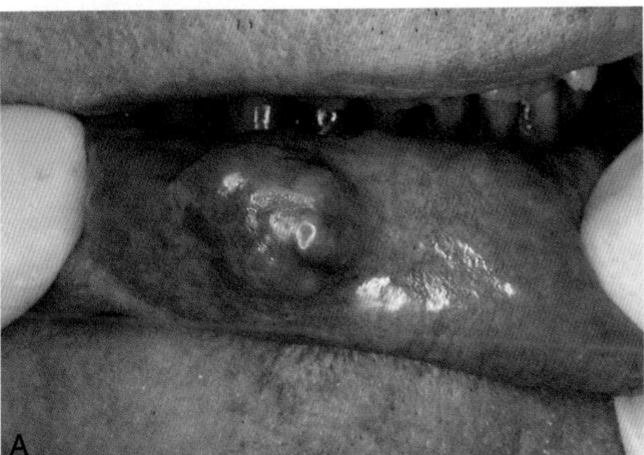

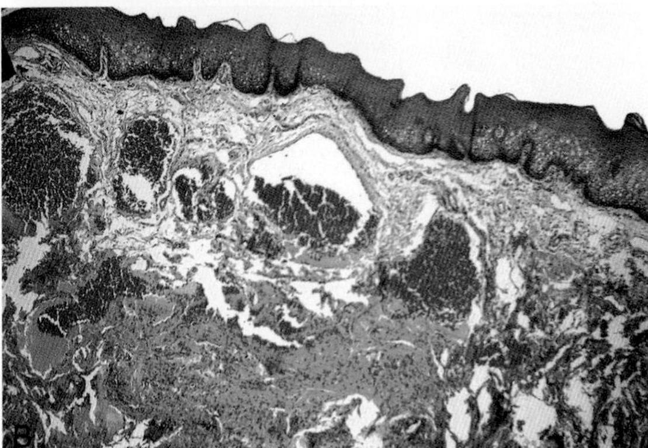

**Fig. 8.4** (A) Clinical appearance of a hemangioma of the lower lip. (B) Photomicrograph of a hemangioma. (From Ibsen OAC, Phelan JA. *Oral Pathology for the Dental Hygienist.* 6th ed. St. Louis: Elsevier Saunders; 2014.)

D. Clinical features (Fig. 8.5A)
   1. Benign tumor of mature fat cells
   2. Single or lobulated, well-defined, painless mass most often <3 cm in size
   3. Sessile or pedunculated base
   4. Soft to palpation
   5. Surface covered with normal colored oral mucosa, yellowish color to submucosal tissues

E. Histologic characteristics (Fig. 8.5B)
   1. Circumscribed mass of mature fat cells with collagen strands, and a few blood vessels
   2. Covered with layer of normal stratified squamous epithelium
   3. When fibrous connective tissue forms a significant part of the lesion, term *fibrolipoma* is applied

F. Treatment and prognosis
   1. Conservative surgical excision
   2. Recurrence is rare

## INFLAMMATORY LESIONS

### General Characteristics

A. Tissue enlargements or growths precipitated by inflammatory response
B. Account for large portion of all oral lesions
C. Benign tissue proliferations

### Pyogenic Granuloma

A. Etiology—chronic irritants or trauma (i.e., plaque biofilm, calculus, poor restorative margins, altered hormone levels)
B. Age and gender—teenagers and young adults; more common in females (3:1) due to increased hormone level fluctuations
C. Location—more common on maxillary labial gingiva than mandibular gingiva; can occur on the lips, tongue, and buccal mucosa
D. Clinical features (Fig. 8.6)
   1. Benign mass containing numerous blood-filled small blood vessels and capillaries
   2. Exuberant tissue response to chronic irritation
   3. Exophytic; pedunculated, sessile, or lobulated base
   4. Deep-red to purple surface which may be ulcerated, bleed easily
   5. Lesions range from a few millimeters to several centimeters in size
   6. In pregnancy, lesions formerly called “pregnancy tumors” or granuloma gravidarum
E. Histologic characteristics
   1. Epithelial covering, if present, often sparse and thin, may be ulcerated
   2. Rich in capillaries initially, later proliferation of connective tissue
   3. Acute and chronic inflammatory cells present, including polymorphonuclear neutrophil leukocytes (PMNs), plasma cells, and lymphocytes
F. Treatment and prognosis
   1. Removal of irritant (most important)
   2. Surgical excision for nonresponsive lesions
   3. Lesions can recur if the irritant persists (e.g., calculus)
   4. Lesions that occur during pregnancy may resolve spontaneously, after delivery when hormone levels return to normal

### Inflammatory Papillary Hyperplasia of the Palate (Palatal Papillomatosis)

A. Etiology—most often associated with complete maxillary or partial denture (considered a type of denture stomatitis); contributing factors include

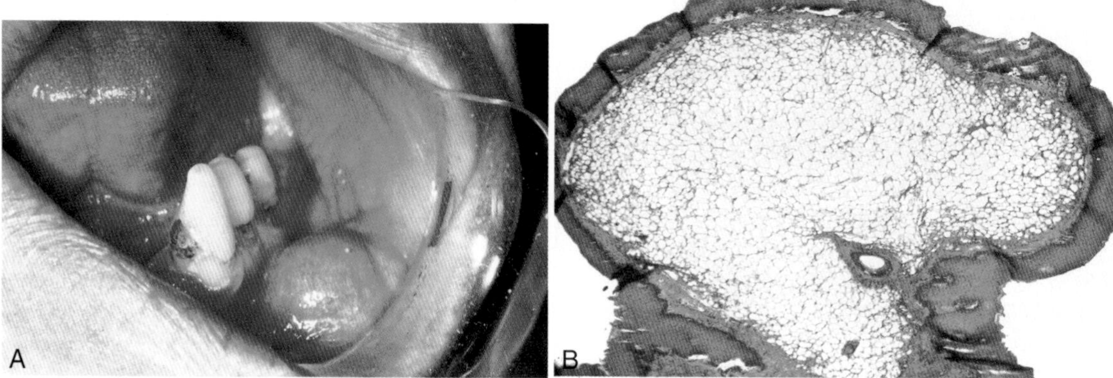

**Fig. 8.5** (A) Clinical appearance of a lipoma. (B) Photomicrograph of a lipoma showing mature fat cells. ((A) courtesy of Dr. Edward V. Zegarelli; from Ibsen OAC, Phelan JA. *Oral Pathology for the Dental Hygienist.* 5th ed. Philadelphia: Elsevier Saunders; 2009.; (B) From Regezi J, Sciubba J, Jordan RCK. *Oral Pathology: Clinical Pathologic Correlations.* 5th ed. St. Louis: Elsevier Saunders; 2008.)

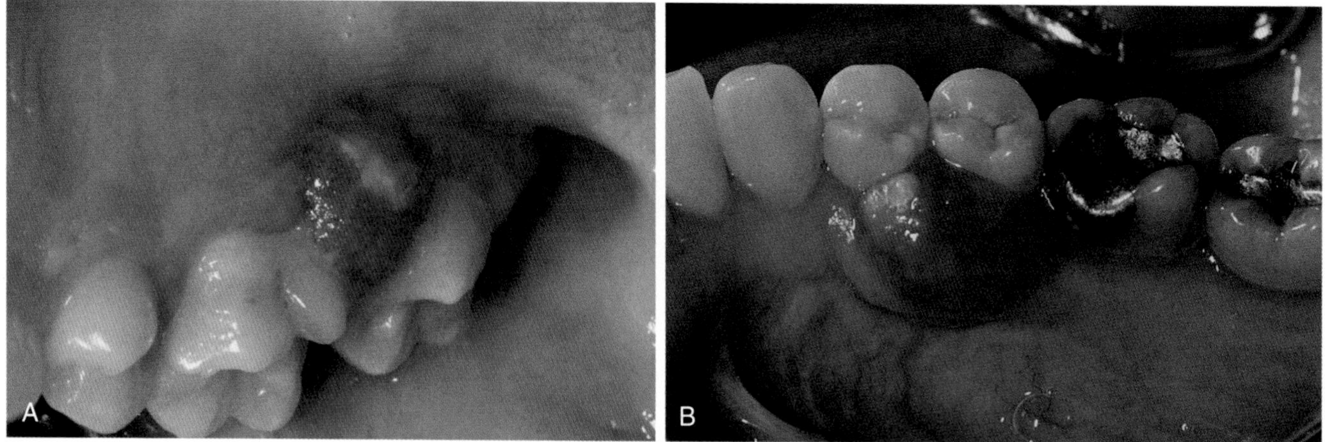

**Fig. 8.6** Pyogenic granuloma. (From Neville B, Damm DD, Allen CM, et al. Color Atlas of Oral and Maxillofacial Diseases. St Louis: Elsevier Inc.; 2019.)

1. Chronic irritation to hard palate related to ill-fitting full or partial denture or orthodontic appliance
2. Poor denture hygiene and/or wearing appliance continuously (24 hours a day)

B. Age and gender—generally adults wearing maxillary dentures, no gender predilection

C. Location—most often hard palate under denture

D. Clinical features (Fig. 8.7)
1. Benign asymptomatic condition composed of closely clustered erythematous papillary projections, small 1 to 4 mm in diameter
2. Round, smooth, glistening red surface; granular appearance
3. Varying degrees of inflammation present

E. Histologic characteristics
1. Small papillary projections of stratified squamous epithelium covering central connective tissue cores
2. Infiltrated with acute and chronic inflammatory cells

F. Treatment
1. Surgical excision of hyperplastic tissue may be indicated before construction of new denture or performing a reline procedure
2. Educate patient on proper denture hygiene, and removal of denture at night to rest oral tissues

G. Prognosis—good

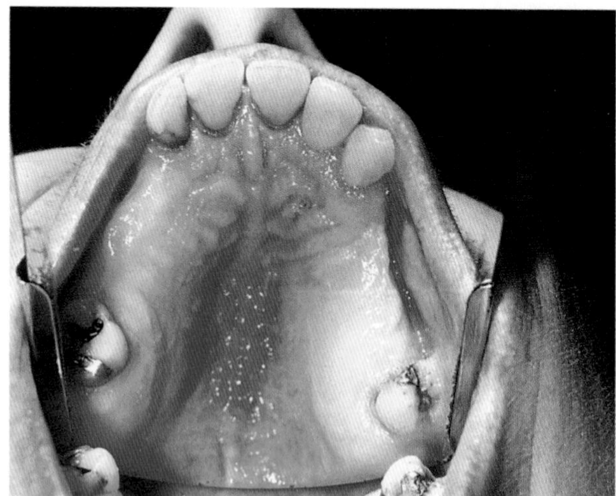

**Fig. 8.7** Papillary hyperplasia of the palate. (Courtesy of Dr. Edward V. Zegarelli; from Ibsen OAC, Phelan JA. *Oral Pathology for the Dental Hygienist.* 6th ed. St. Louis: Elsevier Saunders; 2014.)

## Denture-Induced Inflammatory Fibrous Hyperplasia (Epulis Fissuratum, Inflammatory Hyperplasia)

A. Etiology—irritation caused by ill-fitting denture, produces tissue proliferation along a denture border or flange

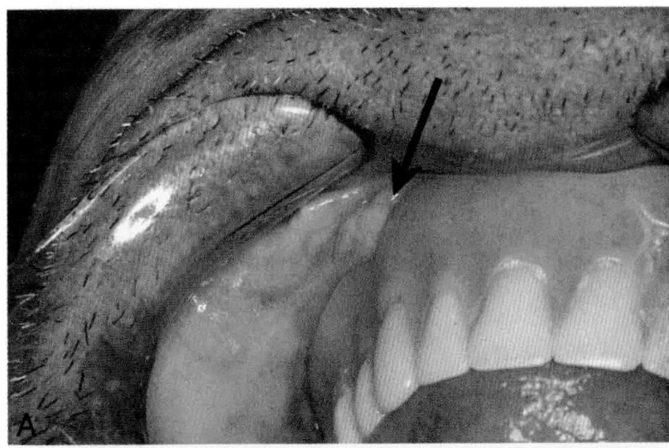


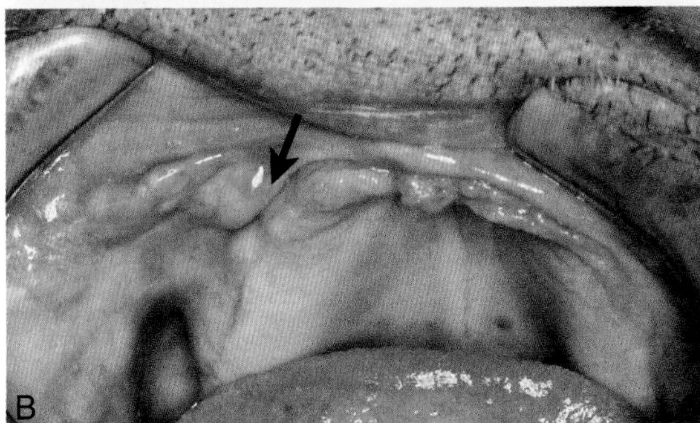


**Fig. 8.8** (A) Denture-induced fibrous hyperplasia (epulis fissuratum) *(arrows)*, shown with denture in place, and (B) denture removed. (From Ibsen OAC, Phelan JA. *Oral Pathology for the Dental Hygienist*. 6th ed. St. Louis: Elsevier Saunders; 2014.)

B. Age and gender—denture wearers; no gender predilection
C. Location—mandibular or maxillary vestibule and alveolar ridge adjacent to denture border
D. Clinical features (Fig. 8.8A and B)
   1. Benign asymptomatic lesion composed of exophytic folds of hyperplastic tissue under or enfolding denture border or flange
   2. Pink to red color (may be ulcerated)
   3. Firm to palpation
   4. Protective response of tissues to impinging denture flange
E. Histologic characteristics
   1. Benign lesion composed of dense fibrous connective tissue covered by stratified squamous epithelium
   2. Connective tissue composed of coarse bundles of collagen fibers
   3. Same type tissue components as seen in irritation fibroma
F. Treatment and prognosis
   1. Surgical removal of excess tissue often indicated to facilitate denture stability and palatal seal
   2. New denture construction or relining procedures may be indicated
   3. Prognosis—good

## Peripheral Giant Cell Granuloma (PGCG)

A. Etiology—unknown but thought to be reactive response to irritation or trauma
B. Age and gender—mean age 30 to 40 years; more common in females (2:1)
C. Location—occurs exclusively on the gingiva or edentulous alveolar ridge, may arise from periodontal ligament or mucoperiosteum
D. Clinical features (Fig. 8.9A)
   1. Exophytic lesion 0.5 to 2.0 cm in diameter
   2. Deep red or red-blue nodular mass
   3. Pedunculated or sessile base
   4. Arises deeper within tissues than does pyogenic granuloma or irritation fibroma
E. Radiographic appearance
   1. Superficial resorption of alveolar bone, "cupping" erosion, may occur
   2. May be difficult to determine if lesion first arose peripherally (within soft tissues) or centrally (within bone)
F. Histologic characteristics (Fig. 8.9B)
   1. Benign lesion composed of proliferating multinucleated giant cells, in a delicate connective tissue stroma, mixed with plump, ovoid, or spindle-shaped cells
   2. Abundant hemorrhage and deposition of hemosiderin pigment
   3. Overlying surface is frequently ulcerated
G. Treatment and prognosis
   1. Surgical removal down to alveolar bone to eliminate recurrence
   2. Prognosis—good

## Central Giant Cell Granuloma (CGCG)

In contrast to peripheral lesions, central lesions occur within bone.

A. Etiology— unknown but thought to be reactive response to irritation or trauma; proposed etiology includes traumatic blow to jaw or tooth extraction
B. Age and gender—children and young adults; more common in females (2:1) age 10 to 30 years
C. Location—75% in the anterior segment of the mandible; also found in the maxilla
D. Clinical features
   1. Benign lesion may be aggressive or nonaggressive
   2. Asymptomatic, often discovered on routine radiographs
   3. Painless expansion of cortical plates
   4. Similar lesion, called "brown tumor," occurs with hyperparathyroidism; resolves without treatment
E. Radiographic appearance (Fig. 8.10A and B)
   1. Well-delineated unilocular or multilocular radiolucent defect with noncorticated margins
   2. Displacement of teeth; divergence and resorption of tooth roots
   3. Radiographic findings are not diagnostic
F. Histologic characteristics
   1. Benign lesion composed of proliferating multinucleated giant cells, in a delicate connective tissue stroma, mixed with plump, ovoid, or spindle-shaped cells
   2. Abundant hemorrhage and deposition of hemosiderin pigment
   3. Histology identical to "brown tumor" of hyperparathyroidism, a systemic condition which must be ruled out
G. Treatment and prognosis
   1. Thorough curettage (more than one treatment may be necessary)
   2. Surgical removal
   3. Radiation therapy is contraindicated

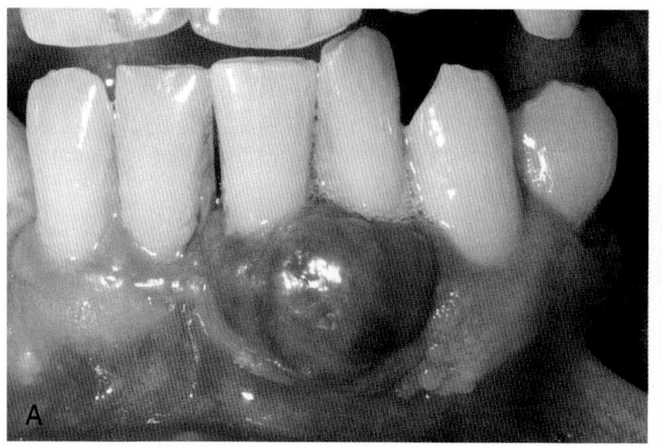


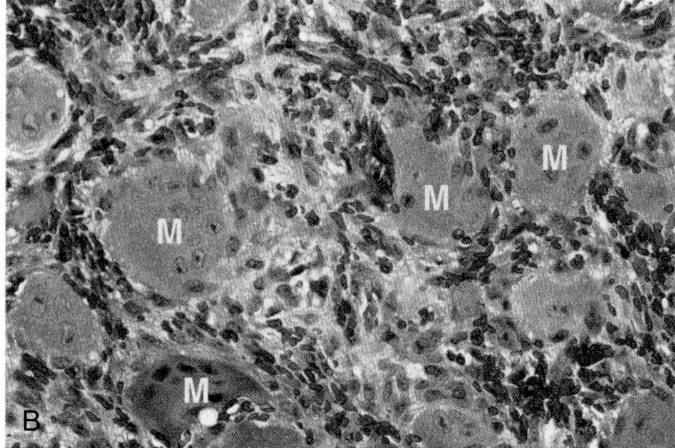


**Fig. 8.9** (A) Peripheral giant cell granuloma. (B) Microscopic appearance of a peripheral giant cell granuloma showing multi-nucleated giant cells *(M)*, capillaries, and fibroblasts. (From Neville BW. *Oral and Maxillofacial Pathology*. 4th ed. St. Louis: Elsevier; 2016.)

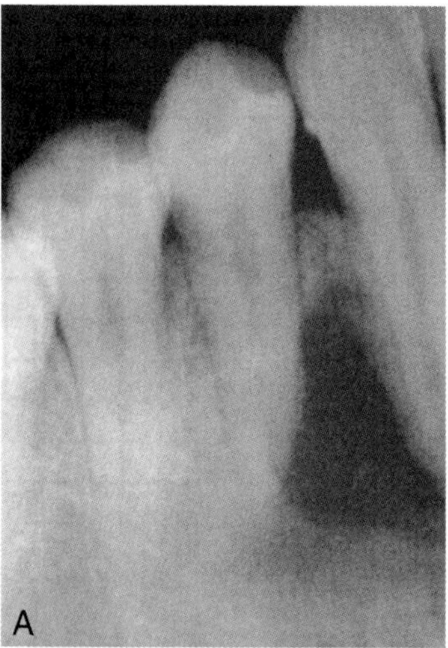


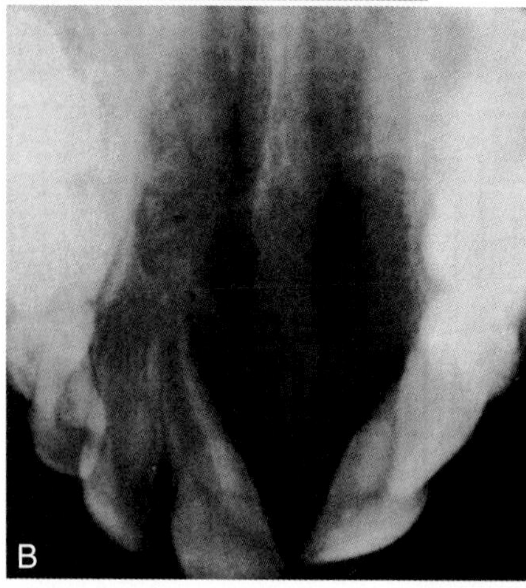


**Fig. 8.10** Radiographs of central giant cell granulomas showing multilocular radiolucencies. (A) The mandible. (B) The maxilla. (From Ibsen OAC, Phelan JA. *Oral Pathology for the Dental Hygienist*. 6th ed. St. Louis: Elsevier Saunders; 2014.)

4. Propensity for recurrence
5. Treatment or removal not indicated in cases of hyperparathyroidism; lesion will resolve when systemic condition resolved

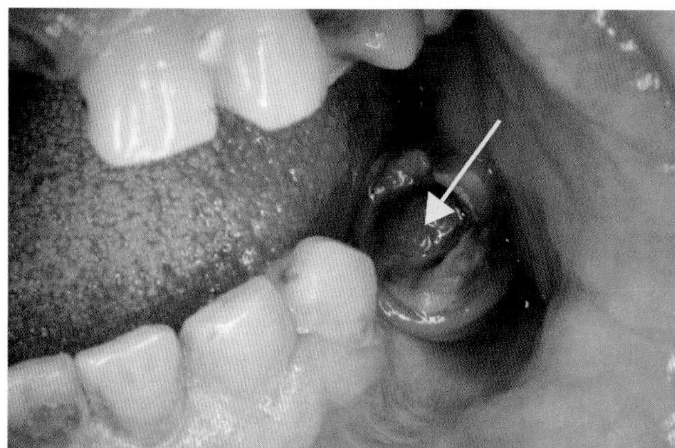

**Fig. 8.11** Chronic hyperplastic pulpitis (pulp polyp) *(arrow)*. (From Neville BW. *Oral and Maxillofacial Pathology*. 4th ed. St. Louis: Elsevier; 2016.)

## Chronic Hyperplastic Pulpitis (Pulpal Granuloma, Pulp Polyp)

A. Etiology—chronically inflamed pulp tissue, in tooth with large open carious lesion
B. Age and gender—children and young adults; no gender predilection
C. Location
   1. Most often in primary molars or permanent first molars
   2. Can occur in any tooth with a large, open, carious lesion
D. Clinical features (Fig. 8.11)
   1. Benign red to pink outgrowth of pulp tissue protruding from occlusal surface
   2. Hyperplastic tissue is asymptomatic
E. Histologic characteristics
   1. Pulp tissue, may be covered with stratified squamous epithelium
   2. Acute and chronic inflammatory cells present
   3. Granulation tissue
F. Treatment and prognosis
   1. Endodontic treatment of involved tooth
   2. Extraction of unrestorable tooth
   3. Prognosis—good

## Internal Resorption

A. Etiology—unknown but may be related to:

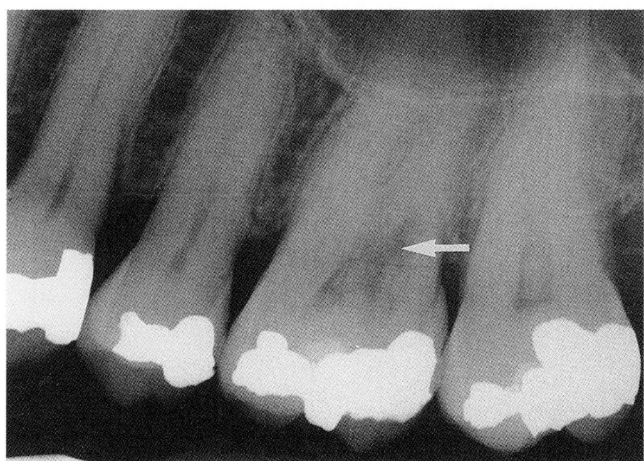

**Fig. 8.12** Radiograph showing an area of internal resorption on the maxillary first molar *(arrow)*. (From Ibsen OAC, Phelan JA. *Oral Pathology for the Dental Hygienist*. 6th ed. St. Louis: Elsevier Saunders; 2014.)

1. Pulpal trauma or injury
2. Inflammatory response to caries

B. Age and gender—any age; no gender predilection
C. Location—within pulp chamber or canal, most frequently in permanent dentition
D. Clinical features
   1. Benign but aggressive process that early on may only be detected radiographically
   2. Crown may display pink spot or coloration ("pink tooth of Mummery") when expanding highly vascularized pulpal tissues approach and show through enamel surface
E. Radiographic appearance—defined radiolucency within enlarging pulp chamber or root canal, reflecting resorption and loss of hard tissue—initially dentin (Fig. 8.12)
F. Histologic characteristics—highly vascularized pulpal tissue with increased odontoclastic activity adjacent to dentin-pulp interface (odontoclasts are tooth resorbing cells), chronic inflammation
G. Treatment—process may perforate through root or crown, results in tooth extraction; endodontic therapy useful to stop process if perforation has not occurred

### Apical Granuloma (Periapical Granuloma, Chronic Apical Periodontitis)

A. Etiology—dental caries, deep restorations, trauma; a response to pulpal necrosis
B. Age and gender—any age; no gender predilection
C. Location—apex of a nonvital tooth
D. Clinical features
   1. Benign condition associated with nonvital tooth
   2. Fistula or parulis may be present if condition is long-standing
   3. Affected tooth most often asymptomatic, may be sensitive to percussion
E. Radiographic appearance—varies from well-defined, circular, radiolucent lesion at apex of involved tooth to diffuse radiolucency or thickening of periodontal ligament space (Fig. 8.13A)
F. Histologic characteristics (Fig. 8.13B)
   1. Inflammatory response: lymphocytes, plasma cells, macrophages
   2. Dense, fibrous connective tissue
   3. Residual epithelial rests (remnants of tooth-forming tissues), but *no* epithelial lining
G. Treatment—endodontic therapy or extraction of affected tooth

## BENIGN BONE LESIONS

### General Characteristics

A. Etiology—most often unknown, but may have hereditary component
B. Onset—gradual, with slow development or enlargement
C. Early stages—asymptomatic
D. Bone expansion may result in malocclusion or thinning of cortical bone

### Osteoma

A. Etiology—unknown, can be associated with autosomal dominant condition; Gardner's syndrome
B. Age and gender—more common in young adults but can be found at any age; no gender predilection
C. Location—most common posterior mandible; rarely seen outside bones of head and neck; most often arises on bone surface
D. Clinical features— benign tumor of compact bone; asymptomatic, grows slowly; detected by palpation
E. Radiographic appearance
   1. Well-circumscribed radiopaque mass
   2. Panoramic or lateral plate radiograph may be needed to view entire lesion (Fig. 8.14)
F. Histologic characteristics—extremely dense, compact bone or coarse, cancellous bone
   1. Compact osteomas—radiopaque, have minimal marrow tissue
   2. Cancellous osteomas—have fibrofatty marrow, may have radiolucent center
G. Treatment and prognosis
   1. Surgical excision for large lesions
   2. Does not recur

### Chondroma

A. Etiology—unknown, multiple chondromas may be associated with inherited disorders
B. Age and gender—ages 30 to 40 years; no gender predilection
C. Location
   1. Rare in oral cavity
   2. Occur in body locations where normal cartilage is found
   3. May involve body of the mandible, coronoid or condylar process
D. Clinical features
   1. Benign tumors of mature cartilage; asymptomatic
   2. Slow, progressive swelling of the jaw may loosen or malposition teeth
   3. Malignant transformation in oral lesions considered rare
E. Radiographic appearance—irregular radiolucent or mottled; may displace surrounding teeth or cause root resorption
F. Histologic characteristics
   1. Composed of well-differentiated hyaline cartilage with foci of calcification
   2. Mature cartilage cells occur individually with lacunae

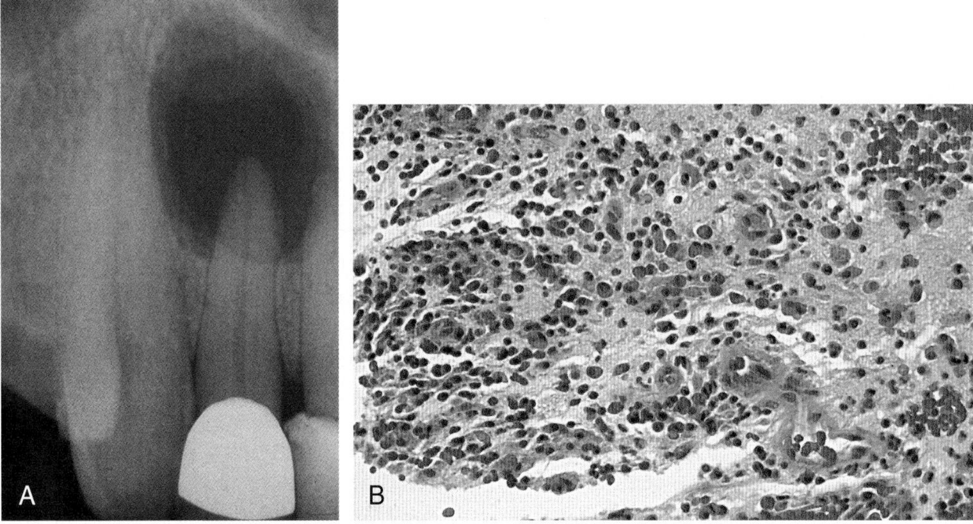


**Fig. 8.13 A,** Radiograph of a periapical granuloma. **B,** Low-power microscopic appearance of a periapical granuloma. (A, From Neville B, Damm DD, Allen CM, et al. Color Atlas of Oral and Maxillofacial Diseases. St Louis: Elsevier Inc.; 2019. B, From Neville B. Oral and Maxillofacial Pathology. 4th ed. St Louis: Elsevier Inc.; 2016.)

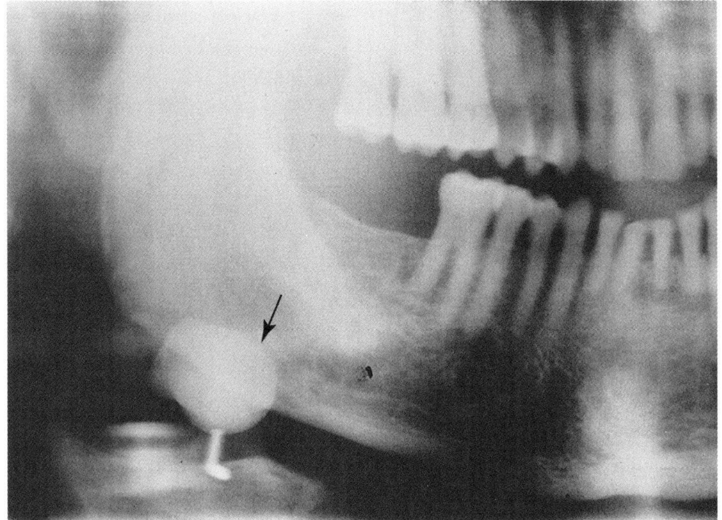

**Fig. 8.14** Radiograph of an osteoma showing a radiopacity *(arrow)* of the posterior mandible. (Courtesy of Dr. Sidney Eisig; from Ibsen OAC, Phelan JA. *Oral Pathology for the Dental Hygienist.* 6th ed. St. Louis: Elsevier Saunders; 2014.)

G. Treatment and prognosis
   1. Surgical removal indicated
   2. Clinical characteristics may mimic malignant chondrosarcoma, requires adequate biopsy sampling to rule out malignant neoplasm
   3. Periodic follow-up evaluation is necessary to detect recurrence, or rare development of chondrosarcoma

## Odontogenic Myxoma

A. Etiology—unknown; odontogenic neoplasm that originates from mesenchymal tissue of tooth germ
B. Age and gender—most often in young adults, ages 10 to 30 years; no gender predilection
C. Location—mandible more often than maxilla
D. Clinical features—benign but aggressive lesion within bone; small lesions asymptomatic, expansion of bone with larger lesions
E. Radiographic appearance (Fig. 8.15)

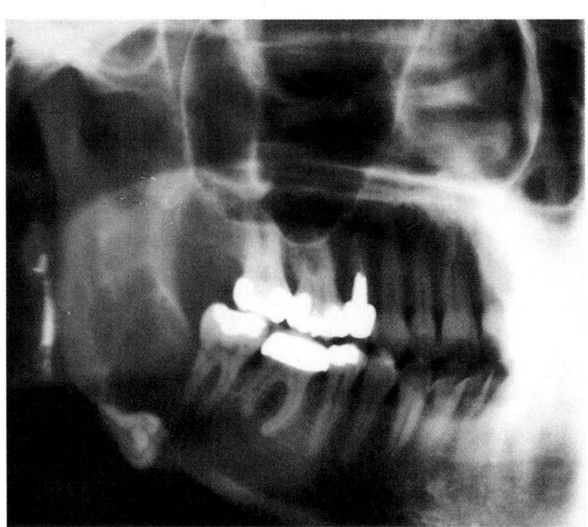

**Fig. 8.15** Radiograph of a myxoma showing multilocular, honeycombed radiolucency. (From Regezi J, Sciubba J, Jordan RCK. *Oral Pathology: Clinical Pathologic Correlations.* 7th ed. St. Louis: Elsevier Saunders; 2017.)

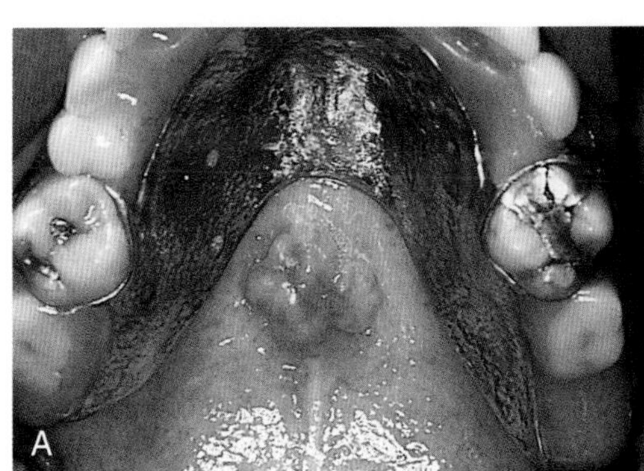
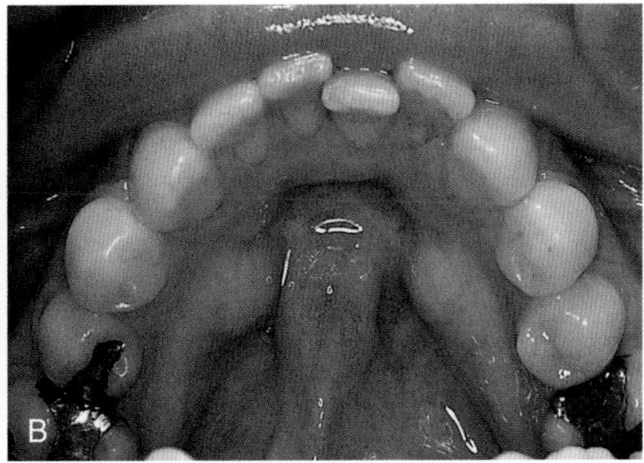

**Fig. 8.16** (A) Clinical appearance of a lobulated torus palatinus. (B) Clinical appearance of bilateral mandibular tori. (From Odell E. *Cawson's Essentials of Oral Pathology and Oral Medicine.* 9th ed. Elsevier; 2017.)

1. Unilocular or multilocular radiolucency, may have "honeycomb" or "soap bubble" appearance
2. Displacement or resorption of adjacent teeth may occur
3. Margins are irregular, diffuse, and not well defined
4. Large lesions may have appearance similar to ameloblastoma

F. Histologic characteristics
1. Loose myxoid stroma containing stellate, spindle-shaped, and round cells
2. Tumor not encapsulated, see infiltration of adjacent tissues

G. Treatment and prognosis
1. Complete surgical excision difficult
2. Recurrence is common (25%), metastasis does not occur

## Torus Palatinus

A. Etiology—inherited, autosomal dominant; genetic and/or environmental factors

B. Age and gender—usually seen by the age of puberty; rarely observed in children, peak incidence occurs before 30 years; more common in females (2:1)

C. Location—midline of the hard palate

D. Clinical features (Fig. 8.16A)
1. Benign hard protuberance of bone in midline of hard palate
2. Variety of shapes—nodular; lobulated; smooth (flat); spindle
3. Occurs in 20% to 35% of US population
4. Torus may appear ulcerated, due to trauma of thin overlying mucosa

E. Radiographic appearance—dense radiopaque area

F. Histologic characteristics—dense lamellar cortical bone

G. Treatment—usually none, surgical removal indicated if interferes with maxillary denture or other prosthodontic appliance

## Torus Mandibularis

A. Etiology—inherited, autosomal dominant; genetic and/or environmental factors

B. Age and gender—first observed in early teen years; slightly more common in males

C. Location—lingual surface of the mandible above the mylohyoid line in area of premolars; most often bilateral

D. Clinical features (Fig. 8.16B)
1. Benign protuberance of bone, varies in size and shape
2. Nodular, lobulated, or smooth; slow growing
3. Most often occur bilaterally (90%)

E. Radiographic appearance—dense radiopaque area

F. Histologic characteristics—dense cortical lamellar bone

G. Treatment—surgical excision if the lesion interferes with mandibular denture or other prosthodontic appliance

## Odontoma

A. Etiology—odontogenic origin, arises from odontogenic epithelium and mesenchyme that gives rise to teeth

B. Age and gender—usually seen in adolescents and young adults, mean age 14 years; no gender predilection

C. Location—more frequently seen in maxilla (especially anterior maxilla for compound type) than in the mandible; usually between the roots of teeth or near apices; complex odontomas seen more often in posterior mandible

D. Clinical features
1. Most common type of benign odontogenic "tumor"
2. Often associated with failure of a permanent tooth to erupt, blocks eruption pathway
3. Asymptomatic
4. Composed tooth hard tissues and pulp, not considered a true neoplasm

E. Radiographic appearance—irregular mass of radiopacities or tooth-like structures surrounded by a narrow radiolucent halo
1. Cyst involvement may occur in association with an odontoma
2. Two types of odontomas
   a. Compound—tooth-like structures ("toothlets") are identified radiographically (Fig. 8.17)
   b. Complex—appears as a radiopaque mass (can be confused with other lesions in bone) (Fig. 8.18)

F. Histologic characteristics—epithelial and mesenchymal differentiation of odontogenic tissues, result is disorganized formation of dental hard tissues and pulp

G. Treatment and prognosis
1. Complete surgical removal (both forms are well encapsulated)
2. Prognosis—good

# GINGIVAL FIBROMATOSES

## General Characteristics

A. Enlargement of gingival tissue, sometimes completely covering tooth crowns

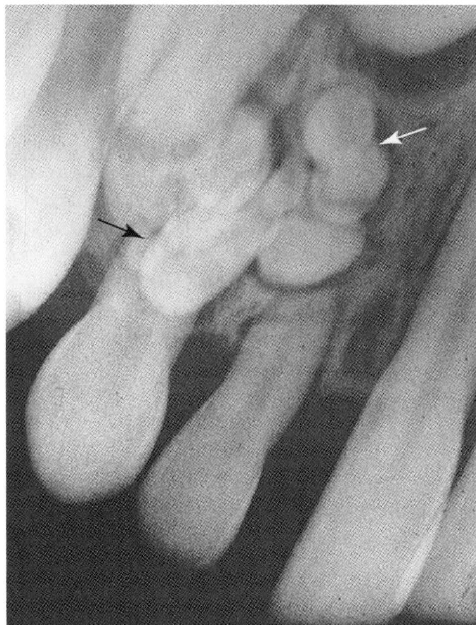

**Fig. 8.17** Radiograph of a compound odontoma, showing a collection of numerous, small, tooth-like radiopacities *(arrows)* surrounded by a radiolucent halo. (From Ibsen OAC, Phelan JA. *Oral Pathology for the Dental Hygienist.* 6th ed. St. Louis: Elsevier Saunders; 2014.)

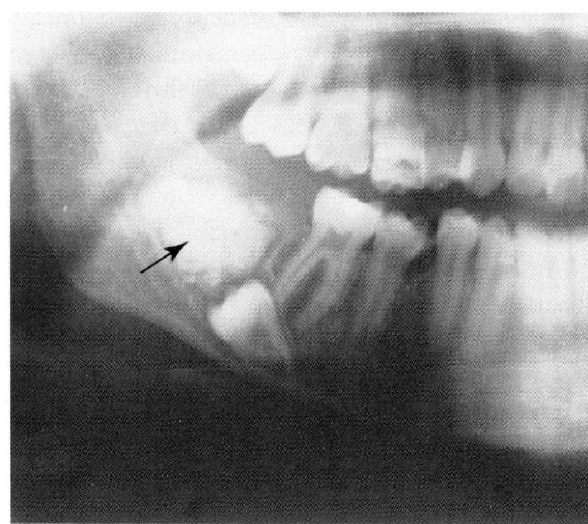

**Fig. 8.18** Radiograph of a complex odontoma showing a radiopaque mass surrounded by a radiolucent halo *(arrow)*. (From Ibsen OAC, Phelan JA. *Oral Pathology for the Dental Hygienist.* 6th ed. St. Louis: Elsevier Saunders; 2014.)

B. Composed of a proliferation of dense fibrous connective tissue
C. Classification includes:
   1. Irritative fibromatosis—localized areas of gingival enlargement, associated with outside irritants
   2. Hereditary fibromatosis—genetic-linked enlargement of gingival tissue
   3. Chemical fibromatosis—drug-influenced enlargement of gingival tissue

## Irritative Fibromatosis

A. Etiology—irritants such as mouth breathing, orthodontic appliances, bacterial plaque biofilm, dental calculus, debris, overhanging restorations, or ill-fitting dental appliances
B. Age and gender—any age; no gender predilection
C. Location—localized areas interproximal papillae; in mouth breathers, on maxillary and mandibular anterior labial gingiva
D. Clinical features—solitary round, smooth-surfaced, pink enlargement of gingival papillae; well attached to surrounding structures
E. Histologic characteristics—proliferation of dense fibrous connective tissue with increased numbers of fibroblasts and inflammatory response
F. Treatment and prognosis
   1. Removal of irritant
   2. Improved oral hygiene
   3. Gingivectomy in severe cases
   4. Prognosis is excellent, once cause is removed

## Hereditary Gingival Fibromatosis (Gingival Enlargement of Genetic Origin)

A. Etiology (see the section on "Genetics" in Chapter 7)
   1. Hereditary, believed to have genetic or developmental origin; or be related to hormonal imbalances; a component of multiple syndromes (e.g., Zimmerman-Laband, Cross, Rutherfurd, Murray-Puretic-Drescher, Cowden)
   2. Contributing factors include poor oral hygiene, food impaction, calculus, and malocclusion
   3. Other associated conditions include growth hormone deficiency, hypothyroidism, epilepsy, intellectual and developmental disabilities (IDDs)
B. Age and gender—appears during the eruption of primary or permanent teeth; slightly more common in females
C. Location—excessive enlargement of interproximal gingival tissues; can be localized; labial and buccal areas are most affected
D. Clinical features
   1. Gingival enlargement may be generalized or localized
   2. Diffuse, smooth-surfaced, pink, firm tissue involving the interproximal papillae
   3. Multiple protruding pink, stippled, firm masses; teeth may be displaced; delays eruption of teeth
E. Histologic characteristics—bundles of fibrous connective tissue with fibroblasts and fibrocytes (depending on the formative stage)
F. Treatment and prognosis
   1. Gingivectomy
   2. Meticulous oral hygiene
   3. Recurrence is common

## Chemical Fibromatosis (Drug-influenced Gingival Enlargement)

A. Etiology—reaction to drugs, specifically phenytoin (Dilantin); calcium channel blockers including nifedipine (Procardia), amlodipine (Norvasc), diltiazem (Cardizem), and verapamil (Calan); cyclosporin, an immunosuppressant drug given in association with organ transplants
B. Age and gender—no gender predilection
C. Location—gingiva, especially gingival papillae
D. Clinical features—smooth, pink, firm enlargement of the gingival papillae (Fig. 8.19A, B, and C)

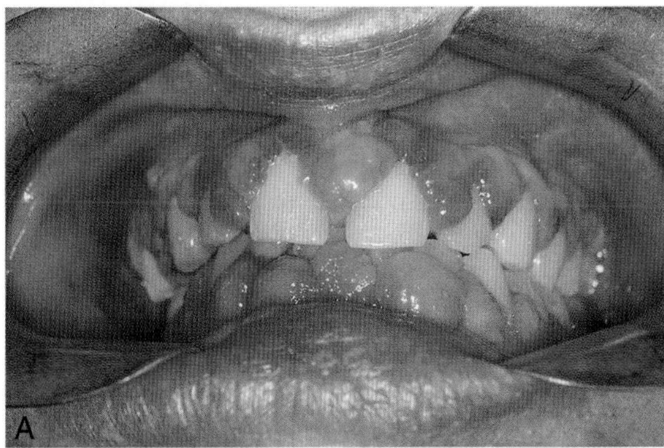


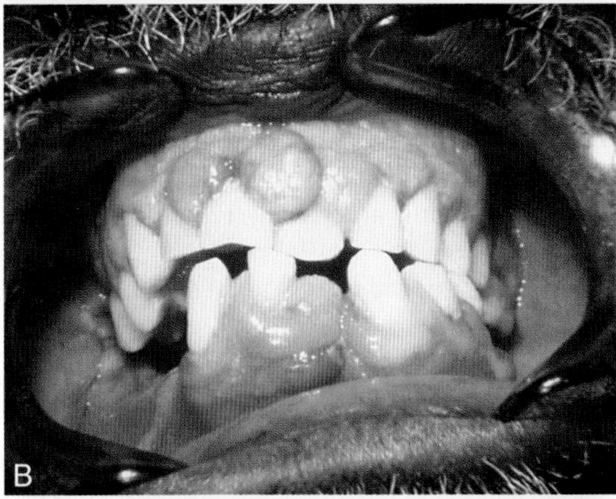


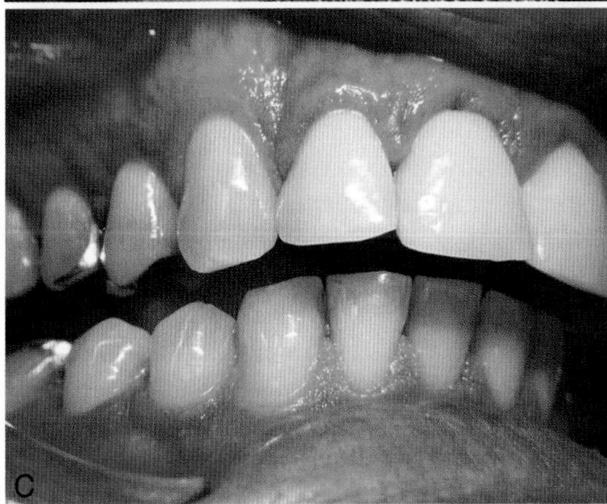


**Fig. 8.19** Drug-influenced gingival enlargement. (A) Gingival enlargement caused by phenytoin (Dilantin). (B) and (C) Gingival hyperplasia caused by nifedipine (Procardia). ((A) courtesy of Dr. Edward V. Zegarelli; (B) and (C) courtesy of Dr. Victor M. Sternberg; (A) to (C) from Ibsen OAC, Phelan JA. *Oral Pathology for the Dental Hygienist.* 6th ed. St. Louis: Elsevier Saunders; 2014.)

E. Histologic characteristics—extensive proliferation of connective tissue
F. Treatment
   1. Change prescribed medication, if possible
   2. Gingivectomy
   3. Improved oral hygiene, self-care

## ULCERS AND ULCERATIVE CONDITIONS

### General Characteristics

A. Ulcer—formed by destruction of surface epithelium and exposure of underlying connective tissue
B. Factors aiding in the diagnosis of ulcerative conditions and ulcer types occurring in the oral cavity include ulcer:
   1. Number and size
   2. Location
   3. Depth
   4. Borders
   5. Clinical history (personal, health, cultural, pharmacologic)
C. Etiology—not always known
D. Can be classified as acute or chronic
   1. Acute ulcerative conditions include traumatic ulcers, aphthous ulcers, allergic reactions, and viral ulcerations
   2. Chronic ulcerative conditions include those caused by or associated with systemic diseases such as leukemia, colitis, malnutrition, tuberculosis, syphilis, sickle cell anemia, and drug toxicity

### Traumatic Ulcer

A. Etiology—various types of trauma; history of lesion plays a significant role in determining the diagnosis
   1. Physical—biting or traumatizing the mucosa, ill-fitting denture, toothbrush injury, sharp tooth or fractured filling rubbing against soft tissue (Fig. 8.20A and B)
   2. Chemical—strong oral rinses, phenol, chemicals used during dental procedures, misuse of toothache medications (placement of aspirin adjacent to tooth may result in soft tissue burn) (Fig. 8.21A and B)
   3. Thermal—hot foods (e.g., soup) (Fig. 8.22A); crack cocaine (Fig. 8.22B)
   4. Electrical—especially in young children, electrical cords often contact commissures of mouth and lips
B. Age and gender—any age; no gender predilection
C. Location—most frequently lateral border of the tongue, buccal mucosa, lips, palate (tori especially vulnerable)
D. Clinical features
   1. Small, single, oval, round, or irregular shape
   2. Flat or slightly depressed
   3. Covered by necrotic debris or fibrinous coat, may be surrounded by erythematous halo
   4. Painful for 2 to 5 days
   5. Most heal within 7 to 14 days
E. Histologic characteristics
   1. Loss of surface epithelium (denuded)
   2. Fibrinous exudate covering exposed connective tissue
   3. Infiltration of PMNs within connective tissue
   4. Fibroblastic activity can be prominent feature
F. Treatment and prognosis
   1. Removal of the irritant or cause
   2. Application of benzocaine to relieve symptoms
   3. Corticosteroids (recommended by some, whereas others suggest corticosteroid medications can delay healing)
   4. Topical dyclonine hydrochloride for temporary relief
   5. Systemic antibiotics may be given in severe cases to prevent secondary infection (surgical debridement may be needed depending on extent of tissue damage)

6. With electrical burns, tetanus immunization advised
7. Caution with persistent chronic ulcerations; may need biopsy to rule out squamous cell carcinoma (SCC)
8. Prognosis—good

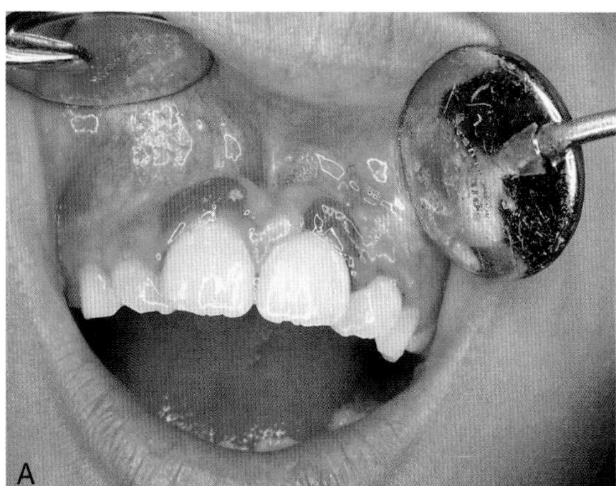

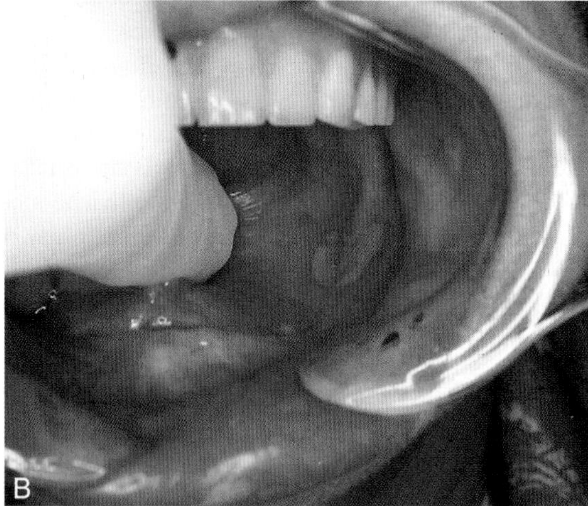

**Fig. 8.20** (A) Traumatic ulceration caused by irritation of gingiva by fingernails. (B) Traumatic ulcer caused by a denture. (From Ibsen OAC, Phelan JA. *Oral Pathology for the Dental Hygienist*. 6th ed. St. Louis: Elsevier Saunders; 2014.)

## Necrotizing Ulcerative Gingivitis (ANUG; Vincent's Infection, Trench Mouth)

The term acute necrotizing ulcerative gingivitis (ANUG) is often applied to this condition, due to its acute clinical presentation and rapid onset.

A. Etiology
   1. Anaerobic bacteria—spirochete and fusiform species, including *Fusobacterium nucleatum* (previously *Bacillus fusiformis*), *Borrelia vincentii*
   2. Recent technology identified involvement and contributions of other bacterial species
   3. Contributory factors
      a. Systemic—strong association between depressed systemic immunity and NUG, stress, fatigue, poor hygiene, malnutrition, recent illness
      b. Local—poor restorations, trauma, gingivitis, poor oral hygiene, heavy smoking

B. Age and gender—any age, usually 17 to 35 years; no gender predilection

C. Location—free gingival margin, crest of gingiva, interdental papillae

D. Clinical features (Fig. 8.23)
   1. Acute gingivitis with extensive tissue necrosis of interdental papillae
   2. Results in blunted, "punched-out," crater-like interdental spaces covered with gray pseudomembrane of necrotic tissue and debris
   3. Foul (fetid) mouth odor, intense gingival pain, spontaneous gingival bleeding, bad taste
   4. Headache, low-grade fever, malaise
   5. Regional lymphadenopathy
   6. May be seen in association with infectious mononucleosis

E. Histologic characteristics
   1. Ulcerated stratified squamous epithelium
   2. Thick fibrinous exudate containing PMNs
   3. Significant bacterial colonization
   4. Connective tissue infiltrated by dense numbers of inflammatory cells

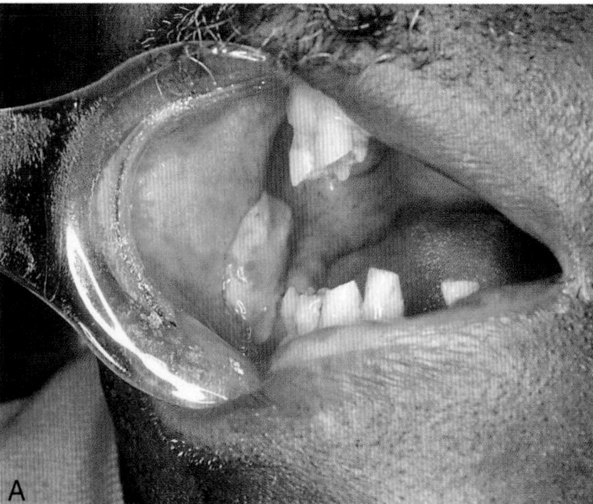

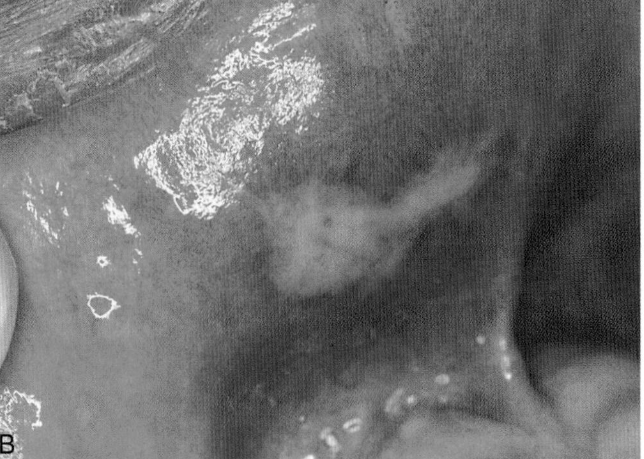

**Fig. 8.21** Mucosal burns. (A) Burns caused by aspirin. (B) Chemical burn caused by contact with caustic material during endodontic treatment. (From Ibsen OAC, Phelan JA. *Oral Pathology for the Dental Hygienist*. 6th ed. St. Louis: Elsevier Saunders; 2014.)

F. Treatment and prognosis
   1. Scaling and debridement (patient may need several visits)
   2. Use of ultrasonic instruments (except when contraindicated)

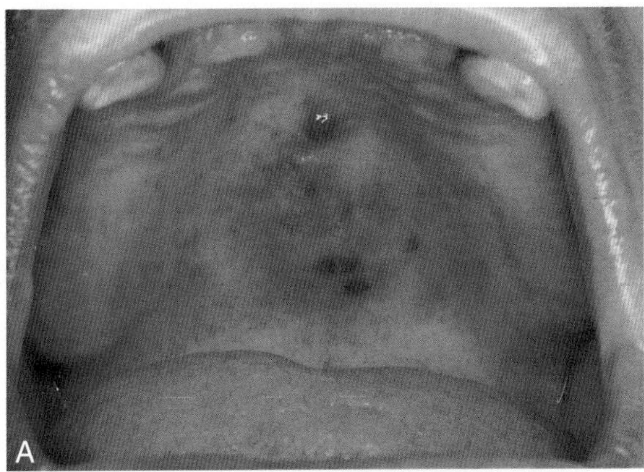

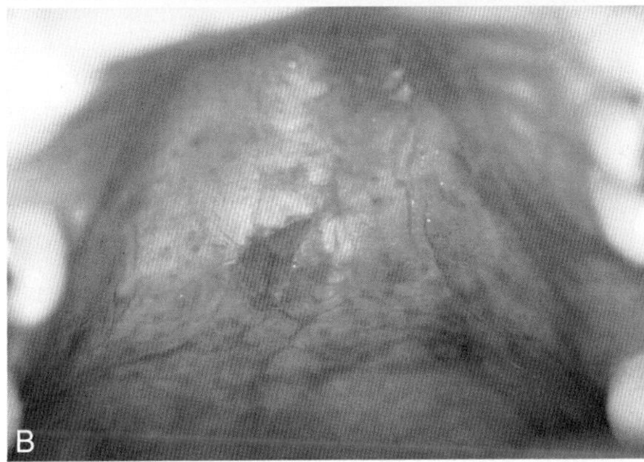

**Fig. 8.22** Mucosal burns. (A) Thermal burn of palate caused by contact with hot soup. (B) Ulcer of midline of palate caused by heat generated during the use of crack cocaine. ((A) from Ibsen OAC, Phelan JA. *Oral Pathology for the Dental Hygienist.* 6th ed. St. Louis: Elsevier Saunders; 2014. (B) from Mitchell-Lewis DA, Phelan JA, Kelly RB, Bradley JJ, Lamster IB. Identifying oral lesions associated with crack-cocaine use. *J Am Dent Assoc.* 1994: 125;1104.)

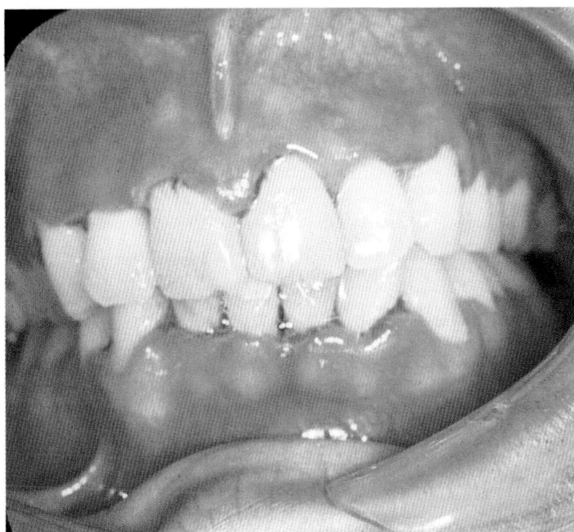

**Fig. 8.23** Necrotizing ulcerative gingivitis. (From Ibsen OAC, Phelan JA. *Oral Pathology for the Dental Hygienist.* 6th ed. St. Louis: Elsevier Saunders; 2014.)

   3. Topical or even local anesthetic may be necessary to perform treatment
   4. Use of an oxygenating rinse four or more times daily for 1 to 2 weeks
   5. Chlorhexidine rinses
   6. Use of systemic antibiotics such as penicillin, tetracycline, or erythromycin, may be indicated if patient has systemic signs or symptoms such as a fever, lymphadenopathy, or both; evaluation for infectious mononucleosis may be indicated
   7. Home care to improve oral hygiene status (e.g., power toothbrush, interdental cleaning)
   8. Follow-up appointments important to evaluate recovery and therapy, and reinforce oral self-care regimens
   9. Recurrences are possible if associated risk factors persist or return

## Recurrent Aphthous Stomatitis (RAU)/Recurrent Ulcerative Stomatitis (RUS)

A. Etiology
   1. Autoimmune inflammatory condition (T cell–mediated response)
   2. Destruction of mucosal tissue barrier, increased antigen exposure
   3. Inherited familial predisposition or acquired immunodysregulation
   4. Systemic disorders associated with aphthous stomatitis:
      a. Hormonal imbalance—premenstrual (incidence increases), pregnancy (incidence decreases)
      b. Psychological—anxiety, depression, acute emotional problems, stress
      c. Allergies—asthma, hay fever, food, drug
      d. Hematologic abnormalities
      e. Infectious agents (microorganisms)
      f. Behçet's disease
      g. Crohn's disease
      h. Ulcerative colitis
      i. Acquired or inherited immunodysregulation disorders such as cyclic neutropenia
      j. Celiac disease (Sprue)

B. Age and gender—childhood to adolescence and young adults; more common in females

C. Location—buccal and labial mucosa, soft palate, pharynx, tongue; more common in the anterior regions

D. Clinical features (Fig. 8.24)
   1. Ulcerations—oval or round in shape with distinct borders; the center of the ulcer has yellowish to white fibrinous surface, surrounded by an erythematous (red) halo
   2. Range from 1 to 12 in number (3 to 10 most common)
   3. Size—3 to 10 mm
   4. Pain out of proportion to small size of lesion, tenderness, discomfort
   5. Interference with functions—speech, eating
   6. Prodromal period of 1 to 2 days; characterized by tingling or burning sensation in area where ulcer will appear
   7. Associated systemic signs can include low-grade fever and localized lymphadenopathy

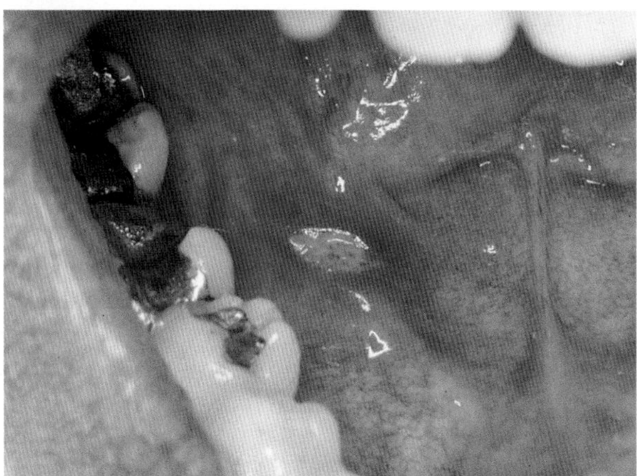

**Fig. 8.24** Example of a minor aphthous ulcer. (From Ibsen OAC, Phelan JA. *Oral Pathology for the Dental Hygienist.* 6th ed. St. Louis: Elsevier Saunders; 2014.)

E. Histologic characteristics
   1. Superficial erosion of mucosal tissue covered by fibrinopurulent layer
   2. Connective tissue demonstrates increased vascularity
   3. Increase in PMNs, lymphocytes, and histiocytes
F. Treatment and prognosis
   1. Self-limiting, healing in 10 to 12 days; recurrent episodes common
   2. Topical corticosteroids; chlorhexidine rinse; topical tetracyclines
   3. Betamethasone syrup (rinse and expectorate)

## Recurrent Major Aphthous Ulcers (Periadenitis Mucosa Necrotica Recurrens; Sutton's Disease)

A. Etiology
   1. Autoimmune inflammatory condition (T cell–mediated response)
   2. Destruction of mucosal tissue barrier, increased antigen exposure
   3. Inherited predisposition or acquired immunodysregulation (e.g., human immunodeficiency virus [HIV], acquired immunodeficiency syndrome [AIDS])
B. Age and gender—usually young adults, onset after puberty; more common in females
C. Location—labial mucosa, buccal mucosa, soft palate, posterior fauces
D. Clinical features (Fig. 8.25)
   1. More common in patients with HIV
   2. Single or multiple large ulcers, 1 to 10 in number and 1 to 3 cm in diameter
   3. Crater-like formations with irregular shapes
   4. Lesions heal in 3 to 6 weeks, may produce scarring
   5. Extremely painful
   6. Occur at frequent intervals; patient is rarely without an ulcer
E. Histologic characteristics
   1. Fibrinopurulent membrane covering large ulcerated area
   2. Necrotic epithelium
   3. Intense inflammatory cell infiltration within connective tissue

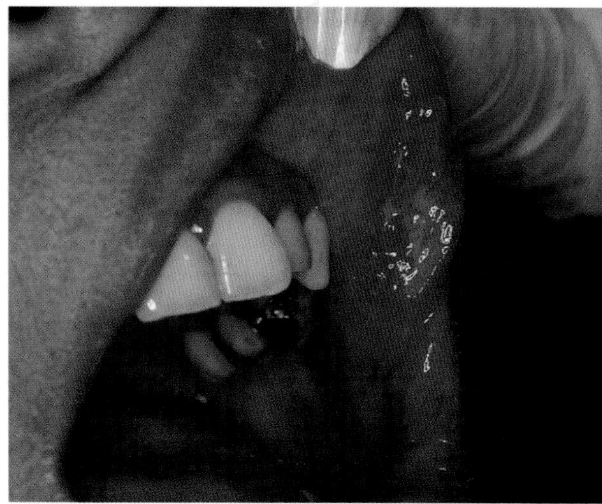

**Fig. 8.25** Example of major aphthous ulcers located on the labial mucosa. (From Ibsen OAC, Phelan JA. *Oral Pathology for the Dental Hygienist.* 6th ed. St. Louis: Elsevier Saunders; 2014.)

   4. Neutrophils and lymphocytes present
   5. Granulation tissue present at base of the lesion
   6. Microscopic picture nonspecific; definitive diagnosis must include clinical and historical data
F. Treatment and prognosis
   1. Corticosteroids (systemic or topical)
   2. Injection of lesion with triamcinolone acetonide
   3. Halobetasol propionate ointment
   4. Healing takes weeks to months
   5. Recurrence is common

## Mucous Membrane Pemphigoid (Cicatricial Pemphigoid, Benign Mucous Membrane Pemphigoid)

A. Etiology—autoimmune disease; type 2 hypersensitivity reaction to specific protein in basement membrane of epithelium (laminins)
B. Age and gender—ages 50 to 65 years; more common in females (2:1)
C. Location
   1. Gingiva
   2. Oral mucous membranes
   3. Eyes, nasal, esophageal, and vaginal mucosa
   4. Skin
D. Clinical features
   1. Vesicles or bullous lesions that rupture, leave denuded (desquamated) painful exposed connective tissue on mucosa or skin
   2. "Desquamative" gingivitis with sloughing of oral mucosa is a generic term, not solely descriptive of this condition
   3. Painful scarring of eye conjunctiva may occur leading to scarring; cicatricial (cicatrix = scar)
E. Histologic characteristics (Fig. 8.26)
   1. Split forms between surface epithelium and underlying connective tissue at basement membrane, subepithelial vesicles and bullae
   2. Epithelium appears to be detached from connective tissue

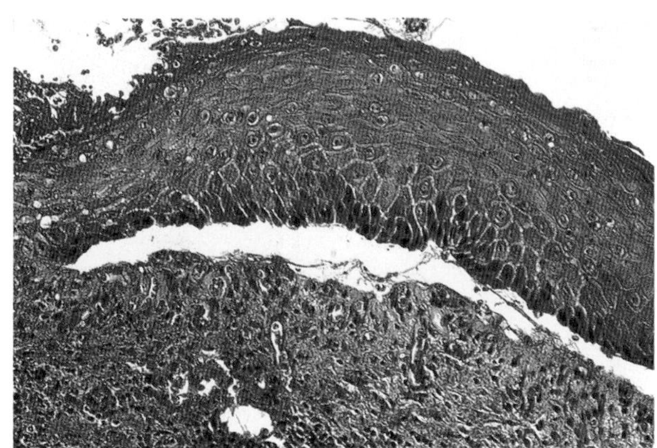

**Fig. 8.26** Histologic appearance of pemphigoid. (From Ibsen OAC, Phelan JA. *Oral Pathology for the Dental Hygienist.* 6th ed. St. Louis: Elsevier Saunders; 2014.)

3. Mild trauma may induce vesicle or bulla formation, phenomenon known as Nikolsky's sign
4. No evidence of acantholysis (degeneration of cohesive elements between epithelial cells, as seen in pemphigus)
5. Inflammatory infiltrate within connective tissue
6. Direct immunofluorescence shows a linear pattern of staining at basement membrane

F. Treatment and prognosis
1. Mild forms—topical corticosteroids, may be applied to oral mucosa in fabricated custom trays
2. High doses of systemic corticosteroids may be indicated with severe bullous eruptions
3. Early referral to ophthalmologist required since eye involvement can evolve to be severe. may not show symptoms in early stages
4. Conjunctiva of eye may be affected with scarring (called symblepharon); can result in blindness
5. Patients go through periods of remission; long-term disease progression

## VIRAL INFECTIONS

### General Characteristics of Herpes Simplex Virus (HSV) Infections

1. Type I: commonly affects face and oral cavity
2. Type 2: sexually transmitted form of virus, mostly genital mucosa
3. Common features: latency, prodromal signs and symptoms

#### Primary Herpetic Gingivostomatitis

A. Etiology
1. Virus—initial infection (first encounter) with HSV
2. Member of the human herpesvirus (HHV) group
3. Transmission—droplet infection; direct contact; highly contagious (amount of virus is highest in the vesicle stage); patients can self-inoculate, spread to other areas of skin or mucous membranes (especially the eyes)

B. Age and gender—ages 6 months to 6 years; no gender predilection

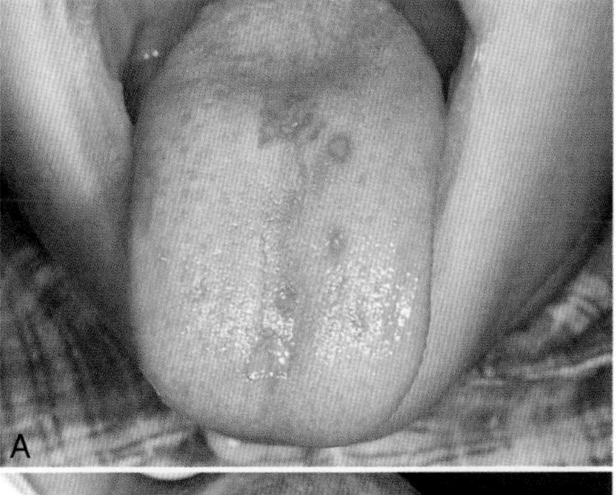

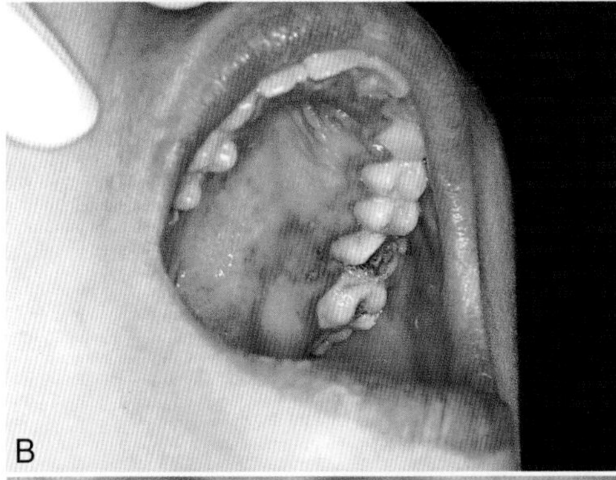

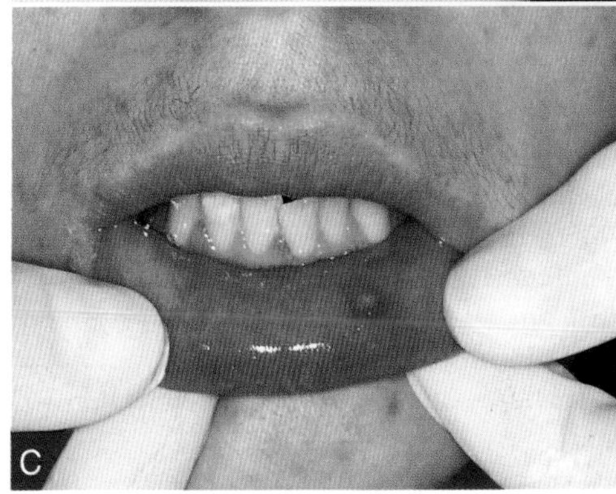

**Fig. 8.27** (A) Example of primary herpetic gingivostomatitis in a child. (B) and (C) Primary herpetic gingivostomatitis in an adolescent. ((A) courtesy of Dr. Edward V. Zegarelli; A to C from Ibsen OAC, Phelan JA. *Oral Pathology for the Dental Hygienist.* 6th ed. St. Louis: Elsevier Saunders; 2014.)

C. Location—lips, gingiva, tongue, pharynx, floor of the mouth, buccal mucosa

D. Clinical features (Fig. 8.27A, B, and C)
1. Systemic signs and symptoms
   a. Abrupt onset of fever
   b. Headache, irritability
   c. Regional lymphadenopathy
2. Oral signs and symptoms
   a. Gingivitis, sore mouth, pain on swallowing
   b. Initially, tiny vesicles (pinhead size) quickly rupture to form ulcerations
   c. Painful ulcers 1 to 3 mm in size; covered by a yellow fibrinous surface
   d. May coalesce to form shallow craters with bright erythematous margins ("halo")
   e. Most acute phase is days 3 to 7

E. Laboratory tests and findings
   1. Cytologic smear (noninvasive and inexpensive test)
   2. Blood test for HSV
   3. Viral isolation from tissue culture (best diagnostic procedure, but up to 2 weeks to obtain results)
F. Histologic characteristics
   1. Intraepithelial vesicles filled with fluid
   2. Cells show "ballooning" degeneration
   3. Acantholysis of epithelium with formation of Tzanck cells
G. Treatment and prognosis
   1. Symptomatic therapy—bed rest, fluids (to prevent dehydration especially very young children)
   2. Antiviral medications such as acyclovir ("swish and swallow") started within first few days
   3. Medications to reduce pain and discomfort
   4. Self-limiting; healing in 7 to 14 days
   5. Virus can remain dormant in (trigeminal or other) ganglion
   6. Recurrence not usual for primary herpes

## Herpes Labialis (Secondary or Recurrent Herpes Simplex, Cold Sore, Fever Blister)

A. Etiology
   1. Reactivation of latent virus (HSV) residing in trigeminal ganglion
   2. Stimuli that can trigger reactivation include
      a. Exposure to sunlight
      b. Trauma (including dental treatment)
      c. Menstruation
      d. Emotional stress, anxiety, fatigue
      e. Allergic reactions
      f. Systemic diseases
B. Age and gender—adults; no gender predilection
C. Location
   1. Lips—most common (hence term: herpes labialis)
   2. Reactivation can also occur intraorally—hard palate, attached gingiva (keratinized mucosa fixed to bone)
D. Clinical features (Fig. 8.28A and B)
   1. Prodromal (before lesion erupts) sensation—burning, tingling, itching, or soreness in area where vesicles eventually will appear
   2. Fluid-filled vesicles (most contagious state); fluid contains virus
   3. Vesicles may appear in clusters, coalesce into a larger blister called a bulla (bullae pl.), eventually rupture and crust
   4. Danger via contaminated dental instruments for spread to fingers, hands of dental personnel (herpetic whitlow)
   5. Contact of virus with eye can lead to herpes eye disease and severe ocular complications
E. Histologic characteristics
   1. Intraepithelial blister (vesicle) filled with fluid; ruptures to leave ulcer
   2. Cells display "ballooning degeneration"
   3. Acantholysis of mucosa with formation of Tzanck cells (used to help diagnose a variety of cutaneous infectious and blistering diseases)

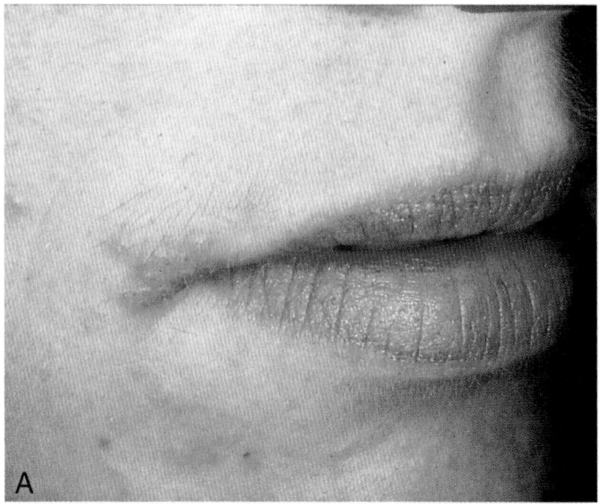


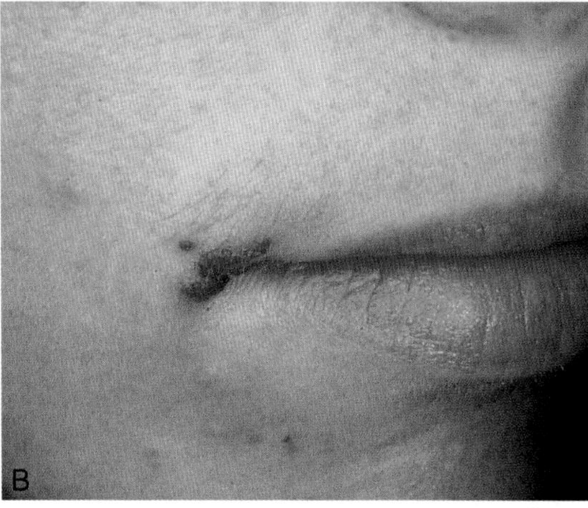


**Fig. 8.28** Herpes labialis. (A) Twelve hours after onset. B, Forty-eight hours after onset. (From Ibsen OAC, Phelan JA. *Oral Pathology for the Dental Hygienist.* 6th ed. St. Louis: Elsevier Saunders; 2014.)

F. Treatment and prognosis
   1. Antiviral drugs (e.g., acyclovir, valacyclovir) especially effective if given during the prodromal period
   2. Prophylactic treatment with antivirals before encountering risk factor
   3. Topical application of 10% n-docosanol cream has been effective
   4. Self-limiting; healing in 7 to 10 days
   5. Sunblock to prevent development on lips
   6. Chlorhexidine rinses, acyclovir suspension, or both can be helpful to treat intraoral recurrent HSV
   7. Recurrence common

## Herpes Zoster (Shingles)

A. Etiology
   1. Reactivation of latent varicella-zoster virus (VZV, HHV-3)
   2. VZV causes chickenpox, which is considered the primary infection with VZV
   3. Depression of cell-mediated immunity
   4. Risk factors important for reactivation of VZV
      a. Systemic disease (malignancies, Hodgkin's disease, leukemia)
      b. Drug toxicity, radiation, alcohol abuse
      c. Advanced age

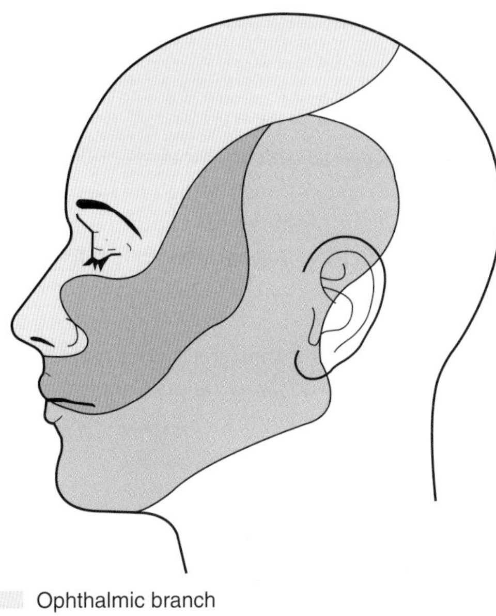


**Fig. 8.29** The divisions of the trigeminal nerve. (From Ibsen OAC, Phelan JA. *Oral Pathology for the Dental Hygienist.* 6th ed. St. Louis: Elsevier Saunders; 2014.)

   d. Extreme fatigue
   e. Immunosuppression

B. Age and gender—any age but more common in adults, usually over 50 years; no gender predilection
C. Location—skin or mucosa, supplied by affected sensory nerve; any of the three branches of trigeminal nerve (Fig. 8.29); most often has distinctive unilateral distribution (considered pathognomonic, meaning virtually diagnostic)
D. Clinical features (Fig. 8.30A, B, and C)
   1. Three phases—prodromal, acute, chronic
   2. Prodromal period 1 to 3 days before eruption of unilateral rash, pain which can be accompanied by systemic features such as fever, severe headaches, malaise, and lymphadenopathy
   3. Acute phase of erythematous rash, evolves into vesicles; pain becomes more intense with burning, tingling, or stabbing sensation
   4. Clusters of vesicles develop along the distribution pathway of a sensory nerve; vesicles contain virus and are considered infectious
   5. Intraoral lesions appear unilaterally as multiple vesicles with white centers, eventually form shallow ulcerations; on movable or attached mucosa
   6. Chronic phase of postherpetic neuralgia possible; residual effect after acute condition resolved
E. Treatment and prognosis
   1. Antiviral medications (acyclovir, valacyclovir, famciclovir)
   2. Postherpetic neuralgia difficult to treat; therapies utilized include analgesics, narcotics, corticosteroids, anticonvulsants; biofeedback, and nerve block
   3. Cutaneous vesicular lesions should be kept clean and dry to prevent secondary infection (antibiotics may be prescribed if secondary infection occurs)

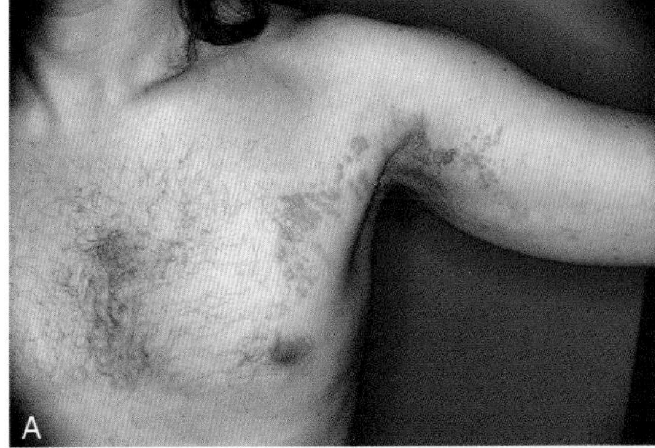


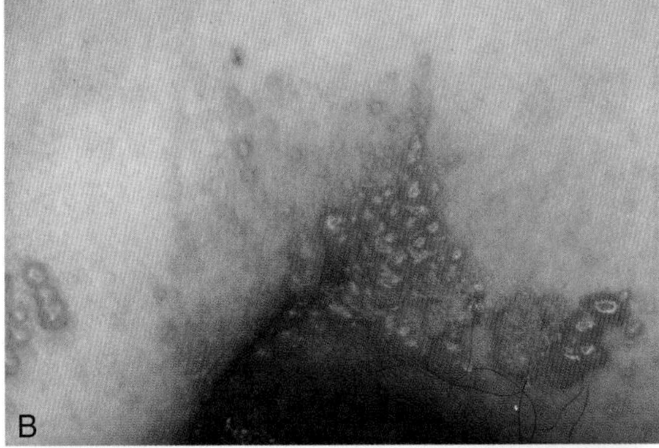


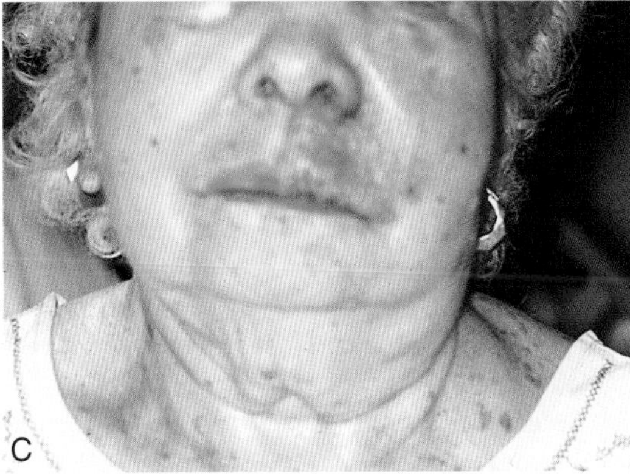


**Fig. 8.30** Herpes zoster. (A) Unilateral distribution of vesicles along the distribution of a sensory nerve. (B) Many vesicles coalesce to form large lesions. (C) Unilateral facial lesions occurring along the distribution of the maxillary branch of the trigeminal nerve. (From Ibsen OAC, Phelan JA. *Oral Pathology for the Dental Hygienist.* 6th ed. St. Louis: Elsevier Saunders; 2014.)

   4. Antibacterial oral rinses for intraoral lesions
   5. Varicella (chickenpox) vaccines are available for children and adults: Varivax for children, Zostavax for individuals 60 years and older; and Shingrix for healthy people over 50
   6. Ocular involvement serious complication when VZV affects maxillary division of trigeminal nerve, can result in blindness
   7. Prognosis is good in healthy individual, with healing in 2 to 3 weeks
   8. Recurrence can occur but not usual

## Herpangina

A. Etiology—coxsackievirus group A, and a number of other enteroviruses

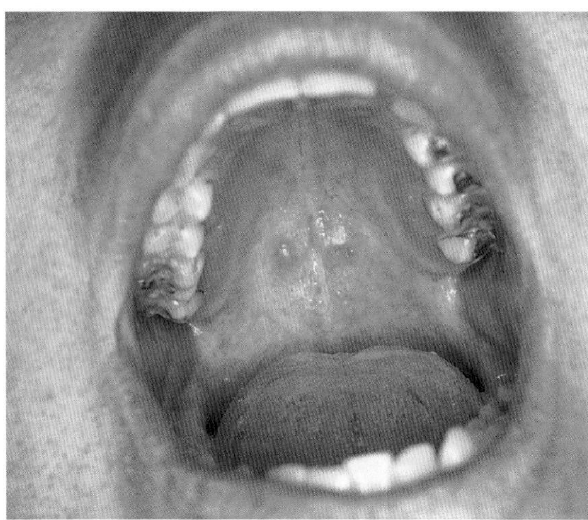

**Fig. 8.31** Herpangina. (From Ibsen OAC, Phelan JA. *Oral Pathology for the Dental Hygienist.* 6th ed. St. Louis: Elsevier Saunders; 2014.)

B. Age and gender—children age 6 months to 5 years; no gender predilection
C. Location—posterior hard or soft palate, fauces (pillars), uvula, tonsils; most likely seen in the summer
D. Clinical features
   1. Systemic symptoms
      a. Comparatively mild and of short duration
      b. Sore throat; dysphagia; headache
      c. Fever
      d. Headache; vomiting; diarrhea
      e. Transmission through fecal-oral route or contact with droplets from sneezing or coughing
   2. Oral symptoms (Fig. 8.31)
      a. Erythematous macules usually on soft palate or tonsillar areas
      b. Become fragile vesicles, rapidly ulcerate to form 2 to 4 mm size ulcers
      c. Vesicles are often overlooked
      d. Two to six small ulcers; ulcers appear with a gray base and inflamed periphery
      e. Slightly painful; the affected person has difficulty swallowing (dysphagia)
      f. Sudden onset—mild to moderate symptoms
      g. Erythematous pharynx
E. Laboratory tests
   1. Viral isolation (throat culture during early stage)
   2. Stool specimens
F. Treatment and prognosis
   1. Self-limiting, with few complications
   2. Nonaspirin pain relievers
   3. Usually resolves within 7 days without treatment
E. Hand, foot, and mouth disease is mild illness, also caused coxsackievirus group A, and a number of other enteroviruses; ulcers similar to herpangina can present in the throat, other locations in the mouth including tongue; skin of hands and feet affected and important for diagnosis

### Infectious Mononucleosis (Glandular Fever, "Kissing Disease")

A. Etiology
   1. Epstein-Barr virus (EBV, HHV-4)
   2. Transmission—via saliva; "kissing disease"; intimate contact, sharing drinking/eating utensils
B. Age and gender—predominantly young adults (15–24 age group); children (transmission through saliva on toys); no gender predilection
C. Clinical features
   1. Systemic signs and symptoms (depending on age)
      a. Fever, chills, prodromal fatigue, malaise
      b. Sore throat, pharyngitis, enlarged tonsils with pus
      c. Headache
      d. Nausea, vomiting
      e. Prominent lymphadenopathy—large tender nodes (however, in adults over 40, less than 30% exhibit lymphadenopathy)
      f. Enlarged spleen (danger of rupture)
      g. Neurologic disorders, including seizures
   2. Oral signs and symptoms
      a. Palatal petechiae (pinpoint hemorrhages)
      b. Pharyngitis, enlarged tonsils with white patches of pus
      c. May occur in association with necrotizing ulcerative gingivitis
      d. Inflamed attached gingiva, soft palate, and uvula
D. Laboratory tests and findings
   1. Increased white blood cells (WBCs) with atypical activated lymphocytes; presence of these atypical lymphocytes in peripheral blood is very characteristic
   2. Increased heterophil antibody titer; positive Paul-Bunnell test in young adults but not in children under 4 years old
   3. Indirect immunofluorescence test for EBV
E. Treatment and prognosis
   1. Bed rest
   2. Nonaspirin antipyretics and nonsteroidal antiinflammatory drugs (NSAIDs)
   3. Benign and self-limiting; fatigue may last longer
   4. Usually resolves in 4 to 6 weeks
   5. Complications can include splenic, hepatic, and neurologic involvement

## MUCOSAL AND SKIN DISORDERS

### General Characteristics

A. Characterized by various forms and sizes of ulcerative eruptions
B. Lesions may appear first or during the course of the disease
C. Reaction may simulate an allergic-type reaction

### Erythema Multiforme

A. Etiology
   1. Exact etiology unknown, thought to be a hypersensitivity reaction

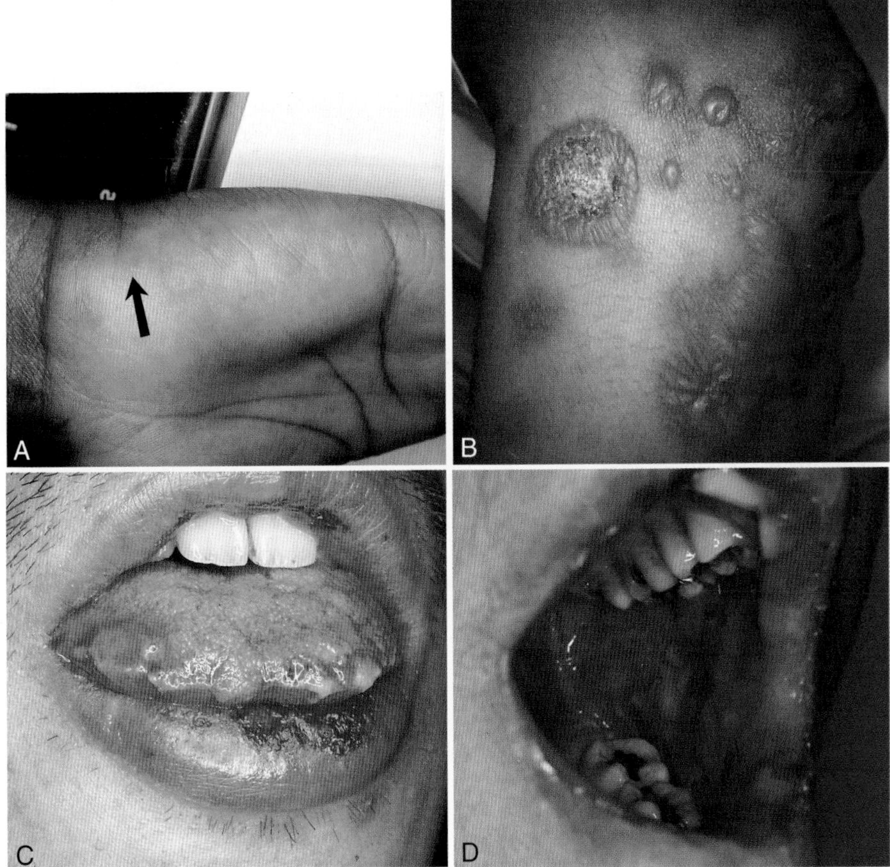


**Fig. 8.32** Skin lesions of erythema multiforme. (A) Target lesion *(arrow)*. (B) Bullae. (C) Crusted lip lesions with edema, ulceration, and erythema. (D) Erythematous and ulcerated lesions of the lips and buccal mucosa. (A courtesy of Dr. Edward V. Zegarelli; A to D from Ibsen OAC, Phelan JA. *Oral Pathology for the Dental Hygienist*. 6th ed. St. Louis: Elsevier Saunders; 2014.)

2. Approximately 50% have exposure to a known trigger such as previous HSV infection, other microorganisms such as *Mycoplasma pneumoniae*; drugs (e.g., antibiotics such as penicillins and cephalosporins, barbiturates, sulfonamides); in 50% specific trigger cannot be identified
3. Immunologic response

B. Age and gender—young adults ages 20 to 30 years; more common in males

C. Location
1. Extremities—hands, feet, arms, legs
2. Skin—macular, papular, or bullous eruptions; characteristic "target" or "bull's-eye" lesions in 50% of cases
3. Oral findings—lips, labial and buccal mucosa, tongue, floor of the mouth, soft palate

D. Clinical features (Fig. 8.32A, B, C, and D)
1. Systemic symptoms
   a. Abrupt onset
   b. Prodromal symptoms (e.g., fatigue, malaise, fever)
   c. May have had previous occurrences
   d. Has been seen in association with other systemic conditions
   e. Characteristic skin lesions referred to as *bull's-eye, target,* or *iris*
2. Oral symptoms
   a. Generally lips, tongue, and buccal mucosa
   b. Red patches develop into multiple, painful ulcerations; onset is explosive
   c. Macules, papules, or vesicles ulcerate and bleed easily
   d. Ulcer with raw tissue base and a grayish, necrotic slough
   e. Irregular shape; surrounded by a band of inflammation; encrustations
   f. Edema and extensive hemorrhagic crusting vermilion of lips

E. Laboratory tests—direct and indirect immunofluorescent studies not useful for definitive diagnosis; may be used to rule-out other vesiculobullous diseases

F. Histologic characteristics
1. Mixed inflammatory infiltrate
2. Intraepithelial or subepithelial vesicle formation
3. Necrotic basal keratinocytes
4. Histopathologic characteristics are nonspecific

G. Treatment and prognosis
1. Removal of the cause, if identified or suspected
2. Topical or systemic applications of corticosteroids
3. Mild antibacterial oral rinses; antibiotics if risk of secondary infection

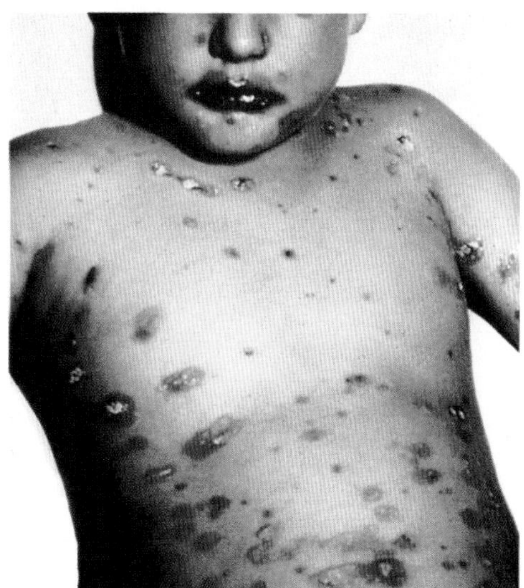

**Fig. 8.33** Stevens-Johnson syndrome. (Courtesy of Dr. Sidney Eisig; from Ibsen OAC, Phelan JA. *Oral Pathology for the Dental Hygienist.* 6th ed. St. Louis: Elsevier Saunders; 2014.)

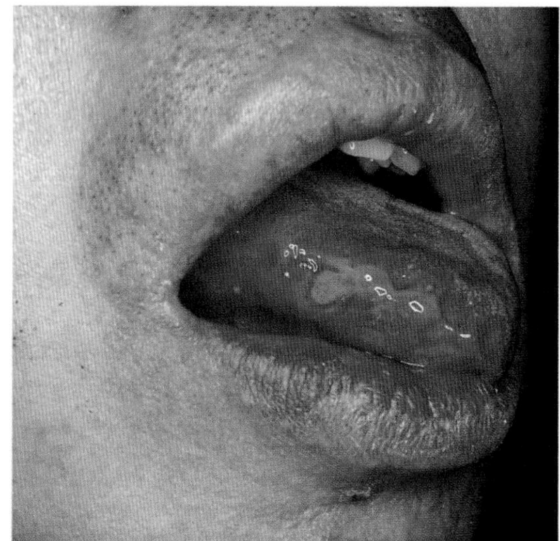

**Fig. 8.34** Oral lesion seen in Behçet syndrome. Aphthous-like oral mucosal ulcer. (From Ibsen OAC, Phelan JA. *Oral Pathology for the Dental Hygienist.* 6th ed. St. Louis: Elsevier Saunders; 2014.)

4. Intravenous rehydration may be necessary if cannot drink fluids or eat due to significant oral pain
5. Condition resolves in 2 to 4 weeks
6. Recurrence is possible

## Stevens-Johnson Syndrome (Erythema Multiforme Major)

A. Severe bullous form of erythema multiforme
B. Etiology—unknown; most often triggered by a drug rather than an infection
C. Age and gender—children and young adults under 25 years; more common in males; history of previous similar illness
D. Location—oral cavity, skin; in addition lesions involving the eyes or genitals must be present for this diagnosis
E. Clinical features (Fig. 8.33)
   1. Oral symptoms—bullae rupture, leaving ulcerations with a raw base; eating becomes impossible; lips are severely encrusted and bleed easily
   2. Skin lesions—severe, numerous; cover wide areas of the body (face, chest, abdomen)
   3. Eye involvement—severe conjunctivitis, photophobia, corneal ulceration, scarring, and potential for blindness
   4. High risk for severe dehydration
F. Treatment and prognosis
   1. Antibiotics and corticosteroids to control severity
   2. Antiviral medications to reduce recurrent episodes if HSV infection a trigger
   3. Duration of 1 to 4 weeks
   4. May require hospitalization
   5. Prognosis is usually good
   6. Mortality rate is 2% to 10% with this form of erythema multiforme

## Behçet's Disease

A. Etiology—rare disease of unknown etiology, persons with HLA-B51 antigen, a gene in immune system, are predisposed to this condition
B. Age and gender—young adults, no gender predilection
C. Location—now considered a multisystem disorder, Behçet's disease is characterized by triad of affected areas: oral, ocular, and genital areas are involved; two of the three areas must be involved for the diagnosis
   1. Oral cavity—oral lesions first manifestation in majority of cases
   2. Eyes are involved in up to 85% of cases, with greater severity in men
   3. Genital lesions occur in 75% of cases, with more symptoms reported in men
D. Clinical features (Fig. 8.34)
   1. Oral lesions
      a. Painful ulcerations similar to minor or major aphthous ulcers, occur in about 40% of Behçet patients (3% of these have herpetiform variety of ulcers)
      b. Large ulcers with gray or yellow center surrounded by a red border
      c. Oral ulcerations involve the soft palate and oropharynx
   2. Eye lesions
      a. Begin with photophobia and irritation
      b. Purulent conjunctivitis and uveitis
      c. Healing may be followed by scar formation and blindness
      d. Hypopyon (pus in anterior chamber of eye between iris and cornea) in severe cases; rare
   3. Genital lesions
      a. In females—painful ulcerations in the vagina, vulval folds, and labia majora
      b. In males—painful ulcerations on the scrotum and base of the penis
   4. Systemic signs and symptoms
      a. Occasionally fever; pallor
      b. Complications can involve the central nervous system (CNS), cardiac, vascular, and pulmonary systems
      c. Arthritis involving knees, wrists, elbows, and ankles

E. Laboratory tests and findings
   1. No laboratory test is diagnostic; however, cutaneous pathergy test is often positive
   2. Definitive clinical criteria for diagnosis have been established
F. Histologic characteristics
   1. Histopathologic features are nonspecific
   2. Endothelial proliferation in lesions
   3. Characteristics similar to those in aphthous stomatitis
G. Treatment and prognosis
   1. Early aggressive therapy for patients with severe clinical manifestations
   2. Systemic and topical corticosteroids
   3. Other immunosuppressive drugs are given for systemic and ocular involvement
   4. Lesions last 2 to 4 weeks
   5. Disease is long lasting with periods of remission
   6. Mortality is low; most often associated with CNS involvement, pulmonary hemorrhage or bowel perforation

## Pemphigus Vulgaris

A. Etiology—severe, progressive autoimmune disease that affects skin and mucous membranes
B. Age and gender—adults, usually between ages 40 and 55 years; no gender predilection
   1. More common in Ashkenazic Jews, South Asians, or persons of Mediterranean descent
C. Location—anywhere on oral mucosa; eyes, or skin
D. Clinical features (Fig. 8.35A and B)
   1. In over 50% of cases, oral lesions appear first; skin lesions can erupt many months or even a year later
   2. Blisters, vesicles, or bullae (caused by an abnormal production of autoantibodies) collapse as soon as they are formed
      a. Vary in shape and size (from several millimeters to several centimeters)
      b. Ragged peripheral borders; flat or shallow; base intensely red and raw; may extend into lips with crusting
   3. Necrotic film or slough of tissue can be detached from underlying tissue
   4. Neighboring soft tissue appears normal
   5. Positive Nikolsky's sign—an intraoral bulla can form under light pressure or slight rubbing with cotton swab or tongue blade; same reaction can occur if pressure is applied to skin
   6. Pain may be severe with inability to eat
   7. Salivation may be profuse; mouth odor
   8. Gingival desquamation (sloughing)
E. Laboratory tests and findings
   1. Biopsy with microscopic analysis
   2. Direct immunofluorescence used to identify antibodies (intercellular)
   3. Indirect immunofluorescence positive in 80% to 90%, shows circulating autoantibodies in serum; may be used to monitor progress of therapy
F. Histologic characteristics

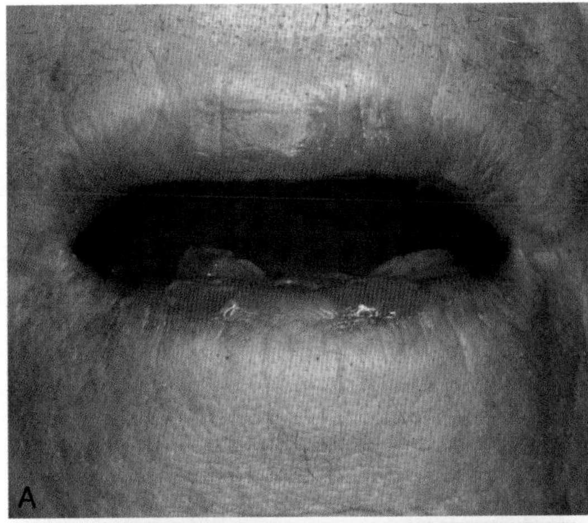


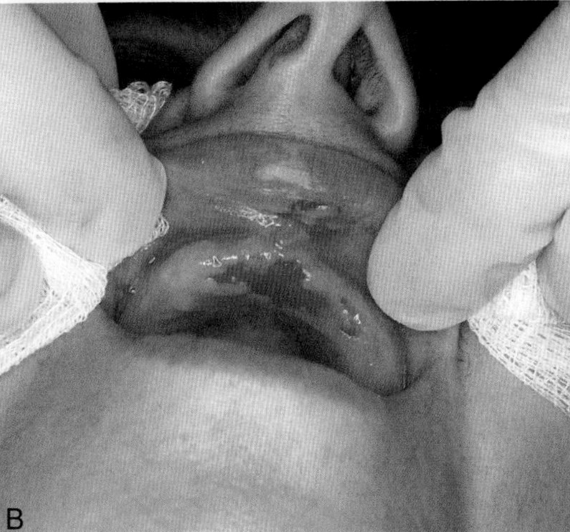


**Fig. 8.35** (A) and (B) Examples of oral lesions in pemphigus vulgaris. ((B) courtesy of Dr. Fariba Younai; (A) and (B) from Ibsen OAC, Phelan JA. *Oral Pathology for the Dental Hygienist*. 6th ed. St. Louis: Elsevier Saunders; 2014.)

   1. Vesicle or bulla entirely intraepithelial, above the basal cell layer, produces a distinctive "split"; basement layer remains attached to underlying connective tissue
   2. Intercellular bridges between epithelial cells disappear, with loss of cohesiveness; epithelial cells separate (acantholysis)
   3. Clumps of enlarged epithelial cells, termed Tzanck cells, are present
   4. Inflammatory cell infiltration in underlying connective tissue
G. Treatment and prognosis
   1. Systemic corticosteroids (prednisone)
   2. Other immunosuppressive drugs such as azathioprine and methotrexate may be used in addition to corticosteroids
   3. Titers of circulating autoantibodies measured using indirect immunofluorescence
   4. Periods of remission; but never a "cure"
   5. Mortality is under 10% and associated with complications from long-term corticosteroid therapy
   6. Potential side effects associated with long-term systemic corticosteroids include type 2 diabetes mellitus, adrenal suppression, and infections

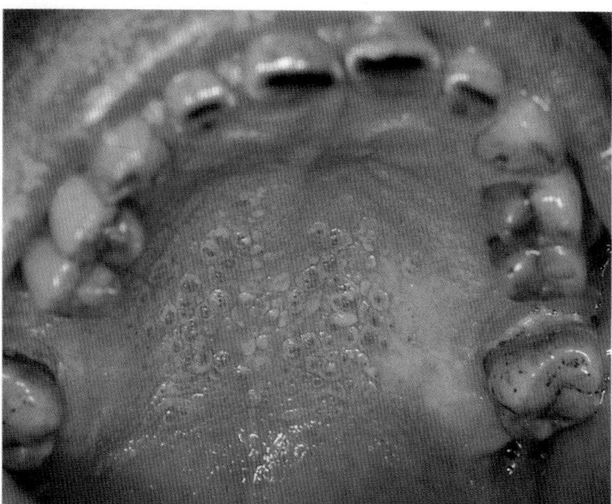

**Fig. 8.36** Nicotine stomatitis. (From Ibsen OAC, Phelan JA. *Oral Pathology for the Dental Hygienist.* 6th ed. St. Louis: Elsevier Saunders; 2014.)

## CONDITIONS ASSOCIATED WITH HYPERKERATOSIS (WHITE LESIONS)

### General Characteristics

A. Build-up of keratin on keratinizing or nonkeratinizing epithelium
B. Clinical term leukoplakia is often associated with *hyperkeratosis*; literally means white patch or plaque
C. Vary from simple localized lesions to diffuse lesions with broad coverage; smooth to rough surfaces; elevated to flat
D. Color—white, grayish white, yellowish white
E. Painless
F. Associated with a variety of conditions (including variants of normal, systemic disease, and premalignant lesions)

### Nicotine Stomatitis

A. Etiology—heavy tobacco smoking using cigarettes, cigars, water pipe (hookah), or pipe; ("pipe smoker's palate")
B. Age and gender—most common in male smokers over 40 years
C. Location—posterior hard and soft palates
D. Clinical features (Fig. 8.36)
   1. Response to irritant (heat, smoke); begins with erythema and inflammation
   2. Result is increased keratinization; turns palate grayish white; scattered erythematous nodules represent inflamed minor salivary duct openings
   3. Thick keratin may form fissures or cracks creating a wrinkled appearance
E. Histologic characteristics
   1. Marked hyperkeratosis and acanthosis
   2. Thickened epithelium surrounding inflamed salivary gland duct openings
F. Treatment and prognosis
   1. Benign condition which is reversible when irritant—smoking—is removed
   2. Not considered precancerous, prognosis good if smoking stopped and tissues return to normal

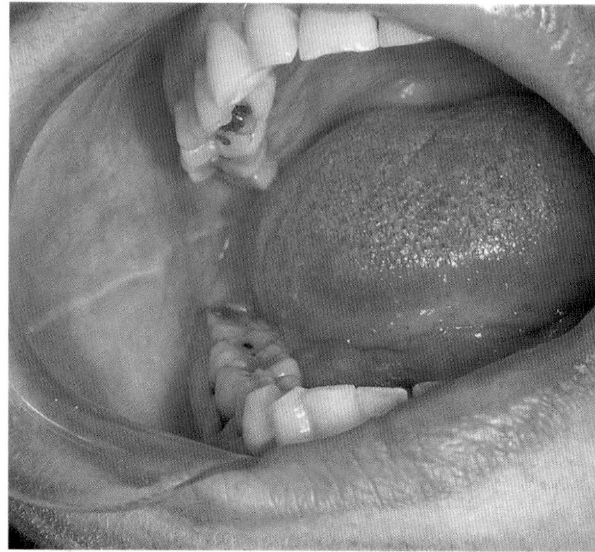

**Fig. 8.37** Linea alba. (From Ibsen OAC, Phelan JA. *Oral Pathology for the Dental Hygienist.* 6th ed. St. Louis: Elsevier Saunders; 2014.)

   3. Biopsy may be indicated for tissues that do not return to normal

### Linea Alba

A. Etiology—impact of occlusion on buccal mucosa creates linear impression of teeth; due to pressure of teeth against buccal mucosa
B. Age and gender—any age; no gender predilection
C. Location—buccal mucosa along the occlusal plane; usually bilateral
D. Clinical features (Fig. 8.37)
   1. "White line" on buccal mucosa, extends anterior to posterior along the line of occlusion
   2. Localized, single line, varies in prominence; usually bilateral
E. Histologic characteristics—hyperorthokeratosis; some localized intracellular edema
F. Treatment and prognosis—no treatment required

### Leukoedema

A. Etiology—unknown; variant of normal
B. Age and gender—average age 45 years; no gender predilection; African Americans are most affected racial group
C. Location—bilateral buccal and labial mucosa
D. Clinical features
   1. Appearance is that of a soft, diffuse, opalescent film over buccal mucosa
   2. Later becomes gray to white with coarsely wrinkled surface
   3. When tissue is stretched, opalescence disappears (this clinical characteristic helps with establishing diagnosis)
   4. Research demonstrates it may be more prominent in smokers
E. Histologic characteristics
   1. Intracellular edema of prickle cells (spinous layer)
   2. Increased thickness of epithelium with a superficial parakeratotic layer several cells thick

3. Broad rete pegs that appear irregularly elongated

F. Treatment and prognosis—no treatment required; considered variant of normal

## Systemic Lupus Erythematosus (SLE)

A. Etiology—unknown, autoimmune disease involving multiple body systems
   1. Cellular and humoral immunity are impaired
   2. Increased activity B lymphocytes; abnormal T lymphocyte function

B. Age and gender—much more common in females (8:1) during childbearing years; African American females more affected than white females (3:1); average age 31 years

C. Location
   1. Buccal mucosa, palate, gingiva (25% to 30% of persons with SLE)
   2. Skin—lesions occur in 85% of persons with SLE; a characteristic erythematous butterfly-shaped rash on the face crossing bridge of nose (malar areas); chest, back, extremities; exposure to sunlight makes rash worse

D. Systemic characteristics
   1. Fever, weight loss, arthritis, muscle pain
   2. Raynaud's phenomenon is seen in up to 15% of persons with SLE
   3. CNS involvement, depression, and seizures
   4. Ocular involvement; retinal nerve damage
   5. Kidney involvement (complications can be fatal)
   6. Cardiac involvement (pericarditis)
   7. Warty vegetations affecting heart valves (Libman-Sacks endocarditis)

E. Clinical features (Fig. 8.38A and B)
   1. Skin lesions—erythematous rash; scales form, scarring in the center; butterfly configuration on the malar areas of the face and nose
   2. Among those with SLE, 25% to 30% have oral manifestations
   3. Erythematous plaques with white striae; can resemble lichen planus but is less defined
   4. Burning mouth; xerostomia; candidiasis

F. Laboratory tests and findings
   1. Direct immunofluorescence of skin lesion (95% effective for SLE)
   2. Direct immunofluorescence of normal skin showing a positive lupus band in 25% to 60% of persons with SLE
   3. Anemia; leukopenia; thrombocytopenia
   4. Positive identification of antinuclear antibodies (ANAs); not very specific for SLE
   5. Anti–double-stranded DNA antibodies, a specific finding in up to 80% of patients with SLE

G. A combination of these test findings, multiorgan involvement, skin lesions, and possible oral lesions can all play a role in establishing the definitive diagnosis

H. Histologic characteristics
   1. Hyperkeratosis; alternating changes within the spinous layer of the epithelium

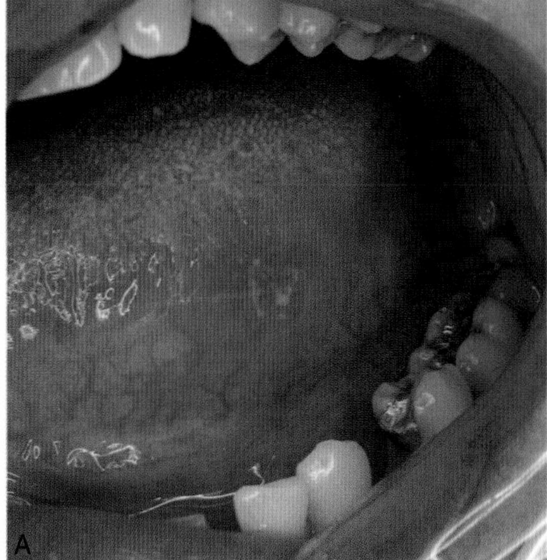


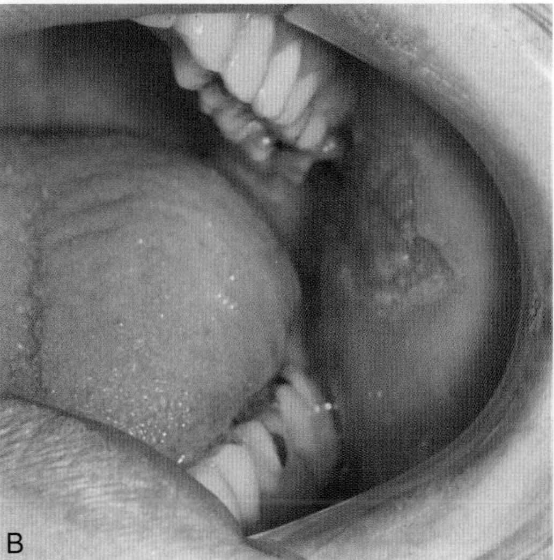


**Fig. 8.38** (A) and (B) Oral lesions in lupus erythematosus. (Courtesy of Dr. Edward V. Zegarelli; from Ibsen OAC, Phelan JA. *Oral Pathology for the Dental Hygienist.* 6th ed. St. Louis: Elsevier Saunders; 2014.)

   2. Necrosis of the basal cell layer
   3. Inflammatory infiltrate around blood vessels in the connective tissue, not in a subepithelial band as seen in lichen planus
   4. Subepithelial edema

I. Treatment and prognosis
   1. Aspirin and NSAIDs
   2. Antimalarial and corticosteroids combined with other immunosuppressive medications
   3. Periods of remission in mild cases, prognosis is good; with significant organ involvement, disease can be fatal, prognosis is worse for men
   4. Consult with patient's physician before dental treatment; prophylactic antibiotic premedication may be necessary (when heart valve involvement)
   5. Patients should avoid exposure to sunlight because ultraviolet light can exacerbate or precipitate disease activity

## White Sponge Nevus (Cannon Disease, Familial White Folded Dysplasia)

A. Etiology—hereditary; autosomal dominant trait; mutation in mucosal keratins K4 or K13; high degree of penetrance with varying degree of expressivity
B. Age and gender—progressive from childhood to adulthood; no gender predilection
C. Location—bilateral buccal mucosa is always affected (sometimes soft palate, ventral tongue, floor of mouth)
D. Clinical features
    1. Asymptomatic white, velvety, thickened, and folded mucosal tissue (especially buccal mucosa)
    2. Diffuse, generalized, and bilateral
    3. Early years—the white mucosa is smooth and flat; becomes corrugated over time
    4. Adolescence—tissues become increasingly folded or corrugated; appear opalescent-white when the condition peaks
E. Histologic characteristics
    1. Thickened epithelium with hyperparakeratosis and acanthosis
    2. Perinuclear condensation of keratin tonofilaments in the superficial cells of the epithelium
    3. Cells of the spinous layer toward the surface exhibit vacuolation (space filled with fluid or air)
F. Treatment and prognosis
    1. Benign condition, no treatment required, no malignant transformation
    2. In adults, important to distinguish from premalignant or malignant lesions
    3. Prognosis excellent

## Lichen Planus

A. Etiology—unknown, immunologically mediated mucocutaneous disorder
B. Age and gender—middle-aged adults; slight predilection for females
C. Location—skin; oral mucosa; especially buccal mucosa, dorsal tongue, gingiva, and palate
D. Clinical features— benign, chronic disease; two forms: reticular and erosive
    1. Reticular lichen planus (most common) (Fig. 8.39A, B, and C)
        a. White, narrow, interconnecting, slightly elevated lines forming a mesh, net, or lace-like pattern (Wickham's striae); lesions can also appear as white papules; cannot be wiped off
        b. Mucosa between white lines appears normal
        c. On dorsal tongue, may appear solid gray to white and plaque-like
        d. Usually asymptomatic
    2. Erosive or ulcerative form
        a. Lesions are symptomatic, pain a feature
        b. Condition begins as an erosive flat lesion
        c. Erythematous area is ulcerated, painful, and surrounded by fine white borders
        d. Slight increased risk for squamous cell carcinoma (SCC) in persons with erosive lichen planus has been reported; frequent reevaluation appointments with extraoral and intraoral examination required
        e. Prominent atrophy and ulceration of gingiva described as "desquamative" gingivitis (Fig. 8.40); this feature is not diagnostic and can appear with other oral conditions
E. Histologic characteristics (Fig. 8.41)
    1. Hyperparakeratosis or hyperorthokeratosis of surface epithelium
    2. Thickened spinous layer (acanthosis)
    3. Intracellular edema of cells in spinous layer
    4. Necrosis or degeneration of basal cell layer
    5. Band-like inflammatory infiltrate of lymphocytes

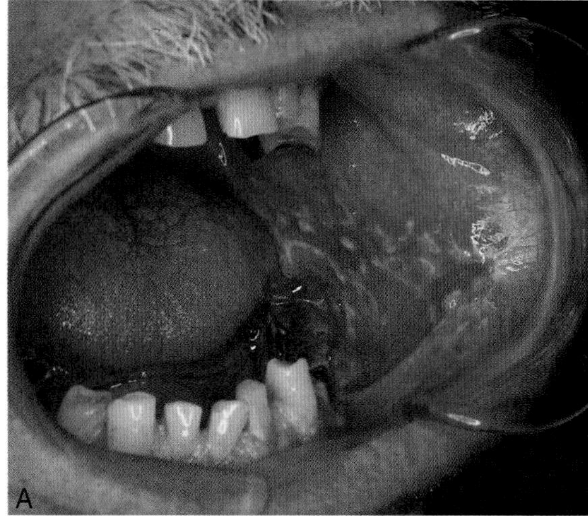


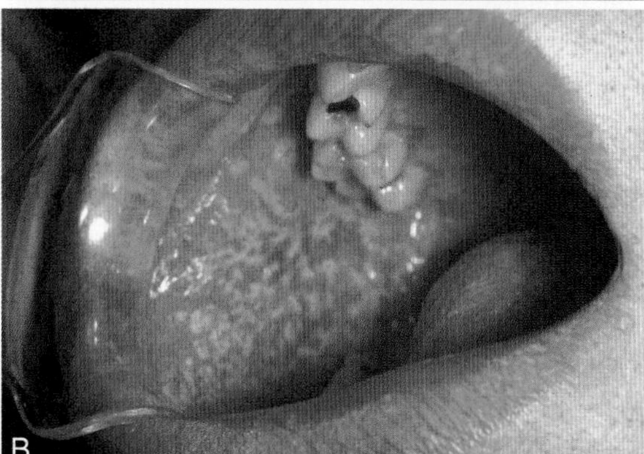


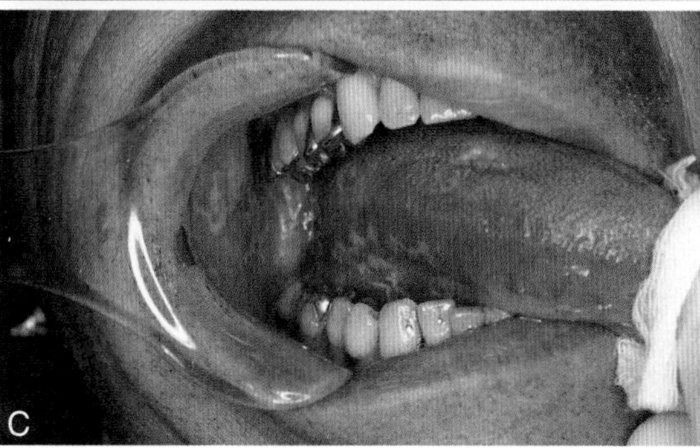


**Fig. 8.39** Lichen planus. (A) Erosion of the mucosa appears as erythema adjacent to white striae. (B) and (C) Two additional examples of the oral lesions of lichen planus. (A courtesy of Dr. Edward V. Zegarelli; A to C from Ibsen OAC, Phelan JA. *Oral Pathology for the Dental Hygienist.* 6th ed. St. Louis: Elsevier Saunders; 2014.)

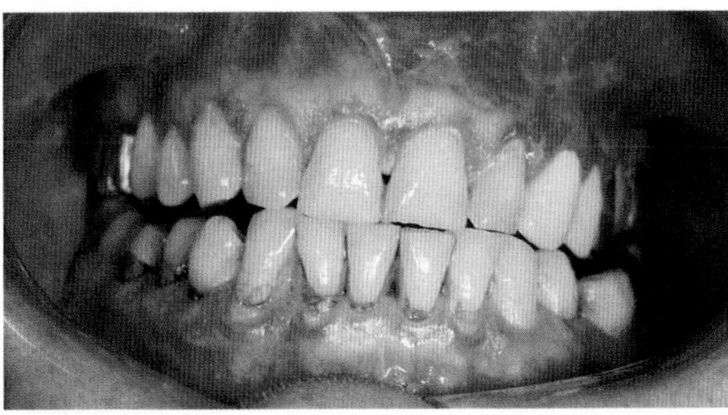

**Fig. 8.40** Lichen planus. The gingival lesions of lichen planus are described clinically as desquamative tissue. (Courtesy of Dr. Edward V. Zegarelli; from Ibsen OAC, Phelan JA. *Oral Pathology for the Dental Hygienist.* 6th ed. St. Louis: Elsevier Saunders; 2014.)

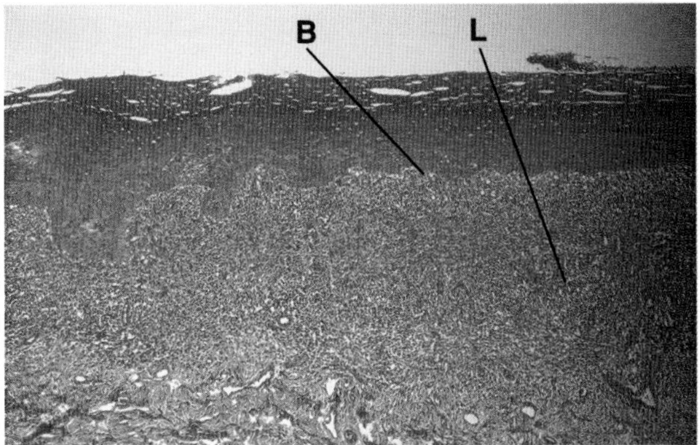


**Fig. 8.41** Lichen planus seen by low-power microscopy. Note the degeneration of the basal cell layer of the epithelium *(B)* and the band-like infiltrate of lymphocytes *(L)*. (From Ibsen OAC, Phelan JA. *Oral Pathology for the Dental Hygienist.* 6th ed. St. Louis: Elsevier Saunders; 2014.)

F. Treatment and prognosis
 1. Treatment for symptomatic cases; often not needed for reticular lichen planus
 2. Corticosteroids to decrease ulcerations and inflammation (local or systemic for severe cases)
 3. Topical corticosteroids (e.g., fluocinonide) applied several times a day
 4. Meticulous oral hygiene
 5. Lesions are self-limiting; most heal in a few weeks with topical corticosteroid therapy
 6. Condition does recur, and reapplication of corticosteroids needed
 7. Frequent reevaluation of patients with erosive lichen planus important

## Hyperkeratosis Due to Irritation

A. Etiology—local factors; constant, low-grade irritation (frictional keratosis; chronic tongue chewing, cheek biting, repetitive irritation); vitamin A deficiency can cause excessive keratinization of skin and mucous membranes
B. Age and gender—usually over age 40 years; more common in males
C. Location—anywhere in the oral cavity; alveolar ridge, buccal mucosa, lateral tongue
D. Clinical features (Fig. 8.42A and B)
 1. Benign reactive phenomenon, attempt to protect underlying tissues from persistent irritation or trauma
 2. Often appears as white flat lesion with a diffuse boundary, may have jagged surface
 3. Three layers of epithelium affected: granular, prickle, and basal cell layers
 4. Fissures or ulcerations rare
E. Laboratory tests—biopsy indicated for persistent or suspicious lesions
F. Histologic characteristics (Fig. 8.42C)
 1. Excessive keratinization of normal mucosa
 2. Normal underlying connective tissue
G. Treatment and prognosis
 1. Removal of cause (irritant)
 2. Tissue should return to normal

# NEOPLASIA

## Oral Squamous Cell Carcinoma (SCC)

A. Etiology—multifactorial etiology, contributions of intrinsic and extrinsic factors is important (e.g. chemicals, viruses, radiation; secondary to genetic mutation; immunosuppression)
 1. Associated risk factors include use of tobacco and alcohol, increasing age
 2. Oncogenic viruses, such as HPV 16 and 18, major risk factor for posterior oropharyngeal cancer including base of tongue and tonsils
 3. Combinations of risk factors can be lethal
 4. Iron deficiency anemia, especially severe form "Plummer-Vinson" syndrome, elevates the risk for SCC in the posterior mouth and esophagus
B. Age and gender—young adults to adults in their 60s, 70s, and beyond
 1. Incidence increases with age
 2. Sixth most common cancer in males and twelfth in females
 3. Ratio of incidence in males and females is 2:1
 4. Highest overall incidence in white males over 65; highest incidence in middle age found in African American males
C. Locations
 1. Tongue—37% to 50%, excluding cancer of the pharynx Posterior third, including lateral borders and ventral surfaces, majority of cases
 2. Floor of the mouth—30% to 35%
 3. Lips—22%; most lower lip; pipe, cigar smokers, patients with fair skin, and persons with an outdoor occupation or hobby who are exposed to sunlight (Fig. 8.43A and B)
 4. Buccal mucosa—6%
 5. Gingiva—6%
 6. Soft palate—4%
D. Clinical features (Fig. 8.44A, B, and C)
 1. SCC accounts for 90% to 95% of oral cancers
 2. Appearance within oral cavity variable, can resemble or mimic other lesions

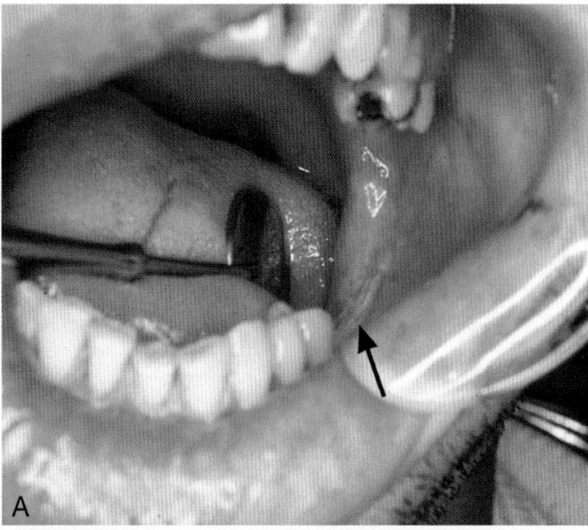


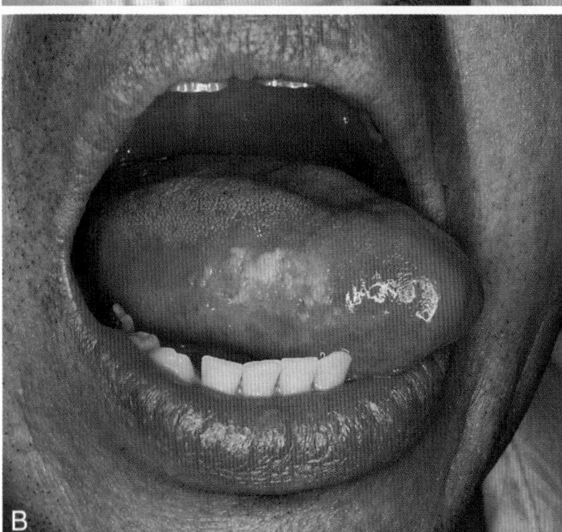


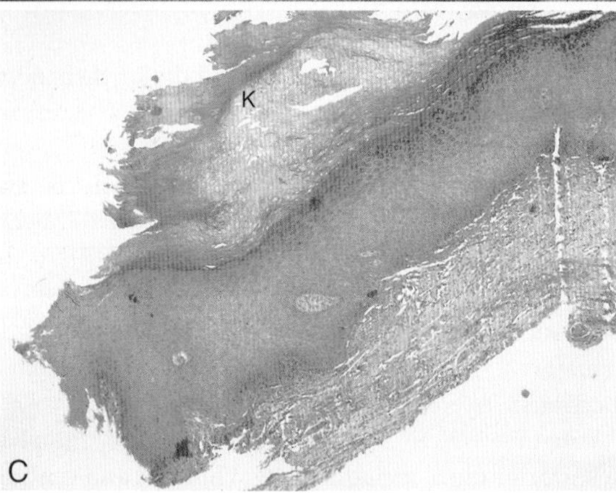


**Fig. 8.42** (A) Frictional keratosis *(arrow)* caused by an opposing third molar. (B) Caused by chronic tongue chewing. (C) Low-power microscopic appearance of hyperkeratosis showing an increase in the amount of surface keratin *(K)*. (From Ibsen OAC, Phelan JA. *Oral Pathology for the Dental Hygienist*. 6th ed. St. Louis: Elsevier Saunders; 2014.)

3. Common features: exophytic, indurated, ulcerated, firm, anchored to underlying tissues
4. Sores or ulcerations that do not heal
5. On lower lip, asymptomatic crusted ulceration mimicking chapped lip, indurated border

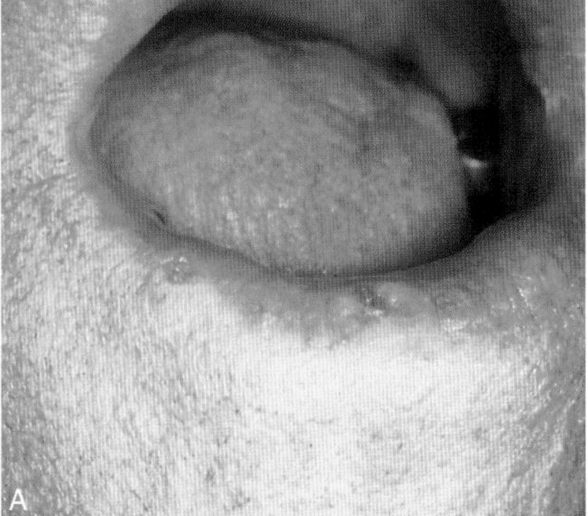


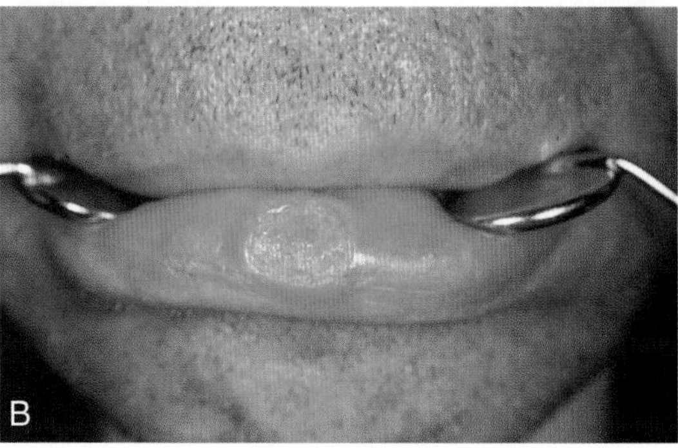


**Fig. 8.43** (A) and (B) Clinical appearance of squamous cell carcinoma of the lower lip. (Courtesy of Dr. Edward V. Zegarelli; from Ibsen OAC, Phelan JA. *Oral Pathology for the Dental Hygienist*. 6th ed. St. Louis: Elsevier Saunders; 2014.)

6. Invasion of tumor cells into adjacent tissues is a feature, can destroy bone, result in paresthesia or dysesthesia of tongue or lips
7. Metastasis (spread of cancerous cells) to regional lymph nodes and distant sites occurs
8. Stages—tumor-node-metastasis (TNM) staging system helps predict patient's prognosis (Box 8.1)
   a. Stage I—early; tumor less than 2 cm in diameter
   b. Stage II—intermediate; tumor 2 to 4 cm in diameter
   c. Stage III—advanced; tumor greater than 4 cm
   d. Stage IV—tumor has metastasized

E. Radiographic appearance (Fig. 8.44D)
   1. Diffuse radiolucency with irregular borders (after significant bone destroyed); penetration into cortex ("moth-eaten appearance")
   2. Resorption and displacement of tooth roots

F. Laboratory tests and findings
   1. Biopsy—biopsy is "gold standard" for definitive diagnosis
      a. Incisional—removal of a segment or piece of lesion for microscopic analysis
      b. Excisional—removal of entire lesion in question for microscopic analysis
   2. Screening tools, in addition to oral examination, that have been used for oral cancer include brush biopsy, ViziLite, and VelScope Vx (for a discussion on these see section on "Diagnostic Tools for Oral Cancer Detection" in Chapter 16)

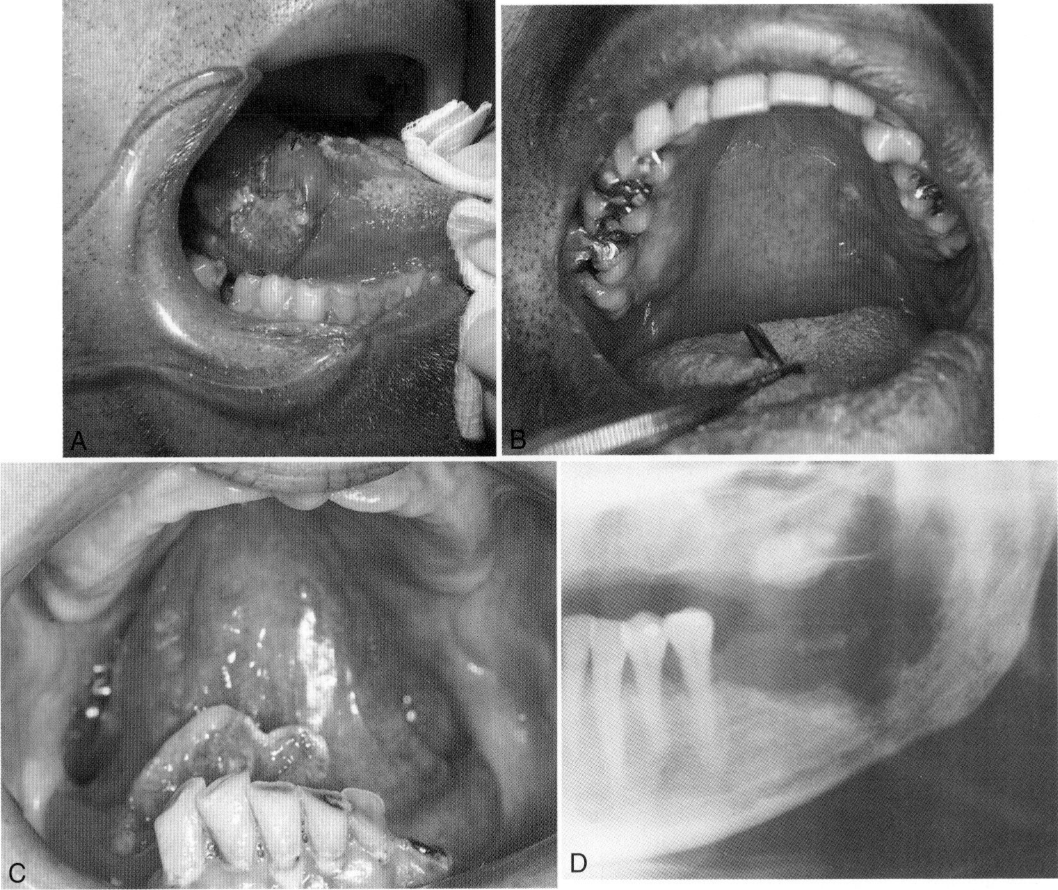


**Fig. 8.44** (A) Clinical appearance of squamous cell carcinoma (SCC) of the posterolateral tongue showing an exophytic, ulcerated mass. (B) Clinical appearance of SCC of the left side of the soft palate and fauces. (C) Clinical appearance of SCC on the floor of the mouth. (D) Left side of a panoramic radiograph showing destruction of the mandible by SCC. (C courtesy of Dr. Edward V. Zegarelli; A to D from Ibsen OAC, Phelan JA. *Oral Pathology for the Dental Hygienist*. 6th ed. St. Louis: Elsevier Saunders; 2014.)

**BOX 8.1 TNM Staging System for Oral Squamous Cell Carcinoma**

T—Tumor
T1—Tumor < 2 cm in diameter
T2—Tumor 2-4 cm in diameter
T3—Tumor > 4 cm in diameter
T4—Tumor invades adjacent structures
N—Node
N0—No palpable nodes
N1—Ipsilateral (same side as primary tumor) palpable nodes (same side as tumor)
N2—Contralateral (opposite side from primary tumor) or bilateral nodes
N3—Fixed palpable nodes
M—Metastasis
M0—No distant metastasis
M1—Clinical radiographic evidence of metastasis

From Regezi JA, Sciubba JJ. *Oral Pathology: Clinical Pathologic Correlations*. 5th ed. Philadelphia: Saunders; 2008.
*TNM*, Tumor-node-metastasis.

G. Histologic characteristics
   1. Islands or sheets of malignant (neoplastic) squamous cells, often invading down from surface into underlying connective tissue
   2. Keratin pearls (cluster of concentrically layered keratinized cells) may be a feature
   3. Malignant cells often display anaplastic features, such as altered size and shape, large hyperchromatic nuclei and increased numbers of abnormal to bizarre mitotic figures

H. Treatment and prognosis
   1. Surgical excision alone or excision with a combination of radiation and chemotherapy; occasionally radiation therapy alone
   2. Tumor size and location influence treatment protocols
   3. Adjunctive chemotherapeutic agents
   4. Metastasis from oral cavity to lymph nodes in neck may require radical neck dissection (procedure to remove lymph nodes)
   5. Prognosis depends on tumor stage and host response to treatment

## Pleomorphic Adenoma (Benign Mixed Tumor)

A. Etiology—exact cause is unknown; benign tumor that accounts for 90% of all salivary gland tumors
B. Age and gender—most common in adults ages 35 to 55 years; female predilection; can occur in children
C. Location
   1. Most common location is parotid gland

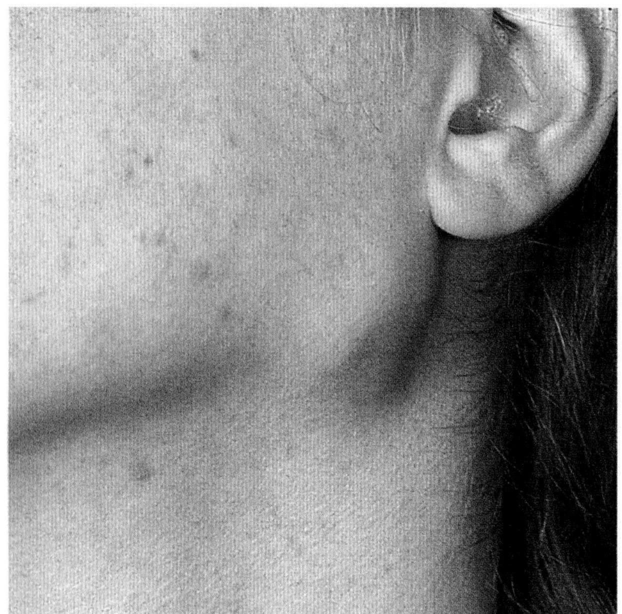

**Fig. 8.45** Benign salivary gland tumor (pleomorphic adenoma). (From Odell E: Cawson's Essentials of Oral Pathology and Oral Medicine. 9th ed. Elsevier; 2017.)

2. Posterior hard or soft palate (most common intraoral site); unilateral

D. Clinical features (Fig. 8.45)
1. Intraoral most common location on either side of the midline, posterior palate
2. Painless, slow growing, firm
3. Smooth, dome-shaped mass, not ulcerated (unless traumatized)
4. Size from a few millimeters to a few centimeters
5. In parotid may arise in close proximity to facial nerve, risk of nerve damage on removal

E. Histologic characteristics
1. Encapsulated tumor composed of variable glandular epithelial, mesenchymal-like stromal components
2. Capsule may be incomplete or show infiltration of tumor cells
3. Most benign; malignant transformation in less than 5% of cases

F. Treatment and prognosis
1. Total surgical excision, conservative enucleation not recommended since it is associated with high reoccurrence rate
2. Partial or complete removal of the parotid gland may be necessary
3. Research reports about 5% risk of malignant transformation
4. Prognosis excellent with total excision

## CYSTS OF THE HEAD AND NECK

### General Characteristics

A. True cyst
1. Sac-like structure lined by epithelium, often contains fluid and/or soft material such as keratin and cellular debris
2. May be surrounded by or enclosed within connective tissue
3. All true cysts are have an epithelial lining; pseudocysts (false cysts) are entities not lined by epithelium

B. Cysts are often classified according to:
1. Etiology, histologic components; location
2. Tissue origin (odontogenic or nonodontogenic or inflammatory)

### Apical Cyst (Radicular Cyst, Periapical Cyst)

A. Etiology
1. Odontogenic origin, most common odontogenic cyst
2. Cyst develops as a response to inflammation associated with a nonvital tooth
3. Contributing factors include dental caries, trauma, deep restorations causing irreversible pulpitis, pulp necrosis

B. Age and gender—any age, but common ages 30 to 60 years

C. Location—apex of a tooth or lateral to tooth root (accessory lateral pulp canals)

D. Clinical features
1. Always in association with nonvital tooth
2. Most often asymptomatic

E. Radiographic appearance
1. Round or ovoid, well-defined radiolucent area attached to apex or lateral to root (Fig. 8.46A)
2. Loss of lamina dura in area; root resorption is possible
3. Radiographic appearance same as apical granuloma

F. Histologic characteristics
1. Lined by epithelium; develops from residual epithelial rests of Malassez (remnants of Hertwig's epithelial root sheath)
2. Cyst wall composed of well-vascularized dense fibrous connective tissue; often with pronounced inflammatory infiltrate (Fig. 8.46B)
3. Lumen may contain fluid or cellular debris

G. Treatment
1. Endodontic therapy
2. Extraction of the tooth with curettage of socket and apical area to remove cystic sac and epithelial remnants
3. Retreatment endodontically if radiolucency persists; apicoectomy may be required
4. Periodic follow-up to ensure resolution

### Residual Cyst

A. Etiology
1. Remnants of apical cyst, left after tooth extraction (apical cyst incompletely removed); odontogenic
2. Open socket with debris and inflammation may act as stimulus

B. Age and gender—most often adults, previous history of apical cyst

C. Location (Fig. 8.47A)
1. Area previous tooth extraction, with prior apical cyst
2. Adjacent to socket area or within alveolar ridge

D. Clinical features—similar to apical cyst, usually asymptomatic

E. Radiographic appearance (Fig. 8.47B)

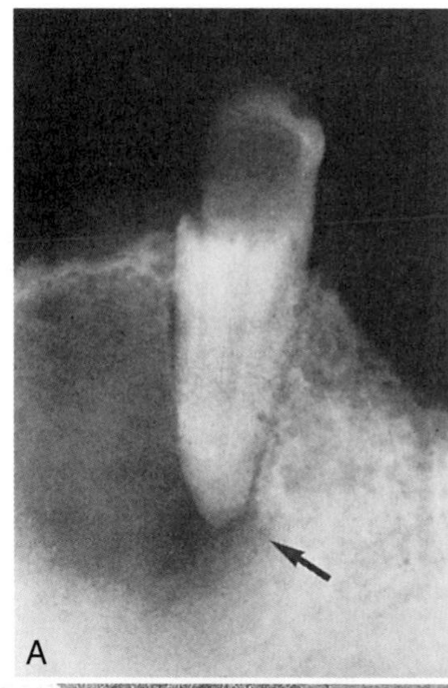


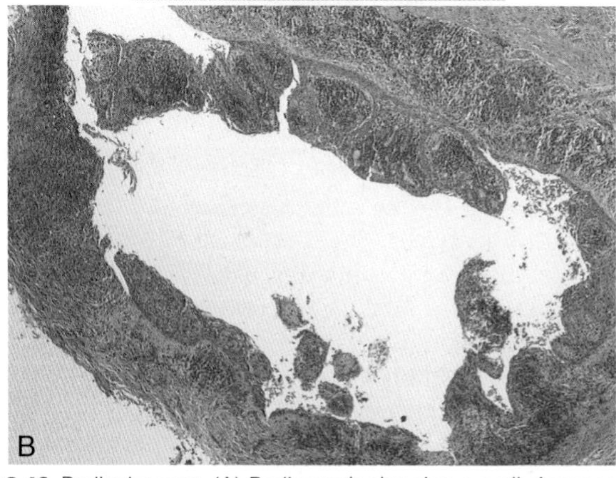


**Fig. 8.46** Radicular cyst. (A) Radiograph showing a well-circumscribed radiolucency around the root of a tooth *(arrow)*. (B) Microscopic features of a radicular cyst. (From Ibsen OAC, Phelan JA. *Oral Pathology for the Dental Hygienist.* 6th ed. St. Louis: Elsevier Saunders; 2014.)

1. Well-defined radiolucent area
2. Round or oval in shape
3. Radiolucency may develop radiopaque rim

F. Histologic characteristics
1. Cyst lined with epithelium
2. Dense fibrous connective tissue wall

G. Treatment—surgical removal

## Developmental Cysts

A. Etiology
1. Median mandibular cyst—cyst in midline of mandible; questionable origin but currently thought to arise from odontogenic epithelium; rare
2. Globulomaxillary cyst—between the maxillary lateral incisor and canine; currently thought to arise from odontogenic epithelium (previously considered a fissural cyst)
3. Nasolabial cyst—soft tissue cyst; develops from the inferior and anterior segments of the nasolacrimal duct; strong female predilection (4:1)
4. Median palatine cyst—fissural cyst arises from trapped epithelial remnants; more posterior location than nasopalatine duct cyst; young adults

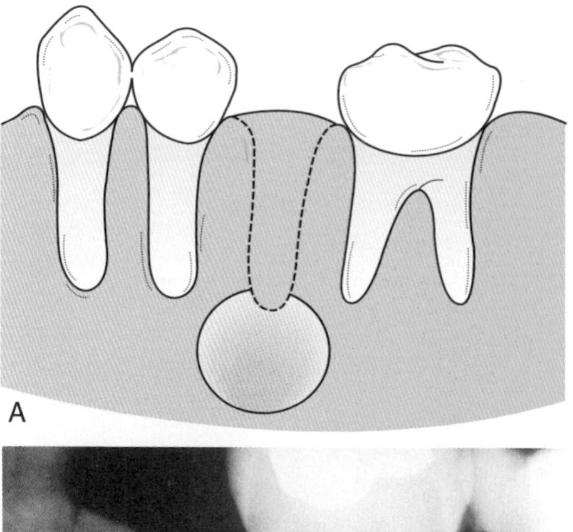


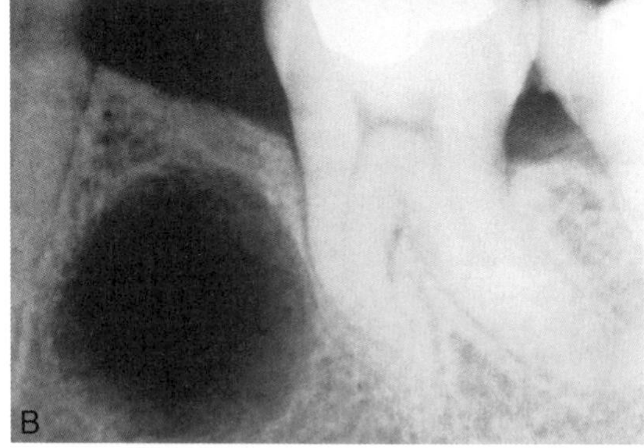


**Fig. 8.47** (A) Schematic of a residual cyst. (B) Radiograph of a residual cyst showing a radiolucency at the site of a previously extracted tooth. (Courtesy of Drs. Paul Freedman and Stanley Kerpel; from Ibsen OAC, Phelan JA. *Oral Pathology for the Dental Hygienist.* 6th ed. St. Louis: Elsevier Saunders; 2014.)

5. Nasopalatine duct cyst (incisive canal cyst)—develops from epithelial remnants of nasopalatine ducts; male predilection

B. Age and gender—adults; no gender predilection

C. Location—cyst names are based on location
1. Median mandibular cyst—midline of anterior mandible
2. Globulomaxillary cyst—appears as a pear-shaped radiolucency between the roots of maxillary lateral incisor and canine
3. Nasolabial cyst—soft tissue of upper lip, lateral to midline; in mucolabial fold near maxillary canine and floor of nose
4. Median palatine cyst—midline of hard palate
5. Nasopalatine duct cyst—within or adjacent to nasopalatine canal or incisive papilla; may appear heart-shaped

D. Clinical features
1. Cysts vary in size from no visible clinical evidence to a bulge or expansion of bone
2. Vitality testing necessary to rule out nonvital pulp, if within bone and located adjacent to teeth

E. Radiographic appearance—well-defined radiolucent area; some have particular shapes due to their anatomical location
1. Globulomaxillary cyst—located between the maxillary lateral incisor and canine; often pear-shaped (Fig. 8.48)
2. Nasopalatine duct (incisal canal) cyst often heart-shaped due to extension between central incisors

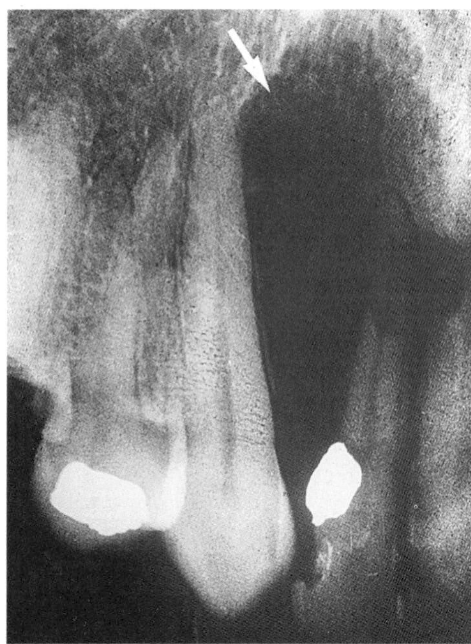

**Fig. 8.48** Radiograph of a globulomaxillary cyst showing a characteristic pear-shaped radiolucency between the maxillary lateral incisor and canine. (From Ibsen OAC, Phelan JA. *Oral Pathology for the Dental Hygienist*. 6th ed. St. Louis: Elsevier Saunders; 2014.)

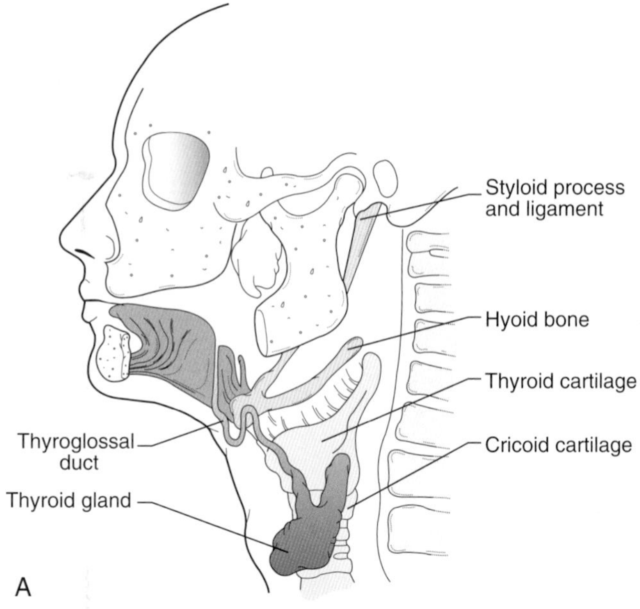


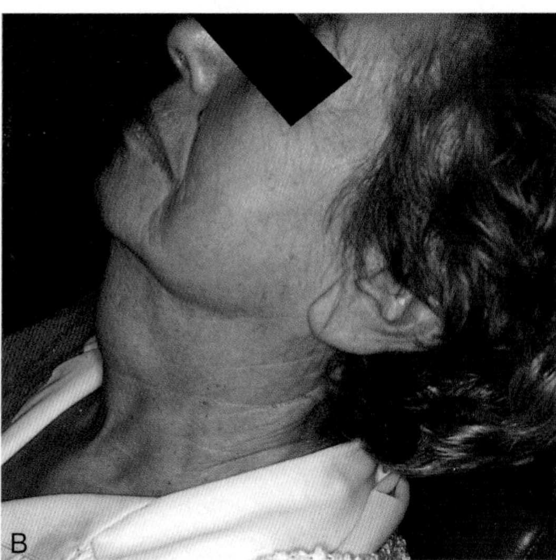


**Fig. 8.49** (A) Thyroglossal tract extends from the area of the foramen cecum, lingual to the lower part of the neck. (B) Thyroglossal tract cyst is the cause of enlargement at the midline of the neck. (From Ibsen OAC, Phelan JA. *Oral Pathology for the Dental Hygienist*. 6th ed. St. Louis: Elsevier Saunders; 2014.)

F. Histologic characteristics
  1. Median mandibular cyst—most often lined by stratified squamous epithelium; few cases of pseudostratified ciliated columnar epithelium
  2. Globulomaxillary cyst—lined by stratified squamous epithelium
  3. Nasolabial cyst—lined by pseudostratified columnar epithelium with goblet cells and cilia
  4. Median palatal cyst—lined by stratified squamous epithelium
  5. Nasopalatine canal cyst—several types of epithelium are found in this cyst along with tissue remnants of nasopalatine duct

G. Treatment and prognosis
  1. Removal of cystic sac and curettage
  2. Prognosis is excellent

## Thyroglossal Tract Cyst (Thyroglossal Duct Cyst)

A. Etiology—develops within embryonic thyroglossal tract; inflammatory stimulus possibly associated with adjacent lymphoid tissue, draining infection from head and neck

B. Age and gender—most often young adults under 20 years; no gender predilection

C. Location—midline of neck along thyroglossal tract, which extends from foramen cecum (posterior tongue) to permanent position of thyroid gland in the neck; cyst can be found as far down as suprasternal notch; 75% of these cysts are below the hyoid bone (Fig. 8.49A)

D. Clinical features (Fig. 8.49B)
  1. Fluctuant (fluid-filled) asymptomatic; movable swelling in midline of neck
  2. Bulge is round or oval shaped; varies in size up to 10 cm diameter
  3. Fistulous tracts to the skin or mucosa can develop
  4. Swallowing becomes difficult (dysphagia) when cyst located adjacent to base of tongue
  5. Inability to extend the tongue may occur

E. Histologic characteristics
  1. Cysts are lined with ciliated columnar epithelium, squamous epithelium or other types of epithelium
  2. Connective tissue wall may contain remnants of residual thyroid tissue

F. Treatment and prognosis
  1. Complete surgical excision of cyst (after a thyroid scan)

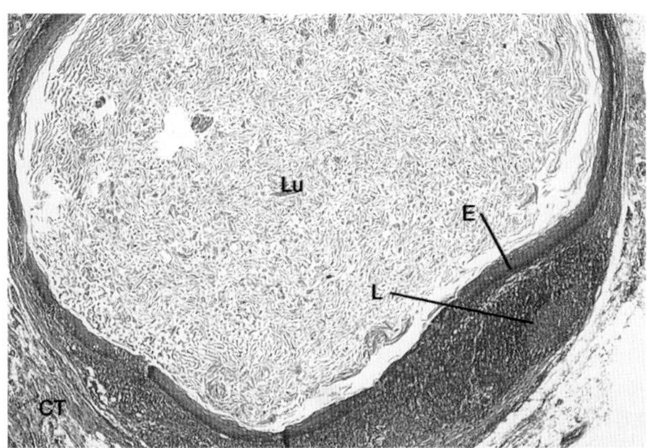


**Fig. 8.50** Low-power microscopic appearance of a lymphoepithelial cyst showing lumen *(Lu)*, epithelial lining *(E)*, surrounding lymphocytes *(L)*, and connective tissue *(CT)*. (From Ibsen OAC, Phelan JA. *Oral Pathology for the Dental Hygienist.* 6th ed. St. Louis: Elsevier Saunders; 2014.)

2. Prognosis is good
3. Malignant transformation rare

## Cervical Lymphoepithelial Cyst (Branchial Cleft Cyst)

A. Etiology
  1. Classic theory is development from epithelial remnants of embryonic branchial arches
  2. About 95% appear to develop in region of second branchial arch
  3. Another theory is possible epithelium entrapped within lymph nodes
B. Age and gender—young adults; no gender predilection
C. Location: can occur both intra- and extra-oral, most often unilateral
  1. Oral lymphoepithelial cyst—posterior floor of mouth, lateral border of tongue
  2. Cervical lymphoepithelial cyst—located on lateral neck near anterior border of sternocleidomastoid muscle
  3. Area from clavicle to parotid gland
D. Clinical features
  1. Slow-growing, fluctuant, movable mass 1 to 10 cm in diameter; asymptomatic
  2. Can have a pink to yellowish color when found intraorally
  3. May be mistaken for parotid swelling or odontogenic infection
E. Histologic characteristics (Fig. 8.50)
  1. Lined by stratified squamous epithelium that may or may not be keratinizing
  2. Lymphoid tissue within connective tissue wall
F. Treatment and prognosis
  1. Surgical removal
  2. Prognosis is good

## Dermoid Cyst

A. Etiology—developmental, from all three germ layers: ectoderm, endoderm, mesoderm; benign cystic form of teratoma (teratomas are a type of germ cell tumor that can contain different types of tissue elements such as hair, muscle, bone, teeth)
B. Age and gender—present at birth or in young children; no gender predilection
C. Location
  1. Within oral cavity, anterior floor of the mouth; can displace tongue
  2. Ovarian teratomas, or "dermoids," may contain actual tooth structures
D. Clinical features
  1. Semifirm, dough-like consistency
  2. Size—a few millimeters to several centimeters
  3. Midline floor of the mouth
E. Histologic characteristics
  1. Lined with orthokeratinized stratified squamous epithelium
  2. Keratin within the lumen
  3. Fibrous connective tissue wall
  4. May contain sebaceous glands, hair follicles, sweat glands
F. Treatment and prognosis
  1. Surgical removal; approach depends on location relative to the geniohyoid muscle
  2. Prognosis is good

## Lateral Periodontal Cyst (LPC)

A. Etiology—odontogenic origin, develops from rests of dental lamina
B. Age and gender—adults over 30 years; common ages 50 to 70 years; male predilection
C. Location—most often lateral root surface of mandibular canine or premolar teeth (occasionally seen in the maxilla in the same areas)
D. Clinical features
  1. Tooth or teeth involved are vital
  2. Asymptomatic, no bone expansion
E. Radiographic appearance
  1. Small; less than 1 cm
  2. Well-defined ovoid or elliptically shaped unilocular radiolucent area found lateral to tooth root (Fig. 8.51A)
  3. Multilocular variant may occur; *botryoid odontogenic cyst* (BOC) is closely related to the LPC, most common in the mandibular cuspid and premolar area
  4. Odontogenic keratocyst (OKC) or keratoystic odontogenic tumor (KCOT) and other inflammatory cysts can have same radiographic features as LPC
F. Histologic characteristics (Fig. 8.51B)
  1. Stratified squamous epithelial lining only a few cells thick; focal epithelial thickening
  2. Thin connective tissue wall
G. Treatment and prognosis
  1. Surgical enucleation of cyst
  2. Few cases of recurrence have been reported
  3. BOC has greater recurrence potential than LPC

## Odontogenic Keratocyst (OKC) and Keratoystic Odontogenic Tumor (KCOT)

A. Etiology—odontogenic developmental cyst, multiple cysts may be associated with autosomal dominant disorder: Nevoid Basal Cell Carcinoma Syndrome (NBCCS or Gorlin Syndrome)

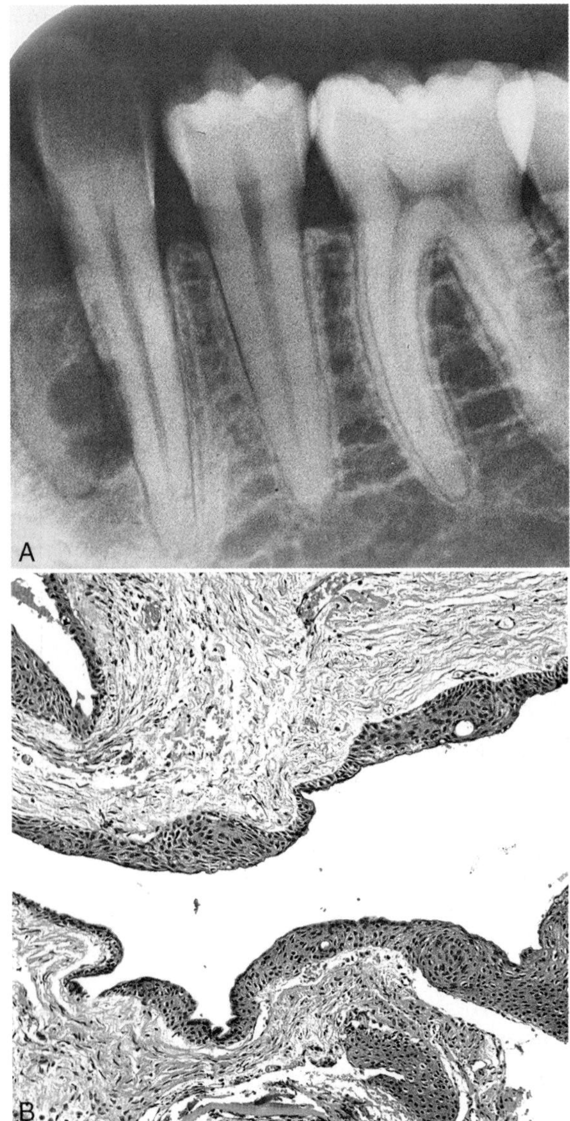


**Fig. 8.51** (A) Radiograph of a lateral periodontal cyst. This biloculated, well-defined radiolucency is located lateral to the tooth root. (B) Microscopic appearance of a lateral periodontal cyst showing a thin epithelial lining with focal epithelial thickenings. (From Ibsen OAC, Phelan JA. *Oral Pathology for the Dental Hygienist*. 6th ed. St. Louis: Elsevier Saunders; 2014.)

B. Age and gender—60% between 10 and 40 years of age; slight male predilection
C. Location—most often posterior mandible
D. Clinical features—may be asymptomatic; does not expand bone, can destroy large amounts of trabecular bone, aggressive behavior with high recurrence rate has led to reclassification as a neoplasm called KCOT
E. Radiographic appearance—well-defined, multilocular radiolucent lesion; can be similar to that of an odontogenic tumor; lesion can move teeth and resorb tooth structure
F. Histologic characteristics
   1. Epithelial lining has a unique histologic appearance
   2. Parakeratinized stratified squamous epithelium with corrugated surface lines lumen
   3. Uniform 8-10 cell thick lining with distinct palisaded basal cell layer
   4. Satellite daughter cysts within connective tissue wall (makes complete removal difficult, increases chance of recurrence)
G. Treatment and prognosis
   1. Aggressive surgical excision and osseous curettage
   2. High recurrence rate
   3. Close follow-up
   4. Evaluation for NBCCS

## Primordial Cyst

A. Etiology—believed to arise from degeneration of tooth germ during development; epithelial remnants of enamel organ; cyst develops in place of a tooth
B. Age and gender—child to young adult; ages 10 to 40 years; slight male predilection
C. Location—posterior mandible; third molar area or posterior to an erupted third molar
D. Clinical features—no obvious intraoral signs or symptoms; affected person most often asymptomatic, lack of tooth development in space occupied by cyst is essential for diagnosis
E. Radiographic appearance
   1. Well-defined radiolucent oval lesion; can be multilocular
   2. Size varies from a few millimeters to a centimeter
   3. Radiographic features not diagnostic, need clinical history of nondevelopment of missing tooth
F. Histologic characteristics
   1. Lining four to eight cell thick stratified squamous epithelium; no rete pegs
   2. Histology often reveals features of an OKC/KCOT
G. Treatment and prognosis
   1. Surgical removal with histologic examination
   2. Recurrence depends on the histologic findings; OKC (KCOT) recur in 30% of cases

## Dentigerous Cyst (Follicular Cyst)

A. Etiology—formed by reduced enamel epithelium after crown of tooth completely formed (unerupted or impacted tooth); accumulation of fluid between the crown and reduced enamel epithelium forms cystic space
B. Age and gender—young adults 20 to 30 years; second most common odontogenic cyst;
C. Location
   1. Most frequent location is mandibular third molar area—around crown of unerupted third molar; may enlarge to extend high into ramus
   2. Maxillary canine region—may compromise the maxillary sinus
D. Clinical features
   1. Always in bone and associated with crown of an unerupted or impacted tooth; asymptomatic
   2. Can be aggressive lesion, causing expansion of bone and extreme displacement of teeth; large cysts thin bone mass and increase risk for pathologic fracture, especially of mandible

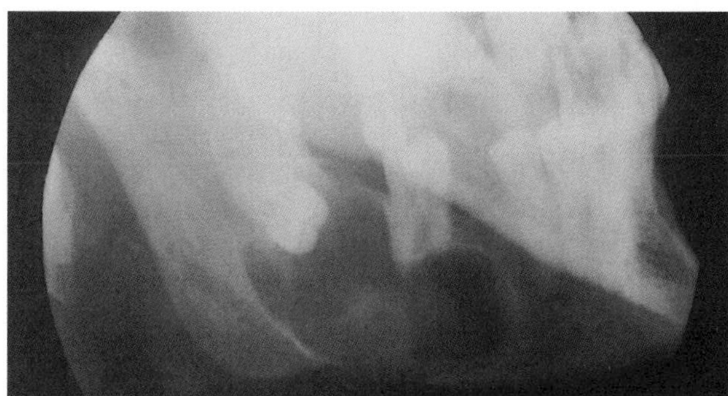

Fig. 8.52 Radiograph of large dentigerous cyst associated with an impacted third molar. (From Odell E: Cawson's Essentials of Oral Pathology and Oral Medicine. 9th ed. Elsevier; 2017.)

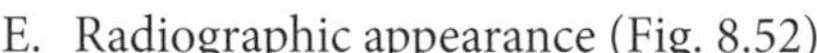

E. Radiographic appearance (Fig. 8.52)
   1. Smooth, unilocular radiolucency associated with crown of unerupted tooth
   2. Radiolucency encircles crown down to cemento-enamel junction (CEJ)
F. Histologic characteristics
   1. Stratified squamous epithelial lining; nonkeratinized
   2. Surrounded by fibrous connective tissue
   3. May see inflammatory infiltrate
G. Treatment and prognosis
   1. Removal of cyst, and sometimes associated tooth
   2. For teeth left in place, orthodontic intervention may be utilized to assist eruption
   3. Rare occurrence of ameloblastoma arising in cyst wall
   4. Prognosis good

## INJURIES TO ORAL SOFT TISSUE

### Ranula

A. Etiology
   1. Trauma to floor of mouth
   2. Blockage or obstruction in duct of major salivary gland (sublingual or submandibular) most often by a salivary "stone" (sialolith)
B. Age and gender—any age, but usually adults; no gender predilection
C. Location—unilaterally in floor of mouth
D. Clinical features (Fig. 8.53)
   1. Term reserved and used for a mucocele that occurs in floor of mouth
   2. Translucent, bluish, round, smooth-surfaced bulge 1 to 3 cm in diameter
   3. Unilateral, semifirm, fluctuant (fluid-filled) mass
   4. Increase and decrease in size associated with eating, stimulation of salivary flow
   5. Located lateral to midline floor of mouth (helpful for diagnosis)
   6. Displacement of tongue may interfere with speech, eating, swallowing
   7. Small lesions can develop along sublingual plica from superficial ducts of Rivini

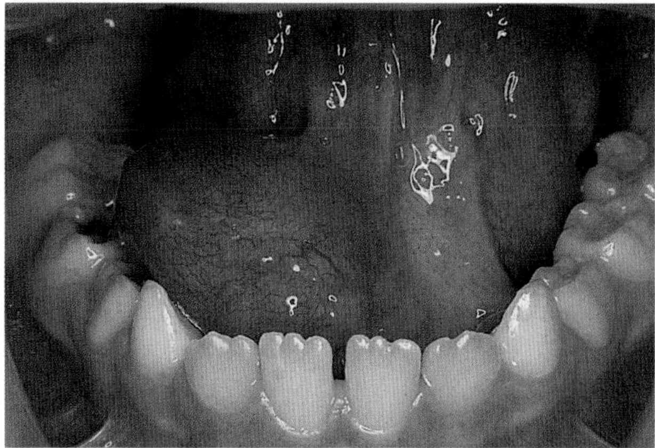

Fig. 8.53 Ranula. (From Odell E: Cawson's Essentials of Oral Pathology and Oral Medicine. 9th ed. Elsevier; 2017.)

E. Radiographic appearance—radiopaque mass present if blockage or obstruction of duct due to sialolith
F. Histologic characteristics
   1. Central cystic space which contains mucin and pseudo cyst wall composed of loose connective (no epithelial lining so not a true cyst)
   2. Inflammatory infiltrate with histiocytes
G. Treatment and prognosis
   1. Surgical excision
   2. Removal of obstruction, if present
   3. May recur

### Mucocele (Mucous Retention or Extravasation Phenomena)

A. Etiology
   1. Trauma to a minor salivary gland duct; mucous secretion spills into connective tissue
   2. Mechanical trauma by lip biting or chewing common
B. Age and gender—all ages but most common in children and young adults; no gender predilection
C. Location—most common site is lower lip mucosa
D. Clinical features
   1. Blister-like, raised subepithelial, circumscribed fluctuant swelling; 1 to 4 mm in size; painless (unless repeatedly traumatized)
   2. Superficial location, bluish translucent hue
   3. Often ruptures and releases mucous secretions
E. Histologic characteristics
   1. Central cystic space which contains mucin and pseudocyst wall composed of loose connective tissue (not lined with epithelium, so not a true cyst)
   2. Inflammatory response present with granulation tissue
F. Treatment and prognosis
   1. Excision of associated minor salivary gland
   2. May rupture, and resolve by itself
   3. Recurrence is possible

### Necrotizing Sialometaplasia

A. Etiology
   1. Trauma results in necrosis of minor salivary glands

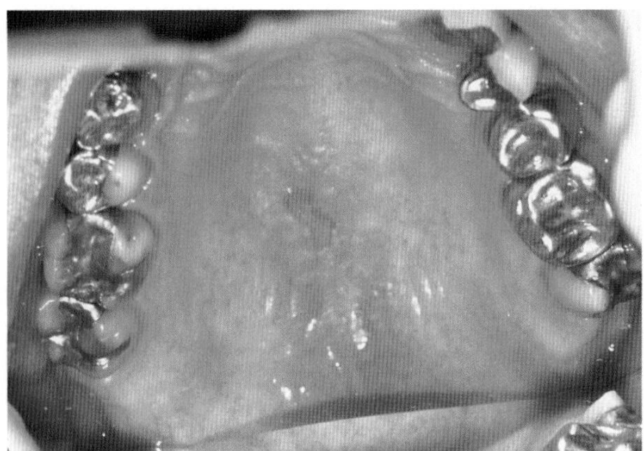

**Fig. 8.54** Necrotizing sialometaplasia. (From Ibsen OAC, Phelan JA. *Oral Pathology for the Dental Hygienist.* 6th ed. St. Louis: Elsevier Saunders; 2014.)

2. Believed due to lack of blood supply to the area, vascular ischemia
3. Trauma due to local events such as dental injection, or adjacent infection

B. Age and gender—adults
C. Location—most often found on palate; however, may be found any site containing minor salivary glands
D. Clinical features (Fig. 8.54)
   1. Initial finding of tenderness and swelling in the area
   2. Well-demarcated crater-like ulcer with rounded borders
   3. Localized pain; can be very painful
   4. Resemblance to other neoplasms (especially malignant) may raise concern
E. Histologic characteristics
   1. Necrotic salivary gland elements
   2. Squamous metaplasia of ductal epithelium
   3. Islands of isolated epithelium within connective tissue
F. Treatment and prognosis
   1. Benign condition, but biopsy to rule out neoplasia and arrive at definitive diagnosis may be needed
   2. Self-limiting with return to normal in about 5-6 weeks
   3. Prognosis good

## PSEUDOCYSTS

### Aneurysmal Bone Cyst

A. Etiology—increase in venous pressure causes dilation and rupture of local vascular network; etiologic theories include:
   1. Arteriovenous shunt—a benign fibro-osseous lesion in area alters blood vessels
   2. Trauma—trauma ruptures blood vessel, blood accumulates outside the vessel wall
B. Age and gender—under 30 years; no gender predilection
C. Location
   1. Long bones or vertebral column
   2. In jaws, mandible is the most common site (2:1)
D. Clinical features
   1. May be asymptomatic or appear as a slight to moderately well-defined bulge

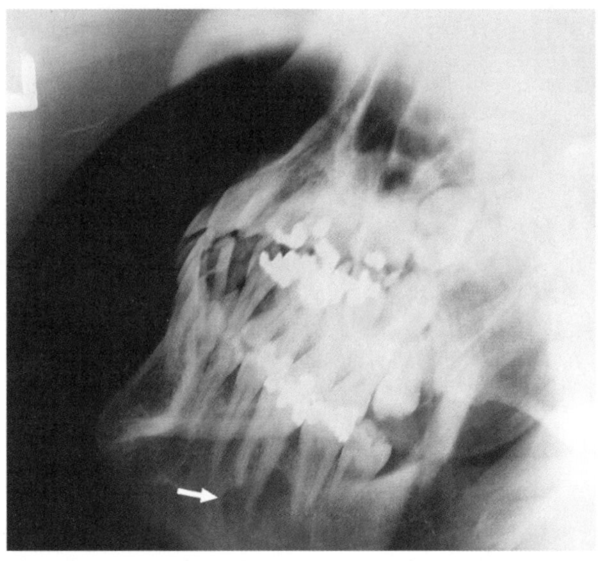

**Fig. 8.55** Extraoral radiograph showing a simple (traumatic) bone cyst *(arrow)* in the mandible, with its unique radiolucent characteristic scalloping around the roots. (Courtesy of Dr. Edward V. Zegarelli; from Ibsen OAC, Phelan JA. *Oral Pathology for the Dental Hygienist.* 6th ed. St. Louis: Elsevier Saunders; 2014.)

   2. Tenderness, in long bones pain on motion; may limit movement
   3. Intraoral may see mobility or migration of teeth
E. Radiographic appearance—hazy, gray, radiolucent area; appears cystic, with a "soap bubble" or honeycomb effect; multi-locular pattern
F. Histologic characteristics
   1. Not a true cyst since no epithelial lining—"pseudocyst"
   2. Fibrous connective tissue separates blood-filled compartments
   3. Blood-filled spaces with scattered multinucleated giant cells
G. Treatment and prognosis
   1. Surgical enucleation and thorough curettage (sometimes with cryosurgery—freezing technique to help control bleeding)
   2. Surgical appearance is that of a "blood-soaked" sponge
   3. Follow-up, on occasion recurs

### Simple Bone Cyst (Simple Bone Cavity, Traumatic Bone Cyst)

A. Etiology—theories include:
   1. Hemorrhage within bone following trauma; resulting blood clot destroyed leaving empty space
   2. Ischemic marrow necrosis
B. Age and gender—ages 10 to 20 years; male predilection
C. Location
   1. More common in mandible than maxilla
   2. Most common in long bones
D. Clinical features—asymptomatic (discovered during radiographic examination); teeth in area of lesion are vital
E. Radiographic appearance (Fig. 8.55)—well-defined radiolucency measuring 1 to 7 cm in greatest dimension; radiolucency projects or "scallops" between roots of teeth, borders may be sharp or diffuse

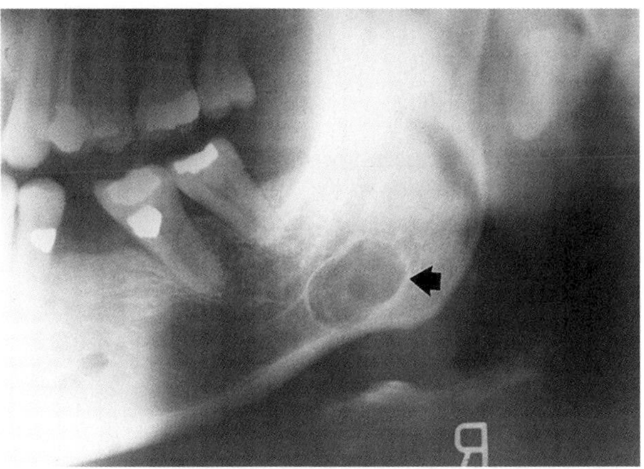


**Fig. 8.56** Part of a panoramic radiograph showing a lingual mandibular bone concavity (Stafne bone cyst). Note the well-circumscribed radiolucency inferior to the mandibular canal *(arrow)*. (From Ibsen OAC, Phelan JA. *Oral Pathology for the Dental Hygienist*. 6th ed. St. Louis: Elsevier Saunders; 2014.)

F. Histologic characteristics
   1. Fragments of vascular fibrous connective tissue may be present along walls of empty space
   2. Not a true cyst since no epithelial lining—"pseudocyst"
G. Treatment and prognosis
   1. Surgical intervention, such as curettage, to establish bleeding and clotting is often sufficient to promote healing
   2. Area fills in with normal bone in 6 months to 1 year after surgical intervention
   3. Prognosis excellent

## Static Bone Cyst (Lingual Mandibular Bone Concavity, Stafne Bone Cyst)

A. Etiology—developmental; lingual concavity in surface of mandible, accommodates position of salivary gland adjacent to mandible
B. Age and gender—young persons; slightly more common in males
C. Location—posterior mandible, anterior to the angle of the ramus, inferior to the mandibular canal
D. Clinical features—asymptomatic; occasionally bilateral, concavity filled with normal salivary gland tissue
E. Radiographic appearance (Fig. 8.56)—sharp, well-defined ovoid radiolucency 1 to 3 cm in diameter, anterior to angle of the ramus, inferior to the mandibular canal
F. Histologic characteristics—lymphoid, fat, normal submaxillary salivary gland tissues; striated muscle (not lined with epithelium, so not a true cyst)
G. Treatment and prognosis
   1. Rare surgical exploration to determine identity, no treatment necessary
   2. Prognosis excellent

# BLOOD DISORDERS

## General Characteristics

A. Benign and malignant diseases with numerous variations

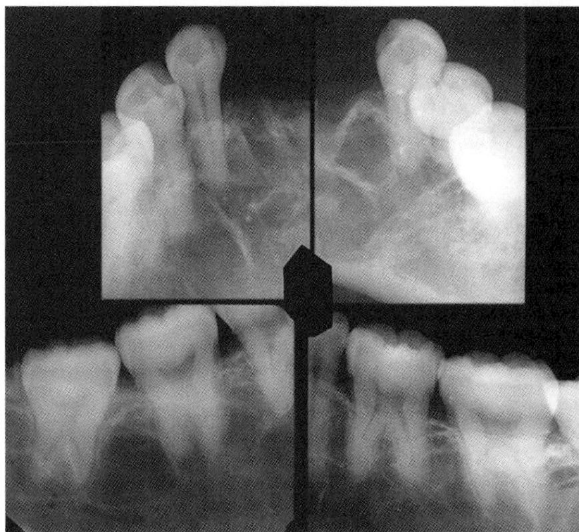

**Fig. 8.57** Sickle cell anemia. The radiograph shows abnormal trabeculation. (Courtesy of Dr. Edward V. Zegarelli; from Ibsen OAC, Phelan JA. *Oral Pathology for the Dental Hygienist*. 6th ed. St. Louis: Elsevier Saunders; 2014.)

B. Blood chemical studies important in making diagnosis
C. Anemias are categorized according to etiology
   1. Blood loss
   2. Congenital or developmental condition
   3. Decreased production of red blood cells (RBCs)

## Sickle Cell Disorder (Sickle Cell Anemia)

A. Etiology—hereditary; genetic disorder involving mutation of beta globin chain of hemoglobin
B. Age and gender—under 30 years; female predilection; 1 in 400 African Americans in United States affected; also persons of Mediterranean or Asian origin
C. Clinical features
   1. Systemic symptoms
      a. Weakness, easily fatigued; pallor of tissues
      b. Shortness of breath; nausea, vomiting
      c. Pain in joints
      d. Sickle cell crisis when oxygen cannot reach tissues, severe systemic complications
      e. Delayed growth and development in children
      f. Cardiac, kidney, CNS, eyes, and pulmonary involvement
      g. Frequent infections due to spleen damage
   2. Oral symptoms
      a. Delayed tooth eruption in children
      b. Pale oral mucosa, oral ulcers and angular cheilitis
      c. Osteomyelitis of mandible
D. Radiographic appearance (Fig. 8.57)
   1. Perpendicular trabeculations radiating outward, giving "hair-on-end" appearance to skull
   2. Decreased trabeculae in the jaws, with large marrow spaces
   3. Lamina dura not affected
E. Laboratory tests and findings (Fig. 8.58)
   1. Anemia; RBC count reduced to 1 million/mm$^3$ (normal is 4 to 6 million/mm$^3$)

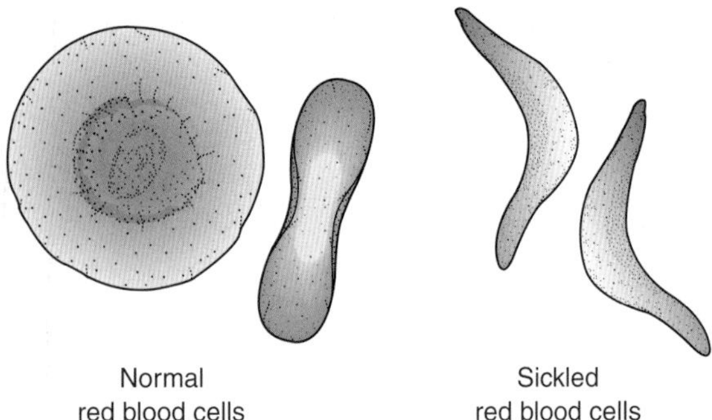


**Fig. 8.58** Normal red blood cells compared with sickled red blood cells. (From Ibsen OAC, Phelan JA. *Oral Pathology for the Dental Hygienist.* 6th ed. St. Louis: Elsevier Saunders; 2014.)

2. Decrease in the hemoglobin level in RBCs (normal in males, 13.5 to 18 g/dL; in females, 12 to 16 g/dL)
3. Blood smear showing sickle-shaped RBCs

F. Histologic characteristics: crescent-shaped erythrocytes, due to abnormal hemoglobin S associated with disorder

G. Treatment and prognosis
1. Symptomatic management; oxygen and intravenous fluids
2. Bone marrow transplantation is only cure, only for younger individuals
3. Hydroxyurea—drug treatment reduces painful crises, but has several side effects
4. Prognosis unpredictable, depends on disease severity and activity

## Pernicious Anemia

A. Etiology
1. Autoimmune disorder in which immune system produces antibodies against parietal cells of stomach
2. Deficiency of intrinsic factor (produced by the parietal cells) necessary to absorb vitamin $B_{12}$ (cobalamin)

B. Age and gender—older adults; rarely before age 30; no gender predilection

C. Clinical features
1. Systemic symptoms
   a. General weakness, dizziness, pallor, anemia (caused by low oxygen in the blood)
   b. Numbness or tingling of extremities
   c. Gastrointestinal (GI) manifestations—nausea, vomiting, diarrhea, abdominal pain
   d. Loss of appetite and weight loss
   e. Shortness of breath
   f. Neurologic changes—severe paresthesias
2. Oral symptoms
   a. Sore, painful, burning tongue; angular cheilitis
   b. Shallow ulcers on the mucosa
   c. Atrophy of tongue papillae; distorted perception of taste
   d. Pallor of the oral mucosa with focal patches of erythema

D. Laboratory tests and findings
1. Diagnosis of pernicious anemia made by laboratory testing; Schilling test is used to determine body's ability to properly absorb an oral dose of vitamin $B_{12}$

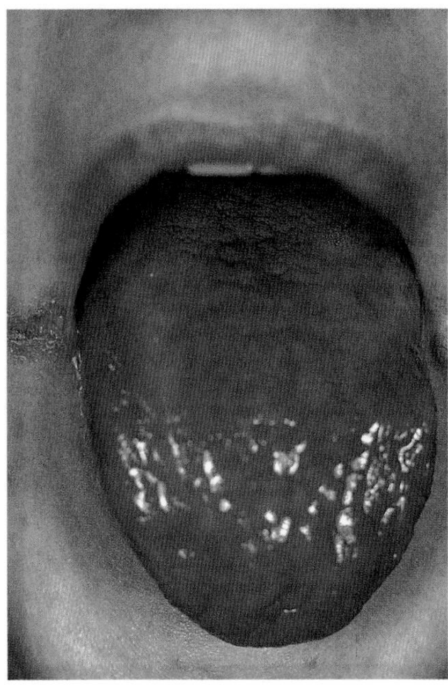

**Fig. 8.59** Iron deficiency anemia. The tongue is devoid of filiform papillae. Angular cheilitis is also present. (From Odell E: Cawson's Essentials of Oral Pathology and Oral Medicine. 9th ed. Elsevier; 2017.)

2. Achlorhydria—lack of gastric hydrochloric acid secretion
3. Megaloblastic anemia—immature, large RBCs

E. Histologic characteristics: macrocytosis of RBCs, megaloblastic anemia

F. Treatment and prognosis
1. Injections of vitamin $B_{12}$
2. Increased dietary intake of folic acid (leafy green vegetables, organ meats, wheat cereals)
3. 1% to 2% of persons with pernicious anemia develop gastric carcinoma

## Iron Deficiency Anemia (Plummer-Vinson Syndrome)

A. Etiology—iron deficiency caused by:
1. Inadequate dietary intake of iron
2. Chronic blood loss
3. Decreased iron absorption
4. Increased iron requirements (e.g., infancy, pregnancy)
5. Long-term chronic iron deficiency can lead to Plummer-Vinson Syndrome; characterized by iron deficiency anemia, dysphagia, and glossitis and increased risk for esophageal and oral cancer

B. Age and gender—ages 40 to 50 years; more common in females (5% to 30% female incidence in the United States)

C. Clinical features
1. Systemic symptoms
   a. Pallor of skin, weakness; fatigue
   b. Difficulty swallowing (dysphagia)
   c. Shortness of breath
   d. Enlarged spleen (splenomegaly) 20% to 30% of cases
   e. Absence of free hydrochloric acid in the stomach
2. Oral symptoms (Fig. 8.59)

a. Angular cheilitis; pallor and atrophy of oral tissues
b. Glossitis with depapillated, smooth, burning, painful tongue
c. Risk for oral candidiasis
d. Predisposition for development of oral cancer

D. Histologic characteristics
1. Altered exfoliated squamous epithelial cells of the tongue and soft tissues
2. Deficiency of keratinized cells
3. Abnormal cell maturation; enlarged nuclei

E. Laboratory findings
1. Complete blood count (CBC) with RBC indices
2. Hypochromatic microcytic RBCs
3. Low number of RBCs
4. Low hemoglobin and hematocrit
5. Plummer-Vinson syndrome esophagus evaluated for mucosal tissue growths that may inhibit swallowing ("webbing" of esophageal walls)

F. Treatment
1. Increase iron intake
2. Dietary supplement
3. Possible parenteral (intravenous [IV] or injection) supplementation

## Aplastic Anemia (Primary Aplastic Anemia)

A. Etiology—many cases unknown; severe depression in bone marrow activity; rare, life-threatening disease
B. Age and gender—young adults; no gender predilection
C. Clinical features
1. Oral symptoms
a. Spontaneous bleeding
b. Petechiae
c. Purpuric spots
d. Gingival infection
e. Pallor of oral tissues
2. Systemic symptoms
a. Fatigue, weakness
b. Tachycardia, dizziness
c. Retinal and cerebral hemorrhages in most severe cases
d. Significant bruising
e. Predisposition to infection

D. Laboratory tests and findings establish the diagnosis
1. Reduction in the number of all blood cells (pancytopenia)
2. Reduction in the number of RBCs (anemia)
3. Reduction in the number of WBCs (leukopenia)
4. Reduction in the number of platelets (thrombocytopenia)
5. Bone marrow changes

E. Treatment and prognosis
1. Blood transfusions
2. Antibiotic drugs to control potential infections
3. Bone marrow transplantation
4. Guarded prognosis, depends on severity
5. Serious medical conditions may lead to fatal outcome

## Secondary Aplastic Anemia

A. Etiology
1. Result of a drug or chemical substance; chemotherapy
2. Exposure to radiant energy—x-rays, radium, or radioactive isotopes

B. Age and gender—any age; no gender predilection
C. Clinical features—same as in primary aplastic anemia
D. Treatment and prognosis
1. Remove the cause
2. Supportive therapy
3. Prognosis is good

## Thalassemia

1. Etiology—inherited blood disorder caused by multiple gene mutations
2. Disorder of hemoglobin production
3. Ethnic predilection—high incidence in Mediterranean, African countries and India

B. Age and gender
1. Thalassemia major
a. Affects individuals within the 1st year of life (homozygous type)
b. More severe type of thalassemia (Cooley Anemia)
2. Thalassemia minor
a. Form appears in later childhood (heterozygous type)
b. Only one gene involved
c. No gender predilection

C. Clinical features
1. Systemic symptoms for thalassemia major
a. Yellow pallor of the skin
b. Enlarged spleen (splenomegaly); enlarged liver (hepatomegaly)
c. Facial features described as "chipmunk facies"
d. Enlargement of the maxilla or mandible and frontal bossing
2. Oral symptoms for thalassemia major
a. Malocclusion; protrusion of the anterior maxillary teeth
b. Pallor of the mucosa

D. Radiographic appearance
1. Peculiar trabecular pattern of the maxilla and the mandible—"salt and pepper" or "hair on end" sign of skull
2. Mild osteoporosis of the jaws
3. Thinning of lamina dura

E. Laboratory tests and findings
1. Elevated WBC count—10,000 to 25,000/mm$^3$
2. Elevated serum bilirubin level
3. Decreased hemoglobin level

F. Histologic characteristics—bone marrow shows cellular hyperplasia
G. Treatment and prognosis
1. Blood transfusions (frequently administered)
2. Frequent transfusions cause significant buildup of iron throughout body (hemochromatosis); these toxic accumulations of iron may be fatal
3. Bone marrow transplantation
4. Prognosis guarded—periods of remission can extend life span

### General Characteristics of Polycythemia

A. Overproduction and increase in number of circulating RBCs
B. Increased hemoglobin level
C. Three forms:
   1. Primary polycythemia (polycythemia vera)
   2. Secondary polycythemia
   3. Relative polycythemia—temporary increase in the number of RBCs; caused by shock, a severe burn, or excessive loss of body fluids

### Primary Polycythemia (Polycythemia Vera)

A. Etiology—in most cases not hereditary (not passed down through family), but is due to gene mutation
B. Age and gender—ages 40 to 60 years; more common in males
C. Clinical features
   1. Systemic symptoms
      a. Headache, dizziness, weakness
      b. Enlarged, painful spleen
      c. Gastric complaints; peptic ulcers
      d. Tips of fingers cyanotic
      e. Nose bleeds (epistaxis)
      f. Itching of skin (pruritus) without the presence of rash
   2. Oral symptoms
      a. Oral mucosa deep red to purple, result of decreased hemoglobin level
      b. Gingiva edematous and spongy; bleeds easily
      c. Submucosal petechiae; ecchymosis
D. Laboratory tests and findings
   1. RBC count elevated to 10 to 12 million cells/mm$^3$ (significant increase)
   2. Increase in:
      a. Hemoglobin content
      b. Blood viscosity
      c. WBC counts
      d. Hematocrit value
   3. Decrease in platelets
E. Treatment and prognosis
   1. Medications and procedures to control platelets
   2. Intermittent phlebotomy
   3. Chemotherapeutic drugs

### Secondary Polycythemia

A. Etiology—increased number of RBCs caused by a physiologic response to decreased oxygen
   1. Bone marrow anoxia (lack of oxygen) caused by:
      a. Pulmonary dysfunction
      b. Heart disease
      c. High altitudes
      d. Carbon monoxide poisoning
   2. Stimulatory factors such as drugs or chemicals
B. Characteristics and features similar to those of primary polycythemia vera

### Relative Polycythemia

A. Etiology—decreased plasma volume (not an increase in RBCs) that may be caused by:
   1. Use of diuretics
   2. Vomiting, diarrhea
   3. Excessive sweating
B. Age and gender—chronic form of relative polycythemia (also called *stress polycythemia*) is more common in white, middle-aged men, who are stressed, overweight, hypertensive and who smoke
C. Treatment—related to cause and risk factors; attempt to remove cause and risk factors

### Agranulocytosis

A. Etiology—significant reduction in or absence of circulating neutrophils in the blood (neutropenia)
   1. Primary form—unknown; immunologic disorder
   2. Secondary form—drug ingestion; chemotherapy; toxic effect of drugs or chemicals
B. Age and gender—any age; more common adults; female predilection in secondary form
C. Clinical features
   1. Systemic symptoms
      a. Sudden onset
      b. High fever, chills, sore throat
      c. Malaise, weakness
      d. Skin is jaundiced
      e. Regional lymphadenopathy
   2. Oral symptoms
      a. Infection (clinical signs affecting gingiva can be similar to NUG)
      b. Ulcerations of the pharynx, palate, buccal mucosa, and tongue
D. Laboratory tests and findings—needed to confirm diagnosis
   1. Severe decrease in or absence of granulocytes or PMNs
   2. Accelerated destruction of neutrophils; bone marrow has few or no granulocytes
   3. WBC count is reduced to less than 1000 cells/mm$^3$
E. Histologic characteristics
   1. Necrosis of involved tissues
   2. Increased bacterial microorganisms
F. Treatment
   1. Removal of causative drug or agent, if possible
   2. Administration of antibiotics to prevent or control infection

### Cyclic Neutropenia

A. Etiology—inherited; autosomal dominant; mutation of the neutrophil elastase *(ELA2)* gene
B. Age and gender related— most frequent infants and young children; no gender predilection
C. Clinical features: regular periodic episodes lasting 3 to 4 days correlating with significant decrease in circulating neutrophils
   1. Systemic symptoms
      a. General weakness, malaise
      b. Recurrent fever, sore throat, headache
      c. Cervical lymphadenopathy
      d. GI mucosal ulcerations
   2. Oral symptoms (Fig. 8.60)

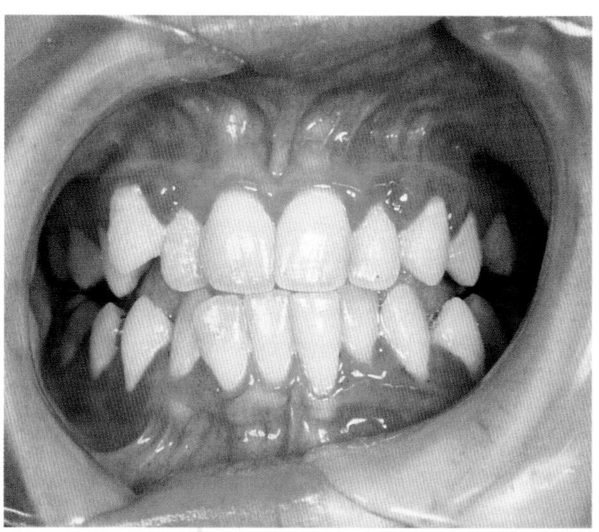

**Fig. 8.60** Marked gingivitis, with areas of gingival recession in a patient with cyclic neutropenia. (From Ibsen OAC, Phelan JA. *Oral Pathology for the Dental Hygienist*. 6th ed. St. Louis: Elsevier Saunders; 2014.)

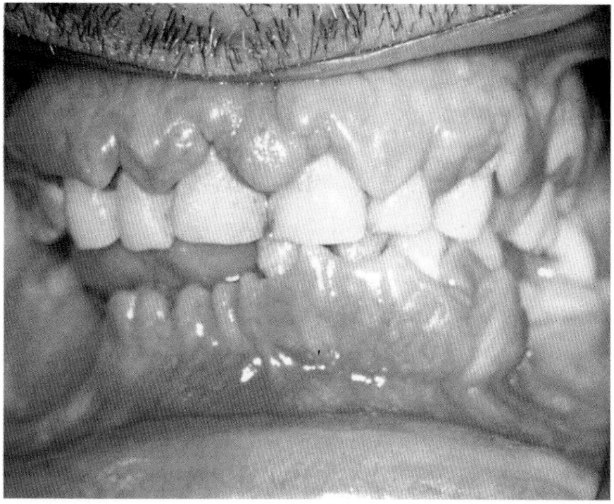

**Fig. 8.61** Generalized gingival hyperplasia in a patient with leukemia. (Courtesy of Dr. Edward V. Zegarelli; from Ibsen OAC, Phelan JA. *Oral Pathology for the Dental Hygienist*. 6th ed. St. Louis: Elsevier Saunders; 2014.)

a. Severe gingivitis, recession, periodontitis
b. Painful chronic ulcerations on oral mucosa especially gingiva, keratinized mucosa severely affected
c. Mild to severe loss of alveolar bone

D. Laboratory tests and findings
1. Neutrophils may completely disappear in acute stage
2. Cycles occur at intervals of 21 to 27 days
3. Sequential blood counts several times a week for several weeks helps determine neutrophil cycle

E. Treatment and prognosis
1. Maintain optimal oral hygiene
2. Perform dental treatment during cycle when circulating neutrophils are normal, this reduces potential for complications and secondary infections
3. Antibiotics to control significant infections
4. Premedication with antibiotics before dental hygiene or surgical procedures may be needed
5. Possible treatment with granulocyte colony-stimulating factor (G-CSF)

## Leukemia

### General Characteristics

A. Malignant neoplastic disorder involving blood-forming cells; originates in bone marrow
B. Excessive proliferation of malignant immature WBCs
C. Etiology—combination of genetic and environmental factors; oncogenic viruses
1. Chronic exposure to chemicals or ionizing radiation
2. Higher incidence among persons with genetic disorders, including Down syndrome and other chromosomal abnormalities, neurofibromatosis, and Klinefelter syndrome (see the section on "Genetics" in Chapter 7)

D. A number of types and subtypes of this condition exist

### Acute Leukemia

A. Two types:
1. Acute myeloid (myelogenous) leukemia (AML)
2. Acute lymphocytic (lymphoblastic) leukemia (ALL)

B. Age and gender
1. AML generally affects adults but can affect children
2. ALL almost always affects children, second peak in old age

C. Clinical features—onset is sudden, rapidly progressing
1. Systemic symptoms
a. Frequent infections
b. Weakness, fever, headache
c. Pale skin
d. Easy bruising of the skin and mucous membranes
e. Unusual bleeding, nosebleeds
f. Enlargement of organs—spleen, liver
g. Bone and joint pain
2. Oral symptoms (Fig. 8.61)
a. Purpuric spots, petechiae
b. Marked gingival enlargement—red, soft, spongy with spontaneous bleeding
c. Gingiva sometimes similar to NUG—characterized by ulcerations, blunted papillae, necrosis, odor
d. Pallor of tissues; nonulcerated edema
e. Candidiasis, herpetic infection, or both
f. Toothache caused by invasion and necrosis of pulp
g. Mobility of teeth due to breakdown of periodontal ligament, supporting bone

D. Laboratory tests and findings
1. Both anemia and thrombocytopenia present
2. Prolonged bleeding and coagulation times; caused by decrease in the number of platelets (thrombocytopenia)
3. WBC count elevated to 100,000/$mm^3$ (many immature cells)
4. Leukemic cells in bone marrow and peripheral blood
5. Tests to identify certain enzymes can help classify leukemia type

E. Treatment and prognosis
1. Chemotherapy depending on type and form of leukemia
2. Antibiotics to control infection
3. Bone marrow or stem cell transplant

4. Transfusions with platelets or packed RBCs
5. Maintain optimal oral hygiene
6. Prognosis depends on multiple factors (e.g., type of leukemia, age at onset)

### Chronic Leukemia

A. Common forms
   1. Chronic myeloid leukemia (CML)—associated with the Philadelphia chromosome (abnormality of chromosome 22)
   2. Chronic lymphocytic leukemia (CLL)—the most common leukemia in adults; asymptomatic for a long time
B. Age and gender—chronic leukemia affects older adults; no gender predilection;
C. Clinical features—slow-growing with slow progression
   1. Systemic symptoms
      a. Very slow onset—disease may be present for weeks to years before symptoms appear and lead to diagnosis
      b. Weight loss, fatigue
      c. Lymph node enlargement and enlarged spleen in the CLL type, not in the CML type
      d. Petechiae on the skin with nodules of leukemic cells
      e. Destructive bone lesions—result in bone fracture
   2. Oral symptoms
      a. Gingival tissues are severely affected; become tender, enlarged, bleed easily
      b. Pallor of gingiva and lips
      c. Purpuric spots; ecchymosis
      d. Cervical lymphadenopathy may be an early sign (underlines importance of lymph node examination)
      e. Oral candidiasis
D. Laboratory tests and findings
   1. Anemia and thrombocytopenia sometimes present
   2. WBC count can increase to 500,000/mm$^3$ (95% of the total number of blood cells)
   3. Shift to the left in the maturity of cells
   4. Differential count of cell type involved elevated
E. Treatment and prognosis
   1. Chemotherapy
   2. Bone marrow transplantation (especially for patients with CML—better survival rates)
   3. Prognosis depends on the stage of the disease; chronic leukemia—2 to 10-year survival depending on stage)

## Purpura

### General Characteristics

A. Purplish discoloration of the skin and mucous membranes caused by spontaneous escape of blood into tissues
B. Caused by:
   1. Defect or deficiency in blood platelets (thrombocytopenic purpura)
   2. Unexplained increase in capillary fragility (vascular or nonthrombocytopenic purpura)

### Thrombocytopenic Purpura

A. Etiology
   1. Primary (idiopathic or immune) thrombocytopenic purpura; cause is unknown
   2. Secondary thrombocytopenic purpura—immune mediated
      a. Drug toxicity
      b. Chemotherapy
      c. Infectious diseases
B. Age and gender—primary form occurs in childhood before age 10 years; secondary form may appear at any age; no gender predilection
C. Clinical features
   1. Systemic symptoms
      a. Spontaneous hemorrhagic skin lesions that vary in size (petechiae, ecchymosis, hematomas)
      b. Patient bruises easily
      c. Bleeding through the urinary tract (hematuria)
      d. Bleeding from the nose (epistaxis)
      e. Spleen not palpable
   2. Oral symptoms
      a. Profuse gingival hemorrhage
      b. Clustered petechiae
D. Laboratory tests and findings
   1. Abnormal platelet count; severe reduction in the platelet count—below 50,000/mm$^3$ (normal, 150,000 to 400,000/mm$^3$)
   2. Bleeding time prolonged to up to 1 hour or more
   3. Positive capillary fragility test
E. Treatment
   1. Discontinue causative drug, if known
   2. Corticosteroid therapy
   3. Blood transfusions (platelets, in particular)
   4. Guarded prognosis
   5. Consult patient's physician prior to any dental or surgical procedure

### Nonthrombocytopenic Purpura

A. Etiology—results from a variety of conditions that produce capillary fragility
   1. Defect in capillary walls (vitamin C deficiency, infections)
   2. Disorder of platelet function (drugs, allergies, autoimmune diseases)
B. Clinical features
   1. Normal platelet count
   2. Other symptoms similar to those of thrombocytopenic purpura
   3. Oral manifestations—spontaneous bleeding, petechiae and ecchymoses
C. Laboratory tests
   1. Platelet count normal
   2. Bleeding time prolonged
D. Treatment
   1. Systemic corticosteroids
   2. Splenectomy
   3. Remove cause

## Hemophilia

A. Etiology—genetic deficiency of clotting factors in the blood; von Willebrand factor, or clotting factors VIII or IX
   1. Von Willebrand's disease; autosomal dominant; affects both males and females

2. Type A hemophilia associated with factor VIII, sex-linked recessive (on X chromosome), occurs almost exclusively in males
3. Type B hemophilia associated with factor IX, sex-linked recessive (on X chromosome), occurs almost exclusively in males
4. Types A and B hemophilia are usually transmitted genetically from asymptomatic carrier mothers to sons; spontaneous gene mutations also occur, up to one-third of cases

B. Age and gender—usually present at birth; symptoms may not appear until later; males are most susceptible, whereas females are carriers of the trait

C. Clinical features
1. Systemic symptoms
a. Prolonged clotting time; persistent bleeding
b. Massive hematomas; hemorrhage
c. Three forms—differ in the deficiency of a blood clotting factor
(1) Type A—(factor VIII) may be mild, moderate, or severe depending on amount of clotting factor in blood; most common type of hemophilia
(2) Type B—(factor IX) also known as Christmas disease; may be mild, moderate or severe depending on amount of clotting factor in blood; second most common type of hemophilia
(3) Von Willebrand's disease—(abnormal von Willebrand's factor) most common inherited bleeding disorder in United States, mild cases may go undetected
2. Oral symptoms
a. Spontaneous gingival bleeding
b. Prolonged bleeding following tooth eruption, exfoliation, scaling, extraction, or surgery

D. Laboratory tests and findings—prothrombin time (PT), factor assays to identify factor deficiency

E. Treatment
1. Main treatment is replacement therapy; injections or infusions of concentrates of missing clotting factor
2. Nonhuman recombinant clotting factor concentrates may be used
3. Genetic counseling
4. Maintain optimal dental and dental hygiene care

## HUMAN IMMUNODEFICIENCY VIRUS (HIV) AND ACQUIRED IMMUNE DEFICIENCY SYNDROME (AIDS)

A. Etiology—HIV is an RNA retrovirus that infects and destroys CD4+ T-lymphocytes resulting in immune deficiency; AIDS is a set of symptoms caused by HIV infection, this is the last stage of HIV infection or late-stage advanced HIV (Box 8.2)

B. Age—any age; virus can be transmitted to anyone

C. Gender and ethnic characteristics
1. Male predilection; however, fastest-growing group of infected persons is women
2. Homosexual or bisexual men
3. Overall increased incidence among IV drug users
4. Others at risk include sex workers, prison inmates, and children of infected mothers

E. Transmission
1. Sexual contact
2. Infected blood or serum; virus has been found in blood and bodily fluids, including saliva and tears, of infected individuals

### BOX 8.2 Definition and Diagnosis of Acquired Immunodeficiency Syndrome (AIDS)

AIDS is an illness characterized by one or more of the following diseases or conditions:

HIV Laboratory Tests Not Performed or Results Inconclusive and the Patient Has No Other Cause of Immunodeficiency

1. Candidiasis of the esophagus, trachea, bronchi, or lungs
2. Cryptococcosis, extrapulmonary
3. Cryptosporidiosis with diarrhea persisting longer than 1 month
4. Cytomegalovirus disease of an organ other than liver, spleen, or lymph nodes in a patient older than 1 month of age
5. Herpes simplex virus infection causing a mucocutaneous ulcer that persists longer than 1 month, or bronchitis, pneumonitis, or esophagitis for any duration affecting a patient older than 1 month of age
6. Kaposi's sarcoma affecting a patient <60 years of age
7. Lymphoid interstitial pneumonia or pulmonary hyperplasia, or both; affecting a child <13 years of age
8. *Mycobacterium avium* or *Mycobacterium kansasii* disease, disseminated
9. *Pneumocystis jiroveci* (formerly *P. carinii*) pneumonia
10. Progressive multifocal leukoencephalopathy
11. Toxoplasmosis of the brain affecting a patient older than 1 month

With Laboratory Evidence for Human Immunodeficiency Virus (HIV) Infection

Less than 200 CD4 + T lymphocytes/mL, or a CD4 + T lymphocyte percentage of total lymphocytes of < 14

Any of the diseases previously listed or those that follow:

1. Multiple bacterial infections of certain types affecting a child <13 years of age
2. Coccidioidomycosis, disseminated
3. HIV encephalopathy (HIV dementia)
4. Histoplasmosis, disseminated
5. Isosporiasis with diarrhea persisting longer than 1 month
6. Lymphoma of the brain at any age
7. Kaposi's sarcoma at any age
8. Certain types of lymphoma
9. Mycobacterial disease, other than tuberculosis, disseminated
10. Extrapulmonary tuberculosis
11. *Salmonella* septicemia, recurrent
12. HIV wasting syndrome
13. Pulmonary tuberculosis
14. Recurrent pneumonia
15. Invasive cervical cancer

Even if HIV laboratory test results are negative, if other causes of immunodeficiency are not ruled out, a diagnosis of AIDS can be made if certain of these diseases are diagnosed.

Modified from Centers for Disease Control and Prevention. 1993 Revised classifications system for HIV infection and expanded surveillance case definition for AIDS among adolescents and adults. *MMWR.* 1992:41(RR-17).

3. Infected mothers can transmit virus to newborns via breast milk
4. Artificial insemination
5. IV drug users
6. Cofactors (e.g., other infections) may influence ability of transmission

F. Clinical features—oral lesions (Box 8.3)
1. Oral findings missing or can be subtle at earliest stage of HIV infection
2. Persistent generalized lymphadenopathy (PGL) may be only initial sign of HIV infection; PGL warns of progression to AIDS (one-third have diagnostic features of AIDS within 5 years)
3. Oral candidiasis occurs in >85% of cases; this is most common intraoral manifestation of HIV and often the presenting sign that leads to initial diagnosis
4. Persistence of active sites of herpes simplex infection for more than one month; severe infections with herpes zoster and human papilloma virus (HPV)
5. Major or herpetiform aphthous ulcers
6. Severe NUG; linear gingival erythema (clinical features similar to marginal gingivitis), highly resistant to oral hygiene care
7. Necrotizing ulcerative periodontitis (NUP); gingival necrosis accompanied by rapid severe bone loss; not responsive to conventional periodontal therapy
8. Hairy leukoplakia (HL); due to Epstein-Barr virus; HL in HIV-infected patient is a strong indicator that AIDS will develop within 2 years
9. Kaposi's sarcoma; considered vascular malignancy; occurs in 15% to 20% of AIDS patients; oral lesions present in 50%; especially hard palate and gingiva
10. HIV-salivary gland disease; parotid enlargement bilaterally, more common in children; may be seen in up to 5% of HIV+ patients

G. Clinical features—general
1. Initially may mimic infectious mononucleosis with lymphadenopathy, fatigue, headache, fever, sore throat
2. Prone to develop multiple opportunistic infections—candidiasis, cytomegalovirus, herpes simplex, herpes zoster, pneumocystis pneumonia (highly suggestive of AIDS and often leads to initial diagnosis)
3. Certain cancers develop more frequently—SCC, Kaposi's sarcoma, and non-Hodgkin's lymphoma
4. Constitutional signs include sudden, unexplained weight loss, persistent lymphadenopathy involving cervical and submandibular nodes

H. Laboratory
1. HIV viral load test looks for actual virus in blood, not routinely used
2. Antigen/antibody test looks for both HIV antibodies and antigens in blood; common test in United States, rapid test available
3. Home testing and collection kits on the market; manufacturer provides confidential counseling and referral for follow-up testing

I. Histologic findings—extremely variable, depending on pathologic condition or disease

J. Treatment—HIV
1. Highly active antiretroviral therapy (HAART); drug combination of reverse transcriptase inhibitors and protease inhibitors; not a cure
2. Disease specific medications to prevent or treat opportunistic infections
3. Prognosis—depends on early diagnosis and therapy

**BOX 8.3 Oral Lesions Associated with Human Immunodeficiency Virus (HIV) Infection**

Candidiasis
Herpes simplex infection
Herpes zoster
Hairy leukoplakia
Human papillomavirus (HPV) lesions
Atypical gingivitis and periodontitis
Other opportunistic infections reported
- *Mycobacterium avium*
- Cytomegalovirus
- *Cryptococcus neoformans*
- *Klebsiella pneumoniae*
- *Enterobacter cloacae*
- *Histoplasma capsulatum*

Kaposi's sarcoma
Non-Hodgkin's lymphoma
Aphthous ulcers
Mucosal pigmentation
Bilateral salivary gland enlargement and xerostomia
Spontaneous gingival bleeding resulting from thrombocytopenia

From Ibsen OAC, Phelan JA. *Oral Pathology for the Dental Hygienist.* 6th ed. St. Louis: Elsevier; 2014.

## BONE DYSPLASIAS

### General Characteristics

A. Etiology—developmental disorder; due defective gene in cells that form bone, not inherited; replacement of bone with fibrous connective tissue
B. Bone enlargement and deformity, fractures, pain
C. Monostotic form affects one bone; polyostotic form affects multiple bones
D. Benign noncancerous disorder, malignant transformation rare

### Monostotic Fibrous Dysplasia

A. Etiology—noninherited developmental disorder, due to defective gene in bone-forming cells
B. Age and gender—early teen and adolescent years during periods of bone growth; often becomes inactive after puberty; boys more often than girls
C. Location
1. Ribs—most common site
2. Craniofacial bones, typically posterior maxilla

D. Clinical features
1. Affects one bone (~70% of cases of fibrous dysplasia)

2. Painless swelling, enlargement or expansion of jaw: buccal plate of maxilla or mandible
3. Result may be malocclusion, tipping, or displacement of teeth
4. Lesions in maxilla may not be clearly outlined due to extension into sinus or floor of orbit

E. Radiographic features
1. Lesion blends into surrounding bone
2. Diffuse radiopacity; "ground glass" appearance
3. Sometimes radiolucency with areas of radiopacity (depending on the degree of calcification)

F. Histologic characteristics
1. Fibrous tissue with irregularly shaped islands of woven bone
2. Irregularly shaped trabeculae give characteristic "Chinese character" or "alphabet soup" appearance

G. Treatment and prognosis
1. Manage pain and stabilize bones
2. Surgical correction of deformed bone, generally postponed until after puberty
3. Radiation therapy contraindicated due to potential for malignant transformation

## Polyostotic Fibrous Dysplasia

A. Etiology—noninherited developmental disorder, due to defective gene in bone-forming cells

B. Age and gender—younger age group than monostotic form; female predilection for McCune-Albright type

C. Location
1. Sometimes more than half of bones in skeletal system involved
2. Bones of the face and skull, thigh bone, upper arm, pelvis, ribs
3. Long bones affected more often than craniofacial bones
4. Unilateral (occurring on one side of body), when multiple bones affected

D. Clinical features (depend on type of polyostotic fibrous dysplasia)
1. Affects multiple bones (~30% of cases of fibrous dysplasia); disease may remain active throughout life
2. Bone fractures, skin lesions; café au lait pigmentation
3. Oral manifestations:
   a. Expansion and deformity of jaws; unilateral enlargement of maxilla or mandible
   b. Disturbed tooth eruption pattern caused by endocrine dysfunction
4. Types of polyostotic fibrous dysplasia
   a. Craniofacial fibrous dysplasia—craniofacial involvement; maxilla often involved, lesion may extend into sinus and surrounding bones
   b. Jaffe-Lichtenstein syndrome—lesions arise in multiple bones; café au lait skin lesions on skin of trunk and upper legs
   c. McCune-Albright syndrome—most severe form of polyostotic fibrous dysplasia
      (1) Multiple bones involved (polyostotic)
      (2) Café au lait skin lesions
      (3) Severe endocrine abnormalities: precocious (early before age 3) puberty; more common in girls than boys

E. Radiographic appearance—lesions blend into surrounding bone; diffuse radiopacity; "ground glass" appearance, sometimes radiolucency with areas of radiopacity

F. Laboratory tests and diagnostic tools
1. Radiographs are the primary tool to diagnose fibrous dysplasia
2. Imaging tests, bone scan, possible bone biopsy

G. Histologic characteristics
1. Fibrous tissue with irregularly shaped islands of woven bone
2. Irregularly shaped trabeculae give characteristic "Chinese character" or "alphabet soup" appearance

H. Treatment and prognosis
1. Some cases treated with drugs such as bisphosphonates to prevent bone loss
2. Surgical correction to treat deformity or fracture
3. Radiation treatment contraindicated because of association with malignant transformation

## Cherubism

A. Etiology—inherited; autosomal dominant; defect in SH3BP2 gene

B. Age and gender—onset as early as 1 year or early childhood (by age 5), males affected over females 2:1

C. Location—maxilla and the mandible

D. Clinical features
1. Painless bilateral facial swelling or enlargement of jaws; firm and hard on palpation
2. Involvement of four quadrants produces chubby cheeks and "cherubic" appearance
3. Condition affects orbital areas creating upturned eyes ("eyes upturned to heaven" appearance)
4. Regional lymphadenopathy, dental malocclusion
5. Early exfoliation of primary dentition
6. Agenesis of permanent second and third molars; lack of or delayed tooth eruption
7. Speech and swallowing problems

E. Radiographic appearance
1. Bilateral multilocular radiolucencies; "soap bubble" appearance
2. Thinning of cortical plates, numerous unerupted or displaced teeth in cyst-like radiolucent spaces
3. Root resorption

F. Laboratory tests and findings—analysis for gene mutation provides definitive diagnosis

G. Histologic characteristics
1. Similar to central giant cell granuloma and hyperparathyroidism; fibrous tissue proliferation
2. Numerous large, multinucleated giant cells in a loose, delicate, fibrous connective tissue stroma

H. Treatment and prognosis
1. Self-limiting; remission at puberty
2. Surgical intervention for severe cases
3. Radiation contraindicated due to risk of sarcoma
4. Prognosis is good

## Periapical Cemento-Osseous Dysplasia (Cementoma)

A. Etiology—unknown; benign fibro-osseous lesion, nonneoplastic type of cemento-osseous dysplasia, believed to be reactive
B. Age and gender—middle age; more common in females (15:1) and African Americans (70%)
C. Location
   1. Anterior mandible; rare in the maxilla
   2. Apices of teeth, surrounding or adjacent to roots
D. Clinical features
   1. Asymptomatic and localized; teeth in the affected area are vital (this feature is critical to diagnosis)
   2. Pulp testing must be part of the diagnostic process
   3. Lesions progress over time through three radiographic stages
   4. Early stage may be mistaken for periapical pathology, presenting diagnostic challenge
E. Radiographic appearance—depends on stage of lesion development
   1. Early stage (osteolytic stage); radiolucent lesion cannot be differentiated from other apical pathology
   2. Middle stage (osteoblastic stage) mixed radiolucent/radiopaque lesions, indicates calcification of connective tissue
   3. Mature or end-stage, lesion uniformly radiopaque with a radiolucent rim, periodontal ligament remains intact
F. Histologic characteristics, depend on stage of lesion
   1. Fibroblast-like cells and collagen with varying amounts of interspersed trabeculae of bone and cementum-like material
   2. Normal bone replaced with abnormal bone/cementum matrix
G. Treatment and prognosis
   1. Self-limiting; no treatment necessary
   2. Prognosis is good

## Paget's Disease (Osteitis Deformans)

A. Etiology—unknown; nonneoplastic disease of bone theories include:
   1. Viral cause
   2. Inflammatory response
   3. Endocrine imbalance
B. Age and gender—most often over 40 years of age; more frequent in Caucasian males
C. Location—may be localized to a few bones or widespread to multiple bones; common sites affected include pelvis, spine, leg, skull
D. Clinical features
   1. Systemic signs and symptoms
      a. Develop slowly over time
      b. Enlargement of bones (bowing of long bones)—spine, femur, tibia; skull (frontal bossing can lead to change in hat size)
      c. Most common symptom is bone pain
      d. Deformities, tingling and numbness in arms or legs, pathologic fractures
      e. Severe headaches, hearing loss
   2. Oral signs and symptoms
      a. Enlargement of jaws and dental arches, may lead to increased spacing between teeth
      b. Edentulous patients may complain their dentures no longer fit
      c. Hypercementosis of teeth, can complicate tooth extractions
E. Radiographic appearance
   1. Initial decreased radiodensity
   2. Irregular radiolucent and radiopaque patches, giving classic "cotton wool" or "cotton ball" appearance
   3. Root resorption; hypercementosis; loss of lamina dura
F. Laboratory tests and findings
   1. Bone scans and skeletal survey, characteristic appearance on radiographs
   2. Elevated level of alkaline phosphatase (significant to the diagnosis)
   3. Normal calcium phosphate and aminotransterase; markers of bone turnover
G. Histologic characteristics—characterized by both bone resorption and bone deposition
   1. Areas of resorption—osteoclast activity
   2. Areas of deposition—osteoblast activity
   3. Areas of both resorption and deposition—osteoclasts and osteoblasts present
   4. Vascular fibrous connective tissue replaces bone marrow
   5. Reversal lines in bone—"mosaic bone"
H. Treatment and prognosis
   1. No treatment, if asymptomatic
   2. Treatment aimed at controlling disease, there is no cure
   3. Bone pain—analgesics
   4. Systemic medications: calcitonin, bisphosphonates
   5. Diet and exercise
   6. Rare complication is osteogenic sarcoma

# ENDOCRINE DISORDERS

## General Characteristics

A. Associated with group of organs controlling metabolism, growth, other tissue functions
B. Occur as a result of hormone excess or deficiency

## Hyperparathyroidism

A. Etiology—excess secretion of parathyroid hormone (PTH) by parathyroid gland
   1. Primary hyperparathyroidism—excessive PTH results from benign or malignant parathyroid pathology
B. Secondary hyperparathyroidism—accompanies other systemic diseases; most common cause is chronic renal failure
C. Age and gender—most often over 60 years of age; female predilection (3:1)
D. Clinical features
   1. Systemic signs and symptoms
      a. Classic signs and symptoms of primary hyperparathyroidism are referred to as "stones, bones, and abdominal groans"

b. Stones refers to kidney stones; caused by increased calcium in urine
c. Bones refers to bone-related pathology; pain, joint stiffness, and resorption of bone with spontaneous fractures
d. Groans refers to discomfort due to GI problems such as ulcers, indigestion, constipation
2. Oral signs and symptoms
a. Jaw swelling due to "brown tumors" of hyperparathyroidism; these resolve without treatment once disorder is under control (brown tumors similar to central giant cell granuloma)
b. Bone loss may result in malocclusion, shifting or mobility of teeth

D. Radiographic appearance (Fig. 8.62A)
1. Loss of bone density results in "ground-glass" appearance
2. Unilocular or multilocular cyst-like radiolucencies in posterior jaws
3. Loss of lamina dura

E. Laboratory tests and findings
1. Blood tests: elevated PTH and calcium levels in blood
2. Skeletal assessment with bone density testing
3. Kidney function assessment

F. Histologic characteristics (Fig. 8.62B)

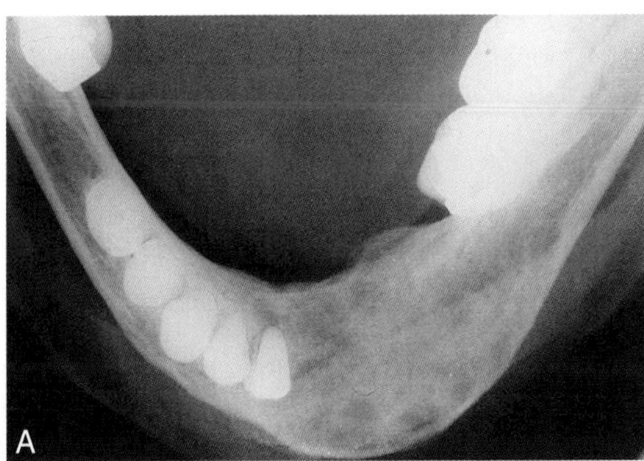


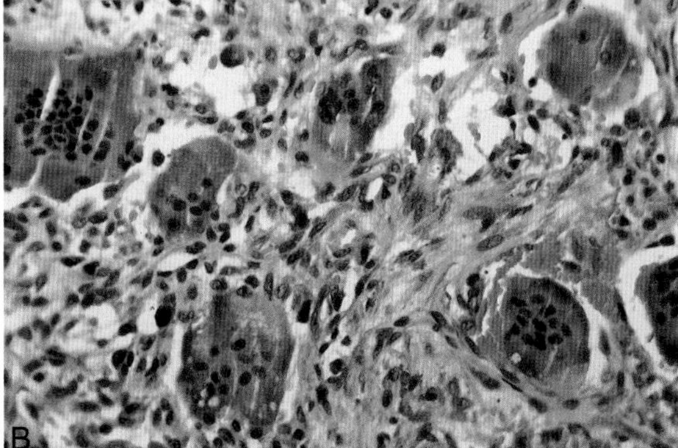


**Fig. 8.62** (A) Radiograph of a mandibular lesion in a patient with hyperparathyroidism. (B) Microscopic appearance of a jaw lesion occurring in a patient with hyperparathyroidism. The histologic appearance is identical to that of a central giant cell granuloma. (A courtesy of Drs. Paul Freedman and Stanley Kerpel; A and B from Ibsen OAC, Phelan JA. *Oral Pathology for the Dental Hygienist.* 6th ed. St. Louis: Elsevier Saunders; 2014.)

1. Osteoclastic activity increased; osteoclasts observed tunneling into bone matrix
2. Increased bone formation and peritrabecular fibrosis
3. "Brown" tumor histologically indistinguishable from central giant cell granuloma

G. Treatment
1. Correct the cause of increased PTH production (tumors, renal disease, vitamin D deficiency)
2. Surgical removal or parathyroidectomy is cure for primary hyperparathyroidism
3. "Brown" tumor resolves without treatment once hyperparathyroidism is controlled

## Osteomalacia

A. Etiology—most often due to severe vitamin D deficiency or impaired absorption of vitamin D (vitamin D deficiency in adults called osteomalacia, in children called rickets)

B. Age and gender—osteomalacia occurs in adults; female predilection, often happens during pregnancy

C. Clinical features
1. Osteomalacia means "soft bones"; loss of mineralization or hardening
a. Easily broken bones
b. Bone pain and tenderness
c. Affects gait, side-to-side or waddling stride when walking
2. Polyuria (urine output greatly increased) and polydipsia (severe thirst) complication of hypercalcemia
3. Oral manifestations may include alveolar ridge resorption and periodontal bone loss

D. Radiographic appearance
1. Generalized demineralization of bone; symmetric stripes in hypocalcified long bones, pelvis and scapula indicate pseudofractures
2. Lamina dura of teeth may be absent
3. Radiopaque stones in kidney

E. Laboratory tests and findings
1. Blood and urine tests to detect low levels of vitamin D, calcium; phosphorus problems
2. Radiographs, bone biopsy

F. Treatment and prognosis
1. Increased dosage of vitamin D; if malabsorption, water-soluble, synthetic vitamin D can be given
2. Calcium supplements
3. Treatment of bone fractures (persons with osteomalacia prone to pathologic fractures)

## Rickets

A. Etiology
1. Due to severe vitamin D deficiency or impaired absorption of vitamin D (called rickets in children, osteomalacia in adults)
2. Failure of cartilage and bone to calcify

B. Age—children, most common in 1st year of life

C. Clinical features
1. Systemic signs and symptoms
a. Delayed growth, spine deformity

b. Muscle weakness, bowed legs or knock knees
c. Protrusion of sternum, "pigeon breast" deformity
d. Prominence of costochondral junctions, "rachitic rosary"
2. Oral signs and symptoms
a. Dentin defects, enamel pits and hypoplasia
b. Large pulp chambers, short roots
c. Hypoplastic alveolar ridge, poorly defined lamina dura

D. Treatment—vitamin D and calcium supplements, other medications and supplements may be indicated; more severe skeletal deformities may require surgical correction

## LANGERHANS CELL HISTIOCYTOSIS

### General Characteristics

A. Etiology—unknown; not inherited, mutations in BRAF gene in about half of cases
B. Age and gender—disorder that primarily affects children, but also all ages
C. Langerhans cells multiply and accumulate in large collections called granulomas
D. Includes a group of three diseases characterized by proliferation of Langerhans cells; a combination of histiocytic cells and eosinophils
E. Three variants:
1. Letterer-Siwe disease (severe, acute disseminated form)
a. Age and gender—first 3 years of life; infants
b. Clinical features
(1) Skin rash on the trunk, scalp, and extremities
(2) Persistent low-grade fever; malaise, irritability
(3) Splenomegaly, hepatomegaly
(4) Anemia
(5) Oral lesions—not common
(6) Most severe form of Langerhans cell histiocytosis
c. Prognosis—poor, early high mortality rate; sometimes responds to chemotherapy
2. Hand-Schüller-Christian disease (intermediate chronic form)
a. Age and gender—mainly children less than 15 years of age
b. Clinical features
(1) Systemic signs and symptoms—classic triad in up to 30%:
(a) Skull and jaws affected—lytic punched-out radiolucencies
(b) Diabetes insipidus—result of pituitary dysfunction
(c) Exophthalmos-bulging of eyes caused by orbital masses of proliferating immature histiocytes and eosinophils
(2) Oral signs and symptoms
(a) Sore mouth, ulcerations, erythema
(b) Halitosis, unpleasant taste, gingivitis
(c) Loose, sensitive teeth
(d) Failure to heal after extractions
c. Radiographic appearance—punched-out radiolucencies in the skull and jaws; teeth appear to be "floating" in bone which has been destroyed around them

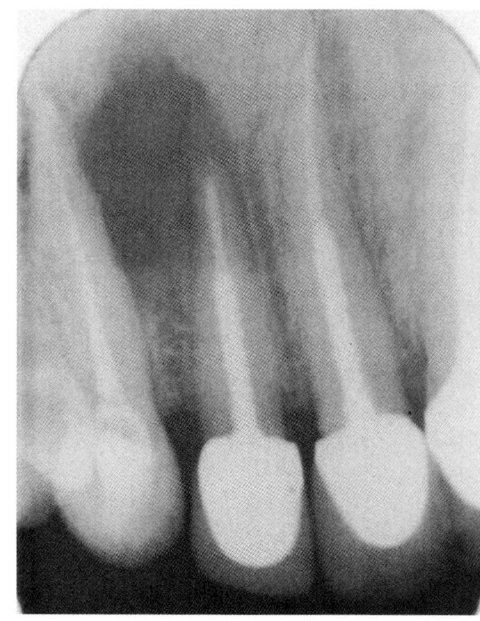

**Fig. 8.63** Radiograph of eosinophilic granuloma. (Courtesy of Drs. Paul Freedman and Stanley Kerpel; from Ibsen OAC, Phelan JA. *Oral Pathology for the Dental Hygienist.* 6th ed. St. Louis: Elsevier Saunders; 2014.)

d. Treatment and prognosis
(1) Curettage of lesions
(2) Radiation therapy
(3) Cytotoxic drugs and adrenocortical hormones
(4) Prognosis is poor; high fatality rate
3. Eosinophilic granuloma (localized less severe form)
a. Age and gender—older children and adults; male predilection (2:1)
b. Clinical features
(1) Most common variant of Langerhans cell histiocytosis
(2) Localized bone destruction; single or multiple lytic skeletal lesions, most often multiple
(3) Any bone can be involved, but skull, mandible, spine, and long bones are frequently involved
(4) Can mimic aggressive periodontitis not responding to periodontal therapy
(5) May see severe ulcerative mucositis
c. Radiographic appearance—lesions are lytic radiolucencies, single or multiple; well defined, resembling a cyst (Fig. 8.63)
d. Treatment and prognosis
(1) Curettage and conservative surgical excision
(2) Radiation therapy
(3) Local injections of corticosteroids
(4) Prognosis is good; recurrence rare

## DEFECTS OF TOOTH STRUCTURE

### Attrition

A. Etiology—wearing away of tooth surfaces by active, physiologic forces
1. Mastication, "tooth to tooth" contact
2. Bruxism, other parafunctional habits such as clenching

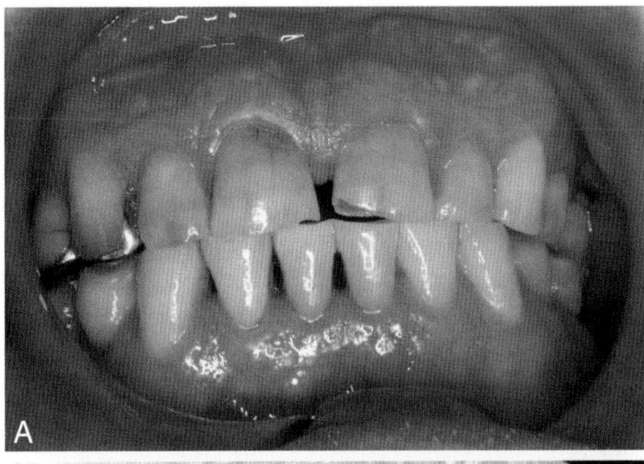


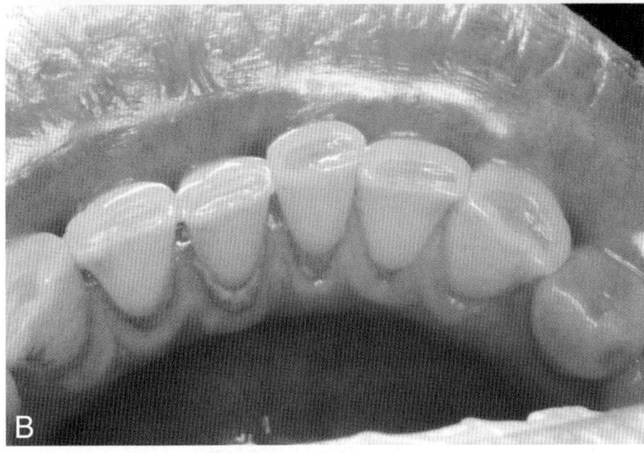


**Fig. 8.64** (A) Attrition. (B) Incisal view of attrition of the adult dentition. (From Ibsen OAC, Phelan JA. *Oral Pathology for the Dental Hygienist.* 6th ed. St. Louis: Elsevier Saunders; 2014.)

3. Occlusion—heavy biting forces
4. Diet—chewing of coarse foods or tobacco accelerates wear

B. Age and gender—occurs in both primary and permanent dentition

C. Clinical features (Fig. 8.64A and B)
1. Occurs almost exclusively on occlusal and incisal surfaces
2. Interproximal tooth contacts can also show attrition
3. Polished facets, flat incisal edges
4. Gradual process over long time, exposed dentin, but pulp exposure rare
5. Result is shortening of clinical crowns

## Abrasion

A. Etiology—wearing away of tooth structure by external force
1. Improper toothbrushing technique; repetitive back-and-forth motion at CEJ
2. Use of hard toothbrush and abrasive toothpastes and powders
3. Occupational exposure to grit or dust; coarse foods in diet are contributors

B. Clinical features (Fig. 8.65)
1. Notching and grooving at cervical margins of teeth; especially over canine eminence, and premolar areas
2. Promotes recession of gingiva, tooth sensitivity
3. Pipe smoking may abrade teeth, where pipe is clenched between teeth

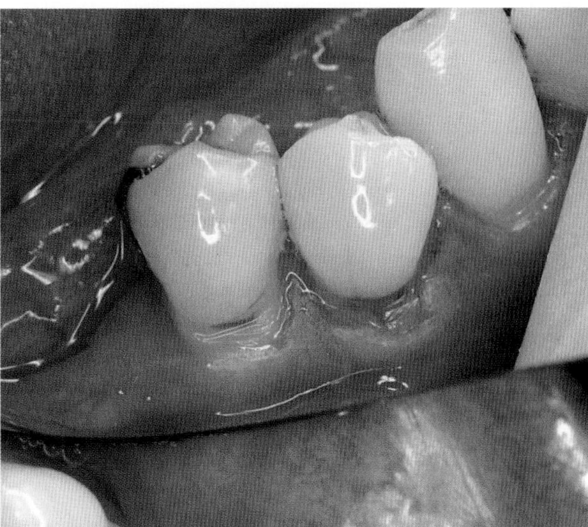

**Fig. 8.65** Abrasion of the cervical area of mandibular premolars caused by aggressive toothbrushing. (From Ibsen OAC, Phelan JA. *Oral Pathology for the Dental Hygienist.* 6th ed. St. Louis: Elsevier Saunders; 2014.)

4. Notching associated with certain occupations or habits; carpenters and tailors who hold tacks, nails, and pins between teeth

## Abfraction

A. Etiology—related to microfracture of tooth structure in areas of focused stress; biomechanical forces due to tooth flexion

B. Age—adults

C. Location
1. Cervical area of teeth
2. Location predisposes the patient to toothbrush abrasion

D. Clinical features—wedge-shaped or V-shaped notch, loss of tooth structure at the CEJ; exposure of dentin

E. Treatment—restorations may be indicated

## Erosion

A. Etiology—loss of tooth structure resulting from chemical action; when caused by stomach acid, it is known as *perimylolysis*
1. GI reflux, vomiting during pregnancy
2. Eating disorders (bulimia)
3. Intake of acidic or low-pH foods such as carbonated or sports drinks
4. Citric acid in lozenges or lemon sucking

B. Clinical features (Fig. 8.66A and B)
1. Pattern of hard tissue loss indicative of etiology
2. Labial or buccal surfaces; due to placement of acidic substance against teeth; may see eroded or washed away enamel/dentin on cervical or occlusal surfaces
3. Dental restorations often appear raised above remaining tooth structure, due to eroded enamel and dentin
4. Erosion affecting maxillary lingual surfaces is indicative of GI reflux or bulimia; often see narrow "picture frame" of remaining enamel on lingual
5. Erosion due to stomach acid occurs rapidly; days to weeks

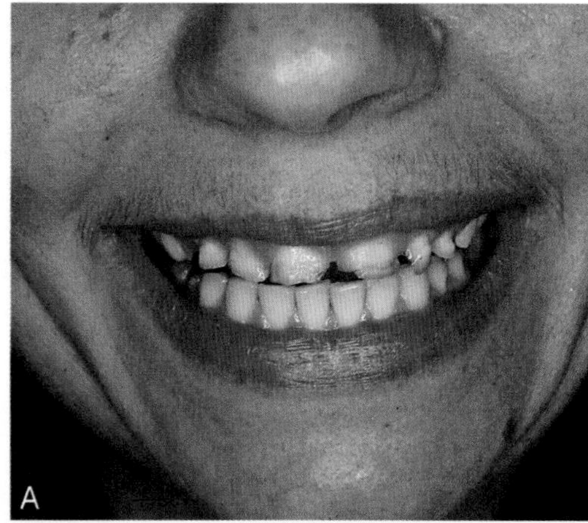


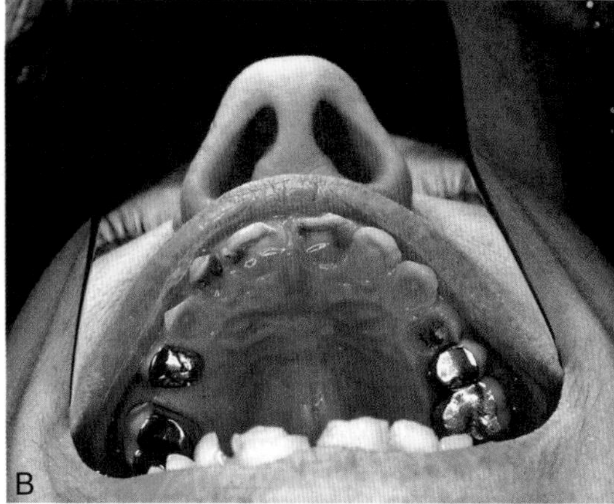


**Fig. 8.66** Erosion caused by bulimia. (A) Decreased tooth size. (B) Erosion of maxillary lingual surfaces. (From Ibsen OAC, Phelan JA. *Oral Pathology for the Dental Hygienist.* 6th ed. St. Louis: Elsevier Saunders; 2014.)

6. Hypersensitivity of affected teeth
7. Home care caution advised; do not follow acidic insult with aggressive brushing and abrasive toothpastes; this can accelerate hard tissue loss; best to rinse with basic rinse or water and allow normal buffering capacity of saliva

## Methamphetamine Abuse and Addiction

A. Street names: meth, speed, crystal, ice, glass, fire
B. Etiology—man-made psychostimulant that can be injected, snorted, inhaled, taken orally, or smoked
   1. Mood alterations depend on how it is taken
   2. Smoking produces a high that can last 10 to 24 hours
C. Demographics
   1. Typical user is Caucasian, 20 to 30 years of age
   2. Increased incidence in college students, young professionals
   3. Usage increasing in females
D. Clinical—general signs and symptoms
   1. Inability to sleep, sometimes for days
   2. Irritability, sudden mood swings
   3. Extreme anorexia (causes a decrease in appetite)
   4. Tremors, repetitive motor activities
   5. Aggressive behavior, uncontrolled and violent
   6. Increased craving for sweets
   7. Scabbing on face, arms, torso, and legs, caused by scratching
   8. Cravings for and high consumption of high-sugar soft drinks with caffeine
E. Clinical—oral signs and symptoms: "meth mouth"
   1. Snorting or smoking produces corrosive vapors; along with self-neglect and consumption of high sugar foods results in significant and rapid damage to teeth and oral tissues
   2. Rampant caries especially facial and proximal surfaces of anterior teeth, resembles radiation caries
   3. Aggressive erosion of enamel, advanced gingival problems and destruction of periodontal tissues
   4. Methamphetamine produces severe xerostomia, loss of protective buffering capacity of saliva
   5. Bruxism and clenching due to feeling anxious and nervous, leads to attrition, fractured teeth
   6. Dangerous interactions with common local anesthetics, nitrous oxide, and pain medications

## Tetracycline and Minocycline Staining of Teeth

A. Etiology—ingested tetracycline medication incorporated into teeth during tooth development; primary or permanent dentitions
B. Clinical—endogenous tooth staining, enamel hypoplasia
   1. Tetracycline incorporated into tissues that are calcifying at time of drug administration; teeth, cartilage, bone
   2. Staining can occur in primary teeth in utero, timing is usually second trimester; after birth to up to crown completion ages 12 to 16
   3. May be seen in association with enamel hypoplasia
   4. Permanent discoloration of teeth from yellow-green to brown-gray; generally discovered when teeth erupt
   5. Minocycline, a semisynthetic derivative of tetracycline, can also stain a variety of soft and hard tissues including teeth
   6. Adult-onset of tooth discoloration has been reported
   7. Black bones, black or green tooth roots, and darkening of crowns of permanent teeth have been reported with minocycline
C. Prevention is key; these medications should not be prescribed to children during tooth formation; restrict use in pregnant and nursing mothers; drug can cross placenta and also enter breast milk

# DEVELOPMENTAL DEFECTS AFFECTING ENAMEL AND DENTIN

Enamel hypoplasia—generic term refers to incomplete or defective development of enamel

A. Etiology—disruption of ameloblasts during enamel production
B. Nonhereditary factors include:
   1. Fever or vitamin deficiency—band-like pattern (contemporaneous enamel hypoplasia)
   2. Local infection or trauma to one or more developing tooth germs (Turner's tooth)
   3. Fluoride ingestion—mottling, rough porous enamel, chalky white, picks up stains

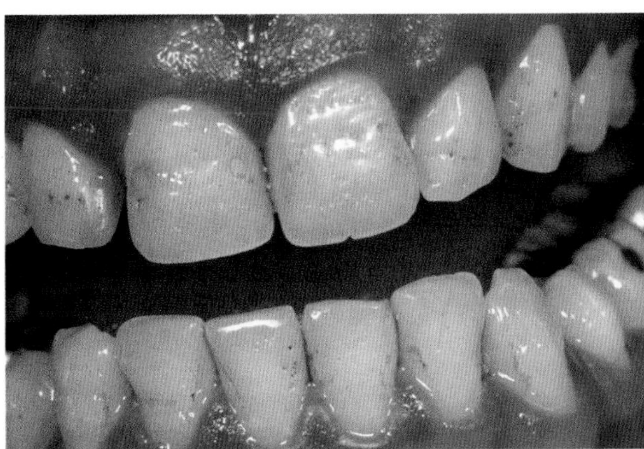

**Fig. 8.67** Pitted autosomal dominant amelogenesis imperfecta. Note the multiple pits on the labial surface of teeth. Some of the pits have been filled with composite. (From Young WG, Sedano HO. *Atlas of Oral Pathology*. Minneapolis: University of Minnesota Press; 1981.)

4. Enamel hypoplasia of congenital syphilis (spirochetes cross placenta, affect ameloblasts: mulberry molars, Hutchinson's incisors)

## Amelogenesis Imperfecta (AI)

A. Etiology—hereditary group of disorders affecting formation of tooth enamel; mutations in genes involved in process of enamel formation (*AMELX, ENAM, or MMP20*)
B. AI can be divided into four basic types:
   1. Hypoplastic— represents majority of all cases of AI; incomplete or arrested development of enamel matrix (Fig. 8.67)
      a. Etiology—hereditary
      b. Clinical features—enamel matrix responsible for crown shape, insufficient matrix leads to smaller teeth with thin enamel; pitting and vertical grooves, yellow to dark-brown color, open contacts, and occlusal wear
      c. Radiographic appearance—enamel may be absent or very thin layer over cusp tips and interproximal areas
      d. Histologic characteristics—thin, defective enamel, dentin normal
      e. Treatment—restorations; crowns; bonding
   2. Hypocalcified—least common type of AI; defect in mineralization of enamel matrix (Fig. 8.68)
      a. Etiology—hereditary
      b. Clinical features—normal teeth on eruption but wear down quickly to expose dentin; enamel soft and uncalcified, chalky appearance, teeth stain rapidly, susceptible to caries, may have open bite; dentin normal
      c. Radiographic appearance—tooth shape normal; enamel less radiopaque so dentin and enamel have similar radiodensity, enamel may appear "moth eaten"
      d. Histologic characteristics—broadening of interprismatic substance; distinct enamel prisms; enamel low in mineral content
      e. Treatment—restorations; crowns; bonding
   3. Hypomaturation—proper matrix deposition, early mineralization, but enamel crystalline structure fails to mature

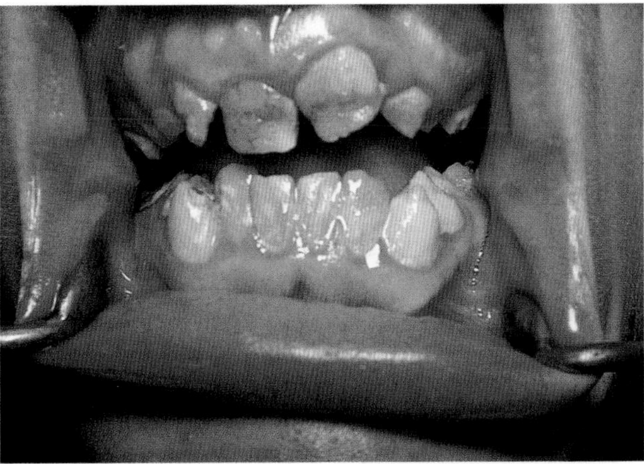

**Fig. 8.68** Note the loss of enamel in the teeth of a patient with hypocalcified amelogenesis imperfecta. (From Odell E: Cawson's Essentials of Oral Pathology and Oral Medicine. 9th ed. Elsevier; 2017.)

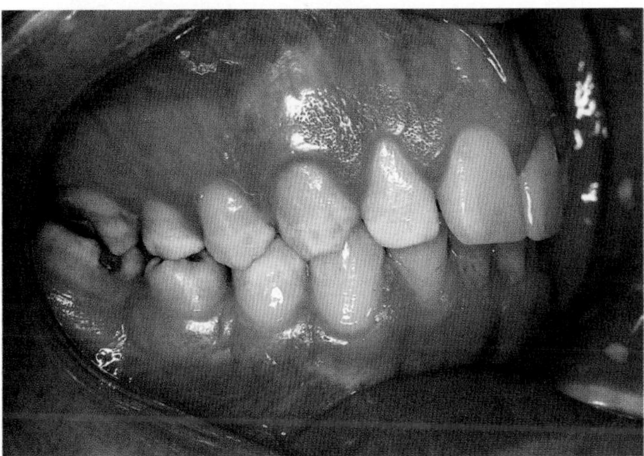

**Fig. 8.69** Note the uniform whitening of incisal edges and occlusal cusps in a case of "snowcapped" amelogenesis imperfecta. (From Odell E: Cawson's Essentials of Oral Pathology and Oral Medicine. 9th ed. Elsevier; 2017.)

      a. Etiology—hereditary
      b. Clinical features—teeth appear mottled and opaque, poorly formed crystals fail to reflect light, results in white appearance
         (1) Malformed enamel, soft and porous; dentin normal
         (2) Enamel easily chips from crowns of teeth
         (3) Rare form of hypomaturation type AI: "snow-capped teeth" (Fig. 8.69)
   4. Hypoplastic/hypomaturation/taurodontism—enamel poorly formed, porous and soft; molars exhibit taurodontism
      a. Etiology—hereditary
      b. Clinical features—small teeth with thin enamel which is pitted, and appears yellow to brown in color; taurodontism of molars; dentin normal

## Dentinogenesis Imperfecta (DI) (Hereditary Opalescent Dentin)

A. Etiology—hereditary group of disorders affecting formation of tooth dentin; affects tissues formed from dental papilla (mesodermal component: forms dentin and pulp), enamel normal

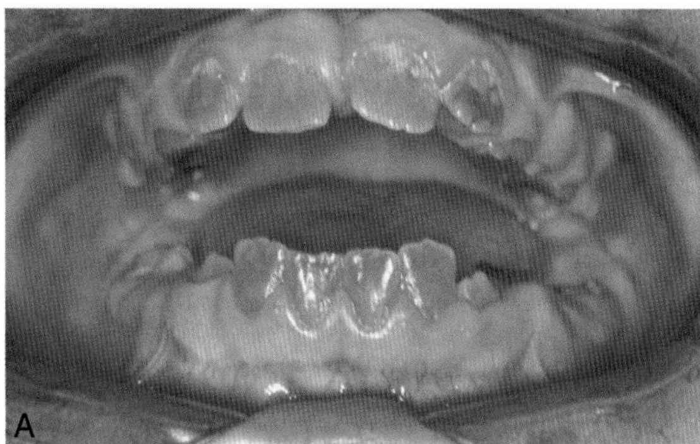


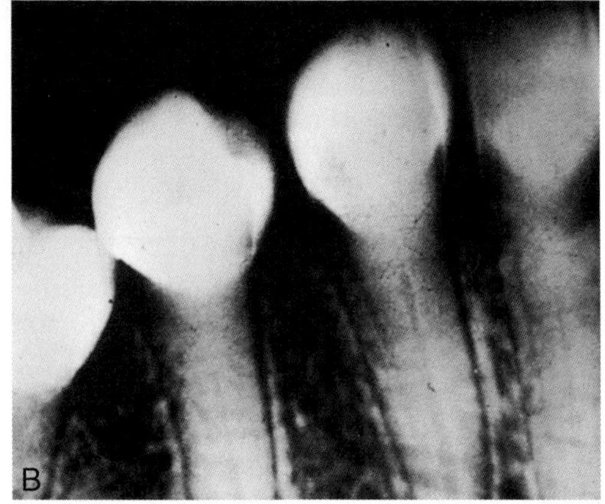


**Fig. 8.70** (A) Clinical view of dentinogenesis imperfecta. (B) Radiographic view. (Courtesy of Dr. Edward V. Zegarelli; from Ibsen OAC, Phelan JA. *Oral Pathology for the Dental Hygienist.* 6th ed. St. Louis: Elsevier Saunders; 2014.)

B. Clinical features (Fig. 8.70A)
   1. Defective pulp formation and mineralization of dentin
   2. Altered dentin gives teeth opalescent hue
   3. Teeth brown to gray to bluish in color
   4. Overlying enamel poorly supported, chips, breaks, and wears away

C. Radiographic appearance (Fig. 8.70B)
   1. Partial or total obliteration of pulp chambers and root canals
   2. Bulbous crowns with distinct constriction at CEJ: "thistle-tube" shaped pulp chamber
   3. Cementum, periodontal membrane, and alveolar bone appear normal

D. Histologic characteristics
   1. Dentin composed of irregular tubules; uncalcified matrix
   2. Odontoblasts degenerate easily within the matrix
   3. Decrease in inorganic content

E. Treatment—full crowns; caution needed with partial appliances due to potential for root fractures

## DEVELOPMENTAL DEFECTS AFFECTING TOOTH SHAPE

### Dilaceration

A. Abnormal sharp bend or curve in tooth root (Fig. 8.71A)

B. Etiology—trauma during tooth development
   1. May occur anywhere from CEJ to tooth apex

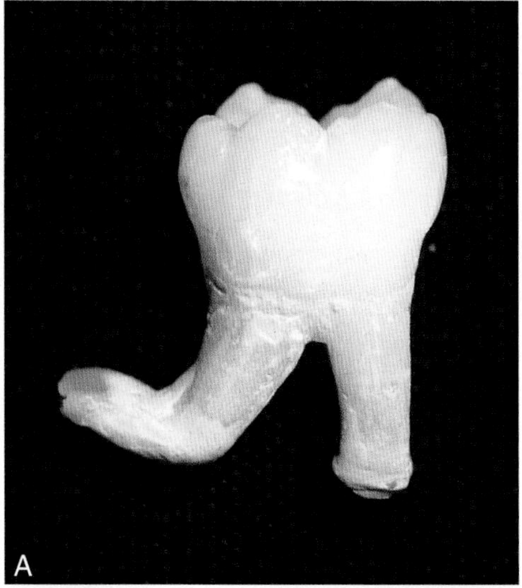


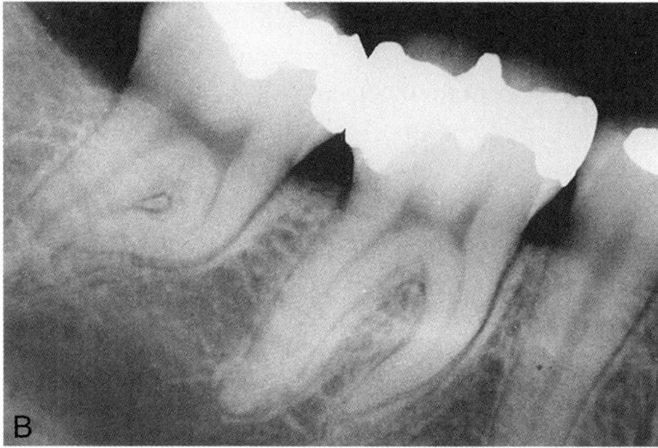

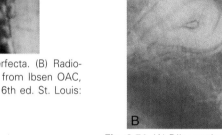

**Fig. 8.71** (A) Dilaceration on the distal root of an extracted tooth. (B) Mesial root dilaceration on a mandibular second molar. (A courtesy of Dr. Rudy Melfi; A and B from Ibsen OAC, Phelan JA. *Oral Pathology for the Dental Hygienist.* 6th ed. St. Louis: Elsevier Saunders; 2014.)

   2. Results from displacement of Hertwig's epithelial root sheath

C. Radiographic appearance—sharp bend or curve in the root (Fig. 8.71B)

D. Treatment—no treatment; may present problem if tooth extracted or requires endodontic treatment

### Fusion

A. Union of two normally separated tooth germs

B. Etiology—physical force or external pressure causes contact between developing teeth

C. Clinical features (Fig. 8.72A and B)
   1. If defect occurs early in development, one large tooth results
   2. If defect occurs later, fusion of roots only
   3. Dentin always confluent (true fusion)
   4. Seen in both primary and permanent dentitions
   5. Occurs between two normal tooth germs or between one normal tooth germ and one supernumerary tooth germ

D. Location—usually anterior region; incisors most often affected

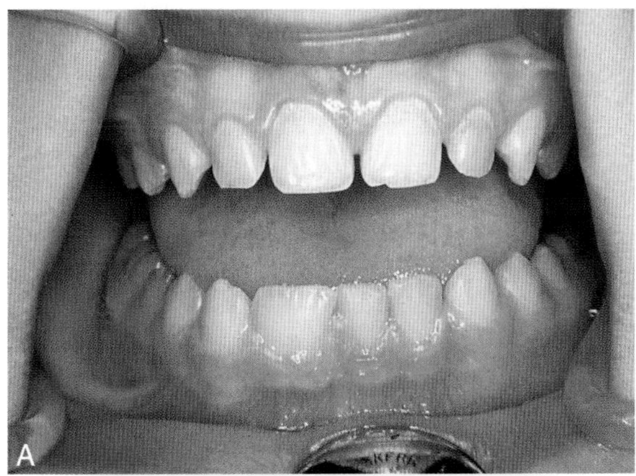
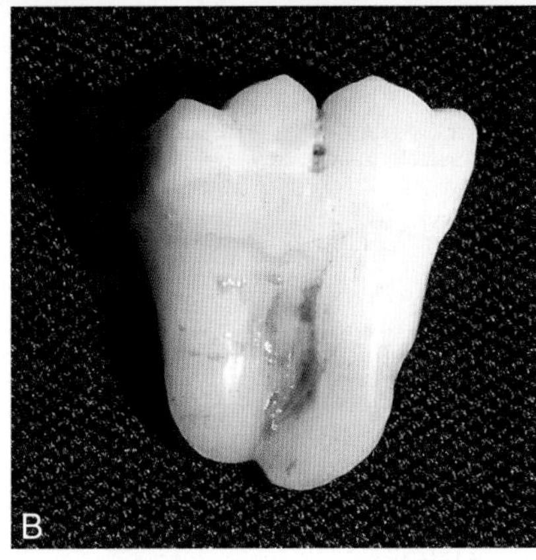

**Fig. 8.72** (A) Clinical view of fusion involving a permanent mandibular lateral incisor. (B) Fusion of mandibular molars. (A courtesy of Dr. George Blozis; B courtesy of Dr. Rudy Melfi; from Ibsen OAC, Phelan JA. *Oral Pathology for the Dental Hygienist.* 6th ed. St. Louis: Elsevier Saunders; 2014.)

E. Radiographic appearance—dentin confluent, can have separate or fused root canals
F. Treatment—usually none

## Gemination

A. Twinning or dividing of a single tooth germ; results in incomplete formation of two teeth (gemination means paired or occurring in twos)
B. Etiology—unknown; possibly trauma
C. Location—can affect the primary or permanent dentition, although it is slightly more common in the primary dentition (e.g., in mandibular incisors or in permanent maxillary incisors)
D. Clinically tooth most often presents with crown which appears to incompletely split in two; with one root, one root canal (Fig. 8.73A and B)
E. Counting tooth crowns can often help distinguish gemination from fusion; in fusion less than the normal number of teeth appear to be present; in gemination more than the normal number of teeth appear to be present

## Concrescence

A. Fusion of tooth roots by cementum only; occurs after root formation is complete; during cementum formation (Fig. 8.74A)
B. Etiology—crowding of teeth with close root proximity; cementum of teeth becomes confluent

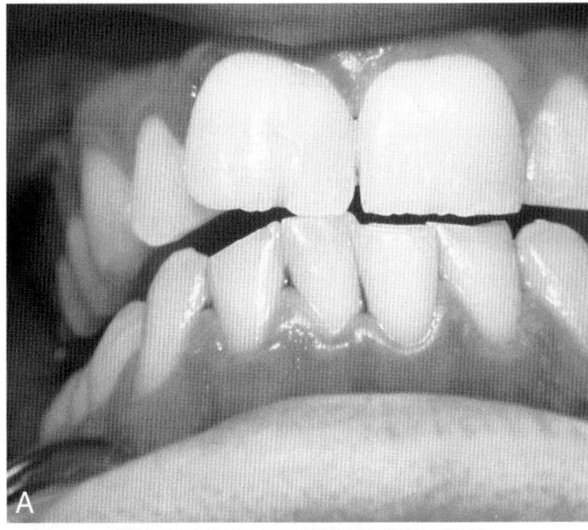
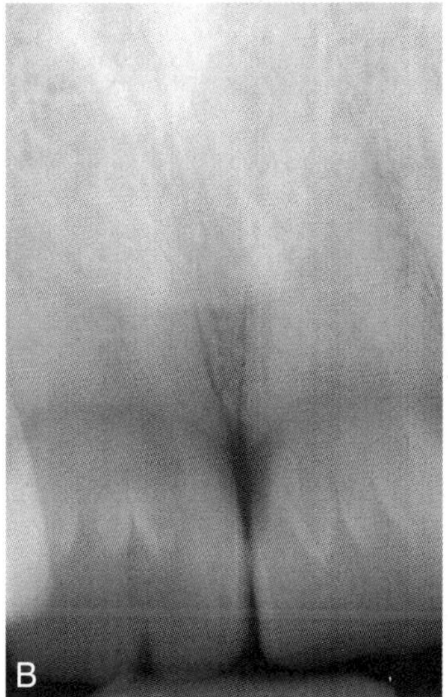

**Fig. 8.73** Clinical (A) and radiographic (B) views of gemination seen in the right maxillary central incisor. (From Ibsen OAC, Phelan JA. *Oral Pathology for the Dental Hygienist.* 6th ed. St. Louis: Elsevier Saunders; 2014.)

C. Location—most often seen in adjacent maxillary molars
D. Radiographic appearance—important in establishing diagnosis; teeth joined (fused together) at root surfaces (Fig. 8.74B)
E. Treatment and prognosis—usually no treatment; significantly complicates tooth extraction

## Dens Invaginatus (Dens in Dente)

A. Also known as "tooth within a tooth"
B. Etiology—invagination (infolding) of enamel organ during crown formation
C. Location—most frequently anterior teeth, may occur bilaterally, usually maxillary lateral incisor, not visible without radiograph (Fig. 8.75)
D. Microportal in cingulum area, forms direct communication with pulp and provides entry for bacteria
E. Apical pathology due to pulpal necrosis often occurs soon after tooth eruption
F. Endodontic treatment

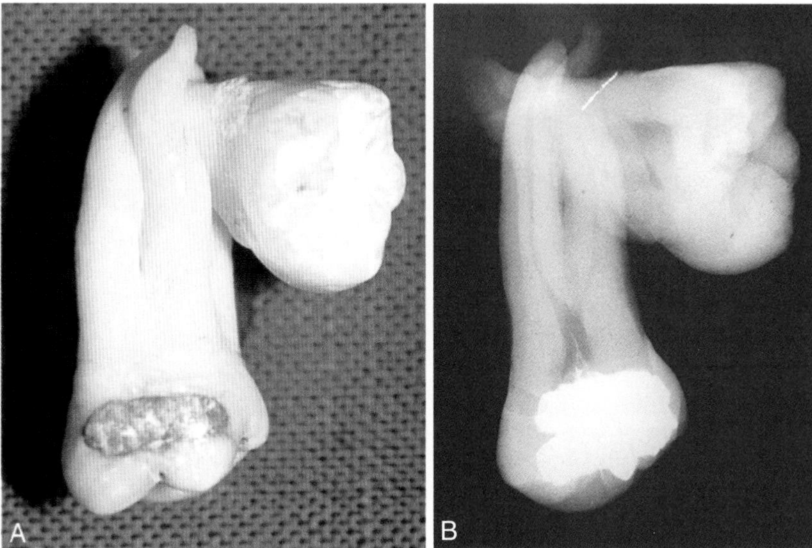


**Fig 8.74** (A) and (B) Example of concrescence seen in extracted teeth and in a corresponding radiograph. (Courtesy of Dr. George Blozis; from Ibsen OAC, Phelan JA. *Oral Pathology for the Dental Hygienist.* 6th ed. St. Louis: Elsevier Saunders; 2014.)

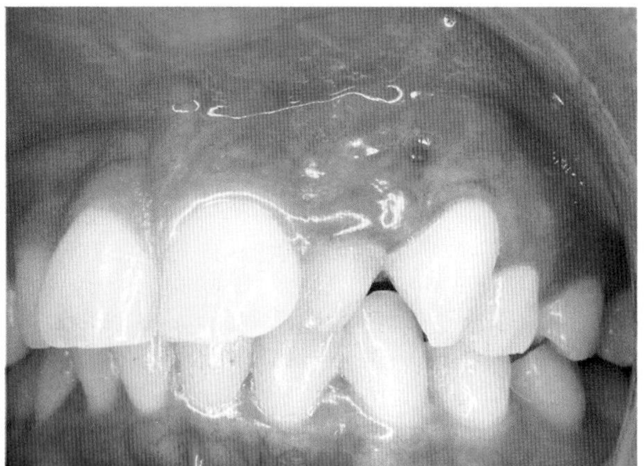

**Fig. 8.75** Clinical view of dens in dente in maxillary lateral incisor. (Courtesy of Dr. George Blozis; from Ibsen OAC, Phelan JA. *Oral Pathology for the Dental Hygienist.* 6th ed. St. Louis: Elsevier Saunders; 2014.)

G. Radiographic appearance—establishes diagnosis, pear-shaped defect projects down into root canal, gives appearance of small tooth within the pulp chamber (Fig. 8.76)
H. Treatment—preventive restoration in cingulum area, early preemptive endodontic treatment important option

## Dens Evaginatus

A. Supernumerary or extra cusp on the occlusal surface
B. Etiology—evagination (outgrowth, proliferation) of enamel organ during crown formation
C. Location—most often occlusal surface of premolars ("tuberculated" premolars), may be unilateral or bilateral
D. Clinical appearance—small, round nodule of enamel forming an extra cusp on the occlusal surface (Fig. 8.77)
E. Frequently contains a slender extension of pulp
F. Cusp wear, fracture, or equilibration may lead to pulp exposure and necrosis

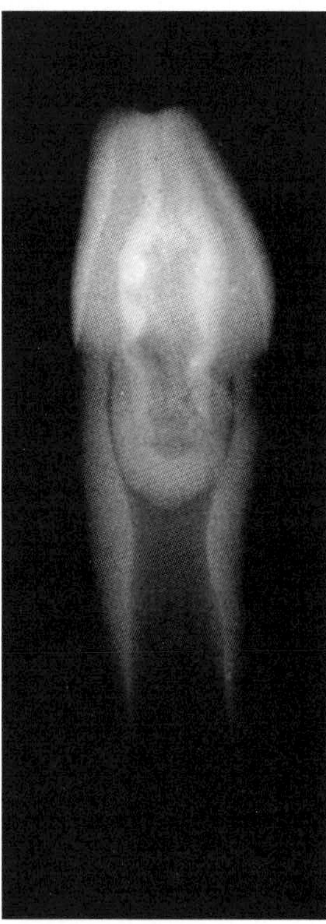

**Fig. 8.76** Radiograph of dens in dente in maxillary lateral incisor. (From Odell E: Cawson's Essentials of Oral Pathology and Oral Medicine. 9th ed. Elsevier; 2017.)

G. Treatment—usually none; caution with restorative procedures and occlusal adjustment
H. "Talon" cusp is considered a form of dens evaginatus

## Natal Teeth

A. Teeth present at birth; neonatal teeth are those that erupt within 30 days after birth
B. Etiology

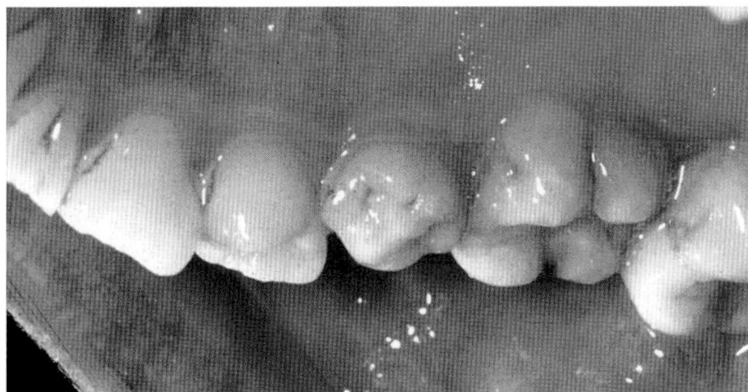

Fig. 8.77 Dens evaginatus of maxillary premolar. (Courtesy of Dr. Margot Van Dis; from Ibsen OAC, Phelan JA. *Oral Pathology for the Dental Hygienist.* 6th ed. St. Louis: Elsevier Saunders; 2014.)

1. Most develop from dental lamina, usually a hollow calcified cap of enamel and dentin without pulp tissue, often little to no root structure
2. Can be associated with other developmental abnormalities and recognized syndromes

C. Location—small conical or normal shaped "tooth"; usually found in mandibular incisor area; may be bilateral

D. Histologic characteristics—thin hollow cap of enamel and dentin or keratinized epithelial structure, without developed root structure

E. Treatment and prognosis
1. Often wobbly due to lack of developed root, potential risk of infant inhaling tooth if dislodged
2. Difficulty in feeding for infant and mother
3. May produce ulceration to ventral surface of tongue (Riga-Fede disease)
4. Removal often performed shortly after birth

## DEVELOPMENTAL DEFECTS AFFECTING THE NUMBER OF TEETH

### Congenitally Missing Teeth

A. Congenital variations in number of teeth

B. Etiology—developmental, may be familial or inherited; failure of dental lamina to form tooth buds

C. Two forms
1. Total anodontia
   a. Complete absence of all teeth to form; abnormality of ectoderm
   b. May involve both primary and permanent dentitions
   c. Most often associated with ectodermal dysplasia, group of inherited syndromes
2. Hypodontia (partial anodontia) (Fig. 8.78A and B)
   a. Failure of some teeth to form; can range from one to multiple teeth
   b. Primary or permanent dentition may be affected
   c. Most frequently seen: third molars, maxillary lateral incisors, mandibular second premolars
   d. May be familial or hereditary and part of a syndrome
   e. Radiographic evaluation required to determine hypodontia versus unerupted teeth
   f. Missing teeth may be unerupted, impacted, and/or malformed; odontodysplasia, "ghost teeth" (Fig. 8.79)

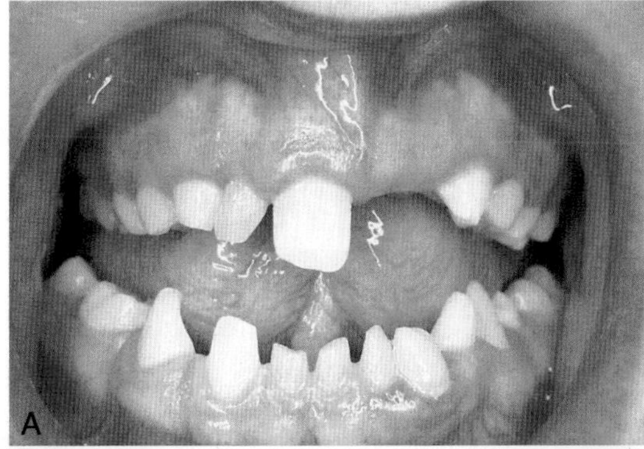


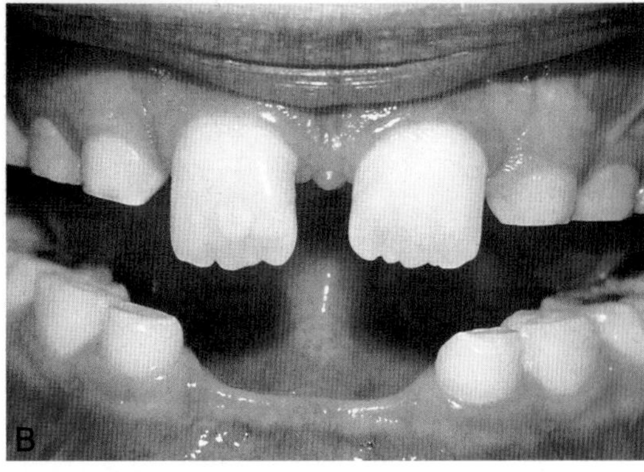


Fig. 8.78 (A) and (B) Hypodontia. The missing teeth were not extracted; they never developed. (A courtesy of Dr. George Blozis; B courtesy of Dr. Margot Van Dis; from Ibsen OAC, Phelan JA. *Oral Pathology for the Dental Hygienist.* 6th ed. St. Louis: Elsevier Saunders; 2014.)

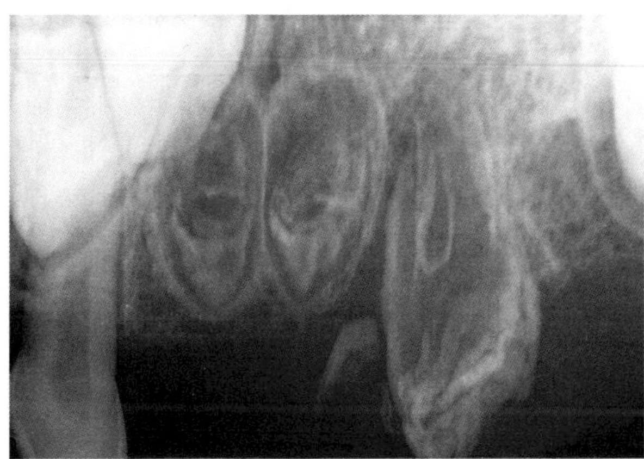

Fig. 8.79 Regional odontodysplasia. (From Regezi J, Sciubba J, Jordan RCK. *Oral Pathology: Clinical Pathologic Correlations.* 7th ed. St. Louis: Elsevier Saunders; 2017.)

D. Treatment for missing teeth
1. Ranges from no treatment to restorative crowns and bridges
2. Orthodontics
3. Space maintainers, partial or complete dentures
4. Dental implants

### Supernumerary Teeth (Hyperdontia)

A. Extra teeth

B. Etiology—developmental, may be familial or inherited, dental lamina produces extra tooth buds

C. Clinical features; varies from one to multiple extra teeth

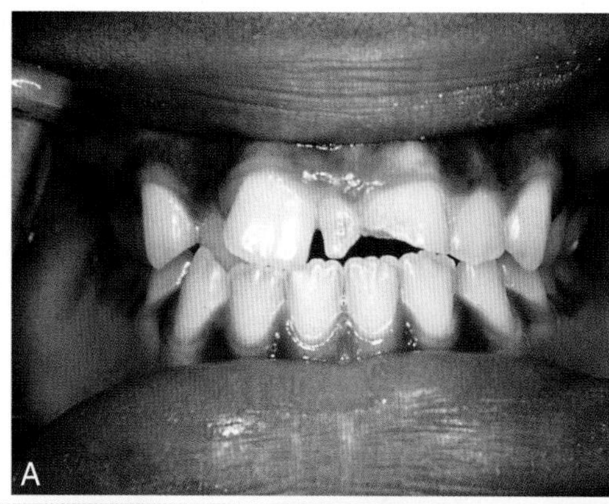


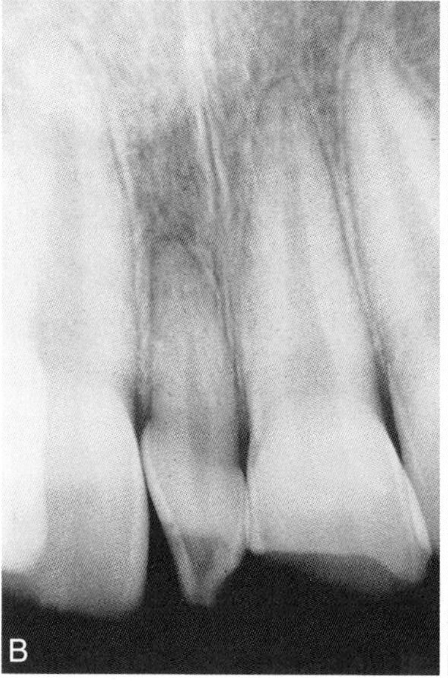


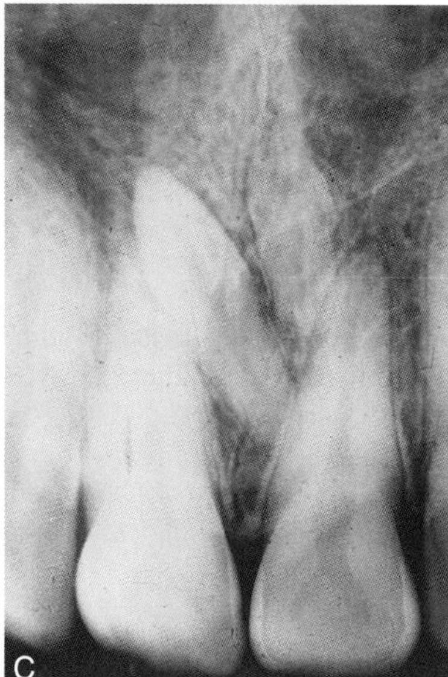


**Fig. 8.80** (A) Mesiodens seen between maxillary central incisors. (B) Radiograph of a mesiodens. (C) Radiograph showing a pair of inverted, impacted mesiodens. (A and B courtesy of Dr. George Blozis; A to C, from Ibsen OAC, Phelan JA. *Oral Pathology for the Dental Hygienist.* 6th ed. St. Louis: Elsevier Saunders; 2014.)

1. May block the eruption path of other teeth
2. Supernumerary teeth are frequently impacted
3. Mesiodens—most common supernumerary tooth; cone-shaped crown; short root; located between maxillary centrals (Fig. 8.80A, B, and C)
4. Other supernumerary teeth include maxillary fourth molar—distal to the third molar; maxillary paramolar—usually a small molar; located buccally or lingually in the area of the maxillary or mandibular molars
5. May be seen in association with inherited disorders such as Cleidocranial dysplasia or Gardner's syndrome

D. Treatment—evaluate unerupted supernumeraries, remove if associated with pathology or interference with normal dentition

## DEVELOPMENTAL DEFECTS AFFECTING TOOTH SIZE

### Macrodontia

A Condition in which a normal tooth or teeth are larger than normal; may be localized to a single tooth or generalized over whole dentition; generalized macrodontia has been associated with gigantism

B Not to be confused with larger-appearing tooth resulting from germination or fusion

### Microdontia

A Condition in which a normal tooth or teeth are smaller than normal; may be localized to a single tooth or generalized over the whole dentition; generalized microdontia has been associated with certain forms of dwarfism

B Maxillary lateral incisor (may be peg-shaped) and third molar most frequently affected (Fig. 8.81)

## ABNORMALITIES OF MUCOUS MEMBRANES OR SKIN

### Amalgam Tattoo

A. Etiology—fragments of dental amalgam embedded in mucosa or gingiva; silver particles leach into surrounding connective tissue and cause discoloration

B. Clinical features—gray to blue submucosal area on gingiva or adjacent mucosa; often located near site of prior amalgam restoration(s) (Fig. 8.82A)

C. Residual fragments left from amalgam removal or carving become trapped in gingival tissues; may also see in tissue over root apex in apicoectomies capped with amalgam
D. "Blue" gingiva may result when slurry of amalgam particles, produced with crown preparation, enters sulcus (retraction cord may embed amalgam particles in sulcus)
E. Radiographic appearance—can aid in diagnosis; amalgam particles appear radiopaque when present (Fig. 8.82B)

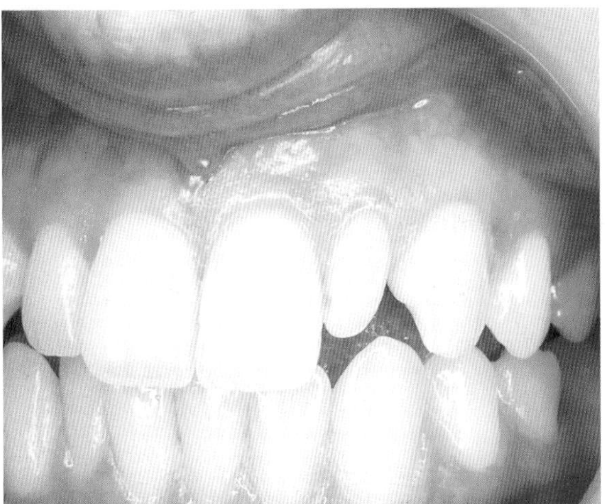

**Fig. 8.81** Peg-shaped lateral incisor. (Courtesy of Dr. George Blozis; from Ibsen OAC, Phelan JA. *Oral Pathology for the Dental Hygienist.* 6th ed. St. Louis: Elsevier Saunders; 2014.)

F. Treatment—none; however, important to differentiate from other pigmented lesions such as blue nevus, melanoma, early Kaposi's sarcoma; biopsy may be needed for definitive diagnosis

## Melanin Pigmentation

A. Wide variation in normal melanin pigmentation of skin and oral mucosa; (Fig. 8.83)
B. Etiology—hereditary: racial pigmentation, those with dark complexions have more melanin than those with lighter complexions; or acquired: result of inflammation or systemic disorder
C. Physiologic (ethnic/racial) pigmentation genetically determined
D. Pathologic melanin pigmentation of oral mucosa can occur with endocrine disorders such as Addison's disease or be drug induced by a variety of medications such as minocycline, bleomycin, cyclophosphamide
E. Postinflammatory pigmentation of skin and oral mucosa can occur after an injury or long-standing inflammatory condition such as lichen planus (Fig. 8.84)
F. Smoking associated melanosis can be seen with tobacco use; especially maxillary anterior facial gingiva

## Angular Cheilitis (Perlèche)

A. Etiology—red cracking, fissuring, patches at corners (angles) of mouth due to:
    1. Decreased vertical dimension of occlusion, lips turn down at corners promotes moisture accumulation, ill-fitting dentures

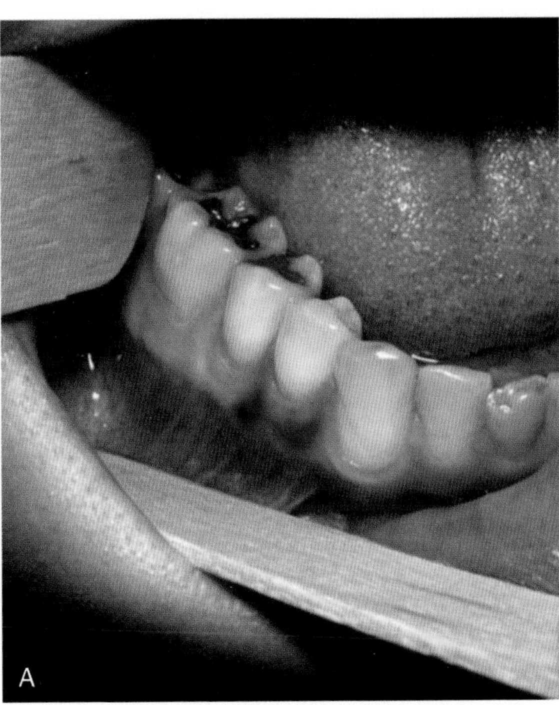


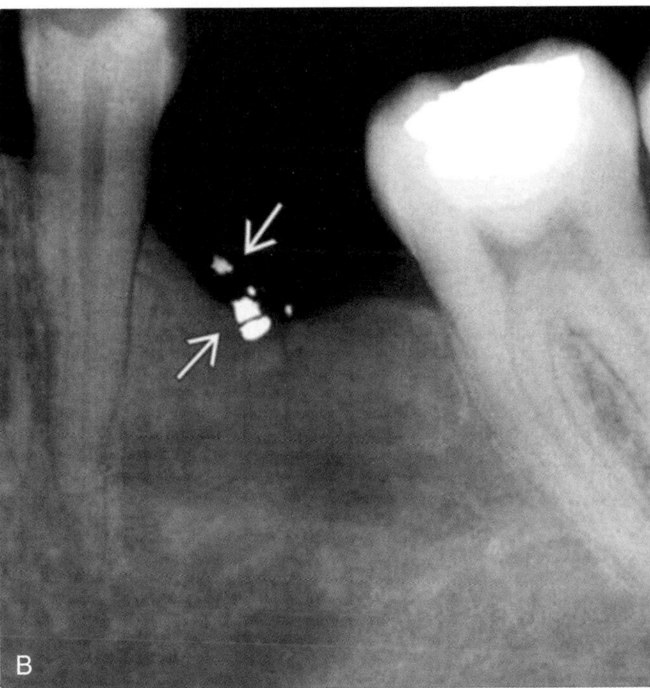


**Fig. 8.82** (A) This blue-gray pigmentation on the gingiva is an amalgam tattoo. (B) Periapical radiograph showing amalgam particles in the gingival tissue. (A from James D, Elston DM, Treat JR, et al. Andrews' Diseases of the Skin: Clinical Dermatology, ed 13, 2020, Elsevier.; B from Koenig LJ, Tamimi DF, Petrikowski CG, et al. *Diagnostic Imaging: Oral and Maxillofacial.* 2nd ed. Philadelphia: Elsevier; 2017.)

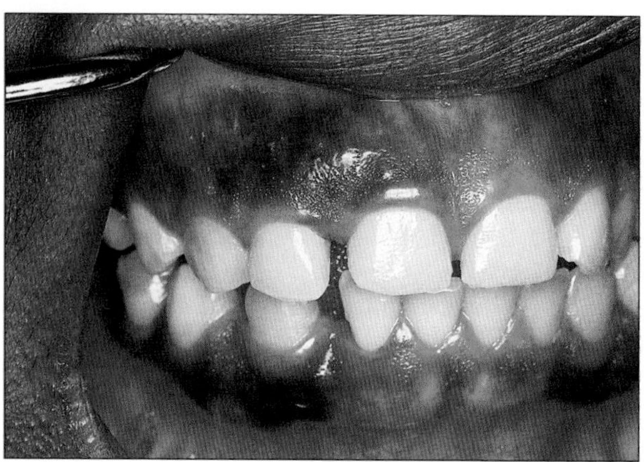

**Fig. 8.83** Melanin pigmentation of the gingiva. (From Eley BM, Soory M, Manson JD: Periodontics, ed 6, Elsevier Ltd.)

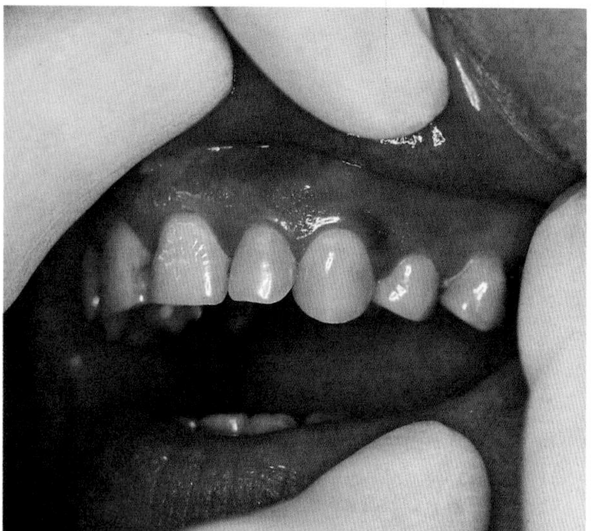

**Fig. 8.84** Posttraumatic melanin pigmentation. This area of melanin pigmentation on the gingiva occurred after the healing of an injury caused by trauma. (From Ibsen OAC, Phelan JA. *Oral Pathology for the Dental Hygienist*. 6th ed. St. Louis: Elsevier Saunders; 2014.)

2. Secondary infection by *Candida albicans* prominent feature
3. Nutritional deficiencies account for 25% of all cases (deficiency of iron and B vitamins ($B_2$, $B_3$, $B_6$, $B_{12}$)
4. Allergic contact dermatitis, especially due to use of lipstick and lip balm
5. Xerostomia, some systemic diseases, and medications contribute

B. Clinical features—erosive inflammation and cracking or fissuring at the corners of the mouth; extends onto facial skin; may be unilateral or bilateral (Fig. 8.85)

C. Histologic characteristics—inflammatory condition often with presence of microorganisms: *Candida albicans or* Staphylococcus aureus *most common*

D. Treatment—depends on the etiology: correction of decreased vertical dimension associated with dentures; *improved intake of B vitamins in diet; remove source of contact dermatitis such as lip balm or lipstick; topical* antifungal or antibacterial ointment if needed

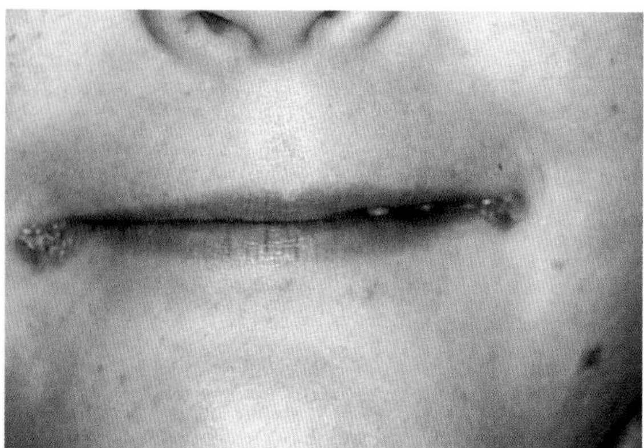

**Fig. 8.85** Angular cheilitis. (From Kliegman RM, St Geme JW III, Blum NJ. *Nelson Textbook of Pediatrics*. 21st ed. Philadelphia: Elsevier, Inc.; 2020)

### Fordyce Granules

A. Etiology—normal developmental soft tissue variation; ectopic sebaceous glands

B. Clinical features (Fig. 8.86)
1. Most commonly observed under buccal mucosa, vermilion border of the lips
2. Yellowish or white papules may be slightly raised, 1 to 5 mm in size
3. Found in 80% to 95% of adults, prominent after puberty
4. Frequently distributed in groups or clusters of 30 to 100

C. Location—buccal mucosa and lips; also reported on genital mucosa

D. Histologic characteristics—normal sebaceous gland architecture without associated hair follicle

E. Treatment—none, unless cosmetic concern

## ABNORMALITIES AFFECTING THE TONGUE

### Geographic Tongue (Benign Migratory Glossitis, Erythema Migrans)

A. Etiology—unknown; tends to run in families; genetics may play a role; seen more frequently in patients with psoriasis and fissured tongue

B. Age and gender—any age, frequently detected in children and young adults; no gender predilection

C. Clinical features (Fig. 8.87A)
1. Patches on tongue of various sizes and shapes, with curved "circinate" raised white to yellow borders
2. Center of patches appears bald due to loss of filiform papillae
3. Repeated cycles of patches developing, regenerating filiform papillae, and migrating on tongue surface (hence term *geographic*)
4. Discomfort may occur when the patient eats spicy or acidic foods
5. Important to differentiate from other pathologic conditions on tongue

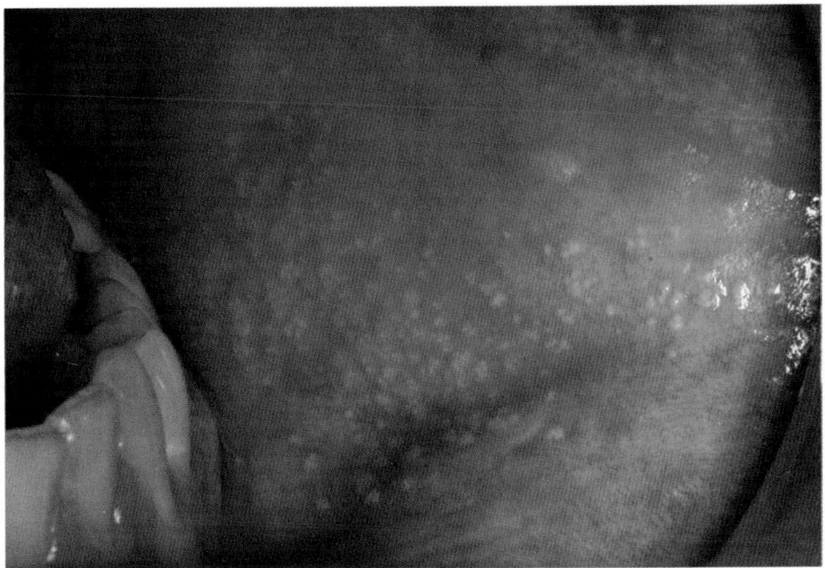

Fig. 8.86 Fordyce granules on the buccal mucosa. (From Neville B, Damm DD, Allen CM, et al. *Color Atlas of Oral and Maxillofacial Diseases*. St. Louis: Elsevier Inc.; 2010)

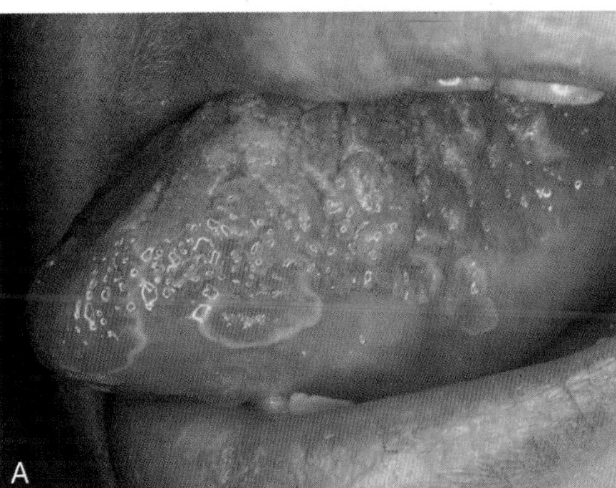

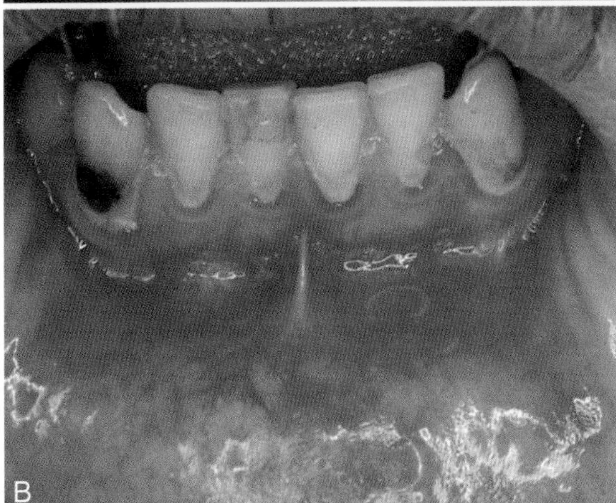

**Fig. 8.87** (A) Geographic tongue. (B) Ectopic geographic tongue observed in the anterior mandibular mucosa. (From Ibsen OAC, Phelan JA. *Oral Pathology for the Dental Hygienist*. 6th ed. St. Louis: Elsevier Saunders; 2014.)

6. Condition can occur on oral mucosa away from tongue (ectopic "geographic tongue") where it goes by name erythema migrans (Fig. 8.87B)

D. Treatment—none; unless symptomatic

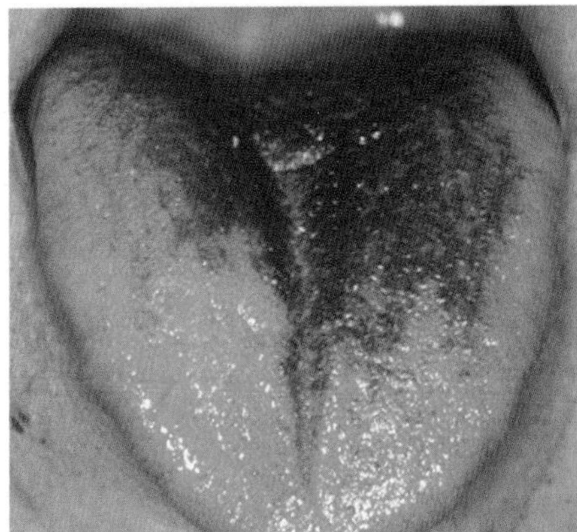

**Fig. 8.88** Black hairy tongue. (From Scully C: Oral and Maxillofacial Medicine: The Basis of Diagnosis and Treatment. 3rd ed. Elsevier; 2013.)

## Hairy Tongue (Lingua villosa)

A. Etiology—filiform papillae on tongue do not shed as they should and grow longer, gives perception of hair; food, bacteria or yeast coat papillae and produce coloration: white, green, black Precipitating factors include:
   1. Certain medications, especially antibiotics
   2. Frequent use of hydrogen peroxide or antimicrobial rinses
   3. Excessive alcohol use
   4. Proton-pump inhibitors (acid reflux)
   5. Radiation to head and neck

B. Clinical features—furry appearance on the dorsal surface of the tongue; white and cream colored to black coloration (lingua villosa nigra) (Fig. 8.88)

C. Treatment and prognosis
   1. Gentle brushing or scraping of the tongue
   2. Condition resolves when contributing factors eliminated

## Website Information and Resources.

| Source | Website Address | Description |
|---|---|---|
| National Institute of Dental and Craniofacial Research | http://www.nidcr.nih.gov/ | News and information related to dentistry and information about the institute's research |
| Mayo Clinic Medicine Center | http://www.mayoclinic.org | Information and links to health conditions and diseases |
| Clinical trials listing service | http://www.centerwatch.com | International listing of clinical research trials and medical centers that perform clinical research and drug therapies newly approved by the U.S. Food and Drug Administration (FDA) |
| National Cancer Institute | http://www.nci.nih.gov | Information about types of cancer, treatments, risk factors, screening, tests, and statistics |
| American Cancer Society | http://cancer.org | Information about cancers and leukemias from both professional and patient points of view |
| American Society of Pediatric Hematology and Oncology | http://www.aspho.org | Information for both professionals and patients about pediatric hematology and oncology |
| Support for People with Oral and Head and Neck Cancers | http://www.spohnc.org | Information and support for those suffering from oral and head and neck cancers |
| Leukemia and Lymphoma Society of America | http://www.leukemia.org | Information about blood-related cancers |

# CHAPTER 8 REVIEW QUESTIONS

Answers and rationales to review questions are available on this text's accompanying Evolve site. See inside front cover for details.

## Case A

Synopsis of Patient History
Age: 30
Sex: M
Height: 6′3″
Weight: 200 lbs
Vital Signs
Blood pressure: 120/80
Pulse rate: 60
Respiration: 16

1. Under the care of a physician: ____ YES x NO
2. Hospitalization within the last 5 years: ____ YES x NO
3. Has or had the following conditions:
   - Rheumatic fever or rheumatic heart disease ____ YES x NO
   - Congenital heart disease (bicuspid aortic valve) ____ YES x NO
   - Heart attack ____ YES x NO
   - Angina pectoris ____ YES x NO
   - Hypertension ____ YES x NO
   - Diabetes mellitus ____ YES x NO
   - Hepatitis ____ YES x NO
   - Bleeding disorder ____ YES x NO
   - Fainting spells, seizures, or epilepsy ____ YES x NO
   - Asthma ____ YES x NO
   - Allergies (medication, food) ____ YES x NO
4. Current medications
   - Anticoagulants ____ YES x NO
   - Insulin ____ YES x NO
   - Antibiotics ____ YES x NO
   - Aspirin ____ YES x NO
   - Nitroglycerin ____ YES x NO
   - High blood pressure ____ YES x NO
   - Corticosteroids ____ YES x NO
   - Oral contraceptives ____ YES x NO
   - Other:
5. Smokes or uses tobacco products ____ YES x NO

### Medical History
Patient is African American and in good health.

### Dental History
Patient is meticulous with his oral hygiene, but has a tendency to brush vigorously.

### Social History
Patient lives with his wife and 3-year-old son.

### Chief Complaint
"I don't like the appearance of my gums pulling away from my teeth, and my teeth are sensitive around my upper canines."

### Supplemental Oral Examination Findings
Patient has a generalized opalescent appearance of the buccal mucosa. Patient has generalized melanin pigmentation of the gingiva. A mucocele is noted.
The gingiva is firm and stippled with no bleeding evident on probing. There is gingival recession on teeth #6 and #11 and mandibular anterior facials, with a 1-mm zone of attached gingiva.

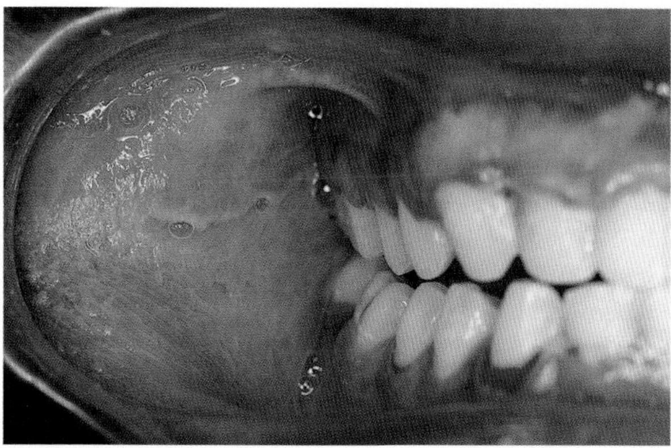

**Fig. 8.89** Case A: The patient wants the areas of gingival recession treated to resolve issues of sensitivity and esthetic problems. The dental care plan includes covering the areas around the canines with soft tissue grafts. The periodontist states that she will perform connective tissue grafts. She explains that the connective tissue taken from an area (donor site) will produce the same type of epithelium at the canine area (recipient site) as the tissue that exists at that donor site. (From Regezi J, Sciubba J, Jordan RCK. *Oral Pathology: Clinical Pathologic Correlations.* 7th ed. St. Louis: Elsevier Saunders; 2017.)

***Use Case A and Fig. 8.89 to answer questions 1 to 11.***

1. What term is used to describe the generalized opalescence covering the buccal mucosa?
   - **a.** Linea alba
   - **b.** Leukoedema
   - **c.** Lichen planus
   - **d.** Leukoplakia
2. The condition in question 1 represents a(an)
   - **a.** Premalignant condition
   - **b.** Infection with *Candida albicans*
   - **c.** Variant of normal
   - **d.** Oral sign of anemia
3. What treatment does this condition require?
   - **a.** Nonsteroidal antiinflammatory drugs
   - **b.** Biopsy and excision
   - **c.** No treatment
   - **d.** Antifungal drugs
4. The patient has a 2-mm probing depth on the facial aspect of tooth #6, and he has 3 mm of recession. What is the clinical attachment level (loss) in this area?
   - **a.** 5 mm
   - **b.** 2 mm
   - **c.** 3 mm
   - **d.** 1 mm
5. Sensitivity of the patient's upper canines is most likely related to:
   - **a.** Hyperkeratosis of sulcular epithelium
   - **b.** Enamel hypoplasia
   - **c.** Fluid entering dentinal tubules
   - **d.** Attrition
6. This patient's vigorous toothbrushing, especially over the canine eminences, can lead to which one of the following conditions?
   - **a.** Attrition
   - **b.** Erosion
   - **c.** Abfraction
   - **d.** Abrasion
7. The type of tissue normally present around the canine area is:
   - **a.** Keratinized, stratified squamous epithelium
   - **b.** Nonkeratinized, stratified squamous epithelium
   - **c.** Keratinized, simple squamous epithelium
   - **d.** Pseudo-stratified columnar epithelium
8. The most appropriate connective tissue donor site is the:
   - **a.** Buccal mucosa
   - **b.** Soft palate
   - **c.** Hard palate
   - **d.** Sublingual area
9. This patient also has a mucocele that is the result of trauma to a minor salivary gland duct. Mucoceles are most commonly found on the:
   - **a.** Lower lip
   - **b.** Soft palate
   - **c.** Dorsal tongue
   - **d.** Opening of Stensen's duct
10. What term is reserved for mucoceles that occur in the floor of the mouth?
    - **a.** Vesicle
    - **b.** Bulla
    - **c.** Pleomorphic
    - **d.** Ranula
11. To prevent further recession, what changes should this patient make in his oral self-care regimen?
    - **a.** More frequent recare appointments
    - **b.** Modify flossing technique
    - **c.** More frequent toothbrushing
    - **d.** Modify toothbrushing technique
12. The radiographs in Fig. 8.90 indicate congenital absence of the:
    - **a.** Mandibular right second premolar and the mandibular left second premolar
    - **b.** Maxillary right first premolar and the maxillary left first premolar
    - **c.** Mandibular right first premolar and the mandibular left first premolar
    - **d.** Mandibular left first premolar and the mandibular right second premolar
13. A benign asymptomatic hard protuberance of bone in the midline of the hard palate, that appears radiopaque on a radiograph, is most likely which one of the following?
    - **a.** Odontogenic myxoma
    - **b.** Torus palatinus
    - **c.** Complex odontoma
    - **d.** Polyostotic fibrous dysplasia

*Use Fig. 8.91 to answer questions 14 to 16.*

14. On the panoramic radiograph in Fig. 8.91, bilateral radiolucent areas are present apical to the mandibular molars, identified by the letter A. These most likely represent?
    a. Stafne bone cysts
    b. Periapical abscesses
    c. Submandibular fossae
    d. Simple (traumatic) bone cysts
15. The radiopaque structure directly above B in Fig. 8.91 is the:
    a. Articular eminence
    b. Maxillary tuberosity
    c. Mandibular condyle
    d. Coronoid process
16. Large bilateral radiolucent areas identified by C in Fig. 8.91 are:
    a. Nasal fossae
    b. Orbits
    c. Frontal sinuses
    d. Maxillary sinuses
17. The most common location for pleomorphic adenomas is the:
    a. Parotid gland
    b. Floor of mouth
    c. Buccal mucosa
    d. Lower lip
18. Which one of the following cysts, by virtue of its location, can create difficulty swallowing?
    a. Branchial cleft
    b. Thyroglossal
    c. Nasopalatine
    d. Dentigerous

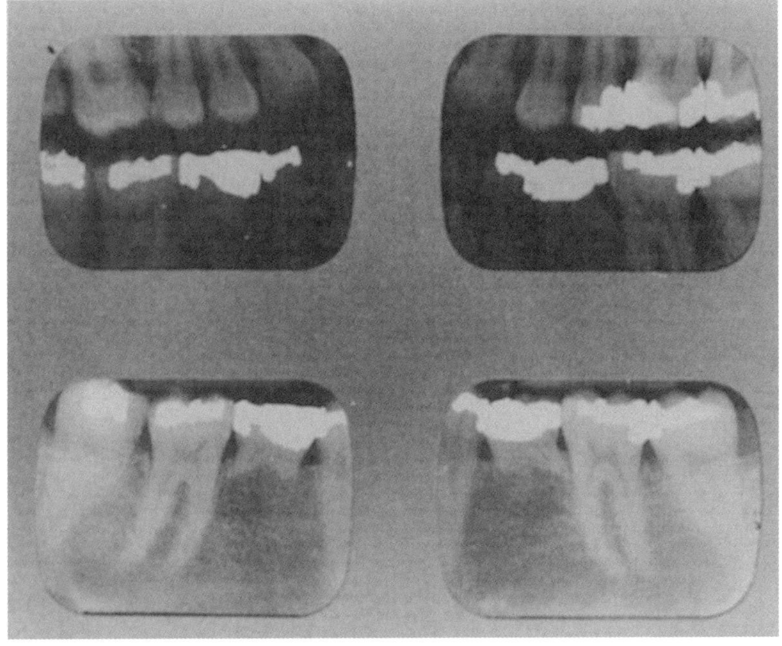

**Fig. 8.90** Radiographs.

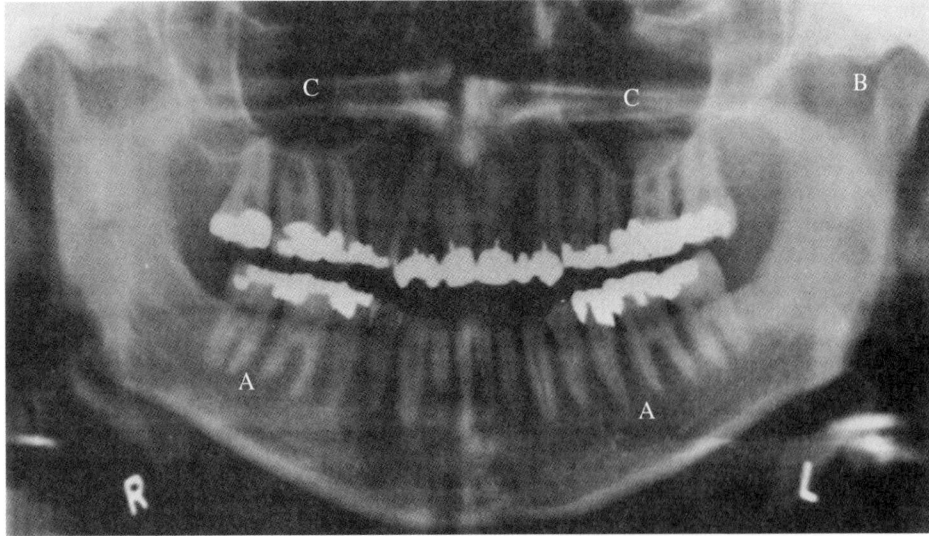


**Fig. 8.91** Panoramic radiograph.

19. Which infectious disease can be associated with (occur in conjunction with) necrotizing ulcerative gingivitis (NUG)?
    a. Primary herpetic gingivostomatitis
    b. Infectious mononucleosis
    c. Acute myelogenous leukemia
    d. Nonthrombocytopenic purpura
20. Intraorally, the most common location for pleomorphic adenomas is the:
    a. Palate
    b. Lower lip mucosa
    c. Buccal mucosa
    d. Floor of the mouth
21. The most common oral malignancy (cancer) in the oral cavity is?
    a. Odontogenic myxoma
    b. Chondroma
    c. Squamous cell carcinoma
    d. Kaposi's sarcoma
22. Fig. 8.92 is a periapical radiograph of the mandibular right quadrant in a 14-year-old. The teeth are asymptomatic. What does the periapical radiolucency (indicated by arrow) on tooth #31 represent?
    a. Root resorption due to traumatic injury
    b. Apical granuloma or cyst
    c. Incomplete root formation
    d. Ankylosis
23. Lack of tooth development in the posterior mandible, in a space occupied by a cyst, is highly suggestive of which one of the following?
    a. Primordial cyst
    b. Dermoid cyst
    c. Odontogenic myxoma
    d. Odontoma
24. The usual location for periapical cemento-osseous dysplasia is:
    a. Mandibular molars
    b. Maxillary anteriors
    c. Mandibular anteriors
    d. Maxillary molars
25. Overproduction of red blood cells with an increased hemoglobin level is characteristic of?
    a. Polycythemia
    b. Thrombocytopenia
    c. Pernicious anemia
    d. Iron deficiency anemia

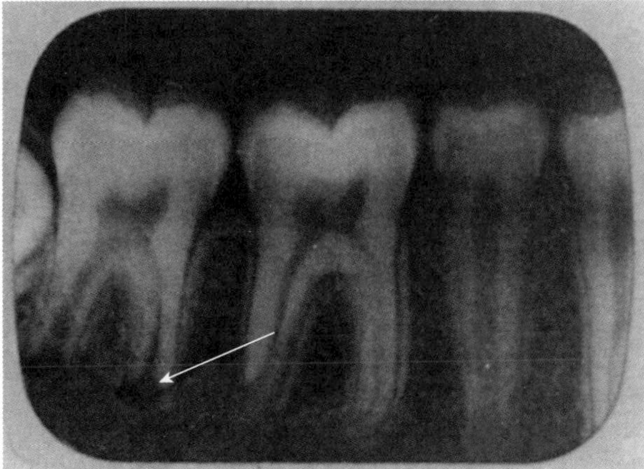

**Fig. 8.92** Periapical radiograph.

26. Which one of the following is the most common inherited bleeding disorder in the United States?
    a. Cyclic neutropenia
    b. Hemophilia Type A
    c. Hemophilia Type B
    d. Von Willebrand's disease
27. Which of the following is the best diagnostic tool to distinguish pemphigus from pemphigoid?
    a. Age of the patient
    b. Sequential blood counts
    c. Immunofluorescence testing
    d. Absence of Nikolsky's sign
28. The Philadelphia chromosome is associated with which one of the following?
    a. Leukemia
    b. Erythema multiforme
    c. HIV/AIDS
    d. Cyclic neutropenia
29. Which of the following is the most common intraoral manifestation of HIV infection, and is often the presenting sign that leads to diagnosis?
    a. Herpangina
    b. Candidiasis
    c. Infectious mononucleosis
    d. White sponge nevus
30. Which of the following pairs of diseases represent different forms of infection resulting from the same virus?
    a. Measles and German measles
    b. Chickenpox and smallpox
    c. Bacterial pneumonia and croup
    d. Shingles and chickenpox
31. A cluster of tiny vesicles is noted on the lower lip of a 40-year-old female. When questioned, the patient reports she "always gets a sore like this" before she develops a cold. The patient most likely has an infection due to which one of the following viruses:
    a. Herpes simplex virus
    b. Coxsackievirus
    c. Herpes zoster virus
    d. Epstein-Barr virus
32. Which one of the following cysts develops from residual epithelial rests of Malassez?
    a. Dentigerous cyst
    b. Apical (periapical) cyst
    c. Primordial cyst
    d. Nasopalatine duct cyst
33. The gingival enlargement shown in Fig. 8.93 was caused by a calcium channel blocker. Which one of the following drugs is implicated?
    a. Phenytoin (Dilantin)
    b. Enalapril (Vasotec)
    c. Fluoxetine (Prozac)
    d. Nifedipine (Procardia)

34. Fig. 8.94 A soft tissue lesion, filled with clear fluid, developed on this patient's lower lip and then suddenly ruptured. This was most likely a?
   a. Ranula
   b. Mucocele
   c. Fibroma
   d. Fibrolipoma
35. All true cysts are characterized by having which one of the following features?
   a. Well delineated round to oval shape
   b. Prominent lumen filled with fluid
   c. Epithelial lining
   d. Clinical evidence of bone expansion
36. Which one of the following clinical procedures is the "gold standard" for determining the definitive diagnosis of squamous cell carcinoma?
   a. Incisional or excisional biopsy
   b. Radiographic evaluation
   c. Sequential blood counts
   d. Capillary fragility test
37. Oral squamous papillomas are caused by which one of the following?
   a. Epstein-Barr virus
   b. Herpes simplex virus

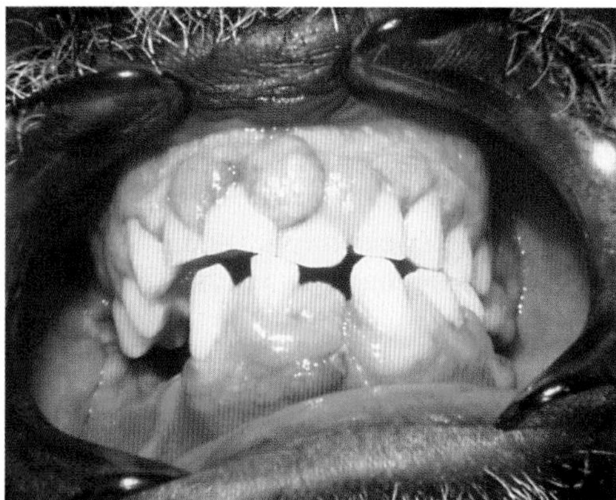

**Fig. 8.93** Gingival enlargement. (Courtesy of Dr. Victor M. Sternberg; from Ibsen OAC, Phelan JA. *Oral Pathology for the Dental Hygienist*. 6th ed. St. Louis: Elsevier Saunders; 2014.)

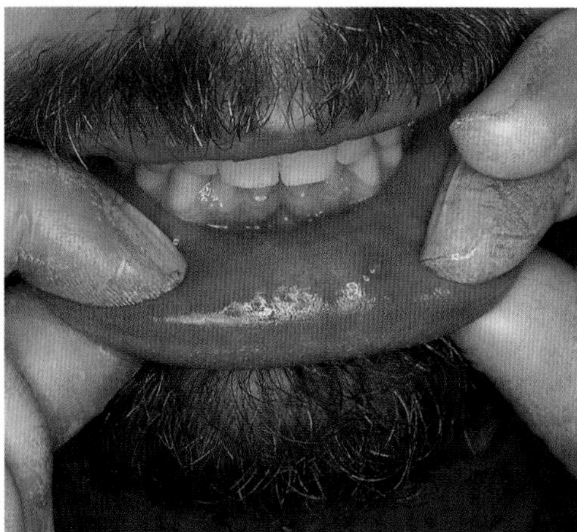

**Fig. 8.94** Soft tissue lesion.

   c. Varicella zoster virus
   d. Human papilloma virus
38. Herpes labialis is due to reactivation of which latent virus residing in the trigeminal ganglion?
   a. Human papilloma virus
   b. Varicella zoster virus
   c. Herpes simplex virus
   d. Epstein-Barr virus
39. A 28-year-old pregnant female presents with a lesion involving the maxillary labial gingiva over teeth #7 and #8. The lesion is bright red, soft, spongy and bleeds easily. Histologic findings reveal a lesion rich in blood-filled capillaries, inflammatory cells and covered with a thin ulcerated epithelium. The lesion described is most likely which one of the following?
   a. Fibrolipoma
   b. Pyogenic granuloma
   c. Peripheral giant cell granuloma
   d. Squamous papilloma
40. Which one of the following cysts is formed by accumulation of fluid between the crown of a tooth and reduced enamel epithelium, after the crown is completely formed?
   a. Lateral periodontal cyst
   b. Odontogenic keratocyst
   c. Simple (traumatic) bone cyst
   d. Dentigerous cyst
41. Wickham's striae are a characteristic of which one of the following?
   a. Erythema multiforme
   b. Behçet's disease
   c. Reticular lichen planus
   d. White sponge nevus
42. Which one of the following is a severe form of erythema multiforme that involves the oral cavity, skin, and eyes or genital mucosa?
   a. Stevens-Johnson syndrome
   b. Pemphigus vulgaris
   c. Necrotizing sialometaplasia
   d. Letterer-Siwe disease
43. An elderly patient presents with exophytic folds of pink hyperplastic tissue, that appear to grow over the flanges of an ill-fitting maxillary denture. This most likely represents which one of the following?
   a. Hyperkeratosis due to irritation
   b. Osteomalacia
   c. Inflammatory papillary hyperplasia of the palate
   d. Denture-induced inflammatory fibrous hyperplasia
44. A 40-year-old female presents with a lesion on the buccal mucosa of many years duration. It is pink, well defined, pedunculated, and soft to palpation. Histologically it consists of dense fibrous connective tissue with sparse small blood vessels, covered with normal oral mucosa. The lesion is most likely which one of the following?
   a. Pyogenic granuloma
   b. Irritation fibroma
   c. Peripheral giant cell granuloma
   d. Hemangioma

45. A radiolucent lesion, in the posterior mandible, anterior to the angle, has the radiographic features of a cyst. Clinical evaluation reveals this is a developmental concavity to accommodate normal salivary gland and not a true cyst. What is the name for this pseudocyst?
   a. Static bone cyst
   b. Traumatic bone cyst
   c. Aneurysmal bone cyst
   d. Median mandibular cyst
46. A unilateral, translucent, bluish, round, smooth-surfaced swelling is present in the floor of the mouth. The lesion increases and decreases in size with eating and stimulation of salivary flow. Which one of the following best describes this lesion?
   a. Pleomorphic adenoma
   b. Mucocele
   c. Ranula
   d. Necrotizing sialometaplasia
47. A 20-year-old male presents with sudden onset of painful ulcerations on his lips, tongue and oral mucosa. He recently completed a 10-day course of antibiotics for a persistent dental infection. Extensive hemorrhagic crusting is observed on the vermilion border of the lips. "Target" or "Bulls-eye" skin lesions are present. What condition does this represent?
   a. Erythema multiforme
   b. Necrotizing ulcerative gingivitis
   c. Major aphthous ulcers
   d. Systemic lupus erythematosus
48. A cigarette smoker presents with a hyperkeratinized white to gray posterior palate with scattered small erythematous nodules. What does this represent?
   a. Squamous cell carcinoma
   b. Nicotine stomatitis
   c. Necrotizing sialometaplasia
   d. Erosive lichen planus
49. A female patient presents for routine dental evaluation. Her medical history is negative for systemic diseases. An erythematous butterfly-shaped rash, crossing the bridge of the nose, is present. She reports recent sun exposure has made this rash worse. Intraorally there are a number of erythematous plaques with white striae, resembling lichen planus. What condition do you suspect may be undiagnosed in this patient?
   a. Sickle cell disorder
   b. Erosive lichen planus
   c. Pemphigus vulgaris
   d. Systemic lupus erythematosus
50. Acute gingivitis with extensive tissue necrosis of the interdental papillae is observed in a young college student. The papillae are blunted or "punched-out" and the interdental spaces are covered with necrotic tissue and debris. There is a foul mouth odor along with intense gingival pain and spontaneous gingival bleeding. What condition must be considered?
   a. Erythema multiforme
   b. Primary herpetic gingivostomatitis
   c. Necrotizing ulcerative gingivitis
   d. Pemphigus vulgaris
51. An autoimmune inflammatory condition is characterized by one or more small oval to round ulcerations, surrounded by an erythematous halo. Pain is out of proportion to the small size of the ulcers, which are self-limiting and heal in 10 to 12 days. Recurrent episodes are common. Which one of the following conditions does this describe?
   a. Mucous membrane pemphigoid
   b. Recurrent aphthous stomatitis
   c. Infectious mononucleosis
   d. Erythema multiforme
52. Which one of the following is a major risk factor for posterior oropharyngeal cancer including base of tongue and tonsils?
   a. Herpes simplex virus
   b. Human papilloma virus
   c. Varicella zoster virus
   d. Epstein-Barr virus
53. Invasion of tumor cells into adjacent tissues and metastasis of tumor cells to regional lymph nodes and distant sites occurs with which one of the following oral neoplasms?
   a. Osteoma
   b. Squamous cell carcinoma
   c. Peripheral giant cell granuloma
   d. Hemangioma
54. Odontogenic keratocysts (OKCs) have recently been reclassified as a neoplasm called keratocystic odontogenic tumor (KCOT) due their aggressive behavior and high recurrence rate. Multiple OKCs have been associated with which one of the following?
   a. Monostotic fibrous dysplasia
   b. Cherubism
   c. Polyostotic fibrous dysplasia
   d. Nevoid basal cell carcinoma syndrome
55. What genetic disorder involves mutation of the beta globin chain of hemoglobin, resulting in crescent shaped red blood cells and a radiographic "hair-on-end" appearance on the skull?
   a. Primary polycythemia
   b. Pernicious anemia
   c. Sickle cell disorder
   d. Thrombocytopenic purpura
56. Severe depression of bone marrow activity can lead to a rare life threatening anemia in which there is a reduction in the number of all blood cells (pancytopenia). What is the name of this disorder?
   a. Aplastic anemia
   b. Iron deficiency anemia
   c. Systemic lupus erythematosus
   d. Primordial cyst
57. A dental hygienist documents the following clinical features in an adult patient: persistent generalized lymphadenopathy, areas of severe necrotizing ulcerative periodontitis (NUP) that are not responsive to home care or periodontal therapy, and white lesions on the tongue suggestive of hairy leukoplakia. Which one of the following conditions are these findings suggestive of?
   a. Eosinophilic granuloma
   b. Osteomalacia

c. Hyperparathyroidism
d. Acquired immune deficiency syndrome

58. Which one of the following describes loss of tooth structure due to chemical action?
a. Abfraction
b. Erosion
c. Attrition
d. Abrasion

59. Clinically the crown of a maxillary incisor displays a pink spot, showing through the enamel, "pink tooth of Mummery." What is the most likely condition?
a. External resorption
b. Internal resorption
c. Dens invaginatus
d. Enamel hypoplasia

60. Overproduction of red blood cells and an increased hemoglobin level are seen in which one of the following conditions?
a. Polycythemia
b. Sickle cell disorder
c. Aplastic anemia
d. Acute leukemia

61. Incomplete or defective development of enamel due to disruption of ameloblasts during enamel formation is known as?
a. Enamel hyperplasia
b. Osteomalacia
c. Enamel hypoplasia
d. Abfraction

62. "Snow-capped teeth" are a result of enamel crystalline structure failing to mature. These teeth are seen in which one of the following?
a. Rickets
b. Monostotic fibrous dysplasia
c. Amelogenesis imperfecta
d. Dentinogenesis imperfecta

63. In which one of the following dental anomalies does apical pathology, due to pulpal necrosis, occur soon after tooth eruption?
a. Dilaceration
b. Dens invaginatus
c. Gemination
d. Concrescence

64. Which one of the following viruses causes herpangina?
a. Varicella zoster virus
b. Coxsackievirus
c. Epstein-Barr virus
d. Herpes simplex virus

65. This noninherited developmental disorder is associated with painless enlargement or expansion of the craniofacial bones causing deformity. The ribs are also commonly affected. Normal bone is replaced with fibrous connective tissue, which radiographically produces a "ground glass" appearance. Which one of the following conditions does this describe?
a. Langerhans cell histiocytosis
b. Osteomalacia
c. Osteoma
d. Fibrous dysplasia

66. Precocious puberty is most characteristic of:
a. Jaffe syndrome
b. Monostotic fibrous dysplasia
c. Cherubism
d. McCune-Albright syndrome

67. Achlorhydria (lack of gastric hydrochloric acid secretion), inability to absorb vitamin $B_{12}$, and a burning, painful tongue are characteristics of:
a. Iron deficiency anemia
b. Leukemia
c. Pernicious anemia
d. Aplastic anemia

68. An elderly male presents with the chief complaint that his dentures no longer fit. He has tingling and numbness in his arms and legs, bone pain, and suffers from severe headaches and hearing loss. What disease of bone is this characteristic of?
a. Paget's disease
b. Monostotic fibrous dysplasia
c. Polyostotic fibrous dysplasia
d. Hyperparathyroidism

69. "Stones, bones, and abdominal groans" are classic signs and symptoms of which one of the following?
a. Hemophilia
b. Thalassemia
c. Agranulocytosis
d. Hyperparathyroidism

70. Severe vitamin D deficiency in children results in?
a. Osteomalacia
b. Hand-Schüller-Christian disease
c. Rickets
d. Cyclic neutropenia

71. Punched-out radiolucencies in the skull and jaws, along with teeth that appear to be "floating" in the bone which has been destroyed around them, is a feature of what form of Langerhans cell histiocytosis?
a. Eosinophilic granuloma
b. Letterer-Siwe disease
c. Hand-Schüller-Christian disease
d. Cyclic neutropenia

72. Snorting or smoking which one of the following drugs produces corrosive vapors that, along with self-neglect and consumption of high sugar foods, results in significant rapid damage to the teeth (erosion, rampant caries) and oral tissues (destruction of periodontal tissues)?
a. Methamphetamines
b. Tobacco (snuff)
c. Marijuana
d. Naloxone

73. Which one of the following medications can be incorporated into the teeth during tooth development and cause permanent endogenous gray-brown staining?
a. Diphenhydramine
b. Tetracycline
c. Tylenol
d. Penicillin

74. Crowding of teeth with close root proximity can result in the joining of teeth by confluent cementum. This is called
 a. Cementoma
 b. Periapical cemental dysplasia
 c. Concrescence
 d. Dilaceration
75. Which form of Langerhans cell histiocytosis is the most common and can mimic an aggressive periodontitis that is not responsive to periodontal therapy?
 a. Letterer-Siwe disease
 b. Hand-Schüller-Christian disease
 c. Eosinophilic granuloma
 d. Peripheral giant cell granuloma
76. Ectopic sebaceous glands on the vermilion of the lips and buccal mucosa are known as?
 a. Fordyce granules
 b. Reticular lichen planus
 c. Erythema migrans
 d. Leukoplakia
77. Patches on the tongue of various sizes with curved "circinate" shapes surrounding center areas that appear bald, due to the loss of filiform papillae, describes what benign condition?
 a. Geographic tongue
 b. Wickham's striae
 c. Erosive lichen planus
 d. Aspirin burn
78. Recurrent major aphthous ulcerations are a common feature in patients with an infection caused by which one of the following viruses?
 a. Herpes simplex virus
 b. Human papilloma virus
 c. Varicella zoster virus
 d. Human immunodeficiency virus
79. What vascular malignancy occurs in 15% to 20% of AIDS patients and intraorally is most often found on the palate and gingiva?
 a. Lymphoma
 b. Kaposi's sarcoma
 c. Squamous cell carcinoma
 d. Chondroma
80. What is the condition called in which filiform papillae on the tongue fail to shed as they should, grow longer, and become coated with microorganisms?
 a. Hypokeratosis
 b. Erythema migrans
 c. Hairy tongue
 d. Hairy leukoplakia
81. Radiographically a mass composed of tooth-like structures, surrounded by a radiolucent rim, is blocking the eruption path of a maxillary lateral incisor. This is a(an)?
 a. Complex odontoma
 b. Odontogenic myxoma
 c. Compound odontoma
 d. Dentigerous cyst
82. An outgrowth of red to pink pulp tissue, protruding from the occlusal surface, in a tooth with a large open carious lesion, is known as?
 a. Apical granuloma
 b. Chronic hyperplastic pulpitis (pulp polyp)
 c. External resorption
 d. Internal resorption
83. Multiple osteomas can be associated with what autosomal dominant syndrome?
 a. Gardner's syndrome
 b. Nevoid basal cell carcinoma syndrome
 c. Polyostotic fibrous dysplasia
 d. Paget's disease
84. Which lesion, thought to be related to trauma and a destroyed blood clot, scallops between tooth roots, and is an empty cavity in bone?
 a. Primordial cyst
 b. Static bone cyst
 c. Aneurysmal bone cyst
 d. Simple bone cyst
85. An elderly female presents with a case of "desquamative" gingivitis. Mild trauma induces vesicle and bulla formation, and a positive Nikolsky's sign. Direct immunofluorescence shows a linear pattern of staining at the basement membrane. What condition doe this patient have?
 a. Pemphigus vulgaris
 b. Mucous membrane pemphigoid
 c. Reticular lichen planus
 d. Stevens-Johnson syndrome
86. Contact of the hands and fingers with contaminated dental instruments can lead to infection with the herpes simplex virus. What is this condition called?
 a. Herpetic whitlow
 b. Herpangina
 c. Hand-foot-and-mouth disease
 d. Herpes zoster

## SUGGESTED READINGS

Ibsen OAC, Phelan JA. *Oral Pathology for the Dental Hygienist*. 7th ed. St. Louis: Elsevier Saunders; 2017.

Neville BW, Damm DD, Allen CM, Bouquot JE. *Oral and Maxillofacial Pathology*. 4rd ed. St. Louis: Elsevier Saunders; 2015.

Regezi J, Sciubba J, Jordan RCK. *Oral Pathology: Clinical Pathologic Correlations*. 7th ed. St. Louis: Elsevier Saunders; 2016.

# 9

# Microbiology and Immunology

*Jessica Peek Scott**

Basic concepts of microbiology and immunology relate to transmissible diseases encountered in client care. Using standard precautions in the dental setting greatly reduces the transmission of pathogens. Dental hygienists must prevent and manage potential occupational exposures from infectious diseases.

## GENERAL MICROBIOLOGY

## MICROORGANISMS

### General Considerations

A. Ubiquitous—found virtually everywhere
B. Only 3% are pathogenic (disease causing); 97% are nonpathogenic
C. Exhibit characteristics common to all biologic systems: reproduction, metabolism, growth, response to stimuli, adaptability, mutation, and organization
D. Medically important microorganisms
   1. Eukaryotes
      a. Protozoa—unicellular, nonphotosynthetic, heterotrophic
      b. Fungi—molds (multicellular) or yeast (unicellular)
         (1) Nonphotosynthetic, heterotrophic
         (2) Classified by type of spores produced, presence or absence of mycelia (singular, mycelium), and mechanisms of sexual and asexual spore formation
         (3) Part of the fungi kingdom
         (4) Identification of infection is accomplished clinically and microbiologically
      c. Helminths
         (1) Multicellular, nonphotosynthetic, heterotrophic
         (2) Generally, macroparasites of the human alimentary tract or hemolymphatic system
         (3) Part of the animal kingdom
         (4) Identification of infection is accomplished on microbiologic and clinical grounds
   2. Prokaryotes (aerobic or anaerobic unicellular bacteria)
      a. Classified by shape
         (1) Cocci (round)
         (2) Bacilli (rod-shaped)
         (3) Vibrio (comma-shaped)
         (4) Spirochete (corkscrew-shaped)
      b. Classified by Gram staining
         (1) Gram-positive (violet on Gram stain)
         (2) Gram-negative (pink on Gram stain)
      c. Classified into two taxa (singular, taxon)
         (1) Eubacteria—"true" bacteria; most important bacteria in medicine
         (2) Archeobacteria—primitive bacteria; can occupy and inhabit extreme environments
   3. Viruses; classification based on
      a. Type and properties of nucleic acid
      b. Morphology of nucleoproteins
      c. Presence and properties of envelopes—the *envelope* is the protein coat that protects the capsid and nucleic acid of the virus
   4. Prion
      a. Type of protein found in brain neurons; contains no genetic material
      b. Not bacterial, viral, or fungal
      c. Improper folding and inability to be degraded allows for accumulation and damage to the nervous system
      d. Transmissible (spongiform encephalopathies)
         (1) Creutzfeldt-Jakob disease (CJD)
         (2) Mad cow disease
      e. Highly resistant to traditional sterilization methods because of the extreme stability of prion proteins
E. Nomenclature—the binomial system
   1. Two-word designation
      a. Genus and species
      b. First word capitalized and both words italicized (e.g., *Escherichia coli*)
   2. Devised by Carolus Linnaeus

### Methods of Measurement and Observation

A. Types
   1. Macroscopic—measurable and observable by the naked eye
   2. Microscopic—too small to be measured or observed by the naked eye; requires a microscope or lens to see
B. Most commonly used units of measurement
   1. Centimeter (cm = $10^{-2}$ m)
   2. Millimeter (mm = $10^{-3}$ m)

*Jessica Peek Scott and the publisher acknowledge the past contributions of Marie Collins to this chapter.

3. Micrometer or micron (μm = $10^{-6}$ m)
4. Nanometer (nm = $10^{-9}$ m)
5. Angstrom unit (Å = $10^{-10}$ m)

C. Light microscopes illuminate objects by visible light
1. Bright-field microscopy
   a. Used to observe the morphology of microorganisms
   b. Used with stained smears
   c. Cannot be used to observe microorganisms less than 0.2 μm, such as viruses and spirochetes
   d. Compound microscopes have at least two lens systems:
      (1) Objective
         (a) Magnifies the specimen and is close to it
         (b) Four powers— × 4, × 10, × 40, and oil immersion (× 100)
      (2) Ocular
         (a) Eyepiece
         (b) Magnifies the image produced by the objective lens
2. Darkfield microscopy
   a. Specimens seen as bright objects against a dark background
   b. Used for the examination of unstained microorganisms and spirochetes and hanging drop preparations
   c. Advantage—allows a view of living bacteria not visible by Gram stain; undisturbed in size or shape by fixing and staining techniques
3. Phase-contrast microscopy
   a. Useful in examining transparent, living cells, including their internal structure, and in determining motility in a fluid medium; can show dense structures
   b. Variations in density between the microbes and the surrounding medium are capitalized on to increase the contrast between the two
4. Fluorescence microscopy
   a. Used to visualize objects that fluoresce or emit light when exposed to light of different wavelengths
   b. Ultraviolet light, fluorescent chemicals, and special filter systems required
   c. Typically used in the medical field to track antigen–antibody reactions and as a diagnostic technique (immunofluorescence)
5. Confocal scanning laser microscopy
   a. A conventional light microscope uses a laser light source to illuminate planes of a fluorochrome-stained specimen
   b. Confocal images combine fluorescent and reflected images
   c. Successive planes are scanned until the entire specimen is scanned
   d. Useful in creating three-dimensional pictures of biofilms
6. Specimen preparation
   a. Viewing living organisms
      (1) Methods
         (a) Hanging drop
         (b) Temporary wet mount
      (2) Advantages
         (a) Maintains the shape of organisms
         (b) Is useful to determine organisms' size, shape, motility, and reactions to chemicals or immune sera
   b. Staining
      (1) Procedure
         (a) Thin films of microorganisms are spread on a glass slide and allowed to dry (smear)
         (b) Films are fixed, either by a chemical fixative or by passing through a flame; this denatures the proteins and kills the cell
         (c) Dyes or stains are applied to the smear to allow for greater visualization; allows for some differentiation of species
         (d) Fixation process tends to reduce the sizes of cells; dye addition tends to increase the sizes of cells
      (2) Types of dyes
         (a) Acidic, or negative, dye is used to stain basic components of the cell (e.g., glycoproteins, matrix)
         (b) Basic, or positive, dye is used to stain acidic components of the cell (e.g., nucleic acid and polysaccharides)
      (3) Simple staining procedures
         (a) Use a single dye (e.g., carbolfuchsin, crystal violet, methylene blue, or safranin)
         (b) Used to show shapes, sizes, and arrangements of bacterial cells
      (4) Differential staining procedures (Table 9.1)
         (a) More than one dye preparation used
         (b) Used for initial bacterial grouping
         (c) Most common methods
            [1] Gram stain—differentiates microorganisms based on color as gram-positive (blue to purple) or gram-negative (pink to red); certain characteristics of microorganisms appear correlated with their staining reactions: cell wall thickness, chemical composition, and sensitivity to penicillin; useful in the diagnosis of infectious diseases
            [2] Acid-fast stain—differentiates between acid-fast and nonacid-fast bacteria; differentiates mycobacteria (e.g., *Mycobacterium leprae*, *M. tuberculosis*) from other bacteria by indicating the presence or absence of special lipids in the cell wall; organisms resist decolorization with an acidic solution of alcohol after being stained with a basic dye

**TABLE 9.1 Comparison of Gram-Positive and Gram-Negative Bacteria**

| | Gram-Positive Bacteria | Gram-Negative Bacteria |
|---|---|---|
| Color after Gram stain procedure | Blue to purple | Pink to red |
| Peptidoglycan layer in cell walls | Thick | Thin |
| Teichoic acid in cell walls | Present | Absent |
| Lipopolysaccharide in cell walls | Absent | Present |

(5) Special staining procedures—used to color and isolate specific parts of microorganisms
(a) Negative staining for capsules—determines if organism is encapsulated
(b) Schaeffer-Fulton spore stain (e.g., *Bacillus, Clostridium*)—determines if organism is a spore former
(c) Flagellar staining—determines if organism has flagella
(d) Toluidine blue-O staining—determines prions, proteoglycans, and glycosaminoglycans in tissues

D. Electron microscopy
1. Electrons used as a source of illumination
2. Higher magnification and better resolving power available than with a light microscope, but because specimens must be dead, dynamic processes cannot be examined
3. Types
a. Transmission electron microscope—used to visualize the ultrastructures of cells and viruses
b. Scanning electron microscope—used to visualize three-dimensional images of surface features of cells and viruses

## Prokaryotic (Bacterial) Cell Structure and Function

A. Bacterial morphology
1. Cocci (singular, coccus)
a. Spherical or ovoid shape
b. Occur in pairs (diplococci), chains (streptococci), four-in-a-square arrangement (tetrad), eight cells in a cubic arrangement (sarcinae), and irregular clusters (staphylococci)
2. Bacilli (singular, bacillus)
a. Cylindrical or rod-like
b. Occur in pairs (diplobacilli); chains (streptobacilli); small, rounded rods (coccobacilli); and with tapered ends (fusiform bacilli)
3. Spirilla (singular, spirillum)
a. Spiral or curved
b. Vary in number and fullness of turns
c. Vibrios are portions of a spiral
4. Palisade arrangement (bacterial cells form weird angles to one another)
a. "Fence post" appearance
b. *Corynebacterium diphtheriae*
5. Pleomorphic (no defined cell shape)
a. Variable in shape
b. *Mycoplasma pneumoniae*

B. External cell structures
1. Appendages
a. Provide motility
(1) Flagella (singular, flagellum)
(a) Threads of protein that extend from the cell surface and move in a whip-like motion
(b) Vectored motility must be distinguished from Brownian movement, which is caused by bacteria randomly hitting molecules in the surrounding medium; flagella enable bacteria to move toward favorable environments and away from adverse ones (chemotaxis)
(2) Axial filaments
b. Allow for movement—spirochetes (e.g., *Treponema pallidum, Borrelia burgdorferi*) move by this method
c. Provide attachments
(1) Pili (singular, pilus)
(a) Hair-like structures often found on gram-negative bacteria; not associated with motility
(b) Longer and fewer in number
(c) Sex pili join bacterial cells in preparation for deoxyribonucleic acid (DNA) transfer (conjugation)
(2) Fimbriae (singular, fimbria)
(a) Shorter and numerous
(b) Enable a cell to adhere to surfaces (e.g., *Neisseria gonorrhoeae, E. coli*)
2. Surface coating (glycocalyx)
a. Capsules
(1) Condensed and well-defined masses of polysaccharides or polypeptides firmly attached to the cell wall
(2) Encapsulation protects pathogenic organisms from drugs, phagocytosis, and bactericidal factors
(3) Some bacteria need capsules to maintain virulence (e.g., *Streptococcus pneumoniae, Streptococcus mutans*)
b. Slime layer (glycocalyx)
(1) Unorganized, soluble mass of polysaccharides or polypeptides loosely attached to the cell wall; polymeric material (glycoprotein)
(2) Protects microorganisms; aids in adherence and gliding motility of organism
3. Cell wall
a. Functions
(1) Determines and maintains the shape of the microorganism
(2) Provides support for flagella
(3) Prevents rupture of the cell resulting from osmotic pressure differences on either side of the cell wall
b. Composed of the macromolecule peptidoglycan
c. Comparison of gram-negative and gram-positive cell walls
(1) Gram-positive cell walls consist of many layers of peptidoglycan and contain teichoic acids
(2) Gram-negative bacteria have a lipoprotein–lipopolysaccharide–phospholipid outer membrane surrounding a thin, peptidoglycan layer
(3) Outer membrane protects gram-negative cells from phagocytosis, penicillin, lysozymes, and other chemicals
(4) Gram-negative cell walls are more easily broken by mechanical forces; susceptible to lysis by antibody, complement, and streptomycin

4. Cytoplasmic (plasma) membrane
   a. Structure—consists of a phospholipid bilayer interspersed with proteins in a mosaic pattern (fluid mosaic)
   b. Functions
      (1) Barrier that regulates movement of materials in and out of the cell
      (2) Active transport
      (3) Excretion of hydrolytic exoenzymes
      (4) Bears enzymes and carrier molecules
      (5) Bears receptors and other proteins of the chemotactic and other sensory transduction systems
   c. Lies adjacent to and beneath the cell wall and encloses the cytoplasm of the cell
5. Cell envelope
   a. Includes all external structures and appendages, including the capsule, pili, flagella, cell wall, and cytoplasmic membrane
   b. May play a role in protection from degradation, maintenance of cell shape, and cell adhesion
   c. Properties confer staining characteristics
   d. Organization and structure different in gram-positive and gram-negative bacteria

C. Internal cell structure
1. Cytoplasm (protoplasm)
   a. Fluid compartment inside the cytoplasmic membrane
   b. Prominent site for many of the cell's biochemical and synthetic activities
   c. Contains chromatin body, ribosomes, and granules
2. Mesosomes—irregular folds of the cytoplasmic membrane resulting from dehydration of cells in preparation for electron microscopy; considered artifacts
3. Genetic material or genome (nucleoid)
   a. Prokaryotes lack the distinct nucleus of eukaryotes
   b. Single chromosome is composed of a single molecule of DNA, existing as a closed loop not enclosed by the nuclear membrane; located in the nucleoplasm of the cell
   c. Additional genetic material is found in plasmids, which are extrachromosomal DNA molecules; they often carry information that determines drug resistance or sensitivity
4. Ribosomes
   a. Function in protein synthesis
   b. Composed of ribosomal protein and ribosomal ribonucleic acid (RNA)
   c. Distributed throughout the cytoplasm
5. Photosynthetic apparatus
6. Inclusions
   a. Accumulations of reserve storage materials
   b. Include polysaccharide granules, metachromatic granules, sulfur granules, lipid inclusions, carboxysomes, and gas vacuoles

D. Endospores (spores)
1. Dormant structures formed within gram-positive bacterial cells as a means of survival
2. Formed during a process called *sporulation*—disintegration of parent cell releases endospore; then called *exposure* or *free spore*
3. Can remain in a spore state for years; exhibit unusual resistance to heat, drying, chemical disinfection, and radiation
4. Can transform back into a vegetative cell through a process called *germination*
5. Ability of bacteria to produce endospores restricted mainly to the genera *Bacillus* and *Clostridium*

## Eukaryotic Cell Structure and Function

See Tables 9.2 and 9.3.

A. More complex than a prokaryotic cell; has a distinct nucleus bounded by a nuclear membrane, a nucleolus, and membrane-bound organelles

B. Animal cells
1. Cell membrane
   a. Surrounds the cell and interconnects with the cell's internal membrane systems
   b. Functions
      (1) Regulates the passage of substances in and out of the cell through active and passive transport
      (2) Involved in phagocytosis, tumor formation, drug sensitivity, and immune response
2. Nucleus
   a. Controls the cell's physiologic and reproductive processes
   b. Composition
      (1) Nuclear membrane
      (2) Nucleoli (involved in RNA synthesis)
      (3) Chromosomes (composed of DNA)
      (4) Nucleoprotein (chromatin)
3. Internal structures
   a. Mitochondria are sites of adenosine triphosphate (ATP), or energy, production
   b. Endoplasmic reticulum
      (1) Network of membranes involved in chemical reactions, storage, and transportation
      (2) Rough endoplasmic reticulum has ribosomes attached
   c. Golgi complex—storage and packaging structure for cellular components
   d. Lysosomes—contain digestive enzymes
   e. Microtubules
   f. Vacuoles

## Microbial Growth and Cultivation

See Fig. 9.1.

A. Definitions
1. Culture media—nutrient preparations used to cultivate microorganisms
2. In vitro techniques—procedures using nonliving materials in a culture vessel
3. In vivo techniques—procedures using living cells or entire animals or plants
4. Colony—accumulation of bacteria on a medium

B. Conditions that affect growth
1. Physical

## TABLE 9.2 Eukaryotic Organelles and Their Functions

| Cell Part or Organelle | Associated Functions and Activities |
|---|---|
| Cell membrane | Transport of substances into and out of cells (selective permeability)<br>In some cells, engulfment of foreign material (phagocytosis)<br>Pinocytosis |
| Cell wall | Found only in plants and certain bacteria; imparts shape and strength to the cell<br>Protection against certain osmotic imbalances |
| Centrioles | Involved in cell division |
| Chloroplast | Photosynthesis |
| Cilium | Motion, or movement of substances, past the ciliated cell |
| Endoplasmic reticulum | Protein synthesis<br>Transport of nutrients to the nucleus |
| Flagellum and cilium | Propulsion |
| Golgi complex | Transfer of proteins and other cellular components to exterior of a secretory cell<br>Storage and packing structure for cellular products |
| Lysosomes | Contain lysozymes and other digestive enzymes<br>Break down foreign material and worn out cell parts |
| Microbody, or peroxisome | Enzymatic activities |
| Microtubule | Cell transport<br>Development and maintenance of cell shape<br>Cell division<br>Ciliary and flagellar movement |
| Mitochondrion | Synthesis of the energy-rich compound adenosine triphosphate (ATP) |
| Nucleolus | Major site for the formation of ribosomal components |
| Nucleus | Control of cellular physiologic process<br>Contains chromosomes<br>Transfer of hereditary factors to subsequent generations |
| Plastids | Contain photosynthetic pigments<br>Sites of photosynthesis<br>Found in plant cells |
| Ribosome | Protein synthesis<br>Attach to outer surface of rough endoplasmic reticulum |
| Vacuoles | Locations of water<br>Storage site for certain amino acids, carbohydrates, and proteins<br>Dumping ground for cellular wastes |

## TABLE 9.3 Major Characteristics of Eukaryotes and Prokaryotes

| | EUKARYOTES | | |
|---|---|---|---|
| **Characteristic** | **Plants** | **Animals** | **Prokaryotes** |
| *Major groups* | Plants, algae, fungi | Animals, protozoa | Bacteria |
| *Size* (approximate) | > 5 μm | > 5 μm | 1 to 3 μm |
| *Nuclear structures* | | | |
| Nucleus | Classic membrane | Classic membrane | No nuclear membrane |
| Chromosomes | Strands of deoxyribonucleic acid (DNA) and protein | Strands of DNA and protein | Single, closed strand of DNA |
| *Cytoplasmic structures* | | | |
| Mitochondria | Present | Present | Absent |
| Golgi complex | Present | Present | Absent |
| Endoplasmic reticulum | Present | Present | Absent |
| Ribosomes (sedimentation coefficient) | 80S | 80S | 70S |
| Cytoplasmic membrane | Contains sterols | Contains sterols | Does not contain sterols |
| Cell wall | Composed of cellulose or chitin | Absent | Complex structure containing protein, lipids, and peptidoglycans |
| *Reproduction movement* | Sexual or asexual<br>Flagella or cilia (complex and similar to centrioles) | Sexual or asexual<br>Flagella or cilia (complex and similar to centrioles) | Asexual (binary fission)<br>Flagella, if present, are simple twisted proteins (no cilia) |
| *Respiration* | Via mitochondria | Via mitochondria | Via cytoplasmic membrane |
| *Photosynthesis* | Present (absent in fungi) | Absent | Present in cyanobacteria and some others |

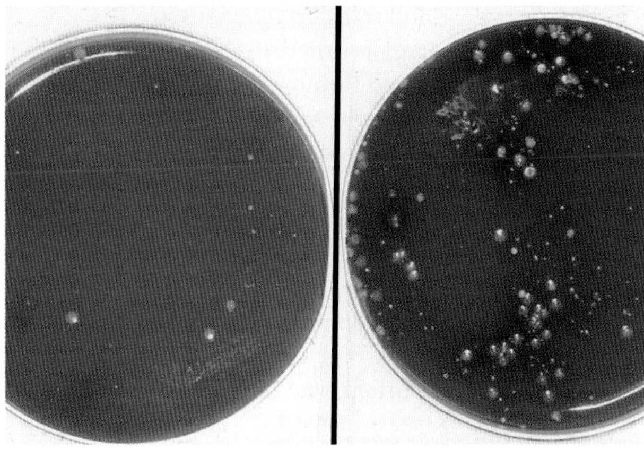

**Fig. 9.1** Bacterial production.

a. Thermal conditions
   (1) Most bacteria grow best over a range of temperatures
      (a) Psychrophiles—0°C to 15°C
      (b) Mesophiles—20°C to 40°C
      (c) Thermophiles—45°C to 60°C
   (2) 30°C is the optimal temperature for many free-living organisms
b. Acidity or alkalinity (pH)—most bacteria prefer a neutral pH, between 7.0 and 7.4
   (1) Acidophiles—pH 0 to 4
   (2) Neutrophiles—pH 5 to 9
   (3) Alkalinophiles—pH greater than 9
c. Osmotic pressure
   (1) Most microorganisms must be grown in an aquatic medium
   (2) Halophilic organisms require high salt concentration
   (3) Osmophilic organisms require high osmotic pressure

2. Chemical
   a. Gaseous requirements
      (1) Aerobes require oxygen
      (2) Micro-aerophilic organisms require low concentrations of oxygen
      (3) Anaerobes do not require oxygen
      (4) Obligate (strict) anaerobes cannot tolerate any free oxygen
      (5) Facultative anaerobes can metabolize aerobically if oxygen is present or anaerobically if it is absent
      (6) Aerotolerant anaerobes metabolize substances anaerobically but are not harmed by oxygen
   b. Nutrition available
      (1) Heterotrophic organisms
         (a) Require organic compounds for growth; obtain carbon from glucose
         (b) Most often cultured on a medium of glucose
      (2) Autotrophic organisms
         (a) Do not require organic nutrients for growth
         (b) Use inorganic compounds such as carbon dioxide
         (c) Thrive in soils and bodies of water
      (3) Hypotrophic organisms
         (a) Obligate intracellular parasites; grow only within a living host cell
         (b) Include viruses and rickettsiae
      (4) Phototrophic organisms
         (a) Use light for energy
      (5) Chemotrophic organisms
         (a) Oxidize chemical compounds for energy
      (6) Nutrients needed include sulfur and phosphorus
      (7) Nitrogen is derived from proteins and their products
      (8) Certain vitamins and growth factors required

C. Types of culture media
   1. Synthetic defined media—exact chemical composition is known
   2. Rich complex media—exact chemical composition varies slightly from batch to batch (e.g., addition of blood or beef extract); contain digested extracts from animal organs, meats, fish, yeasts, and plants
   3. Differential media
      a. Contain combinations of nutrients and pH indicators to produce visual differentiation between several microorganisms
      b. Examples
         (1) Blood agar is an enriched medium that allows streptococci to leave different signs on the medium; green discoloration around colonies indicates α-hemolytic streptococci, clear zone signifies β-hemolysis, and no effect denotes γ-hemolysis
         (2) Chocolate agar is even more enriched than blood agar
   4. Selective media
      a. Allow interference with or prevention of the growth of certain microorganisms while permitting others to grow
      b. Dyes and antibiotics make the media selective
      c. Examples
         (1) Sabouraud dextrose agar is selective for fungi
         (2) Thayer-Martin agar is selective for *Neisseria gonorrhoeae*
   5. Selective and differential media
      a. Combine properties of the preceding two types of media
      b. Examples—mannitol, salt agar, and MacConkey agar
   6. Enriched media—similar to selective media but designed to increase the numbers of particular microbes to detectable levels
   7. Reducing media
      a. Contain ingredients that chemically combine with and deplete oxygen in the culture medium
      b. Used for anaerobes

D. Pure culture techniques
   1. Used to isolate and identify a bacterial species
   2. Methods
      a. Pour-plate technique
         (1) Cool the melted agar-containing medium

(2) Inoculate the medium
(a) Use the loop or needle to transfer the organism
(b) Pass the loop through the flame and heat to redness
(c) Flame the edges of tubes from which cultures are taken before and after removal of the organism
(3) Pour the inoculated medium into a sterile Petri dish
(4) Allow the medium to solidify
(5) Incubate at the desired temperature
b. Streak-plate technique
(1) Spread a loopful of material containing organisms over the surface of the solidified agar
(2) Various streaking directions or patterns are possible

E. Bacterial growth
1. Most bacteria reproduce through binary fission (i.e., two new cells are produced by one parent cell)
2. Growth on the culture medium
a. Typical growth curve results
b. Phases
(1) Lag phase—period of intense metabolic activity but no increase in cell number
(2) Log phase or exponential growth phase—cell number increases in an exponential manner; generation time is the average time for the cell to divide; phase when cells are most metabolically active
(3) Stationary phase—total number of viable cells is constant; metabolic activity slows
(4) Phase of decline (death phase)—number of viable cells decreases
3. Measurement of growth
a. Population growth curve—made by observing an increase in mass or numbers over time
b. Cell mass can be measured by dry weight, chemical analysis, and turbidity
c. Population counts—cell numbers can be measured by viable platelet counts; estimates are expressed as colony-forming units (CFU) for bacteria or plaque-forming units (PFU) for viruses

## Microbial Metabolism and Cell Regulation

A. Metabolism
1. Definition—set of chemical reactions by which cells maintain life
2. Phases
a. Anabolism—biosynthetic reactions that use energy (ATP)
(1) Energy-consuming phase in which macromolecules such as nucleic acids, proteins, lipids, and polysaccharides are synthesized
b. Catabolism—degradative reactions that release energy (ATP)
(1) Energy-releasing phase in which complex compounds are broken down, creating energy in the form of ATP
3. Energy storage and transfer
a. Chemical energy is stored as ATP
b. May be generated through the transport of electrons (electron transport system)
c. Energy produced through oxidation-reduction reactions
(1) Aerobic oxidation (respiration)
(2) Anaerobic oxidation (fermentation)
4. Metabolic pathways
a. Series of steps to complete biochemical process
b. Glycolytic pathway (glycolysis)
(1) Most important way carbohydrates are metabolized
(2) Converts glucose to pyruvic acid
(3) Anaerobic fermentation process
(4) Tricarboxylic acid (Krebs) cycle
c. Occurs inside mitochondria
(1) Follows the glycolytic pathway
(2) Responsible for further oxidation of glucose and the production of other biochemically important intermediates
(3) Important to aerobic bacteria
5. Protein synthesis
a. DNA directs the formation of proteins aided by various types of RNA
b. Transcription—synthesis of messenger RNA (mRNA) from a DNA template
c. Translation—synthesis of protein from an mRNA template
d. Three stages of protein synthesis occurring at the ribosome:
(1) Initiation
(2) Elongation
(3) Termination

B. Metabolic control
1. Largely by enzymatic control
2. Types of regulation
a. Feedback inhibition
(1) Allosteric enzymes—end product binds to the enzyme and lowers its affinity for its substrate, thus preventing further product formation
(2) When more end product is needed, the enzyme is released
b. Genetic regulation—regulated by a specific unit of DNA called an *operon*
(1) Enzyme repression—when the level of end product is sufficient, the genetic synthesis of the enzyme is suppressed
(2) Enzyme induction—enzymes are genetically synthesized only when substrates are present

## Microbial Genetics

A. Eukaryotic genome
1. Almost all the eukaryotic genome is diploid
2. Gene expression can be recessive or dominant
3. Mitochondria and chloroplasts have a single, circular DNA; function of DNA is related to that organelle

B. Prokaryotic genome
   1. Most prokaryotes have a single, circular chromosome
   2. Additional genes are present on plasmids (small circles of DNA)
C. Some viruses (phage) multiply in bacteria
D. Genetic recombination (see the section on "Genetics" in Chapter 7)
   1. Conjugation
      a. Transfer of genetic material between two living bacteria that are in physical contact
      b. Plasmids are most frequently transferred
   2. Transduction—a bacterial virus (bacteriophage) transfers genetic material
   3. Transformation—the direct uptake of donor DNA by a recipient cell
E. Genetic rearrangement—*transposons* are small segments of DNA that can move from one region of a chromosome to another region of the genome
F. Mutations
   1. Result in changes in DNA sequence
   2. Can be caused by agents such as ultraviolet light, radiation, nitrous acid, and carcinogens

## Microbial Relationships

A. Syntrophism
   1. Organisms are not intimately associated with each other but benefit from each other
   2. Examples—yogurt production, organisms feeding in soil where decaying plant material is found
B. Competition
   1. Interaction between organisms resulting from a demand for a finite supply of nutrients and other resources
   2. Example—molds such as *Penicillium* compete by secreting substances toxic to other organisms
C. Predation—interaction that controls the population by predators feeding on another species, the prey
D. Symbiosis—interaction in which two different species live in a mutually beneficial coexistence
E. Commensalism—interaction in which only one organism benefits and the other neither benefits nor is harmed
F. Parasitism—interaction in which one organism benefits at the expense of the other

## Bacteria

A. Firmicutes—gram-positive eubacteria
B. Gracilicutes
   1. Gram-negative eubacteria
   2. Largest group of bacteria
   3. Contain many medically significant microorganisms
C. Tenericutes (mycoplasmas)
   1. Eubacteria lacking cell walls—because they lack cell walls, they are highly pleomorphic
   2. Enclosed by the plasma membrane—plasma membranes have lipids called *sterols* that aid in resisting lysis
   3. Mycoplasmas are the smallest self-replicating microorganisms
D. Mendosicutes (archaeobacteria)
   1. Conventional peptidoglycan in the cell wall is replaced with pseudomurein
   2. Often live in extreme environments
   3. Carry out atypical metabolic processes
   4. No known medically significant species

## Fungi

A. Description
   1. Eukaryotic
   2. Nonphotosynthetic
   3. Heterotrophic saprophytes—use preexisting organic products, either living or dead
   4. Grow well in dark, moist environments
   5. Few species are pathogenic to humans
B. Forms
   1. Molds (mycelial forms)
      a. Long filaments are structural units called *hyphae*; multicellular hyphae result in a cobweb-like growth called a *mycelium*
      b. Reproduce by sexual or asexual spores
   2. Yeasts
      a. Oval or spherical single cells
      b. Produce moist, shiny colonies
      c. Reproduce asexually by producing new buds or daughter cells
   3. Dimorphic fungi—some fungi exhibit characteristics of both molds and yeasts, depending on growth conditions
C. Classification of medically important fungi
   1. Zygomycota (the phycomyces)—include the common bread molds *Rhizopus* and *Mucor*
   2. Ascomycota (sac fungi)—include *Histoplasma, Microsporum, Aspergillus, Trichophyton, Penicillium* (a source of antibiotics), and *Saccharomyces* (leavened bread and fermented beer and wine)
   3. Basidiomycota—include *Cryptococcus neoformans*
   4. Deuteromycota (the imperfect fungi)—include *Candida, Pneumocystis, Coccidioides, Sporothrix,* and *Epidermophyton*; do not produce sexual spores
D. Fungal diseases (mycoses)
   1. Generally long-lasting infections
   2. Classification
      a. Systemic—involving a number of tissues and organs
      b. Subcutaneous—beneath the skin
      c. Cutaneous (superficial)—involving only the epidermis, hair, and nails
         (1) Tinea infections caused by *Microsporum, Trichophyton,* and *Epidermophyton*
      d. Opportunistic—generally harmless; can become pathogenic in a debilitated host

## Protozoa

A. Description
   1. Unicellular
   2. Eukaryotic
   3. Heterotrophic
   4. Most have a motile feeding stage called *trophozoite*
   5. Many can form cysts
      a. Protective resting stage

b. Can serve as a site for division or spreading of pathogenic protozoans (e.g., *Entamoeba histolytica,* which causes amoebic dysentery)

6. Reproduce asexually by fission, budding, or schizogony (multiple fission); reproduce sexually by conjugation

B. Four phyla (Sarcomastigophora, Mastigophora, Ciliophora, Microspora)

### Viruses

A. Properties of a mature virus particle, or virion
  1. Has a single type of nucleic acid, RNA or DNA, that contains genetic material, or a genome
  2. Nucleic acid is surrounded by an outer protein coat, the capsid; nucleic acid and capsid compose the nucleocapsid
  3. Capsids may or may not be covered by an envelope
  4. Viral nucleic acid contains the necessary information for programming an infected host cell
  5. Absence of cellular structures
  6. Lack components for energy production and protein synthesis
  7. Obligate intracellular parasites

B. Bacteriophages (bacterial viruses)
  1. Contain either RNA or DNA
  2. Life cycles: lytic and lysogenic
     a. Lytic cycle—virus enters a host cell, takes over cell replication mechanism, makes viral DNA and protein, then lyses (breaks open) the cell; this allows newly produced viruses to leave host cell and infect other cells (destroys host cell)
     b. Lysogenic cycle—virus attaches to host cell's DNA and replicates when host cell divides; once integrated, the virus is referred to as a *prophage,* and a stable association is established between the host cell and the virus (no harm done to host cell)

C. Human viruses
  1. Classified by structure and type of nucleic acid, mode of replication, and morphology
  2. Destructive effects on cells are termed *cytopathic*
  3. Prions
     a. Proteinaceous infectious particles believed to cause kuru and CJD
     b. Organization, replication, and how they cause disease are unknown

D. Viral replication
  1. Uses biosynthetic mechanisms of the host cell
  2. Phases
     a. Attachment, penetration, and uncoating
     b. Synthesis of viral components
     c. Morphogenesis and release

E. Modes of viral transmission
  1. Direct transmission from person to person
  2. Transmission from animal to animal
  3. Transmission by an arthropod vector

F. Role of virus in cancer
  1. Oncogenous viruses can induce various types of cancers (RNA-type or DNA-type viruses)
  2. Proto-oncogenes are highly conserved, "friendly" transforming genes
  3. Mechanisms of oncogene activation
     a. Transduction by a virus
     b. Insertional mutagenesis
     c. Translocation
     d. Gene amplification
     e. Mutation
  4. Role oncogenes play in the development of cancer is unclear

## MICROBIAL VIRULENCE AND DISEASE TRANSFER

A. Bacteria that produce disease or pathologic changes in humans (Table 9.4)

B. Definitions
  1. Pathogen—agent producing disease or pathologic changes
  2. Opportunist—commensal bacterium that invades the host under favorable conditions
  3. Virulence—the degree of pathogenicity; properties that determine pathogenicity of an organism include invasiveness (transmissibility), ability to multiply in the host, and toxin production
  4. Infection—invasion of the tissue by a pathogenic microorganism and multiplication of the organism
     a. Localized—organism remains in a particular area of the body
     b. Generalized or systemic—microorganism invades the bloodstream and the lymphatic system
     c. Acute—runs a rapid course; terminates abruptly (less than 6 months)
     d. Chronic—slow onset; infection of long duration
     e. Primary—original infection
     f. Secondary—infection that follows a primary infection and is often caused by an opportunistic organism
     g. Toxemia—presence of toxin in the blood
     h. Subclinical—lacking recognizable symptoms
     i. Focal—localized in one area and spreading elsewhere in the body from that point
     j. Bacteremia—presence of bacteria in the bloodstream
     k. Latent—causative agent remains inactive for a time but then becomes active to produce symptoms of the disease
     l. Sequelae—long-term or permanent damage to diseased tissues or organs
     m. Nosocomial—acquired during a hospital stay
     n. Sign—objective changes that a healthcare provider can observe and measure
     o. Symptom—subjective changes in body experienced by the patient or client
  5. Infectious disease—interference with the normal functioning of the host; proof by Koch's postulates:
     a. Microorganisms are present in every case of disease
     b. Microorganisms grow in pure culture from the diseased host
     c. Same disease is reproduced when pure culture is inoculated into a healthy host
     d. Microorganism is recovered from the inoculated host

TABLE 9.4 **Bacteria of Human Importance**

| Organism | Diseases | Other Features |
|---|---|---|
| **Gram-Positive Cocci** | | |
| *Staphylococcus aureus* | Boils, carbuncles, septicemia, food poisoning, pneumonia | Common skin commensal; phage typing identifies virulent strains; enterotoxin causes food poisoning |
| *Streptococcus pyogenes* | Tonsillitis, scarlet fever, erysipelas, septicemia, strep throat, rheumatic fever | Also causes glomerulonephritis and rheumatic fever, with immunopathologic basis |
| *Streptococcus viridans* group (*Streptococcus sanguinis*, etc.) | Infective endocarditis | Oral commensals settle on abnormal heart valves during bacteremia |
| *Streptococcus mutans* | Dental caries | Regular inhabitant of mouth; initiates plaque on tooth surface |
| *Streptococcus pneumoniae* | Pneumonia, otitis, meningitis | Normal upper respiratory tract commensal; can spread to infected or damaged lungs |
| **Gram-Negative Cocci** | | |
| *Neisseria gonorrhoeae* | Gonorrhea | Obligate human parasite |
| *Neisseria meningitidis* | Meningitis, nasopharyngitis | Obligate human parasite; increased upper respiratory carriage in epidemics |
| **Gram-Positive Bacilli** | | |
| *Corynebacterium diphtheriae* | Diphtheria | Natural host humans; noninvasive disease caused by toxin |
| *Bacillus anthracis* | Anthrax | Pathogen of herbivorous animals that ingest spores; occasional human infection |
| *Clostridium* spp. | Tetanus, gas gangrene, botulism | Widely distributed in soil and intestines |
| **Gram-Negative Bacilli** | | |
| *Escherichia coli* | Urinary tract infections, infantile gastroenteritis | Normal intestinal inhabitant (humans and animals); many antigenic types |
| *Salmonella* spp. | Enteric fever, food poisoning, gastroenteritis | *Salmonella typhi*—natural host is humans; invasive<br>Other *Salmonella*—1000 species, mainly animal pathogens |
| *Shigella* spp. | Bacillary dysentery (shigellosis) | Obligate parasites of humans; local invasion only |
| *Proteus* spp. | Urinary tract infection, gastroenteritis, wound infection | Common in soil, feces; occasionally pathogenic |
| *Klebsiella* spp. | Urinary tract and wound infection, otitis, meningitis, pneumonia | Present in vegetation, soil, sometimes feces; pathogenic when host resistance lowered |
| *Pseudomonas aeruginosa* | Urinary tract, respiratory and wound infection | Common human intestinal bacteria; resists many antibiotics |
| *Haemophilus influenzae* | Pneumonia, meningitis | Human commensal; invades damaged lung |
| *Bordetella pertussis* | Whooping cough | Specialized human respiratory parasite |
| *Yersinia pestis* | Plague | Flea-borne pathogen of rodents; transfer to humans as greatest infection in history |
| *Brucella* spp. | Undulant fever, brucellosis | Pathogens of goats, cattle, and pigs with secondary human infection |
| **Acid-Fast Bacilli** | | |
| *Mycobacterium tuberculosis* | Tuberculosis | Chronic respiratory infection in humans; 10 to 15 million active cases in the world; enteric infection with bovine type via milk |
| *Mycobacterium leprae* | Leprosy (Hansen's disease) | Obligate parasite of humans; attacks skin, nasal mucosa, and nerves; 15 million people with leprosy in the world |
| **Miscellaneous** | | |
| *Vibrio cholerae* | Cholera | Obligate parasite of humans; noninvasive intestinal infection |
| *Treponema pallidum* | Syphilis | Obligate human parasite; sexual transmission; related nonvenereal human bacteria |
| *Actinomyces israelii* | Actinomycosis | Normal inhabitant of the human mouth |
| *Leptospira* spp. | Leptospirosis (Weil's disease, etc.) | Mostly pathogens of animals; human infection from urine of rats, etc. |
| *Legionella pneumophila* | Legionnaires disease | Respiratory pathogen of humans, often acquired from contaminated air-conditioning units |

C. Transmission of disease
1. Reservoir of infection—contains potential sources of the disease-causing agent
   a. Human
      (1) Active cases of infectious disease
      (2) Carriers—persons (asymptomatic) harboring infectious agents potentially pathogenic for other members of the population
      (3) Endogenous infection—the causative organism is derived from the host's own microflora
   b. Animal—zoonosis; disease transmitted from animal to human
   c. Insects and arthropods—flies, mosquitoes, fleas, lice, ticks, and mites
   d. Nonliving—water, food, soil, and dust
2. Portals of exit are sources of infectious body fluids

a. Gastrointestinal (GI) tract
b. Genitourinary system
c. Oral region
d. Respiratory tract
e. Blood and blood derivatives
f. Skin lesions
g. Conjunctiva

3. Routes of transmission
   a. Contact
      (1) Direct
      (2) Indirect—involves nonliving reservoir (fomite)
      (3) Droplet transmission (short distance)
   b. Vehicles
      (1) Waterborne transmission
      (2) Foodborne transmission
      (3) Airborne transmission
   c. Vectors—insects and arthropods
4. Basic path of an infectious disease
   a. Exposure to the pathogen
   b. Incubation period
   c. Prodromal period
   d. Appearance of the signs and symptoms of the disease
   e. Outcome of the disease (e.g., convalescence, disability, or death)

## Microbial Virulence Factors

A. Capsules *(Streptococcus pneumoniae)*—resist the host's defenses by impairing phagocytosis
B. Enzyme production—includes coagulases, kinases, hyaluronidases, collagenases, mucinases, lecithinases, leukocidins, and hemolysins
C. Toxin production
   1. Exotoxins
      a. Soluble substances secreted by gram-positive bacteria
      b. Clinically significant exotoxins are associated with botulism, tetanus, diphtheria, gas gangrene, scarlet fever, staphylococcal food poisoning, toxic shock syndrome, and traveler's diarrhea
   2. Endotoxins
      a. Heat-stable lipopolysaccharides—toxic component associated with cell wall
      b. From gram-negative bacteria
      c. Pathologic effects
         (1) Fever
         (2) Interference with hemostatic mechanisms of blood
         (3) Activation of the complement system
         (4) Leukopenia
         (5) Hypotension and shock
         (6) Organ dysfunction
         (7) Activation of complement system
         (8) Death

## Disease Barriers

A. Normal or indigenous flora
   1. Most highly specialized bacteria; highly adapted to commensal life; cause minimal damage under normal conditions
   2. Includes beneficial microorganisms and pathogens
   3. When ecologic balance is disturbed, infection can occur (e.g., antibiotic therapy may result in *Candida albicans* infection)
B. Nonspecific immunity
   1. Physical and chemical barriers
      a. Intact skin
      b. Mucous membranes and their secretions
      c. Gastric acid barrier
   2. Blood and lymphatics
      a. Leukocytes—proportionate number changes in response to infection
         (1) Granulocytes (basophils, eosinophils, and neutrophils [polymorphonuclear leukocytes; PMNs])
         (2) Agranulocytes (lymphocytes and monocytes)
      b. Lymphatic system transports white blood cells and removes foreign cells and tissue debris
   3. Phagocytosis
      a. Digestion of the invading matter
      b. Accomplished by neutrophils and mature monocytes, or macrophages
   4. Inflammation
      a. Produced by disease agents or irritants such as chemicals, heat, or mechanical injury
      b. Cardinal signs include heat, pain, redness, swelling, and loss of function
      c. Pus formation possible
   5. Fever
      a. Inhibits the growth of some microorganisms
   6. Antimicrobial substances
C. Specific immunity—the immune system (Fig. 9.2 and Box 9.1)
   1. Humoral immunity—B lymphocyte production and release of specific antibodies into the circulating blood or body fluids; antibodies then interact with foreign antigens; defends primarily against bacteria, toxins, and viruses; antibodies protect the host as follows:
      a. Recognize an organism or its toxin by binding to it
      b. Opsonize or coat bacteria, which enhances ingestion by macrophages or natural killer (NK) cells
      c. Cause antigens to clump or agglutinate, which enhances phagocytosis
      d. Activate complement system, resulting in cell lysis
   2. Cell-mediated (cellular) immunity—stimulation of T lymphocytes to activate a variety of effector T cells in response to foreign organisms or tissues (antigens); defends primarily against bacteria, viruses, fungi, protozoa, helminths, foreign tissue, and cancerous cells
   3. Acquired immunity
      a. Natural
         (1) Active—person is exposed to an antigen and the body produces antibodies
         (2) Passive—antibodies of a mother are passed to her infant
      b. Artificial
         (1) Active—vaccination with killed, inactivated, or attenuated microorganisms or toxoid

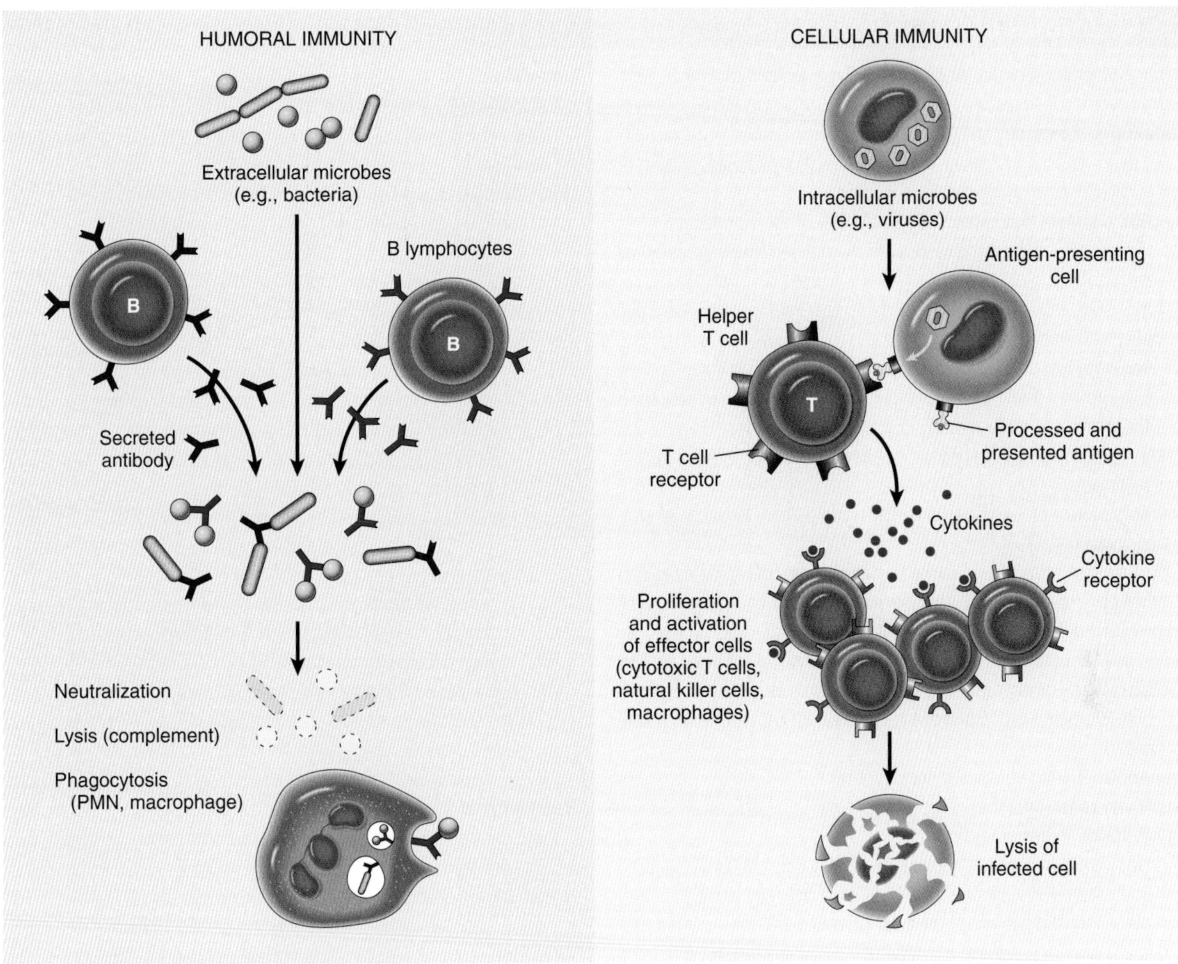


**Fig. 9.2** The duality of the immune system. *Left,* Humoral immunity mediated by soluble antibody proteins produced by B lymphocytes. *Right,* Cellular immunity mediated by T lymphocytes. (Modified from Kumar V, Cotran R, Robbins S. *Basic Pathology.* 7th ed, Philadelphia: Saunders; 2005.)

(2) Passive—injection of immune serum or γ-globulin

D. Hypersensitivity or allergy is an exaggerated response to specific substances; the inciting agent is the allergen (Fig. 9.3; see Box 9.1)

## Cells of Immune System

A. Leukocytes
   1. PMNs: phagocytic, first-responders, short-lived.
   2. Monocytes/Macrophages: slower to arrive at infection, present antigen to T cell
B. Lymphocytes
   1. B lymphocytes: make antibodies
   2. Antibodies (immunoglobulins): neutralize bacterial toxins, coat bacteria for phagocytosis, implement complement system.
   3. T lymphocytes: intensify the immune response, release cytokines

## Immunodeficiency

See the section on "Human Immunodeficiency Virus" in Chapter 8.

A. Inability of the immune system to perform normally; properly functioning system recognizes and destroys all that is foreign or "nonself"
B. Results in increased susceptibility to infection
C. Autoimmune disease (autoallergic)
   1. "Self" antigens stimulate the production of antibodies or sensitized lymphocytes; antigen–antibody complex
   2. Mechanisms
      a. May be caused by the release of sequestered antigens; escape of tolerance to the "self" antigen at the T-cell level; diminished suppressor T-cell function
      b. Intolerance of self-antigen because of cross-reactions
      c. Decreased function of suppressor T cells
   3. Includes systemic lupus erythematosus, rheumatoid arthritis, myasthenia gravis, and Graves' disease
D. Immunodeficiencies in B cells or T cells
   1. Hypergammaglobulinemias—overabundance of immunoglobulin
   2. Hypogammaglobulinemias—decreased catabolism, or loss of immunoglobulins
   3. Thymic aplasia (DiGeorge syndrome)—congenital absence of thymus gland
E. Drug-induced immunosuppression
   1. Used as an adjunct to organ transplantation and other organ grafts; also used for the treatment of immunologically mediated disease

## BOX 9.1 Immunology Terms

Modified from Stites DP, Stobo JD, Wells JV, eds. *Basic and Clinical Immunology.* 8th ed. East Norwalk, CT: Appleton & Lange; 1984.

**Anaphylatoxin:** a substance produced by complement activation (especially C3a, C5a) that results in increased vascular permeability through release of pharmacologically active mediators from mast cells

**Antibody (Ab):** a protein that is produced as a result of the introduction of an antigen and has the ability to combine with the antigen that stimulated its production

**Antigen (Ag):** a substance that can induce a detectable immune response when introduced into an animal

**B cell (B lymphocyte):** strictly, a bursa-derived cell in avian species and, by analogy, a cell derived from the equivalent of the bursa in nonavian species; B cells are the precursors of plasma cells that produce antibody

**Chemotaxis:** a process whereby phagocytic cells are attracted to the vicinity of invading pathogens

**Complement:** a system of serum proteins that is the primary mediator of antigen-antibody reactions

**Cytokine:** a factor such as a lymphokine or monokine produced by cells that affect other cells (e.g., lymphocytes and macrophages) and have multiple immunomodulating functions; cytokines include interleukins and interferons

**Cytolysis:** the lysis of bacteria or of cells such as tumor cells or red blood cells by the insertion of the membrane attack complex derived from complement activation

**Hapten:** a molecule that is not immunogenic by itself but can react with a specific antibody

**Histocompatible:** sharing transplantation antigens

**Hypersensitivity reactions:** these occur in four types:

**Antibody-mediated hypersensitivity**

*Type I. Anaphylactic* ("immediate"): immunoglobulin E (IgE) antibody is induced by allergen and binds via its Fc receptor to mast cells and basophils; after encountering the antigen again, the fixed IgE becomes cross-linked, inducing degranulation and release of mediators, especially histamine (e.g., in asthma, hay fever, hives, anaphylactic shock)

*Type II. Cytotoxic:* antigens on a cell surface combine with antibody, which leads to complement-mediated lysis (e.g., transfusion or Rh reactions) or other cytotoxic membrane damage (e.g., in autoimmune hemolytic anemia)

*Type III. Immune complex:* antigen-antibody immune complexes are deposited in tissues, complement is activated, and polymorphonuclear cells are attracted to the site, causing tissue damage (e.g., in serum sickness, Arthus reactions)

**Cell-mediated hypersensitivity**

*Type IV. Delayed:* T lymphocytes, sensitized by an antigen, release lymphokines on second contact with the same antigen; the lymphokines induce inflammation and activate macrophages (e.g., in contact dermatitis, poison ivy, graft rejection, tuberculin skin reaction)

**Immune response:** development of resistance (immunity) to a foreign substance (e.g., infectious agent); it can be antibody mediated (humoral), cell mediated (cellular), or both

**Immunoglobulin:** a glycoprotein composed of H and L chains that functions as an antibody; all antibodies are immunoglobulins, but not all immunoglobulins have an antibody function

**Immunoglobulin class:** a subdivision of immunoglobulin molecules based on unique antigenic determinants in the Fc region of the H chains; five immunoglobulin classes in humans

1. IgG: principal immunoglobulin of the secondary immune response; the only immunoglobulin capable of crossing placental barriers
2. IgM: first immunoglobulin to appear in a given immune response
3. IgA: principal immunoglobulin in external secretions of mucosal surfaces, tears, saliva, bile, urine, and colostrum
4. IgD: thought to activate the B cell
5. IgE: plays important role in immediate hypersensitivity reactions and parasitic infections

**Interferon:** one of a heterogeneous group of low-molecular-weight proteins elaborated by infected host cells that protect noninfected cells from viral infection; interferons, which are cytokines, also have immunomodulating functions

**Interleukin (IL):** a cytokine that stimulates or otherwise affects the function of lymphocytes and some other cells

IL-1: induces T helper cell synthesis of IL-2; activates T cells; induces chemotaxis for neutrophils
IL-2: stimulates antibody synthesis, T cytotoxic cells, and natural killer cells
IL-3: stimulates hematopoiesis
IL-4: induces isotype switching
IL-5: promotes the growth and differentiation of B cells
IL-6: stimulates B cell differentiation; activates T cells
IL-7: promotes pre–B-cell growth and pre–T-cell growth
IL-8: stimulates chemotaxis of neutrophils
IL-9: promotes T-cell growth; enhances mast cell
IL-10: inhibits T helper cell 1 (TH1) and cytokine release; stimulates mast cell growth
IL-11: stimulates development of B cells; stimulates hematopoiesis
IL-12: activates T cells; stimulates TH1 cell development
IL-13: antiinflammatory activity; B-cell growth and differentiation
IL-14: induces proliferation of activated B cells
IL-15: stimulates growth of intestinal epithelium, T cells, and natural killer cells
IL-16: lymphocyte chemoattractant factor

**Lymphocyte:** a mononuclear cell 7 to 12 μm in diameter containing a nucleus with densely packed chromatin and a small rim of cytoplasm; lymphocytes include T cells and B cells, which have primary roles in immunity

**Lymphokine:** a cytokine that is a soluble product of a lymphocyte; lymphokines are responsible for multiple effects in a cellular immune reaction

**Macrophage:** a phagocytic mononuclear cell derived from bone marrow monocytes and found in tissues and at the site of inflammation; macrophages serve accessory roles in cellular immunity

**Major histocompatibility complex (MHC):** a cluster of genes located close to each other; this determines the histocompatibility antigens of the members of a species

**Membrane attack complex (MAC):** the end product of activation of the complement cascade, which contains C5, C6, C7, and C8 (and C9); the MAC makes holes in the membranes of gram-negative bacteria, killing them and, in red blood cells or other cells, resulting in lysis

**Monocyte:** a circulating phagocytic blood cell that develops into tissue macrophages

**Opsonin:** a substance capable of enhancing phagocytosis; antibodies and complement are the two main opsonins

**Opsonization:** the coating of an antigen or particle (e.g., infectious agent) by substances such as antibodies, complement components, fibronectin, and so on, that facilitate uptake of the foreign particle into a phagocytic cell

**Polymorphonuclear cell (leukocyte, PMN):** also known as a neutrophil or granulocyte; a PMN is derived from a hematopoietic cell of bone marrow and is characterized by a multi-lobed nucleus; PMNs migrate from the circulation to a site of inflammation by chemotaxis and are phagocytic for bacteria and other particles

**T cell (T lymphocyte):** a thymus-derived cell that participates in a variety of cell-mediated immune reactions

TH1 (helper) or CD4 cell: activates macrophages and cytotoxic and other T cells
TH2 (helper) or CD4 cell: activates B cells to secrete immunoglobulin
TC (cytotoxic) or CD8 cell: destroys target cells
TD (delayed hypersensitivity) cell: causes inflammation associated with allergic reactions and tissue transplant rejectionTS (suppressor) or CD8 cell: regulates the immune response

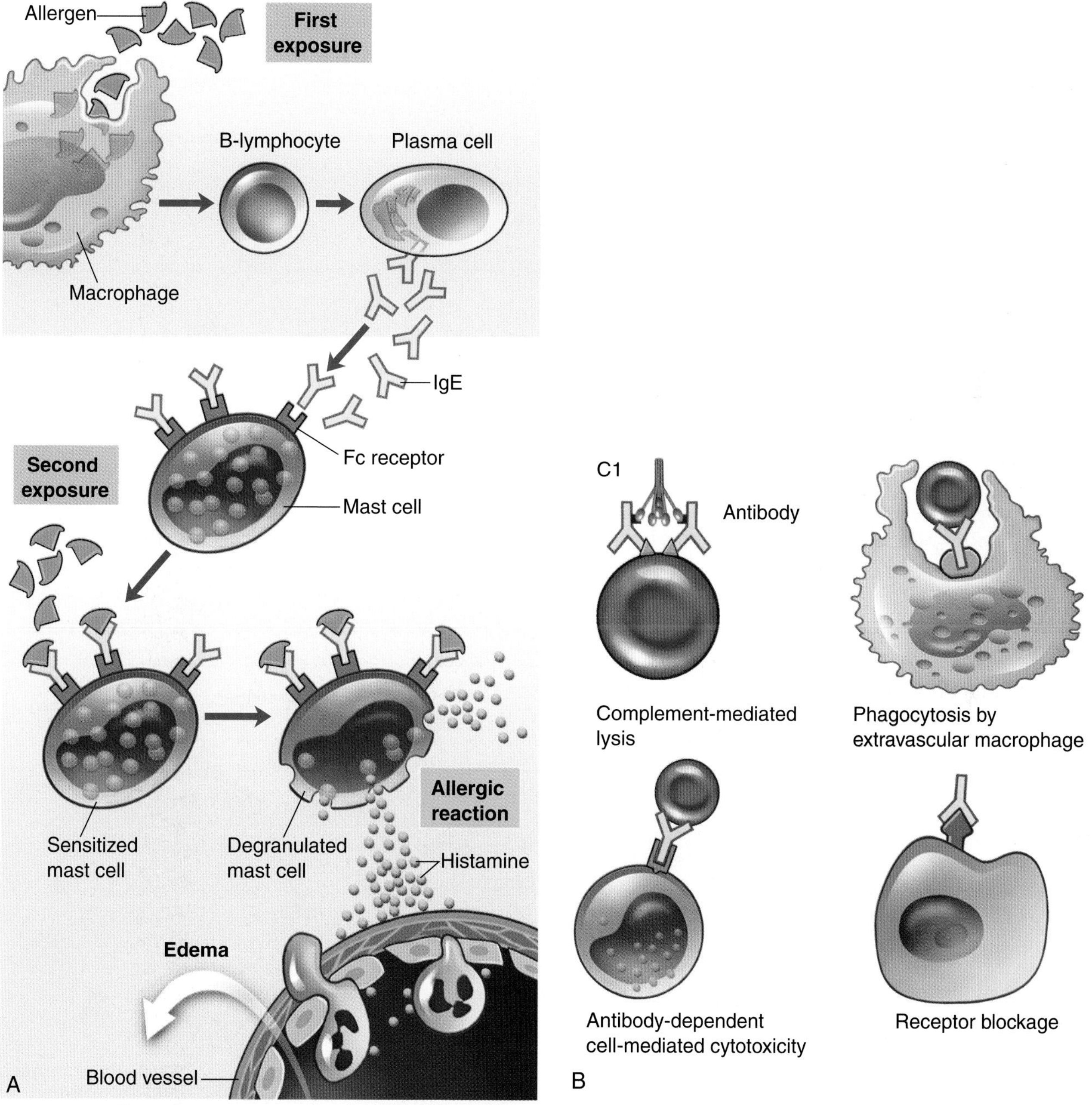


**Fig. 9.3 Hypersensitivity reactions are secondary responses to antigens that occur in an exaggerated or inappropriate form.** These reactions have been classified into four major types. (A) Type I reaction (antibody mediated). (B) Type II reaction (antibody mediated).

*Continued*

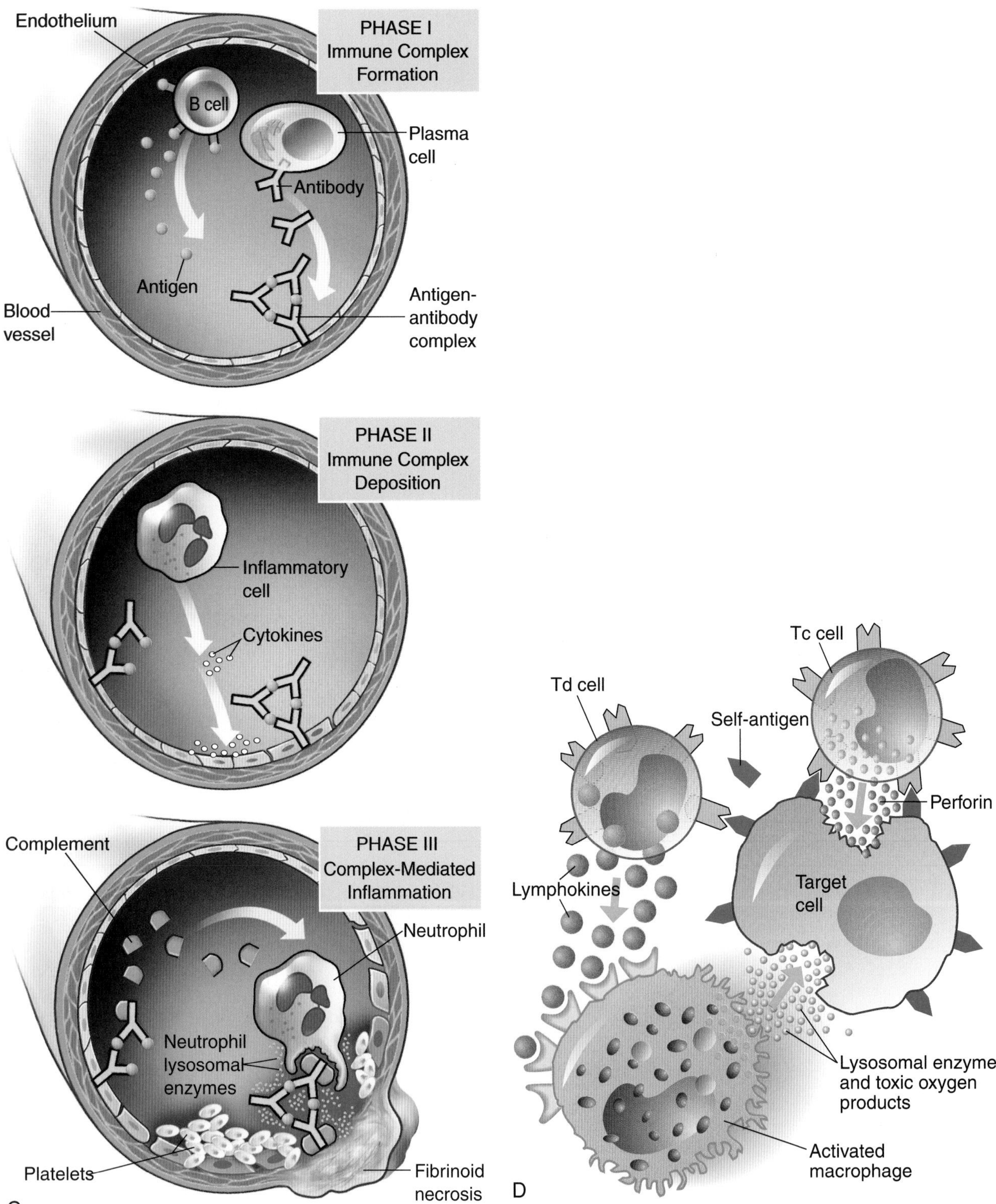


**Fig. 9.3, CONT'D** (C) Type III reaction (antibody mediated). (D) Type IV reaction (cell mediated). (Modified from Huether SE, McCance KL. *Understanding Pathophysiology.* 6th ed, St. Louis: Elsevier; 2017.)

F. Acquired immunodeficiency syndrome (AIDS)
1. Definition
   a. US Centers for Disease Control and Prevention (CDC) surveillance case definition includes all human immunodeficiency virus (HIV)–infected persons with a CD4 + T lymphocyte count of less than 200 cells/mm$^3$ of blood
   b. AIDS diagnosis can also be established by the development of one or more opportunistic infections regardless of CD4 + count[1]
2. Irreversible acquired defect
3. Etiology
   a. Lentivirus subfamily of human retroviruses
4. Virus isolated from blood, semen, vaginal secretions, rectal fluid, saliva, breast milk, cerebrospinal fluid, amniotic fluid, and urine
5. Transmission
   a. Susceptible exposure to infected blood (e.g., intravenous [IV] drug use, blood transfusion)
   b. Sexual contact
   c. Mother to newborn (perinatal)
7. CDC classification system for HIV-infected adolescents and adults categorizes persons based on CD4 + T lymphocyte counts and clinical conditions associated with HIV infection
   a. CD4 + T lymphocyte categories
      (1) Three CD4 + T lymphocyte categories:
         (a) Category 1—500 or more cells/µL
         (b) Category 2—200 to 499 cells/µL
         (c) Category 3—less than 200 cells/µL
   b. Clinical categories of HIV infection
      (1) Category A—consists of one or more of the conditions listed below in an adolescent or adult (at least 13 years old) with documented HIV infection; conditions listed in categories B and C must not have occurred
         (a) Asymptomatic HIV infection
         (b) Persistent generalized lymphadenopathy
         (c) Acute (primary) HIV infection with accompanying illness or history of acute HIV infection
      (2) Category B—consists of symptomatic conditions in an HIV-infected adolescent or adult that are not included among conditions listed in clinical category C and that meet at least one of two criteria: the conditions are attributed to HIV infection or are indicative of a defect in cell-mediated immunity, or the conditions are considered by physicians to have a clinical course or to require management that is complicated by HIV infection; examples of conditions in clinical category B include, but are not limited to:
         (a) Bacillary angiomatosis
         (b) Candidiasis, oropharyngeal (thrush)
         (c) Candidiasis, vulvovaginal; persistent, frequent, or poorly responsive to therapy
         (d) Cervical dysplasia (moderate or severe) or cervical carcinoma in situ

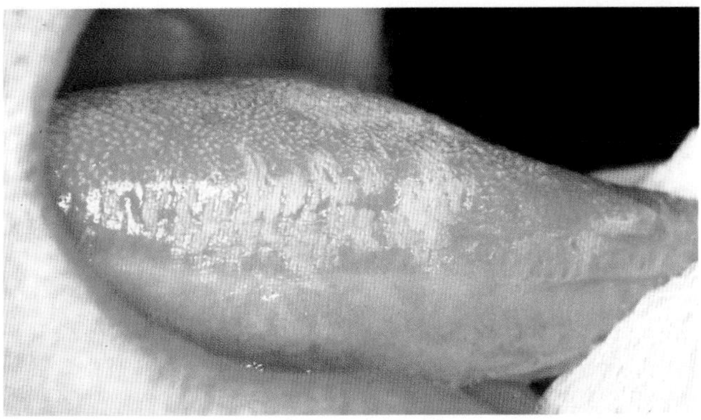

**Fig. 9.4** Hairy leukoplakia.

         (e) Constitutional symptoms such as fever (38.5°C) or diarrhea lasting longer than 1 month
         (f) Hairy leukoplakia, oral (Fig. 9.4)
         (g) Herpes zoster (shingles), involving at least two distinct episodes or more than one dermatome
         (h) Idiopathic thrombocytopenic purpura
         (i) Listeriosis
         (j) Pelvic inflammatory disease, particularly if complicated by tubo-ovarian abscess
         (k) Peripheral neuropathy
      (3) Category C—includes the clinical conditions listed in the AIDS surveillance case definition; for classification purposes, once a category C condition has occurred, the person will remain in category C
8. Secondary neoplasms
   a. Kaposi's sarcoma—skin lesions; may be oral; multiple small, reddish blue, purple, or hyperpigmented brown papules, plaques, or nodules; associated with human herpesvirus 8 (HHV-8) (Fig. 9.5)
   b. B-cell lymphomas
9. Opportunistic infections
   a. Cytomegalovirus—frequently involves the eye, causing retinal lesions
   b. Tuberculosis
   c. Oral and esophageal infection from *Candida albicans*
   d. Herpes simplex viruses (HSV) 1 and 2
10. Incidence and prevalence
   a. Approximately 1.1 million people have been diagnosed with HIV infection in the United States
   b. Risk factors
      (1) Unsafe sexual practices
      (2) Exposure to blood or blood products
      (3) IV drug use
      (4) Infant of infected individual
   d. Transmission to health care personnel providing care to infected individuals is rare
11. Treatment (see the section on "Antiviral Agents" in Chapter 11)
   a. No known cure or vaccine yet available
   b. Food and Drug Administration (FDA)–approved antiretroviral drugs used for the treatment of HIV:
      (1) Multiclass combination products (e.g., Atripla)

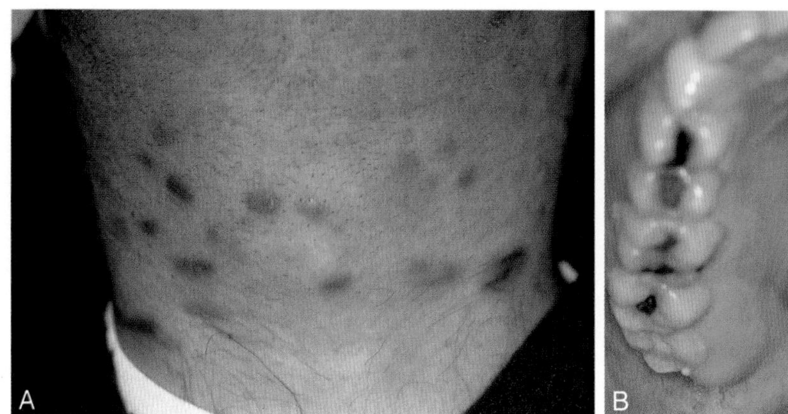


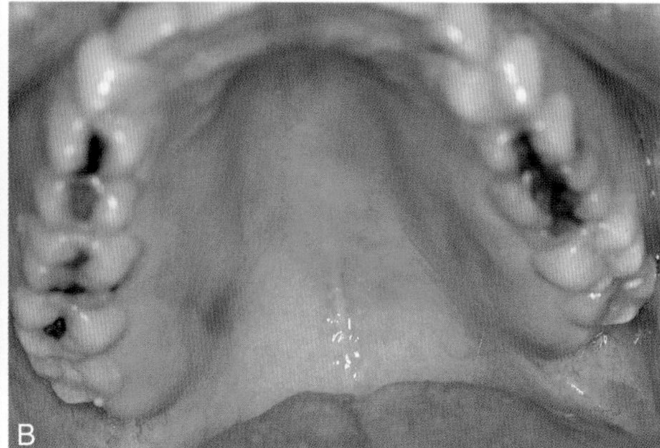


**Fig. 9.5** (A) Kaposi's sarcoma of the neck ; (B) presenting as a dark macule in the right posterior palate. (From Regezi JA, Sciubba JA, Jordan CK. *Oral Pathology: Clinical Pathologic Correlations*. 7th ed. St. Louis: Elsevier; 2017.)

(2) Nucleoside reverse transcriptase inhibitors (NRTIs) (e.g., zidovudine [AZT], didanosine [ddI], stavudine [d4T], lamivudine [3TC])
(3) Nonnucleoside reverse transcriptase inhibitors (NNRTIs) (e.g., nevirapine [NVP], efavirenz [EFV])
(4) Protease inhibitors (PIs) (e.g., amprenavir [AP], indinavir [IDV], darunavir, atazanavir sulfate [ATV])
(5) Fusion inhibitors (e.g., enfuvirtide [T-20])
(6) Entry inhibitors (e.g., maraviroc [Selzentry, Celsentri])
(7) HIV integrase strand transfer inhibitor (e.g., raltegravir)

c. Prophylactic Treatment Options
   a. Pre-exposure prophylaxis (PrEP)
      i. Taken daily to prevent HIV infection in high risk individuals
      ii. Truvada® and Descovy®
   b. Post exposure prophylaxis (PEP)
      i. Antiretroviral medications taken after potential exposure to HIV to prevent from becoming infected
      ii. Must be started within 72 hours after possible exposure to HIV

12. Oral manifestations
   a. Hairy leukoplakia
   b. Herpetic lesions
   c. Oral and esophageal candidiasis
   d. Kaposi's sarcoma
   e. Linear gingival erythema and necrotizing ulcerative periodontitis
   f. Human papillomavirus
   g. Lymphoma
   h. Recurrent aphthous ulcers

## Infections of the Skin, Nails, and Hair

A. Bacterial infections
   1. Tetanus
      a. Etiology—*Clostridium tetani*
      b. Pathogenesis and transmission—by spores that germinated in the wound and produce tetanus-causing toxin
      c. Clinical findings and symptoms
         (1) Trismus (stiff jaw); eventually, locked jaw
         (2) Spasms of facial muscles
         (3) Dysphagia
         (4) Difficulty breathing
   2. Leprosy
      a. Etiology—*Mycobacterium leprae*
      b. Pathogenesis and transmission—transmitted via prolonged direct contact or inhalation of organisms
      c. Clinical findings and symptoms
         (1) Skin lesions
         (2) Oral lesions are tumor-like masses of tissue that involve the oral lining, tongue, lips, or palate
   4. Staphylococcal infections
      a. Etiology—*Staphylococcus aureus* and *Staphylococcus epidermidis*
      b. Pathogenesis—determined by extracellular factors and invasive properties of the strain
      c. Clinical findings and symptoms
         (1) Most *S. aureus* strains are resistant to penicillin
         (2) Causes furuncles (boils), carbuncles, impetigo, and cellulitis
   5. Streptococcal infections
      a. Etiology—*Streptococcus pyogenes* (group A β-hemolytic)
      b. Pathogenesis
         (1) Determined by portal of entry
         (2) Diffuse and rapidly spreading infection
      c. Clinical findings and symptoms
         (1) Scarlet fever
            (a) Acute inflammation of the upper respiratory tract
            (b) Generalized rash caused by erythrogenic exotoxin
            (c) Oral mucosa is red; "strawberry tongue"
            (d) Sequelae from group A streptococcal infection include rheumatic fever and hemorrhagic glomerulonephritis

B. Fungal infections
   2. Candidiasis
      a. Etiology—*Candida albicans*

b. Pathogenesis
   (1) Dissemination and sepsis in compromised patients (opportunistic infection)
   (2) Normal inhabitant of the skin and mucosal surfaces
   (3) Predisposing factors include diabetes mellitus, pregnancy, obesity, vitamin deficiency, use of broad-spectrum antibiotics, and immunologic defects
c. Clinical findings and symptoms—vary with site

C. Viral infections
1. Herpes simplex
   a. Etiology—HSV
   b. Pathogenesis
      (1) Transmission through oral and ocular secretions
      (2) Virus is present in saliva, even in apparent good health
      (3) Indirect contact (e.g., fomites)
      (4) Infects epithelial cells
      (5) Establishes a latent infection from retroviruses
   c. Clinical findings and symptoms
      (1) Types
         (a) HSV-1—generally above the waist; usually found in and around the mouth
         (b) HSV-2—herpes genitalis
      (2) Frequently asymptomatic
      (3) Most often, acute gingivostomatitis; usually in children—fever, malaise, irritability, local lymphadenopathy, and anorexia; red, edematous gingiva and adjacent mucosa; lesions are vesicles with yellowish contents that rupture and ulcerate; bright margin of erythema; sharply defined; pain may be severe; duration of about 7 days; self-limiting
      (4) Herpetic whitlow infection of fingers; can be caused by HSV-1 or HSV-2; abrupt onset; local irritation; tenderness, edema, erythema, and vesicles; difficult to differentiate from bacterial pyoderma caused by staphylococci
      (5) Recurrent secondary infections by HSV-1
         (a) Virus now latent but permanently established in nerve ganglia (carrier)
         (b) Infections may be induced by stress, sun, or colds
      (6) Herpes labialis (Fig. 9.6) is the most common clinical manifestation of recurrent infection
         (a) Cold sores, fever blisters
         (b) Vesicles on an erythematous base
         (c) Prodromal burning and hyperesthesia
         (d) Swollen lymph nodes
      (7) Intraoral lesions
         (a) Usually found on the mucosa or hard palate overlying bone
         (b) Small, discrete lesions; vesicles of clear fluid; ulcerate with a red base
2. Chickenpox
   a. Etiology—varicella-zoster virus (VZV)
   b. Pathogenesis
      (1) Route of infection through the mucosa of the upper respiratory tract
      (2) Highly infectious
      (3) Virus probably circulates in the blood and localizes on the skin
      (4) Incubation period 2 weeks
      (5) Vaccine available
   c. Clinical findings and symptoms
      (1) Earliest symptoms are malaise and fever, followed by a rash and formation of vesicles
      (2) Oral lesions may occur throughout the mouth and appear as small canker sores or aphthae; vesicles rupture quickly
3. Shingles
   a. Etiology—VZV
   b. Pathogenesis
      (1) Reactivation of latent virus in dorsal root ganglion
      (2) Closely follows area of innervation
      (3) Chickenpox and shingles represent different forms of infection by the same agent
      (4) Virus resides in ganglia; usually affects sensory nerves (thoracic area most often involved; ophthalmic division of trigeminal nerve next most involved)
      (5) Vaccine available
   c. Clinical findings and symptoms
      (1) Mostly found in adults
      (2) Malaise, fever, followed by severe pain in area
      (3) Rash and vesicles along the nerve trunk
4. Warts
   a. Etiology—papillomaviruses
   b. Pathogenesis—affects epithelial cells of skin and mucous membranes
   c. Clinical findings and symptoms
      (1) Skin warts, plantar warts, flat warts, genital condylomas, laryngeal papillomas
      (2) Oral warts are papular or nodular lesions covered with papilliferous projections; also may look like common warts
5. Measles
   a. Etiology—rubeola virus
   b. Pathogenesis
      (1) Transmission through the respiratory tract
      (2) Spreads to regional lymphoid tissue
      (3) Primary viremia disseminates the virus
      (4) Secondary viremia seeds the epithelial surfaces of the body
   c. Clinical findings and symptoms
      (1) Koplik's spots
         (a) Small, bluish white spots with a red surrounding zone; cannot be wiped off
         (b) Occur on the buccal mucosa opposite the molars
      (2) Followed by a diffuse skin rash and fever
      (3) Bacterial secondary infections occur, such as middle ear infections or pneumonia

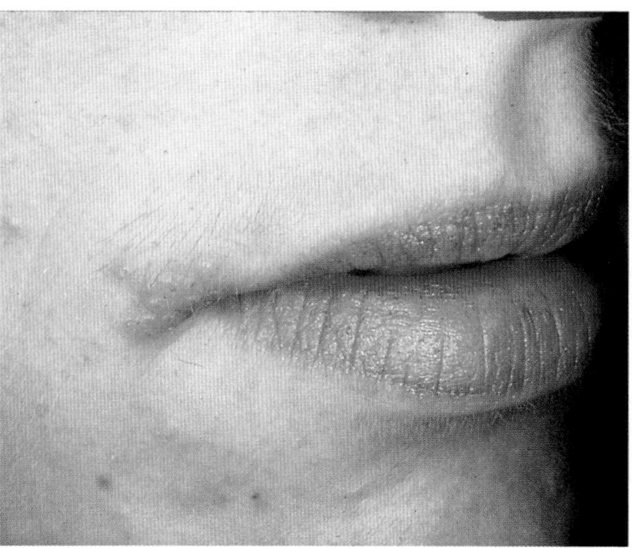

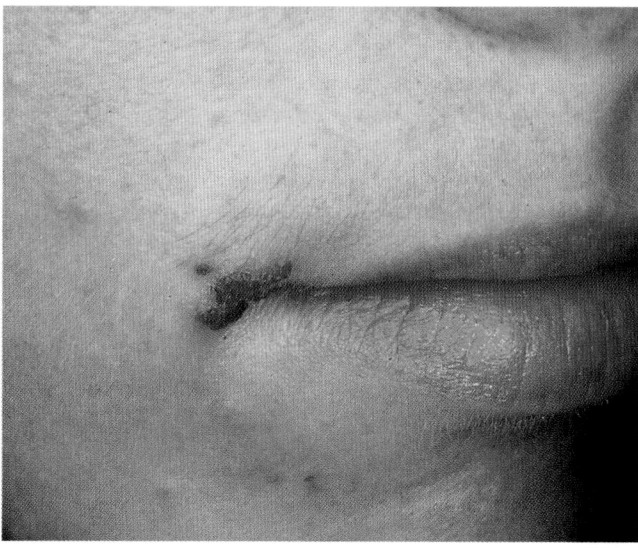

**Fig. 9.6** Herpes labialis.

## Infections of the Respiratory Tract

### Upper Respiratory System Infections

A. Bacterial infections
  1. Diphtheria
    a. Etiology—*Corynebacterium diphtheriae*
    b. Pathogenesis
      (1) Droplets or by contact with susceptible individuals
      (2) Bacilli grow on mucous membranes or in skin abrasions
      (3) Damage caused by the systemic distribution of toxin
    c. Clinical findings and symptoms
      (1) Enlarged lymphadenopathy of the neck; possibly edema
      (2) Pseudomembrane forms on tonsils
  2. Streptococcal pharyngitis ("strep throat")
    a. Etiology—*Streptococcus pyogenes* (group A)
    b. Pathogenesis—transmitted by the respiratory route and contaminated food, water, and milk
    c. Clinical findings and symptoms: severe inflammation of the throat and tonsils; fever
B. Viral infections—common cold

### Lower Respiratory System Infections

A. Bacterial infections
  1. Pneumococcal pneumonia
    a. Etiology—most common agent is *Streptococcus pneumoniae*
    b. Pathogenesis
      (1) Spread by droplets from nasal or pharyngeal secretion
      (2) Person may contract the disease or become an asymptomatic carrier
      (3) Predisposing factors include age, impaired resistance, and bacteremia
    c. Clinical findings and symptoms: symptoms include sudden onset of high fever, chills, chest pain, dry cough, and rust-colored sputum
  2. Bacterial pneumonia
    a. Etiology—several species—*Streptococcus pyogenes, Staphylococcus aureus, Klebsiella pneumoniae, Haemophilus influenzae*
    b. Pathogenesis is similar to that caused by *S. pneumoniae*
    c. Inflammation of the lungs
  3. Legionnaires disease
    a. Etiology—*Legionella pneumophila*
    b. Pathogenesis
      (1) Inhalation of bacteria from aerosols
      (2) Bacteria multiply in lungs and produce pneumonia
    c. Clinical findings and symptoms
      (1) Influenza-like illness with pneumonia
      (2) Complications include renal failure, GI hemorrhage, and respiratory failure
  4. Tuberculosis
    a. Etiology—*Mycobacterium tuberculosis*
    b. Pathogenesis
      (1) Transmitted by inhalation of droplets, ingestion, or direct inoculation; disseminated by coughing, sneezing, or contaminated dust
      (2) Predisposing factors include advanced age, chronic alcoholism, poor nutrition, diabetes mellitus, and prolonged stress
      (3) Incubation period is generally 28 to 47 days; can be as long as 6 months
    c. Clinical findings and symptoms
      (1) Symptoms vary but include fever, general discomfort, weight loss, tubercle formation (nodule in lung tissue), night sweats, and persistent cough
      (2) Oral lesions may appear as an ulcerated lesion on the tongue or mucosa (rare)
      (3) Diagnosis by a skin test and a radiograph
  5. Whooping cough (pertussis)
    a. Etiology—*Bordetella pertussis*
    b. Pathogenesis—transmitted by inhalation of droplets; produce toxins

c. Clinical findings and symptoms—spasmodic coughing and gasping noise with inhalation
6. Mycoplasmal pneumonia
   a. Etiology—*Mycoplasma pneumoniae*
   b. Pathogenesis—transmitted in airborne droplets; binds respiratory epithelium and inhibits ciliary action
   c. Clinical findings and symptoms—mild symptoms of low fever, cough, and headache that persist for 3 weeks or longer

B. Fungal infections
1. Histoplasmosis
   a. Etiology—*Histoplasma capsulatum*
   b. Pathogenesis—transmitted by inhalation of spores, especially in excreta of wild birds, poultry, and bats
   c. Clinical findings and symptoms
      (1) Skin lesions are common
      (2) Meningitis

C. Viral infections
1. Influenza virus infection
   a. Etiology—orthomyxoviruses
   b. Pathogenesis
      (1) The genome can undergo sudden genetic reassortment
      (2) Spread by airborne droplets or contact with contaminated objects
      (3) Virus attaches to the respiratory epithelium
   c. Clinical findings and symptoms
      (1) Chills, headache, dry cough, fever, malaise, muscular ache, and inflammation of the soft palate
      (2) Secondary infection by *S. aureus, H. influenzae, S. pyogenes,* and *S. pneumoniae*; may result in bronchitis and pneumonia
      (3) Reye syndrome may be a complication
2. Coronavirus Disease (COVID-19)
   a. Etiology – Severe Acute Respiratory Syndrome Coronavirus 2
   b. Pathogenesis – transmission occurs through contact, droplet, airborne, fomite transmission.
   c. Clinical findings and symptoms – cough, fever, chills, shortness of breath, difficulty breathing, fatigue, muscle or body aches, headache, new loss of taste or smell, sore throat, congestion, nausea, diarrhea

## Infections of the Gastrointestinal Tract

A. Bacterial infections
1. Cholera
   a. Etiology—*Vibrio cholerae*
   b. Pathogenesis
      (1) Transmitted as a result of unsanitary living conditions and through ingestion of the organisms
      (2) Organisms attach to microvilli of epithelial cells; produce toxin
   c. Clinical findings and symptoms—dehydration, nausea, vomiting, profuse diarrhea, and abdominal and leg cramps
2. Salmonellosis
   a. Etiology—several species of *Salmonella*
   b. Pathogenesis—organisms enter by the oral route usually through contaminated food or drink
   c. Clinical findings and symptoms—organisms cause enteric fevers, bacteremia, followed by focal lesions or endocarditis
4. Enteric infections caused by *Escherichia coli*
   a. Etiology
      (1) Enterotoxigenic *E. coli* (ETEC)—traveler's diarrhea
      (2) Enteroinvasive *E. coli* (EIEC)
      (3) Enteropathogenic *E. coli* (EPEC)
      (4) Enterohemorrhagic *E. coli* (EHEC)—serotype O157: H7
      (5) Enteroaggregative *E. coli* (EaggEC)
   b. Pathogenesis
      (1) Acquired by ingestion of contaminated food or water or through contact with contaminated persons
      (2) Factors responsible for the different ways in which *E. coli* produces disease vary with strain
   c. Clinical findings and symptoms—abdominal pain, malaise, loss of appetite, diarrhea, and dehydration; diarrhea may be watery or bloody, depending on the strain of *E. coli*
5. Typhoid fever
   a. Etiology—*Salmonella typhi*
   b. Pathogenesis—transmitted through contaminated food or water
   c. Clinical findings and symptoms
      (1) Fever, severe headache, abdominal pain, and abdominal rash
      (2) Complications include carrier state, relapses, inflammation of the gallbladder, and intestinal bleeding
7. Food poisoning
   a. Botulism
      (1) Etiology—*Clostridium botulinum*
      (2) Pathogenesis
         (a) Regularly contaminates human, plant, and animal food products
         (b) Produces a deadly toxin that acts on nerves
         (c) Transmitted through improperly preserved foods and uncooked fish and meats; foods do not appear contaminated
      (3) Clinical findings and symptoms
         (a) Difficulty speaking, blurred vision, inability to swallow, heart failure, and respiratory paralysis
         (b) Infant botulism may be one of the causes of sudden infant death syndrome
   b. Staphylococcal food poisoning
      (1) Etiology—toxin produced by staphylococci (usually *S. aureus*) in unrefrigerated foods such as dairy products, custard, cream-filled products, fish, or processed meats
      (2) Pathogenesis
         (a) Caused by ingestion of preformed enterotoxin

**TABLE 9.5 Characteristics of the Various Types of Viral Hepatitis**

| Characteristic | Hepatitis A | Hepatitis B | Hepatitis C | Hepatitis D | Hepatitis E | Hepatitis G[a] |
|---|---|---|---|---|---|---|
| Transmission | Fecal-oral (ingestion of contaminated food, ice, and water) | Parenteral (injection of contaminated blood or other body fluids) | Parenteral | Percutaneous, permucosal, or parenteral (host must be co-infected with hepatitis B or as a superinfection in persons with chronic HBV infection) | Fecal-oral (contaminated drinking water most common) | Bloodborne and co-infection with HCV |
| Agent | Hepatitis A virus (HAV); single-stranded (ss) ribonucleic acid (RNA); no envelope | Hepatitis B virus (HBV); double-stranded deoxyribonucleic acid (DNA); envelope | Hepatitis C virus (HCV); ss RNA; envelope | Hepatitis D virus (HDV); defective ss RNA, envelope from HBV | Hepatitis E virus (HEV); ss RNA; no envelope | Hepatitis G virus, although causal association remains to be confirmed |
| Incubation period | 15 to 50 days | 45 to 160 days | 2 to 26 weeks | Uncertain | 15 to 60 days | Acute disease spectrum unknown |
| Manifestations or symptoms | Children under age 6 years may not have signs of illness; severe cases: fever, headache, malaise, jaundice, fatigue, loss of appetite, nausea, dark urine | Clinical manifestations are age dependent; anorexia, nausea, malaise, vomiting, jaundice, dark urine, clay-colored stools, abdominal pain, and more likely to progress to severe liver damage | Similar to HBV | Severe liver damage; high mortality rate | Similar to HAV, but pregnant women may have high mortality rate; less common symptoms include arthralgia, diarrhea, pruritus, and urticaria | |
| Chronic liver disease | No | Yes | Yes | Yes | No | No |
| Vaccines | A sterile suspension of inactivated virus | Genetically engineered | None | HBV vaccine is protective because coinfection is required | None | None |

[a]Information on hepatitis G, from the Centers for Disease Control and Prevention: *Guidelines for Viral Hepatitis Surveillance and Case Management.* Atlanta, 2005. Available at https://www.cdc.gov/hepatitis/statistics/surveillanceguidelines.htm.
From Tortora GJ, Funke BR. Case DL. *Microbiology: an Introduction.* 8th ed. Menlo Park, CA: Benjamin/Cummings; 2003.

(b) Incubation period is from 1 to 8 hours
(c) Symptoms include nausea, violent vomiting, diarrhea; no fever
(d) Rapid convalescence; self-limiting

B. Viral infections
1. Hepatitis A (Table 9.5)
a. Etiology—hepatitis A virus (HAV)
b. Pathogenesis
(1) Oral-fecal route in unsanitary conditions; contaminated food and water; close, intimate contact with infected person
(2) Rarely through the blood
(3) The incubation period is 15 to 50 days
(4) Usually occurs in children and young adults
c. Clinical findings and symptoms
(1) Preicteric (before jaundice appears)—similar to influenza; fever, headache, nausea, vomiting, fatigue, abdominal pain, loss of appetite, dark urine
(2) Icteric—jaundice (rare in children); other symptoms continue
(3) Anicteric—without jaundice; two or three times more prevalent than the icteric state; symptoms resemble those of influenza
d. Active immunization
(1) Hepatitis A vaccine (Havrix) at least 2 weeks before expected exposure; booster dose recommended 6 to 12 months later for adults
(2) The vaccine may be administered concomitantly with immunoglobulin in persons exposed to HAV

2. Hepatitis B (see Table 9.5)
a. Etiology—hepatitis B virus (HBV)
b. Pathogenesis
(1) Infected blood or serum through parenteral inoculation (e.g., blood transfusions, contaminated dental or medical instruments, needles and syringes used by IV drug abusers, accidental self-inoculation by health care professionals)
(2) Other body fluids, including saliva, semen, tears, urine, sweat, and nasopharyngeal secretions
(3) Oral or sexual contact or other close, personal contact
(4) Coughing, sneezing, and aerosols
(5) Salivary transmission by way of hands, instruments, and other equipment is an important consideration in the practice of dental hygiene
d. Symptoms
(1) Similar to hepatitis A
(2) Slower onset; longer duration
(3) Asymptomatic to severe and debilitating
(4) Patient may have subclinical disease and remain undiagnosed
(5) May result in chronic liver disease; strong evidence for link between chronic HBV infection and hepatocellular carcinoma (liver cancer)

f. Risk factors
 (1) Exposure to virus at birth (e.g., infants born to mothers infected with HBV)
 (2) Exchange of blood or blood products (e.g., during hemodialysis, blood transfusions, or IV drug use)
 (3) Exposure to blood or blood products (e.g., in the case of health care workers)
 (4) Close, intimate contact with infected person
 (5) Unsafe sexual practices
 (6) Institutionalization (e.g., in the case of some individuals with Down syndrome and prisoners)
 (7) Immunosuppressive therapy
g. Immunization
 (1) Two types of hepatitis B surface antigen (HBsAg) vaccines
  (a) Obtained from HBsAg-positive carriers (Heptavax)
  (b) Obtained from recombinant DNA in yeast cells (Recombivax)
 (2) Passive immunization results from hepatitis B immune globulin (HBIg); used for postexposure prophylaxis; preferably within 24 to 48 hours; partially effective
 (3) Given as a series of three or four shots

3. Hepatitis type C (see Table 9.5)
 a. Etiology—hepatitis C virus
 b. Pathogenesis
  (1) Originally named "non-A, non-B" hepatitis virus
  (2) Risk factors include blood transfusion, IV drug use, and heterosexual transmission
 c. Clinical findings and symptoms
  (1) Mild symptoms; most asymptomatic
  (2) Development of chronic hepatitis in 50%; may develop into cirrhosis and hepatocellular carcinoma
4. Hepatitis D (formerly delta hepatitis) (see Table 9.5)
 a. Etiology—hepatitis D virus
 b. Pathogenesis
  (1) Similar to HBV
  (2) Infection dependent on HBV replication
 c. Clinical findings—may produce acute exacerbations of chronic HBV and fulminant hepatitis
5. Hepatitis type E (see Table 9.5)
 a. Etiology—hepatitis E virus
 b. Pathogenesis
  (1) Originally named "non-A, non-B" hepatitis virus
  (2) Enteric transmission
  (3) Epidemic outbreaks occurring in developing countries
6. Hepatitis G (see Table 9.5)
 a. Etiology—hepatitis G virus
 b. Pathogenesis
  (1) Bloodborne transmission and coinfection with HCV
  (2) Acute disease spectrum unknown
7. Norwalk virus and Norwalk-like virus
 a. Pathogenesis—disease spread via the fecal-oral route
 b. Clinical findings and symptoms—nausea, vomiting, abdominal cramps, lethargy, and diarrhea in older children and adults

## Infections of the Circulatory System

### Diseases of the Heart

A. Rheumatic fever
 1. Etiology—β-hemolytic group A streptococcal infection
 2. Pathogenesis
  a. Rheumatic fever—hypersensitivity state developing after streptococcal infection; associated with β-hemolytic group A streptococci
  b. Heart valves become inflamed; subsequent abnormal growths of connective tissue; scarring of valves occurs, resulting in rheumatic heart disease
 3. Clinical findings and symptoms
  a. Fever, malaise, polyarthritis, inflammation of the heart
  b. Defective heart valves are a result of carditis
  c. Heart valve damage
   (1) Stenosis—narrowing of the valve opening
   (2) Valvular insufficiency—failure of the valve to close completely
 4. Prophylactic antibiotic premedication is necessary before dental and dental hygiene treatments
B. Infective endocarditis
 1. Etiology—most often associated with the normal flora of the respiratory or intestinal tract
 2. Pathogenesis
  a. Inflammatory condition of the heart; microbial colonization of the endothelial membrane that covers the inner surface of the heart and the heart valves
  b. Predisposing factors
   (1) Artificial heart valves
   (2) Congenital heart defects
   (3) History of endocarditis
   (4) Damaged heart valves
   (5) History of IV drug use
  c. Dental and dental hygiene procedures may allow bacteria to enter the bloodstream (bacteremia) and lodge in the heart valves
 3. Clinical findings and symptoms
  a. Fever, anemia, weakness, and heart murmur
  b. Inflammation of the heart
  c. May result in death

### Other Microbial Diseases of the Circulatory System

A. Bacterial infections
 1. Rickettsial infections
  a. Etiology—obligate intracellular parasites
  b. Pathogenesis
   (1) Transmitted by arthropods such as fleas, lice, mites, and ticks
   (2) Rocky Mountain spotted fever (tick vector)
   (3) Typhus (flea-borne, common in rats)
   (4) Rickettsialpox (mouse-mite vector)—usually involves fever, rash, and vasculitis

B. Viral infections
   1. Infectious mononucleosis
      a. Etiology—Epstein-Barr virus (EBV)
      b. Pathogenesis
         (1) Transmitted by kissing or sharing drinking glasses with an infected person
         (2) Involves lymph nodes and the spleen; increase in lymphocytes
      c. Clinical findings and symptoms
         (1) Acute leukemia-like infection
         (2) Primarily found in young adults
         (3) Symptoms include mild jaundice, fever, enlarged and tender lymph nodes, sore throat, bleeding gingiva, and general weakness

## Infections of the Reproductive and Urinary Systems

### Reproductive System Infections

A. Bacterial infections
   1. Gonorrhea
      a. Etiology—*Neisseria gonorrhoeae,* a gram-negative aerobic bacterium; often coinfection with *Chlamydia trachomatis*
      b. Pathogenesis
         (1) Grows primarily in the genitourinary tract; possesses pili that allow attachment to mucosal cells and resist phagocytosis; can infect the eye, rectum, and throat
      c. Clinical findings and symptoms
         (1) Sometimes found in the pharynx; localized yellow or gray-white raised patches or generalized lesions with a gray membrane; the membrane sloughs, leaving a bright area; seen on the gingiva, tongue, and soft palate; may have itching or burning
         (2) Gonococcal glossitis (Fig. 9.7)
         (3) The newborn's eyes may be infected while the baby is passing through the birth canal (ophthalmia neonatorum); use of silver nitrate or antibiotic after birth alleviates the condition
         (4) Men experience painful and frequent urination and discharge containing mucus and pus

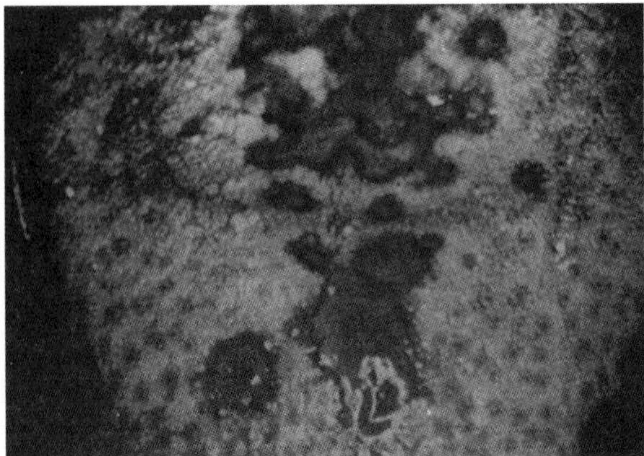

**Fig. 9.7** Gonococcal glossitis. (Courtesy of Beverly Entwistle Isman, formerly with the Department of Applied Dentistry, University of Colorado School of Dentistry, Denver.)

         (5) Women often do not have symptoms; may have urethral or vaginal discharge, backache, or abdominal pain (pelvic inflammatory disease)
         (6) Oral infection results in pharyngitis, glossitis, or stomatitis, including some areas of ulceration
         (7) Complications include sterility, disseminated infection, and meningitis
   2. Syphilis (Fig. 9.8)
      a. Etiology—*Treponema pallidum*; spirochete, anaerobic
      b. Pathogenesis
         (1) Usually transmitted by sexual contact with skin or mucous membrane lesions of an infected person
         (2) Infection limited to the human host
         (3) Congenital syphilis occurs when the organism crosses the placenta
         (4) *T. pallidum* can pass through abraded skin and can probably pass through intact mucous membranes
         (5) If the organisms gain access to the circulatory system, they can affect all organs and spread rapidly to the lymphatic system and bloodstream
      c. Clinical findings and symptoms (Fig. 9.9)
         (1) Primary stage—chancre, a single granulomatous lesion; often asymptomatic; common on the lips; may involve the tongue and oral mucosa; highly contagious; occurs 2 to 3 weeks after exposure and lasts 3 to 5 weeks; red, small, elevated nodule; heals spontaneously; no scarring
         (2) Secondary stage
            (a) Appears 6 to 8 weeks after exposure; patient can be asymptomatic for 2 to 6 months, and then secondary lesions appear
            (b) Flu-like symptoms
            (c) Skin rashes—maculopapular rash on the face, hands, and feet
            (d) Mucous patches on the lips, soft palate, and tongue—painless shallow ulcers; grayish white areas may be removed, leaving red areas of erosion; highly contagious
            (e) Swollen lymph nodes
         (3) Tertiary stage
            (a) Gumma—inflammatory granulomatous lesion with a central zone of necrosis; may be on the tongue, palate (perforation), or facial bones; soft, swollen areas or tumors; not contagious and usually asymptomatic
            (b) Often takes 5 to 20 years to develop
            (c) Involvement of the central nervous system (CNS) and spinal cord leads to paresis, loss of fine muscle coordination, and personality changes
            (d) Involvement of the cardiovascular system—major cause of death
         (4) Congenital syphilis
            (a) Hutchinson's incisors—notched, bell shaped (Fig. 9.10)

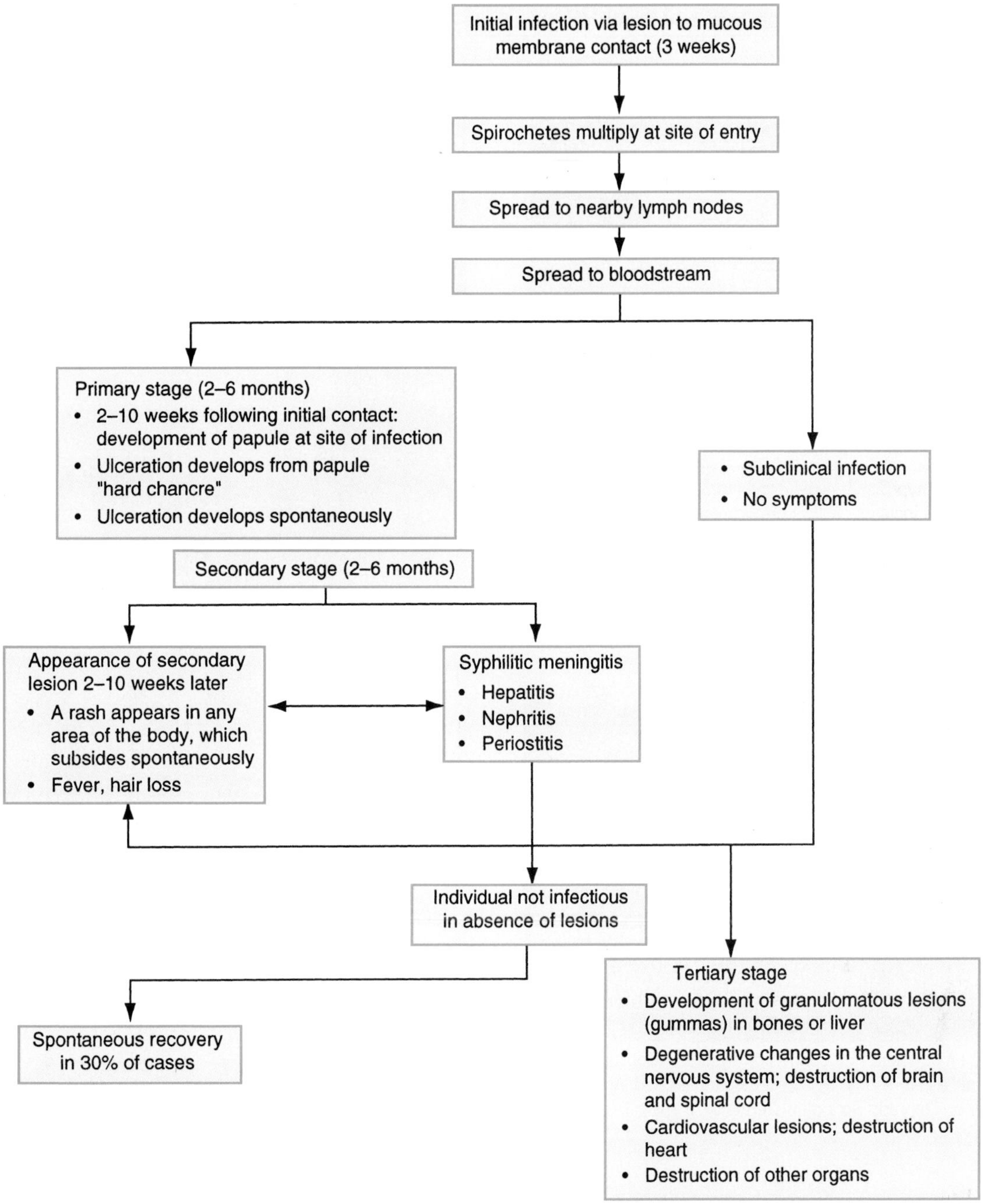

Initial infection via lesion to mucous membrane contact (3 weeks)

↓

Spirochetes multiply at site of entry

↓

Spread to nearby lymph nodes

↓

Spread to bloodstream

↓

Primary stage (2–6 months)

- 2–10 weeks following initial contact: development of papule at site of infection
- Ulceration develops from papule "hard chancre"
- Ulceration develops spontaneously

- Subclinical infection
- No symptoms

Secondary stage (2–6 months)

Appearance of secondary lesion 2–10 weeks later

- A rash appears in any area of the body, which subsides spontaneously
- Fever, hair loss

Syphilitic meningitis

- Hepatitis
- Nephritis
- Periostitis

Individual not infectious in absence of lesions

Spontaneous recovery in 30% of cases

Tertiary stage

- Development of granulomatous lesions (gummas) in bones or liver
- Degenerative changes in the central nervous system; destruction of brain and spinal cord
- Cardiovascular lesions; destruction of heart
- Destruction of other organs

**Fig. 9.8** Primary, secondary, and tertiary stages of syphilis.

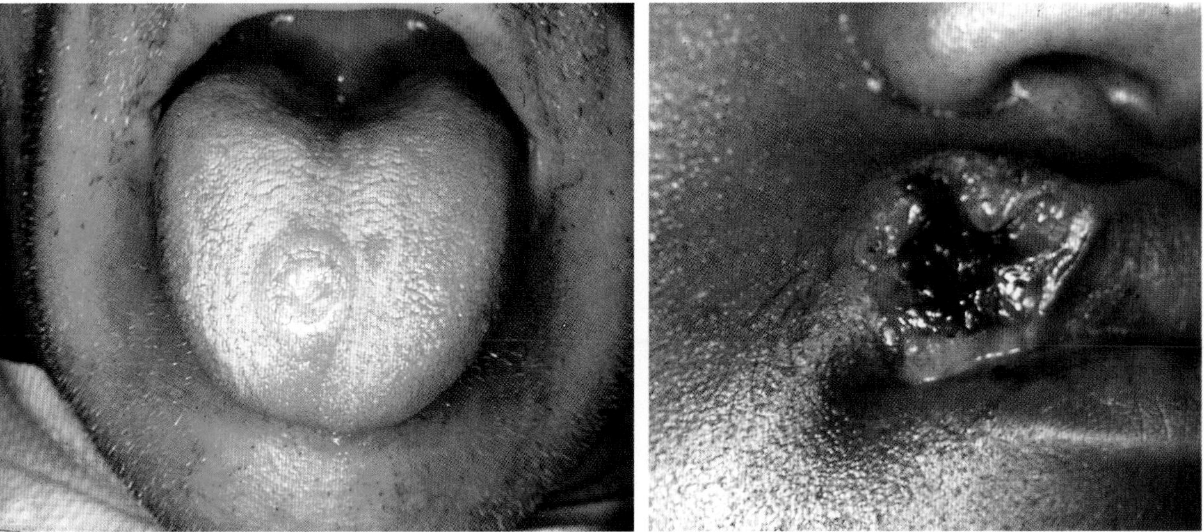

**Fig. 9.9** Chancre lesion of primary syphilis. (From Sapp JP, Eversole LR, Wysocki GP. *Contemporary Oral and Maxillofacial Pathology.* 2nd ed. St. Louis: Mosby; 2004.)

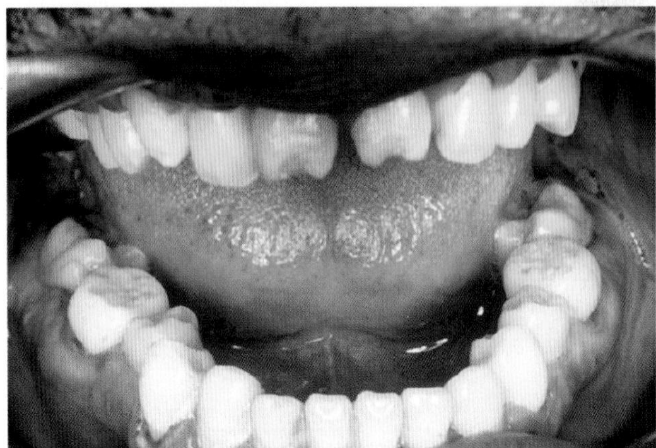

**Fig. 9.10** Congenital syphilis. The patient exhibits anomalously shaped teeth, consisting of incisors with screwdriver-shaped crowns and notched incisal edges and molars with constricted crowns and a lack of cuspal development (mulberry molars). (From Sapp JP, Eversole LR, Wysocki GP. *Contemporary Oral and Maxillofacial Pathology.* 2nd ed. St. Louis: Mosby; 2004.)

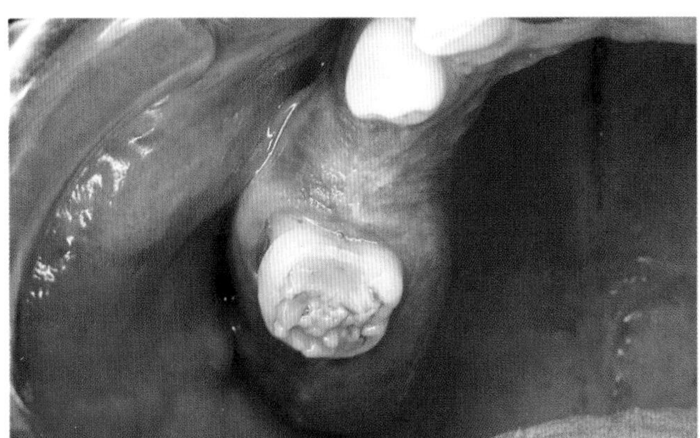

**Fig. 9.11** "Mulberry molars" of congenital syphilis. (Courtesy of Beverly Entwistle Isman, formerly with the Department of Applied Dentistry, University of Colorado School of Dentistry, Denver.)

(b) "Mulberry molars"—first molars are irregular with poorly developed cusps (Fig. 9.11)
(c) Skin, mucous membrane lesions
(d) High mortality

B. Viral infections (Fig. 9.12)
1. Genital herpes
a. Etiology
(1) Herpesvirus
(2) HSV-2—herpes genitalis (genital herpes)
b. Pathogenesis—transmitted by sexual contact
c. Clinical findings and symptoms
(1) Lesions appear 2 to 7 days after exposure
(2) Lesions appear in or on the genitalia and skin
(3) Lesions may ulcerate early and be painful or crust over
(4) Fever, lymphadenopathy, malaise, anorexia
(5) Initial lesions subside and heal in 2 to 3 weeks
(6) Recurrent lesions have a milder course
(7) Highly infectious
(8) Primary and recurrent infections

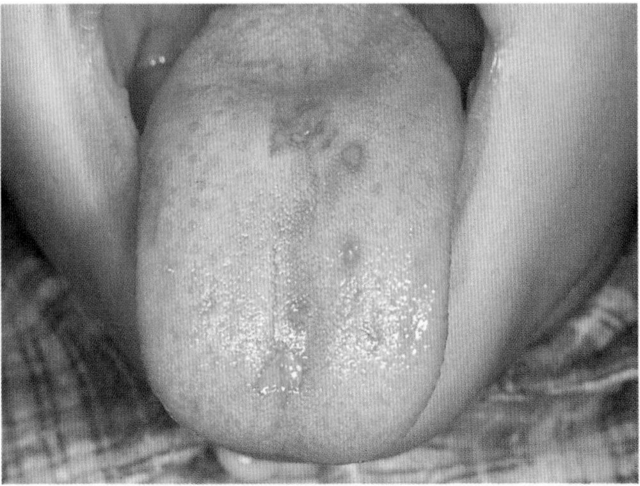

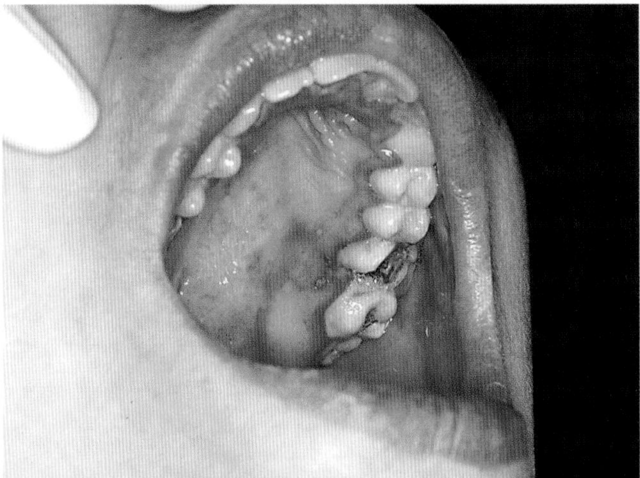

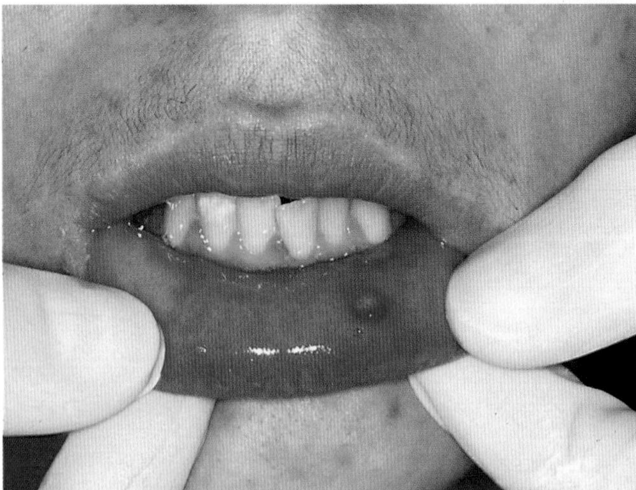

**Fig. 9.12** Primary herpetic gingivostomatitis.

(a) Most (90%) primary infections are subclinical
(b) Recurrent infections in women often serve as a source of neonatal herpes

## Infections of the Central Nervous System

A. Bacterial infections
1. Meningitis
a. Etiology

(1) Meningococcal meningitis—caused by *Neisseria meningitidis*

b. Pathogenesis—transmitted by droplet inhalation

c. Clinical findings and symptoms

(1) Meningococcal meningitis produces headache, vomiting, stiff neck, and coma within a few hours

B. Viral infections

1. Poliomyelitis

a. Etiology—poliomyelitis virus

b. Pathogenesis—virus transmitted through the mouth and intestines

c. Clinical findings and symptoms

(1) Flaccid paralysis; destruction of motor neurons in the spinal cord

(2) Acute inflammation of the meninges

(3) May range from mild illness to paralysis

### Infections of the Eye

A. Viral infections

1. Adenovirus infection

a. Etiology—adenoviruses

b. Pathogenesis

(1) Hand-to-eye contact is the most significant factor

(2) Swimming pool conjunctivitis most likely transmitted by the waterborne route

c. Clinical findings and symptoms—inflammation of the conjunctiva, excessive lacrimation, periorbital edema

2. Herpetic keratitis

a. Etiology—primarily caused by HSV-1; occasionally by HSV-2

b. Pathogenesis—cytolytic, herpetic infection of the cornea

c. Clinical findings and symptoms

(1) Severe keratoconjunctivitis; corneal ulcers or vesicles on the eyelids

(2) May recur

(3) May cause blindness

## MICROBIOLOGY OF THE ORAL CAVITY

### Normal Oral Flora

A. Composition and distribution—different types of surfaces create distinct habitats within the mouth, so the distribution of microflora is not uniform throughout the mouth (Table 9.6)

1. Lips—predominantly facultatively anaerobic streptococci; *Streptococcus vestibularis* found in the vestibule

2. Palate—predominantly *Actinomyces* spp. and *Streptococcus* spp.

3. Cheek—predominantly *Streptococcus* spp. and *Haemophilus* spp.; 5 to 25 bacteria per epithelial cell

a. Majority of streptococci are *Streptococcus oralis* and *S. mitis,* and fewer are *S. sanguinis*

b. *Simonsiella* spp. isolated primarily from human cheek cells

**TABLE 9.6 Bacterial Genera Found in the Oral Cavity**

| | Gram-Positive | Gram-Negative |
|---|---|---|
| Cocci | *Abiotrophia* | *Moraxella* |
| | *Enterococcus* | *Neisseria* |
| | *Peptostreptococcus* | *Veillonella* |
| | *Staphylococcus* | |
| | *Stomatococcus* | |
| | *Streptococcus* | |
| Rods | *Actinomyces* | *Aggregatibacter* |
| | *Bifidobacterium* | *Campylobacter* |
| | *Corynebacterium* | *Cantonella* |
| | *Eubacterium* | *Capnocytophaga* |
| | *Lactobacillus* | *Centipeda* |
| | *Propionibacterium* | *Desulfovibrio* |
| | *Pseudoramibacter* | *Desulfobacter* |
| | *Rothia* | *Eikenella* |
| | | *Fusobacterium* |
| | | *Haemophilus* |
| | | *Johnsonii* |
| | | *Leptotrichia* |
| | | *Porphyromonas* |
| | | *Prevotella* |
| | | *Selenomonas* |
| | | *Simonsiella* |
| | | *Tannerella* |
| | | *Treponema* |
| | | *Wolinella* |

Insert Color Complexes (attached in site)

4. Tongue (100 bacteria per tongue epithelial cell)—papillae allow for a large surface area for colonization, resulting in higher bacterial density and diverse microflora

a. Predominantly *S. oralis, S. mitis,* and *Streptococcus salivarius*

b. *Stomatococcus mucilagenosus* is found exclusively on the tongue

c. *Veillonella* spp., *Actinomyces naeslundii, Actinomyces odontolyticus,* and *Haemophilus* spp. also isolated

d. Increased numbers of *Porphyromonas, Prevotella, Fusobacterium,* and *Treponema* spp. lead to halitosis resulting from an increase in volatile sulfur compound production

5. Saliva—108 to 109 bacteria/mL of saliva; normal salivary flow ensures that bacteria do not multiply in saliva; so saliva does not contain resident flora but rather bacteria from other surfaces—primarily from the dorsum of the tongue and dental plaque

6. Tooth surfaces (plaque)

a. Pits and fissures

(1) Morphologic condition allows for proliferation

(2) Predominantly *Streptococcus mutans* and *A. naeslundii*

(3) Common sites for caries

b. Interproximal surfaces

(1) Inaccessible to routine oral hygiene care

(2) Bacteria in biofilm can proliferate in microcolonies undisturbed

(3) Predominantly *A. naeslundii, Actinomyces israelii, and Streptococcus, Veillonella,* and *Prevotella* spp.
(4) Majority of streptococci are *S. sanguinis*
(5) Common site for caries

c. Smooth coronal surfaces
(1) Can be covered with plaque if oral hygiene is not practiced
(2) Plaque formation limited by the cleaning action of saliva, the movement of soft tissue, and the action of food particles
(3) Oral bacteria colonize in a predictable succession

B. Factors that influence microbial composition
1. Temperature 35°C to 36°C (95°F to 96.8°F)
a. Temperature may influence proportions of bacterial species
b. Periodontal pockets with active disease have higher temperatures—up to 39°C (102.2°F)
2. Nutrient sources
a. Exogenous sources include the host's diet, especially dietary sugar, which is needed for acid and polysaccharide production
b. Endogenous sources
(1) Saliva
(2) Gingival exudate
(3) Epithelial cells and leukocytes
(4) Continuing existence of flora even when humans and animals are fed by a stomach tube
(5) Certain bacteria use metabolic by-products from other bacteria
3. pH requirements
a. The pH of most surfaces regulated by saliva (pH 6.75 to 7.25)
b. Dietary sugars provide a selective force favoring predominance of certain organisms that tolerate an acidic medium (pH 5)
c. Strains of *S. mutans,* related streptococci, and lactobacilli are both acidogenic (produce acid) and aciduric (tolerate low pH values)
d. Dairy products can elevate pH
e. The pH of the gingival sulcus becomes alkaline during the host inflammatory response in periodontal disease (pH 7.2 to 7.8)
f. Alkaline pockets favor the growth of the pathogen *Porphyromonas gingivalis*
4. Oxygen concentration
a. Distribution of microorganisms in the mouth is related to the redox potential at a particular site
b. The majority of organisms are micro-aerophilic, facultative, or obligate anaerobes
5. Microbial interactions
a. Microbial aggregation
(1) Certain species undergo reactions between host cell surfaces (adhesion receptor)
(2) Bacterial cells can attach to each other (coaggregation)
(3) Some bacteria produce extracellular polysaccharides (glucans, fructans, heteropolysaccharides) that provide structural and energy sources for plaque
6. Saliva
a. Nonspecific factors
(1) Flow of saliva removes planktonic bacteria from oral surfaces
(2) Flow rate bears some relationship to caries susceptibility
(3) Rate of secretion is correlated to buffering capacity
(4) Proteins and glycoproteins form acquired pellicles on teeth; bacteria can attach to the pellicle
(5) Proteins and glycoproteins act as nutrient source for microflora
(6) Proteins and glycoproteins can aid in coaggregation of bacteria, thus facilitating their clearance
(7) Antibacterial components include lysozymes, lactoperoxidase, lactoferrin, salivary thiocyanate, and peptides
b. Specific factors—secretory immunoglobulin A inhibits microbial attachment
7. Host factors that affect microflora
a. Oral hygiene—antimicrobial agents in toothpaste and mouth rinses; mechanical force of toothbrush and interdental care
b. Gender and race
c. Age
d. Alterations in the food web
e. Long-term use of antibiotics and development of antimicrobial resistance
f. Scratches and grooves on tooth surfaces or restorations, or margins between dental restorations and tooth surface that enhance biofilm formation
g. Genetics

## Development of Oral Microflora

A. The oral cavity is usually sterile at birth
B. Initial colonization of the infant's mouth by the microflora of the mother, milk, water, and saliva of those in close contact
1. Oral microflora consist of aerobic and facultatively anaerobic gram-positive species
2. *S. salivarius, S. oralis,* and *S. mitis* predominate by the first month of the infant's life
C. The microflora diversify in the next few months with several gram-negative anaerobes—*Prevotella melaninogenica, Fusobacterium nucleatum,* and *Veillonella* spp.
D. At 12 months, most children have the following organisms:
1. Streptococci
a. *S. salivarius, S. oralis,* and *S. mitis* predominate
b. *S. mutans* and *S. sanguinis* are not established until tooth eruption
2. Staphylococci
3. *Veillonella* spp.
4. *Neisseria* spp.
5. *Actinomyces* spp.
6. Lactobacilli
7. *Nocardia* spp.
8. *Fusobacterium* spp.
E. Preschool-age child
1. Adult-like microflora

2. *P. melaninogenica* and spirochetes not common at age 5 years, but increase in numbers by age 13 years

F. Age-related changes in oral microflora
   1. Increase in numbers of yeast *(C. albicans)* may be associated with increased denture wear, changes in the oral mucosa, blood glucose level, and malnutrition
   2. Increased use of medications common with aging; may decrease salivary flow

## BACTERIAL PLAQUE

See the section on "Bacterial Dental Biofilm" in Chapter 14.

A. Definition
   1. Deposit formed by the colonization of teeth by members of the normal oral flora
   2. Complex of bacteria in the matrix mainly of bacterial polysaccharides; biofilm
   3. Bacteria embedded in an exopolymeric matrix that provides a protective environment for bacteria

B. Stages of formation
   1. Cell-free pellicle
      a. High-molecular-weight salivary glycoproteins
      b. Quickly colonized by bacteria
   2. Plaque formation
      a. Days 1–2
         (1) Gram-positive cocci and short rods show early dominance
         (2) Streptococci (aerobe)
      b. Days 2–4
         (1) Cocci still dominate, but gram-positive rods and gram-negative cocci begin to appear
         (2) *Streptococcus sanguinis, S. oralis,* or *S. mitis* usually first colonizer, but *Haemophilus* and *Neisseria* spp. may also be early colonizers
      c. Days 4–7
         (1) After 7 days, streptococci remain the dominant organism, but by day 8, their numbers decrease, filaments increase
      d. Days 7–14
         (1) Vibrios and spirochetes appear (*Veillonella* and *Actinomyces* spp.)
         (2) Gingival inflammation present
      e. Days 14–21
         (1) Vibrios and spirochetes prevalent, anaerobic, gram-negative, motile bacteria
         (2) Gingivitis clinically present

C. Microbial composition of plaque
   1. Bacterial composition of supragingival (supramarginal) plaque
      a. Gram-positive cocci and rods dominate
      b. Other species found include *A. israelii, S. mutans, Veillonella* and *Fusobacterium* spp., *Treponema* spp., and *Capnocytophaga* spp.
   2. Bacterial composition of subgingival plaque
      a. Filamentous dominate, cocci and rods present
      b. *S. sanguinis,* S. mitis, *A. naeslundii, S. oralis, S. intermedius, P. gingivalis, P. intermedia, T. forsythis, Eubacterium and F. nucleatum*
   3. Bacterial composition of normal gingival crevicular plaque
      a. Gingival crevice—an area of stagnation and bacterial proliferation—environmental influences include an increase in crevicular fluid, desquamation of epithelial cells, and bacterial acid products
      b. Quantity of species relatively constant; proportions of species vary among people and even within the same mouth
      c. Predominant organisms are *S. mitis, S. sanguinis, A. naeslundii, A. odontolyticus, A. meyeri, A. georgiae, Rothia dentocariosus,* and *Eubacterium, Fusobacterium,* and *Treponema* spp.
   4. Calculus
      a. Inorganic salts, 70% to 90%
      b. Microbes similar to those of the gingival crevicular area
      c. Main role in periodontal disease is to serve as a collection site for more bacteria

## DENTAL CARIES

See Fig. 9.13.

A. Prerequisites for caries development
   1. Cariogenic bacteria
   2. Supply of substrate for acid production
   3. Susceptible host/tooth
   4. Time

B. Cariogenic bacteria
   1. Essential properties
      a. Acidogenic and aciduric; acid must be produced and a low pH maintained for a long period
      b. Ability to attach to tooth surfaces
      c. Formation of a protective matrix

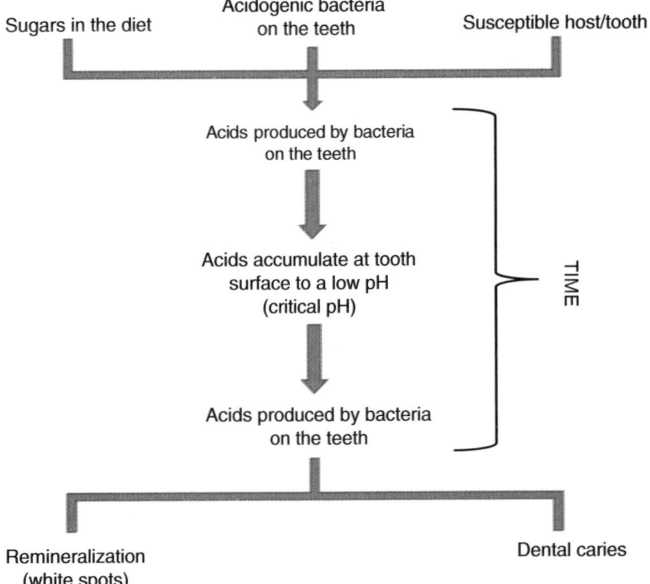


**Fig. 9.13** Formation of dental caries.

2. Streptococci
   a. *Streptococcus mutans*
      (1) Initiates caries process
      (2) Most strongly cariogenic bacteria in animals
      (3) Hard surfaces are a prerequisite for its presence; the organisms disappear if teeth are extracted and reappear with dentures
      (4) Homofermentive lactic acid former
      (5) Produces insoluble and soluble glucans
      (6) A high-sucrose diet is generally associated with an increase in the *S. mutans* population
      (7) Usually found in the early stages of plaque formation
   b. *Streptococcus sobrinus*
      (1) A *mutans* streptococcus
      (2) Possible roles in caries are still evolving
   c. *Streptococcus sanguinis*
      (1) Produces glucans
      (2) Some strains cariogenic in animals
      (3) Colonizes tooth enamel
      (4) Is present in plaque and sometimes cheek
   d. *Streptococcus mitis*
      (1) Cariogenic in animals
      (2) Found on oral soft tissues
   e. *Streptococcus salivarius*
      (1) Produces fructans
      (2) Usually has a strong affinity for oral soft tissues, especially the tongue
      (3) Some strains cariogenic in animals
3. Lactobacilli
   a. Contributes to progression of caries
   b. Present in small numbers in plaque
   c. Increase in number in the mouth when the sugar content in the diet is high
      (1) Present in the mouth where sugar is retained
      (2) Carious lesions act as retention sites
   d. Strongly acidogenic and aciduric
   e. May have important role in the progression of caries
2. *Actinomyces*
   a. *Actinomyces naeslundii* primary cause of root-surface caries
   b. Plaque-forming organisms
   c. Ferment glucose to produce mostly lactic acid
   d. *A. naeslundii* present on tongue, tooth surfaces, and plaque

C. Acid production in plaque
1. Enamel demineralization occurs at pH of 4.5–5.5
2. Root surface demineralization occurs at pH of 6.0–6.7
3. Important features of the acid production process
   a. Amount of plaque
   b. Predominant microflora
   c. Rate of salivary flow
   d. Substrate characteristics
   e. Location of plaque
4. More lactic acid present than any other acid

D. Bacterial substrates and diet
1. Sucrose
   a. Main substrate for cariogenic bacteria
   b. Important in the formation of smooth-surface caries
   c. Metabolized to form acids and glucans
   d. Essential for caries production in animals
   e. Epidemiologic evidence has established its role in human caries
   f. Increase in the frequency of sucrose consumption is associated with an increase in caries
   g. High cariogenic effect when retained on teeth for a long period
2. Starches
   a. Low cariogenicity
   b. Probably influences plaque microflora

E. Host/Tooth Factors
1. Tooth surface
   a. Caries formation influenced by tooth morphology and arch form
   b. Enamel surfaces are probably more caries resistant than the subsurface
2. Saliva
   a. Functions that affect the carious process
      (1) Clearance of food
      (2) Buffer activity
      (3) Bacterial aggregation
      (4) Antibacterial function (e.g., immunoglobulin A, lysozymes, salivary peroxidase)
   b. Amount of ambient calcium, phosphate, and fluoride ions in the saliva for remineralization of tooth structure
   c. Rate of flow and buffering abilities
      (1) As flow rate increases, pH rises
      (2) High salivary flow rates and buffering are associated with low caries activity

## PERIODONTAL DISEASES

See the section on "Diseases of the Periodontium" in Chapter 14.

A. Classification of periodontal diseases
1. Periodontal health and gingival health
   a. Clinical gingival health on intact periodontium
   b. Clinical gingival health on reduced periodontium
      (1) Stable periodontal patient
      (2) Nonperiodontitis patient
2. Dental biofilm–induced gingivitis
   a. Associated with biofilm alone
   b. Mediated by systemic or local risk factors
   c. Drug-influenced gingival enlargement
   d. Predominant microflora include: *S. sanguinis, S. mitis, Fusobacterium spp., Actinomyces viscosus*
3. Nondental Biofilm–induced gingivitis
   a. Genetic/developmental disorders, specific infections, inflammatory and immune conditions, reactive processes, neoplasms, endocrine, nutritional and metabolic diseases, traumatic lesions, gingival pigmentation

B. Periodontitis
1. Necrotizing periodontal diseases
   a. Necrotizing gingivitis

(1) Anaerobic infection of gingival margins causes ulceration; if allowed to progress, destruction of gingivae and underlying bone occurs; onset is sudden and acute
(2) The interproximal areas are affected first
(3) Appears to be an opportunistic infection based on predisposing factors (e.g., plaque formation, depression of PMN function, stress, poor diet, immunocompromise)
(4) Predominant microflora include *P. intermedia,* spirochetes, and fusiform bacteria

b. Necrotizing periodontitis
(1) Appearance—necrosis of gingival tissues, periodontal ligaments, and alveolar bone
(2) Indications—client presents with pain and excessive necrosis
(3) Severe and rapid periodontal destruction; lack of deep-pocket formation
(4) Occurs in persons infected with HIV and those undergoing immunosuppressive therapies
(5) Predominant microflora include *C. albicans, Haemophilus actinomycetemcomitans, F. nucleatum,* and *Porphyromonas gingivalis*

c. Necrotizing stomatitis

2. Periodontitis)
a. Stages
(1) I. Initial periodontitis
(2) II. Moderate periodontitis
(3) III. Severe periodontitis with potential for additional tooth loss
(4) IV. Severe periodontitis with potential for loss of dentition

b. Extent and Distribution
(1) Localized, generalized, molar–incisor distribution

c. Grades
(1) Grade A: slow rate of disease progression
(2) Grade B: moderate risk of disease progression
(3) Grade C: rapid rate of disease progression

d. Predominant microflora in periodontitis: *A. actinomycetecomitans, P. gingivalis, T. forsythia, P. intermedia, T. denticola, C. rectus, P. micros, F. nucleatum, Selenomonas.*

3. Periodontitis as a manifestation of systemic diseases
4. Socransky complexes (table of microbial complexes)
a. Not grouped periodontal pathogens: *A. actinomycetecomitans, Selenomas*
b. Red complex: high risk for developing periodontitis: *T. forsythia, P. gingivalis, T. denticola*
c. Orange complex: moderate risk for developing periodontitis: *C. rectus, F. nucleatum, P. intermedia, P. micros*
d. Yellow complex: low risk of developing periodontitis: *S. gordonii, s. intermedius, S. mitis, S. oralis, S. sanguinis*
e. Green and purple found in subgingival plaque: *Capnocytophaga, E. corrodens, A. odontolyticus, Veillonella*

C. Other conditions affecting the periodontium
1. Systemic diseases or conditions affecting the periodontal supporting tissues
2. Periodontal abscesses and endodontic periodontal lesions
3. Mucogingival deformities and conditions
4. Traumatic occlusal forces
5. Tooth and prosthesis related factors

D. Peri-implant diseases and conditions
1. Peri-implant health
2. Peri-implant mucositis
3. Peri-implantitis
4. Peri-implant soft and hard tissue deformities

## PERIAPICAL INFECTIONS AND ORAL-FACIAL TISSUE INFECTIONS

A. Infections
1. Abscesses (periodontal and periapical)
2. Postsurgical and postextraction wound infections
3. Endodontically involved infections
4. Sinus tract infections
5. Cellulitis
6. Traumatic injuries
7. Osteomyelitis
8. Postextraction alveolar osteitis (dry socket)
9. Pericoronitis
10. Periodontally involved infections

B. Bacteria cultivated from such infections
1. Polymicrobial and opportunistic in nature
2. Obligate anaerobic bacteria predominate in acute endodontic infections

C. Ludwig's angina
1. Mixed infection
a. *Fusobacterium* spp., *Prevotella* spp., *Porphyromonas* spp., and streptococci
b. Often caused by the normal oral flora gaining access through the infected tooth
2. Symptoms
a. Rapidly spreading, diffuse bilateral cellulitis of the floor of the mouth and neck
b. Swelling that may block air passages
c. Fever and malaise
3. Predisposing factors
a. Infected mandibular molars
b. Thin lingual cortical plate of the mandible

## OPPORTUNISTIC INFECTIONS OF THE ORAL CAVITY

A. Definition—opportunistic organisms take advantage of a compromised situation in the host and subsequently invade and cause infections of the oral cavity

B. Actinomycosis
1. Etiology
a. *Actinomyces israelii* most common
b. *A. naeslundii* and *Arachnia propionica* found in some lesions

2. Pathogenesis
   a. Gram-positive bacteria; member of the normal oral flora
   b. Infection may follow injury with introduction of contaminated debris into tissue
3. Clinical findings and symptoms
   a. Facial swelling, most frequently in soft tissue below the angle of the jaw
   b. Small, chronic, superficial mass
   c. Abscess with sinus and chronic discharge develops

C. Oral candidiasis—four clinically distinct forms:
1. Pseudomembranous candidiasis
   a. A removable soft, creamy, white plaque; red or bleeding base
   b. Predominantly found on the buccal and labial mucosa, tongue, hard and soft palates
2. Erythematous candidiasis
   a. A smooth, flat, red lesion on the dorsum of the tongue; associated with loss of papillae
   b. Can also be found on the hard palate
3. Angular cheilitis—cracking or redness around the corners of the mouth
4. Hyperplastic candidiasis
   a. A raised, white, nonremovable plaque
   b. Appears on the buccal mucosa, hard palate, or dorsum of the tongue

D. Staphylococci
1. Etiology—*S. aureus* and *S. epidermidis*
2. Pathogenesis—normal flora of the skin, oral cavity, and anterior nares
3. Clinical manifestations
   a. Mandibular osteomyelitis
   b. Acute suppurative parotitis

E. Other oral diseases
1. Mumps
   a. Etiology—mumps virus
   b. Clinical findings and symptoms
      (1) Painful, swollen parotid or submaxillary glands
      (2) Fever and malaise
      (3) Red and swollen papilla of Stensen's duct
   c. Prevention through vaccine
2. Herpangina (vesicular pharyngitis)
   a. Etiology—coxsackievirus A
   b. Pathogenesis
      (1) Transmitted by ingestion of contaminated materials
      (2) Primarily occurs in children
   c. Clinical findings and symptoms—fever and vomiting; vesicles and later ulcers on the mucous membrane of the throat, palate, or tongue
   d. Recovery in 7 to 10 days; complications rare
3. Recurrent aphthous ulcers
   a. Etiology—unknown; evidence suggests immunologic etiology
   b. Clinical findings and symptoms
      (1) Canker sore, small ulcer
      (2) Covered by pseudomembrane
      (3) Surrounding erythematous halo
      (4) Occur on nonkeratinized mucosa
4. Hand-foot-and-mouth disease
   a. Etiology—coxsackievirus A
   b. Pathogenesis
      (1) Highly infectious
      (2) Typically affects many children, particularly in schools
   c. Clinical findings and symptoms
      (1) Vesicular stomatitis and rash
      (2) Affects the buccal mucosa, tongue, gingiva, lips, hands, and feet
      (3) Pain

## WEBSITE INFORMATION AND RESOURCES

| Source | Website Address | Description |
|---|---|---|
| Bergey's Taxonomic Outline | https://www.bergeys.org/ | Online publication, updated approximately six times per year and is free to registered users |
| Centers for Disease Control and Prevention (CDC) | http://www.cdc.gov/ | One of the 13 major operating components of the Department of Health and Human Services (HHS), which is the principal US government agency for protecting the health and safety of all Americans and for providing essential human services, especially for persons who are least able to help themselves |
| Organization for Asepsis and Safety Procedures (OSAP) | http://www.osap.org/ | Promotes infection control and related science-based health and safety policies and practices through quality education and information dissemination |
| *Morbidity and Mortality Weekly Report (MMWR)* | http://www.cdc.gov/mmwr/ | The *MMWR* series is prepared by the CDC and provides data regarding a variety of health and safety concerns |

## CHAPTER 9 REVIEW QUESTIONS

Answers and rationales to review questions are available on this text's accompanying Evolve site. See inside front cover for details.

1. What cellular structure is involved in protein synthesis?
   a. Golgi complex
   b. Ribosome
   c. Mitochondrion
   d. Nucleus
2. What is the type of microscopic technique used to examine living cells?
   a. Phase-contrast microscopy
   b. Darkfield microscopy
   c. Bright-field microscopy
   d. Scanning electron microscopy
3. Identify the type of staining used to determine if an organism is a spore former.
   a. Flagellar stain
   b. Acid-fast stain
   c. Gram staining
   d. Schaefer-Fulton stain
4. What is the CORRECT morphologic name for bacteria that do appear in irregular clusters?
   a. Staphylococci
   b. Diplococci
   c. Sarcinae
   d. Pleomorphic
5. The type of microbial relationship in which one organism benefits and the other neither benefits or is harmed.
   a. Symbiosis
   b. Predation
   c. Commensalism
   d. Parasitism
6. Which immunoglobulin is the first to appear in immune response?
   a. IgG
   b. IgM
   c. IgA
   d. IgE
7. An infection in which the causative agent remains inactive for a time, but then becomes active to produce symptoms of the disease?
   a. Latent
   b. Primary
   c. Toxemia
   d. Nosocomial
8. A chancre is present during which stage of a syphilis infection?
   a. Primary
   b. Secondary
   c. Tertiary
   d. Quaternary
9. The structure that is responsible for regulating movement of materials into and out of the cell:
   a. Ribosome
   b. Plastid
   c. Cytoplasmic membrane
   d. Vacuole
10. In prokaryotes, respiration occurs through what cellular structure?
    a. Cytoplasmic membrane
    b. Mitochondria
    c. Ribosomes
    d. Lysosomes
11. Shingles are caused by this virus:
    a. Rubella virus
    b. Human parvovirus B19
    c. Varicella-zoster virus
    d. Papillomavirus
12. The cardinal signs of inflammation include all of the following except one. Which one is the exception?
    a. Heat
    b. Pain
    c. Swelling
    d. Pus formation
13. The bacterial species primarily responsible for root caries is:
    *a. Streptococcus mitis*
    *b. Streptococcus sanguinis*
    *c. Streptococcus salivarius*
    *d. Actinomyces naeslundii*
14. The type of immunity acquired when a mother passes antibodies to her infant is called:
    a. Natural active
    b. Artificial active
    c. Natural passive
    d. Artificial passive
15. Herpes viruses are responsible for the formation of:
    a. Cold sores
    b. Warts
    c. Chickenpox
    d. Measles
16. The causative agent of syphilis is:
    a. Neisseria gonorrhoeae
    b. Epstein-Barr virus
    c. Treponema pallidum
    d. Rubella virus
17. The primary organism in necrotizing ulcerative gingivitis is:
    *a. Streptococcus mutans*
    *b. Aggregatibacter actinomycetemcomitans*
    *c. Candida albicans*
    *d. Prevotella intermedia*
18. The causative agent of tuberculosis is:
    *a. Chlamydia psittaci*
    *b. Treponema pallidum*
    *c. Treponema tuberculosis*
    *d. Mycobacterium tuberculosis*
19. All of the following are gram-negative bacteria except one. Which one is the exception?
    a. *Neisseria* spp.
    b. *Veillonella* spp.
    c. *Fusobacterium* spp.
    d. *Streptococcus* spp.

20. The bacterial species commonly responsible for smooth surface caries is:
    *a. S. sobrinus*
    *b. S. salivarius*
    *c. S. mitis*
    *d. S. mutans*
21. Enamel demineralization typically occurs at this pH:
    a. 2.0–3.0
    b. 4.5–5.5
    c. 6.0–6.7
    d. None of the above
22. During the first month of an infant's life all of the following bacteria are typically present except one. Which one is the exception?
    *a. F. nucleatum*
    *b. S. salivarius*
    *c. S. mitis*
    *d. S. oralis*
23. Phase of bacterial growth where the number of viable cells decrease is called:
    a. Lag phase
    b. Stationary phase
    c. Phase of decline
    d. None of the above
24. The presence of bacteria in the bloodstream is termed:
    a. Toxemia
    b. Nosocomial
    c. Symptom
    d. Bacteremia
25. Each of the following oral microorganisms could colonize soft tissues except one. Which one is the exception?
    *a. Streptococcus mitis*
    *b. Candida albicans*
    *c. Streptococcus mutans*
    *d. Streptococcus salivarius*
26. Which of the following bacteria are MOST commonly found in supragingival plaque?
    a. Gram-negative cocci
    b. Gram-positive cocci
    c. Spirochetes
    d. Vibrios
27. All of the following are prerequisites for caries development except one. Which one is the exception?
    a. Cariogenic bacteria
    b. Supply of substrate for acid production
    c. Susceptible host
    d. Portal of exit
28. The causative agent of aphthous ulcers is:
    a. Coxsackievirus A
    b. S. mutans
    c. C. albicans
    d. None of the above
29. A 21-year-old woman presented for her dental cleaning. Upon examination the dental hygienist noticed a raised, white, nonremovable plaque on the hard palate. Which of the following fungal infections is likely present?
    a. Pseudomembranous candidiasis
    b. Erythematous candidiasis
    c. Angular cheilitis
    d. Hyperplastic candidiasis
30. Which type of organism uses light for energy?
    a. Hypotrophic
    b. Chemotrophic
    c. Phototrophic
    d. None of the above
31. The microbial relationship that results in an interaction in which two different species live in a mutually beneficial coexistence?
    a. Syntrophism
    b. Symbiosis
    c. Commensalism
    d. Parasitism
32. All of the following statements are true regarding innate immunity except one. Which one is the exception?
    a. Present at birth
    b. Does not improve with repeated exposure
    c. Not antigen specific
    d. Antigen specific
33. The human immunodeficiency virus is transmitted in all of the following ways except one. Which one is the exception?
    a. Semen
    b. Blood
    c. Saliva
    d. Breast milk
34. Risk factors for acquiring the human immunodeficiency virus include:
    a. Unsafe sexual practices
    b. Exposure to infected blood or blood products
    c. Intravenous drug use
    d. All of the above
35. The causative agent of chickenpox is:
    a. Varicella-zoster
    b. Herpes simplex virus
    c. Papillomavirus
    d. Rubeola virus
36. All of the following microorganisms are transmitted via droplet transmission except one. Which one is the exception?
    a. Corynebacterium diphtheriae
    b. Streptococcus pneumonia
    c. Mycobacterium tuberculosis
    d. Hepatitis A virus
37. The causative agent of syphilis is:
    a. Herpes simplex virus-2
    b. Treponema pallidum
    c. Neisseria gonorrhoeae
    d. None of the above
38. All of the following are periodontal pathogens except one. Which one is the exception?
    *a. P. gingivalis*
    *b. T. forsythia*
    *c. S. mutans*
    *d. A. actinomycetecomitans*
39. All of the following organisms are gram-negative, facultative anaerobes except one. Which one is the exception?

a. *P. gingivalis*
b. *A. actinomycetecomitans*
c. *E. corrodens*
d. None of the above

40. All of the following bacteria are found in tooth-associated plaque biofilms except one. Which one is the exception?
a. *S. mitis*
b. *S. sanguinis*
c. *P. gingivalis*
d. *A. viscosus*

## CASE A

**Patient Profile:** patient is a 32-year-old Caucasian female, 5'6", and weighs 168 lbs.
**Chief Complaint:** "I have a painful sore on the inside of my cheek and my back tooth is hurting."
**Dental History:** her last dental visit was 5 years ago for a dental cleaning.
**Medical History:** the patient reported that she has been diagnosed with anxiety and depression. She currently takes Lexapro and Wellbutrin. Her blood pressure was recorded at 130/80.
**Extraoral Exam:**
- No significant findings.

**Intraoral Exam:**
- Dental decay on #3-O
- Generalized bleeding on probing
- Generalized light to moderate plaque
- Generalized moderate subgingival calculus
- Localized moderate bone loss in the mandibular anterior and between #18 and #19
- 2mm by 3mm round, greyish-white lesion with erythematous halo on right buccal mucosa

**Supplemental Information:**
- Patient reports she is stressed out financially.
- Patient reports flossing 1x/month.

**Bleeding Index:** 55%

***Use Case A to answer questions 41 to 44.***

41. The bacteria most likely responsible for decay on #3-0 is:
a. *A. actinomycetecomitans*
b. *S. mutans*
c. *A. naeslundii*
d. None of the above

42. The 2mm x 3mm round, greyish-white lesion with the erythematous halo is likely a/an:
a. Cold sore
b. Aphthous ulcer
c. Erythematous candidiasis
d. Angular cheilitis

43. The etiology most likely responsible for the greyish-white lesion with an erythematous halo is:
a. Coxsackievirus
b. T. pallidum
c. Herpes simplex virus 2
d. None of the above

44. The predominant bacteria most likely to be found in the gingival crevicular fluid of this patient is:
a. Gram + cocci
b. Gram + rods
c. Gram – rod
d. None of the above

## CASE B

**Patient Profile:** patient is a 39-year-old African American male, 6'3", and 275lbs.
**Chief Complaint:** "My gums bleed all the time and I haven't had my teeth cleaned in 15 years."
**Dental History:** his last dental appointment was 15 years ago. He had his #2 extracted due to decay.
**Medical History:** the patient reported he has AIDS. He also reported that he has a history of cold sores and depression. His recent CBC panel indicated: CD4 T-lymphocyte count was 189. He currently takes Lorazepam, Retrovir, Sustiva, and Prozac. His blood pressure was recorded at 130/85.
**Extraoral Examination:**
- Three purplish 2mm x 3mm spots on face (mid-forehead, distal to left eye, left cheek bone)

**Intraoral Examination:**
- Class V dental decay on #8
- Ulcerated and necrotic papilla with a punched-out appearance
- Gray pseudomembranous slough
- Generalized moderate to heavy plaque
- Generalized moderate to heavy calculus
- White nonremovable plaque on the hard palate

**Supplemental Information:**
- Previous IV drug user.

**Bleeding Index:** 65%

***Use Case B to answer questions 45 to 50.***

45. The patient's reported history of cold sores is MOST likely caused by:
a. Herpes simplex virus
b. Herpes zoster
c. Epstein-Barr virus
d. None of the above

46. The 2mm x 3mm purplish spots found during the extraoral exam is likely:
a. Koplik spots
b. Herpetic lesions
c. Kaposi's sarcoma
d. Aphthous ulcers

47. The bacteria most likely responsible for the class V decay on #8 is:
a. *A. actinomycetecomitans*
b. *S. mutans*
c. *A. naeslundii*
d. None of the above

48. The white nonremovable plaque on the palate is likely:
a. Cold sore
b. Aphthous ulcer
c. Hyperplastic candidiasis
d. Angular cheilitis

49. The periodontal condition that is most likely present is:
    a. Periodontal abscess
    b. Gingivitis
    c. Necrotizing ulcerative periodontitis
    d. None of the above

50. The medication that is indicated for depression is:
    a. Wellbutrin
    b. Retrovir
    c. Sustiva
    d. Lorazepa

## REFERENCES

1. Centers for Disease Control and Prevention. *About HIV/AIDS*; 2019. http://www.cdc.gov/hiv/statistics/basics.html.
2. Centers for Disease Control and Prevention. *Symptoms of Coronavirus*; 2020. Accessed August 27, 2020 https://www.cdc.gov/coronavirus/2019-ncov/symptoms-testing/symptoms.html.
3. World Health Organization. *Transmission of SARS-CoV-2: Implications for Infection Prevention Precautions*; 2020. Accessed August 27, 2020 https://www.who.int/news-room/commentaries/detail/transmission-of-sars-cov-2-implications-for-infection-prevention-precautions.
4. Papapanou PN, Sanz M, Buduneli N, Dietrich T, Feres M, Fine DH, Greenwell H. Periodontitis: Consensus report of workgroup 2 of the 2017 World Workshop on the Classification of Periodontal and Peri–Implant Diseases and Conditions. *Journal of periodontology*. 2018;89:S173–S182. https://doi.org/10.1111/jcpe.12936.
5. Caton JG, Armitage G, Berglundh T, Chapple IL, Jepsen S, Kornman KS, Tonetti MS. A new classification scheme for periodontal and peri–implant diseases and conditions–Introduction and key changes from the 1999 classification. *Journal of periodontology*. 2018;89:S1–S8. https://doi.org/10.1111/jcpe.12935.

10

# Infection Control and Prevention of Disease Transmission in Oral Health Care

*Darnyl M. Palmer*

Preventing disease transmission in dental hygiene practice requires an understanding of microbial transfer, infection, and disease in the oral health care environment. Implementing and practicing the elements of standard precautions is essential.

## DISEASE TRANSMISSION

See the section on "Microbial Virulence and Disease Transfer" in Chapter 9.

A. Development of an infectious disease
   1. Source of microbe or pathogen (capable of causing infectious disease)
      a. Primarily originating from a patient's mouth
      b. May originate from dental health care personnel (DHCP) (this mode less likely than from a patient's mouth)
      c. Microbes may be present in saliva, blood, respiratory secretions, and other bodily fluids
   2. Portal of exit—escape of microbe from a person
      a. Coughing, sneezing, and talking
      b. Contaminated dental equipment, instruments, and supplies used in a patient's mouth
      c. Spatter droplets and aerosol particles generated by using power instrumentation, low-speed and high-speed handpieces, and air/water syringe
         (1) Spatter droplets—large, visible particles that settle quickly, contaminating the clinician and the surfaces of the treatment area
         (2) Aerosol particles—small, invisible particles that remain airborne for an extended period and may be inhaled
   3. Transfer of microbes to another person
      a. Direct contact—person to person exposure of microbes
      b. Indirect contact—exposure to items contaminated by a patient's microbes, including sharps (all items that can puncture skin), instruments, surfaces, hands, and equipment
      c. Droplet infection— contact with spatter, spray, splashes containing microbes
      d. Airborne infection—contact with aerosol particles containing microbes
   4. Portal of entry—entry of microbes into a person
      a. Inhalation—breathing aerosol particles
      b. Ingestion—swallowing droplets of saliva or blood spattered into the mouth
      e. Through mucous membranes—droplets of saliva or blood spattered into the eyes, nose, or mouth (ocular, nasal, oral)
      c. Through breaks in the skin—touching patient tissues or contaminated objects, spattering of microbes onto nonintact skin, or punctures with contaminated sharps
         (1) Percutaneous injury—injury that penetrates the skin
         (2) Parenteral—intravenous or by injection
   5. Infection
      a. The infectious agent has a portal of entry into a susceptible (not immune) host
      b. Establishment, multiplication, and survival of microbe in the body
   6. Damage to the body—the disease occurs when microbes multiply to a harmful level
   7. Pathogenic agents and diseases associated with oral health care (Table 10.1)

B. Infection control
   1. Goal—to prevent oral health care–related infections, injuries, and illnesses among patients, DHCP, and community
   2. Reducing the numbers of microorganisms that may be transmitted from person to person or from persons to the oral health care environment, and vice versa
   3. Preventing disease transmission includes reducing circulating microbes while increasing immunity of the body
   4. Infection control protocols seek to reduce or eliminate the likelihood of disease transmission by eliminating one or more factors required for disease transfer (Fig. 10.1)
      a. Asepsis—absence of infectious materials; achieved by removing or killing microorganisms
      b. Disinfection—reducing the number of pathogenic organisms in or on an object, thereby minimizing the potential for disease transmission
         (1) Disinfectants are applied to inanimate objects
         (2) Antiseptics are applied to living tissues

**TABLE 10.1 Pathogenic Agents Important in Oral Health Care**

| Disease | Pathogen |
|---|---|
| **Bloodborne Diseases** | |
| ***Viral*** | |
| Hepatitis B | Hepatitis B virus (HBV) |
| Hepatitis C | Hepatitis C virus (HCV) |
| Hepatitis D | Hepatitis D virus (HDV) |
| Acquired immunodeficiency syndrome (AIDS) | Human immunodeficiency virus (HIV) |
| **Oral Diseases** | |
| ***Bacterial*** | |
| Gonococcal pharyngitis | *Neisseria gonorrhoeae* |
| Streptococcal pharyngitis and scarlet fever | *Streptococcus pyogenes* |
| Syphilis | *Treponema pallidum* |
| ***Viral*** | |
| Primary herpetic gingivostomatitis | Human herpesvirus 1 or 2 |
| Recurrent herpes (e.g., herpes labialis) | Human herpesvirus 1 or 2 |
| Hand-foot-and-mouth disease | Coxsackievirus |
| Herpangina | Coxsackievirus |
| Hairy leukoplakia | Human herpesvirus 4 |
| ***Fungal*** | |
| Candidiasis (thrush) | *Candida albicans* |
| Denture stomatitis | *Candida albicans* |
| **Systemic Diseases with Oral Lesions** | |
| ***Bacterial*** | |
| Secondary syphilis | *Treponema pallidum* |
| ***Viral*** | |
| Chickenpox | Human herpesvirus 3 (varicella-zoster virus) |
| Infectious mononucleosis | Human herpesvirus 4 (Epstein-Barr virus) |
| **Other Diseases Spread by Respiratory or Oral Fluids** | |
| ***Bacterial*** | |
| Tuberculosis | *Mycobacterium tuberculosis* |
| Diphtheria | *Corynebacterium diphtheriae* |
| Pneumonia | *Streptococcus pneumoniae, Staphylococcus aureus, Mycoplasma pneumoniae, Chlamydia pneumoniae, Moraxella catarrhalis, Haemophilus influenzae* |
| Meningitis, sinusitis, conjunctivitis | *Haemophilus influenzae* type B |
| Meningitis | *Neisseria meningitidis* |
| Bronchitis | *Haemophilus influenzae, Moraxella catarrhalis* |
| ***Viral*** | |
| Common cold | Rhinoviruses and several others |
| Influenza | Influenza viruses |
| Bronchitis | Influenza A, parainfluenza virus, coronavirus |
| Pneumonia | Influenza virus, adenovirus, respiratory syncytial virus |
| Cytomegalovirus (CMV) disease | Cytomegalovirus |
| Infectious mononucleosis | Human herpesvirus 4 (Epstein-Barr virus) |
| Erythema infectiosum (fifth disease) | Human parvovirus B19 |
| Measles | Rubeola (measles) virus |
| Rubella | Rubella virus |
| Mumps | Mumps virus |
| Middle eastern respiratory syndrome (MERS) | Coronavirus (MERS-CoV) |
| COVID-19 | SARS-CoV-1 (Coronavirus) |
| Severe acute respiratory syndrome | SARS-CoV-2 |

Modified from Miller CH. *Infection Control and Management of Hazardous Materials for the Dental Team*. 6th ed. St Louis: Elsevier; 2018.

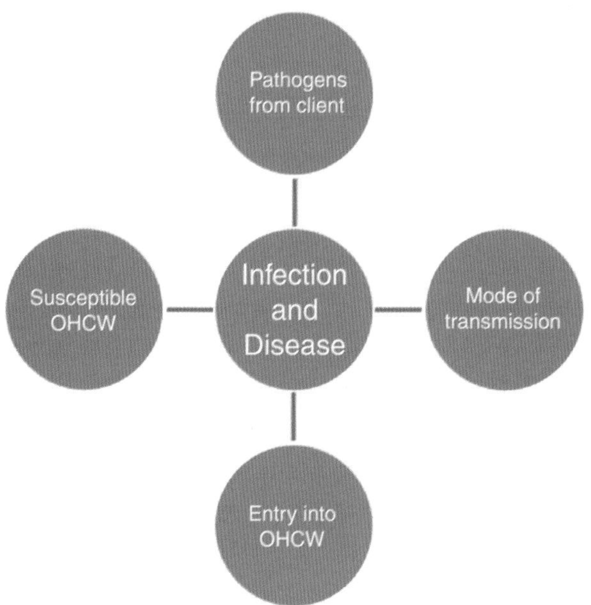


**Fig. 10.1** Factors related to infection and disease transfer. *OHCW,* Oral health care worker.

c. Engineering controls—devices that reduce the risk of exposure to potentially infectious materials (e.g., self-sheathing needles and instrument cassettes)
d. Personal protective equipment—items designed to protect DHCP from exposure to bloodborne and other pathogens (e.g., gloves, masks, N95 respirators, safety glasses, face shields, barrier gowns)
e. Standard precautions—treating all blood and bodily fluids (including secretions and excretions, except sweat), nonintact skin, and mucous membranes as potentially infectious in all patients
   (1) In the oral health care setting, saliva is an important source of contamination; although invisible, it is capable of containing infectious agents that can survive on surfaces for a long period
f. Transmission-based precautions—additional measures beyond standard precautions provided during urgent care to patients with certain diseases having multiple modes of transmission (e.g., tuberculosis [TB]); in this situation, care would be provided in a facility equipped with a respiratory protection program including an airborne infection isolation room (AIIR)
g. Sterilization—the destruction or removal of all microorganisms in or on an object
h. Work practice controls—procedures that reduce the chance of exposure to potentially infectious materials (e.g., using a one-handed technique to recap needles; maintaining a 14-inch to 18-inch working distance to reduce exposure to droplets; fulcruming one to four teeth away from tooth being treated)
i. DHCP-related controls
   (1) Maintaining a healthy lifestyle and immune status
   (2) Receiving recommended vaccinations
   (3) Obtain a baseline tuberculin skin test (TST)
   (4) Abiding by the recommended US Public Health Service work restrictions for DHCP in the case of certain infections and after exposure to some diseases (Box 10.1). Consult with department of public health, CDC, and healthcare provider for return to work guidance
j. Patient-related controls
   (1) Prophylactic antibiotic premedication to reduce the possibility of infection in individuals with systemic health-related conditions, especially those with immune deficiencies
   (2) Preprocedural rinse to decrease the microbial load in spatter and aerosols and to help protect against autogenous (self-derived) infection
   (3) Avoiding treatment of patients with known communicable illnesses (e.g., influenza) or contagious lesions (e.g., herpes)

**BOX 10.1 Summary of Work Restrictions for DHCP**

Conjunctivitis
Diarrheal disease
Enteroviral infection
Hepatitis A
Hepatitis B and HIV (consult expert review panel)
Herpes on the hands
Measles
Meningococcal infection
Mumps
Pediculosis
Pertussis
Rubella
Viral respiratory infection (acute, febrile) (example: COVID-19)
Active *Staphylococcus aureus* infection
Group A streptococcal infection
Active tuberculosis
Varicella (chickenpox)
Zoster (shingles)

From Guidelines for Infection Control in Dental Health-Care Facilities 2003, https://www.cdc.gov/mmwr/preview/mmwrhtml/rr5217a1.htm#tab1.

5. Infection control protocols are designed to reduce or prevent the spread of pathogens from:
   a. Patient to DHCP
   b. DHCP to patient
   c. Patient to patient
   d. Dental office to community, including families of DHCP
   e. Community to patient
6. Table 10.2 outlines the mechanisms of the spread and the prevention of diseases

## INFECTION CONTROL PROCEDURES FOR DENTAL HEALTH CARE PERSONNEL

A. Health history
   1. Obtain, review, and update patients' health histories at all visits. Obtain vital signs including blood pressure, pulse, respiration, and temperature
   2. Address specific questions related to present health status, physician care, hospitalizations, surgery, diseases, medications, allergies, current or chronic illness, review of major organ systems, and recent overseas travel

TABLE 10.2 **Mechanisms of Disease Spread and Prevention**

| Pathway of Cross-Contamination | Source of Microorganism | Mode of Disease Spread | Mechanism or Site of Entry into Body | Infection Control Procedure |
|---|---|---|---|---|
| Patient to DHCP | Patient's mouth | Direct contact | Through breaks in skin of dental team | Gloves and handwashing<br>Immunizations |
| | | Droplet infection | Inhalation by DHCP | Facemask/N95 respirator<br>Rubber dam<br>Preprocedural rinse<br>Face shield<br>Avoid aerosol-generating procedures (AGPs) |
| | | | Through breaks in skin of DHCP | Gloves and handwashing<br>Protective clothing<br>Face shield<br>Rubber dam<br>Preprocedural rinse |
| | | | Through mucosal surfaces of DHCP | Facemask/N95 respirator<br>Eyewear<br>Face shield<br>Rubber dam<br>Preprocedural rinse<br>Immunizations |
| | | Airborne infection | Inhalation by DHCP | Facemask/N95 respirator<br>Face shield<br>PPR<br>Rubber dam<br>Avoid aerosol-generating procedures (AGPs) |
| | | Indirect contact | Cuts, punctures, or needlesticks in DHCP | Needle safety and waste management<br>Utility gloves for cleanup<br>Ultrasonic cleaning rather than hand scrubbing<br>Instrument cassettes to reduce direct handling during cleaning<br>Antimicrobial holding solution<br>Antimicrobial cleaning solution |
| | | | Through breaks in skin of DHCP | Utility gloves for cleanup<br>Protective clothing<br>Immunizations |
| | Patient's skin lesions | Direct contact | Through breaks in skin of DHCP | Gloves and handwashing<br>Immunizations |
| DHCP to patient | DHCP hands (lesions or bleeding) | Direct contact | Through mucosal surfaces of patient | Gloves and handwashing<br>Care in handling sharp objects<br>Immunizations |
| | | Indirect contact | Bleeding on items used in patient's mouth | Gloves and handwashing<br>Instrument sterilization<br>Surface disinfection<br>Immunizations |
| | DHCP mouth (oral or respiratory fluids) | Droplet infection | Inhalation by patient | Facemask/N95 respirator<br>Face shield |
| | | | Through oral mucosal surfaces of patient | Facemask/N95 respirator<br>Face shield |
| Patient to patient in light of COVID-19 | Patient's mouth<br>Patient's nose and mouth, inhalation | Indirect contact (instruments, surfaces, hands) | Through oral mucosal surfaces of patient | Instrument and handpiece sterilization<br>High volume evacuation systems<br>Air filtration systems<br>Avoid aerosol generating procedures (AGPs)<br>Sterilization monitoring<br>Surface covers<br>Surface disinfection<br>Handwashing and proper gloving<br>Changing mask<br>Decontaminating protective eyewear<br>Changing protective clothing when needed<br>Use of sterile or clean supplies<br>Flushing dental unit water lines<br>Monitoring water line antiretraction valves<br>Use of disposable items<br>Use of one-way valves for slow-speed suction |

**TABLE 10.2 Mechanisms of Disease Spread and Prevention—cont'd**

| Pathway of Cross-Contamination | Source of Microorganism | Mode of Disease Spread | Mechanism or Site of Entry into Body | Infection Control Procedure |
|---|---|---|---|---|
| OHC setting to community | Preprocedural rinse (PPR)<br>Patient's mouth | Indirect contact | Anyone entering OHC setting may be exposed to COVID-19 including caregivers, interpreters, dental product/equipment representatives, repair and cleaning personnel, consultants and continuing education providers<br>Cuts, punctures, breaks in skin of dental laboratory worker, waste disposal, or laundry personnel | Waste management<br>Disinfection of impressions and appliances<br>Proper management of contaminated laundry<br>Handwashing |
| DHCP to DHCP's family | DHCP bodily fluids | Direct or indirect contact | Intimate contact | Immunization |
| Community to patient | Municipal water | Direct contact or airborne | Patient's mouth or lungs | Independent water reservoir<br>Periodically disinfecting inside of dental unit water lines<br>Quarantine/isolation<br>Use of water containing an approved antimicrobial agent<br>Filtering the water |

*DHCP,* Dental health care personnel; *OHC,* oral health care.
Modified from data from US Department of Labor. Occupational Safety and Health Administration. *Controlling Occupational Exposure to Bloodborne Pathogens.* Washington, DC: OSHA 2001, 3127 (revised).

3. Be aware that obtaining health histories will not identify all infectious patients; patients may suppress information purposely or unknowingly (many persons with hepatitis B virus [HBV], hepatitis C virus [HCV], and human immunodeficiency virus [HIV] are asymptomatic)
4. Health history may identify conditions requiring:
   a. Diagnostic evaluation and laboratory testing
   b. Medical consultations
   c. Prophylactic antibiotic premedication to reduce the incidence of autogenous infections, that is, conditions caused by introducing the microflora of patients into injured tissues (e.g., bacteremia, abscess)
5. The US Centers for Disease Control and Prevention (CDC) recommends conducting a TB risk assessment for an oral health care setting and then formulating a prevention program appropriate for its designated risk category; most dental settings will be low or very low risk

B. Immunizations are recommended for DHCP
1. Essential component of an infection control program
2. Most effective method to prevent contracting a vaccine-preventable disease
3. Immunizations are recommended for the following diseases, unless evidence of past infection and immunity: hepatitis A and B, varicella, influenza, measles, mumps, rubella, tetanus, diphtheria, pertussis, meningococcal disease, and COVID-19 vaccine when available
4. The US Occupational Safety and Health Administration (OSHA) policies regarding hepatitis B vaccination
   a. OSHA requires employers within 10 working days to make the hepatitis B vaccine available at no cost to employees who are or may be exposed by occupation to bloodborne pathogens
   b. Employers must provide information about the vaccine and ensure that all medical records concerning the vaccination are kept confidential
   c. Employees have the right to refuse vaccination but must read and sign an OSHA declination statement
   d. Employers cannot request employees be serologically prescreened before vaccination
5. Hepatitis B vaccine
   a. Three single-antigen vaccines available:
      (1) Recombivax HB (Merck & Co., Inc.)
      (2) Engerix-B (GlaxoSmithKline)
      (3) Heplisav-B (Dynavax Technologies)
   b. One combination-antigen (hepatitis A and B) vaccine available:
      (1) Twinrix (GlaxoSmithKline)
   c. Process
      (1) Serologic screening for antibodies to hepatitis B surface antigen (HBsAg) before vaccination is not recommended, unless infection is suspected
      (2) Pregnancy is not a contraindication for vaccination
      (3) A series of three injections in the deltoid muscle given at 0, 1, and 6 months
      (4) Seroconversion rates are 95% to 97% in healthy younger adults; lower rates (approximately 70%) in persons over 40 years old, smokers, overweight persons, and those receiving injections in the buttocks
      (5) Genetic factors may influence seroconversion rates
      (6) Testing for antibody (anti-HBsAg) is recommended after vaccination to ensure protection against HBV; testing should be conducted 1 to 2 months after the final injection
      (7) With successful seroconversion, protective antibodies have been sustained for at least 20 years
      (8) Failure to seroconvert requires a second series of three injections
      (9) Continued failure to seroconvert could signal chronic HBV infection in a person who is unable

**TABLE 10.3 Frequency of TB Testing**

| Risk classification | Frequency of testing |
|---|---|
| Low | Baseline; then test if TB exposure occurs |
| Medium | Baseline, then annually |
| Potential ongoing transmission | Baseline, then every 8–10 weeks until evidence of transmission has ceased |

Health care facilities have different TB testing requirements. Facilities should conduct staff TB testing based on risk classification.
From: https://www.cdc.gov/tb

to produce antibodies; nonresponders should be evaluated by a medical provider
(10) The CDC currently does not recommend a booster injection
(11) Minimal side effects of vaccine include injection site soreness, headache, and fever
(12) Individuals with allergies to yeast or iodine (vaccine preservatives) should consult their primary care provider before the vaccination
6. Recommended screenings for DHCP
a. Hepatitis B blood testing to determine anti-HBsAg titer
b. TB testing in health care workers
(1) Initial baseline testing upon hire: two-step testing with Mantoux TST or TB blood test
(a) Blood test: may be given to DHCP born outside the US that have been given a vaccine called Bacille Calmette-Guérin (BCG). BCG vaccine may cause a false positive TST. Blood tests are not affected by prior BCG vaccination and are not expected to give a false-positive result
(2) Annual or serial screening: determined by state regulations or risk assessment outcomes (Table 10.3)
c. Majority of dental offices are at low risk for DHCP contracting TB
(3) Oftentimes, a positive test indicates previous infection with *Mycobacterium tuberculosis* but not active disease
d. Anti-TB drug therapy advised to prevent future active disease
(4) Protocols should be in place to identify patients with active disease so they may be referred for treatment in a hospital-based facility
(5) TB is acquired by inhaling respiratory droplets from an infected person
(6) Only 10% of individuals infected will eventually develop disease
(7) TB has become problematic for certain populations, including the homeless, drug abusers, and persons infected with HIV
(8) Multiple drug-resistant TB has emerged in hospitalized and institutionalized individuals and those with AIDS

C. Hand hygiene
1. Extremely important disease prevention practice
2. Hands are a primary source of microorganisms capable of disease transmission
3. Rationale
a. Handwashing reduces both resident and transient flora on skin
(1) *Resident flora* are permanent residents that colonize several skin layers and cannot be completely removed; this type is less important and less likely to transmit disease than transient flora
(2) *Transient flora* contaminate hands when hands touch contaminated surfaces; this type colonizes the outer layers of skin, only survive for a limited time, and can be easily removed by routine handwashing
b. Protects patients and DHCP by reducing the spread of microorganisms and subsequent infections by the hands
c. Unwashed, contaminated hands can transfer microbes to sterile instruments, dental equipment, and environmental surfaces
4. Use of gloves is *not* a substitute for routine handwashing
5. Hands must be washed before gloves are put on to minimize organisms that can multiply rapidly when enclosed in a moist, warm environment; bacteria and yeast growth can cause skin irritation
6. Hands must be washed after removal of gloves because defects, tears, and punctures may occur in gloves, permitting microbes to be transferred to hands; this also helps remove glove powder, which contains latex protein and other glove chemicals that can elicit irritant contact dermatitis or an allergic reaction in sensitized individuals
7. Watches, bracelets, and rings must be removed to prevent harboring of microorganisms; also, rings may perforate glove materials
8. Nails must be kept short and clean and the cuticles well maintained; artificial nails and nail jewelry should not be worn, since research has implicated them in disease transmission in hospitals
9. Intact skin is the best protection against infection; this can be achieved by:
a. Minimizing trauma to hands (e.g., cuts, scrapes) while outside the dental setting
b. Protecting hands from drying and chapping during cold weather
c. Frequent use of lubricating hand lotions
(1) When at work, use hand lotion containing petroleum or oil emollients at the end of the day, because these ingredients can negatively affect the integrity of latex gloves
10. DHCP who have open or weeping lesions or dermatitis on hands should not provide patient care until the condition resolves, since dermatitis reduces the effectiveness of handwashing, and nonintact skin provides a portal of entry for microorganisms
11. Hand hygiene procedures for routine dental hygiene care include:
a. Vigorous lathering of hands using an interlacing finger motion with either antimicrobial or plain soap for at least 20 seconds
(1) Plain soap will remove soil and transient microbes
(2) Antimicrobial soap will remove or destroy transient microorganisms and reduce resident flora

(3) Disposable soap containers should not be refilled, and when empty should be discarded and replaced
(4) Soap dishes accumulate microorganisms and are not recommended
(5) Sinks and soap dispensers should be electronically operated or have foot controls; if not, paper towels should be used to turn off sink faucet

b. Rinsing with cool to lukewarm water while rubbing hands together for 10 seconds
c. Drying hands with single-use paper towels
d. Using alcohol-based hand sanitizers as an alternative to handwashing
(1) Used when no visible soil appears on the hands
(2) Have been shown to be effective, sometimes reducing bacterial counts more effectively than soap and water
(3) Most effective at inactivating microorganisms at 60% to 95% alcohol concentrations
(4) May increase the frequency of hand hygiene because of ease of use
(5) According to manufacturer's directions, place an adequate amount of alcohol-based hand sanitizer in hand and then vigorously rub hands until dry
(6) Alcohol-based hand sanitizers may cause dry skin (choose ones that contain emollients)

e. Washing hands between patients, before and after lunch, before and after restroom visits, or any time hands become contaminated
f. Maintaining asepsis by touching only sterile instruments or disinfected surfaces

12. For surgical procedures, use an antimicrobial soap with persistent or residual activity (inhibits growth and survival of microorganisms); chlorhexidine digluconate or triclosan

D. Personal protective equipment (PPE)
1. Protective barriers used to reduce exposure of mucous membranes, hands, and body of DHCP to microorganisms and also to prevent injury from chemicals and particles of debris
2. Used during patient treatment, laboratory procedures, operatory disinfection, and instrument processing
3. PPE includes gloves, masks, protective eyewear, and protective clothing
4. Sequence for donning PPE: protective clothing, then mask and eyewear, and finally, after handwashing, gloves
5. The employer is responsible for providing and maintaining appropriate PPE for employees
6. Gloves
a. The use of gloves provides a high level of protection for both DHCP and patients
(1) Prevents direct contact with microbes in the patient's mouth and on contaminated surfaces (bare hands often will have areas of nonintact skin providing portals of entry for pathogenic microbes)
(2) Prevents saliva and blood from being retained under fingernails; saliva and blood have been shown to persist for several days even with handwashing
(3) Protects against contact with disinfecting and cleaning chemicals and radiograph processing solutions
(4) Protects patients from the microorganisms on the hands of DHCP
(5) Examination gloves provide minimal protection against sharps injuries; utility gloves provide more protection; however, injuries still can occur

b. Risks associated with not routinely wearing gloves
(1) DHCP exposure to potentially infectious patient tissues and contaminated surfaces—most likely route by which DHCP have acquired HBV from patients
(2) Patient exposure to infectious agents originating from the DHCP
(a) Documented source of transmission of HBV from ungloved dentist to patients
(b) Documented case in which an ungloved hygienist transmitted herpes to 20 of her patients
(3) Skin irritation from contact with disinfecting chemicals
(4) Burns resulting from contact with hot items from sterilizer

c. Protocol for glove use
(1) Wear during intraoral procedures and when in contact with contaminated items or surfaces (e.g., contaminated laundry or waste)
(2) Exam gloves are single use and disposable (SUD)
(a) New gloves are worn for each patient
(b) When removing gloves, both pairs should be removed without contamination of hand, wrist, or arm
(c) Previously removed gloves should not be reworn but disposed of immediately after removal
(d) Removing only one contaminated glove and later regloving will result in contamination of DHCP skin
(3) If it is necessary to leave the chairside during patient care, remove gloves, and after hand hygiene, don a new pair on returning (prevents contamination of additional surfaces one may touch and also prevents contamination of the patient with microbes that already may be present on those surfaces)
(4) Ensure that gloves cover the cuff of a long-sleeved gown
(5) Change gloves during long appointments because defects in gloves increase with use beyond 60 minutes
(6) Change gloves when heavily soiled with blood
(7) Do not wash or disinfect gloves; may cause "wicking" or enhanced penetration of liquids through undetected defects in gloves
(8) Remove torn or punctured gloves as soon as possible; wash hands and don new gloves
(9) If using latex gloves, do not use petroleum or oil-based hand lotion or apply petroleum-based lubricants to patient's lips

d. Types of gloves—Table 10.4 outlines glove materials
(1) Nonsterile, ambidextrous gloves in sizes extra-small, small, medium, and large are adequate for most procedures; proper glove fit is important to ensure efficient instrumentation and to prevent hand fatigue and possibly carpal tunnel syndrome

**TABLE 10.4 Types of Gloves Used in Oral Health Care**

| Type | Material |
|---|---|
| Nonsterile (examination) gloves | Latex<br>Nitrile<br>Neoprene<br>Vinyl<br>Polyurethane<br>Styrene-based co-polymer<br>Butadiene methyl methacrylate |
| Sterile (surgical) gloves | Latex<br>Nitrile<br>Neoprene<br>Polyurethane<br>Styrene-based co-polymer<br>Synthetic polyisoprene |
| Utility gloves | Latex<br>Nitrile<br>Neoprene<br>Butyl rubber<br>Fluoroelastomer<br>Polyethylene and ethylene vinyl<br>Alcohol copolymer |
| Overgloves | Thin copolymer<br>Thin plastic ("food handlers") |

(2) Majority of DHCP are wearing latex-free gloves due to possible DHCP and patient latex allergy
(3) Sterile gloves are recommended for surgical procedures
(4) Use puncture-resistant and chemical-resistant utility gloves to prepare chemicals, handle contaminated instruments, and clean and disinfect surfaces
 (a) Utility gloves are reusable and can be disinfected or sterilized in an autoclave
 (b) Replace utility gloves when they show any signs of wear (e.g., cracks, punctures, discoloration)
(4) Overgloves are worn over treatment gloves to prevent cross-contamination of items and surfaces such as pens, charts, and drawers
(5) Heat-resistant gloves or oven mitts are worn when handling hot items (e.g., unloading sterilizers)

e. Dermatitis and latex allergy
 (1) Irritant contact dermatitis
  (a) Nonimmunologic (nonallergic) reaction of skin to chemicals used in glove manufacturing
  (b) Skin on hands becomes dry, red, itchy, and cracked
  (c) The condition is aggravated by soaps, not rinsing or drying hands completely, perspiration, or cornstarch powder
  (d) Most skin reactions from wearing gloves are caused by irritant contact dermatitis and are not true allergic reactions
 (2) Allergic contact dermatitis
  (a) Type IV, or delayed, hypersensitivity occurring within hours or days because of allergy to glove chemicals
  (b) Limited to area of contact, causing itching, redness, and vesicles to appear within 24 to 48 hours, followed by dry skin, fissures, and sores
  (c) Patch test identifies sensitivity to specific chemical
 (3) Latex allergy
  (a) Type I, or immediate, hypersensitivity within minutes or hours
  (b) Allergy to naturally occurring latex proteins
  (c) Symptoms: skin (hives, swelling, burning, tightness, itching, redness, tingling), lungs (asthma, wheezing, constriction, coughing, sneezing, rhinitis, angioedema), and other (nausea, vomiting, diarrhea, cramps, hypertension, tachycardia, shock)
  (d) Anaphylactic shock and death can occur with subsequent exposures to latex
  (e) High-risk individuals for latex allergy include: persons who have had multiple surgeries and persons with spina bifida, urogenital anomalies, spinal cord injuries, and allergies to bananas, kiwis, chestnuts, or avocados
  (f) Reductions in exposure to latex proteins are known to decrease sensitivity (important for DHCP to reduce their daily exposure to airborne latex proteins by wearing latex-free gloves)
  (g) The CDC indicates that DHCP need to be educated about skin problems that can occur with frequent hand hygiene and the use of gloves
  (h) Latex-free environment should be provided to patients and DHCP with a latex allergy
 (4) Procedures for management of persons with latex allergy
  (a) Include questions in health history appropriate for identifying possible latex allergy
  (b) Document latex allergy in health history record in a way that will ensure observation by DHCP
  (c) Schedule allergic patients for the first appointment of the day, when airborne latex proteins are at their lowest levels (still risky)
  (d) Ensure that DHCP uses latex-free gloves for treatment area preparation and for touching all items that will come in contact with the patient
  (e) Use latex-free gloves and dental materials during patient care

7. Masks
 a. Purpose
  (1) Worn to protect the mucous membranes of the nose and mouth from spatter of oral fluids
  (2) Provide a lesser degree of protection from inhalation of aerosol particles
   (a) Surgical masks will not provide protection from airborne infections (e.g., TB and severe acute respiratory syndrome [SARS])
   (b) The N-95 respirator is needed to protect against airborne infections, i.e., COVID-19
  (3) May provide some protection to patient from nasal or oral secretions of DHCP

b. Types of exam masks
   (1) Dome mask with elastic band
   (2) Tie-on or ear-loop mask
c. Composed of synthetic material that should filter at least 95% of small particles
   (1) National Institutes for Occupational Safety and Health (NIOSH) certifies three classes of filters (N-95%, R-99%, & P-99.97%)
   (2) American Society for Testing and Materials (ASTM International) has developed standard specifications for facemask materials in five areas (bacterial filtration efficiency, particulate filtration efficiency, fluid resistance, breathability, and flammability)
      (a) ASTM 1—low amounts of fluid exposure
      (b) ASTM 2—moderate amounts of fluid exposure
      (c) ASTM 3—heavy amounts of fluid exposure (should be used during ultrasonic instrumentation with a face shield when a N95 respirator is unavailable)
      (d) N95 respirator used with a face shield for aerosol generating procedures. Using an exam mask over N95 is not recommended because it can alter the fit and allow inhalation of aerosols around the edges. N95 requires medical clearance and fit test before use
d. Maximizing effectiveness and minimizing cross-contamination
   (1) N95 should be changed when it becomes moist/soiled. Reuse of N95s is only acceptable when there is a shortage of PPE
   (2) Change the mask if it becomes moist; moistness compromises its effectiveness by increasing the passage of unfiltered air around the edges of the mask and may wick contaminants through the mask. Refrain from twisting ear loops because this practice will cause gaping of mask and prevent it from fitting snugly against the face
   (3) Don a new mask every 20 to 30 minutes to maintain high filterability
   (4) Select mask that fits the face well and adjust it to fit snugly against the face, covering the nose and mouth to minimize leakage around the margins
   (5) Avoid touching the mask during the appointment
   (6) Keep the mask on after completing the procedure to reduce inhalation of aerosols
   (7) When removing the mask, handle it by its strings or elastic
   (8) Do not leave the mask on the head, dangling around neck, or in your pocket

8. Protective eyewear
   a. Purpose—protect the eye from microbial invasion, chemicals, physical projectiles, ultraviolet (UV) light, and lasers
   b. Risks for unprotected eyes
      (1) Conjunctivitis
      (2) Ocular herpes (can cause blindness)
      (3) Hepatitis B (eye as portal of entry)
      (4) Eye injury (physical or chemical)
   c. Types of eyewear
      (1) Regular glasses offer limited side or top protection and are not recommended
      (2) Safety glasses, goggles, or magnification loupes
         (a) Cover entire eye orbit (providing protection on all sides)
         (b) Goggles may be worn over prescription glasses
         (c) Are more shatter resistant than regular glasses
         (d) Provide minimal visual distortion
         (e) Are able to withstand disinfection (should be cleaned and disinfected between patients)
         (f) Should meet American National Standards Institute (ANSI) guidelines for spatter and impact protection
      (3) Face shields
         (a) Worn over eyewear for maximum protection
         (b) Should be chin-length and provide top and side protection
         (c) Masks should still be worn to reduce inhalation of aerosols
         (d) Combination eye shield with attached mask is available
         (e) Provide maximum coverage of face for high-spatter procedures (e.g., air polishing, power scaling)
         (f) Face shields made of thin plastic may have limited impact resistance
      (4) Protective eyewear should be provided to patients
         (a) Protection against damage from UV (curing) light and lasers
         (b) Protection against physical and chemical injury to the patient's eyes during treatment
         (c) Documented case where patient lost an eye due to anesthetic needle penetrating eye and resultant infection

9. Protective (barrier) clothing
   a. Purpose
      (1) Protects nonintact skin from contamination by microorganisms
      (2) Reduces the risk of bringing contaminants on unprotected clothing beyond dental setting
      (3) May protect patient from microorganisms on street clothing or may provide protection against disease transmission when soiled protective clothing is changed between patients (*fomites*—clothing and paper that can absorb and transmit infectious agents)
      (4) Microorganisms adhere to clothing; however, lack of evidence exists to support the extent to which barrier clothing protects against disease transmission
   b. Characteristics of protective clothing
      (1) Reusable or disposable. During pandemics or in other situations when the recommendation is to change gowns after each patient, disposable gowns are more convenient
      (2) Gowns, aprons, laboratory coats, or uniforms used as a covering for street clothing or scrub uniforms
      (3) High collar that fits closely around the neck
      (4) Long-sleeved garments with fitted cuffs allow gloves to extend over them for complete coverage

(5) Type of protective clothing required based on OSHA levels of exposure and procedures being performed
(a) Low level— soiled (laboratory coats)
(b) Medium level—splashed, splattered, or sprayed (fluid-resistant garments)
(c) High level—soaked (fluid-proof garments)
c. To maximize effectiveness and minimize cross-contamination
(1) Use fabric made of synthetic material, which is more fluid resistant
(2) Do not wear protective clothing outside treatment area (remove before going out [e.g., to lunch] or leaving the dental setting)
(3) Change protective clothing daily or when visibly soiled
(4) Avoid touching clothing during patient care and throughout the day
(5) Roll protective clothing inside out to minimize contact with exposed surface
10. Additional barrier protection used when cleaning or performing surgery
a. Plastic aprons or other fluid-proof garments
b. Head covers
c. Shoe covers
11. Laundering of reusable clothing
a. Laundered in the office following the manufacturer's instructions
b. Sent to a laundry service in a leak-proof bag labeled with the biohazard symbol
c. It is against OSHA regulations for DHCP to take contaminated protective clothing home for laundering

## ORAL HEALTH CARE ENVIRONMENT AND PROMOTION OF INFECTION CONTROL

A. Design and equipment selection emphasizes:
1. Smooth construction—eliminates knobs, hooks, and crevices
2. Design of patient chairs and operator stools that:
a. Minimize buttons and seams
b. Use vinyl upholstery instead of cloth
c. Provide foot-control operation
3. Avoidance of fabric-covered, coiled, or mechanically retracted tubings
4. Sink faucets and soap dispensers with foot or electronic controls
5. Paper towel dispenser designed to avoid touching hardware or electronically controlled
6. Plastic-lined waste containers recessed under cabinet, with opening on countertop
7. Surfaces that are compatible with disinfectants and detergents
8. Plastic laminate instead of wood for cabinets and countertops
9. Vinyl flooring and walls that are smooth and seamless
10. Carpeting or wallpaper not recommended
11. Dental unit water lines (DUWLs) that provide:
a. Antiretraction valves to prevent the aspiration of microorganisms into water lines
b. Equipment, devices, and treatments for DUWLs
(1) Filtration unit
(2) Sterile-water delivery system
(3) Flushing the lines with antimicrobial agents
(4) Scheduled testing and monitoring equipment (off-site lab or on-site kit)
(5) Periodic testing of water quality either on-site or off-site
12. Reduction of airborne microbes
a. Air circulation exchange system or single-room filtration units
b. Ventilation systems to control noxious sterilization and laboratory vapors
c. Prevention of recirculation of contaminated air or transport of microbes
d. Cooling and heating system filters that prevent transfer of microbes
13. Housekeeping surfaces are surfaces that are not contaminated by hands or equipment (e.g., walls, floors) and should be cleaned and disinfected routinely or when visibly soiled with detergents or low-level hospital disinfectants
a. Clean mops and cloths after use and allow to dry before reuse, or use single-use items
b. Periodically clean walls, blinds, and window treatments in patient care areas
c. Perform cleaning with a wet cloth or mop to prevent distribution of microorganism-laden dust particles
14. Keep treatment area free of unnecessary or seldom-used equipment and items

### Maintaining Asepsis in the Oral Health Care Environment

A. Items associated with oral health care are classified as:
1. Critical—instruments that penetrate oral soft tissue or bone, enter the bloodstream, or enter other sterile tissues of the mouth (e.g., curette); must be heat-sterilized or a SUD
2. Semicritical—items that come in contact with mucous membranes (used in the mouth) but will not penetrate soft tissue, contact bone, enter the bloodstream, or enter other sterile tissues of the mouth (e.g., radiographic positioning devices)
a. Preferably heat-sterilized or a SUD
b. If heat sensitive, decontaminate using a chemical sterilant or cover the device with a Food and Drug Administration (FDA)–approved barrier to prevent contamination (e.g., digital radiography sensors)
3. Noncritical—items that contact intact skin (e.g., blood pressure cuff)
a. If contamination is possible, cover the device to prevent contamination
b. If the device is contaminated, clean and disinfect
(1) If contaminated by blood, use intermediate-level disinfectant
(2) If not contaminated by blood, use low-level disinfectant
c. Noncritical items should be stored after use to prevent contamination
B. Maintaining asepsis with the use of chemicals and surface covers
1. Categories of disinfecting or sterilizing chemicals (Table 10.5)
a. Sterilant—destroys all microbes, including high numbers of bacterial spores

**TABLE 10.5 Categories of Disinfecting or Sterilizing Chemicals**

| Category | Definition | Examples | Use |
|---|---|---|---|
| Sterilant[a] | Destroys all microorganisms, including high numbers of bacterial spores | Glutaraldehyde, glutaraldehydephenate, hydrogen peroxide, hydrogen peroxide with peracetic acid, peracetic acid | Heat-sensitive reusable items: immersion only |
| High-level disinfectant[a] | Destroys all microorganisms, but not necessarily high numbers of bacterial spores | Glutaraldehyde, glutaraldehydephenate, hydrogen peroxide, hydrogen peroxide with peracetic acid, peracetic acid, orthophthaldehyde | Heat-sensitive reusable items: immersion only |
| Intermediate-level disinfectant | Destroys vegetative bacteria, most fungi, and most viruses; inactivates *Mycobacterium tuberculosis* var. *bovis* (is tuberculocidal) | Environmental Protection Agency (EPA)–registered hospital disinfectant[b] with label claim of tuberculocidal activity (e.g., chlorine-based products, phenolics, iodophors, quaternary ammonium compounds with alcohol, bromides) | Clinical contact surfaces, noncritical surfaces with visible blood |
| Low-level disinfectant | Destroys vegetative bacteria, some fungi, and some viruses; does not inactivate *M. tuberculosis* var. *bovis* (is *not* tuberculocidal) | EPA-registered hospital disinfectant with no label claim of tuberculocidal activity (e.g., quaternary ammonium compounds) | Housekeeping surfaces (e.g., floors, walls); noncritical surfaces without visible blood; clinical contact surfaces[c] |

[a]Some, but not all, of these products can serve as high-level disinfectants and sterilants, depending on the immersion time used.
[b]A hospital disinfectant is one that has been shown to kill *Staphylococcus aureus, Pseudomonas aeruginosa,* and *Salmonella choleraesuis.*
[c]The Centers for Disease Control and Prevention (CDC) indicates that low-level disinfectants can be used on clinical contact surfaces if the product has a label claim of killing human immunodeficiency virus (HIV) and hepatitis B virus (HBV) in addition to being an EPA-registered hospital disinfectant.
Modified from Centers for Disease Control and Prevention. Guidelines for infection control in dental health -care settings. *MMWR.* 2003; 52(RR-17):1–66.

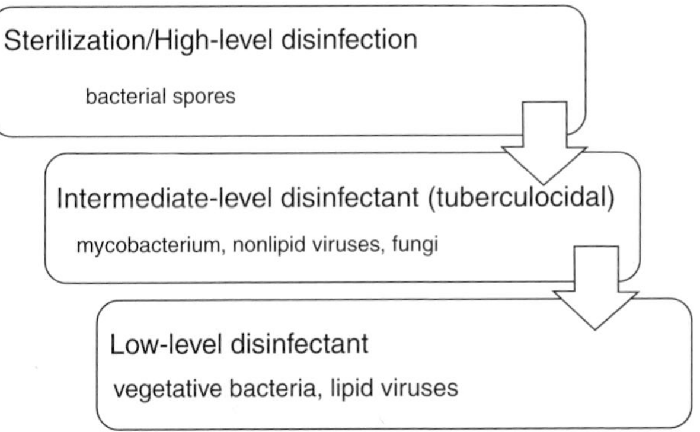


**Fig. 10.2** Decreasing order of resistance of microorganisms to germicidal chemicals. (Modified from Centers for Disease Control and Prevention. Guidelines for infection control in dental health-care settings. *MMWR.* 2003; 52(RR-17):1–68.)

b. High-level disinfectant—destroys all microorganisms but may not destroy bacterial spores (depending on contact time, can be either a disinfectant or sterilant)
c. Intermediate-level disinfectant—destroys vegetative bacteria, most fungi, and most viruses; inactivates *Mycobacterium tuberculosis* var. *bovis*
d. Low-level disinfectant—destroys vegetative bacteria, some fungi and viruses; does *not* inactivate *M. tuberculosis* var. *bovis* (Fig. 10.2)

C. Surface disinfection of clinical contact surfaces
1. Any surface that is touched by contaminated hands, instruments, devices, or other items during the provision of oral health care (e.g., light handles, dental equipment)
2. Identify and list surfaces that will be contaminated during treatment
3. Post the list in the treatment area to increase effectiveness and efficiency of decontamination procedures
4. Approaches to clinical contact surface asepsis
a. Avoid unnecessarily contaminating surfaces during treatment by:
(1) Using unit doses of materials to avoid contamination of multiple-use containers
(2) Using prearranged tray setups and cassettes containing a complete selection of instruments needed for a particular procedure
(3) Gathering the needed supplies and equipment at the beginning of treatment to eliminate the need to open drawers and cabinets or to leave the treatment area to retrieve supplies during patient care
(4) Having sterile pliers, overgloves, gauze, and paper towels available for use as barriers between contaminated gloved hands and uncontaminated objects (e.g., drawer handle, dental record)
b. Prevent contamination by using a surface cover or barrier protection
(1) Surface covers protect surfaces that are difficult to preclean adequately
(2) May be less time-consuming than precleaning or disinfecting surfaces before and after patient care
(3) Surface covers include clear plastic wrap, bags, and tubing
(4) May be placed using cleaned bare hands on cleaned and disinfected surfaces
(5) Should be placed to protect the entire surface and to ensure that the barrier protection will not come off when the surface is touched
(6) Reduce the use of chemicals that may stain or corrode and are hazardous to DHCP and the environment
c. Disinfection of surfaces not covered by barriers
(1) Requires purchase and proper use of disinfecting chemicals
(2) Chemical use requires that Safety Data Sheets (SDSs) be filed on site and that DHCP be provided

information and training on the hazards and proper use of chemicals
   (3) Disinfection is best reserved for surfaces that are difficult to cover, smooth surfaces, and those not involving electricity
   d. A dual approach consisting of both barrier protection and disinfection with chemicals is most often used in oral health care settings
5. Clinical contact surfaces to be covered or disinfected
   a. Mobile cart, master control unit, countertop, and radiographic equipment
   b. Air/water syringe, high-volume and low-volume evacuators (parts of these may be sterilized or disposable, which is preferred because these items come in contact with mucous membranes)
   c. Hoses, tubing, and controls attached to handpieces
   d. Supports for handpieces, air/water syringe, and suction devices
   e. Chairs, including switches and levers
   f. Control switches
   g. Light handles
   h. Faucet handles and soap dispenser (if manually operated)
   i. Instrument tray (if it cannot be sterilized)
   j. Stethoscope earpieces
   k. Floss dispenser, hand mirror, pens, pencils
   l. Chairside computers and keyboards
   m. Phones, intercoms
6. Factors influencing effectiveness of surface disinfection with chemicals
   a. Numbers and types of organisms present; some organisms have a higher resistance to destruction by chemicals (e.g., *Mycobacterium* species)
   b. Amount of *bioburden* (blood, saliva, and microorganisms)
      (1) Organic materials in blood and saliva insulate microorganisms from chemicals
      (2) May partially inhibit the active ingredient in the disinfectant
   c. Selection of an Environmental Protection Agency (EPA)–registered disinfectant that is tuberculocidal (sterilant or high-level disinfectant should *not* be used for clinical contact surfaces)
   d. Use of a water-based disinfectant is reported to clean organic material better than alcohol-based disinfectants
   e. Performing procedures carefully and following manufacturer's instructions by using appropriate disinfectant concentration, use life, and contact time
      (1) Do not store gauze squares or other materials moistened in disinfectant; instead, wet material before use
      (2) If using container of disinfectant towelettes, keep lid closed to prevent drying
   f. Clean surfaces with a combination of a detergent and a disinfectant to maximize the removal of bioburden before the disinfection step
      (1) The detergent or disinfectant used for the cleaning step must contain a surfactant
         (a) Surfactant—an agent that loosens, emulsifies, and holds soil in suspension, allowing for easier removal of debris and for more thorough cleaning
      (2) An advantage to using a combination agent is that a chemical disinfectant starts the killing process during the cleaning step and reduces the opportunity for contaminants to spread to other surfaces
7. Cleaning or disinfection technique for clinical contact surfaces
   a. Exercise care when using disinfectants, and wear PPE, including utility gloves
      (1) To prevent irritation or injury to eyes, mucous membranes, and skin
      (2) To avoid breathing in noxious vapors
   b. Step 1—clean; spray the detergent or disinfectant, or apply with a premoistened wipe
   c. Step 2—wipe; vigorously wipe surfaces with a paper towel or premoistened wipe to remove stuck-on debris
   d. Step 3—reapply the disinfectant by spraying or applying with premoistened wipe
      (1) Leave surfaces undisturbed for a specified contact time, usually 10 minutes
      (2) Wipe any remaining wet areas with a paper towel
8. Chemical disinfectants for surface disinfection (Table 10.6)—selection criteria
   a. EPA-registered intermediate-level disinfectant that is tuberculocidal (kills *M. tuberculosis* var. *bovis*)
   b. Effective within 10 minutes or less

**TABLE 10.6 Chemical Agents for Surface Disinfection**

| Chemical Classification | Advantages | Disadvantages |
|---|---|---|
| Chlorines | Rapid acting<br>Broad spectrum<br>Economical | Prepare solution daily<br>Diminished activity by organic matter<br>Corrosive<br>Strong odor |
| Iodophors | Broad spectrum<br>Few reactions<br>Residual biocidal activity | Unstable at high temperatures<br>Dilution and contact time critical<br>Prepare solution daily<br>Discoloration of some surfaces<br>Inactivated by hard water |
| Synthetic phenolics | Broad spectrum<br>Residual biocidal activity<br>Compatible with most metals | Degrades certain types of plastic over time<br>Difficult to rinse<br>Film accumulation<br>Alcohol-based products are only fair to poor in cleaning ability |
| Dual or synergized quaternaries | Broad spectrum<br>Contains detergent for cleaning | Easily inactivated by anionic detergents and organic matter<br>Damaging to some materials |
| Oxidizers | Broad spectrum, Fast acting, Breaks down to nonhazardous components | Corrosive to some materials |

c. Does not have an offensive odor
d. Reasonable cost
e. Provides persistent or residual effect on treated surfaces
f. Retains stability and effectiveness in the presence of bioburden, preferably water-based
g. Good penetrating and cleaning ability
h. Compatible with and innocuous to equipment and clinical surfaces (consult product manufacturer for recommendations)
i. The CDC does not recommend alcohol, household bleach, or early-generation quaternary ammonium compounds as surface disinfectants

D. Dental unit water line asepsis
1. High concentrations of bacteria have been found in untreated DUWLs (e.g., power instrumentation, air-polishing units, high-speed handpieces, air/water syringes)
a. Municipal water entering the dental unit is not sterile and contains 0 to 500 colony-forming units per milliliter (CFU/mL) of heterotrophic bacteria
b. Water exiting untreated DUWLs may contain more than 100,000 CFU/mL
(1) Consists of waterborne bacteria of low pathogenicity or opportunistic pathogens, which pose the greatest risk to immunocompromised individuals
(2) Organisms of greatest concern are *Pseudomonas, Legionella,* and *Mycobacterium* species
2. Microorganisms attach to and accumulate on the inside of the water line tubing, creating biofilm colonies (an organized, protected, and highly resistant colony of live microorganisms attached to a surface) (see the section on "Bacterial Dental Biofilm" in Chapter 14); formation of biofilm:
a. Biofilm includes naturally occurring waterborne bacteria and may include oral microbes from previously treated patients
b. Stagnation of water and small-diameter tubing in DUWLs encourages biofilm formation
c. Incoming water brings a continuous source of nutrients to bacteria
d. As water flows past the biofilm in the water line, it picks up detached bacteria before exiting through dental equipment
3. Dental unit water and infection control
a. No epidemiologic evidence of a widespread public health problem caused by dental unit water
(1) In 2011, one confirmed case of an 82-year-old woman in Italy who died after contracting Legionnaires' disease from aspirating *Legionella*-contaminated dental unit water at her dental office
(2) In 2015 and 2016, pediatric patients developed infections after having pulpotomies with DUWLs contaminated with *M. abscessus*—a common inhabitant of water, soil, and dust
b. Using water that does not meet the standards for drinking water (potable) increases patient and DHCP exposure to microorganisms (immunocompromised individuals most at risk)
c. CDC recommendations for potable water is no more than 500 CFU/mL of aerobic mesophilic heterotrophic bacteria
d. Oral health care facility water should meet the CDC standard for routine dental care
e. Dental unit water from a municipal supply should not be used for oral surgery or in the treatment of immunocompromised persons (sterile water delivery systems must be used)
f. Boil water notices in the community
(1) Do not use dental unit or faucet water until the notice is lifted
(2) After the notice is lifted, flush all water lines for 1 to 5 minutes, and disinfect them following manufacturer's recommendations
4. Improving the quality of dental unit water
a. Routinely check antiretraction valves (valves can become stuck in the open position with age)
b. Flush water lines for 3 to 5 minutes at the beginning of each day; flush for 30 seconds between patients
(1) Flushing does not remove biofilm but may temporarily reduce planktonic (free-floating) microbes
(2) Flushing may help remove patient materials that have entered the turbine, air, and water lines
c. Use an independent water reservoir—a bottle that supplies treated water to the dental unit
d. Chemical treatment of DUWLs is still necessary to control biofilm formation, even when an independent water reservoir is used
e. Test periodically quality of water as needed to ensure compliance

## Maintaining the Treatment Area During Patient Care

A. Spatter and aerosol management to reduce the number of microorganisms escaping from the source
1. Use a preprocedural, antimicrobial rinse containing chlorhexidine, diluted hydrogen peroxide, essential oils, or iodophor to reduce microbial counts in spatter and aerosols
2. Use air and water separately instead of a combination spray
3. High-volume evacuation (HVE) is strongly recommended for aerosol-generating procedures. A wide variety of HVE systems are available
a. When using the saliva ejector without a one-way valve, do not allow the patient to close the lips around the tip since previously suctioned fluids might enter a patient's mouth by reverse flow in the vacuum line
b. Use one-way valve attached to saliva ejector to prevent backflow of oral fluids
4. Use a rubber dam to reduce spatter and aerosols and to lessen the chance of a patient's saliva retracting into the dental handpiece and the air/water syringe

B. Reducing the risk of contamination and disease transmission
1. Limit the areas of contamination; use overgloves when touching clinical contact surfaces
2. Disinfect anything not covered with barriers when touched by contaminated hands
3. Avoid accessing drawers, cabinets, and other storage areas with contaminated gloves; ask for assistance if additional supplies are needed

4. Protect dental records from contamination
   a. Ask for the help of a hygiene assistant or other personnel to record
   b. Use overgloves
   c. Record data on audio, and make manual entries in patient record after glove removal
   d. Generate patient record with voice-activated computer software
5. Eating, drinking, smoking, applying of cosmetics or lip balm, and handling of contact lenses are prohibited in patient care areas
6. Food and drink cannot be stored in refrigerators, freezers, or cabinets or on shelves and countertops where blood or saliva is present

C. Waste disposal during treatment
1. Immediately discard blood-soaked items in a small biohazard bag taped to the mobile cart or the cabinet
2. Do not allow contaminated waste to accumulate on trays (e.g., exam gloves)

D. Precautions and care in handling syringes or sharp instruments
1. Needlestick injuries are a major cause of disease transmission to health care personnel
   a. Never permit "sharps" to be directed toward the body
   b. Do not allow uncovered needles to remain on tray
   c. Never recap a needle using a two-handed technique
      (1) Using one hand, the cap is scooped up from the tray
      (2) Use the sheath holder
      (3) Use self-sheathing disposable needles
   d. Never bend, break, or otherwise manipulate a needle
   e. DHCP giving an injection should appropriately recap the needle to eliminate the danger of passing an uncovered needle to another worker for recapping
   f. Sharps containers should be located in each treatment area
2. Instrument sharpening
   a. Sharpening contaminated instruments poses risk of disease transmission
      (1) Avoid sharpening during a procedure
      (2) Instead, include duplicates of most-used instruments in the cassette for difficult cases
   b. The ideal method involves sharpening sterile instruments and then sterilizing again before use
3. Avoid injury with contaminated instruments during patient care (i.e., curettes and scalers)
   a. Avoid fulcruming on the same tooth being treated
   b. Never wipe instruments on gauze held in your hand or wrapped around your finger
   c. Instruments should be organized and lying flat (instruments should not be on top of each other, sticking up, or balancing crosswise on the edges of cassettes)
   d. Never grab instruments by the working end
   e. Avoid holding more than one instrument in each hand
   f. Do not adjust dental light while holding an instrument

E. Exposure incident protocol (Box 10.2)
1. Includes all needlesticks, puncture wounds, cuts, and scrapes with contaminated instruments and all nonintact skin and mucous membrane exposure to blood and saliva
   a. In DHCP, 90% of exposures result from sharps penetrating the hands and fingers
2. Immediately wash the injured area with antimicrobial soap and water or flush with water for a mucous membrane exposure (eye)
3. Inform the employer about the incident
4. If the source individual can be identified, request his or her consent for blood testing for HBV, HCV, and HIV as soon as possible (if the source individual's disease status is not already known)
5. Results of the source individual's tests are confidential and are revealed only to the exposed employee, not to the employer
6. The employer is responsible for providing to the exposed employee laboratory testing for HBV, HCV, and HIV (30-minute rapid test available), medical evaluation, and counseling by a preselected, qualified, licensed health care provider (HCP)
7. HCP should be familiar with most current United States Public Health Service recommendations for testing and postexposure prophylaxis (PEP)
8. Within 2 hours of exposure, the employee should seek medical care allowing PEP, if indicated, which offers the greatest chance of success in preventing disease transmission (seroconversion)
   a. Seroconversion depends on dose of blood transferred, titer of virus (viral load), resistant viral strain, depth of injury, and host factors
   b. PEP may reduce the risk of infection by 80%
9. If the employee declines testing, a blood sample from the employee may be preserved for 90 days in case the employee later consents to testing
10. The HCP informs the employee about both his or her own test results and the source patient's test results and of any conditions that require further evaluation and treatment
11. The employer receives a written report from the HCP confirming that the employee was tested, informed of results, and counseled if further evaluation or treatment was needed

**BOX 10.2 Recommendations for Contents of the Occupational Exposure Report**

Date and time of exposure

Details of the procedure being performed, including when and how the exposure occurred
- If related to a sharps device, the type and brand of device and how and when in the course of handling the device the exposure occurred

Details of the exposure, including the type and amount of fluid or material and the severity of exposure; for example:
- For a percutaneous exposure, depth of injury and whether fluid was injected
- For a skin or mucous membrane exposure, the estimated volume of material and the condition of the skin (e.g., chapped, abraded, intact)

Details about the exposure source; for example:
- Whether the source material contained hepatitis B virus (HBV), hepatitis C virus (HCV), or human immunodeficiency virus (HIV)
- If the source is HIV-infected, the stage of disease, history of antiretroviral therapy, viral load, and antiretroviral resistance information, if known

Details about the exposed person (e.g., hepatitis B vaccination and vaccine response status)

Details about counseling, postexposure management, and follow-up

a. Report notes if hepatitis B vaccine was administered
b. Report does *not* include test results, diagnoses, or treatment because this information is confidential and protected employee health information

F. Prevention of disease transmission during radiographic procedures
1. Although radiographic procedures are generally noninvasive, the potential for disease transmission does exist
2. The use of barriers on equipment will prevent contamination and promote efficiency
   a. Plastic bag to cover position-indicating device (PID), tubehead, and swivel arms
   b. Plastic cover for exposure control switch
   c. Cover for headrest and chair controls
   d. FDA-approved plastic barrier for digital sensor
   e. Plastic barrier underneath exposed films and on countertop
3. If contamination occurs, disinfect
   a. Use EPA-registered intermediate-level disinfectant
   b. Disinfect all touched surfaces that are unprotected by barriers
   c. Do not directly spray disinfectant on the control panel because it has electrical components
   d. Follow manufacturer's directions for digital sensors (most cannot be disinfected)
4. Radiographic film holders—use reusable film holders that can be heat-sterilized, or use disposable items (SUDs)
5. Radiographic film options
   a. Digital radiographs (sensor—immediate image with no processing necessary; phosphor plates (PSP) require nonchemical processing)
   b. Film in plastic covering or pouch (best option when using film)
   c. Film without plastic covering (during processing, special handling is necessary when removing the film from the packet to avoid contaminating the film)
6. Aseptic procedure for imaging and processing dental radiographs in plastic pouches
   a. Drape the patient with lead apron and thyroid shield, and position the patient's bib to act as a barrier; if shields become contaminated, disinfect with an intermediate-level disinfectant
   b. Wear PPE
   c. After exposing the film, drop it into a disposable cup
   d. Remove the plastic pouches, and drop the film packet into a new cup without contaminating the film packet or the outside of the cup
   e. Remove gloves, and wash hands before transporting the film to the processing area
   f. With ungloved hands, unwrap the film and put it into the automatic processor
7. Aseptic procedure for processing dental radiographs without plastic covering
   a. After exposure, contaminated film should be placed in a plastic cup without contaminating the outside of the cup
   b. Don a new pair of gloves before transporting the film to the darkroom
   c. Open the film packet, and drop the film on a paper towel (proceed carefully to avoid contaminating the film)
   d. Remove gloves, wash hands, and with bare hands, feed the film into the automatic processor
8. Aseptic technique for processing phosphor plate covered with disposable barrier
   a. After exposure, contaminated plates should be placed in a cup
   b. Don a new pair of gloves before transporting cup to PSP processor
   c. Tear disposable barrier and squeeze plate into open PSP box without contaminating inside of box
   d. Dispose of contaminated barriers and gloves
   e. Place plates into processor
   f. After plates have exited processor, don gloves and replace barriers

G. Infection control for the dental laboratory
1. Prevention of disease transmission between the treatment area and the dental laboratory
2. OSHA regulations include measures for the protection of dental laboratory personnel from bloodborne pathogens
3. Impression materials, prostheses, and appliances are exposed to oral microflora
4. Protective attire and barrier techniques
   a. When performing laboratory procedures, PPE should be worn; use caution with lathes because gloves can become caught and cause injury
   b. Masks and eyewear protect against chemicals, aerosols, spatter, and projectiles
5. Preparation of materials and transport to laboratory
   a. Clean and disinfect impressions, prostheses, and casts before transport
   b. Always disinfect prostheses before sending them to another location or returning to the patient
   c. Use new packing material every time the prosthesis is transported between the laboratory and the oral health care facility to prevent contamination of shipping materials
   d. Communicate the infection control protocol to the laboratory and DHCP
6. Minimizing contamination of common areas in laboratory
   a. Use paper covers on countertops
   b. Place plastic barriers on frequently touched areas
   c. Procedures for using the lathe
      (1) Use fresh pumice each time
      (2) Use disposable trays
      (3) Use sterile or disposable ragwheels (polishing device made of cloth)
7. Use a shielding device and air-suction motor with the polishing lathe, model trimmer, or grinding bench to minimize aerosol spray
8. An EPA-registered intermediate-level disinfectant should be used to disinfect contaminated laboratory materials (e.g., impressions, fixed and removable prostheses, retainers, crowns)

a. Spray the chemical or, preferably, immerse the material in the chemical using minimal effective exposure time (at least 15 minutes) to prevent damage to the material
b. Consult with the manufacturer to determine which chemicals are compatible with the item to be disinfected and the immersion time required

9. Professional cleaning of removable prostheses
   a. Use of denture-cleaning solutions is *not* a substitute for disinfection
   b. To prevent microbial contamination:
      (1) Use resealable plastic bags
      (2) Do not reuse the denture-cleaning solution or plastic bags
      (3) Place sealed bags in a disinfected beaker in the ultrasonic unit
      (4) Sterilize or dispose of the equipment used in cleaning (e.g., brushes)
   c. Rinse the prosthesis with water to remove any residual chemical, and place it in a mouthwash solution to ensure a pleasant taste for the patient

## Maintaining the Oral Health Care Environment After Patient Care

A. Decontamination of the treatment area
   1. Wear PPE, including utility gloves
   2. Seal and transport the biohazard bag (that is taped to the mobile cart) containing blood-soaked gauze to the biohazard waste container
   3. Deliver contaminated instruments and cassettes to the instrument-processing area on a tray or in a puncture-resistant container
   4. Remove surface barriers carefully to avoid contamination of the surfaces underneath, and dispose of in a trash receptacle
   5. Remove and dispose of SUDs (air/water syringe tip, saliva ejector)
   6. Using air/water syringe, flush low-volume and high-volume (if used) evacuator tubing for 30 seconds
   7. Flush all other water lines for 30 seconds between patients (ultrasonic unit)
   8. If instrument sterilization is delayed, place the instruments in a holding solution to prevent bioburden from drying on the instruments
   9. At the end of the workday, flush high-volume and low-volume evacuator tubing with a cleaning and disinfecting solution; at least weekly, clean the trap of the evacuation system, or preferably, replace with a disposable trap

B. Regulated infectious waste
   1. Medical waste that has the potential for disease transmission and requires special handling and disposal
   2. OSHA regulates the handling of infectious waste; EPA regulates the disposal of infectious waste for three categories:
      a. Sharps (e.g., needles, scalpel blades, instruments)
      b. Tissue and extracted teeth; CDC allows extracted teeth to be returned to the patient

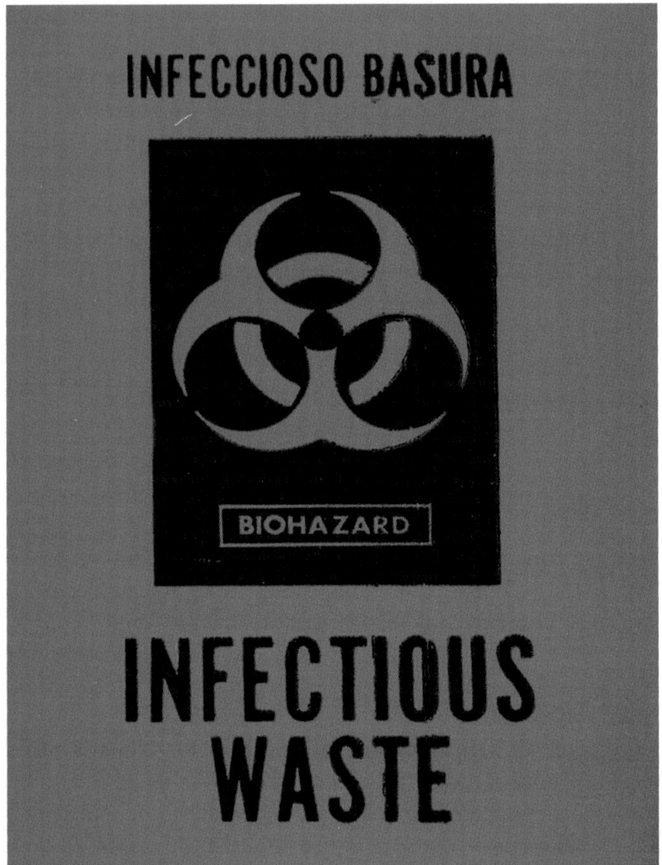


**Fig. 10.3** Biohazard symbol. (From Kelly R. *Mosby's Textbook for Long-Term Care Nursing Assistants.* 7th ed. St Louis: Elsevier; 2014.)

      c. Blood, items soaked or caked with blood, or items that could release potentially infectious materials when compressed; CDC considers saliva as infectious material but not as regulated medical waste
   3. Unregulated medical waste—solid waste that is generated, including all disposable items other than sharps, tissues, extracted teeth, and blood-soaked items (e.g., gloves, saliva ejectors, cups, surface barriers); unregulated medical waste may be potentially infectious; however, it is unregulated and may be disposed of as common trash unless restricted by state and local laws
   4. Contact state and local governments for regulations on the disposal of regulated and unregulated medical waste

C. Waste management
   1. Line trash receptacles with plastic bags
   2. Sharps containers should be placed in each treatment area

D. Waste disposal
   1. Regulated infectious waste must be separated from other waste, put in a color-coded ("red bagged") container, and labeled with the biohazard symbol (Fig. 10.3)
      a. Sharps must be in a closed, leakproof, and puncture-resistant sharps container
      b. Nonsharp items must be placed in a leakproof container (e.g., biohazard bag)
   2. Disposal options

a. Sterilization on-site and disposal according to local and state regulations
(1) Do not process instruments and waste in same load
(2) Properly perform biologic monitoring during sterilization
(3) Extracted teeth, to be used for educational purposes, with amalgam restorations must not be heat-sterilized because this will generate toxic vapors; use a chemical sterilant instead; teeth without restorations must be heat-sterilized
b. Hazardous waste removal service by an EPA-approved waste hauler
(1) The oral health care facility is ultimately responsible for the proper disposal of infectious waste; therefore the waste hauler's credentials should be checked carefully
(2) A manifest should be provided by the waste hauler indicating the method by which the waste was treated and its final disposal site

E. Instrument processing
1. Organization of sterilization area
a. For efficiency, the instrument-processing area should be centrally located
b. The area is designed to allow for linear progression of instrument processing and for the separation of contaminated and clean or sterile items
c. The area should be divided into three designated areas:
(1) Decontamination area—receiving area for contaminated instruments (soaking and waste disposal), ultrasonic cleaning, rinsing, and drying
(2) Packaging area—instruments are arranged in sets; chemical and biologic indicators (BIs) are added; instruments are wrapped or bagged, sealed, and labeled
(3) Sterilization and storage area—instruments are processed and stored
2. Decontamination area procedures
a. Use PPE, including utility gloves
b. If a delay occurs before decontamination, soak instruments in a holding solution to prevent the drying of saliva and blood
(1) Extended soaking is not recommended because it can damage the instruments
(2) The holding solution can be water, enzyme solution, heparin solution (dissolves blood), or detergent
c. Cleaning instruments in an ultrasonic unit or instrument washer is an important step; otherwise, stuck-on blood or other organic material will remain on the instruments even after sterilization (instruments with adhered debris are not sterile)
d. Ultrasonic cleaning
(1) Vibrations dislodge and dissolve organic material
(2) The safest and most efficacious method of cleaning
(3) Eliminates the need for hand scrubbing and potential for injury with contaminated instruments
(4) Procedure for using ultrasonic instrument cleaner
(a) Use solution specifically designed for ultrasonic cleaners; may contain antimicrobial properties
(b) Time—4 to 16 minutes, depending on the unit, the instruments, and the amount of material on the instruments (instruments in cassettes require longer exposure time)
(c) Keep the unit covered to prevent exposure to aerosols
(d) Rinse the instruments, and let excess water drain from the cassettes
(e) Open cassette and inspect instruments to ensure absence of debris
(f) Drain ultrasonic solution, disinfect unit, and replace with new solution daily
(g) Periodically test the unit (aluminum foil test)
e. Manual scrubbing technique—used rarely when bioburden remains on instruments or when ultrasonic exposure would cause damage to instruments or devices (ultrasonic inserts, some handpieces)
(1) Scrub with a long-handled, stiff brush; wear utility gloves
(2) Scrub the item, holding it low in the sink to minimize spatter
(3) Manual scrubbing is not advised because it poses an increased risk for injury
f. Asepsis for high-speed and low-speed dental handpieces
(1) Refer to the manufacturer's instructions for cleaning, lubrication, and sterilization
(2) Some handpieces can be cleaned ultrasonically; all handpieces must be able to withstand heat sterilization and must be sterilized before reuse
(3) Flush the water lines of high-speed handpieces for 30 seconds after use
g. Prophylaxis angles; should be heat-sterilized or SUDs; consult the manufacturer's instructions for cleaning, lubrication, and sterilization
3. Packaging area procedures
a. Surgical and hinged instruments
(1) Instruments can be dipped in surgical milk to prevent rusting and to lubricate hinged instruments (rusted instruments should be discarded and never used because sterility of these instruments cannot be ensured)
(2) Hinged instruments should be opened before packaging
b. The instruments to be bagged should be dry to avoid penetrating the packaging, and excess moisture can interfere with sterilization
c. Packaging materials vary according to the type of sterilization method (Table 10.7)

TABLE 10.7 **Comparison of Heat Sterilization Methods**

| Method | Sterilizing Conditions[a] | Packaging Materials | Advantages | Precautions |
|---|---|---|---|---|
| Steam Autoclave | | Paper wrap<br>Nylon "plastic" tubing | Time-efficient<br>Good penetration | No closed containers<br>Damage to plastic and rubber |
| Standard cycles | 20 to 30 minutes at 250°F | Paper or plastic peel pouches<br>Thin cloth<br>Wrapped, perforated cassettes | | Non–stainless steel items corrode<br>Use of hard water may leave deposits<br>Items may be wet after cycle |
| Flash cycles | 3 to 10 minutes at 273°F | No packaging (unwrapped) | Quick turn-around | Unwrapped items quickly contaminated after processing |
| Unsaturated chemical vapor | 20 minutes at 270°F | Paper wrap<br>Paper or plastic peel pouches<br>Wrapped, perforated cassettes | Time-efficient<br>No corrosion<br>Items dry quickly after cycle | No closed containers<br>Damage to plastic and rubber<br>Must use special solution<br>Predry instruments<br>Provide adequate ventilation<br>Cannot sterilize liquids<br>No cloth wrap (absorbs too much chemical vapor) |
| Dry heat | 60 to 120 minutes at 320°F | Paper wrap | No corrosion | Some paper may get charred<br>Predry instruments |
| Oven type (static-air) | | Appropriate nylon "plastic" tubing<br>Closed containers<br>Wrapped, perforated cassettes | Can use closed containers[b]<br>Low-cost<br>Items are dry after cycle | Long sterilization time (oven type)<br>Damage to plastic and rubber<br>Door cannot be opened during cycle<br>Cannot sterilize liquids |
| Rapid heat transfer (forced air) | 12 minutes at 375°F (wrapped)<br>6 minutes at 375°F (unwrapped) | Aluminum foil[c] | No corrosion<br>Short cycle<br>Items are dry after cycle | Unwrapped items quickly contaminated after processing |

[a]These conditions do not include warm-up or cool-down time, and they may vary, depending on the contents and volume of the load and brand of the sterilizer.
[b]Biologic indicator must be used to ensure sterility.
[c]Tears or punctures easily.
Modified from Miller CH. *Infection Control and the Management of Hazardous Materials for the Dental Team*. 6th ed. St. Louis: Elsevier; 2018.

d. Packaging materials include plastic or paper pouches, plastic tubing, cassettes, or trays to be wrapped with paper or cloth, sealed with appropriate tape, dated, and labeled with the date, type of instrument setup, and sterilizer used (in the case of more than one sterilizer)
   (1) With more than one sterilizer in use, if one was to malfunction, it would be important to identify the packages that had been processed in that sterilizer
e. To maintain package integrity, do not seal the package using staples, pins, or paper clips
f. Packages should be folded on the perforation (autoclave bags) and tightly sealed to eliminate gaps
g. Autoclave bags are designed for single use because of pores in the paper that open during sterilization, allowing steam to penetrate, and then close on cooling to inhibit microbes from entering into package
h. The packaging materials used must NOT:
   (1) Melt or char
   (2) Prevent the sterilizing agent from penetrating
   (3) Be easily torn by sharp instruments
i. Instruments should be packaged loosely to allow for maximum contact with steam or chemical vapors; overloaded packages can lead to incomplete sterilization
j. Biologic and chemical indicators are added during packaging procedures

4. Sterilization area procedures
5. Sterilization methods (see Table 10.7)
   a. Steam (moist heat under pressure) sterilization—autoclave
      (1) Types based on how air is removed the chamber
         (a) Gravity displacement
         (b) Vacuum pump (type B sterilizer)—perform air removal test (Bowie-Dick) at the beginning of each day to ensure complete air removal from the chamber
         (c) Pressure pulse
      (2) Moist heat denatures and coagulates microbial proteins; pressure serves to elevate temperature
      (3) Periodically check gasket on door to ensure a tight fit
      (4) Steam must be able to penetrate the instrument package; pack loosely to allow for free passage of steam
      (5) Packages and cassettes should be placed on their edges, not laid flat
      (6) Avoid the package coming in contact with chamber walls

(7) Use distilled or deionized water to prevent deposits on instruments

b. Dry-heat sterilization
   (1) Sterilizes by oxidizing cell parts
   (2) Keeps air spaces between packages
   (3) If the sterilizer is opened, timer must be restarted

c. Unsaturated chemical vapor sterilization
   (1) Alcohols, formaldehyde, ketone, acetone, and water are heated under pressure to produce the gas that permeates and destroys microbes

d. Ethylene oxide gas sterilization
   (1) Used mostly in hospitals and large clinics
   (2) Operation
      (a) Sterilize at room temperature, 75°F (25°C), for 10 to 16 hours
      (b) Alternatively, sterilize at 120°F (49°C) for 2 to 3 hours
      (c) Aerate plastic and rubber materials for at least 16 hours after sterilization to remove gas molecules
      (d) *Warning:* residual gas can cause tissue burns

e. Liquid chemical sterilants
   (1) Used for heat-sensitive, semicritical items when ethylene oxide gas is not available
      (a) Should not be used as a substitute for heat sterilization of semicritical items that are not heat sensitive
      (b) Should be avoided because mostly heat tolerant, or SUDs are available
      (c) Biologic monitoring is not possible, so this method cannot ensure sterility
   (2) Follow the manufacturer's instructions for dilution, temperature, and contact time
   (3) Ensure that the instruments are dry to avoid diluting the solution
   (4) Remove the instruments with sterile forceps, rinse with sterile water, and package or cover with sterile towel
   (5) Chemicals used for sterilization (see Table 10.6); the disadvantages of chemicals are:
      (a) They produce toxic fumes and are irritating to tissues
      (b) BIs are not available with the use of chemical sterilants; therefore, the sterility of items cannot be verified
      (c) When removed from chemicals, items are exposed to the environment and can easily become contaminated because of lack of packaging
      (d) Chemical sterilization requires an extended contact time of 3 to 12 hours, depending on the chemical

6. Verification of sterilization
   a. Failure of sterilization can occur as a result of operator or mechanical failure
      (1) Overloading—the reason for failure in the majority of cases
      (2) Improper packaging
      (3) Improper timing
      (4) Improper unit operation
      (5) Unit malfunction
      (6) Improper maintenance of equipment
   b. The CDC recommends routine use of BIs (spore tests) for verification of sterility
      (1) Biologic monitoring is a process in which highly resistant spores are passed through the sterilizer and then cultured to determine whether they have been killed
         (a) If spores have been killed, all the less-resistant microorganisms exposed to the same conditions will also have been destroyed
         (b) Primary method to ascertain sterility
         (c) Biologic monitoring with BIs can be done in the dental setting or in a processing facility
      (2) Types of BIs
         (a) Spore strips—paper strips containing one or two types of spores enclosed in a glassine envelope
            [1] After sterilization, remove the spore strip aseptically, place it in a culture medium, and incubate for 7 days
            [2] If spores are present, they will grow and change the color of the growth medium, indicating sterilization failure
            [3] Strips can be used for all methods of heat sterilization
         (b) Self-contained vial—contains spore strip with an ampule of growth medium in a plastic vial
            [1] After sterilization, squeeze the vial to break the internal ampule, which would mix the growth medium with the spores
            [2] Incubate the vial; if spores are present, they will multiply and change the color of the growth medium, indicating sterilization failure
            [3] Vials can only be used in a steam autoclave
         (c) Specific bacterial endospores used in BIs
            [1] Steam autoclave and chemical vapor sterilizer—spores of *Geobacillus stearothermophilus*
            [2] Dry heat and ethylene oxide gas sterilizer—spores of *Bacillus atrophaeus*
      (3) Use of BIs
         (a) Place a strip inside one of each type of package (e.g., autoclave bag, cassette)
         (b) Incubate a control BI that has not been sterilized, along with the test BI
         (c) Growth of spores from the control BI confirms that live spores were present
         (d) No growth from the test BI indicates that sterilization has been achieved

(4) Use BIs once a week to test sterilization equipment and when:
(a) The equipment has been repaired
(b) New packaging material is used
(c) A new sterilizer is operated
(d) Training new staff
(e) The loading procedure is changed
(f) Sterilizing an item to be implanted
(5) Sterilization failure (growth on the BI test, or positive spore test)
(a) Review the procedures to determine any operator error
(b) Take the sterilizer out of operation, and retest with mechanical, chemical, and biologic monitors
(c) If the repeat BI test is negative, put the sterilizer back in service
(d) If the repeat BI test is positive, determine the cause of failure, and repeat the BI test three times before putting the sterilizer back into service
(e) Withdraw the instruments, and repeat the process
(6) Documentation
(a) Record the results of biologic monitoring in a log book
(b) Necessary for compliance with federal regulations
(c) Serves quality assurance and risk management purposes

c. Chemical monitoring
(1) Chemical indicators—items containing heat-sensitive chemicals that change color when exposed to certain temperatures to assess conditions during the sterilization process (e.g., autoclave tape, special markings on autoclave bags, chemical indicator strips)
(2) Chemical monitoring does not provide proof of sterilization
(3) Types of chemical indicators
(a) Integrated indicator (class V)—changes color slowly when exposed to a combination of time, temperature, and steam; placed inside each instrument package to confirm whether instruments have been exposed to sterilizing conditions
(b) External chemical indicator—changes color after a certain temperature has been reached (e.g., autoclave tape)
[1] Distinguishes those instruments that have been in the sterilizer from those that have not, preventing accidental use of unprocessed items
[2] Should be present on packaging material or applied on the outside of every instrument package and cassette

d. Mechanical monitoring
(1) Observation of sterilizer gauges, including temperature, pressure, and exposure time
(2) Incorrect reading indicates a functional problem

7. Storage area procedures
a. After sterilization, allow the instrument packages to cool and dry before storage
(1) Microorganisms and instrument tips can penetrate wet packaging material and compromise sterility
(2) Microorganisms on contaminated surfaces can wick through wet packaging
b. Instruments must not be stored unwrapped or unpackaged (unpackaged instruments are immediately contaminated when exposed to the environment)
c. Packaged instruments should not be stored above the sterilizers and should be stored away from treatment areas to lessen chances of contamination
d. Sealed packages should be kept on shelves protected by doors for dry, low-dust storage
e. Sealed instrument packages have been shown to maintain sterility for up to 6 months; however, to err on the side of caution, repackage and sterilize after 30 days
f. Instrument packages should be rotated so that the oldest dated instrument pack is used first
g. Packages that are dropped on the floor, punctured, torn, or wet are considered contaminated and must be reprocessed
h. Wrapped cassettes are ideal for storing and then serving as sterile instrument trays

## GOVERNMENTAL AGENCIES AND INFECTION CONTROL

A. FDA
1. Regulates all medical devices
a. Examples in oral health care include liquid sterilants, biologic and chemical indicators, ultrasonic cleaners, PPE, dental instruments, and sterilizers
2. Ensures products are safe and effective
3. Ensure devices fulfill performance standards before marketing

B. EPA
1. Mission to protect human health and the environment
2. Ensures the safety and effectiveness of chemical disinfectants (EPA registration number displayed on container)
3. Regulates medical and chemical waste after leaving the oral health care (OHC) setting

C. CDC
1. Under the auspices of the US Department of Health and Human Services
2. Health and quality-of-life promotion mitigating injury, disability, and disease
3. Infection control guidelines and recommendations for dentistry (infection procedures used in oral health care

settings are based on 2003 recommendations and 2016 enhancements)

4. Regulatory agency only; does not have authority to enforce guidelines

D. OSHA

1. Within the US Department of Labor (federal and state divisions)
2. Ensuring a safe and healthy working environment for employees
   a. Instrument sterilization is *not* covered by OSHA regulations because it is considered a procedure involved in patient protection instead of DHCP (employee) protection
3. OSHA formulates and has the authority to enforce regulations related to occupational safety and health
4. Protection of DHCP against exposure to bloodborne pathogens, other contagions, and workplace hazards
5. COVID-19 pandemic guidance
   a. Inform DHCP about their risks of exposure to SARS-CoV-2, what employer site-specific measures enacted to protect them, and how they can protect themselves
   b. Recommendations for administrative, work, and engineering controls following CDC guidelines
   c. Recommendations for return-to-work guidance
6. OSHA Bloodborne Pathogens Standard
   a. The most important infection control regulation in dentistry for the protection of DHCP
   b. The final Bloodborne Pathogens Standard was published in 1991 and became effective in 1992
   c. The Needlestick Safety and Prevention Act was added to the Standard in 2001
      (1) On an annual basis, employers must solicit input from DHCP to identify, evaluate, and select safer medical devices to minimize or eliminate occupational exposures (e.g., self-sheathing needles)
   d. Employers are responsible for staff compliance with the Standard; this includes:
      (1) Review of the Standard and ensuring that a copy is available on-site
      (2) Formulation of a written exposure control plan that contains:
         (a) Clarification of which employees face a potential risk for occupational exposure and will be covered under the Standard
         (b) Description of how and when provisions will be implemented (i.e., communication of the hazards to employees, hepatitis B vaccination, postexposure evaluation and follow- up, record keeping, use of PPE, engineering and work practice controls, and housekeeping)
         (c) Prevention and evaluation of exposure incidents (sharps injuries)
         (d) In 2005, OSHA determined that oral health care settings are of low hazard and are exempt from keeping an injury and illness log
         (e) Employers still must report any workplace incident that results in the hospitalization of three or more employees or a fatality
      (3) Training of employees
         (a) Training that provides information about the hazards and preventive measures related to occupational exposure to bloodborne pathogens
         (b) Training to be completed at the initial time of assignment and annually thereafter
         (c) Person conducting the training must be qualified and knowledgeable
         (d) Training must provide an opportunity for interactive questions and answers with the person conducting the training
      (4) Providing employees with necessary materials to comply with the Standard
         (a) Offer and pay for hepatitis B vaccination
         (b) Provide, maintain, and ensure use of PPE and engineering controls
         (c) Establish appropriate work practices and decontamination procedures in the oral health care setting to ensure the safety of DHCP (appropriate decontamination, laundry handling, and infectious waste disposal)
         (d) Establish and provide postexposure medical evaluation and follow-up without any cost to employees
         (e) Provide appropriate biohazard communication by posting signs, biohazard waste labels, and red containers that indicate infectious waste on-site
      (5) Maintain appropriate records
         (a) Training sessions (participants, trainers, summary of content, evaluations)
         (b) Employee medical records to include: name and social security number of employee, HBV immunization status, postexposure evaluation from health care professional limited to whether the employee has been informed of the results of the evaluation and has been told about any medical conditions resulting from exposure to blood or other potentially infectious materials that require further evaluation or treatment
         (c) Employers must keep employee records for the duration of employment plus an additional thirty years
7. Inspections conducted by OSHA
   a. Initiated by employee complaints or other interested parties
   b. Programmed inspections of randomly selected worksites employing 11 or more people
   c. Noncompliance with any provision in the Standard can result in the imposition of fines

**TABLE 10.8 Evaluating Infection Control Programs**

| Program Element | Evaluation Activity |
|---|---|
| Appropriate immunization of dental health care personnel (DHCP) | Conduct annual review of personnel records to ensure up-to-date immunization. |
| Assessment of occupational exposures to infectious agents | Report occupational exposures to infectious agents. Document the steps that occurred around the exposure, and plan how such exposure can be prevented in the future. |
| Comprehensive postexposure management plan and medical follow-up program after occupational exposures to infectious agents | Ensure the postexposure management plan is clear, complete, and available at all times to all DHCP. All staff should understand the plan, which should include toll-free phone numbers for access to additional information. |
| Adherence to hand hygiene before and after patient care | Observe and document circumstances of appropriate or inappropriate handwashing. Review findings in a staff meeting. |
| Proper use of personal protective equipment (PPE) to prevent occupational exposures to infectious agents | Observe and document the use of barrier precautions and careful handling of sharps. Review findings in a staff meeting. |
| Routine and appropriate sterilization of instruments using a biologic monitoring system | Monitor paper log of steam cycle and temperature strip with each sterilization load, and examine results of weekly biologic monitoring. Take appropriate action when failure of sterilization process is noted. |
| Evaluation and implementation of safer medical devices | Conduct an annual review of the exposure control plan, and consider new developments in safer medical devices. |
| Compliance of water in routine dental procedures with current drinking U.S. Environmental Protection Agency water standards (fewer than 500 colony-forming units [CFU] of heterotrophic water bacteria) | Monitor dental water quality as recommended by the equipment manufacturer, using commercial self-contained test kits or commercial water-testing laboratories. |
| Proper handling and disposal of medical waste | Observe the safe disposal of regulated and nonregulated medical waste, and take preventive measures if hazardous situations occur. |
| Health care–associated infections | Assess the unscheduled return of patients after procedures, and evaluate them for an infectious process. A trend might require formal evaluation. |

From Centers for Disease Control and Prevention. Guidelines for infection control in dental health-care settings. *MMWR*. 52(RR-17):1–68; 2003.

**BOX 10.3 Legal and Ethical Guidelines in Disease Prevention**

- Treat all patients regardless of disease status
- Practice infection control according to the standard of care
  - Adhere to the Centers for Disease Control and Prevention (CDC) and the Occupational Safety and Health Administration (OSHA) guidelines
  - Adhere to state and federal laws
  - Use evidence-based protocols
  - Follow state board of dentistry laws and regulations
  - Follow expert opinion related to infection control
  - Stay current of new protocols and guidelines
- Abide by US Public Health Service (PHS) guidelines for employee work restrictions
- Adhere to local department of public health guidelines
- Participate in contact tracing to help identify people exposed to contagious diseases

## Evaluation of Infection Control Programs

Table 10.8 lists program elements with corresponding activities in the evaluation of infection control programs. The websites listed in the Website Information and Resources table provide the oral health care professional with immediate access to current recommendations and regulations concerning infection control.

## Legal and Ethical Issues in Disease Prevention

Box 10.3 lists recommendations to address legal and ethical considerations in infection control measures.

**WEBSITE INFORMATION AND RESOURCES**

| Source | Website Address | Description |
|---|---|---|
| Association for Professionals in Infection Control and Epidemiology (APIC) | http://www.apic.org | Infection control organization for health care |
| Centers for Disease Control and Prevention (CDC) | http://www.cdc.gov | US government agency that provides resources and recommendations for numerous health and safety topics |
| Organization for Safety, Asepsis, and Prevention (OSAP) | http://www.osap.org | Organization that promotes infection control and safety policies to the dental community |
| Occupational Safety and Health Administration (OSHA) | http://www.osha.gov | US government agency responsible for ensuring the health and safety of employees at workplaces |
| National Institutes for Occupational Safety and Health (NIOSH) | http://www.cdc.gov/niosh | US government agency that provides national and world leadership to prevent illness and injury |

## CHAPTER 10 REVIEW QUESTIONS

Answers and rationales to review questions are available on this text's accompanying Evolve site. See inside front cover for details.

### CASE A

Isabelle Sanchez, a registered dental hygienist (RDH), has been practicing dental hygiene for 7 years and has decided to return to college to pursue her master's degree in dental hygiene. She has moved to another state and is currently working during the summer as a temporary hygienist to earn money for living expenses. For the last two consecutive Mondays, she has been working in the same practice, substituting for a hygienist who is on maternity leave. Today, when she reports to work, Isabelle is told by the dental assistant that the elderly man whom Isabelle treated last Monday is in the hospital and has been diagnosed with Legionnaires' disease. During the last week, he had only left his house to go to his dental visit, and the water tested in his house was negative for *Legionella.* In hindsight, Isabelle realizes that in her treatment room, she did not see a water bottle attached to the master control unit that would have indicated use of an independent water system. She just assumed that the dental unit water lines were being treated with another method.

***Use Case A to answer questions 1 to 6.***

1. Which of the following pathways of disease transmission is depicted in this case?
   **a.** Patient to DHCP
   **b.** DHCP to patient
   **c.** Patient to patient
   **d.** Community to patient
2. Which of the following modes of disease transmission is depicted in this case?
   **a.** Direct contact
   **b.** Indirect contact
   **c.** Droplet infection
   **d.** Airborne infection
3. What is the source of the microbes in this case?
   **a.** Patient's oral cavity
   **b.** Hygienist's hands
   **c.** Contaminated instrument
   **d.** Dental unit water
4. In this case, which of the following infection control procedures likely would have prevented disease transmission?
   **a.** Using barriers
   **b.** Cleaning the housekeeping surfaces
   **c.** Treating dental unit water lines
   **d.** Wearing proper PPE
5. Which of the following microorganism types is responsible for Legionnaires' disease?
   **a.** Bacterium
   **b.** Prion
   **c.** Virus
   **d.** Fungus
6. What was the portal of entry of *Legionella* into the elderly patient's body?
   **a.** Breathing in contaminated water vapor
   **b.** Swallowing contaminated water
   **c.** Infiltrating microbes into nonintact mucosa
   **d.** Splashing of droplets on mucous membranes

### CASE B

After dismissing his last patient of the day, Preston Miller, RDH, returns to his treatment room. He is in a rush because his daughter's softball team has a game tonight and he is the coach. Preston hurriedly closes his instrument cassette, not taking care to arrange the instruments beforehand. In the instrument-processing area, he lifts the cassette off the metal tray to place it into the ultrasonic unit. Unknowingly, an explorer tip is protruding from a hole in the cassette and penetrates his finger through the exam glove. He removes his gloves and sees a small amount of blood forming on his index finger. Additionally, Preston has received the HBV vaccine and has verified immunity to HBV.

***Use Case B to answer questions 7 to 13.***

7. What should Preston the dental hygienist do next?
   **a.** Scrub the finger using a stiff brush
   **b.** Squeeze the finger to let out the contaminants
   **c.** Wash the finger with antimicrobial soap
   **d.** Immerse the finger in bleach for 1 minute
8. Preston, the employee, has sustained a percutaneous injury and may have been exposed to a bloodborne pathogen. In this situation, what is the responsibility of his employer according to OSHA?
   **a.** None; an employee works at his own risk
   **b.** Pay for the treatment of any acquired disease
   **c.** Give the employee the following day off with pay
   **d.** Arrange for a consultation with a qualified HCP
9. Which of the following modes of disease transmission is depicted in this case?
   **a.** Direct contact
   **b.** Indirect contact
   **c.** Droplet infection
   **d.** Airborne infection
10. What is the source of the microbes in this case?
    **a.** Contaminated droplets
    **b.** Hygienist's hands
    **c.** Contaminated instrument
    **d.** Dental unit water
11. The dental hygienist elects to be tested for bloodborne pathogens (HCV and HIV), and he is informed of the results by a qualified health care professional. Which of the following actions is he then required to take?
    **a.** Inform his employer of the results
    **b.** Document the results in his employee file
    **c.** Inform the CDC and OSHA
    **d.** None of the above is required
12. According to OSHA, which of the following does NOT need to be included in a dental office's record keeping?
    **a.** Employee vaccine declination statements
    **b.** Records of annual staff trainings on infection control
    **c.** Log of employee injuries and illnesses
    **d.** Employees' Social Security numbers
13. What is the level of risk related to the transmission of HCV or HIV from this exposure?
    **a.** High
    **b.** Moderate

c. Low
d. Very low

14. All the following viruses are bloodborne pathogens EXCEPT:
a. Human immunodeficiency virus
b. Hepatitis B virus
c. Hepatitis C virus
d. Varicella-zoster virus

15. Which term is used for the practice of treating a patient's blood, body fluids, nonintact skin, and mucous membranes as potentially infectious?
a. Standard precautions
b. Pervasive precautions
c. Universal precautions
d. Protective precautions

16. Glutaraldehyde is a high-level disinfectant; therefore it can be used to sterilize critical items.
a. Both statements are TRUE
b. Both statements are FALSE
c. The first statement is TRUE; the second statement is FALSE
d. The first statement is FALSE; the second statement is TRUE

17. A dental health care employee has occupationally acquired tuberculosis. Which of the following modes of disease transmission would be implicated in this case?
a. Direct contact
b. Indirect contact
c. Droplet infection
d. Airborne infection

18. Which of the following methods will achieve sterilization?
a. Dry heat at 320°F for 50 minutes
b. Steam autoclave at 200°F for 30 minutes
c. Chemical vapor at 270°F for 20 minutes
d. Ethylene oxide gas for 5 hours

19. The CDC recommends disinfecting clinical contact surfaces with an intermediate-level disinfectant that is tuberculocidal, because *Mycobacterium tuberculosis* var. *bovis* is a resistant microbe and all other, less resistant microbes would also be killed.
a. Both the statement and the reason are TRUE
b. Both the statement and the reason are FALSE
c. The statement is TRUE, but the reason is FALSE
d. The statement is FALSE, but the reason is TRUE

20. What is the ultimate goal of disease prevention in the oral health care (OHC) setting?
a. Prevent pathogens from entering the OHC setting
b. Sterilize clinical contact surfaces between patients
c. Prevent OHC-related infections and diseases
d. Eliminate all microbes in the OHC setting

21. Alcohol-based sanitizers may be used instead of handwashing when no visible soil is present, because hand sanitizers have been found to be at least as effective as handwashing.
a. Both the statement and the reason are TRUE
b. Both the statement and the reason are FALSE
c. The statement is TRUE, but the reason is FALSE
d. The statement is FALSE, but the reason is TRUE

22. All the following are TRUE related to using instrument cassettes EXCEPT:
a. Unwrap the cassette in view of the patient
b. Sterilized cassettes are used as instrument trays
c. Exposure to sharps is decreased
d. Using cassettes is less time-efficient

23. Many DHCP experience skin problems on their hands related to the use of gloves. In most cases, these problems are caused by an allergic response to latex proteins in gloves.
a. Both statements are TRUE.
b. Both statements are FALSE.
c. The first statement is TRUE; the second statement is FALSE.
d. The first statement is FALSE; the second statement is TRUE.

24. Which of the following indicators is used to determine sterility?
a. External indicator
b. Integrated indicator
c. Biologic indicator
d. Chemical indicator

25. Which of the following is OSHA primarily concerned with protecting?
a. Employee
b. Employer
c. Patient
d. Community

26. Which of the following characteristics is an advantage of chemical-vapor sterilization?
a. A ventilation system is not required
b. It can sterilize closed containers
c. Extra drying time is not needed
d. It is the least costly method of sterilization

27. All the following are vaccine-preventable illnesses EXCEPT:
a. Hepatitis B virus (HBV)
b. Hepatitis A virus (HAV)
c. Hepatitis C virus (HCV)
d. Varicella-zoster virus (VZV)

28. Which of the following statements BEST characterizes the resident flora on hands?
a. They colonize the deeper layers of the skin
b. They are less resistant to removal by handwashing
c. They are the primary source of disease transmission
d. They are associated with allergic contact dermatitis

29. Which of the following statements is TRUE regarding the handling of regulated infectious waste?
a. Containers of infectious waste must be identified with the biohazard symbol
b. Infectious waste can be disinfected and then combined with the regular trash
c. Infectious waste must be sterilized before leaving the oral health care setting
d. Infectious waste does not require any special handling in some states

30. Examination gloves to be used intraorally should be donned immediately prior to:

a. Dental operatory setup
b. Unwrapping the cassette
c. Taking the blood pressure
d. Entering the patient's mouth

31. Which of the following packaging materials should NOT be used with chemical vapor sterilization?
a. Paper wrap
b. Paper pouches
c. Plastic pouches
d. Cloth wrap

32. Which of the following characteristics BEST describes the use of protective barriers for clinical contact surfaces?
a. They need to be changed only when visibly soiled
b. They should be used after sterilization of the surface
c. They are ideally used for surfaces that are difficult to disinfect
d. They decrease the cost of maintaining asepsis

33. All following characteristics describe EPA-registered intermediate-level disinfectants EXCEPT:
a. Must inactivate *Mycobacterium tuberculosis* var. *bovis*
b. Will kill vegetative bacteria and most viruses
c. Must be used on surfaces with visible blood
d. Will achieve sterilization if long contact time is used

34. All DHCP who are vaccinated for hepatitis B will become immune to the virus. Therefore, the CDC does not recommend booster injections.
a. Both statements are TRUE
b. Both statements are FALSE
c. The first statement is TRUE; the second statement is FALSE
d. The first statement is FALSE; the second statement is TRUE

35. Face shields provide maximum coverage for the face and protection from spatter during oral health care procedures. Therefore, wearing a facemask is not required when using a face shield.
a. Both statements are TRUE
b. Both statements are FALSE
c. The first statement is TRUE; the second statement is FALSE
d. The first statement is FALSE; the second statement is TRUE

36. Which of the following pathogens has been identified in the biofilm that accumulates inside dental unit water lines?
a. *Pseudomonas aeruginosa*
b. *Neisseria meningitidis*
c. *Candida albicans*
d. *Treponema pallidum*

37. Which of the following governmental agencies is responsible for approving the safety and effectiveness of small office sterilizers and ultrasonic units?
a. EPA
b. FDA
c. CDC
d. OSHA

38. An individual should be tested for antibodies to HBV 1 to 2 months after receiving the last dose of the hepatitis B vaccine. The reason for this testing is that not all individuals will seroconvert.
a. Both statements are TRUE
b. Both statements are FALSE
c. The first statement is TRUE; the second statement is FALSE
d. The first statement is FALSE; the second statement is TRUE

39. In which of the following methods are biologic monitors containing spores of *Geobacillus stearothermophilus* used to verify sterilization?
a. Steam autoclave
b. Dry-heat oven
c. Ethylene oxide gas
d. Rapid heat transfer

40. Which of the following is NOT considered a safe work practice control?
a. Using an instrument cassette instead of autoclave bags
b. Hand scrubbing instruments using exam gloves
c. Using a one-handed technique to recap needles
d. Instrumenting a tooth using a fulcrum one tooth away

41. Sterilization failure is most often caused by:
a. The autoclave not working properly
b. Improper packaging materials used
c. Overloading the office sterilizer
d. Inadequate sterilization time

42. A chemical indicator is used on the outside of packaging to identify the items that have been processed through the sterilizer. The chemical indicator changes color when the packages are sterile.
a. Both statements are TRUE
b. Both statements are FALSE
c. The first statement is TRUE; the second statement is FALSE
d. The first statement is FALSE; the second statement is TRUE

43. Dental handpieces are considered semicritical items, and therefore they can be disinfected by wiping with an intermediate-level disinfectant.
a. Both statements are TRUE
b. Both statements are FALSE
c. The first statement is TRUE; the second statement is FALSE
d. The first statement is FALSE; the second statement is TRUE

44. What is the maximum level of bacteria that the CDC has recommended for water exiting dental unit waterlines?
a. 400 CFU/mL
b. 500 CFU/mL
c. 600 CFU/mL
d. 700 CFU/mL

45. In most cases, what is the number of bacteria in the water exiting from an untreated dental unit water line?
a. Lower than in drinking water
b. The same as in drinking water
c. Slightly higher than in drinking water
d. Much higher than in drinking water

46. All the following materials are considered regulated infectious waste EXCEPT:
   a. Extracted tooth
   b. Blood-soaked gauze
   c. Anesthetic needle
   d. Saliva coated exam gloves
47. The primary reason for patients to perform a preprocedural rinse before undergoing oral health care is to:
   a. Remove malodorous breath
   b. Remove adherent food debris
   c. Reduce the microbes in aerosols
   d. Eliminate oral infections
48. Using biologic indicators to test sterilizing equipment, biologic monitors should be used once every:
   a. Day
   b. Week
   c. Month
   d. Quarter
49. All the following methods inhibit the formation of biofilm in dental unit water lines EXCEPT:
   a. Flushing water lines for 2 minutes
   b. Independent water reservoir
   c. Chemical disinfection of water lines
   d. Sterile water delivery systems
50. The practice of using a cotton roll taped to the bracket tray for wiping instruments, instead of a gauze square wrapped around the finger, is considered by OSHA as a/an:
   a. Standard bioburden control
   b. Safe practice control
   c. Engineering control
   d. Work practice control
51. Considering the COVID-19 pandemic, which of the following masks is now recommended for use during aerosol generating procedures?
   a. N95
   b. Level 1
   c. Level 2
   d. Level 3
52. Based on the CDC Interim Infection Prevention and Control Recommendations for Patients suspected of COVID-19, the new definition of fever is:
   a. 99.0°F or higher
   b. 99.5°F or higher
   c. 100.0°F or higher
   d. 100.4°F or higher
53. A patient presenting for a routine prophylaxis has symptoms consistent with a respiratory infection (cough, low grade fever), but has not been tested for COVID-19. The patient says that they will be okay, it's probably just a "cold", and to proceed with treatment. Which of the following actions should a dental hygienist take?
   a. Provide patient care using standard precautions
   b. Use an isolation room and respiratory precautions
   c. Dismiss and reschedule patient for a future time
   d. Wear a N95 respirator while providing care

## SUGGESTED READINGS

Centers for Disease Control and Prevention. Guidelines for infection control in dental health-care settings. *MMWR (Morb Mortal Wkly Rep)*. 2003;52, RR-17.

Centers for Disease Control and Prevention. Guidelines for disinfection and sterilization in healthcare facilities. Updated 2019, pages 1–163.

Centers for Disease Control and Prevention. Summary of Infection Prevention Practices in Dental Settings: Basic Expectations for Safe Care. Atlanta, GA: Centers for Disease Control and Prevention, US Dept of Health and Human Services; October 2016.

Miller CH. *Infection Control and Management of Hazardous Materials for the Dental Team*. 6th ed. St Louis: Elsevier; 2018.

US Department of Labor. *Occupational Safety and Health Administration. Controlling Occupational Exposure to Bloodborne Pathogens*. Washington, DC, 2012, https://www.osha.gov/laws-regs/regulations/standardnumber/1910/1910.1030.

# 11

# Pharmacology

*Elena Bablenis Haveles*

As a health care provider responsible for patient assessment and care, a dental hygienist must understand drugs, the conditions for which these drugs are used, and the actions, range of effects, and interactions of the drugs. The health, dental, and pharmacologic histories are the foundation on which decisions regarding patient care rest. For example, some patients may need prophylactic antibiotic premedication before dental and dental hygiene care. Therefore, before care is planned, the patient's medical conditions and medications used to manage them are assessed and recorded in the patient's permanent record. Contraindications to professional care or precautions concerning these drugs are determined using appropriate references and consultations. Through this knowledge, medical emergencies may be prevented; and, if an emergency occurs, the oral health care team can act within the standard of care.

## GENERAL CONSIDERATIONS

### Definitions

A. Pharmacology—the study of drugs and their effects on living organisms
B. Pharmacotherapy—the use of medications to treat different disease states
C. Pharmacodynamics—the action of drugs on living organisms
D. Pharmacokinetics—what the body does in response to the drugs (e.g., absorption, distribution, metabolism, excretion)
E. Pharmacy—the practice of compounding, preparing, and dispensing drugs and of counseling patients about their medications
F. Toxicology—the study of the harmful effects of drugs on living organisms
G. Drugs—biologically active substances that can modify cellular function; used in the prevention, diagnosis, treatment, and cure of disease or in the prevention of pregnancy
H. Nomenclature—each drug has several names
   1. Chemical name—based on the drug's chemical formula (e.g., *N*-acetyl para-amino phenol)
   2. Trade (proprietary) name—each drug company makes up its own product trade name (e.g., Tylenol, Peridex, Atridox, Arestin)
   3. Brand name—technically, the name of the drug company itself, but often used interchangeably with the trade name (e.g., either Astra [company that makes Xylocaine] or Xylocaine can be considered the brand name)
   4. Generic name—official name of the drug determined by the US Adopted Names Council that is used by all manufacturers of a particular drug (e.g., acetaminophen, chlorhexidine gluconate)
I. Table 11.1 lists the Latin abbreviations used in prescription writing

### Agencies and Legislation

A. US Food and Drug Administration (FDA)—determines drugs to be marketed in the United States; after considering safety, efficacy, and physical and chemical data, the FDA requires quality control of manufacturing facilities, determines what drugs are sold by prescription, and regulates the advertising and labeling of prescription drugs
B. US Drug Enforcement Administration (DEA)—branch of the Department of Justice; determines the degree of control for substances with abuse potential; controlled substances used in dentistry are classified under schedules I to V (Table 11.2) It should be noted that individual states may change the schedule of a drug, which could impact on prescription handling. Consult with the National Association of State Controlled Substance Authorities for update information on a state-to-state basis.

### Drug Action

A. Log dose–response curve—as the dose of a drug increases (*x* axis), the percentage of maximum response increases (*y* axis) until increasing the dose further produces no increase in the percentage of response (the effect of the drug reaches a plateau) (Fig. 11.1)
B. Definitions
   1. Effective dose (ED) 50—dose that produces 50% of the maximum response, or the dose of a drug that produces a specific response in 50% of the subjects
   2. Lethal dose (LD) 50—dose that is lethal to (kills) 50% of the subjects; laboratory animals are used to derive LD
   3. Therapeutic index (TI)—$LD_{50}$ divided by $ED_{50}$; a measure of the safety of a drug
   4. Onset—time required for a drug's effect to begin; onset is short if the drug is given intravenously, longer if administered orally
   5. Duration—length of time a drug's effect lasts; related to a drug's half-life
   6. Half-life (t½)—time required for a drug's serum concentration to decrease by 50%; five half-lives are required for a drug to be eliminated from the body

7. Potency—amount of drug (e.g., in milligrams) needed to produce an effect; the more potent an agent is, the lower is the dose needed to produce an effect (Fig. 11.2)
8. Efficacy—the desired effect elicited by a drug, independent of dose (see Fig. 11.2)
9. Tolerance—physiologic response to the same dose produces less effect, or a higher dose is required to achieve the same effect
10. Therapeutic effect—desired pharmacologic effect

C. Routes of administration
1. Oral (PO)—by mouth; easiest to use; good patient acceptance; however, a latency period exists
2. Rectal—administration by suppository or enema; produces either local or systemic effect
3. Parenteral—a route other than an oral route; usually refers to an injection
4. Intravenous (IV)—administration into a vein; shortest onset of action and higher risk of adverse events compared with other routes of administration
5. Intramuscular (IM)—administration into the muscle; sometimes painful
6. Subcutaneous (SC, SQ)—injected beneath the skin (e.g., insulin)
7. Oral or nasal—particles, volatile liquids, or gasses that are inhaled (e.g., nitrous oxide–oxygen [$N_2O$-$O_2$] analgesia; as are some medications used to treat allergies and asthma)
8. Topical—ointments or creams applied to the skin or mucous membranes (e.g., hydrocortisone)
9. Sublingual (SL)—a tablet that dissolves or a solution that is sprayed under the tongue (for systemic effect)

D. Dosage forms
1. Capsule—gelatin shell
2. Tablet—compressed or molded dosage form
3. Ointment or cream—semisolid for topical application
4. Suppository—penile, rectal, or vaginal; systemic or local
5. Solution—single-phase system consisting of more than one constituent
6. Suspension—insoluble particles in liquid (e.g., milk of magnesia)

E. Dosage
1. Varies depending on the patient's:
   a. Age—older adults may require lower doses because they may metabolize and excrete drugs more slowly
   b. Weight—total body weight, muscle-to-fat ratio, and body size can affect drug absorption
   c. Condition (disease)—many different disease states can affect drug absorption, metabolism, or excretion (e.g., congestive heart failure slows down metabolism; hyperthyroidism speeds up metabolism)
   d. Route of administration
2. Pediatric dose
   a. Less than the adult's dose
   b. Based on:
      (1) Manufacturer's recommendations—best method
      (2) Surface area—good method
      (3) Weight—adequate method
      (4) Age—very poor method

**TABLE 11.1 Common Latin Abbreviations Used in Prescription Writing**

| Abbreviation[a] | Interpretation |
|---|---|
| a., ante | Before |
| a.c., ante cibum | Before meals |
| A.D., aurisdextra | Right ear |
| A.L., aurislaeva | Left ear |
| b.i.d., bis in die | Twice per day or twice daily |
| gt., gutta | Drop (plural gtt.) |
| h., hora | Hour |
| h.s., hora somni | At bedtime |
| o.d., oculus dexter | Right eye |
| o.s., oculus sinister | Left eye |
| o.u., oculus uterque | Each eye |
| p.c., post cibum | After meals |
| p.o., per os | By mouth |
| p.r. | By rectum |
| p.r.n., pro re nata | As needed |
| q.d., quaque die | Once per day or once daily |
| q.i.d., quater in die | Four times per day |
| q.o.d. | Every other day |
| q.h. | Every 6 hours |
| sl. | Sublingual |
| supp. | Suppository |
| t.i.d., ter in die | Three times per day |
| u.d. | As directed |

[a]Periods usually omitted (e.g., bid, po) when abbreviations used (as with dosages).

**TABLE 11.2 Drug Enforcement Administration Schedules Used in Dentistry (I Through V)**

| Schedule | Abuse Potential | Examples | Handling |
|---|---|---|---|
| I | High | Heroin, phencyclidine (PCP) | Prescriptions may not be sent by telephone |
| II | High | Morphine, meperidine, oxycodone mixtures (Percodan, Percocet), hydrocodone mixtures (Vicodin) | Prescriptions must be signed by the prescriber; may not be telephoned to pharmacist; emergency prescriptions may be phoned; however, signed original prescription order must be delivered to the pharmacy within 72 hours of the phone order; no refills |
| III | Some | Codeine mixtures (Tylenol and codeine), "weaker" stimulants and sedatives | Prescriptions may be telephoned to pharmacy; may be refilled five times within 6 months |
| IV | Low | Dextropropoxyphene (Darvon), diazepam (Valium) | Same as schedule III |
| V | Very low | Some cough syrups containing codeine | Same as schedule III |

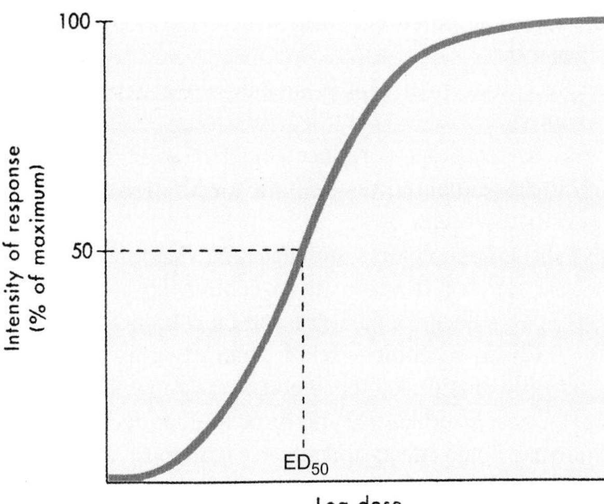

Fig. 11.1 Log dose-effect curve. *ED,* Effective dose.

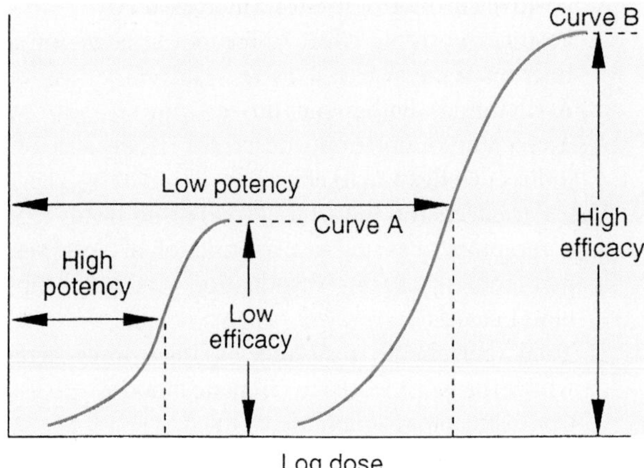

Fig. 11.2 Potency and efficacy of a drug. *Curve A* has high potency and low efficacy; *Curve B* has low potency and high efficacy.

## Adverse Reactions

### Side Effect

A. Side effect on a nontarget organ—effect on an organ other than that intended to be altered (e.g., insomnia resulting from a $\beta_2$-agonist or theophylline); dose-related and often predictable
B. Toxic reaction—predictable and dose-related effect on a target organ (e.g., insulin can lower blood glucose levels to the point of hypoglycemia)
C. Allergic reaction—varies from mild rash to anaphylaxis; involves an antigen-antibody reaction (e.g., rash from penicillin); can include urticaria, soft tissue swelling, and difficulty breathing; not predictable and not dose-related
D. Idiosyncrasy—abnormal drug response that is genetically related
E. Interference with natural defense mechanisms—body is less able to fight infection (e.g., steroids weaken the immune system)
F. Teratogenic effect—adverse effect on a fetus (e.g., alcohol intake during pregnancy produces fetal alcohol syndrome)

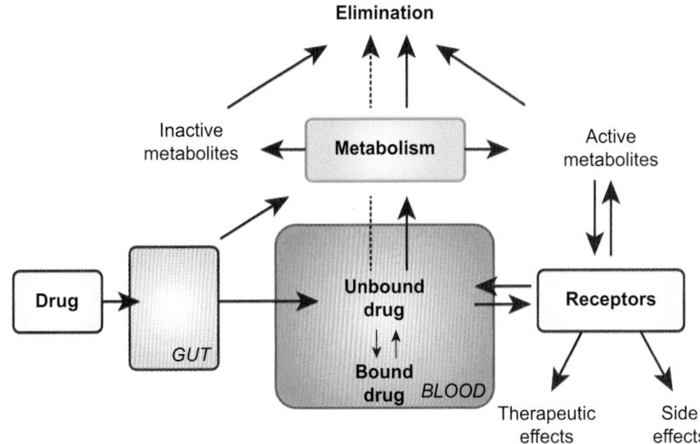

Fig. 11.3 Protein binding and drug distribution (From: Vuignier K, Schappler J, Veuthy J-L, Carrupt P-A, Martel S. Drug-protein binding: a critical review of analytical tools. *Anal Bioanal Chem.* 2010;398:53–66.)

## Pharmacokinetics

Pharmacokinetics is the way in which the body responds to drugs through the four processes of absorption, distribution, metabolism, and excretion (ADME).

A. Absorption depends on:
   1. Degree of ionization—the more ionized (charged) the drug, the less it will be absorbed; conversely, the less ionized the drug, the more it will be absorbed; with weak acids or bases, this is a function of pH
   2. Lipid solubility—the more lipid soluble the drug, the more readily it will be absorbed; the less lipid soluble it is, the less readily it will be absorbed
   3. Factors that affect absorption
      a. Patient compliance
      b. Age
      c. Gender
      d. Other disease states
      e. Genetic variations
      f. Placebo effect
B. Distribution of the drug (Fig. 11.3)[1]
   1. Drugs are transported to the site of action
   2. Only the free, or unbound, drug can cross cell membranes (indicated by arrows between boxes in Fig. 11.3)
   3. In each cellular compartment, equilibrium is reached between the bound and unbound (free) drug
   4. Redistribution—the drug moves from one tissue (where it exerts an effect) to another tissue (where it is inactive); this is one method of terminating a drug's effect
   5. Protein binding—drugs bind to protein receptors to varying degrees; once the drug binds to a protein receptor, it cannot exert its pharmacologic effect; when more than one drug is present in the system, the drugs may compete for the same receptor site; the drug with the stronger affinity will bind to the receptor site, and the drug with the weaker affinity will then exert its pharmacologic effect
   6. Tissue binding—some drugs can also bind to body tissues and cause significant chemical effects (e.g., tetracycline has an impact on developing bones and teeth of the fetus and of a young child)

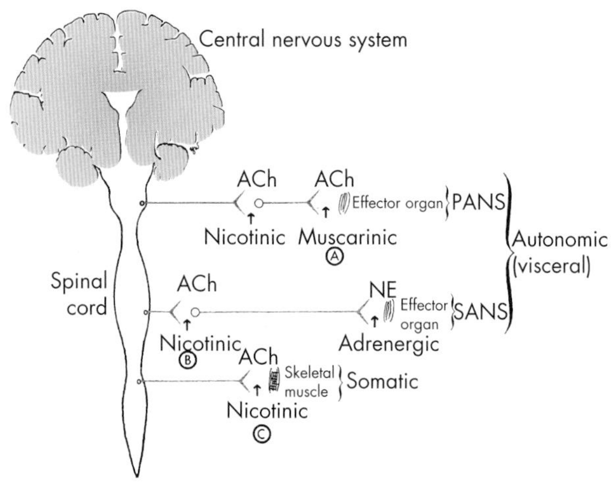


**Fig. 11.4** Typical neurons with neurotransmitters (*ACh*, acetylcholine; *NE*, norepinephrine), and the typical parasympathetic nervous system (*PANS*); the sympathetic nervous system (*SANS*); somatic nerves; and muscarinic (*A*) and nicotinic (*B* and *C*) receptors.

C. Metabolism (biotransformation)—takes place mainly in the liver by hepatic microsomal enzymes; metabolites are more polar, less protein bound, and more easily excreted; drugs metabolized by microsomal enzymes can affect their own metabolism or that of other drugs (e.g., either increasing [as with barbiturates] or decreasing [as with cimetidine, erythromycin] the rate of metabolism); biotransformation is a source of drug interactions
D. Excretion—usually by way of kidneys (urine); can also occur through feces (enterohepatic circulation), sweat, tears, or lungs (e.g., $N_2O$ is exhaled)

### Receptors

A receptor site is an area in the body to which a drug binds.

A. Agonist—a drug that has an affinity for a receptor site and binds to it, producing an effect (e.g., opioid [narcotic] analgesic agent)
B. Antagonist—a drug has an affinity for a receptor site and binds to it but produces no effect; competitively blocks the effect of an agonist (e.g., naloxone, an opioid [narcotic] antagonist blocks the effect of the agonist, an opioid)

## AUTONOMIC NERVOUS SYSTEM AGENTS

Agents affecting the autonomic nervous system (ANS) are divided into four groups: parasympathetic (P) nervous system stimulation (P+) and inhibition (P−), and sympathetic (S) nervous system stimulation (S+) and inhibition (S−).

### Sympathetic (Adrenergic) Agents

Mimic the action of the sympathetic autonomic nervous system (SANS); act like norepinephrine (NE) in the SANS, producing stimulation of the SANS; epinephrine produces the same effect (Fig. 11.4)

A. Adrenergic agonists
   1. The SANS is activated by fear (the "fight-or-flight" response)
   2. Catecholamine—chemical structure of some adrenergic agents
   3. Receptors in the SANS include alpha (α) and beta (β) types:
      a. $\alpha_1$-receptors—produce constriction of smooth muscles and blood vessels (vasoconstriction)
      b. β-receptors
         (1) $\beta_1$-receptors—stimulate the heart, increase heart rate (HR), increase the contractility and conduction velocity of the heart, and cause bronchodilation
         (2) $\beta_2$-receptors—relax smooth muscles, causing dilation of the blood vessels of skeletal muscle (vasodilation) and bronchodilation
B. Pharmacologic effects and adverse reactions
   1. The central nervous system (CNS)—stimulation produces increased alertness; may also cause anxiety, anorexia
   2. Stimulation of the heart—S+, produces
      a. Positive chronotropic effect (increased HR)
      b. Positive inotropic effect (increased strength of contraction of the heart)
      c. Arrhythmias, with higher doses
      d. α-receptor stimulation—decreases HR because of the indirect (reflex vagal) effect
   3. Vascular effects (on the arterial tree) result from
      a. α-receptors—causing vasoconstriction of blood vessels
      b. β-receptors—causing vasodilation of skeletal muscle blood vessels
      c. Total peripheral resistance (TPR)—force against which the heart works to circulate blood
         (1) α-receptors—increased TPR
         (2) β-receptors—decreased TPR
   4. Mydriasis (pupil dilation) and reduced intraocular pressure; useful in treating glaucoma
   5. Bronchodilation (by action of β2-agonist); useful in treating patients with asthma
   6. Production of thick, viscous saliva
C. Drug interactions—examples of interactions caused by adrenergic agents:
   1. Tricyclic antidepressants (TCAs; e.g., amitriptyline [Elavil], imipramine [Tofranil])—interaction increases blood pressure (BP); produces dysrhythmias
   2. β-blockers (e.g., propranolol [Inderal])—produce hypertension and bradycardia (slowed HR)
   3. Antidiabetic agents (e.g., insulin, glipizide [Glucotrol], glyburide (DiaBeta)—increase the blood glucose level
   4. Monoamine oxidase inhibitors (MAOIs)—no problem with epinephrine; indirect-acting amines (e.g., pseudoephedrine) must be avoided
   5. General anesthetics—halogenated hydrocarbons (e.g., halothane [Fluothane]) sensitize the myocardium to catecholamines; epinephrine is a catecholamine; increase the risk of arrhythmia/dysrhythmias
D. Dental hygiene considerations—the patient's pulse and BP must be checked; all these medications can increase HR and BP

**TABLE 11.3 Adrenergic Agents and Their Use**

| Adrenergic Agent | Receptor Stimulated | Comments |
|---|---|---|
| Epinephrine (Adrenalin) | Aβ | Endogenous catecholamine; local anesthetic additive |
| Methylphenidate (Ritalin) | A | Attention deficit hyperactivity disorder (ADHD) |
| Phenylephrine (Neo-Synephrine) | A | Nasal decongestant |
| Levonordefrin (Neo-Cobefrin) | $\alpha > \beta$ | Local anesthetic additive |
| Amphetamine | Aβ | Diet pill (abused) |
| Pseudoephedrine (Sudafed) | Aβ | Orally active nasal decongestant |

E. Therapeutic uses (Table 11.3)
  1. Medical purposes—treatment of:
    a. Anaphylaxis
    b. Cardiac arrest
    c. Nasal congestion—decongestant
    d. Asthma (β2-agonist)
    e. Attention deficit hyperactivity disorder (ADD) or attention deficit disorder (ADD)
    f. Glaucoma
  2. Dental purposes
    a. Local anesthetic additive (vasoconstrictor)
    b. Hemostatic additive to reduce bleeding; provides adequate tissue retraction (cord)

F. Adrenergics as vasoconstrictors are contained in local anesthetic solutions
  1. Examples
    a. Epinephrine (Adrenalin)
    b. Levonordefrin (Neo-Cobefrin)
  2. Advantages of adrenergic vasoconstriction
    a. Prolongs duration of anesthesia
    b. Reduces systemic toxicity
    c. Provides hemostasis
    d. Reduces absorption (vasoconstriction)
    e. Increases concentration of anesthetic at the nerve membrane
  3. Disadvantages of adrenergic vasoconstriction
    a. Excessive amount produces systemic toxicity
    b. In persons with cardiovascular disease:
      (1) Reasonable amounts can be used in local anesthetic additives for patients whose cardiovascular conditions are stable
      (2) Avoid using epinephrine-impregnated retraction cords
      (3) Maximum (safe) dose (MD) varies for normal patients and patients with cardiovascular disease
        (a) Epinephrine—dose for normal patients, 0.2 mg; for patients with cardiovascular disease, 0.04 mg
        (b) Levonordefrin (Neo-Cobefrin)—dose for normal patients, 1 mg; for patients with cardiovascular disease, 0.2 mg (some sources state 1.0 mg)
    c. Hyperthyroidism—vasoconstrictors may produce a thyroid storm in patients who have not received treatment and in those receiving drug therapy
      (1) *Thyroid storm* or *thyroid crisis* is characterized by an acceleration of all body processes (e.g., increases in HR, BP, respiration, body temperature, and pulse)
      (2) Pulmonary edema and congestive heart failure can occur
  4. Minimize toxicity by:
    a. Injecting slowly
    b. Aspirating before injecting
    c. Calming the patient
    d. Using the lowest ED
  5. Dental hygiene considerations
    a. Use is contraindicated in patients with uncontrolled cardiovascular disease
    c. Check BP and pulse

## α-Adrenergic Blockers (α-Blockers)

See the section on "Cardiovascular Agents" for a more detailed discussion.

A. Mechanism of action—block α-receptors, which block action of the SANS
B. Used to treat hypertension (e.g., Raynaud disease)
C. Examples (note generic names ending with "-sin")
  1. Prazosin (Minipress)
  2. Terazosin (Hytrin)
  3. Doxazosin (Cardura)

## β-Adrenergic Blocker (β-Blocker) Antagonists

See the section on "Cardiovascular Agents" for more information.

A. Mechanism of action—drug blocks SANS action (β-receptors); some β-blockers are more selective for the $\beta_1$-receptor than $\beta_2$-receptor; some drugs are formulated to target $\beta_1$-receptors, others to $\beta_2$-receptors; other drugs target both $\beta_1$- and $\beta_2$-receptors
B. Used to treat hypertension, angina, arrhythmias; also congestive heart failure, anxiety, and glaucoma; used to prevent myocardial infarction (MI, heart attack)
C. Examples (note generic names ending with "-olol")
  1. Propranolol (Inderal)—nonselective $\beta_1$- and $\beta_2$-blocker
  2. Metoprolol (Lopressor)—selective $\beta_1$-blocker
  3. Atenolol (Tenormin)—selective $\beta_1$-blocker
D. Dental hygiene considerations
  1. Check the patient's BP and pulse—these medications can increase or decrease HR
  2. Raise the dental chair slowly, and allow the patient to remain seated for a few minutes to minimize the risk of orthostatic hypotension

## Adrenergic Neuronal Agonists and Antagonists

A. Pharmacologic effects—affect the release of NE from nerve endings and the level of adrenergic activity; influence α-receptor and β-receptor activities
B. Therapeutic use—treatment of hypertension; use is limited by adverse effects (e.g., can cause xerostomia and sedation)

C. Examples
   1. Reserpine (Serpasil)
   2. Methyldopa (Aldomet)
   3. Clonidine (Catapres)

## Parasympathomimetic (Cholinergic) Agents

A. Cholinergic agonists—mimic the action of the parasympathetic autonomic nervous system (PANS); stimulation of the PANS
   1. Receptors—see Fig. 11.4 for an illustration of a typical cholinergic nerve
      a. Muscarinic—receptor stimulated by the compound found in the poisonous mushroom *Amanita muscaria* (Fig. 11.4, *A*)
         1. Areas affected (*A*)
            (a) Smooth muscle
            (b) Cardiac muscle
            (c) Gland cells
         2. Neurotransmitter—acetylcholine (ACh)
         3. Location—the synapse between the postganglionic fiber and the neuroeffector organ in the PANS
         4. Stimulated by muscarine
         5. Blocked by atropine
      b. Nicotinic—receptor stimulated by nicotine; found in cigarettes (Fig. 11.4, *B* and *C*)
         1. Areas affected
            (a) Postganglionic neurons (*B*)
            (b) Skeletal muscle end plates (*C*)
         2. Neurotransmitter—ACh
         3. Location—autonomic ganglia (*B*) and neuromuscular junction (*C*)
         4. Stimulated by nicotine
         5. Blocked by hexamethonium (autonomic, *B*) and *d*-tubocurarine at the neuromuscular junction (*C*)
   2. Acetylcholine—the following diagram illustrates synthesis and inactivation of ACh

$$\underset{\text{(CoA)}}{\overset{\text{A}}{\text{Acetyl}}} + \overset{\text{Ch}}{\text{Choline}} \underset{\substack{\text{Acetylcholinesterase} \\ \text{(AChE)}}}{\overset{\substack{\text{Choline} \\ \text{acetyltransferase}}}{\rightleftharpoons}} \overset{\text{ACh}}{\text{Acetylcholine}}$$

   3. Classification and mechanism of action
      a. Direct-acting drugs—act just as ACh at the receptor site, such as:
         (1) Choline derivatives
         (2) Pilocarpine (Salagen)
      b. Indirect-acting drugs—increase the amount of ACh indirectly; block ACh inactivation by inhibiting acetylcholinesterase (AChE), the enzyme that normally destroys ACh
         (1) "Reversible" cholinesterase inhibitors—drugs that block action of AChE, but whose action is terminated (ACh is then destroyed)
            (a) Edrophonium (Tensilon)
            (b) Physostigmine (Eserine)
            (c) Neostigmine (Prostigmin)
         (2) "Irreversible" cholinesterase inhibitors—drugs that attach to and inactivate AChE (e.g., organophosphates used as insecticides [malathion, parathion])
   4. Pharmacologic effects—similar to stimulation of the PANS
      a. Smooth muscle stimulation
         (1) Increase in gastrointestinal (GI) motility—diarrhea may result; advantageously used to treat postoperative GI and genitourinary (GU) retention
         (2) Bronchoconstriction—causes constriction of bronchial smooth muscle, an adverse reaction
      b. Glands—increased secretion of saliva; used to treat dry mouth (xerostomia)
      c. Eye—decreased intraocular pressure; used to treat glaucoma
   5. Toxic reactions—symptoms of overdose are extensions of the pharmacologic effects; the "too much" effect
      a. SLUD—excessive salivation, lacrimation (tearing), urination, and defecation
      b. Treatment of overdose
         (1) Pralidoxime (2-PAM, Protopam)—regenerates AChE
         (2) Atropine—antimuscarinic; blocks the muscarinic effects of ACh excess (not nicotinic effects)
   6. Dental hygiene considerations
      a. Oral forms can cause increased salivation and may cause hypotension and bradycardia
      b. Patients should maintain good oral hygiene
      c. Have patient rise slowly from the dental chair to minimize orthostatic hypotension
   7. Dental use—treatment of xerostomia; pilocarpine tablets may increase salivary flow.

B. Anticholinergic agents—block muscarinic actions of the PANS
   1. Basic principles
      a. Decreased salivary flow; used advantageously to dry up saliva
      b. Many drugs can have an anticholinergic, atropinic, or atropine-like effect
      c. Anticholinergic agents block the muscarinic receptors
   2. Pharmacologic effects on the:
      d. Heart—tachycardia (increased HR; useful during general anesthesia when HR may fall too low)
      e. Eye—produces:
         (1) Mydriasis—dilation of pupils; results in photophobia
         (2) Cycloplegia—paralysis for distant vision; patient cannot focus or read up close
         (3) Avoid repeated doses in patients who have narrow-angle glaucoma (this is the only autonomic drug group relatively contraindicated in certain forms of glaucoma)
      f. Salivary secretions—salivary flow reduced; useful in dentistry (Table 11.4 lists several drug groups that produce xerostomia)
      g. CNS—can cause sedation or excitation

TABLE 11.4 Xerostomia-Producing Drug Groups With Examples

| Drug Group | Examples |
|---|---|
| Antiacne | Isotretinoin |
| Anticholinergics[a] (P-) | Atropine |
| Anticonvulsants | Carbamazepine, felbamate, gabapentin, lamotrigine |
| Antidepressants | Amitriptyline, imipramine, fluoxetine, fluvoxamine |
| Antihistamines | Astemizole, brompheniramine, chlorpheniramine, loratadine |
| Antihypertensives[a] | Clonidine, guanethidine, methyldopa, captopril |
| Antinauseants | Cyclizine, diphenhydramine, meclizine |
| Antiparkinson drugs | Benztropine mesylate, biperiden, carbidopa, levodopa, trihexyphenidyl |
| Antipsychotics | Chlorpromazine, clozapine, fluphenazine, haloperidol, thioridazine |
| Antispasmodics | Dicyclomine, propantheline |
| Antidiarrheal | Diphenoxylate, loperamide |
| Benzodiazepines | Diazepam, alprazolam, lorazepam |
| Decongestants | Pseudoephedrine |
| Diuretics | Hydrochlorothiazide, furosemide |
| Muscle relaxants | Baclofen, orphenadrine |
| Nonsteroidal antiinflammatory drugs (NSAIDs) | Diflunisal, ibuprofen, naproxen |

[a]More likely to produce xerostomia; effect still dose-related.

3. Adverse reactions and toxicity—contraindications to use
   a. Xerostomia, dry skin, and dry eyes—caution in persons wearing contact lenses; reduces lactation in nursing mothers
   b. Eyes—blurred vision; avoid use in patients with narrow-angle glaucoma; careful use of eyedrops in persons with wide-angle glaucoma is usually acceptable
   c. Urinary retention—avoid use in persons with prostatic hypertrophy (enlarged prostate)
   d. Dizziness and fatigue—toxic levels can cause delirium, hallucinations, coma, and convulsions
   e. Tachycardia—monitor persons with cardiovascular disease
   f. Reduced GI motility—avoid in persons with gastric retention or intestinal obstruction
4. Clinical uses—effects offer advantageous treatment in:
   a. GI activity—has antispasmodic properties (reduced GI overactivity) and reduces secretions (e.g., stomach acid)
   b. Overactive bladder - inhibit acetylcholine/muscarinic receptors in the detrusor muscle of the bladder; preventing contractions thereby allowing the bladder to completely fill up, reduces frequency and urgency
   c. Ophthalmology—dilates eyes and paralyzes the muscles of accommodation (the person can see only distant objects); used for eye examinations
   d. Parkinson's disease
   e. Drug-induced Parkinson's disease
   f. Dental
      (1) Used before general anesthesia to dry up saliva and to prevent vagal slowing of the heart
      (2) Used to prepare the mouth for procedures that require a drier field
5. Dental hygiene considerations
   a. Xerostomia—instruct the patient to drink plenty of water, suck on tart sugarless gum or candy with xylitol or ice chips, avoid products containing alcohol and caffeine, and avoid juices and soft drinks to reduce the risk of dental caries; saliva substitutes (Xero-lube, Salivart) can also be recommended
   b. Tachycardia—check the patient's BP and pulse
   c. Sedation—an increased risk of sedation exists if combined with other sedating agents; patient should be instructed to avoid driving or operating heavy machinery or any task that requires thinking or concentration
6. Examples of anticholinergic agents
   a. Atropine
   b. Benztropine mesylate (Cogentin)
   c. Dicyclomine (Bentyl)
   d. Fesoteradine (Toviaz)
   e. Methantheline (Banthine)
   f. Oxybutyin (Detrol)
   g. Propantheline (Pro-Banthine)
   h. Solifenacin (VESIcare)
   i. Trihexyphenidyl hydrochloride (Artane)
   j. Trospium chloride (Sanctura)

## LOCAL ANESTHETIC AGENTS

A. Pharmacokinetics
   1. Absorption
      a. Effect on the vasculature—LAs produce vasodilation (except cocaine); vasoconstrictors are added to counteract dilation
      b. Absorption and distribution of LAs are determined by the pH of the environment, as shown in the following reaction:

$$\text{Inflammation} \rightarrow \downarrow \text{pH} \rightarrow \uparrow [\text{H}^+] \rightarrow \uparrow \text{charged form}$$
$$\text{(more acide) (more hydrogen ions)}$$
$$\text{S} \rightarrow \downarrow \text{un} - \text{ionized form B} \rightarrow \updownarrow \text{:chraged distribution}$$

      c. Solubility
         (1) Lipid-soluble—the nonionized form penetrates membranes
         (2) Water-soluble—the ionized form crosses the cell membrane and exerts its effect at the nerve
      d. Rate of absorption
         (1) The faster the rate of absorption, the greater the chance of systemic toxicity and the shorter the duration of action

(2) Route of administration alters the rate of absorption; the topical anesthetic agent can be absorbed quickly

2. Distribution—the level of the LA in the blood is determined by movement of the LA around the body; side effects occur if the LA reaches a high enough level in other organs (e.g., CNS, heart); blood level is determined by:
   a. Rate of injection
   b. Speed of absorption (depends on proximity to blood vessels)
   c. Speed of distribution to other tissues
   d. Speed of metabolism and excretion
3. Metabolism (biotransformation)
   a. Esters—hydrolyzed by plasma pseudo-cholinesterases
   b. Amides—metabolized in the liver
      (1) Procaine—metabolized to PABA—allergenic
      (2) Congenital cholinesterase deficiency—LAs containing esters are absolutely contraindicated
      (3) Liver dysfunction—LAs containing amides should be given cautiously; they may be metabolized more slowly; toxic levels can build up if repeated doses are administered
      (4) Prilocaine—metabolized to orthotoluidine, which can produce methemoglobinemia, a condition in which excess methemoglobin in the blood results in lowered oxygen-carrying capacity; not usually a problem in healthy clients
         (3) Excretion capacity
            a. Esters are almost completely metabolized before they are excreted
            b. Amides are mostly metabolized before they are excreted
            c. The presence of significant renal disease can cause all LA metabolites to accumulate

B. Adverse reactions
   1. Factors influencing toxicity:
      a. Drug
      b. Concentration
      c. Route
      d. Tissue inflammation
      e. Vasoconstriction
      f. Body weight
      g. Rate of metabolism and excretion
   2. Symptoms of LA toxicity—the CNS and the cardiovascular system (CVS) are affected most; the severity of effects is related directly to the amount of the LA in blood
      a. CNS response—stimulation followed by depression
      b. CNS stimulation (excitatory)—produces restlessness, shivering, tremors, convulsions
      c. CNS depression—results in sedation, drowsiness, respiratory and cardiovascular depression, coma; can occur without previous excitation
      d. CVS response
         (1) Antidysrhythmic action—lidocaine used intravenously to treat dysrhythmias
         (2) Vasodilation produces hypotension; releases vascular smooth muscle; lowers resistance
   3. Malignant hyperthermia—life-threatening complication associated with the administration of general anesthesia, characterized by tachycardia, tachypnea, cardiac dysrhythmia, muscle rigidity, and extreme increase in body temperature; LA agents containing amide administered in standard doses in oral health care appear to be safe for individuals susceptible to malignant hyperthermia
   4. Allergic reactions
      a. Range of reactions—mild rash to anaphylaxis

## LOCAL ANESTHETIC REVERSAL AGENT

Information pertaining to this topic is covered in Chapter 18.

## GENERAL ANESTHETICS

Information pertaining to this topic is covered in Chapter 18.

## SEDATIVE-HYPNOTIC MEDICATIONS

### General Considerations

A. Used to treat anxiety disorder, situational anxiety, and insomnia
B. Other drugs, in addition to sedative–hypnotics, can cause sedation; all can increase a patient's risk for sedation when used together (Box 11.1)
C. Dental concerns
   1. Additive CNS depressant effects when taken with alcohol, opioid analgesics, or other CNS depressants
   2. The patient should be instructed to avoid driving or operating heavy machinery or any task that requires thinking or concentration

### Benzodiazepines

A. Mechanism of action—potentiates the inhibitory neurotransmitter $\gamma$-aminobutyric acid (GABA); GABA-ergic neurotransmission increases sedation
B. Wide TI when ingested alone; much safer than barbiturates
C. Adverse reactions
   1. Sedation—the patient should be instructed to avoid driving or operating heavy machinery or any task that requires thinking or concentration
   2. Addiction potential—some potential exists but less than that for barbiturates
   3. Teratogenicity—increased incidence of birth defects if taken during the first trimester
   4. Thrombophlebitis—when administered intravenously; local irritation may occur with diazepam because of the use of propylene glycol as diluent; midazolam (Versed) is soluble in water, so no propylene glycol is used
   5. Overdose—treated with flumazenil (Mazicon), a benzodiazepine antagonist
D. Specific agents

**BOX 11.1 Select Pharmacologic Groups Producing Sedation**

Alcohol, ethyl
Antihistamines
Antipsychotics (phenothiazines)
Barbiturates
Benzodiazepines
Centrally acting muscle relaxants
Nonbarbiturate sedative-hypnotics
Nonsteroidal antiinflammatory drugs (NSAIDs)
Opioid (narcotic) analgesic agents
Tricyclic antidepressants

**TABLE 11.5 Examples of Benzodiazepines**

| Drug | Usual Dose (oral) (mg/day) |
|---|---|
| Alprazolam (Xanax) | 0.25–4.0 |
| Chlordiazepoxide (Librium) | 15.0–100.0 |
| Diazepam (Valium) | 4–40 |
| Flurazepam (Dalmane) | 15–30 |
| Lorazepam (Ativan) | 2–9 |
| Midazolam (Versed) | Intravenous |
| Oxazepam (Serax) | 45–120 |
| Temazepam (Restoril) | 7.5–30 |
| Triazolam (Halcion) | 0.125–0.25 |

1. Examples of benzodiazepines and typical doses for both anxiety and insomnia are provided in Table 11.5 (see also Table 11.4)
2. Differences between benzodiazepines
3. Drug interactions—the presence of cimetidine reduces the metabolism of oxidized benzodiazepines; patients who smoke experience less sedation (smoking induces liver enzymes)
   a. Equivalent dose—usual dose varies with agent
   b. Duration—varies from a few hours to a few days
   c. Metabolism
      (1) Most benzodiazepines are metabolized by oxidation to active metabolites
      (2) Oxazepam, lorazepam, and temazepam are inactivated by glucuronidation
      (3) The patient's age is a factor that can reduce the metabolism of oxidized benzodiazepines

E. Dental hygiene considerations
   1. Can cause anterograde amnesia (limited to events occurring after drug administration); patients should be cautioned about making life-changing decisions after taking a benzodiazepine
   2. All other *dental hygiene considerations* are the same as the general considerations

## Nonbarbiturate Nonbenzodiazepines

A. Nonbenzodiazepine receptor hypnotics—agonist effects at $GABA_A$ receptors, decrease sleep latency, little effect on sleep stages
   1. Zolpidem (Ambien)
   2. Zaleplon (Sonata)
   3. Eszopiclone (Lunesta)

B. Nonbenzodiazepine–nonbarbiturate sedative hypnotic
   1. Buspirone (Buspar)
      a. Mechanism of action is unknown, thought to interact with serotonin, dopamine, cholinergic, and α-adrenergic receptors
      b. Does not appear to cause much sedation
      c. Used for anxiolytic effects, not for insomnia
      d. 2 to 4 weeks to see effects

C. Melatonin receptor agonist—ramelteon (Rozerem); used to treat insomnia characterized by difficulty falling asleep

D. Orexin Receptor Antagonist - competitively inhibits the neuropeptides orexin A and B, which promote wakefulness
   1. Suvorexant (Belsomra)
   2. Lemborexant (Dayvigo)

E. Centrally acting muscle relaxants
   a. Carisoprodol (Soma)—Class 2 (CII) drug
   b. Chlorzoxazone (Paraflex)
   c. Methocarbamol (Robaxin)
   d. Orphenadrine (Norflex)
   e. Baclofen (Lioresal)
   f. Tizanidine (Zanaflex)
   g. Dantrolene (Dantrium)

F. Dental hygiene considerations—same as earlier "General Considerations"

# ANALGESICS

See Table 11.6.

## General Considerations

A. Pain is characterized by:
   1. Perception—experienced uniformly through the nerve (signal from the site of pain to the CNS)
   2. Reaction—varies greatly from person to person (interpretation of the signal within the CNS)

B. Variables—patient's age, gender, race, ethnic group, fatigue, and pain threshold

## Salicylates (Aspirin)

A. Mechanism of action—primarily peripheral; prostaglandin synthesis inhibitor functions by inhibiting the enzyme cyclooxygenase (COX) or prostaglandin synthetase

B. Pharmacologic effects—"the three As"
   1. Analgesic—reduces pain
   2. Antipyretic—therapeutic dose reduces elevated body temperature
   3. Antiinflammatory—higher dose reduces inflammation

C. Adverse reactions
   1. GI upset—minimized by ingesting the drug with food, water, or antacids
   2. Alteration in bleeding
      a. Platelet adhesiveness—reduced platelet adhesion for the life of the platelet (4 to 7 days); normal clotting

**TABLE 11.6 Analgesic Summary**

| Pharmacologic Effects and Adverse Reactions | Aspirin | NSAIDs | Acetaminophen | Opioids (Narcotics) |
|---|---|---|---|---|
| Analgesic | + | ++ | + | ++++ |
| Antipyretic | + | +/0 | + | 0 |
| Antiinflammatory | + | ++ | 0 | 0 |
| Central nervous system (CNS) effects (drowsiness) | ++[a] | ++ | 0[b] | ++ |
| Gastrointestinal (GI) effects | ++[c] | +[c] | 0 | +[d] |
| Bleeding | ++ | +[e] | 0 | 0 |
| Hepatotoxic | +[f] | + | +[g] | 0 |
| Nephrotoxic | +[e] | +[e] | +[e] | 0 |
| Addicting effects | 0 | 0 | 0 | ++++ |

+, Very low; ++, low; +++, moderate; ++++, high; 0, no effect.
[a]Poisoning—salicylism.
[b]Very high doses.
[c]Upset stomach, ulcers, pain.
[d]Nausea, constipation.
[e]Aspirin or nonsteroidal antiinflammatory drugs (NSAIDs) and acetaminophen.
[f]Hepatitis in persons with systemic lupus erythematosus or rheumatoid arthritis.
[g]With acute overdose.

reappears 72 hours after ingestion; reduced clotting effect requires only a low single dose; useful in low doses to prevent clotting
   b. Hypoprothrombinemia—reduced prothrombin levels; requires several consecutive doses to reduce prothrombin levels
3. Salicylate toxicity ("salicylism")—symptoms include tinnitus, hyperthermia (increased body temperature), electrolyte and glucose problems, and altered sensorium
4. Allergic reactions—true allergy is uncommon; if person is allergic, some cross-reactivity exists with other agents (e.g., nonsteroidal antiinflammatory drugs [NSAIDs]); can produce an acute asthma attack; persons with asthma and nasal polyps are more susceptible
5. Reye syndrome—children with chickenpox or influenza should not be given aspirin; avoid aspirin in children and adolescents up to 18 years of age

D. Drug interactions—adverse reactions occur with aspirin used in conjunction with:
   1. Warfarin (Coumadin)—used as an anticoagulant; bleeding or hemorrhage
   2. Probenecid (Benemid)—used to treat gout; acute attack of gout
   3. Tolbutamide (Orinase)—used to control diabetes; altered blood glucose level
   4. Methotrexate (MTX)—used to treat cancer or control arthritis; MTX toxicity in bone marrow
   5. Alcohol—can increase bleeding or hemorrhage
   6. Other antiinflammatory drugs—can increase bleeding or hemorrhage

E. Dental hygiene considerations
   1. Avoid drugs that can cause GI upset or prolong bleeding time
   2. Check for aspirin allergies
   3. If taken before procedure, patient may experience more bleeding than normal

## Nonsteroidal Antiinflammatory Agents (NSAIAs) and Drugs (NSAIDs)

A. Mechanism—similar to that of aspirin, drug inhibits prostaglandin synthesis (COX)

B. Pharmacologic effects—"the three As" (similar to aspirin)
   1. Analgesic
   2. Antipyretic
   3. Antiinflammatory

C. Adverse reactions
   1. GI—more severe than aspirin; abdominal problems range from discomfort to ulcers; treated or managed with prostaglandin—misoprostol (Cytotec); increased risk for severe GI events, including bleeding and ulcers
   2. CVS—may increase the risk for serious cardiovascular thrombotic events, stroke, and MI
   3. CNS—dizziness, sedation; the patient should be instructed to avoid driving or operating heavy machinery, or any task that requires thinking or concentration
   4. Blood coagulation—reduction in platelet aggregation and possible prolongation of bleeding time; alteration is reversible, unlike the effect of aspirin, which is not reversible
   5. Oral—can produce stomatic gingival ulceration and xerostomia
   6. Renal—can result in renal failure or cystitis
   7. Hypersensitivity—ranges from mild rash to anaphylaxis

D. Drug interactions
   1. Lithium—can increase lithium levels
   2. Digoxin—can increase the effects of digoxin
   3. MTX—can increase the effects of MTX
   4. Antihypertensives—can reduce the antihypertensive effects of diuretics, angiotensin-converting enzyme (ACE) inhibitors, and β-blockers

5. Other inflammatory drugs—can increase bleeding and hemorrhage
6. Alcohol—can increase bleeding or hemorrhage

E. Contraindications
1. Contraindicated in patients that have experienced asthma or allergic reaction to aspirin therapy
2. Fluid-retention problems
3. Coagulation problems
4. Peptic ulcer disease
5. Ulcerative colitis
6. Renal disease; especially in patients at risk for renal disease or for patients taking ACE inhibitors or angiotensin receptor blockers (ARBs)

F. Dental hygiene considerations
1. Same as for aspirin
2. CNS sedation—the patient should be instructed to avoid driving or operating heavy machinery or any task that requires thinking or concentration

G. Therapeutic uses
1. Pain control—analgesic; stronger than aspirin, equal to or stronger than some opioids; strength of effect is dose dependent; antiinflammatory effect makes NSAIDs especially useful in dentistry
2. Arthritis—antiinflammatory action
3. Dysmenorrhea (painful menstruation)—effective because the mechanism of action is specific for the problem of excess prostaglandins caused by excessive uterine contractions

H. Examples
1. Ibuprofen (Motrin-IB, Rufen, Nuprin, Advil); naproxen sodium (Anaprox; Aleve); available without a prescription
2. Naproxen (Naprosyn)
3. Indomethacin (Indocin)—prescription only
4. Celecoxib (Celebrex)—prescription only
   a. Caution should be exercised because COX-2 inhibitors can increase the risk of a heart attack
   b. Caution should be exercised because of an increased risk for significant GI bleeding

## Acetaminophen (*N*-Acetyl-*p*-Aminophenol [NAPAP]; Tylenol [Available Over the Counter])

A. Pharmacologic effects—"the two As"
1. Analgesic
2. Antipyretic
3. Not an antiinflammatory

B. Adverse reactions
1. Analgesic nephropathy—adversely affects the kidneys; more likely to occur if used chronically in combination with aspirin or NSAIDs
2. Hepatotoxicity—may occur with acute overdose or chronic use; delayed reaction; treated with *N*-acetylcysteine; may be fatal without liver transplantation

C. Drug interactions—alcohol increases the risk of acetaminophen toxicity

D. Contraindications
1. Hepatotoxicity
2. Renal toxicity
3. Patients with alcohol-abuse problems

E. Dental hygiene considerations—avoid use in patients with hepatotoxicity, renal toxicity, or alcohol abuse problems

## Opioid (Narcotic) Analgesic Agents

A. Pharmacologic effects—proportional to the "strength" of the opioid
1. Analgesia
2. Sedation (anxiety relief)
3. Euphoria
4. Dysphoria
5. Cough suppressant
6. GI effects
7. Respiratory effects

B. Examples of agonists (combine with opioid receptor and produce an effect) are provided in Table 11.7)

C. Examples of agonist–antagonist agents: pentazocine (Talwin-NX)
1. Can precipitate withdrawal in opiate addicts
   a. Maintain analgesic properties
   b. Have lower abuse potential

D. Antagonists
1. Example—Naloxone (Narcan), Naltrexone (Vivitrol), Nalmefene (Revex)
2. Combine with opioid receptor; produces no effect; reverses opioid overdose
3. Therapeutic uses
   a. Treat opioid overdose
   b. Counteract respiratory depression
   c. Include in any dental emergency kit

E. Adverse reactions—proportional to the "strength" of the opioid
1. CNS effects—sedation, euphoria, dysphoria
2. Respiratory depression—dose related; overdose can result in death; reversed with naloxone
3. GI—nausea, vomiting, constipation; diphenoxylate can be useful therapeutically
4. Abuse—can occur with all opioid analgesics; tolerance develops to all pharmacologic effects except miosis (pupillary constriction) and constipation; withdrawal produced if the drug is abruptly stopped
5. Miosis
6. Urinary retention

**TABLE 11.7 Examples of Agonists**

| Drug | Usual Dose (Oral) (mg/day) | "Strength" |
|---|---|---|
| Morphine | 10–30 po q4h | Stronger |
| Hydromorphone (Dilaudid) | 1–6 q4–6 h | |
| Meperidine (Demerol) | 50–150 po q4h | |
| Oxycodone (in Percodan) | 5 q6h | |
| Hydrocodone (in Vicodin) | 5–10 po q4–6 h | |
| Codeine (in Tylenol No. 3, Empirin No. 3) | 30–60 q4–6 h | Weaker |

*po,* By mouth; *q4h,* every 4 hours; *q4–6 h,* every 4 to 6 hours; *q6h,* every 6 hours.

7. Cardiovascular effects—orthostatic hypotension

F. Therapeutic uses
1. Pain relief—this is the central mechanism; agent affects a person's perception of pain; some opioids can relieve severe pain
2. Sedation and anxiety relief—not the main use of opioids; used preoperatively
3. Cough suppression—antitussive action (cough suppressant); low dose needed (e.g., codeine-containing cough syrups)
4. Diarrhea—symptomatic relief only; reduce GI motility by increasing tone and spasm; diphenoxylate (in Lomotil)

G. Drug interactions
1. Increase sedation when used with other CNS depressant drugs
2. Increase constipation when combined with anticholinergic drugs

H. Dental hygiene considerations
1. Increased risk for sedation—as with other CNS depressant drugs
2. Increased risk for xerostomia—as with anticholinergic drugs

### Drugs Used for Gout

A. Disease—gout is a metabolic condition involving increased serum uric acid, with episodes of acute attacks of pain in joints (big toe, knee) and severe inflammation caused by deposition of monosodium urate

B. Prevention
1. Probenecid (Benemid)—uricosuric (promotes uric acid excretion); aspirin interferes with this effect of probenecid
2. Allopurinol (Zyloprim)—xanthine oxidase inhibitor (inhibits uric acid synthesis); also used in patients with cancer before chemotherapy or radiation therapy when many cells are killed and release their amino acids, which leads to accumulation of uric acid and attacks of gout

C. Treatment
1. Colchicine—binds to microtubular protein tubulin (prevents leukocyte migration and phagocytosis); inhibits formation of leukotrienes; GI toxicity—nausea, vomiting, diarrhea are end points of treatment and adverse reactions
2. NSAIDs—antiinflammatory action ameliorates symptoms (e.g., indomethacin)

### Drugs for Arthritis

A. Disease - Rheumatoid arthritis (RA) is an autoimmune disorder characterized by chronic inflammation of the body's joints causing painful inflammation and swelling

B. Treatment
1. Disease-Modifying Antirheumatic Drugs
   a. Immunosuppressives - interfere with the formation of immune cells by damaging the RNA and DNA necessary for cell replication
      1. Include azathioprine (Imuran), methotrexate, cyclophosphamide, auranofin (Ridaura), hydroxychloroquine (Plaquenil), leflunomide (Arava), and sulfasalazine (Azulfidine)
      2. Can weaken the immune system
   b. Tumor Necrosis Factor (TNF)-α inhibitor
      1. TNF is a cytokine that is released by cells when the body senses a foreign invasion. High levels of TNF are found in people with RA. Blocks the inflammatory process of RA
      2. Include adalimumab (Humira), etanercept (Enbrel)
      3. Can weaken the immune system
2. Biologic Response Modifiers
   a. Work by inhibiting or modifying the body's immune response system
   b. Examples include rituximab (Rituxan), tofacitinib (Xeljanz)
   c. Can weaken the immune system

## ANTIINFECTIVES (ANTIBIOTICS)

### General Considerations

A. Prevention of infection (see the section on "Disease Transmission" in Chapter 10)
1. Sterilization measures prevent infection
2. Many infections—treat with local measures (e.g., incision and drainage), antibiotics are often not needed; the patient's resistance and the development of resistant strains of bacteria must be considered
3. Antibiotic administration carries risks
4. Prophylaxis is rarely indicated except for decreasing the likelihood of infective endocarditis in persons who have the highest risk, prosthetic joint infection, or when patient is immunosuppressed[2] (see Chapter 15, Table 15-2)

B. Definitions
1. Antimicrobial—agent that acts against microbes
2. Anti-infective—agent that acts against the organisms that cause infections
3. Antibacterial—agent that acts against bacteria
4. Antiviral—agent that acts against viruses
5. Antifungal—agent that acts against fungi
6. Antibiotic—agent that is effective in low concentrations; produced by microorganisms; kills or suppresses growth of other organisms
7. Spectrum—range of an antibiotic's anti-infective properties; can be narrow (acting on few organisms) to wide or broad (acting on many organisms); may include effectiveness against gram-positive and gram-negative bacteria
8. Resistance—the organism is unaffected by an anti-infective; the resistance may be natural (always has been resistant) or acquired (resistance has developed); prolonged exposure to antibiotics allows for the organism to develop resistance towards the antibiotic
9. Suprainfection (superinfection)—onset of a new infection from an organism other than the original organism; occurs after taking an antimicrobial agent; the new infection is usually more difficult to treat, and commonly occurs when

the spectrum is the widest; for example, Candida infection may arise in person taking tetracycline

10. Synergism—agent's effect is more than additive (1 + 1 > 2)
11. Antagonism—agent's effect is less than additive (1 + 1 < 2)
    a. Bactericidal—kills bacteria
    b. Bacteriostatic—retards or incapacitates bacteria (reversible)

C. General side effects
  1. GI side effects—variable, depending on antibiotic; includes nausea, vomiting, diarrhea, dyspepsia
  2. Suprainfection from antibiotic-resistant bacteria is possible, usually in the form of a vaginal yeast infection
  3. Drug interactions
     a. Oral contraceptives—some antibiotics may reduce effectiveness; inform the patient that alternative forms of birth control should be used for the duration of the prescription, plus an additional 7 days or until the end of their menstrual cycle
     b. Warfarin (Coumadin)—antibiotics alter the GI flora that make vitamin K, which then can potentiate warfarin's effect

D. Treatment versus prophylaxis
  1. Treatment—the antiinfective is used to treat an infection that is present
  2. Prophylaxis—used to prevent some potential future infection; only proven beneficial in a few instances

E. General dental concerns for all antibiotics—make sure that the patient:
  1. Knows the name of the antibiotic and how to take it
  2. Understands the need to complete the full course of therapy
  3. Understands the rationale for prophylactic antibiotic medication
  4. Takes all antibiotics with a full glass of water
  5. Takes antibiotics on an empty stomach; if the medicine causes nausea, it should be taken with food

## Penicillins

A. Mechanism—inhibit cell wall synthesis; bactericidal

B. Spectrum—three penicillin subgroups:
  1. Penicillin G, penicillin V
  2. Penicillinase-resistant penicillin
  3. Extended-spectrum penicillins
     a. Ampicillin-like
     b. Carbenicillin-like

C. Stability
  1. Acid labile—degrades in stomach acid; therefore administered parenterally (e.g., penicillin G, methicillin, carbenicillin)
  2. Acid stable—may be used orally (e.g., penicillin VK, amoxicillin)

D. Pharmacokinetics
  1. Peak—penicillin blood levels peak between 30 minutes and 1 hour when administered by the oral or IM route; peak immediately when administered intravenously
  2. Half-life (t½)—between 30 minutes and 1 hour
  3. Excretion very rapid, actively secreted; duration prolonged by concomitant probenecid (Benemid) administration

E. Adverse effects
  1. GI—mild GI upset to nausea and vomiting
  2. Allergic reactions—range from mild rash to anaphylaxis
  3. Nephrotoxicity—occurs occasionally; kidney damage more likely with broader-spectrum penicillins

### Penicillin G and Penicillin V

A. Examples
  1. Penicillin G potassium
  2. Penicillin G procaine (Wycillin, Crysticillin)
  3. Penicillin G benzathine (Bicillin)
  4. Penicillin VK (V-Cillin K, Pen-Vee K)

B. Spectrum—potent against many gram-positive aerobic organisms, such as *Streptococcus* and *Staphylococcus,* certain gram-negative aerobic cocci, such as *Neisseria gonorrhoeae,* and some anaerobic organisms; not resistant to penicillinase

C. Penicillin G—parenteral administration
  1. Dose specified in units (e.g., 5 million units [MU])
  2. IM salts (procaine and benzathine) provide longer duration of action than do sodium and potassium salts

D. Penicillin V—more acid stable than penicillin G, thus, can be used orally; potassium salt better absorbed; therefore, penicillin VK is the most frequently used antibiotic in dentistry; 400,000 units (U) = 250 mg

### Extended-Spectrum ("Broader-Spectrum" or "Wider-Spectrum") Penicillins

A. Ampicillin-like
  1. Examples
     a. Ampicillin (Omnipen, Totacillin, Polycillin)
     b. Amoxicillin (Amoxil, Larotid, Polymox)
  2. Spectrum—effective against many gram-positive and some gram-negative bacteria such as *Haemophilus influenzae, Escherichia coli,* and *Proteus mirabilis*
  3. Not penicillinase resistant
  4. Augmentin—amoxicillin combined with clavulanic acid, which binds with penicillinase, so amoxicillin is not inactivated; can be used with penicillinase-producing organisms

## Macrolides

A. Mechanism—interfere with protein synthesis by binding to the 50S ribosomal subunit; provide bacteriostatic action

B. Spectrum
  1. Erythromycin
     a. Effective primarily against gram-positive microorganisms; ineffective against anaerobes
     b. Used against certain strains of *Rickettsia, Chlamydia,* and *Actinomyces*; drug of choice for treating infections caused by *Mycoplasma pneumoniae* and *Legionella pneumophila*
  2. Azithromycin (Zithromax)
     a. Recommended by the American Heart Association (AHA) for use in the prevention of bacterial

endocarditis before certain dental procedures, in persons who are allergic to penicillin[2]
   b. Adverse effects—stomatitis, candidiasis, angioedema (allergic reaction), heart palpitations, chest pain, nausea, vomiting, diarrhea, abdominal pain, hepatotoxicity, heartburn, flatulence
   c. Alternative drug of choice for mild infection caused by susceptible organisms in persons allergic to penicillin
3. Clarithromycin (Biaxin)
   a. Recommended by the AHA for use in the prevention of bacterial endocarditis prior to certain dental procedures in persons who are allergic to penicillin[2]
   b. Adverse effects—abnormal taste, candidiasis, stomatitis, nausea, abdominal pain, diarrhea, hepatotoxicity, heartburn, anorexia, vomiting, vaginitis, moniliasis, urticaria, rash, pruritus
   c. Alternative drug of choice for mild infection caused by susceptible organisms in persons allergic to penicillin

C. Pharmacokinetics of erythromycin
   1. Erythromycin—high acid lability (instability) requires enteric coating (does not dissolve in the stomach; dissolves in the intestine) or formulation as an ester to protect against stomach acid (e.g., ethylsuccinate, erythromycin ethylsuccinate [EES])
   2. Effect peaks in 2 to 4 hours

D. Adverse effects
   1. GI upset is very common; must be taken with food to decrease
   2. Cholestatic jaundice is primarily associated with the estolate ester

E. Drug interactions—theophylline and erythromycin; increase theophylline levels

F. Examples—erythromycin
   1. Erythromycin base (E-mycin)
   2. Erythromycin estolate (Ilosone)
   3. Erythromycin ethylsuccinate (EES, Pedia-mycin)
   4. Erythromycin stearate (Erythrocin)

G. Therapeutic uses
   1. Treatment of dental infections in persons allergic to penicillin
   2. Specific suspected infections (see earlier B. Spectrum)

## Cephalosporins

A. Mechanism—similar to penicillins; inhibits cell wall synthesis; bactericidal

B. Chemistry similar to penicillins

C. Spectrum—effective against many gram-positive and gram-negative bacteria; the third-generation cephalosporins and the newest fourth-generation cephalosporins have the widest spectrum of action

D. Adverse reactions
   1. GI upset common (33%)
   2. Other—similar to those of the broader-spectrum penicillins (e.g., nephrotoxicity, suprainfection)
   3. Allergy—some cross-hypersensitivity (10%) with penicillin allergy (possess a similar chemical structure)

E. Examples
   1. Cefuroxime (Ceftin)
   2. Cephalexin (Keflex)
   3. Cephradine (Velosef, Anspor)

F. Suggested oral antibiotic regimen for the patient with joint prosthesis less than 2 years after surgery, only if the patient is immunocompromised[2]

## Clindamycin (Cleocin)

A. Mechanism—inhibits protein synthesis (binds to the 50S ribosomal subunit); bacteriostatic protection

B. Spectrum—effective against gram-positive organisms and many anaerobes such as *Bacteroides*

C. Adverse reactions
   1. GI—diarrhea; pseudomembranous colitis (PMC) or antibiotic-associated colitis (AAC, incidence up to 10%); drug must be discontinued if bloody stools with mucus occur
   2. The FDA states that this agent should be "reserved for serious anaerobic infections"

D. Dental use—used against certain anaerobic infections thought to be caused by *Bacteroides* species (spp.), jaw infections, and periodontal infections; and for the prophylaxis of infective endocarditis[2]

## Tetracyclines

A. Mechanism—inhibit protein synthesis by binding to the 30S ribosome; provide bacteriostatic action

B. Spectrum—truly broad spectrum; effective against many gram-positive and gram-negative bacteria

C. Pharmacokinetics
   1. Tetracyclines—divalent and trivalent cations (e.g., calcium [$Ca^{+2}$; in dairy products], magnesium [$Mg^{+2}$] and aluminum [$Al^{+3}$] in antacids, iron [$Fe^{+2}$]); inhibit the absorption of tetracycline by chelation
   2. Doxycycline (Vibramycin) and minocycline (Minocin)—less affected by food or dairy products than is tetracycline; avoid taking antacids or $Ca^{+2}$ supplementation concomitantly

D. Resistance—cross-transference can occur; organisms can become resistant without being exposed to drug

E. Adverse effects
   1. GI upset—relatively common
   2. Suprainfection—very common because of the wide spectrum of action; drug alters normal flora (e.g., may result in vaginal candidiasis)
   3. Photosensitivity—exaggerated sunburn with exposure to ultraviolet (UV) light
   4. Teeth—both hypoplasia and intrinsic stain can occur if the drug is taken during enamel development; primary

teeth affected from the last half of the pregnancy to age 4 to 6 months; permanent teeth are affected from age 2 months to 7 to 12 years

F. Examples
   1. Doxycycline (Vibramycin, Atridox)
   2. Minocycline (Minocin, Arestin)
   3. Tetracycline (Achromycin-V)
   4. Tetracycline fibers (Actisite)
G. Therapeutic uses
   1. Medical—treatment of acne, respiratory tract infections in patients with COPD (emphysema or bronchitis), certain sexually transmitted diseases (STDs)
   2. Dental—management of periodontal diseases; drug placed in periodontal pocket (e.g., tetracycline fibers [Atridox, Actisite, Arestin])
H. Dental hygiene considerations
   1. Must be taken 1 hour before or 2 hours after eating
   2. Should be taken with crackers if stomach upset occurs
   3. Should not be taken with antacids or dairy products
   4. Patients must be counseled about photosensitivity

## Quinolones

A. Mechanism—inhibition of bacterial gyrase so that the daughter segment of deoxyribonucleic acid (DNA) cannot acquire the proper configuration to divide
B. Spectrum—effective against gram-negative bacteria, including *Enterobacter* spp., *Escherichia coli,* and *Morganella morganii*
C. Adverse reactions—abdominal pain, nausea, vomiting, diarrhea, rash, urticaria, angioedema
D. Dental concerns—the patient must avoid direct light (e.g., dental light); offer the patient dark glasses to be worn during dental procedures; the patient must also avoid direct sun exposure
E. Examples
   1. Ciprofloxacin (Cipro)
   2. Enoxacin (Penetrex)
   3. Ofloxacin (Floxin)

## Sulfonamides ("Sulfa" Drugs)

A. Mechanism—competitive antagonist of PABA; prevents the use of PABA to make the folic acid needed in an organism
B. Adverse reactions
   1. Allergic reactions—rash
   2. Photosensitivity
C. Examples
   1. Sulfisoxazole (Gantrisin)
   2. Trimethoprim-sulfamethoxazole (TMP-SMX; Bactrim, Septra)
D. Therapeutic uses
   1. Urinary tract infections (UTIs)
   2. Otitis media (children's ear infections)
   3. Respiratory infections
   4. Dental use unclear; probably not useful

## Metronidazole (Flagyl)

A. Mechanism—breaks DNA structure, which inhibits protein synthesis; provides bactericidal action
B. Spectrum
   1. Trichomonicidal (effective against *Trichomonas vaginalis*)
   2. Bactericidal (effective against anaerobes such as *Bacteroides* spp.)
C. Adverse reactions
   1. GI—anorexia, nausea, vomiting, headache, dizziness
   2. CNS—disulfiram (Antabuse)-like reaction; concurrent alcohol ingestion produces nausea and vomiting
   3. Carcinogenic in animals; mutagenic in bacterial organisms; however, significance with regard to cancer is unknown
D. Dental use—management of periodontal patients with anaerobic infections; effective against organisms; inexpensive
E. Dental hygiene considerations
   1. Patients must avoid alcohol-containing products, including beverages, foods cooked with alcohol, colognes, aftershaves, perfumes
   2. Patients must avoid mouth rinses with alcohol; recommend alcohol-free mouth rinses

## Antituberculosis Agents

A. Tuberculosis (TB)—a chronic disease
   1. Resistant organisms develop easily
   2. Treatment is difficult, so drug combinations are frequently required; multidrug-resistant (MDR) organisms are common
   3. Requires drug treatment regimen of 6 to 9 months
B. Drugs
   1. Isoniazid (INH)—used alone as prophylaxis; used in combination with other agents; hepatitis is an adverse side effect
   2. Rifampin (Rifadin, Rimactane)
   3. Pyrazinamide
   4. Ethambutol (Myambutol)
C. Dental hygiene considerations—use standard precautions; affected persons are treated for 6 weeks to 2 months; the patient is generally not contagious if compliant with TB treatment regimen; direct observation and monitoring of the patient are needed

## Antifungal Agents

A. Disease—candidiasis (*Candida albicans*), called thrush in infants
B. Nystatin (Mycostatin, Nilstat)—dosage forms: oral suspension or pastille (rubbery lozenge)
C. Clotrimazole (Mycelex)—lozenges available
D. Ketoconazole (Nizoral)
   1. Tablets—dose: once per day
   2. An acid stomach environment is required for adequate absorption—be alert to histamine ($H_2$)-blockers
   3. Adverse reactions
      a. Nausea and vomiting
      b. Hepatocellular dysfunction

c. Teratogenic potential
d. Drug interactions

E. Fluconazole (Diflucan)
1. Tablets, oral suspension, and IV administration
2. Therapeutic use—systemic fungal infections
3. Adverse reactions—headache, abdominal pain, nausea, diarrhea, hepatic toxicity

F. Itraconazole (Sporanox)
1. Capsules
2. Therapeutic use—indicated for the treatment of certain fungal infections in both immunocompromised patients and those who are not
3. Adverse reactions—nausea, vomiting, diarrhea, abdominal pain, anorexia, edema, rash, fatigue, fever, malaise

### Antiviral Agents

A. Acyclovir (Zovirax)
1. Topical, oral, and IV forms available
2. Therapeutic uses
a. Treatment of initial genital herpes in patients who are not immunocompromised
b. Treatment of recurrent genital herpes in immunocompromised patients
c. Oral administration is recommended with continuous use as a prophylactic

B. Docosanol (Abreva)
a. Treatment of oral herpes simplex labialis (cold sores)
b. Available without a prescription
c. Adverse effects—stinging at the site of application
d. L-lysine (an amino acid) is often recommended with docosanol to aid in tissue repair and growth

C. Ganciclovir (Cytovene)
1. Inhibits replication of most herpesviruses
2. Therapeutic use—prevention and treatment of cytomegalovirus (CMV) in persons with acquired immunodeficiency syndrome (AIDS)
3. Adverse effects—fever, coma, chills, confusion, abnormal thoughts, dizziness, bizarre dreams, headaches, psychosis, tremors, paresthesia, dysrhythmia, hypertension, hypotension, hemorrhage, anorexia, blood dyscrasia

D. Antiretroviral drugs—indications: HIV-positive patients and those with AIDS (see Table 11.8)

E. Dental hygiene considerations—use standard precautions

**TABLE 11.8 Examples of Drugs Used to Treat Human Immunodeficiency Virus (HIV)**

| Drug Class | Drug Name | Comments |
|---|---|---|
| Nucleoside analogs or nucleoside/nucleotide reverse transcriptase inhibitors | Abacavir (Ziagen)<br>Didanosine (Videx)<br>Emtricitabine (Emtriva)<br>Lamivudine (Epivir)<br>Stavudine (Zerit)<br>Tenofovir (Viread)<br>Zalcitabine (Hivid)<br>Zidovudine (Retrovir) | Monitor for adverse drug reactions<br>Use caution to prevent instrument and needle sticks<br>Antibiotic prophylaxis when polymorphonuclear leukocyte count <500 PMNs/mm; delay elective treatments until normal<br>Anticipate oral candidiasis<br>Encourage meticulous oral hygiene<br>Frequent oral maintenance therapy needed |
| Nonnucleoside analogs or Nonnucleoside reverse transcriptase inhibitors | Delavirdine (Rescriptor)<br>Efavirenz (Sustiva)<br>Etravine (Intelence)<br>Nevirapine (NVP) (Viramune)<br>Rilpivirine (Edurant) | Encourage meticulous plaque control to minimize, prevent, and control inflammation<br>Used in combination with other anti-HIV therapy |
| Protease inhibitors | Amprenavir (Agenerase)<br>Atazanavir (Reyataz)<br>Darunavir (Prezista)<br>Fosamprenavir (Lexiva)<br>Indinavir (Crixivan)<br>Nelfinavir (Viracept)<br>Tipranavir (Aptivus)<br>Ritonavir (Norvir)<br>Saquinavir (Invirase, Fortovase) | |
| Fusion/entry inhibitors | Enfuvirtide (Fuzeon)<br>Maraviroc (Selzentry) | Used in combination with other anti-HIV therapy |
| Integrase inhibitors | Dolutegravir (Tivicay)<br>Elvitegravir (Vitekta<br>Raltegravir (Isentress) | Used in combination with other antiretroviral agents |
| Pharmacokinetic Enhancer | Cobicistat (Tybost) | Used in combination with other antiretroviral agents |

## CARDIOVASCULAR AGENTS

See Chapters 8 and 19 for contraindications and cautions involving dental treatment in persons with cardiovascular disease.[3]

### Digitalis Glycosides

A. Pharmacologic effects—heartbeats are stronger (positive chronotropic effect) but usually slower (bradycardia); therefore, efficiency is increased

B. Adverse reactions
1. GI disturbances—nausea, vomiting
2. CVS—arrhythmias/dysrhythmias
3. CNS—yellow-green vision; halos around lights

C. Therapeutic uses—heart failure, certain arrhythmias

D. Dental hygiene considerations
1. Hypokalemia—decreased potassium levels because of diuretics; digitalis toxicity may exacerbate dysrhythmias; epinephrine exacerbates dysrhythmias
2. Epinephrine—use of epinephrine may increase the risk for arrhythmias (dysrhythmias)
3. Pulse rate must be monitored
4. Tetracycline and erythromycin can increase the levels of digoxin in blood, causing digoxin toxicity (signaled by nausea, vomiting, and copious salivation)

E. Example—digoxin (Lanoxin)

## Antiarrhythmics

A. Pharmacologic effects—suppress arrhythmias
B. Dental considerations—in patients with cardiac problems, use caution when administering LAs with epinephrine
C. Examples
  1. Lidocaine (Xylocaine)—local anesthetic agent can be used parenterally as an antidysrhythmic agent
  2. Procainamide
  3. Propranolol (Inderal)
  4. Quinidine
D. Dental hygiene considerations
  1. Review health history to determine the patient's state of health
  2. Check BP and pulse

## Antianginal Agents

A. Pharmacologic effects—reduce the "work" of the heart because these agents function as nonspecific vasodilators, thereby reducing the amount of blood returning to the heart (preload) which lowers the heart's workload. Arterial dilation reduces the resistance which the heart must pump (afterload) which reduces workload both leading to decrease oxygen demand on the heart
B. Adverse reactions—hypotension and severe headache are common; patient should be in the sitting position to take nitroglycerin (NTG)
C. Drug interactions—phosphodiesterase-5 inhibitors (sildenafil, tadalafil, vardenafil)
D. Therapeutic use—angina pectoris
E. Dental hygiene considerations
  1. Storage—unstable products; must be stored properly; heat, light, and moisture cause further degradation; discard opened containers after 2 months or on the basis of the expiration date on the original vial, whichever comes first
  2. Acute anginal attack—administer NTG sublingually
  3. Routes of NTG administration
  4. Anxiety about the dental appointment may cause the angina attack; the patient can take tablet prophylactically
    a. SL—tablets or spray
    b. Transdermal—patches applied to chest or arm
    c. Ointment—in ointment applied to skin
F. Examples
  1. NTG (Nitrostat), SL tablet or spray (Nitrolingual SL spray)
  2. Isosorbide dinitrate (Isordil) or mononitrates

## Antihypertensives

See Table 11.9.

A. Pharmacologic effects—reduce elevated BP
B. Adverse reaction—CNS depression, fatigue, xerostomia, orthostatic hypotension, constipation and diarrhea, sexual dysfunction, upset stomach
C. Therapeutic use—treatment of hypertension
D. Dental hygiene considerations
  1. Take BP reading to ensure it is normal
  2. Xerostomia—instruct the patient to drink plenty of water; suck on tart sugarless gum or candy that contains xylitol, or ice chips; avoid products containing alcohol and caffeine; and avoid juices and soft drinks to reduce the risk of dental caries; saliva substitutes (Xero-lube, Salivart) can also be recommended
  3. Have the patient rise slowly from the dental chair
  4. Some calcium channel blockers can cause drug-influenced gingival enlargement; patients should perform meticulous oral hygiene and obtain frequent periodontal maintenance care
  5. CNS sedation—several antihypertensive medications can cause sedation; the patient is at an increased risk for sedation if an opioid analgesic or benzodiazepine is prescribed; the patient should be instructed to avoid driving or operating heavy machinery, or any task that requires thinking or concentration
  6. GI effects—several antihypertensives can cause GI irritation; NSAIDs may increase the risk of GI irritation; these agents must be taken with food, milk, or an antacid
  7. Constipation—may be further aggravated by the addition of an opioid analgesic; have the patient drink plenty of water and eat fruits, vegetables, and other high-fiber foods

## Anticoagulants

### Warfarin (Coumadin)

A. Mechanism—interfere with vitamin K–dependent clotting factors (II, VII, IX, X)
B. Pharmacologic effects—reduce the ability of blood to clot; latent time required before full effect is seen (several days); a certain amount of time is required for the effect to subside after discontinuation of treatment
C. Adverse reactions—bleeding, hemorrhage
D. Therapeutic uses—used after MI, thrombophlebitis, atrial fibrillation, emboli, valve replacement (any condition in which too much blood clotting occurs)
E. Dental hygiene considerations
  1. Excessive bleeding may result; assess health history at every appointment
  2. Monitoring—performed using international normalized ratio (INR);[4,5] older test is prothrombin time (PT)—patients with INR of 3 or less can safely receive periodontal debridement
F. Examples—warfarin (Coumadin)
G. Drug interactions—occur with warfarin given with:
  1. Aspirin or NSAID—potentiates bleeding problems; do not use concomitantly; alternative is acetaminophen
  2. Vitamin K—helps blood clot; used to treat overdose or to reduce the latent period for improving the clotting status; antibiotics may reduce vitamin K levels by altering the intestinal flora that would potentiate the anticoagulant's effect

### Factor XA Inhibitors

A. Rivaroxaban (Xarelto); Apixaban (Eliquis); Edoxaban (Savaysa)
B. All can prolong bleeding times; increased risk for bleeding
C. Antidotes available for all three drugs

**TABLE 11.9 Selected Antihypertensives: Examples, Mechanisms, and Adverse Reactions**

| Drug Group | Examples | Mechanism | Adverse Reactions |
|---|---|---|---|
| Diuretics–thiazides | Hydrochlorothiazide (HCTZ) | Inhibits sodium (Na) resorption, direct vasodilator, moderate potency | Hypokalemia<br>Hyperuricemia<br>Hyperglycemia<br>NSAIDs ↓ effect |
| Loop diuretic | Furosemide (Lasix) | Loop of Henle, high potency | Similar to thiazides |
| Thiazides combined with potassium ($K^{+2}$) sparing | Maxzide<br>Dyazide | K-sparing, low potency | Hyperkalemia |
| α-Adrenergic selective blockers | Terazosin (Hytrin)<br>Doxazosin (Cardura)<br>Prazosin (Minipress) | Blocks $\alpha_1$-receptor in arterioles/venules | Sedation<br>D/C gradually<br>Also used for benign prostatic hypertrophy |
| β-Adrenergic blockers (select drugs) | Atenolol (Tenormin)<br>Betaxolol (Kerlone)<br>Bisoprolol (Zebeta)<br>Metoprolol (Lopressor)<br>Metoprolol (Toprol-XL)<br>Nadolol (Corgard)<br>Propranolol (Inderal [LA])<br>Timolol (Generic) | Blocks sympathetic effect on heart (↓ CO); ↓ PVR, inhibits stimulation of rennin | NSAIDs ↓ effect |
| Angiotensin-converting enzyme (ACE) inhibitor | Benazepril (Lotensin)<br>Captopril (Capoten)<br>Enalapril (Vasotec)<br>Fosinopril<br>Lisinopril (Zestril, Prinivil)<br>Moexipril (Generic)<br>Perindopril (Generic)<br>Quinapril (Accupril)<br>Ramipril (Altace)<br>Trandolapril (Mavik) | Inhibits ACE, angiotensin II (vasoconstriction; aldosterone secretion) production inhibited | Neutropenia<br>Bone marrow depression<br>Cough<br>Dysgeusia (altered taste)<br>NSAIDs ↓ effect |
| Angiotensin receptor blocker | Azilsartan (Edarbi)<br>Candesartan (Atacand)<br>Eprosartan (Teveten)<br>Irbesartan (Avapro)<br>Losartan (Cozaar)<br>Olmesartan (Benicar)<br>Telmisartan (Micardis)<br>Valsartan (Diovan) | Blocks the binding of angiotensin I to angiotensin II receptors; blocks vasoconstriction and aldosterone-secreting effects of angiotensin II | Oral lesions, nausea, vomiting, dyspepsia |
| Calcium channel blocking agents | Verapamil (Isoptin, Calan)<br>Diltiazem (Cardizem)<br>Nifedipine (Procardia)<br>Nisoldipine (Sular)<br>Isradipine (Dynacire) | Blocks calcium channel: relaxes vascular smooth muscle, decreases myocardial contractility (force) | Gingival enlargement<br>Hyperkalemia<br>Renal failure<br>Dysgeusia |
| Centrally acting antiadrenergic agents | Clonidine (Catapres)<br>Methyldopa (Aldomet) | Stimulates arteriolar and the central nervous system (CNS; medulla) α-receptors | Transdermal patch<br>Xerostomia |
| Postganglionic sympathetic blockers | Guanethidine (Ismelin)<br>Reserpine (Serpasil) | Inhibits release of NE, replaces NE (false neurotransmitter)<br>Blocks uptake and storage of amines | Postural hypotension<br>Diarrhea<br>Impaired ejaculation<br>Mental depression<br>Sedation |
| Vasodilators | Hydralazine (Apresoline)<br>Minoxidil (Loniten) | Relaxes smooth muscles of arterioles | Combined with sympathetic blockers, β-blockers, and diuretics<br>Hirsutism |

*CO*, Cardiac output; *D/C*, discontinue; *NE*, norepinephrine; *NSAIDs*, nonsteroidal antiinflammatory drugs; *PVR*, peripheral vascular resistance.

**TABLE 11.10 Antiepileptic Drugs of Choice for Seizures**

| Seizure Disorder | Drugs | |
|---|---|---|
| | *FIRST CHOICE* | *ALTERNATIVES* |
| **Primary Generalized Seizures** | | |
| Tonic-clonic | Lamotrigine<br>Levetiracetam<br>Valproate[a] | Perampanel<br>Topiramate<br>Zonisamide |
| Absence | Ethosuximide<br>Valproate | Clonazepam<br>Lamotrigine<br>Levetiracetam<br>Zonisamide |
| Atypical absence, atonic, myoclonic | Lamotrigine<br>Levetiracetam<br>Valproate[a] | lobazam<br>Clonazepam<br>Felbamate<br>Rufinamide<br>Topiramate<br>Zonisamide |
| Status epilepticus | Diazepam (Valium) IV<br>Phenytoin (Dilantin) IV<br>Phenobarbital (Luminal) IV | |
| **Partial Seizures** | | |
| Simple<br>Complex<br>Secondarily generalized | Carbamazepine<br>Lamotrigine<br>Levetiracetam<br>Oxcarbazepine | Brivaracetam<br>Clobazam<br>Eslicarbazepine<br>Gabapentin<br>Lacosamide<br>Perampanel<br>Phenytoin<br>Pregabalin<br>Topiramate<br>Valproate<br>Zonisamide |

*IV*, Intravenous.
[a]Not approved by US Food and Drug Administration (FDA) for this indication.

### Direct Thrombin Inhibitor

A. Dabigatran (Pradaxa)
B. Can prolong bleeding time; at risk for increased bleeding
C. Antidote available

### Others (All prolong bleeding time; at risk for increased bleeding)

A. Ticlopidine (Ticlid)
B. Clopidogrel (Plavix)
C. Prasugrel (Effient)
D. Ticagrelor (Brilinta)

## ANTICONVULSANTS

A. General properties of anticonvulsants (Table 11.10)
   1. Pharmacologic effects—reduction of frequency or elimination of seizures (see Table 11.10)
   2. GI upset—common side effect
   3. Teratogenicity—variable teratogenic potential (pregnant women with epilepsy need to be treated)
   4. Sedation—tolerance to sedative effect occurs without tolerance to anticonvulsant effect
   5. Blood dyscrasias—sudden and drastic drops in either white blood cell (WBC) count or red blood cell (RBC) count, or both, which can be serious; laboratory monitoring is important
   6. Dental Hygiene Considerations
      a. Sedation—patient should be instructed to avoid driving or operating heavy machinery, or any task that requires thinking or concentration
      b. GI upset—need to avoid NSAIDs and aspirin because they increase the risk of GI upset
      c. Increased risk for sedation with CNS depressants or sedating drugs
      d. CNS stimulant effects—may be difficult to treat a patient who cannot sit still
      e. Xerostomia—instruct the patient to drink plenty of water; suck on tart sugarless gum or candy containing xylitol, or ice chips; avoid products containing alcohol and caffeine; and avoid juices and soft drinks to reduce the risk of dental caries; saliva substitutes (Xero-lube, Salivart) can also be recommended
B. Phenytoin (Dilantin)—adverse effects
   1. Drug-influenced gingival enlargement—meticulous oral hygiene reduces the enlargement
   2. Vitamin deficiencies—may induce deficiency in vitamins D and folate
   3. Fetal hydantoin syndrome—associated with teratogenic conditions
      a. Wait 1 year after medication change before performing surgical interventions
C. Valproic acid (Depakene, Depakote)—adverse effects
   1. Hepatic failure—liver function tests are required to monitor the patient's liver status
   2. Thrombocytopenia—bleeding; use caution when combining with aspirin, NSAIDs, or warfarin
   3. GI—nausea, vomiting
   4. CNS—sedation, drowsiness; hyperactivity, aggressiveness in children
D. Carbamazepine (Tegretol)—adverse effects
   1. Induces metabolism of itself and other drugs
   2. CNS—drowsiness, dizziness
   3. GI—nausea and vomiting
   4. Hematologic—can cause agranulocytosis; frequent monitoring of WBC count is necessary; signs and symptoms of a low count include fever, chills, aches, and pains
   5. Hepatic—liver function tests are necessary
   6. Indications—various seizures and trigeminal neuralgia
   7. Drug interactions—carbamazepine increases the metabolism of warfarin, theophylline, and doxycycline; the drug's metabolism is inhibited by erythromycin, verapamil, and diltiazem; increases the effect of lithium
E. Ethosuximide
   1. Used to treat absence seizures
   2. GI—anorexia, GI upset, nausea, vomiting

3. CNS—drowsiness, dizziness, lethargy, hyperactivity
4. Oral adverse drug reactions—drug-influenced gingival enlargement, swollen tongue

F. Newer agents (see Table 11.10)

## PSYCHOTHERAPEUTIC AGENTS

### Antipsychotics

A. Pharmacologic effects
1. Antipsychotics—used in the management of psychoses; the patient may perceive comments as threats (paranoia)
2. Sedation and drowsiness—additive CNS depression with other CNS depressants
3. Antiemetics—depress the chemoreceptor trigger zone (CTZ); reduce nausea and vomiting

B. Adverse reactions
1. Orthostatic hypotension—dizziness or fainting on rising from a supine position
2. Extrapyramidal effects—areas in the brain affecting body movements
3. Anticholinergic—xerostomia increases the risk of dental caries
   a. Dyskinesia—uncontrollable movements of the tongue or face
   b. Tardive dyskinesia—abnormal involuntary movements that occur with prolonged use of conventional antipsychotic agents
   c. Parkinsonian symptoms—tremors and rigidity resembling Parkinson's disease
   d. Akathisia—motor restlessness (e.g., swinging legs)
   e. Acute dystonic reaction—difficulty in opening the mouth; jaw muscles are contracted; dislocation of the jaw might occur

C. Drug interactions—occur with antipsychotic agent given with:
1. CNS depressants—additive CNS depression
2. Anticholinergic—additive anticholinergic toxicity

D. Dental hygiene considerations
1. Dyskinesia, akathisia, and tardive dyskinesia—the patient may not be able to perform self-care
2. Acute dystonic reaction—can occur during a procedure; the patient needs to be treated with an anticholinergic drug
3. Orthostatic hypotension—raise the dental chair slowly; have the patient remain seated for a few minutes before standing to prevent a fall
4. Xerostomia—instruct the patient to drink plenty of water; suck on tart sugarless gum or candy containing xylitol, or ice chips; avoid products containing alcohol and caffeine; and avoid juices and soft drinks to reduce the risk of dental caries; saliva substitutes (Xero-lube, Salivart) can also be recommended

E. Therapeutic uses
1. Treatment of psychosis (e.g., schizophrenia) and bipolar disorder
2. Antiemetic—for nausea or vomiting
3. Opioid potentiation—combined with an opioid to potentiate analgesia and sedation; reduce the dose of the opioid if an antipsychotic is added

F. Table 11.11 provides examples of select antipsychotic agents

**TABLE 11.11 Selected Antipsychotic Drugs**

| Group | Drug |
|---|---|
| **First Generation** | |
| High potency | Haloperidol (Haldol) |
| Medium potency | Trifluoperazine (Stelazine) |
| | Thiothixene (Navane) |
| Low potency | Chlorpromazine (Thorazine) |
| | Thioridazine (Mellaril) |
| **Second Generation** | |
| Aripiprazole (Abilify) | |
| Asenapine (Saphris) | |
| Brexiprazole (Rexulti) | |
| Cariprazine (Vraylar) | |
| Clozapine (Clozaril) | |
| Iloperidone (Fanapt) | |
| Lurasidone (Latuda) | |
| Olanzapine (Zyprexa)<br>Orally disintegrating (Zyprexa Zydis) | |
| Paliperidone (Invega) | |
| Quetiapine (Seroquel)<br>Extended release (Seroquel XR) | |
| Risperidone (Risperdal)<br>Orally disintegrating (Risperdal M-TAB) | |
| Ziprasidone (Geodon) | |

### Antidepressants

A. Pharmacologic effects
1. Affect NE and serotonin levels in the brain (require 4 to 6 weeks to be effective)
2. Adverse reactions
   a. Cardiotoxic in overdose— arrhythmias (mainly with TCAs); usual cause of death when used in a suicide attempt
   b. Xerostomia (anticholinergic action)
   c. Sedation
   d. GI—nausea resulting from selective serotonin reuptake inhibitors (SSRIs)
   e. Orthostatic hypotension

B. Drug interactions—occur with TCAs given with:
1. Epinephrine—results in hypertension (increased vasopressor response); low doses contained in local anesthetic solutions can be used safely in normotensive persons (those with normal BP)
2. Anticholinergic—results in additive anticholinergic action and excessive xerostomia

C. Therapeutic uses

1. Treatment of depression
2. Migraine headache prophylaxis
3. Treatment of nocturnal enuresis (bedwetting) in children
4. Chronic pain treatment adjuvant

D. Drugs
1. Select TCAs
   a. Amitriptyline (Elavil)
   b. Imipramine (Tofranil)
2. MAOIs—phenelzine (Nardil); tranylcypromine (Parnate)
   a. Infrequently used for depression
   b. Potential for numerous severe drug-food interactions (e.g., wine, sausage, cheese; indirect-acting adrenergic agents, meperidine)
3. Dopamine-NE reuptake inhibitors
   a. Bupropion (Wellbutrin, Zyban)
   b. Bupropion, sustained release (Wellbutrin SR)
   c. Bupropion, extended release (Wellbutrin ER)
4. Select SSRIs
   a. Fluoxetine (Prozac)
   b. Sertraline (Zoloft)
   c. Paroxetine (Paxil)
   d. Citalopram (Celexa)
   e. Escitalopram (Lexapro)
5. Serotonin and NE reuptake inhibitors
   a. Venlafaxine (Effexor)
   b. Venlafaxine, extended release (Effexor XR)
   c. Desvenlafaxine (Pristiq)
   d. Duloxetine (Cymbalta)
   e. Levomilnacipran (Fetzima)
6. Other antidepressants
   a. Nefazodone (Serzone)
   b. Trazodone (Desyrel)
   c. Vilazodone (Viibryd)
   d. Vortioxetine (Trintellix)
   e. Mirtazapine (Remeron)

### Other Psychotherapeutic Agents

A. Lithium—for treating bipolar-affective disorder (manic depression); blood level is difficult to maintain; NSAIDs increase serum lithium levels

B. Carbamazepine, valproate—these drugs are also used to treat seizure disorders; drug interactions and dental concerns are the same as those in the treatment of seizure disorders

## ENDOCRINE AGENTS

### Adrenocorticosteroids (Steroids)

A. Classification
1. Glucocorticoids—regulate glucose metabolism and have an antiinflammatory effect
2. Mineralocorticoids—regulate sodium (minerals) and water

B. Pharmacologic effect—antiinflammatory, antiallergenic, involved in carbohydrate metabolism, and have catabolic effects

C. Adverse reactions
1. Cushing syndrome—long-term, high-dose steroids produce symptoms including:
   a. Metabolic effects—"moon face," "buffalo hump," truncal obesity
2. Peptic ulcers—exacerbation or stimulation of stomach acid secretion
3. Skin conditions—bruising, striae, delayed healing
4. Mental changes—euphoria, depression, psychosis, mood swings
5. Infection—caused by suppression of immunity, symptoms may be masked; close observation and aggressive treatment are necessary
6. Osteoporosis—bones break more easily
7. Hypertension—elevated water and sodium retention (mineralocorticoid action)
8. Hyperglycemia—exacerbation of diabetes
9. Adrenal crisis (thyroid storm)—abrupt withdrawal or stress (e.g., a dental appointment) can precipitate a crisis; can be prevented by premedicating with additional steroids; potentially serious situation

D. Contraindications and cautions
1. Ulcers—ulcerogenic
2. Cardiovascular disease—can precipitate congestive heart failure, edema (result of mineralocorticoid effect)
3. Acute psychoses
4. Infection—increased susceptibility to bacterial, fungal, or viral infections
5. Diabetes—hyperglycemia is induced

E. Dental hygiene considerations
1. Check BP before procedure or administration of a vasoconstrictor
2. Avoid NSAIDs, aspirin, and opioid analgesics because of the increased risk of GI upset
3. Steroids can delay wound healing and mask the symptoms of infection; consider administration of prophylactic antibiotic before procedure
4. Osteoporosis may be evident on dental radiographs
5. The steroid-dependent patient may need short-term increase in steroid dose before a dental procedure to avoid an adrenal crisis

F. Therapeutic uses
1. Medical—treatment of many inflammatory conditions (e.g., arthritis, asthma, dermatitis)
2. Dental—treatment of:
   a. Aphthous lesions—palliative treatment; topical or intralesional therapy
   b. Oral lesions secondary to collagen vascular diseases—respond to topical, intralesional, or systemic therapy
   c. Temporomandibular joint disease—intraarticular injection (into the joint) if the patient has arthritis

G. Table 11.12 provides examples of steroid agents

### Agents for Diabetes Mellitus

See also the section on "Diabetes Mellitus" in Chapter 19.

A. Definition
1. Symptoms
   a. Polyuria—increased urination
   b. Polydipsia—increased thirst
   c. Polyphagia—increased hunger

**TABLE 11.12 Common Steroids**

| Steroid | Comments | Equivalent Dose (mg/day) |
|---|---|---|
| Hydrocortisone | Some mineralocorticoid action | 20–240 |
| Prednisone | Most commonly used orally | 5–60 |
| Triamcinolone (Kenalog) | Used topically and injected into joints | 2–20 |
| Dexamethasone (Decadron) | Very potent, thus lower dose used | 0.75–9.0 |

d. Weight loss
e. Xerostomia

2. Classifications
   a. Type 1 diabetes (insulin-dependent diabetes mellitus)—circulating insulin is absent; usually is a result of autoimmune destruction of pancreatic beta (β-) cells; requires insulin therapy
   b. Type 2 diabetes (noninsulin–dependent diabetes mellitus)—decreased tissue sensitivity to insulin and impaired β-cell response to glucose; controlled by diet, oral hypoglycemic agents, and insulin, alone or in combination
3. Microvascular and macrovascular complications
   a. Cardiovascular problems—circulation and heart problems, MI, stroke
   b. Retinopathy—vision problems, cataracts, blindness
   c. Neuropathy—reduced sensations in the extremities
   d. Renal failure—nephropathy (kidney problems)
   e. Immunity—reduced ability to fight infections
   f. Healing—slower or delayed
   g. Oral manifestations—reduced immunity caused by WBC dysfunction; reduced vascular supply (small-vessel disease), and other alterations in immune system function; predisposes a patient to periodontal disease; loss of alveolar bone is characteristic

B. Dental hygiene considerations
1. Reinforce the importance of good oral hygiene to minimize the risk of xerostomia, candidiasis, and dental caries
2. Keep at hand a source of glucose that will act quickly (e.g., tube of cake frosting or orange juice) in case the patient experiences hypoglycemia
3. Patients with diabetes are at increased risk for periodontal disease and disease progression
4. These patients are at a higher risk for delayed wound healing and infection; those with poorly controlled diabetes may require prophylactic antibiotic premedication
5. Epinephrine, steroids, and opioid analgesics can decrease insulin release or increase insulin requirements; therefore must be used with caution in patients with diabetes

C. Adverse reactions
1. Hypoglycemia—too much drug or too little food (intakes are not balanced)
   a. Symptoms—nervousness, sweating, tremulousness, compulsive talking, mental confusion, nausea, convulsions, coma
   b. Treatment—administer glucose orally if the patient is conscious and able to swallow; if the patient is unconscious, administer glucose intravenously, or administer glucagon subcutaneously or intramuscularly
2. Hyperglycemia—less common cause of problems in the person with diabetes; treated in the emergency room with insulin and fluids
3. Lipodystrophy—occurs when insulin is injected into the same site for a prolonged period.

D. Examples of hypoglycemic agents:
1. Insulin
   a. Rapid-acting—insulin lispro, insulin aspart
   b. Short-acting—regular insulin (Humulin R, Novolin R) and prompt insulin zinc suspension (Semilente, Semilente Insulin, Semitard)
   c. Intermediate-acting—insulin time suspension (Lente, Humulin L); isophane insulin suspension (Humulin, WPH, Novolin N)
   d. Long-acting—extended insulin zinc suspension (Ultralente, Humulin U Ultralente)
   e. Mixed preparations—isophane insulin suspension and regular insulin injection (Humulin 70/30)
2. Use and sources
   a. Combined regular and neutral protamine Hagedorn (NPH) insulin—given one to two times per day
   b. Human insulin—from gene splicing (made from *E.coli*) or altered pork insulin
3. Oral hypoglycemic agents (sulfonylureas)
   a. First-generation agents
      (2) Chlorpropamide (Diabinese)
   b. Second-generation agents
      (1) Glyburide (DiaBeta, Micronase)
      (2) Glipizide (Glucotrol)
      (3) Glimepiride (Amaryl)
4. Biguanides-metformin (Glucophage)
5. α-glucosidase inhibitors—acarbose (Precose); miglitol (Glyset)
6. Thiazolidinediones—pioglitazone (Actos); rosiglitazone (Avandia)
7. Meglitinides—nateglinide (Starlix); repaglinide (Prandin)
8. GLP-1 receptor agonist—exenatide (Byetta); albiglutide (Tanzeum); dulaglutide (Trulicity); liraglutide (Victoza, Saxenda); semaglutide (Ozempic)
9. Bile acid sequestrant—colesevelam (Welchol)
10. DPP-4 inhibitors—alogliptin (Nesina); linagliptin (Tradjenta); saxagliptin (Onglyza); sitagliptin (Januvia)
11. SGLT-2 inhibitors - canagliflozin (Invokana); dapagliflozin (Farxiga); empagliflozin (Jardiance)
12. Amlinonmymetic agent—pramlintide (Symlin)

## Thyroid Agents

A. Hypothyroidism—also hypothyroidosis, athyroidosis, hypothyrosis, thyroid insufficiency; deficient thyroid activity results in lowered metabolism, fatigue, lethargy; more common in women than in men; can lead to cretinism in infants
1. Thyroid replacements used; leads to a euthyroid condition (normal thyroid)
2. Examples of hypothyroidism agents
   a. Levothyroxine (Synthroid, Levothroid)
   b. Liotrix (Euthroid, Thyrolar)

3. The patient requires no special handling if the dose is adequate
4. Dental hygiene considerations
   a. Carefully examine children suspected of having hypothyroidism and children diagnosed with hypothyroidism; the patient with hypothyroidism must maintain good oral health
   b. Patients with hypothyroidism are more sensitive to medications that depress the CNS; lower doses may therefore be necessary; counsel the patient about the CNS side effects

B. Hyperthyroidism—also Graves' disease; various causes lead to the excessive production of thyroid hormones; produces goiter, cardiopulmonary dysfunction (atrial fibrillation, palpitations, widened pulse rate), skin and behavioral conditions (tremor, excessive sweating, heat intolerance, nervousness, fatigue), and ocular symptoms (exophthalmos)
1. Partial thyroidectomy (treated surgically or with radioactive iodine [$^{131}I$]) ablates part of the thyroid gland—the patient requires supplemental thyroid hormone therapy; no unusual dental considerations if the patient is taking drug treatment
2. Patients awaiting surgery or those who are poor surgical candidates are maintained on a regimen of thyroid suppressants
3. Drugs suppress thyroid function—propylthiouracil (PTU)
4. β-blockers are given to bring down elevated HR (e.g., propranolol)
5. Dental hygiene considerations—avoid epinephrine because it can trigger a thyroid storm; patients have a lower pain threshold and may require higher doses of local anesthetic agents or higher doses of CNS-depressing medications

## Estrogens and Progesterone

### Estrogen

A. Responsible for female sex characteristics, reproduction development, and preparing for conception

B. Adverse reactions
1. Nausea, vomiting
2. Uterine bleeding, vaginal discharge
3. Edema
4. Thrombophlebitis
5. Weight gain
6. Headache
7. Hypertension

C. Dose forms
1. Oral tablets
2. Creams
3. Transdermal patches

D. Clinical uses include treatments for:
1. Symptoms of menopause
2. Menstrual disturbances
3. Osteoporosis

### Progesterone

A. Responsible for preparing the uterus for implantation of the fertilized egg

B. Adverse reactions
1. Abnormal menstrual bleeding
2. Breakthrough bleeding
3. Spotting between menstrual periods
4. Change in amount of menstrual blood flow
5. Amenorrhea

C. Dose forms
1. Oral
2. Parenteral

D. Clinical uses include treatments for:
1. Dysfunctional uterine bleeding
2. Endometriosis
3. Dysmenorrhea
4. Premenstrual tension

## Oral Contraceptives

A. Pharmacologic activity—inhibits the release of follicle-stimulating hormone (FSH) and luteinizing hormone (LH), which prevent ovulation and pregnancy

B. Contain either progesterone alone or a combination of estrogen and progesterone; both come in varying doses

C. Adverse reactions
1. Nausea, dizziness, weight gain, headache, breast tenderness
2. Hypertension, liver damage, thrombophlebitis, thromboembolism
3. Oral—increased gingival fluid, susceptibility to gingivitis, gingival inflammation, increased risk of dry socket after extraction (newer formulations contain less hormone and therefore are less likely to cause these conditions)

D. Dental hygiene considerations
1. Review with the patient the importance of good oral hygiene because of the potential for gingivitis
2. Extractions should be performed on days 23 to 28 of the oral contraceptive cycle to reduce the risk of dry socket
3. Check BP at each appointment because of the risk of hypertension
4. During long procedures, have scheduled breaks to minimize risk of thrombophlebitis; have the patient stretch the legs and walk around, if possible
5. Instruct patients to use a contingent method of birth control if they require antibiotic therapy

# RESPIRATORY SYSTEM AGENTS

## Agents for Asthma and COPD

A. Disease—dyspnea, cough, and wheezing, secondary to bronchospasm (hyperirritable bronchioles), inflammation of bronchioles with secretions

B. Drugs
1. Adrenergic agonists (sympathomimetics)—see the earlier section on "Autonomic Nervous System"
   a. Dose forms—oral inhalers, tablets, liquid
   b. Inhalers—$\beta_2$-adrenergic agonists
      (1) Short-acting $\beta_2$-agonists
         (a) Albuterol (Proventil, Ventolin)
         (b) Metaproterenol (Alupent, Metaprel)
      (2) Long-acting $\beta_2$-agonists

(c) Salmeterol (Serevent)
(d) Formoterol (Foradil Aerolizer)

c. Epinephrine—administered intravenously for an acute attack
d. Used for maintenance and prophylactic therapy
e. Adverse reactions—nervousness, tachycardia, insomnia, xerostomia with oral inhalers
f. Dental hygiene considerations for short-acting and long-acting $\beta_2$-agonists
   (1) Measure the patient's BP and pulse rate before the procedure because of the potential for tachycardia
   (2) Have the patient "rinse, swish, and expectorate" after each inhaler use to reduce xerostomia
   (3) Instruct the patient to maintain good oral hygiene, especially with the use of oral inhalers

2. Methylxanthines
   a. Examples
      (1) Theophylline (Theo-dur, Slo-bid)
   b. Pharmacologic effects
      (1) Bronchodilation (smooth muscle relaxation) helps reduce the symptoms of asthma
      (2) CNS stimulation—alertness, insomnia
      (3) Diuresis—increased urination
3. Cromolyn sodium (Intal, Nasalcrom)
   a. Used for asthma prophylaxis by inhalation, for allergic rhinitis, and for maintenance therapy for asthma
   b. Adverse reactions—nausea, vomiting, restlessness, anxiety
   c. Dental hygiene considerations—same as with $\beta_2$-adrenergic agonists
4. Ipratropium bromide (Atrovent); tiotropium bromide (Spiriva)
   a. Anticholinergic bronchodilator; used mainly to treat emphysema
   b. Adverse reactions—xerostomia and bad taste
   c. Dental hygiene considerations
      (1) Counsel the patient to rinse well and expectorate after each use
      (2) Counsel the patient about the importance of good oral hygiene
5. Adrenocorticosteroids
   a. Used for acute and maintenance therapy
   b. Dose forms—oral, parenteral, metered-dose inhaler (MDI), tablets
   c. Adverse reactions with MDI—dysphonia (hoarseness), xerostomia, cough, and candidiasis
   d. Dental hygiene considerations
      (1) MDI—same as with other oral inhalers
   e. Examples
      (1) Flunisolide (Aerobid)
      (2) Fluticasone (Flovent)

C. Dental hygiene considerations
   1. Disease considerations
      a. Degree of control—avoid elective treatment if the asthma is poorly controlled
      b. The patient's anxiety may precipitate an acute attack; an antianxiety agent may be useful (e.g., benzodiazepine)
   2. Analgesic selection—sometimes difficult to make Aspirin-containing compounds—may precipitate an attack
      a. NSAIDs—if aspirin causes bronchospasm, NSAIDs are contraindicated
      b. Acetaminophen—best choice; may be used in combination with a weak opioid (e.g., Tylenol No. 3)

## GASTROINTESTINAL AGENTS

### Agents Affecting GI Motility

A. Laxatives—increase GI motility; symptomatically used to treat constipation (e.g., milk of magnesia)
B. Antidiarrheals—reduce GI motility; symptomatically used to treat diarrhea (e.g., Lomotil, Imodium, any opioid)
C. Dental hygiene considerations
   1. CNS sedation—the patient should be instructed to avoid driving or operating heavy machinery, or anything that requires thinking or concentration
   2. Xerostomia—instruct the patient to drink plenty of water; suck on tart sugarless gum or candy containing xylitol, or ice chips; avoid products containing alcohol and caffeine; and avoid juices and soft drinks to reduce the risk of dental caries; saliva substitutes (Xero-lube, Salivart) can also be recommended

### Agents for Gastroesophageal Reflux Disease and Peptic Ulcer Disease

#### Histamine ($H_2$-) Blockers

A. Mechanism of action—block stomach acid secretion; pain subsides and no further damage occurs from esophageal exposure to stomach acid
B. Examples (all available OTC)
   1. Cimetidine (Tagamet HB)
   2. Famotidine (Pepcid AC)
   3. Nizatidine (Axid AR)
   4. Ranitidine (Zantac 75)
C. Dental hygiene considerations
   1. These agents interfere with the absorption of drugs that need acid for absorption (e.g., ketoconazole [Nizoral])
   2. Avoid ulcerogenic medications unless absolutely necessary (e.g., aspirin, NSAIDs, glucocorticoids)
   3. Cimetidine
      a. Reduces hepatic blood flow
      b. Inhibits the metabolism of certain drugs (diazepam, warfarin)

#### Proton Pump Inhibitors

A. Mechanism—irreversibly bind to the proton pump, resulting in acid suppression lasting more than 24 hours
B. Examples
   1. Omeprazole (Prilosec)
   2. Lansoprazole (Prevacid)
   3. Esomeprazole (Nexium)
C. Adverse reactions
   1. Esophageal candidiasis
   2. Mucosal atrophy of the tongue
   3. Xerostomia

**COMMON MULTIDRUG REGIMENS FOR *HELICOBACTER PYLORI***

| Drug | Daily Dose | Duration | Comments |
|---|---|---|---|
| **Triple Therapy** | | | No longer preferred. Consider if no prior macrolide exposure and clarithromycin resistance <15%. |
| Clarithromycin + | 500 mg bid | 14 days | |
| amoxicillin | 1 gm bid | 14 days | |
| *Or* | | | |
| Metronidazole + | 500 mg tid | 14 days | |
| a PPI | standard PPI dose | 14 days | |
| **Bismuth Quadruple Therapy** | | | Preferred first line therapy. Good for prior macrolide exposure or true penicillin allergy. |
| Bismuth subsalicylate (Pepto-Bismol) + | 262 or 525 mg qid | 10–14 days | |
| Metronidazole + | 250 mg qid or 500 mg tid or qid | 10–14 days | |
| Tetracycline + | 500 mg tid or qid | 10–14 days | |
| PPI | Standard dose | 10–14 days | |
| **Concomitant Quadruple Therapy** | | | Preferred first-line, more convenient dosing. |
| Clarithromycin + | 500 mg bid | 10–14 days | |
| Amoxicillin + | 1 gm bid | 10–14 days | |
| Metronidazole + | 500 mg bid | 10–14 days | |
| PPI | Standard dose | 10–14 days | |

*bid,* Twice a day; *PPI,* proton pump inhibitor; *qid,* four times a day; *tid,* three times a day.

D. Dental hygiene considerations
   1. Evaluate for adverse oral reactions
   2. Xerostomia—instruct the patient to drink plenty of water; suck on tart sugarless gum or candy that contains xylitol, or ice chips; avoid products containing alcohol and caffeine; and avoid juices and soft drinks to reduce the risk of dental caries; saliva substitutes (Xero-lube, Salivart) can also be recommended

### Emetics and Antiemetics

A. Emetics—induce vomiting; used to treat most poisonings (e.g., syrup of ipecac, which is available without a prescription); abused by persons with bulimia
B. Antiemetics
   1. Reduce nausea or vomiting
   2. Examples
      a. Benzquinamide (Emete-Con)
      b. Prochlorperazine (Compazine)
      c. Trimethobenzamide (Tigan)
C. Dental hygiene considerations
   1. CNS sedation—the patient should be instructed to avoid driving or operating heavy machinery or performing any task that requires thinking or concentration
   2. Xerostomia—instruct the patient to drink plenty of water; suck on tart sugarless gum or candy containing xylitol, or ice chips; avoid products containing alcohol and caffeine; and avoid juices or soft drinks to reduce the risk of dental caries; saliva substitutes (Xero-lube, Salivart) can also be recommended

## ANTINEOPLASTIC AGENTS

A. Mechanism—interfere with the metabolism or reproductive cycle of malignant cells; also affect normal cells
B. Drugs
   1. Alkylating agents
      a. Nitrogen mustards
         (1) Cyclophosphamide (Cytoxan)
         (2) Chlorambucil (Leukeran)
         (3) Melphalan (Alkeran)
      b. Nitrosureas—carmustine (BiCNU)
      c. Busulfan (Myleran)
   2. Antimetabolites
      a. Folic acid analog—MTX
      b. Purine antagonists
         (1) Mercaptopurine (6-MP)
         (2) Thioguanine (6-TG)
      c. Pyrimidine antagonists
         (1) 5-Fluorouracil (5-FU)
         (2) Cytarabine (Cytosar-U, ara-C)
   3. Other antineoplastics
      a. Plant alkaloids
         (1) Vinblastine (Velban)
         (2) Vincristine (Oncovin)
   4. Antibiotics
      a. Dactinomycin (actinomycin D, Cos-megen)
      b. Daunorubicin (Cerubidine)
      c. Doxorubicin (Adriamycin)
      d. Mitomycin (Mitocin-C)
   5. Hormones
      a. Adrenocorticosteroids
      b. Androgens
      c. Estrogens
      d. Progestin
      e. Tamoxifen (Nolvadex)—antiestrogen
   6. Aminobisphosphonates
      a. Alendronate (Fosamax)
      b. Ibandronate (Boniva)
      c. Pamidronate (Aredia)

d. Risedronate (Actonel)
e. Zoledronic acid (Zometa)
7. Miscellaneous
a. Asparaginase (Elspar)
b. Bleomycin (Blenoxane)
c. Cisplatin (Platinol)
d. Hydroxyurea (Hydrea)

C. Adverse reactions
1. Lack of specificity against tumor cells because normal cells are also destroyed; cells with the fastest life cycle are affected first
2. Bone marrow activity suppression
a. Leukopenia—lowered WBC count; infections are more likely
b. Thrombocytopenia—lowered platelets; risk of bleeding is increased
c. Anemia
3. GI—stomatitis, mucosal sloughing
4. Infection—reduced immunity and ability to fight infection
5. Skin and hair—rash, alopecia (baldness)
6. Oral effects
a. Symptoms—pain, ulcers, dryness, impaired taste, gingival hemorrhage, sensitivity of teeth and gingivae
b. Treatment—avoid mouth rinses with alcohol; substitute saline or sodium bicarbonate; avoid alcohol
c. Candidiasis—use antifungal agents (e.g., Nystatin)
d. Xerostomia—instruct the patient to drink plenty of water; suck on tart sugarless gum or candy with xylitol, or ice chips; avoid products containing alcohol and caffeine; and avoid juices and soft drinks to reduce the risk of dental caries; saliva substitutes (Xero-lube, Salivart) can also be recommended
7. Osteonecrosis of the jaw (ONJ)
a. In cancer, primarily breast cancer, patients receiving IV bisphosphonates, 94% of cases with ONJ have been reported; the incidence is much lower in patients taking oral bisphosphonates for osteoporosis
b. Prolonged use may suppress bone turnover—leads to microdamage
c. Most cases of ONJ occur after tooth extractions or other procedures that cause trauma to the jawbone
d. Very difficult to treat once it occurs
e. Oral health examinations and other dental procedures should be performed before starting bisphosphonate therapy and continued every 3 months thereafter
f. Any dental procedures that are performed should involve minimal trauma to the jaw and adjacent tissue
g. ONJ treatment by oral and maxillofacial surgeons; treatment varies according to size of the lesion
h. If clinically necessary, 0.12% chlorhexidine gluconate rinses, systemic antibiotics, and analgesics can be used

D. Dental hygiene considerations
1. Have patients improve their oral hygiene before chemotherapy, if possible
2. Avoid elective procedures during chemotherapy; timing is important; the best time for procedures are the days before chemotherapy begins
3. Check the coagulation status before any emergency surgery
4. Use of prophylactic antibiotic premedication is controversial
5. If xerostomia is a problem, patient will need custom-fitted mouth trays for at-home, self-administered fluoride therapy

## SUBSTANCE ABUSE

See the section on "Chemical Dependency" in Chapter 19.

### Definitions

A. Tolerance—increasingly higher doses are required to produce the same effect; the same dose produces less effect; occurs with repeated administration
B. Physical dependence—symptoms of withdrawal occur if the drug is abruptly discontinued
C. Psychological dependence—craving occurs if the drug is stopped; no physical withdrawal syndrome; however, psychological dependence is just as likely to result in relapse (e.g., cocaine)
D. Abuse—improper or excessive self-administration of a drug that results in an adverse outcome
E. Addiction—pattern of abuse that continues despite medical or social complications
F. Withdrawal—a physical reaction attributable to physical dependence
G. Abstinence—drug-free state
H. Enabling—a pattern of coping methods (e.g., making excuses for absences) used by the associates of those addicted, which allows the addicted person to continue the drug use

### Drugs of Abuse

A. Depressants
1. Alcohol—impaired judgment, slurred speech, ataxia, seizures, coma, death; withdrawal produces autonomic hyperactivity, hallucinations, or seizures; cirrhosis with chronic use
2. Opioids (hydrocodone, heroin, codeine, morphine)—euphoria, abscesses, constipation, respiratory depression; withdrawal produces "cold turkey" syndrome; methadone maintenance and naltrexone (acts similar to orally active naloxone) used to suppress a "high"
3. Barbiturates—secobarbital, pentobarbital
4. Volatile solvents—glue sniffing and paint solvent inhaling; called "huffing"
5. Benzodiazepines—diazepam
6. Anesthetics—$N_2O$-$O_2$ analgesia

B. Stimulants
1. Amphetamines—methamphetamine; highly addictive; street name "ice"
2. Cocaine—most psychologically addicting drug; produces euphoria, hyperactivity, paranoia; risk of acute MI; street names include coke and crack
3. Nicotine—in e-cigarettes, chewing tobacco, and cigars
4. Caffeine—in soft drinks, coffee, and tea

C. Psychedelics
   1. Lysergic acid diethylamide (LSD)—flashbacks occur (without the drug); called "bad trip"
   2. Psilocybin—hallucinogen derived from mushrooms of the genus *Psilocybe*
   3. Phencyclidine (PCP)—disorientation, seizures; treatment consists of "talking down"
   4. Marijuana (cannabis)—active ingredient is tetrahydrocannabinol (THC); causes silliness, relaxation, euphoria, paranoia, confusion, chronic amotivational syndrome; entrance drug (used first before trying other addictive drugs)

D. Dental hygiene considerations
   1. Cocaine—cardiac stimulant effect; causes addictive effect on heart with local anesthetic agents with vasoconstrictors
   2. Nitrous oxide ($N_2O$)—sense of euphoria; incidence of dental personnel abuse (unsupervised use); abuse produces neuropathy (sometimes irreversible); without adequate $O_2$, hypoxia is produced
   3. Addicts—"shopper" patients attempt to obtain prescriptions for controlled substances from several dental offices; feign dental pain but refuse definitive treatment; suspicion is warranted
   4. Caffeine—increased HR and BP with excessive caffeine intake
   5. Nicotine—check for oral manifestations of tobacco use (e.g., nicotine stomatitis, periodontal disease, oral leukoplakia, precancerous lesions, hairy tongue, halitosis)

## DRUG USE DURING PREGNANCY

A. General—pregnant women must:
   1. Avoid any unnecessary drugs
   2. Consult with an obstetrician

B. Pregnancy and professional oral health care
   1. First trimester—period of highest risk for drug effects on the fetus; negative organogenic effects possible
   2. Second trimester—best for elective dental treatment
   3. Third trimester—use of any unnecessary drugs must be avoided because of patient comfort and proximity to delivery

C. Drugs used in dental practice that are probably safe
   1. Amoxicillin
   2. Penicillin
   3. Erythromycin
   4. Lidocaine
   5. Epinephrine (limit dose)

D. Drugs used in dental practice that must be avoided
   1. Aspirin
   2. NSAIDs
   3. Metronidazole
   4. $N_2O$—dental personnel who are pregnant should be especially careful
      a. Women exposed to high levels of $N_2O$ (more than 5 hours per week) were significantly less fertile than unexposed women; levels of allowable exposure vary from state to state
      b. Dental practices should improve room air circulation and cleaning procedures and use an air evacuation system to reduce adverse outcomes[5,6]
      c. More information is available at http://www.osha.gov/dts/osta/anestheticgases/index.html#C1

### Smoking Cessation

A. Nicotine reduction systems
   1. Nicotine is a ganglionic cholinergic receptor agonist
   2. Nicotine reduction (also known as *replacement*) therapies reduce the withdrawal symptoms associated with smoking cessation
   3. Smoking cessation reduces the risk of oral and lung cancers, heart disease, and other lung diseases

B. Types of nicotine reduction systems
   1. Chewing gum—Nicorette 2 or 4 mg; available without a prescription
   2. Transdermal systems—all available without a prescription
      a. Habitrol
      b. Nicoderm
      c. Nicotrol
      d. Prostep
   3. Nasal spray—Nicotrol NS
   4. Adverse effects
      a. Chewing gum—sore mouth, hiccups, dyspepsia, jaw ache, nausea
      b. Chewing gum can stick to dentures and dental work
      c. Transdermal systems—nausea, hypersalivation, abdominal pain, vomiting, diarrhea, perspiration, headache, dizziness, hearing and visual disturbances, confusion, weakness
      d. Nasal spray—runny nose, throat irritation, watery eyes, sneezing, cough
   5. Dental hygiene considerations
      a. Follow protocol: Ask Assess Advise Assist Arrange
      b. Evaluate the patient who smokes for oral benign and malignant changes
      c. Stress the importance of nicotine cessation
   6. Evaluate patients using the chewing gum for any problems (e.g., gum sticking to dentures or dental work); recommend using another form of nicotine cessation aid

C. Bupropion (Zyban)
   1. Antidepressant used to reduce nicotine cravings
   2. Also called Wellbutrin; the pills are identical and made by the same manufacturer, but coded differently for insurance purposes
   3. Concomitant treatment modalities are encouraged (behavior modification)
   4. Recommended dosing—150 mg once daily for 3 days, followed by 150 mg twice daily for 2 to 3 months if the patient is experiencing success

D. Varenicline (Chantix)
   1. Nicotine receptor blocker; amount of dopamine released into the brain is reduced; thereby blocking the feelings of pleasure associated with nicotine use
   2. Dosing—once daily for the first 3 days, twice daily thereafter for the full course of therapy (usually 12 weeks)
   3. Taken after meals and with a full glass of water
   4. Adverse effects include nausea, sleep problems, constipation, gas, vomiting, and changes in mood and behavior
   5. Cannot be used in conjunction with other nicotine cessation products

## WEBSITE INFORMATION AND RESOURCES

| Source | Website Address | Description |
|---|---|---|
| RxList, The Internet Drug Index | http://www.rxlist.com | A HealthCentral.com Network site providing information about medications, indications, contraindications, dosages, and patient information |
| Drug Topic | https://www.drugtopics.com/ | Current news on drug-related topics |
| FDA – Drugs | http://www.fda.gov/drugs | Information on new drug development and regulatory issues |
| Med Watch | https://www.fda.gov/safety/medwatch-fda-safety-information-and-adverse-event-reporting-program | Safety information |
| American Herbal Products Association | http://www.ahpa.org | Current information on herbal remedies |
| Malignant Hyperthermia Association of the United States | http://www.mhaus.org | Online brochures, including an explanation of malignant hyperthermia as a concern in dentistry and oral and maxillofacial surgery |

# CHAPTER 11 REVIEW QUESTIONS

Answers and rationales to review questions are available on this text's accompanying Evolve site. See inside front cover for details.

## CASE A

**Synopsis of Patient History**
Age:70
Sex: M
Height: 5′7″
Weight: 162 lbs (73.6 kg)

**Vital Signs**
Blood pressure: 117/80 mm Hg
Pulse rate: 70 bpm
Respiration rate: 22 rpm

1. Under care of physician: _x_ YES ___ NO
   Condition: chronic obstructive pulmonary disease (COPD), Seasonal allergies
2. Hospitalized within the last 3 years: ___ YES _x_ NO

**Current Medications**
Albuterol inhaler: as needed
Montelukast (Singulair) 10 mg: one tablet daily
Fluticasone furoate, umeclidinium, vilanterol (Trelegy) inhaler: one inhalation once daily
Multivitamin: once daily
Cetirizine (Zyrtec) 10 mg daily
Aspirin 81 mg; daily

**Medical History**
Patient has a history of COPD and is under the care of his general physician. Patient also has seasonal allergies.
Coronary artery disease

**Dental History**
Visits the dental office for regular examination and cleaning.

**Social History**
He lives with his wife.
He enjoys playing golf, watching soccer, movies, and traveling.
He is a retired shipyard contractor.

**Chief Complaint**
Sore and dry throat

***Use Case A to answer questions 1 to 10.***

1. Which of the following drugs could be causing the sore throat and dry mouth?
   a. Albuterol
   b. Montelukast
   c. Fluticasone
   d. Aspirin
2. Albuterol is a short-acting bronchodilator that can be administered via a metered-dose inhaler. It is recommended for treating sudden breathing problems in patients with COPD.
   a. Both statements are TRUE
   b. Both statements are FALSE
   c. The first statement is TRUE; the second statement is FALSE
   d. The first statement is FALSE; the second is TRUE
3. Which one of the following drugs can result in oral candidiasis?
   a. Cetirizine
   b. Naproxen
   c. Aspirin
   d. Fluticasone furoate
4. All the following are recommendations that you should make to patients with asthma EXCEPT one. Which one is the *exception*?
   a. Bring your rescue inhaler (albuterol) to the dental appointment
   b. Rinse after using corticosteroid/anticholinergic/β-adrenergic agonist inhaler
   c. Avoid ibuprofen
   d. Avoid naproxen
   e. Avoid acetaminophen

5. Patients with COPD are at higher risk for developing pneumonia and this patient is using Trelegy, a combination drug inhaler. Which of the following drugs in his inhaler would weaken his immune system and put him at higher risk for developing pneumonia?
   a. Vilanterol
   b. Umeclidinium
   c. Fluticasone furoate
   d. Albuterol
6. Which of the following orally inhaled drugs should the patient bring with him to each appointment in case of sudden breathing problems?
   a. Flulticasone
   b. Albuterol
   c. Vilanterol
   d. Umeclidinium
7. Each drug in the combination inhaler Trelegy works differently to treat COPD. How does the drug umeclidinium work?
   a. It is an anticholinergic drug that blocks acetylcholine receptors in the lungs that blocks the smooth muscles in the lungs from tightening
   b. Umeclidinium is a corticosteroid that reduces lung inflammation
   c. This drug is a corticosteroid that blocks the smooth muscles in the lungs from tightening
   d. Drugs such as umeclidinium work by stimulating β-receptors thereby relaxing smooth muscle airways in the lungs
8. Patients using the fluticasone furoate/umeclidium/vilanterol (Trelegy) inhaler should be instructed about all the following EXCEPT:
   a. Rinse, swish, and spit after each use of the inhaler
   b. The inhaler must be discarded 2 months from the expiration date listed on the inhaler
   c. It is a good idea to floss your teeth after each inhaler use
   d. This inhaler should be used for maintenance therapy only
9. Patients taking montelukast should be counseled about all the following EXCEPT:
   a. Mood changes
   b. Headache
   c. Gastrointestinal upset
   d. Sedation
10. Histamine-1 ($H_1$)–blocking drugs such as cetirizine are preferred over drugs such as fexofenadine because they are less sedating. Cetirizine is a nonsedating $H_1$-blocking drug.
   a. Both statements are TRUE
   b. The first statement is TRUE; the second statement is FALSE
   c. The first statement is FALSE; the second statement is TRUE
   d. Both statements are FALSE

## CASE B

**Synopsis of Patient History**
Age: 62
Sex: M
Height: 5′10″
Weight: 220 lbs (100 kg)

**Vital Signs**
Blood pressure: 130/85 mm Hg
Pulse rate: 75 bpm
Respiration rate: 25 rpm

1. Under care of physician: X YES ___ NO
   Condition: Hypertension, high cholesterol, type 2 diabetes, coronary artery disease, depression

2. Hospitalized within the last 3 years: X YES ___ NO
   Rule out myocardial infraction (MI)

**Current Medications**
Lisinopril (Zestril)
Hydrochlorothiazide
Baby aspirin
Rivaroxaban (Xarelto)
Atorvastatin (Lipitor)
Glipizide (Glucotrol) 10 mg bid
Metformin (Glucophage)
Citalopram (Celexa) 40 mg qd
Sublingual nitroglycerin as needed

**Medical History**
Patient has a history of cardiovascular disease, type 2 diabetes, depression, and high cholesterol. Patient is being treated by a cardiologist and his general physician.

**Dental History**
Visits the dental office for regular examination and cleaning.

**Social History**
Married with three children.
Enjoys golf, football, television, and good meals.
Currently employed as a government contractor.

**Chief Complaint**
Presents for routine oral health examination.

*Use Case B to answer questions 11 to 20.*

11. Eating a banana or drinking a glass of orange juice when taking a thiazide diuretic will:
   a. Increase sodium levels
   b. Increase the rate of diuresis
   c. Replenish potassium
   d. Increase the drug's absorption
12. One of the main differences between angiotensin-converting enzyme (ACE) inhibitors and thiazide diuretics, in terms of side effects, is that ACE inhibitors increase potassium levels. Thiazide diuretics lower potassium levels.
   a. Both statements are TRUE
   b. The first statement is TRUE; the second statement is FALSE

c. The first statement is FALSE; the second statement is TRUE
d. Both statements are FALSE

13. Patients taking antihypertensive agents who have been supine for some time can rise from that position at a regular rate. There is no need for them to dangle their legs over the side of the chair and wiggle them before rising to the standing position.
a. Both statements are TRUE
b. Both statements are FALSE
c. The first statement is TRUE; the second statement is false
d. The first statement is FALSE; the second statement is true

14. Which of the following drugs inhibits hydroxymethylglutaryl coenzyme A (HMG-CoA) reductase?
a. Atorvastatin
b. Niacin
c. Gemfibrozil
d. Cholestyramine

15. Which agent reduces serum cholesterol by increasing its use for bile acid synthesis?
a. Clofibrate
b. Ezitimibe
c. Icosapent ethyl
d. Cholestyramine

16. Which class of drugs is recommended in persons with diabetes to help lower the progression to diabetic nephropathy?
a. Alpha blockers
b. Diuretics
c. Angiotensin-converting enzyme (ACE) inhibitors
d. Calcium channel blocker

17. All the following drugs inhibit platelet function EXCEPT:
a. Ticagrelor
b. Rivaroxaban
c. Apixaban
d. Evolocumab

18. Patients taking nitroglycerine (NTG) sublingual tablets should be instructed to:
a. Store their NTG in a clear glass container
b. Keep their NTG in the bathroom
c. Use NTG once every 10 minutes until the anginal attack has stopped
d. Bring their NTG to the dental appointment and make it available to the practitioner in the event the patient experiences an acute anginal attack

19. Your patient complains of chest pain while sitting in the dental chair. Even though the information is not recorded on his health history or pharmacologic history form, it is a good idea for you to ask if he has taken tadalafil (Cialis) within the last 24 hours. The use of nitroglycerine is contraindicated if tadalafil has been taken within 24 hours because the nitroglycerine-tadalafil combination can precipitate significant orthostatic hypotension.
a. Both statements are TRUE
b. Both statements are FALSE
c. The first statement is TRUE; the second statement is FALSE
d. The first statement is FALSE; the second statement is TRUE

20. Which oral antidiabetic agent produces lactic acidosis as a significant adverse effect?
a. Empagliflozin
b. Metformin
c. Dulaglutide
d. Linagliptin

21. Patients taking glipizide should be instructed to do all of the following when scheduling a dental appointment EXCEPT one. Which one is the exception?:
a. Have their most current HgA1C levels available
b. Schedule their dental appointments around the time they take their glipizide and their meals
c. Schedule their dental appointments around mealtimes in addition to when they take the glipizide
d. Schedule their dental appointment any time, as the timing of the appointment is not a significant factor as long as the patient factors in when they take their glipizide and when they eat

22. Which antidepressant is MOST likely to cause xerostomia?
a. Fluoxetine
b. Citalopram
c. Amitriptyline
d. Venlafaxine

23. Selective serotonin reuptake inhibitors (SSRIs) tend to produce central nervous system (CNS) depression rather than CNS stimulation. Therefore, SSRIs are more sedating.
a. Both statements are TRUE
b. The first statement is TRUE; the second statement is FALSE
c. The first statement is FALSE; the second statement is TRUE
d. Both statements are FALSE

24. Patients should be warned that an acute overdose with acetaminophen can result in damage to the:
a. Stomach
b. Liver
c. Esophagus
d. Ears

25. Alcohol consumption in combination with acetaminophen slows the breakdown of acetaminophen, thereby decreasing the toxic potential of acetaminophen use.
a. Both statements are TRUE
b. Both statements are FALSE
c. The first statement is TRUE; the second statement is FALSE
d. The first statement is FALSE; the second statement is TRUE

26. Patients with hypertension should avoid all of the following drugs EXCEPT for one. What is the exception?
a. Naproxen
b. Ibuprofen
c. Acetaminophen
d. Celecoxib

27. Which of the following drugs is best suited to treat dental pain in a person taking lithium?
   a. Naproxen
   b. Ibuprofen
   c. Acetaminophen
   d. Celecoxib
28. Patients taking ibuprofen should be counseled about all the following EXCEPT one. What is the exception?
   a. Gastrointestinal upset
   b. Insomnia
   c. Sedation
   d. Fluid retention
29. Both opioid and nonopioid analgesics relieve pain by blocking the pain pathways. Lowering the pain threshold decreases one's reaction to pain.
   a. Both statements are TRUE
   b. The first statement is TRUE; the second statement is FALSE
   c. The first statement is FALSE; the second statement is TRUE
   d. Both statements are FALSE
30. A patient was given a prescription for acetaminophen with codeine following a dental procedure. The patient developed itching and urticaria after taking her acetaminophen with codeine at home. This response MOST likely represents a:
   a. Pharmacologic action of codeine
   b. Hypersensitivity reaction to codeine
   c. Pharmacologic action of acetaminophen
   d. Hypersensitivity reaction to acetaminophen
31. Patients that overdose on opioid analgesics, such as hydrocodone, are best treated with?
   a. Naloxone
   b. Flumenazil
   c. Codeine
   d. Epinephrine
32. For pain control, patients are best treated with ibuprofen. NSAIDS, such as ibuprofen are most effective in treating dental pain and inflammation.
   a. Both statements are TRUE
   b. The first statement is TRUE; the second statement is FALSE
   c. The first statement is FALSE; the second statement is TRUE
   d. Both statements are FALSE
33. Lorazepam is often used to treat acute dental anxiety, thereby resulting in a calmer patient who does not experience cognitive impairment.
   a. Both statements are TRUE
   b. Both statements are FALSE
   c. The first statement is TRUE; the second statement is FALSE
   d. The first statement is FALSE; the second statement is TRUE
34. Patients taking zolpidem (Ambien) for sleep may experience:
   a. Insomnia
   b. Agitation
   c. Sleep-driving
   d. Headache
35. A drug effect that is predictable and dose-related and acts on a target organ is called a:
   a. Therapeutic effect
   b. Toxic reaction
   c. Side effect
   d. Allergic reaction
36. The combination of alcohol and metronidazole can result in:
   a. Sedation
   b. Mild headache
   c. Antabuse-like reaction
   d. Significant insomnia
37. All of the following organs are responsible for drug excretion except for one. What is the EXCEPTION?
   a. Kidney
   b. Lungs
   c. Saliva
   d. Spleen
38. NSAIDs, such as ibuprofen, carry cautions for the following side effects except for one. What is the EXCEPTION?
   a. Myocardial infarction
   b. Sedation
   c. Severe GI bleeding
   d. Renal function impairment
39. Chewable carbamazepine is palatable to children because of its high sugar content. Children and anyone using the chewable dose form should practice good oral hygiene after each dose.
   a. Both statements are TRUE
   b. Both statements are FALSE
   c. The first statement is TRUE; the second statement is FALSE
   d. The first statement is FALSE; the second statement is TRUE
40. Gingival hyperplasia is an adverse effect of phenytoin. Valproate can also cause gingival hyperplasia.
   c. Both statements are TRUE
   d. Both statements are FALSE
   e. The first statement is TRUE; the second statement is FALSE
   f. The first statement is FALSE; the second statement is TRUE

For each mechanism of action listed below, select the correct drug from the list provided:

41. Blocks the conversion of angiotensin I to angiotensin II
42. Irreversibly bind to the proton pump, resulting in acid suppression lasting >24 hours
43. Increases hepatic and peripheral insulin sensitivity, resulting in decreased hepatic glucose production
44. Lowers plasma glucose levels by blocking the reabsorption of glucose in the kidneys, causing excess glucose to be eliminated in the kidneys
45. Block the reuptake of serotonin
46. Block the angiotensin II receptor
47. Inhibit calcium ion movement into the cell and lowers blood pressure
48. Inhibits the intestinal absorption of cholesterol

**49.** Binds to bile acids and produces an insoluble product that is lost through the gastrointestinal tract. Formation of new bile acids uses up cholesterol which reduces cholesterol levels

**50.** Blocks histamne$_2$ receptors in the stomach

**A.** Ezetimibe (Zetia)
**B.** Niacin
**C.** Cholestyramine (Questran)
**D.** Citalopram (Celexa)
**E.** Venlafaxine (Effexor)
**F.** Metformin (Glucophage)
**G.** Canaglifozin (Invokana)
**H.** Linagliptin (Tradjenta)
**I.** Nifedipine (Procardia XL)
**J.** Enalapril (Vasotec)
**K.** Atenolol (Tenormin)
**L.** Candesartan (Atacand)
**M.** Esomeprazole (Nexium)
**N.** Ranitidine (Zantac)
**O.** Vilazodone (Viibryd)

## REFERENCES


1. Vuignier K, Schappler J, Veuthy J-L, Carrupt P-A, Martel S. Drug-protein binding: a critical review of analytical tools. *Anal Bioanal Chem*. 2010;398:53–66.
2. Wilson W, Taubert KA, Gewitz M, et al. Prevention of infective endocarditis: guidelines from the American Heart Association. *Circulation*. 2007;116:1736. 11.
3. Sollecito TP, Abt E, Lockhart PB, et al. The use of prophylactic antibiotics prior to dental procedures in patients with prosthetic joints. Evidence-based clinical practice guideline for dental practitioners—a report of the American Dental Association Council on Scientific Affairs. *JADA*. 2015;146:11–16.
4. Kearon C, Akl EA, Ornelas J, et al. Antithrombotic therapy for VTE disease: CHEST guideline and expert panel report. *Chest*. 2016;149(2):315–352.
5. *American Hospital Formulary Service*. Bethesda, MD: *Drug Information*. American Society of Hospital Pharmacists; 2018.
6. Allaert SEG, Carlier SPK, Weyne LPG, Vertommen DJ, Dutré PEI, Desmet MB. First trimester anesthesia exposure and fetal outcome. A review. *Acta Anaesth. Belg.* 2007;58:119–123.

12

# Biochemistry, Nutrition, and Nutritional Counseling

*Lisa F. Mallonee*

Humans require specific chemicals or nutrients from food to grow, maintain homeostasis, and achieve optimal health. An understanding of cellular biochemistry and nutrition is essential for preventing and treating disease and for promoting health. Nutrition science includes the intake of food and the processes involved in digestion, absorption, transportation, metabolism of nutrients, and excretion. As an applied science, it involves counseling people to adapt food patterns to nutritional needs within the cultural, economic, and psychosocial environment. Nutrition assessment counseling, when performed effectively, motivates individuals to modify eating behaviors so that optimal health can be achieved.

This chapter reviews the six major nutrient groups and their metabolic activities in mammalian cells, dietary modifications for diseases, nutritional diseases and disorders, and oral manifestations of nutritional deficiencies and toxicities. The effects of nutrients on oral tissues and the dietary assessment tools and techniques available for counseling individuals with various types of oral diseases are also described. Because nutritional problems in the developed countries are a result of overeating and undereating, a review of energy balance and weight control is included. Cellular biochemistry is fundamental to the study of nutrition; therefore the reader is referred to the section on "General Histology" in Chapter 2 for a review of structural and functional similarities in cells.

## SIX MAJOR CLASSES OF ESSENTIAL NUTRIENTS

### Carbohydrate

A. Definition—polyhydroxy aldehydes or ketones that serve as the body's primary sources of quick energy; carbohydrates (CHO) are composed of monosaccharides, basic units that contain carbon, hydrogen, and oxygen
B. Basic chemical structure
  1. The ratio of carbon, hydrogen, and oxygen is 1:2:1
  2. The reactive portion of the molecule may be in a ketose form or an aldose form
  3. The position of the hydroxyl (–OH) groups determines properties such as sweetness and absorbability
C. Classification
  1. Simple carbohydrates
    a. Monosaccharides
      (1) Trioses (C3) and tetroses (C4)—usually formed during intermediary metabolism and are not important dietary components
      (2) Pentoses (C5)—important in nucleic acids and coenzymes; do not occur in free form (uncombined); not important dietary components (e.g., ribose)
      (3) Hexoses (C6)—most important group physiologically
        (a) Glucose—blood sugar; primary energy source
        (b) Galactose—seldom found free; but found in lactose
        (c) Fructose—fruit sugar; sweetest-tasting sugar; found in honey and fruits
    b. Disaccharides—composed of two monosaccharide units
      (1) Sucrose—glucose plus fructose (e.g., cane and beet sugar)
      (2) Lactose—glucose plus galactose (e.g., milk sugar)
      (3) Maltose—glucose plus glucose (intermediate of starch hydrolysis [digestion])
D. Oligosaccharides—composed of two to six monosaccharide units
  1. Complex carbohydrates
    a. Homopolysaccharides—made up of more than six identical monosaccharide units
      (1) Starch—plant storage form of glucose; source of half of dietary carbohydrates
        (a) Amylose—straight chain
        (b) Amylopectin—branched chain
      (2) Glycogen—animal storage form of glucose; found in the liver and muscle of living animals; insignificant source of dietary carbohydrates
      (3) Cellulose—chief constituent of the framework of plants; glucose units are in β-linkages, not capable of being hydrolyzed by human digestive enzymes; provides bulk and fiber in the diet
    b. Heteropolysaccharides—carbohydrates associated with noncarbohydrates or carbohydrate derivatives
      (1) Pectin, lignin—important contributors to fiber in the diet
      (2) Glycoproteins—carbohydrate and protein in a specific, functional arrangement (e.g., blood group substances and many hormones)
      (3) Glycolipids—carbohydrate and lipid, as in gangliosides
      (4) Mucopolysaccharides—protein and carbohydrate in a loose binding

TABLE 12.1 Digestive Action at Various Points Along the Gastrointestinal Tract

| | Carbohydrates | Proteins | Fats |
|---|---|---|---|
| Mouth | Salivary amylase: starch → maltose | No enzymatic action | No enzymatic action |
| Stomach | No enzymatic action | Hydrochloric acid (HCl): denatures proteins → activates pepsinogen → pepsin → hydrolysis of peptide bonds → peptides + proteoses | Gastric lipase[a]: → short- and medium-chain triglycerides → fatty acids + monoglycerides |
| Small intestine<br>Pancreatic enzymes | Pancreatic amylase: starch → dextrin<br>dextrin → maltose | Trypsin → chymotrypsin + aminopeptidase + carboxypeptidase → hydrolysis of peptide bonds | Pancreatic lipase: fatty acids → triglycerides → diglycerides + monoglycerides |
| Bile salts | No action | No action | Bile salts: emulsification of fats |
| Brush-border enzymes | Disaccharidases → monosaccharides:<br>Sucrase → glucose → fructose<br>Lactase → lactose → glucose + galactose<br>Maltase → maltose → glucose | Dipeptidases → dipeptides → amino acids | Lecithinase: lecithin → monoglyceride + fatty acid + $PO_4$ + choline |
| Large intestine | Some fermentation of undigested nutrients but with negligible absorption of the fermentation products | | |

[a]A minor role in total fat digestion.

(a) Hyaluronic acid—vitreous humor and joint lubricant
(b) Heparin—anticoagulant
(c) Chondroitin sulfate—cartilage, skin, bone, and teeth
(d) Keratin sulfate—nails and teeth

E. Digestion, absorption, and transport
1. Digestion (Table 12.1)
a. Mouth
(1) Teeth and tongue—mechanical breakdown and mixing of food
(2) Saliva—hydration and lubrication of food
(3) Salivary amylase (ptyalin)—initial enzymatic hydrolysis of starch
b. Stomach—no digestive enzymes for carbohydrates; initial enzymatic hydrolysis of starch by salivary amylase may continue
c. Small intestine
(1) Pancreatic juices—pancreatic amylases
(2) Intestinal villi (brush border) enzymes—disaccharidases
(a) Sucrase—converts sucrose to glucose and fructose
(b) Lactase—converts lactose to glucose and galactose
(c) Maltase—converts maltose to glucose
d. Large intestine—bacterial "fermentation" of some undigested carbohydrates
(1) No significant contribution to absorbable carbohydrates
(2) May be the cause of gas production and bloating during primary or secondary disaccharidase deficiency (e.g., "lactose intolerance")
2. Absorption (Fig. 12.1)
a. Factors affecting absorption
(1) Intestinal motility
(2) Type of food mixture
(3) Integrity of intestinal mucosa
(4) Endocrine activity
b. Mechanism
(1) Passive diffusion along the osmotic gradient—when the intestinal concentration of carbohydrates is greater than the level of carbohydrate in the blood
(2) Facilitated diffusion—only certain molecules allowed to pass across a membrane using an ion channel or a carrier protein
(3) Active transport—requires energy and allows molecules to pass against a concentration gradient with the aid of an ion channel or a carrier protein at the brush border
c. Route
(1) Carbohydrates are water soluble and are absorbed directly into the capillaries of the intestinal mucosa
(2) Carried by the portal circulation to the liver

F. Metabolism—glucose is the main immediate source of energy for the body; a glucose level of 70 to 120 mg/100 mL blood is maintained by most healthy persons (Fig. 12.2)
1. Sources of blood glucose
a. Dietary carbohydrates—sugars, starches
b. Stored liver glycogen breakdown—glycogenolysis
c. Synthesis from intermediary metabolites such as pyruvic acid—glyconeogenesis
d. Synthesis from noncarbohydrate sources— gluconeogenesis
(1) Deaminated (glucogenic) amino acids
(2) Glycerol portion of lipids
2. Reactions of blood glucose—"burned" (oxidized) for energy
a. Glycolysis—end product is pyruvate or lactic acid in the absence of oxygen (anaerobic conditions) or acetyl-coenzyme A (acetyl-CoA) in the presence of oxygen (aerobic conditions)
b. Tricarboxylic acid cycle (TCA) or Krebs cycle—oxidation of acetyl-CoA with the release of carbon dioxide ($CO_2$)
c. Oxidative phosphorylation and electron transport—production of adenosine triphosphate (ATP a high-energy molecule) and water

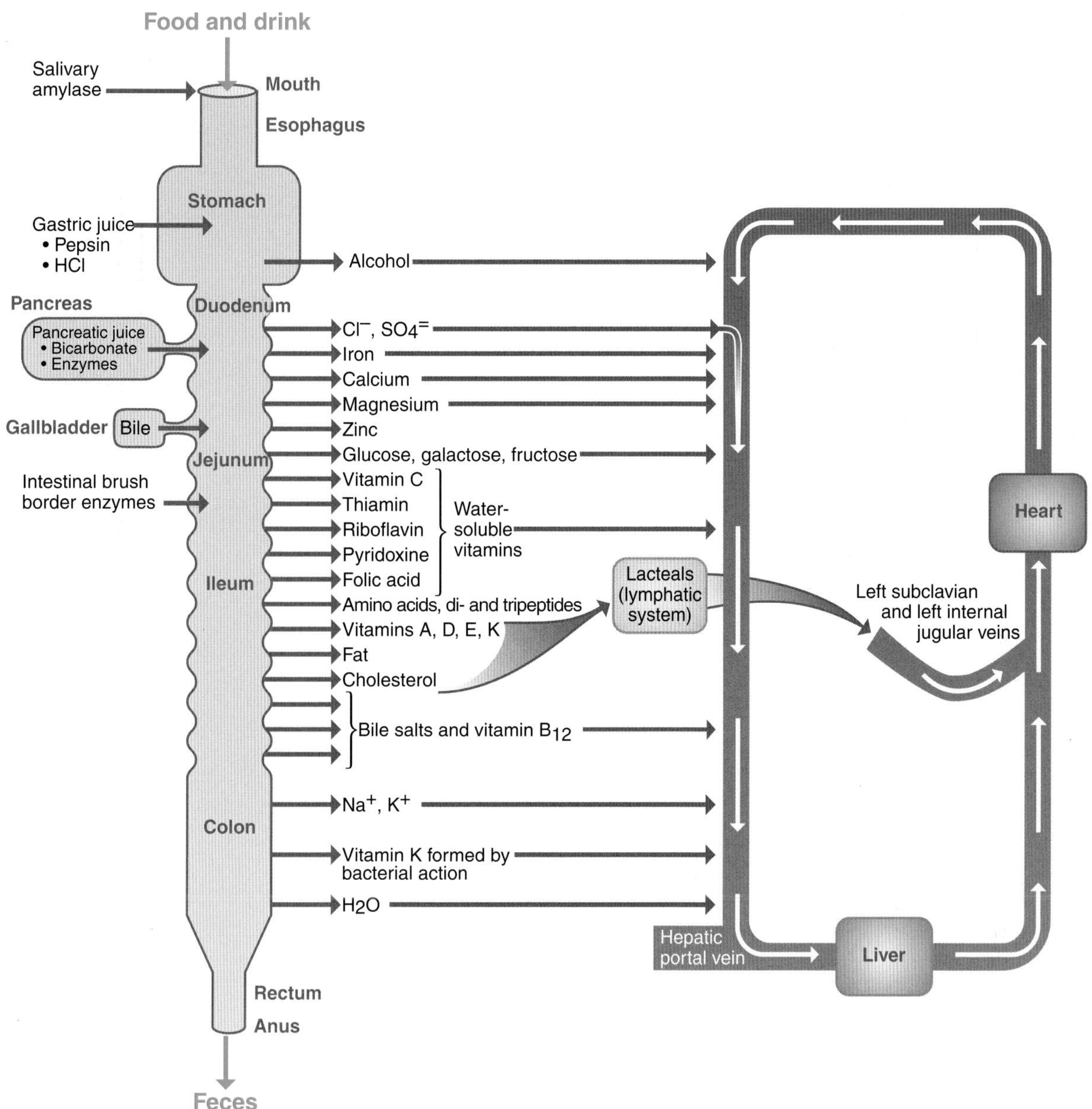


**Fig. 12.1** Absorption of major nutrients, vitamins, and minerals. (Adapted from Mahan LK, Raymond JL. *Krause's Food and the Nutrition Care Process.* 14th ed. St. Louis: Saunders; 2017.)

3. Storage for reserve use
   a. Glycogenesis—glycogen is the short-term storage form of glucose in the liver and muscle (6 to 18 hours)
   b. Lipogenesis—excess carbohydrate in the diet is converted to fat to be stored in adipose tissue as a long-term energy storage form
4. Conversion to other molecules, such as:
   a. Other carbohydrates needed for structural or functional roles
   b. Keto acids to be used in protein synthesis

G. Metabolic regulators
1. Anabolic hormones—lower the blood glucose level (e.g., insulin)
   a. Increase the entry of glucose into cells
   b. Increase glycogenesis
   c. Increase lipogenesis
2. Catabolic hormones—raise the blood glucose level
   a. Glucagon—stimulates glycogenolysis
   b. Steroid hormones—stimulate gluconeogenesis
   c. Epinephrine—stimulates glycogenolysis
   d. Growth hormone and adrenocorticotropic hormone (ACTH)—act as insulin antagonists
   e. Thyroxine—increases insulin breakdown, intestinal absorption of glucose, and epinephrine release
3. Coenzymes—B-complex vitamins are important precursors of the coenzymes involved in the catabolism of carbohydrates

H. Fiber
1. Definition—substance, usually nonstarch polysaccharide, found in plants; not broken down by human digestive enzymes; some of it is digested by bacteria in the gastrointestinal (GI) tract

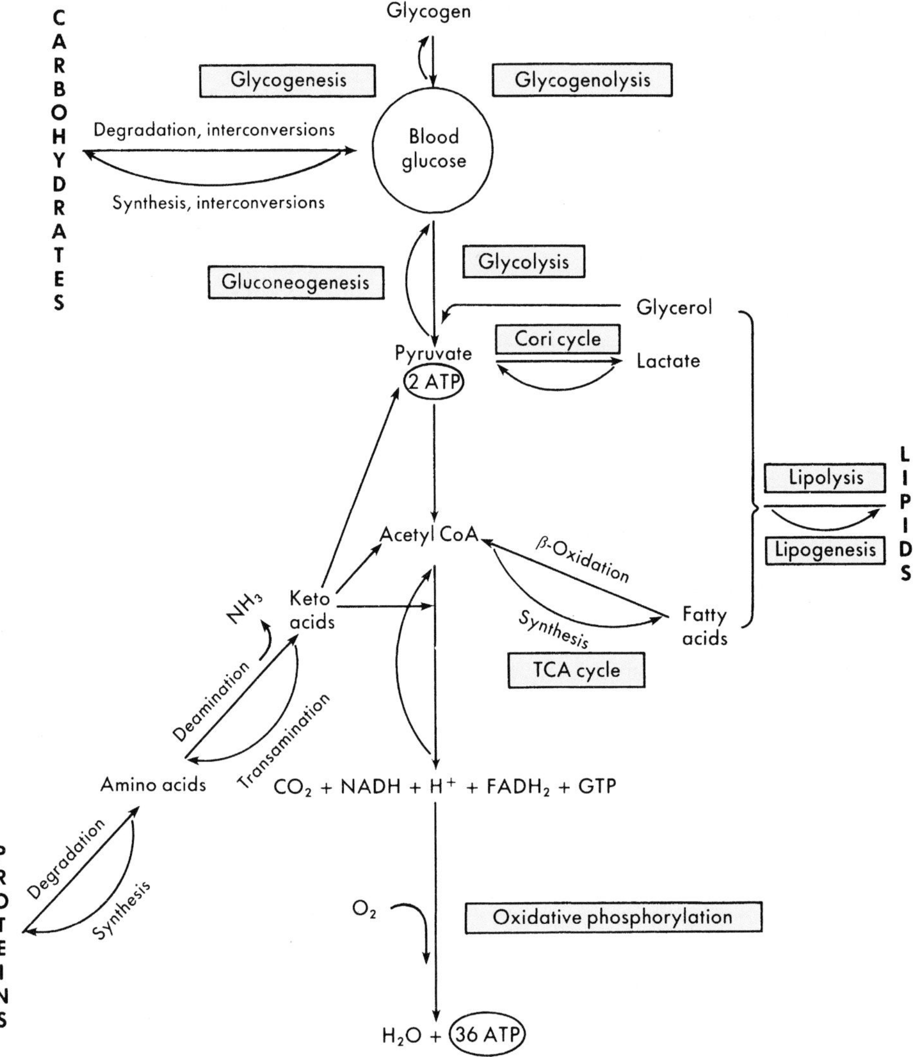


**Fig. 12.2** An overview of metabolism.

a. Insoluble fiber—substance (e.g., cellulose, hemicellulose, lignin) that gives structure to plant cell walls; adds bulk and softness to stools; reduces contact with possible carcinogens by decreasing transit time through the colon; foods high in insoluble fiber include wheat bran, raw fruits, and vegetables
b. Soluble fibers—substances (e.g., gums, mucilages, pectin, oat bran) that dissolve to become gummy or viscous; lower blood cholesterol; regulate the use of sugars and slow down gastric emptying; foods high in soluble fiber include legumes, raw apples, and whole oats

2. Epidemiologic studies indicate that individuals whose diets include a significant amount of fiber have a low incidence of chronic "Western" diseases, such as coronary heart disease (CHD), diabetes, atherosclerosis
3. Specific fibers are believed to play roles in decreasing the incidence of obesity, irregularity, hemorrhoids, appendicitis, diverticulosis, colon cancer, hyperlipidemia, and fluctuations in blood glucose
4. Excessive dietary fiber
   a. For persons with a limited intake, diets high in fiber bulk may cause nutritional deficiency
   b. Use of large doses of purified fiber may inhibit absorption of calcium, potassium, zinc, and iron
   c. Phytic acid, often found in high-fiber foods such as cereal grains, can bind and prevent absorption of minerals such as iron, calcium, and zinc
5. Recommended fiber intake—for adults, 21 to 38 grams per day (g/day), depending on age and gender

I. Biologic role and functions of carbohydrates
   1. Provide precursors of structural and functional molecules (e.g., gangliosides)
   2. Energy source (4 kilocalories per gram [kcal/g])
   3. Spare protein
   4. Provide bulk and palatability to the diet

J. Role in oral biology
   1. Preeruptive effect on teeth
      a. Energy source for growth and development
      b. Protein-sparing nutrient
   2. Posteruptive effect on teeth

**TABLE 12.2 Dietary Sweeteners**

| Common Category | Chemical Structure and Category | Examples | Caries Promoting Potential | Relative Sweetness in Comparison to Sucrose[a] | Food Sources |
|---|---|---|---|---|---|
| Sugars | Monosaccharide | Glucose, dextrose | Yes | 74 | Most foods |
| | | Fructose, high-fructose corn syrup | Yes | 100–110 | Fruits, honey, condiments, soft drinks |
| | | Galactose | Yes | 60 | ____ |
| | Disaccharide | Sucrose, granulated, powdered or brown sugar, turbinado, molasses | Yes | 100 | Fruits, vegetables, table sugar |
| | | Lactose | Yes | 16 | Milk |
| | | Maltose | Yes | 50 | Beer |
| Other carbohydrates | Polysaccharide | Starch | Yes | N/A | Potatoes, grains, rice, legumes, bananas, cornstarch |
| | Fiber | Cellulose, pectin, gums, β-glucans, fructans | No | N/A | ____ |
| Sugar alcohols | Polyol-monosaccharide | Sorbitol, mannitol, xylitol, erythritol | No | 60–100 | Grains, fruits, vegetables |
| | Polyol-disaccharide | Lactitol, isomalt, maltitol | No | 30–90 | Fruit, seaweed, exudates of plants or trees |
| | Polyol-polysaccharide | Hydrogenated starch, hydrolysates (HSH) or maltitol syrup | No | 70 | Derived from lactose, maltose, or starch |
| Nutritive Sweeteners | Aspartame | Nutrasweet, Equal | No | 200 | ____ |
| Non-nutritive Sweeteners | Saccharin | Sweet' n Low | No | 200–700 | Derived from monosaccharides |
| | Acesulfame-K | Sunett | No | 200 | ____ |
| | Sucralose | Splenda | No | 600 | ____ |
| | Neotame | Newtame | No | | ____ |
| | Advantame | | No | | ____ |
| | Lu han guo | Monk fruit | No | 100–250 | ____ |
| | Rebaudioside A | Truvia, Stevia | No | 200–400 | ____ |

[a]Sucrose has a relative sweetness value of 100%.
*N/A*, Not applicable.
Relative sweetness values for various sweeteners. https://owlsoft.com/pdf_docs/WhitePaper/Rel_Sweet.pdf. Accessed April 9, 2019. High-intensity sweeteners permitted for use in the US. https://www.fda.gov/food/ingredientspackaginglabeling/foodadditivesingredients/ucm397725.htm. Accessed April 9, 2019.
Stegeman CA, Davis. JR. *The dental hygienist's guide to nutritional care.* 5th ed. St. Louis, MO: Elsevier; 2019, and Palmer CA, Boyd LD. *Diet and Nutrition in Oral Health.* 3rd ed. Upper Saddle River, NJ: Pearson; 2016.

a. Energy source for oral cariogenic bacteria (e.g., *Streptococcus mutans*)
b. Acidogenic bacteria metabolize monosaccharides and disaccharides, particularly sucrose, for the production of energy through glycolysis that results in the formation of lactic acid, pyruvate, and other acetyl-CoA, dependent on the conditions
c. *S. mutans* synthesizes polysaccharides (glucans, levans, and glycogen) from sucrose
   (1) Polysaccharides are used for energy when sucrose is unavailable
   (2) Glucans form insoluble complexes with *S. mutans* and have a strong affinity for enamel, thus enhancing bacterial biofilm formation
   (3) The organic acids are liberated into the interface between the bacterial biofilm and surface enamel
   (4) At pH of 5.5, decalcification and demineralization begin
d. The firm texture of some complex carbohydrates, as found in raw fruits and vegetables, can help to remove food debris retained between teeth; the chewing action can also stimulate salivary flow

3. Dietary sweeteners (Table 12.2)
   a. Nutritive sweeteners are used by the body as an energy source; they provide calories
      (1) Sugar alcohols (xylitol, sorbitol, and mannitol) are noncariogenic nutritive sweeteners that are slowly fermented through anaerobic metabolism by oral bacteria; excessive intake of these polyols can cause diarrhea because of the osmotic transfer of water into the bowel
      (2) Xylitol is found naturally in plants and is equal to or sweeter than sucrose; consumption of xylitol-containing products after eating food has been shown to interfere with the metabolism of *S. mutans* and decrease the demineralization of enamel

(3) Aspartame is classified as a nutritive sweetener by the United States Food and Drug Administration (FDA)

b. Nonnutritive sweeteners are calorie-free and have no nutritive value; saccharin, acesulfame-K, sucralose, neotame and advantame are nonnutritive sweeteners approved by the FDA; are noncariogenic

c. Aspartame should be avoided by patients who have phenylketonuria, a genetic disorder characterized by an inability to metabolize the amino acid phenylalanine

d. Food labels often list sugar content in its various forms (e.g., invert sugars, dextrose, fructose, corn sweeteners) to give an appearance of lower sugar content

4. Cariogenicity factors of diet habits (from *most* important to *least* important)

a. Intake frequency of simple sugars—the more frequent the exposure to sugar, the more cariogenic is the diet; six candy bars eaten at six different times during the day are more harmful in terms of acid and bacterial biofilm formation than six candy bars consumed at the same time. Likewise, frequent consumption of acidogenic foods and beverages contributes to demineralization and increased risk of caries

b. Form of simple sugars (liquid, retentive or slow dissolving)—liquid sweets clear the oral cavity faster than solid retentive sweets or slow-dissolving sweets. Slow-dissolving sugars are the most cariogenic along with retentive solid foods. Liquids are less cariogenic but can still contribute to increased risk of demineralization of the tooth structure

c. Time of ingestion of simple sugars—combining sticky, starchy foods and sweets with liquids and other noncariogenic foods during a meal is less cariogenic than a concentrated exposure to sweets between meals as a snack. It is recommended that these types of foods and acidic beverages be consumed within 20 to 30 minutes

d. Total intake of simple sugars—average daily intake of sugar is 22 teaspoons (tsp); the majority of our simple sugar intake comes from soft drinks, fruit drinks, desserts, candies, and ready-to-eat cereals; the American Heart Association (AHA) recommends limiting added sugar intake to 6 tsp/day for women and 9 tsp/day for men[1]

e. Starch-rich foods that are retained on the teeth for prolonged periods are ultimately degraded to organic acids and can contribute to the production of dental caries

f. Combining cariogenic foods with noncariogenic foods— cariogenic foods simple carbohydrates and starchy foods are less cariogenic when combined with noncariogenic food (e.g., cheese, foods high in protein and fat)

5. Importance of carbohydrates in periodontal health

a. Energy source for the growth and repair of periodontal tissues

b. Protein-sparing nutrient

c. Firm texture of complex carbohydrates can promote circulation in gingival tissue

d. Dietary monosaccharides and disaccharides enhance supragingival bacterial growth and biofilm formation; these bacteria set the stage for the growth and development of subgingival bacteria and biofilm, which are responsible for the destructive effects of periodontitis

K. Requirements

1. The recommended daily allowance (RDA) of digestible carbohydrate is 130 g/day for adults and children

a. Minimum adult intake (50 to 100 g) prevents use of body protein as an energy source

b. Pregnant and lactating women need additional carbohydrates to prevent ketosis

2. Recommendations

a. The Food and Nutrition Board recommends that 45% to 65% of calories should come from carbohydrates[2]

b. Calories from simple carbohydrates (monosaccharides and disaccharides)—10% or less of the total caloric intake

c. The majority of calories should come from complex carbohydrates (including fiber)

L. Dietary modifications for persons with disease conditions

1. Obesity—reduce total calories and percentage of simple carbohydrates (concentrated sweets) to increase the nutrient density of a lower-calorie diet

2. Genetic defects

a. Lactose intolerance (inability to hydrolyze lactose)—eat fewer milk products, use fermented products, or add a commercial lactose enzyme (lactase) to milk

(1) Yogurt with active bacteria culture is recommended because the lactose is digested by the yogurt

(2) The main concern for oral and systemic health is an inadequate intake of calcium and vitamin D; a hydrogen breath test can be used for diagnosis

(3) Types of lactose intolerance

(a) Primary—congenital absence of lactase (a brush-border enzyme)

(b) Secondary—temporary or permanent loss of lactase activity resulting from intestinal injury, diseases (e.g., Crohn), or infections which cause injury to the GI mucosa

b. Galactosemia—congenital inability to metabolize galactose; lactose and milk products should be removed from the diet

c. Fructose intolerance—congenital inability to metabolize fructose; fructose and sucrose should be removed from the diet; individuals with fructose intolerance have significantly fewer dental caries

3. Dental caries and periodontal disease—a protective diet should be implemented

a. A diet that is low in retentive carbohydrates

b. Avoidance of cariogenic snacks

c. A diet that is adequate in all nutrients (Table 12.3)

d. Inclusion of foods of firm or hard texture

**TABLE 12.3 Dietary Reference Intake, Adequate Intake, and Tolerable Upper Limits of Nutrients Specific to Bone Health**

| Nutrient | Dietary Reference Intake (DRI)/ Recommended Dietary Allowance (RDA)[a] | Adequate Intake (AI) (Therapeutic Range)[b] | Tolerable Upper Limit (UL)[c] |
|---|---|---|---|
| Calcium (mg/d) | 700–1300 mg/d for most healthy adults and children | 200–260mg/d for infants | 1000–3000 mg/d for most healthy adults and children |
| Phosphorus (g/d) | 460–1250 g/d for most healthy adults and children | 100–275 g/d for infants | 3–4 g/d for most healthy adults and children; no determined tolerable UL for infants |
| Magnesium (mg/d) | 80–420 mg/d for most healthy adults and children | 30–75 mg/d for infants | 65–350 mg/d for most healthy adults and children; no determined tolerable UL for infants. |
| Vitamin D (μg/d) | 10–15 μg/d for most healthy adults and children | — | 25–100 μg/d for most healthy adults and children |
| Fluoride (mg/d) | No established daily value | 0.01–4 mg/d | 0.7–10 mg/d |

[a]Recommended dietary allowance values meet the needs of 97% of individuals in a group. Daily reference intake values are groups of values that provide quantitative estimates of nutrient intake for planning and assessing diets for all healthy individuals.
[b]Adequate intake (AI), also known as a therapeutic range, is the mean intake for healthy individuals that is used when an RDA value cannot be determined. The lower number represents the adequate intake for infants and children, and the higher range of numbers will vary depending on life stage and gender group. Refer to the National Academies Press website (http://nap.edu/) for more in-depth information. The therapeutic range (AI) is the dose at which physiologic benefits for healthy individuals and decreased risk for toxicity may exist.
[c]The lower number represents the upper limits for infants and children, and the higher number represents upper limits for males and females (pregnant and lactating). The tolerable upper limit is the highest level of daily nutrient intake that is likely to pose no risk of adverse health effects.

4. Diabetes (inability to regulate glucose because of insufficiency or relative ineffectiveness of insulin)—dietary treatment (see the section on "Diabetes Mellitus" in Chapter 19)
   a. Two major forms
      (1) Type 1 diabetes—persons with type 1 diabetes require:
         (a) Daily injections of insulin
         (b) Routine blood testing to monitor blood sugar levels
         (c) Routine urine testing to monitor ketone levels
      (2) Type 2 diabetes—persons with type 2 diabetes require:
         (a) Medication to facilitate glucose metabolism
         (b) Specialized diet to help control the disease
         (c) Routine blood testing to monitor blood sugar levels
   b. Signs and symptoms of diabetes mellitus
      (1) Frequent urination (polyuria)
      (2) Excessive thirst (polydipsia)
      (3) Recurring gingival infections
      (4) Extreme hunger (polyphagia)
   c. Dietary recommendations
      (1) Type 1 diabetes
         (a) Is managed primarily with insulin therapy
         (b) A regular pattern of three meals per day, with one or more snacks between meals
         (c) A diet that is rich in complex carbohydrates and dietary fiber
         (d) A diet high in carbohydrates replaced with unsaturated fat and dietary fiber, if elevated triglycerides are present
      (2) Type 2 diabetes
         (a) Regular meal patterns
         (b) Regular physical activity
         (c) Monitoring carbohydrate intake and increasing the consumption of unsaturated fat and dietary fiber, if elevated triglycerides are present
5. Reactive hypoglycemia—rare; symptoms of dizziness, hunger, and heart palpitations are lessened with a low-carbohydrate diet
6. Dumping syndrome—occurs after gastric surgery; postprandial symptoms of nausea, dizziness, cramping, and diarrhea are lessened by a low-monosaccharide, low-disaccharide diet
7. Alcoholism—overconsumption of alcohol may cause malnutrition
   a. Depresses the appetite
   b. Empty-calorie food—provides energy but few other nutrients (e.g., concentrated sweets, alcohol, and fats)
   c. Causes vitamin B depletion because the liver needs niacin and thiamine to metabolize alcohol
   d. Causes folate and iron deficiency
   e. Depresses antidiuretic hormone (ADH), causing loss of magnesium, potassium, and zinc in urine
8. Alcohol consumption during pregnancy—has a direct teratogenic effect on the developing fetus: fetal alcohol syndrome (see the section on "Fetal Alcohol Spectrum Disorders" in Chapter 19)
9. Carbohydrate regulation in some hyperlipoproteinemias—total carbohydrate and alcohol intake is controlled; concentrated sweets are restricted

## Proteins

A. Definition—complex biologic compounds of high molecular weight that contain nitrogen, hydrogen, oxygen, carbon, and small amounts of sulfur; each protein has a specific size and is made up of amino acid building blocks linked through peptide bonds in a specific arrangement

B. Classifications
   1. Chemical
      a. Simple proteins—contain amino acids only
      b. Compound (conjugated) proteins—contain simple proteins and a nonprotein group
         (1) Nucleoproteins
         (2) Metalloproteins
         (3) Phosphoproteins
         (4) Lipoproteins
      c. Derived proteins—fragments produced during digestion or hydrolysis (e.g., peptides, peptones, proteases)
   2. Biologic
      a. Complete proteins contain sufficient amounts of the essential amino acids for normal metabolic reactions; found in foods of animal origin
         (1) A total of 20 essential amino acids that cannot be synthesized by humans and must be provided in the diet in sufficient amounts to meet the body's needs
            (a) Adult—histidine, isoleucine, leucine, lysine, methionine, phenylalanine, threonine, tryptophan, and valine
            (b) Infant—all the above plus taurine
            (c) Premature infant—all the above plus cysteine
         (2) Nonessential amino acids can be synthesized by the body and need not be provided by the diet but are necessary for normal metabolic reactions; include alanine, arginine, aparagine, aspartic acid, cysteine, glutamic acid, glutamine, glycine, proline, serine, and tyrosine
      b. Incomplete proteins have insufficient quantities of one or more essential amino acids to support protein synthesis in humans; plant proteins are often incomplete (e.g., corn protein is low in lysine; legume protein is low in methionine)
      c. Complementary proteins are proteins that are incomplete when ingested singly but, when combined, provide sufficient essential amino acids
         (1) In a "vegan" (or strict vegetarian) diet, the complementing of plant proteins can be accomplished by combining appropriate incomplete proteins
            (a) The amino acids in different foods can complement one another, even when eaten at different meals
            (b) Persons on a strict vegetarian diet are at the greatest risk for developing deficiencies in calcium, iron, zinc, and vitamin $B_{12}$ because the major food sources of these nutrients come from animal products
         (2) In an "ovo-lacto" vegetarian diet, milk and egg proteins can provide the essential amino acids that are inadequate in incomplete plant proteins; however, this diet still may be deficient in iron
      d. Protein quality is a measure of a protein's ability to support protein synthesis; it is measured by comparing the test protein with a reference protein, usually egg protein
         (1) Amino acid or protein chemical score (CS)—compares the essential amino acid content in a dietary protein to that of a reference protein
         (2) Protein efficiency ratio (PER)—measures a protein's ability to support growth
         (3) Biologic value (BV)—expression of the percentage of nitrogen retained for maintenance and growth compared with the amount absorbed
         (4) Net protein utilization (NPU)—expression of the percentage of retained nitrogen compared with the amount ingested; differs from BV because it takes into account the protein's digestibility
         (5) Protein digestibility-corrected amino acid score (PDCAAS)—preferred method for measurement of protein value in human nutrition; compares the amino acid balance of a food protein with the amino acid requirements of preschool-aged children and then corrects for digestibility; used by the FDA for labeling

C. Structure
   1. Primary—linear sequence of the component amino acids
   2. Secondary—steric interaction of amino acids that are close to one another in the linear sequence (e.g., the α-helix and β-sheet)
   3. Tertiary—steric interaction between amino acids that are far apart in the linear sequence, which causes folding and the ultimate functional structure of the protein (e.g., disulfide bonds)
   4. Quaternary—steric interaction between subunits of proteins with more than one polypeptide chain (e.g., hemoglobin)

D. Digestion, absorption, and transport (see Table 12.1 and Fig. 12.1)
   1. Mouth—mechanical breakdown and moistening
   2. Stomach
      a. Hydrochloric acid from parietal cells denatures or unfolds proteins and activates pepsinogen to give pepsin
      b. Pepsin begins the hydrolysis of the peptide bonds of proteins to form peptides and proteoses
   3. Small intestine
      a. The pancreas secretes bicarbonate into the duodenum to neutralize the acidic products from the stomach and proteolytic enzymes into an inactive form; enzymes activated by trypsin through a hormonal feedback mechanism are chymotrypsin, aminopeptidase, and carboxypeptidase; each hydrolyzes peptide bonds formed by different classes of amino acids
      b. Enzymes of the brush border are dipeptidases that hydrolyze dipeptides to amino acids
   4. Absorption—at the brush border of the microvilli of the small intestine, absorption occurs both by simple diffusion along a concentration gradient and by active transport at specific amino acid sites involving carrier enzymes, a sodium-ATP pump, and vitamin $B_6$
   5. Transport—absorbed amino acids collected by the portal blood system and transported to the liver

E. Metabolism (see Fig. 12.2)
1. Amino acid pool—a collection of amino acids in a dynamic equilibrium in the liver, blood, and other cells that provides the raw material for the body's protein and amino acid needs
   a. Input into the pool comes from proteins in the diet, breakdown of body proteins, and synthesis of nonessential amino acids
   b. Output from the pool is for synthesizing body structures, specialized substances (e.g., melanin from tyrosine), and energy, as needed
2. Anabolism
   a. De novo synthesis—requires deoxyribonucleic acid (DNA), messenger ribonucleic acid (mRNA), and ribosomal ribonucleic acid (rRNA)
      (1) In the nucleus, DNA carries the genetic information in groups of three bases that provide the code for the individual amino acids comprising a specific protein
      (2) mRNA transports a copy of the code from DNA into the cytoplasm
      (3) mRNA attaches to a ribosome and acts as a template for the alignment of amino acids that are attached to transfer RNA (tRNA)
      (4) If the proper amino acids are in the correct proportions and the synthetic enzymes and energy are available, the polypeptide chain is synthesized
   b. Transamination
      (1) Nonessential amino acids can be synthesized from the corresponding α-keto acids, an α-amino acid (as the $NH_3^+$donor), a specific transaminase enzyme, and the coenzyme pyridoxal phosphate (vitamin $B_6$)
      (2) The intermediate complex formed in this reaction is called a *Schiff base*
3. Catabolism—amino acids in excess of those needed for the synthesis of proteins and other biomolecules cannot be stored or excreted; they may, however, be deaminated and the α-keto acid used as a metabolic fuel for immediate energy needs or for long-term energy storage as fat
   a. Amino group
      (1) Deamination—loss of the α-amino group, usually in the liver, through transfer to α-ketoglutarate to form glutamate; glutamate is then oxidatively deaminated to yield ammonia ($NH_3$)
      (2) Urea cycle—series of steps whereby the ammonia produced during deamination is converted to urea for excretion
   b. α-Keto acid
      (1) Ketogenic amino acids are those whose carbon skeleton, after deamination, yields acetyl-CoA or acetoacetyl-CoA, which then yields ketone bodies; high concentrations of ketone bodies lead to some of the undesirable side effects of high-protein, low-carbohydrate diets (e.g., ketoacidosis)
      (2) Glucogenic amino acids are those that yield pyruvate, α-ketoglutarate, and other intermediates of the citric acid cycle that, if needed, can be converted to glucose
4. Nitrogen balance—comparison measurement of the amount of nitrogen ingested with the amount excreted (e.g., urinary nitrogen plus approximately 1 g/day for nail, hair, skin, and perspiration losses) made to determine whether net protein catabolism, anabolism, or equilibrium exists
   a. Positive balance—intake is greater than output; indicates net protein synthesis and is the normal situation for anyone building protein-containing tissue, such as during childhood, pregnancy, and recovery from undernutrition, surgery, or illness
   b. Negative balance—intake is less than output; indicates net protein breakdown, when the body must break down its own protein to meet energy or metabolic needs; can result from insufficient protein (or essential amino acids) or energy intake or from fever, infection, anxiety, or prolonged stress

F. Metabolic regulation
1. Hormones
   a. Anabolic—growth hormone, insulin, normal thyroid hormone, and sex hormones
   b. Catabolic—adrenocortical hormones and large amounts of thyroid hormone
2. Vitamins—pyridoxine and riboflavin are necessary for protein synthesis; when they are deficient in the diet, synthesis may be limited

G. Functions
1. Structural—formation of:
   a. Collagen and elastin
   b. Bone and tooth matrix
   c. Myosin fibrils
   d. Keratin
2. Dynamic
   a. Transport of nutrients by:
      (1) Lipid-soluble and fat-soluble vitamins
      (2) Iron—transferrin
      (3) Hemoglobin and myoglobin—oxygen
      (4) Protein-bound molecules
      (5) Membrane transport
   b. Regulation and control by:
      (1) Immunoglobulins
      (2) Buffers
      (3) Hormones
      (4) Enzymes
      (5) Blood coagulation—fibrin
      (6) Muscle contraction—actin and myosin
3. Energy source (4 kcal/g)
4. Role of proteins in oral biology
   a. Preeruptive effects on teeth—essential for all cells and therefore necessary for normal tooth bud and pulp formation and synthesis of protein matrix for enamel and dentin
   b. Posteruptive effects on teeth
      (1) Essential for maintaining the integrity of pulpal tissue throughout life
      (2) Chemical nature of protein foods can neutralize acids produced by oral bacteria

c. Periodontal health and disease
   (1) Essential for all cells in the growth, development, and maintenance of the periodontium
   (2) Essential for the normal function of cellular defenses against subgingival bacteria and toxins
   (3) Necessary in the healing and repair of injured tissues from periodontitis or periodontal surgery

H. Requirements
1. Determination and estimates of protein requirements
   a. Studies of nitrogen balance are used to determine the lowest protein intake that will support homeostasis or equilibrium
   b. Average requirement for reference proteins of 0.8 g/kg/day for young adult males; other groups by extrapolation or interpolation
   c. Estimates for growth needs in infants are based on the amount of protein provided by that quantity of human milk that ensures a satisfactory growth rate
2. Recommended dietary allowances—developed by the National Research Council; based on 1985 World Health Organization (WHO) recommendations, which use nitrogen balance data; these allowances assume ingestion of good-quality protein in a mixed diet; adjustments are made for growth, pregnancy, and lactation
3. Food sources—protein needs of an average adult can be met by choosing two or more servings per day of meats, poultry, fish, eggs, dried beans, and nuts

I. Dietary modifications for disease
1. Genetic disorders
   a. Phenylketonuria (PKU)—inherited enzyme defect in which individuals cannot metabolize the phenylalanine found in almost all proteins; the prescribed diet provides only enough phenylalanine to meet growth and maintenance needs; dietary protein is restricted, but amino acids are provided by a synthetic formula from which the phenylalanine has been removed
   b. Other genetic disorders—maple syrup urine disease, homocystinuria, tyrosinemia, methylmalonic aciduria, propionic acidemia, and isovaleric acidemia are genetic disorders in which amino acid metabolism is altered; treated with low-protein diets and synthetic amino acid formulas
   c. Gout—characterized by excessive uric acid production leading to the formation of urate crystals deposited in the joints; treatment often includes restriction of protein to limit purine and uric acid production
2. Protein needs are increased during fever, after severe injury and surgery, and by intestinal malabsorption, increased protein loss from the kidneys, or diminished protein synthesis by the liver
3. Dietary protein must be restricted when the kidneys can no longer remove nitrogenous wastes from the body or in severe liver disease when the nitrogenous byproducts of protein catabolism can no longer be synthesized
4. Protein-energy (or protein-calorie) malnutrition (PEM or PCM)
   a. Kwashiorkor (classic)—failure of the young child to grow because of insufficient protein intake (usually following weaning from mother's milk); edema often masks muscle wasting
   b. Marasmus (classic)—failure of the infant or young child to grow because of partial starvation; total caloric and protein intakes are insufficient
   c. Adult PEM or PCM—seen even in the developed countries among alcoholic persons and long-term hospitalized patients with acquired immunodeficiency syndrome (AIDS), tuberculosis, or anorexia nervosa

## Lipids (Fats)

A. Definition—biochemical compounds composed of carbon, hydrogen, oxygen, and small amounts of phosphorus; insoluble in water and soluble in fatty substances and organic solvents

B. Classification
1. Simple lipids
   a. True fats—contain fatty acids attached to glycerol (a trihydroxy alcohol) through an ester linkage; these may be monoglycerides, diglycerides, or triglycerides, depending on the number of glycerol-hydroxyl groups esterified; chemical and biochemical characteristics of glycerides depend on the number, order, and types of fatty acids attached
      (1) Saturated fatty acids—contain no double bonds and are found in lipids from animal sources; are solids at room temperature (high melting point)
      (2) Unsaturated fatty acids—contain one or more double bonds and come from plant sources; are usually liquids at room temperature (low melting point)
      (3) Hydrogenation—addition of hydrogen to some or all of the double bonds; used in the manufacture of margarine or butter substitutes from vegetable oils; in partial hydrogenation, some trans bonds are formed and may present a health risk
      (4) Rancidity—addition of oxygen to some of the double bonds of fatty acids that contributes to spoilage; occurs spontaneously in foods and can be reduced by the addition of antioxidants, such as butylated hydroxytoluene (BHT)
      (5) Iodine number—chemical indication of the degree of unsaturation of a fatty acid; the more molecules of iodine bound by the fatty acid, the more unsaturated and the higher the iodine number
   b. Waxes—esters of a fatty acid and an alcohol other than glycerol; the body is unable to use waxes because digestive enzymes do not hydrolyze their ester linkage
2. Compound lipids contain compounds added to the glycerol and fatty acids
   a. Phospholipids (glycerol + 2 fatty acids + phosphate group = R group)
      (1) Water-soluble emulsifiers (e.g., lecithin, with choline as the R group)

(2) Membrane constituents (e.g., sphingomyelin)
(3) Active intermediates in metabolism of lipid compound (e.g., CoA)

b. Glycolipids—contain a carbohydrate component and are found in the brain and nervous tissue (e.g., cerebrosides)

c. Lipoproteins—are water soluble and responsible for carrying lipids throughout the body
(1) Chylomicrons—approximately 2% protein; carry exogenous (absorbed from the diet) triglycerides throughout the body
(2) Very-low-density lipoproteins (VLDLs)—9% protein; carry endogenous triglycerides around the body
(3) Low-density lipoproteins (LDLs)—21% protein; carry mostly cholesterol from the liver to peripheral sites
(4) High-density lipoproteins (HDLs)—50% protein; carry cholesterol back to the liver; can be elevated by exercise

3. Derived lipids are compounds whose synthesis begins like fatty acid synthesis, with acetyl groups added on one at a time
a. Sterols—all have a polycyclic nucleus
b. Cholesterol is a precursor for the synthesis of many steroid compounds and a constituent of cell membranes
(1) Sources
(a) Exogenous—average dietary intake is 400 to 600 milligrams (mg) from foods of animal origin
(b) Endogenous—average synthesis in the body is 1 to 2 g/day
(2) Regulation of cholesterol—dietary cholesterol, percentage of fat, ratio of polysaturated to monosaturated to unsaturated fat, and amount of certain fibers in the diet
c. Steroids—similar to sterols but with side-chain modification (e.g., bile acids, sex hormones, adrenocortical hormones, vitamin D)

4. Artificial fats—substances developed for use in foods; have the flavor, appearance, and feel of dietary fats without their physiologic effects
a. Olestra—a zero-kilocalorie (0-kcal) artificial fat made from an indigestible combination of sucrose and fatty acids; may help serum cholesterol levels by directly interfering with cholesterol absorption; may increase the requirement for vitamin E; approved for use in snack foods
b. Simplesse—has approximately 15% of the kilocalorie of the fat it replaces; made by microparticulation of whey protein; the small protein particles have the feel of fat; not suitable for use in cooking but used in fat-free dairy products and salad dressings
c. Oatrim and maltodextrim—carbohydrate-based fat replacements; mimic the texture and feel of fat by forming gels; are digestible and contribute some calories

C. Digestion, absorption, and transportation (see Table 12.1 and Fig. 12.1)
1. Digestion
a. Mouth—no enzymatic action; mechanical and moistening action only
b. Stomach—gastric lipase hydrolyzes some short-chain and medium-chain fatty acids from triglycerides
c. Small intestine
(1) Gallbladder—bile salts emulsify fats before digestion
(2) Pancreas—pancreatic lipase hydrolyzes fatty acids from triglycerides to form diglycerides and monoglycerides
(3) Intestinal mucosa—lecithinase converts lecithin to fatty acids, monoglyceride, phosphate, and choline

2. Absorption and transport
a. Short-chain fatty acids can be absorbed into the portal system
b. Medium-chain and long-chain fatty acids are water insoluble, require bile as a carrier (emulsifier), and are absorbed in stages
(1) Bile separated out at the intestinal wall and recirculated
(2) Complete breakdown of triglycerides within the mucosal cells by mucosal lipase
(3) Resynthesis of new triglycerides that combine with protein carriers to form chylomicrons
(4) Passage into the lymph system (lacteals) and blood through the thoracic duct
(5) At its destination, lipoprotein lipase hydrolyzes the triglycerides, clearing chylomicrons from blood
(6) Lipoprotein carriers (VLDLs, LDLs, and HDLs) carry endogenous lipids and cholesterol

D. Metabolism (see Fig. 12.2)
1. Anabolism
a. Lipogenesis—synthesis of triglycerides for long-term storage of energy; starting material is acetyl-CoA, which can come from glucogenic amino acids, carbohydrates, or breakdown of dietary lipids; lipogenesis takes place in almost all cells but is most active in adipose cells
b. Synthesis of steroids occurs in all cells
c. Synthesis of lipoproteins occurs mainly in the liver

2. Catabolism
a. β-Oxidation—fatty acids are broken down in a stepwise manner to yield one molecule of acetyl-CoA for every two carbon atoms; acetyl-CoA can be catabolized further by means of the TCA and oxidative phosphorylation
b. Ketone production—when the body's supply of carbohydrates is low, the TCA is depressed and acetyl-CoA from β-oxidation accumulates; alternative route for acetyl-CoA is ketone production; acetoacetone, acetone, and β-hydroxybutyrate are the ketone bodies; excess ketone production can cause ketosis, ketonuria, and ketoacidosis (which is sometimes fatal)

E. Metabolic regulators
   1. Vitamins as coenzyme precursors
      a. Anabolism—biotin, riboflavin (in flavin adenine dinucleotide [FAD]), niacin (in nicotinamide adenine dinucleotide [NAD]), and pantothenic acid (in CoA) (see Fig. 12.2)
      b. Catabolism—riboflavin, niacin, and pantothenic acid
   2. Hormones
      a. Anabolism—insulin
      b. Catabolism—ACTH, thyroid-stimulating hormone (TSH), epinephrine, and glucagon
   3. Enzymes necessary for the metabolism of lipids are synthesized or inhibited in response to the relative amounts of substrates and products available
F. Biologic role and functions of lipids
   1. Structural components of cell membrane
   2. Energy source
      a. Provide 9 kcal/g (compared with 4 kcal/g for protein or carbohydrates)
      b. Long-term storage of energy
   3. Carrier medium of fat-soluble vitamins
   4. Protective padding for body organs
   5. Insulation for the maintenance of body temperature
   6. Role of lipids in oral biology
      a. Cariostatic properties
         (1) Lipids provide a coating on the tooth's surface and form a protective pellicle on the tooth
         (2) Lipids act by neutralizing the acids produced by bacterial metabolism of the plaque biofilm; they raise the pH and decrease risk of the demineralization of enamel
      b. Consumption of less saturated fats in the diet and more monounsaturated and polyunsaturated fats may result in reduced inflammation and improved periodontal health. [3]
G. Nutritional requirements
   1. Essential fatty acids (EFAs)—cannot be synthesized in sufficient amounts to meet the body's needs; must be supplied in the diet; for humans the only EFAs are linoleic (ω-6) and linolenic (ω-3; omega fatty acids); requirement is approximately 3% of total kilocalories
      a. Function—necessary for the synthesis of membranes and prostaglandins (local hormone)
      b. Deficiency symptoms—seen in infants on low polyunsaturated fatty acid (PUFA) diets and in adults receiving total parenteral nutrition feedings without lipids; the deficiency is characterized by slow growth, reproductive failure, and skin lesions
   2. Recommendations (dietary goals as recommended by the AHA)
      a. Total fats: 30% or less of total kilocalories; majority of calories should come from monounsaturated and PUFAs
      b. Cholesterol: 300 mg/day or less; 200 mg/day for high-risk individuals
      c. Saturated fats—avoid saturated and *trans* fatty acids (found in processed foods); less than 10% of total kilocuries should come from saturated fatty acids
      d. Two weekly servings of fatty fish such as tuna or salmon
H. Dietary modifications for disease
   1. Cardiovascular disease (CVD)—blood vessel lumens become narrower and sometimes completely blocked because of the plaques caused by the accumulation of fatty substances, cellular debris, and calcium; blood pressure and the work required of the heart increase; formation of clots increase, and the result may be a heart attack (myocardial infarction) or stroke (cerebrovascular accident)
      a. Hyperlipoproteinemias—for diagnosis, elevation of serum VLDL, LDL, and chylomicron levels indicates that a patient is at risk for CVD; a genetic predisposition for certain hyperlipoproteinemias exists; elevated HDL levels may exert a protective effect against CVD; routine exercise elevates HDL levels in most people
      b. Dietary factors that may increase serum lipids—high intake of cholesterol, saturated fats, total fats, sucrose, fructose, and ethanol (alcohol)
      c. Dietary factors that may decrease serum lipids—monounsaturated fatty acids and PUFAs, omega fatty acids (fish oils), and pectin; ethanol in moderate amounts may have a protective effect by increasing HDL levels; unidentified substances in garlic, yeast, onions, and some wines may also have a protective effect
   2. Obesity—because fats are a concentrated source of calories (9 kcal/g), most reducing diets recommend a decrease in fat intake; fat should not be too severely restricted because it adds to the palatability and satiety of the diet
   3. Gallbladder disease and chronic pancreatitis—often cause pain after lipid ingestion; diet may have to be restricted in fats until the conditions are corrected
   4. Cystic fibrosis and malabsorption disorders—often treated with synthetic medium-chain triglyceride formulas that are more easily absorbed
   5. Dumping syndrome and gastric ulcers—often treatment involves increasing fat in the diet to delay gastric emptying
   6. Epilepsy—children with some types of epilepsy may be effectively treated with a ketogenic diet that is high in fats, is low in carbohydrates, and causes a ketotic condition

## Vitamins

A. Definition—organic substances that are essential to life and are needed in very small amounts; serve in regulatory functions and often act as coenzymes or precursors of coenzymes; some vitamins can be produced in precursor form or activated in the body
B. Classification
   1. Water-soluble vitamins
      a. Vitamin C
      b. B-complex vitamins

2. Fat-soluble vitamins
   a. Vitamin A
   b. Vitamin D
   c. Vitamin E
   d. Vitamin K

C. Chemistry and general properties
1. Water-soluble vitamins
   a. Soluble in water
   b. Sensitive to heat, light, and oxygen
   c. Contain the elements carbon, hydrogen, oxygen, and nitrogen, and, in some cases, other elements such as cobalt or sulfur
   d. Absorbed into blood by both active and passive transport from the upper portion of the digestive tract (see Fig. 12.1); vitamin $B_{12}$ requires the intrinsic factor for absorption
   e. Transported free and unbound to cells by blood
   f. Minimal storage of excess dietary vitamins except for:
      (1) Vitamin C—stores may last 30 to 90 days
      (2) Vitamin $B_{12}$—stores may last many years in those without pernicious anemia
      (3) Folic acid—stores may last 4 to 5 months
   g. Are excreted in urine
   h. Should be supplied in the diet almost every day
   i. Deficiency symptoms often develop rapidly
   j. Are relatively nontoxic with excessive dietary intake, although the increased use of over-the-counter (OTC) "megavitamin" preparations has caused the appearance of toxic symptoms
2. Fat-soluble vitamins
   a. Soluble in fat and fat solvents (some water-soluble derivatives are available)
   b. More stable than water-soluble vitamins in light, heat, and oxygen
   c. Contain only elements of carbon, hydrogen, and oxygen
   d. Must be emulsified and carried across the membranes of the intestinal cells in the presence of fat and bile (see Fig. 12.1); any conditions that decrease the digestion, absorption, or transport of lipids will lower the usable amount of fat-soluble vitamins
   e. Absorbed into the lymphatic system and transported by attachment to protein carriers
   f. Not readily excreted
   g. Not absolutely necessary in the diet every day
   h. Amount ingested in excess of the daily need is stored in the liver and fatty tissues
   i. Deficiency symptoms slow to develop
   j. Toxic with chronic excessive intake

D. General functions
1. Water-soluble vitamins
   a. Form coenzymes for energy metabolism
   b. Synthesis of red blood cells and DNA
2. Fat-soluble vitamins—play a role in:
   a. Vision
   b. Maintenance of the body's mucosal linings and epithelial cells
   c. Integrity of mineralized tissues of bone and teeth by regulating the calcium and phosphorus levels in the body
   d. Cellular antioxidant
   e. Normal blood clotting

E. Nutritional requirements—dietary reference intake (DRI) and RDA are based on vitamin and mineral intake from food, not supplements; for an elaboration of DRI and RDA, see the section on "Methods for Assessment of Dietary Intake" later in this chapter. Refer to the National Institutes for Health, Office of Dietary Supplements website, https://ods.od.nih.gov/Health_Information/Dietary_Reference_Intakes.aspx; also see Website Information and Resources table at the end of this chapter

F. Dietary sources, specific body functions, and symptoms of deficiencies and toxicities (Table 12.4)

G. Role of vitamins in oral biology
1. Functions
   a. Tooth formation (Table 12.5)
   b. Periodontium (Table 12.5)
2. Oral manifestations of deficiencies and toxicities (see Table 12.4)

## Minerals

A. Definition—inorganic elements that are essential to life; serve both structural and regulatory functions

B. Classification (see Table 12.4)
1. Macrominerals—present in relatively high amounts in body tissues
2. Trace elements—present at less than 0.005% of body weight

C. Chemistry and general functions
1. Exist as inorganic ions
2. Chemical identity not altered in the body or in food
3. Indestructible
4. Soluble in water and tend to form acidic or basic solutions
5. Vary in amounts absorbed and in pathways of excretion (see Fig. 12.1)
6. Some readily absorbed into blood and transported freely
7. Some require carriers for absorption and transportation
8. Excessive intake can be toxic

D. General functions
1. Maintenance of acid-base balance
2. Coenzymes or catalysts for biologic reactions
3. Components of essential body compounds
4. Maintenance of water balance
5. Transmission of nerve impulses
6. Regulation of muscle contraction
7. Growth of oral and other body tissues

E. Nutritional requirements (see information on the National Academies Press website)

F. Dietary sources, specific body functions, and symptoms of deficiencies and toxicities (see Table 12.4)

G. Role of minerals in oral biology
1. Function (see Table 12.5)
   a. Tooth formation
   b. Periodontium
2. Oral manifestations of deficiencies and toxicities (see Table 12.4)

**TABLE 12.4 Nutrients and Their Related Effects on the Oral Cavity**

| Nutrient | Dietary Sources | Major Body Functions | Oral Manifestations of Nutrient Deficiency | Oral Manifestations of Nutrient Excess |
|---|---|---|---|---|
| **Vitamins** | | | | |
| Vitamin A | Fortified dairy foods, orange, yellow and green vegetables, fruit, and protein foods | Antioxidant<br>Constituent of rhodopsin<br>Maintains epithelial tissue involved in bone growth and remodeling | Ameloblast atrophy<br>Faulty bone and tooth formation<br>Enamel hypoplasia<br>Xerostomia<br>Cleft lip<br>Increased risk of candidiasis<br>Decreased taste sensitivity | Hypertrophy of bone<br>Cracking and bleeding lips<br>Cheilosis<br>Erythemic gingivae |
| Vitamin D | Sunlight, oily fish, eggs, fortified dairy foods, cheese, egg yolks, beef liver | Promotes growth and mineralization of bones and teeth<br>Increases absorption of calcium at intestine | Loss of alveolar and mandibular bone<br>Delayed eruption<br>Increased caries rate; hypomineralization<br>Loss of lamina dura around roots of tooth | Pulp calcification<br>Enamel hypoplasia |
| Vitamin E | Vegetable oils, seeds, green leafy vegetables, whole-grain or fortified cereals, wheat germ, nuts | Antioxidant<br>Involved in cellular respiration and synthesis of body compounds<br>Prevents hemolysis of red blood cells (RBCs) | Loss of resistance to inflammation in peridontium | No effect noted |
| Vitamin K | Green and orange vegetables, microflora in the gut, soy foods | Important in blood clotting<br>Involved in the formation of active prothrombin | Gingival hemorrhage<br>Increased risk of candidiasis | No effect noted |
| Vitamin C | Citrus fruits, tomatoes, green and red peppers, broccoli, strawberries, kiwi | Important in collagen synthesis<br>Important in the body's use of iron, $B_{12}$, and folic acid | Odontoblast atrophy<br>Atypical dentin formation<br>Gingival inflammation<br>Cyanotic gingival tissues<br>Ulceration and necrosis<br>Slow wound healing<br>Defects in collagen formation | No effect noted |
| Thiamin | Pork, whole grains, nuts, legumes | Coenzyme in reactions involving removal of carbon dioxide in carbohydrate metabolism<br>Synthesized by intestinal bacteria in large intestine | Increased sensitivity and burning sensation of oral mucosa<br>Loss of taste and appetite | No effect noted |
| Riboflavin | Dairy products, whole grains | Functions as a coenzyme in the metabolism of carbohydrate, protein, and fat<br>Synthesized by intestinal bacteria in the large intestine | Angular cheilosis<br>Atrophy of filiform papillae<br>Enlarged fungiform papillae<br>Shiny, red lips<br>Painful tongue<br>Glossitis | No effect noted |
| Niacin | Beef liver, beef, fish, poultry, fortified cereals, legumes, peanuts | Coenzyme in energy (ATP) production | Angular chelosis<br>Loss of filiform and fungiform papillae<br>Mucositis<br>Stomatitis<br>Glossitis<br>Ulcerative gingivitis<br>Glossodynia | No effect noted |
| Pyridoxine | Beef, beef liver, poultry, fish, vegetables, fortified or whole-grain cereals | Coenzyme involved in amino acid metabolism<br>Converts tryptophan to niacin<br>Role in hemoglobin synthesis | Angular cheilosis<br>Sore, burning mouth<br>Glossitis<br>Glossodynia<br>Stomatitis<br>Deficiency usually occurs in combination with other B vitamins | No effect noted |
| Pantothenic acid | Organ meats, whole-grain cereals, broccoli, avocados | Constituent of coenzyme A, which plays a central role in energy metabolism | No effect noted | No effect noted |

**TABLE 12.4 Nutrients and Their Related Effects on the Oral Cavity—cont'd**

| Nutrient | Dietary Sources | Major Body Functions | Oral Manifestations of Nutrient Deficiency | Oral Manifestations of Nutrient Excess |
|---|---|---|---|---|
| Cobalamin | Clams, beef liver, beef, poultry, eggs, fish, shellfish, dairy products | Coenzyme involved in synthesis of single carbon units in nucleic acid metabolism<br>Important in RBC formation and myelin synthesis | Stomatitis<br>Hemorrhagic gingiva<br>Pale to yellow mucosa<br>Atrophy of filiform papilla<br>Glossopyrosis<br>Glossitis<br>Atrophy and burning tongue<br>Altered taste<br>Halitosis<br>Oral paresthesia<br>Detachment of periodontal fibers<br>Bone loss<br>Xerostomia<br>Aphthous ulcers | No effect noted |
| Folate | Fortified grain products, beef liver, kidney beans, yeast, leafy green vegetables, black-eyed peas | Coenzyme involved in RNA and DNA synthesis<br>Important in the proper formation of neural tubes during fetal development | Glossitis<br>Enlargement of fungiform papillae<br>Ulcerations along edge of tongue<br>Gingivitis<br>Neural tube defects: cleft palate and lip | Excess can mask cobalamin deficiency<br>Pale mucosa<br>Angular cheilosis |
| Biotin | Beef liver, canned pink salmon 2% milk, whole egg, sunflower seeds | Coenzyme required for the synthesis and oxidation of fats and carbohydrates and for deamination of proteins | Glossitis<br>Gray mucosa<br>Atrophy of lingual papillae | No effect noted |
| **Minerals** | | | | |
| Calcium | Milk, cheese, dark-green vegetables, fortified breads, juices and cereals, canned salmon | Bone and tooth formation<br>Blood clotting<br>Nerve transmission<br>Muscle contraction | Incomplete calcification of teeth<br>Risk of hemorrhage<br>Increased susceptibility to caries and periodontal disease | No effect noted |
| Phosphorus | Milk, cheese, meat, poultry, whole-grain breads and cereals, eggs | Bone and tooth formation<br>Acid-base balance<br>Release of energy: adenosine triphosphate (ATP), adenosine diphosphate (ADP) | Incomplete calcification of teeth<br>Failure of dentin formation<br>Increased susceptibility to caries during tooth development<br>Increased susceptibility to periodontal disease | No effect noted |
| Sulfur | Meat, fish, poultry, legumes | Important in oxidation reduction reactions<br>Body water balance | No effect noted | No effect noted |
| Potassium | Meats, milk, many fruits, fish, eggs | Acid-base balance<br>Body water balance<br>Nerve function<br>Affects heart muscle contraction | No effect noted | No effect noted |
| Chlorine | Table salt, cured and pickled foods, water | Formation of gastric juice<br>Body water balance<br>Acid-base balance | No effect noted | No effect noted |
| Sodium | Table salt; cured, processed, canned, and pickled foods; broth | Acid-base balance<br>Body water balance<br>Nerve function | Decrease in salivary flow | Dry, sticky tongue and oral mucous membranes |
| Magnesium | Whole grains, green leafy vegetables, nuts, beans, bananas | Activates enzymes involved in energy metabolism<br>Maintains calcium homeostasis | Alveolar bone fragility<br>Gingival hyperplasia<br>Enamel hypoplasia<br>Widening of periodontal ligament | No effect noted |
| Iron | Egg yolk, meats, liver, whole grains, dark-green vegetables, dried fruits | Constituent of hemoglobin and enzymes involved in energy metabolism | Angular cheilosis<br>Pallor of lips or oral mucosa<br>Atrophy of filiform papillae<br>Decreased resistance to infection<br>Glossitis<br>Increased risk of candidiasis<br>Salivary gland dysfunction | No effect noted |

*Continued*

**TABLE 12.4 Nutrients and Their Related Effects on the Oral Cavity—cont'd**

| Nutrient | Dietary Sources | Major Body Functions | Oral Manifestations of Nutrient Deficiency | Oral Manifestations of Nutrient Excess |
|---|---|---|---|---|
| Fluoride | Drinking water, tea, seafood | Important in the maintenance of bone structure<br>Forms strong apatite crystals during tooth formation | Decreased resistance to dental caries | Enamel fluorosis; mottled enamel |
| Zinc | Lamb, beef, oysters, eggs, peanuts, whole grains | Required for synthesis of DNA, RNA, and protein<br>Bone growth and metabolism | Impaired taste<br>Loss of tongue sensation<br>Delayed wound healing<br>Impaired keratinization of epithelial cells<br>Increased susceptibility to periodontal disease<br>Flattened filiform papillae | No effect noted |
| Copper | Shellfish, oysters, organ meats nuts, whole grains, dried fruits, legumes | Important catalyst in hemoglobin synthesis | Decreased trabecular pattern<br>Decreased tissue vascularity<br>Fragility of tissue | No effect noted |
| Selenium | Seafood, kidney, liver, dairy products, whole grains, nuts | Antioxidant | No effect noted | Associated with increased dental caries |
| Manganese | Whole grains, legumes, nuts, tea, green leafy vegetables | Normal skeletal development<br>Involved in fat synthesis, urea formation, and energy release | No effect noted | Associated with increased dental caries |
| Iodine | Marine fish and shellfish, table salt, eggs | Constituent of thyroid hormones<br>Regulates energy metabolism | Delayed tooth eruption | No effect noted |
| Molybdenum | Legumes, whole-grain cereals, organ meats | Constituent of enzymes involved in uric acid formation and oxidation of aldehydes | No effect noted | No effect noted |
| Chromium | Vegetables, whole grains, wheat germ, nuts, mushrooms, beer and wine | Involved in carbohydrate and lipid metabolism | No effect noted | No effect noted |
| Cobalt | Liver, kidney, fish, poultry eggs, tempeh | Important in RBC formation as a component of $B_{12}$ | No effect noted | No effect noted |
| **Other Nutrients** | | | | |
| Carbohydrates | Breads, cereals, and grains, starchy vegetables, fruits | Source of energy | Decrease in caries rate as carbohydrate intake decreases in population and individuals | Cariogenic; causative risk factor for dental caries<br>Form, frequency, and total contact time influence cariogenicity |
| Fats | Cooking oils, butter, fats found in meat, fish, poultry with skin, dairy products | Source of energy<br>Cariostatic; antimicrobial action that produces an oily film on enamel and protects against cariogenic challenges | Difficult to develop a deficiency | Cariostatic: antimicrobial action that produces an oily film on enamel and protects against cariogenic challenges |
| Protein | Beef, fish, poultry, eggs, lentils, legumes, tofu, dairy products, peanut butter, quinoa | Source of energy<br>Cariostatic | Defects in composition, eruption pattern, and resistance to decay during periods of tooth development<br>Increased susceptibility to soft tissue infection, poor healing, and tissue regeneration | No effect noted |
| Water | Tap water, bottled water, water used in coffee and tea; some fruits and vegetables contain water | Source of hydration | Dehydration<br>Fragility of epithelial tissues<br>Decreased muscle strength for chewing<br>Xerostomia<br>Fissured tongue | No effect noted |

Adapted from Touger-Decker R, Rigassio-Radler D, DePaola DP. Nutrition and dental medicine. In Ross AC, et al, eds. *Modern Nutrition in Health and Disease.* 11th ed. Baltimore: Wolters Kluwer Health/Lippincott Williams & Wilkins; 2014; Davis JR, Stegeman CA. *The Dental Hygienist's Guide to Nutritional Care.* 5th ed 5. St. Louis: Elsevier; 2019; and Palmer CA, Boyd LD. *Diet and Nutrition in Oral Health.* 3rd ed. Upper Saddle River, NJ: Pearson Prentice Hall; 2017.

**TABLE 12.5 Effects of Nutrients on Oral Tissues and Their Role in Tooth Formation**

| Nutrients | Effects on Oral Soft and Hard Tissue | Role in Tooth Formation |
|---|---|---|
| Vitamin A | Synthesis and function of epithelial cells<br>Maintenance of the integrity of the sulcus<br>Normal growth and function of salivary glands<br>Essential for activity of epiphyseal cartilage cells and normal endochondral bone growth | Normal growth of dentin and enamel<br>Normal growth of periodontal tissues and maintenance of epithelium |
| Vitamin D | No effects noted | Controls calcification of dentin and enamel by regulating calcium absorption in the intestines |
| Vitamin C | Synthesis of connective tissue<br>Essential for integrity of capillaries and oral mucosa<br>Needed for normal bone matrix formation<br>Needed for normal phagocytic function and antibody synthesis in host defense system | Integrity of blood vessels in gingival and pulpal tissues<br>Hydroxylation of proline and lysine in collagen synthesis<br>Normal formation of dentin |
| **B-Complex Vitamins** | | |
| Thiamin (Vitamin B1) | Normal energy metabolism during development and maintenance of oral tissue | No effects noted |
| Riboflavin (Vitamin B2) | Energy metabolism of oral tissues | No effects noted |
| Niacin (Vitamin B3)_ | Integrity of oral tissues | No effects noted |
| Pyridoxine (Vitamin B6) | Normal carbohydrate metabolism and hemoglobin synthesis in oral tissues | No effects noted |
| Folate (Vitamin B9); formerly Folacin | Normal synthesis of protein compounds in oral tissues (e.g., hemoglobin and enzymes) | No effects noted |
| Cobalamin (Vitamin B12) | Integrity of nerve tissue and normal red blood cell formation in oral tissues | No effects noted |
| **Other Nutrients** | | |
| Calcium/phosphorus ratio | No effects noted | Normal tooth and bone mineralization |
| Fluoride | No effects noted | Forms dentin and enamel |
| Iron | Normal hemoglobin formation and carbon dioxide transport to tissue | No effects noted |
| Fiber | Stimulates salivary flow and integrity of periodontal tissues | No effects noted |
| Protein | Synthesis of antibodies and leukocytes<br>Synthesis of epithelial and connective tissues in the healing process<br>Maintains integrity of periodontal tissues | Formation of matrix of dentin and enamel<br>Collagen formation<br>Tooth eruption<br>Tooth size |

Adapted from Touger-Decker R, Rigassio-Radler D, DePaola DP. Nutrition and dental medicine. In Ross AC et al, eds. *Modern Nutrition in Health and Disease*. 11th ed. Baltimore: Wolters Kluwer Health/Lippincott Williams & Wilkins; 2014.

## Water

A. Definition—essential nutrient abundantly found in foods and beverages; makes up 50% to 60% of total body weight; survival without water is possible only up to 2 or 3 days

B. Total body water
   1. Body water, as a percentage of body weight, decreases with age, ranging from 69% in newborn infants to 49% in women
   2. Distribution—majority is intracellular, with the remainder being extracellular in serum, cerebrospinal fluid, tissue spaces, and saliva
      a. Intracellular
         (1) Enclosed within the cell membrane
         (2) Accounts for two-thirds of the total
         (3) Increases with increased body cell mass
      b. Extracellular compartment
         (1) Intravascular
            (a) Approximately 3 liters (L)
            (b) Includes water in blood vessels
         (2) Intercellular (interstitial)
            (a) Approximately 12 L
            (b) Fluids that leave blood vessels
            (c) Fluids present in spaces between and surrounding each cell

C. Biologic role and functions
   1. Is the medium in which most of the body's reactions take place
   2. Is the means for transporting vital materials to cells and waste products away from cells
   3. Regulates a constant body temperature
   4. Maintains a constant composition of elements in body fluids (e.g., calcium, sodium, fluoride)
   5. Is part of the chemical structure of compounds that form cells (e.g., proteins)
   6. Is active in many chemical reactions (e.g., digestion of a disaccharide)
   7. Serves as a solvent (e.g., amino acids dissolve in water); this permits their transport to body cells
   8. Lubricates and protects sensitive tissue around joints and mucosal linings

D. Water balance
1. Intake—controlled by thirst sensations; total daily intake need ranges from 1 to 3 L at a minimum to replace daily water losses; sources of water intake are:
a. Ingested liquids and foods—1200 to 2000 milliliters (mL) per day
b. Metabolic water from the oxidation of foods—300 to 350 mL/day
2. Elimination—total water output is 1500 to 3000 mL/day
a. Sensible or measurable losses—occur through the kidneys as urine and through the bowel as feces; constant daily losses amount to 500 to 800 mL
b. Insensible or unmeasurable losses—occur through the lungs with expired air and through the skin as perspiration; daily losses vary considerably, with an average of 850 to 1200 mL

E. Regulation
1. Potassium and sodium concentrations are responsible for maintaining water balance; when extracellular sodium equals intracellular potassium, water will not move into or out of the cell
2. Mechanisms of regulation
a. Thirst response—when sodium increases, it stimulates the hypothalamus and increases the urge to drink
b. Excretion regulation
(1) Increased sodium stimulates the hypothalamus to signal the pituitary to release ADH, and water is resorbed in the kidney tubules
(2) Decreased sodium causes the release of aldosterone, which causes resorption of sodium at the kidney tubules

F. Requirements—include water from liquids and food
1. For men, the adequate intake (AI) is 15 to 16 cups (3.7 L) per day
2. For women, the AI is 11 to 12 cups (2.7 L) per day

G. Causes of water deficiency and conditions of toxicity
1. Dehydration
a. Malfunction of kidneys
b. Blood loss
c. Vomiting
d. Diarrhea
e. Inadequate fluid intake
2. Water intoxication
a. Edema
b. Hypertension
c. Sodium retention

## SPECIALIZED CELLS OF ORAL TISSUES: EFFECTS OF NUTRIENTS

A. Epithelial cells
1. Important in tooth formation during the embryonic period
2. Make up the outer layers of tissue in the oral mucosa
a. Rapid cell renewal, especially in the sulcular area
b. Cell renewal more frequent with increasing age
3. Important in the normal development of salivary glands
4. Vitamin A and protein are essential for the normal proliferation of epithelial cells

B. Fibroblasts
1. Synthesize collagen fibrils in connective tissues of the gingiva, periodontal ligament, and pulp
2. Throughout life, fibroblasts maintain a rate of collagen synthesis equal to that of collagen breakdown; nutrient deficiencies can interfere with this equilibrium and cause a net loss of collagen tissue
3. Vitamin C, zinc, copper, and protein are important in collagen formation

C. Cementoblasts and cementocytes
1. Synthesize the protein matrix for cementum; vitamin C, zinc, copper, and protein are essential
2. Calcify the protein matrix; protein, calcium, phosphorus, and vitamin D are essential
3. Cementum is avascular and part acellular
4. Cellular cementum consists of cementocytes that depend on diffusion from the periodontal ligament for their nutrient supply

D. Ameloblasts
1. Synthesize the protein matrix for enamel; vitamins A and C, zinc, copper, and protein are essential
2. Calcify the protein matrix; protein, calcium, phosphorus, and vitamin D are essential; fluoride improves the quality of the apatite crystals formed
3. Once enamel is formed, no metabolic cells are present

E. Odontoblasts
1. Synthesize the protein matrix for dentin; vitamins A and C, zinc, copper, and protein are essential
2. Calcify the protein matrix; protein, calcium, phosphorus, and vitamin D are essential; fluoride improves the quality of the apatite crystals formed
3. Once dentin is formed, no metabolic cells are present, except in reaction to trauma; with trauma, new odontoblasts can form (possibly from pulpal tissue), and secondary dentin can be laid down

F. Osteocytes—osteoblasts and osteoclasts
1. Function in the synthesis of the alveolus
2. Function in the lifelong process of bone apposition (osteoblasts) and resorption (osteoclasts) in the alveolus
3. Nutrients important in the formation and maintenance of the alveolus are protein; vitamins A, C, and D; zinc; copper; calcium; and phosphorus

## ENERGY BALANCES AND WEIGHT CONTROL

A. Definition—energy balance is a dynamic state in which the calories from food are equal to the caloric needs of the body; changes in energy balance result in a relative gain or loss in body weight
1. Lean body mass is highly metabolically active; basal metabolism is generally higher in people with greater amounts of lean body mass

2. In older adults, increases in body weight and body fat are not attributed to increased intake but are related to decrease in energy expenditure from loss of lean body mass

B. Measurement of energy
   1. By calorimetry—food sample is burned in oxygen in an enclosed vessel surrounded by water; 1 kcal is the amount of heat produced sufficient to raise the temperature of 1 kg of water to 1°C; the commonly used term *calorie* has the same definition
   2. In the body—carbon, hydrogen, and oxygen (from protein, carbohydrates, alcohol, or fats) are converted to carbon dioxide, water, and energy; energy is produced in the form of ATP; when needed, each ATP molecule loses a high-energy phosphate bond and becomes adenosine diphosphate (ADP) with a release of approximately 7.3 kcal/mole

C. Energy-producing systems
   1. Blood glucose—immediate and preferred source of energy for cellular metabolism; glycogen stores provide glucose through glycogenolysis during the short periods of fasting between meals and in response to hormonal signals during sudden movement or intense exercise
      a. Protein—can be used as an energy source when the blood glucose level falls; glucogenic amino acids are converted to glucose after deamination by gluconeogenesis; in a starvation state, body proteins are used for energy, which may cause irreversible damage if the essential protein components of the body are catabolized
      b. Fat—mobilized from adipose tissue; triglycerides are broken down into glycerol and fatty acids in the liver; fatty acids are catabolized by β-oxidation to acetyl-CoA
      c. Ethanol (alcohol)—can be oxidized to acetaldehyde, which is then converted into acetyl-CoA
   2. Acetyl-CoA—enters the TCA from many sources
   3. ATP—made during the process of oxidative phosphorylation in the mitochondria; proteins, carbohydrates, and fats do not yield the same number of ATP molecules per molecule of starting material because of their difference in molecular structure; to estimate the stored energy of foods, use these approximations: protein, 4 kcal/g; carbohydrate, 4 kcal/g; fat, 9 kcal/g; and ethanol, 7 kcal/g

D. Energy-using systems—ATP produced during catabolism is used by the body for biosynthetic activities, muscle contraction, ion transport, nerve conduction, and maintenance of body temperature
   1. Energy for basal metabolism—*basal metabolic rate* (BMR) is a measure of the energy required to maintain a living state while at rest and without food; includes respiration, circulation, maintenance of body temperature, muscle tone, glandular activities, and cellular metabolism
      a. Conditions for BMR measurement—postabsorptive state; muscles totally relaxed; awake; environmental temperature between 20°C and 25°C (68°F and 77°F); free of emotional stress; not during ovulation
      b. Factors influencing the BMR—age, genetics, gender, body size, nutritional state, muscular training, pathologic conditions, thyroid gland activity, climate, and altitude
   2. Energy for activity—the activity component of the energy requirement is for voluntary physical activity and varies from 20% of the BMR for sedentary activity to 50% or more of the BMR for heavy activity; factors influencing energy needs for the activity component include the size of the individual and the intensity and duration of the activity
   3. Thermic effect of food (TEF)—energy required to digest, absorb, and metabolize food; also called *nonshivering thermogenesis* because a slight elevation in body temperature occurs after a meal; not a clearly defined phenomenon; believed to include the energy needed to increase muscular contractions of the digestive tract, increases the synthesis of digestive enzymes and transports molecules; amounts to about 5% to 10% of the BMR and activity energy components

E. Nutritional requirements: determined by intake of food energy that allows the maintenance of ideal weight; data have been gathered from animal studies, balance studies, and intake surveys
   1. Recommendations represent the average needs of people in each age group and within a given activity category
   2. Recommendations are influenced by body size, gender, climate, age, and activity level

F. Weight management and control
   1. Calculating caloric intake needs—body mass index (BMI) and ideal body weight (IBW); see the section on "Complete Nutritional Assessment" later in this chapter
      a. BMI—approximate positive correlation of height and weight with body fat ($r = +0.7–0.8$); used to assess obesity and as an indicator of optimal weight for health (Table 12.6); for example, overweight adults with a BMI greater than 25 are at risk for comorbid diseases
         (1) Calculate BMI by dividing body weight in kilograms (kg) by the height in square meters ($m^2$); for example, a man weighing 270 pounds (122.7 kg) who is 6 feet (3.34 $m^2$) tall has a BMI of approximately 37
         (2) BMI does not differentiate between lean body mass and fat mass; thus could inaccurately label an individual as "obese"
      b. Waist circumference is a more accurate method of determining central obesity, also known as *abdominal obesity* in an individual; puts an individual at greater risk of CVD
         (1) Women with waist measurements greater than 35 inches are at risk for comorbid conditions
         (2) Men with waist measurements greater than 40 inches are at risk for comorbid conditions
         (3) Waist circumference standards used for the general population may not apply to individuals under 5 feet in height or with a BMI of 35 or greater

**TABLE 12.6 Body Mass Index and Waist Circumference Overweight and Obesity Classification Chart**

| | Obesity Class | Body Mass Index (BMI) (1 kg/m²) | Waist Circumference Women > 35 inches Men > 40 inches |
|---|---|---|---|
| Underweight | — | < 18.5 | |
| Normal | — | 18.5–24.9 | |
| Overweight | — | 25.0–29.9 | Increased (W) to High (M) |
| Obesity | I | 30.0–34.9 | High (W) to Very High (M) |
| | II | 35.0–39.9 | Very High |
| Extreme obesity | III | ≥ 40 | Extremely High |

Modified from National Institute of Health: Classification of Overweight and Obesity by BMI, Waist Circumference, and Associated Disease Risks. https://www.nhlbi.nih.gov/health/educational/lose_wt/BMI/bmi_dis.htm. Accessed April 9, 2019.

c. Determining IBW
   (1) Male IBW = 106 + (6 × inches over 5 feet tall)
   (2) Female IBW = 100 + (5 × inches over 5 feet tall)
   (3) For individuals under 5 feet, subtract 2 lb for each inch below 5 feet
d. Alternative method—decreasing usual caloric intake by 500 kcal/day usually allows a weight loss of 1 lb per week; this loss may reach a plateau as the body adjusts to a new BMR
e. Refer to https://www.choosemyplate.gov/MyPlatePlan to determine individual caloric needs based on age, height, weight, gender, and activity level.

2. Types of diet modifications
   a. Balanced, low-calorie diet—the safest and healthiest reducing diet if calories are approximately 1200 kcal/day and the intake is balanced and varied (e.g., Weight Watchers diet)
   b. Low-carbohydrate, high-protein diet—risk of development of ketosis (e.g., Atkins diet, Ketogenic diet, Paleo diet)
   c. Low-fat diet—may deprive the individual of EFAs and fat-soluble vitamins; causes rapid emptying of the stomach (low satiety) and may make food seem flavorless; most individuals can decrease their usual fat intake without any harmful effects (e.g., Pritikin diet)
   d. High-fiber diet—increases fiber and bulk in the diet and allows a more rapid transit time for food in the GI tract; fiber also binds other nutrients, so they are not completely absorbed; moderate increases in the fiber content of the diet appear to be helpful in treating diabetes, diverticulosis, and hypercholesterolemia as well as in decreasing the total caloric intake of reducing diets; very-high-fiber diets cause GI discomfort and may induce mineral deficiencies (e.g., in well-designed vegetarian diets, Pritikin diet)
   e. Single-food (monotonous) diet—no one food by itself can provide a balance of nutrients; diets that promote a single food with unrealistic claims are not recommended (e.g., the grapefruit diet, the cabbage soup diet)
   f. Liquid formulas (protein)—very-low-calorie diets; have been successfully used in treating morbidly obese persons in carefully monitored hospital settings but are not recommended for the individual (e.g., Optifast)
3. Prescription drugs used for weight loss are recommended for individuals with a BMI of 30 or greater with no obesity-related risk factors or for those with a BMI of 27 to 29.9 with obesity-related risk factors; adverse side effects have been observed in long-term use of such drugs; FDA approved prescription drugs for overweight and obesity treatment include:
   a. Noradrenergic drugs for short-term weight loss
      (1) Diethylpropion
      (2) Phentermine (e.g., Adipex-P, Suprenza)
      (3) Phentermine-topiramate (Qsymia)
      (4) Mazindol
   b. Serotonergic drugs
      (1) Fenfluramine (also phentermine plus fenfluramine, or Phen-Fen) and dexfen-fluramine (Redux) were removed from the US market because of reports of primary pulmonary hypertension, heart valve abnormalities, and death associated with their use
      (2) Belviq (Lorcaserin) promotes a feeling of fullness or satiety
   c. Sibutramine (Meridia) is an approved combination of serotonin and adrenergic drugs; centrally acting agent that increases satiety but has little effect on hunger
   d. Orlistat (Xenical prescription or Alli OTC) is a lipase inhibitor; interferes with fat digestion; taking the drugs with meals inhibits fat absorption by 30%
   e. Bupropion hydrochloride (Contrave) suppresses appetite, increases metabolism
   f. Liraglutide (Saxenda) proposed mode of action is that it regulates areas of brain involved in appetite
4. Activity in weight management—even moderate activity such as walking will increase caloric expenditure and should be considered in every weight loss program; moderate exercise also improves muscle tone, stimulates circulation, increases BMR, and often creates a sense of well-being
5. Behavior modification—eating habits and attitudes often must be changed to prevent weight regain; many successful diet programs combine decreased food intake and increased activity with an analysis and modification of eating behaviors; group programs such as Weight Watchers help make behavioral changes
6. Dietary aids—represent a multimillion-dollar business, and although they may help cause an initial rapid weight loss, they are no more effective than mere calorie cutting in long-term weight maintenance; moreover, most diet drugs have the potential for serious side effects if used habitually over a long period or by persons with certain medical conditions; types most often used are

appetite suppressants, stimulants, laxatives, diuretics, and bulk-producing agents

7. Surgical therapy—gastric bypass surgery may be recommended to individuals with BMI of 40 or greater and for those with BMI greater than 35 and comorbid conditions
   a. This surgical approach is used to reduce the size of the stomach to decrease its reserve capacity
   b. Bloating, nausea, vomiting, dumping syndrome, anemia, and nutrient deficiencies may result if diet instructions are not followed after surgery
   c. Fluids are consumed separately from meals; more frequent small meals throughout the day are recommended
   d. Increased risk of caries due to alterations in eating habits

G. Eating disorders
1. Treatment
   a. Correction of any underlying physiologic causes of weight loss
   b. Increased caloric intake with foods that are concentrated sources of energy; several small meals per day
   c. Limiting weight gain goals to 1 to 2 lb per week
   d. Team approach; physician, registered dietitian, psychotherapist, or all should be involved in the treatment
2. Signs and symptoms of disordered eating
   a. Erosion of tooth enamel (perimylolysis)
   b. Halitosis
   c. Severe weight loss
   d. Dental caries
   e. Lanugo
   f. Enlarged tongue
   g. Angular cheilosis
   h. Enlarged parotid glands
   i. Xerostomia
   j. Glossitis
3. *Anorexia nervosa*—state of protein-energy malnutrition brought on by voluntary starvation; also may use diet aids, laxatives, diuretics, intense exercise, and self-induced vomiting as additional methods of weight loss
   a. Seen most often in middle-income and upper-income adolescent females, who are typically described as perfectionists, overachievers, and models of good behavior; they begin dieting because they have a distorted perception of body shape and weight
   b. Death may occur from failure of multiple organ systems
   c. Treatment usually includes specially tailored counseling and hospitalization before voluntary weight gain is possible; treatment encourages regular mealtimes, varied and moderate intake, and gradual introduction of feared foods
   d. The patient should be referred to a physician, a registered dietitian, or a psychologist for treatment
4. *Bulimia*—condition of alternate food gorging and purging by vomiting; occasional use of laxatives, diuretics and excessive exercise to maintain weight
   a. Most often found in adolescent females who appear to be of normal weight
   b. Is more prevalent than anorexia nervosa
   c. Treatment involves counseling; self-induced vomiting can cause swelling of the salivary glands and esophagus and the destruction of tooth enamel by acid that results in sensitive teeth
   d. The patient should be referred to a physician, a registered dietitian, or a psychologist for treatment
5. *Obesity*—an individual with a BMI of 30 or higher is considered obese.
   a. Not specifically an eating disorder; however, much like anorexia and bulimia obesity often stems from body dissatisfaction and unhealthy dieting practices
   b. Almost 40% of adults in the United States are obese and 18.5% of children aged 2–19 years old are obese.[4]
   c. A review of the literature on obesity and periodontal disease suggests that they both confound each other; obesity itself has been recognized as a major risk factor for periodontal disease. Hypersecretion of proinflammatory cytokines and various other bioactive substances are attributed to increased presence of adipocytes (fat cells) resulting in adverse effects on the periodontium such as increased bleeding on probing, increased pocket depths, and heightened inflammation
6. *Other Specified Eating or Feeding Disorder(OSFED); formerly known as Eating disorders not otherwise specified* (EDNOS)—a broad category established to ensure treatment for individuals who do not meet the strict diagnostic criteria for anorexia nervosa, bulimia, or binge-eating disorder despite multiple indicators of an eating disorder

## NUTRITIONAL ASSESSMENT AND COUNSELING

### Malnutrition

A. Overconsumption of nutrients such as:
1. Fat—can result in excess weight gain; associated with CHD, obesity, and certain types of cancers
2. Sugar—can result in excess weight gain; associated with obesity, dental caries, and biofilm-induced gingivitis
3. Salt or sodium—can result in retention of excess body fluid; associated with high blood pressure; increased sodium may also decrease calcium levels
4. Excess calories—can result in obesity; associated with CHD, hypertension, and diabetes mellitus type 2
5. Vitamin and mineral supplements—"megadoses" may result in toxicity of one or many nutrients and inhibition of others

B. Nutrient deficiencies—the health of a person is at risk because of the unavailability of nutrients for cellular activities; end result of deficiencies is the same, but the multiple causes can be classified as primary or secondary
1. *Primary deficiency* is a result of an inadequate food intake and can result from the following conditions:
   a. Fad diets—low-calorie or imbalanced diet plans
   b. Economics—inadequate resources to obtain a healthy diet
   c. Illness—loss of appetite

d. Improper food preparation—destruction of nutrients because of delayed storage and overcooking of foods
e. Accessibility to food—nutritious foods unavailable because of problems with transportation or market supplies encountered by individuals
f. Ignorance—lack of nutritional knowledge
g. Flavor preferences—palatability of sweets and fats can lead to a diet high in empty-calorie foods
h. Time constraints—inadequate time for food preparation can lead to the use of highly processed convenience foods, which tend to have low nutrient density
i. Poor oral health—inability to masticate food because of edentulism or oral disease; altered taste perceptions result from oral disease

2. *Secondary deficiency* is the result of inability to digest, absorb, and use foods consumed; an individual may eat a balanced diet, but other factors interfere with the body's use of nutrients in foods; examples of these conditioning factors include:
   a. Disease—any GI or metabolic disease can interfere with the digestion and use of foods and nutrients (e.g., ulcers, lactase deficiency, partial obstruction of the GI tract, inborn errors of metabolism)
   b. Drug-nutrient interactions—certain drugs can interfere with and reduce the absorption, transportation, and metabolism of nutrients (e.g., grapefruit juice with high blood pressure medication)
   c. Nutrient-nutrient interactions—excess or deficiency of certain nutrients can affect the absorption of other nutrients (e.g., vitamin C and iron)
   d. Allergies—sensitivity to certain foods or chemicals in foods can lead to malabsorption syndromes (e.g., gluten sensitivity, as in celiac disease)
3. Manifestations of primary and secondary deficiencies
   a. Gradual decreases in the tissue level of nutrients
      (1) Earliest sign of malnutrition
      (2) Determined by blood and urine analyses for each nutrient
   b. Biochemical disturbances
      (1) Occur if duration of deficiency is long enough to deplete the body's stores and interfere with cellular metabolism
      (2) Determined by blood and urine analyses for alterations in cellular levels of enzymes and metabolites
   c. Anatomical lesions
      (1) Signs of chronic and severe malnutrition, leading to destruction of body tissues
      (2) Determined by clinical examination of body tissues

## Complete Nutritional Assessment

A. Health and pharmacologic history
   1. Factors that influence food intake
      a. Socioeconomic conditions—food-purchasing power
      b. Home environment—culture, family values, and eating practices
      c. Patient motivation and education—interest and awareness of the principles of a nutritious diet
      d. Prescriptive drugs and nonprescriptive drugs or supplements that may suppress appetite, alter taste perception, or negatively interact with foods
   2. Factors that influence food use
      a. Oral health—ability to masticate, saliva production, and presence of oral disease
      b. Systemic health—ability to digest, absorb, and metabolize nutrients in food; therapeutic diets for disease control
      c. Mental health—desire to eat
      d. Drug use—alcohol abuse and illegal drugs

B. Assessment of dietary intake
   1. Collection of objective data on what a person eats
      a. Assessment tools—screening questionnaire for food intake frequency, 24-hour recall method, and food record or diary
         (1) Food-frequency questionnaires—ask how often food items are consumed; elicit specific details; work better with large groups in the community setting
         (2) A 24-hour recall method—mental recall of everything eaten in the previous 24 hours; useful for individual counseling in a clinical setting; does not represent "usual" diet
         (3) Food record diary—exact record of everything eaten in a specific period; more accurate account
         (4) Combining 3- to 7-day food record with a 24-hour recall method presents a more accurate measure of intake
      b. Specific amounts or quantities of foods eaten must be recorded to use assessment tools effectively
   2. Analysis and evaluation of food intake
      a. Methods of analysis—the US Department of Agriculture (USDA) MyPlate (Fig. 12.3)
      b. Methods of evaluation—comparing results of diet analysis with standards of adequacy
   3. Diet modifications
      a. Adding foods to the diet to correct for nutrient deficiencies
      b. Eliminating or reducing excessive nutrient intake for disease control and prevention (e.g., sugar, fat, oils, sodium)
      c. Collaborate with a registered dietitian for in-depth analysis and modification of dietary intake

C. Biochemical analysis and immune function
   1. Blood and urine analyses
      a. Most objective and precise assessment data
      b. Determine marginal nutritional deficiencies before overt clinical signs appear by measuring either the concentration of a nutrient or the functional activity of the nutrient
   2. Delayed cutaneous hypersensitivity skin tests
      a. Assessment of host defense mechanisms by evaluating the patient's reaction to common skin test antigens as a nonspecific indicator of malnutrition
      b. Most useful for evaluating the critically ill patient's ability to withstand the stresses of surgery

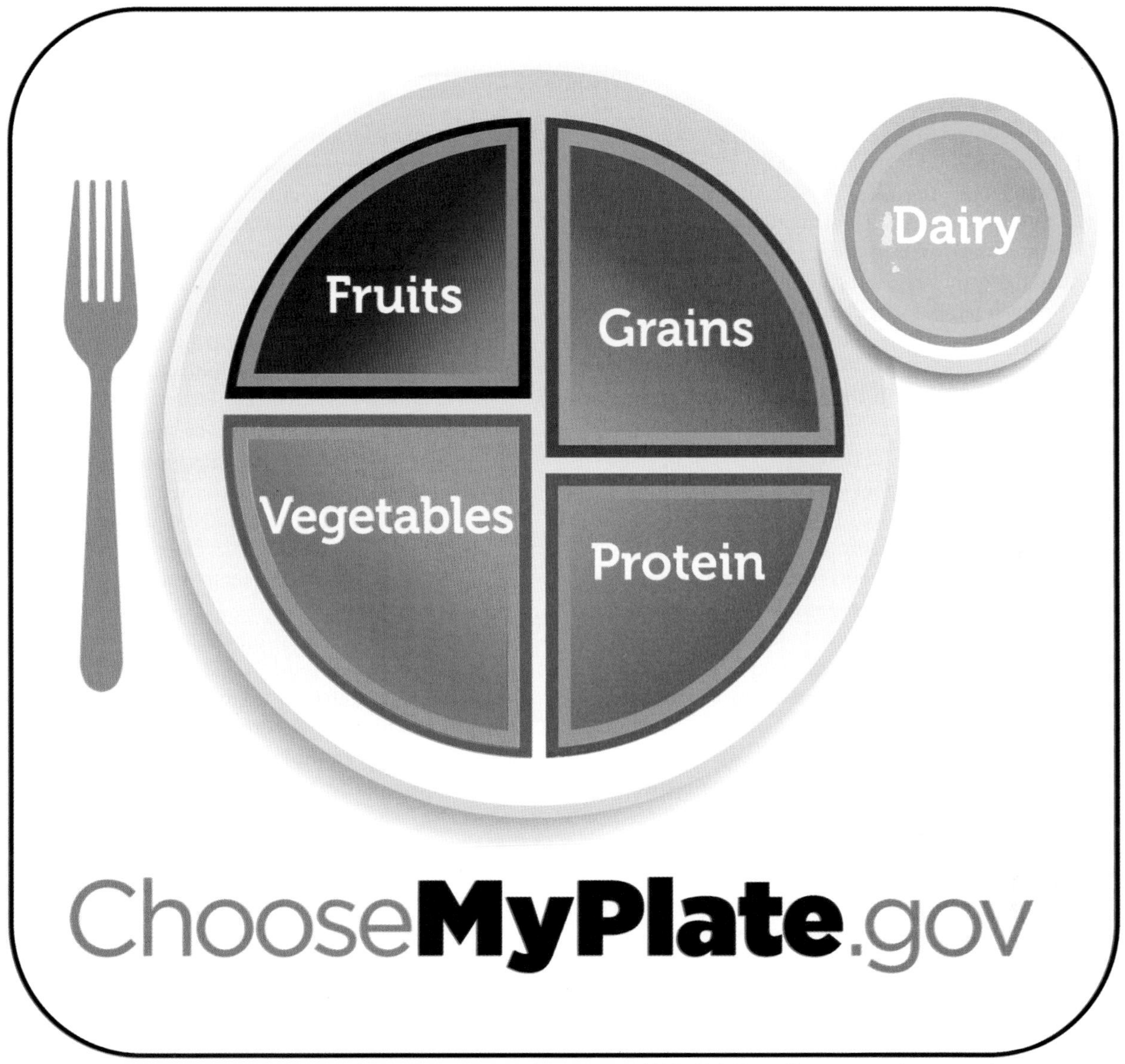


**Fig. 12.3** Anatomy of United States Department of Agriculture (USDA) MyPlate. (From www.choosemyplate.gov. Accessed April 8, 2019.)

D. Clinical examination of body tissues—indicator of systemic health and nutritional status (see Table 12.4)
   1. Oral tissues
      a. Dental caries—excessive sugar or acid exposure (supports *S. mutans* and *Lactobacillus acidophilus*)
      b. Gingivitis and periodontal disease—excessive sugar intake (supports growth of biofilm and nutritional deficiencies)
      c. Glossitis—nutritional deficiencies affecting the papillae and color of the tongue
      d. Stomatitis—nutritional deficiencies affecting oral soft tissues
      e. Cheilosis—nutritional deficiencies affecting the lips and the corners of the mouth
      f. Necrotizing ulcerative gingivitis (NUG)—excessive sugar and caffeine intake, smoking, stress, and poor oral hygiene combined with nutritional deficiencies result in lowered host resistance to bacterial plaque biofilm and bacterial challenges
   2. Anthropometric analysis—determines the body structure, form, and composition (e.g., content of lean body mass and fat tissue); the following tools are useful, but each has its limitations:
      a. BMI, IBW, and waist circumference (see the earlier section on "Energy Balances and Weight Control")
      b. Skinfold thickness measurements
         (1) Obtained by using skinfold calipers to measure subcutaneous fat in millimeters in selected areas (e.g., triceps and subscapular regions)
         (2) Measurements are compared with standards to estimate total body fat composition
      c. Arm muscle circumference
         (1) Sensitive indicator of the muscle mass that reflects protein stores
         (2) Determined by measuring the arm circumference at the midpoint of the upper arm and by measuring triceps skinfold

d. Bioelectrical impedance and ultrasound methods
    (1) Potential predictors of total body fat
    (2) Lean body mass conducts electricity better than fat mass
e. Underwater weighing
    (1) Measures body weight when the person is under water
    (2) One of the most accurate methods used to determine body volume
f. Dual-energy x-ray absorptiometry (DEXA)—can distinguish fat mass, fat-free mass, and bone mineral loss; most accurate method to determine body fat

## Methods for Assessment of Dietary Intake

A. Dietary intake standards
  1. DRI and RDA
    a. Published by the Panel on Micronutrients of the Food and Nutrition Board (FNB), Institute of Medicine, National Academy of Sciences; principally used as measurement tools by nutrition professionals who plan and evaluate food supplies for groups; to establish guidelines for new food products; used as the basis for regulatory standards in determining nutritional quality; and used to set standards for nutritional labeling (e.g., percentage of daily value)
    b. DRIs were established by the FNB at the Institute of Medicine of the National Academies; DRI values are used to plan and assess the nutrient intake of healthy people. They vary by age and gender.
      (1) Unlike RDA values, DRI values aim to prevent nutrient deficiency as well as reduce the likelihood of chronic disease
      (2) DRI includes five sets of standards:
        (a) RDA—intake level sufficient to meet nutrient requirements of almost all healthy individuals
        (b) AI—value based on approximation of nutrient intake by a group of healthy people, used when an RDA value cannot be determined
        (c) UL (upper limit)—highest level of daily nutrient intake that is likely to pose no risk of adverse health effects to almost all individuals in the general population; risk of adverse effects increases as intake increases above the UL
        (d) EAR (estimated average requirement)—nutrient intake value that is estimated to meet the requirements of half the healthy individuals in a group
        (e) EER (estimated energy requirement)—average calorie need estimates for various life stage groups and genders
      (3) A useful tool for calculation of DRI based on height, weight, gender, activity level can be found USDA Website's Food and Nutrition Center https://www.nal.usda.gov/fnic/dri-calculator/
  2. *Dietary Guidelines for Americans* are issued by the USDA and the US Department of Health and Human Services (HHS) and are revised every 5 years[5]
    a. The *Dietary Guidelines for Americans* evolves to address pressing public health concerns and the nutrition needs of specific populations
    b. Specific populations include children and adolescents, women capable of becoming pregnant, pregnant women, women who are breastfeeding, older adults, and adults at high risk of chronic disease
    c. Previously, the Dietary Guidelines have concentrated on Americans ages 2 years and older but future guidelines will also include guidance for infants and toddlers.
    d. Key recommendations of the current guidelines include the following[5]:
      (1) Follow a healthy eating pattern across the lifespan
      (2) Focus on variety, nutrient density, and amount of foods consumed
      (3) Limit added sugars to less than 10% of total daily calories
      (4) Limit sodium intake to 2300 mg/day for adults and children 14 years and older
      (5) Limit alcohol to no more than 1 drink daily for women and 2 drinks daily for men
      (6) Make healthier food and beverage choices
      (7) Support healthy eating patterns at home, in schools, at work, and in the community
  3. Dietary guidelines for oral health
    a. Eat a balanced diet representing moderation and variety as shown by MyPlate food guidance system, and follow the recommendations of the *Dietary Guidelines for Americans*[5]
    b. Combine and eat foods in sequence to enhance mastication, saliva production, and oral clearance; for example, combine dairy foods with sweet or starchy foods, or combine protein-rich foods with cooked or processed starches
    c. Plan eating intervals that allow time for the pH of the biofilm to return to neutral; for example, up to 120 minutes may be needed for the biofilm pH to return to neutral after exposure to a fermentable carbohydrate
    d. Take care not to replace other foods needed to maintain optimum health with sweets and soft drinks; obtain most calories from whole grains, fruits and vegetables, low-fat or nonfat dairy products, and lean meats or meat alternatives
    e. Drink water often; consume sweetened and acidic beverages *with* meals to allow for a buffering action, rather than consuming soft drinks *between* meals
    f. Limit the consumption of sugar-free beverages and sports drinks; demineralization of tooth structure can still occur as a result of the low pH of these beverages; consume these with meals
  4. The FNB's recommendations for healthy adult Americans
    a. Maintain a healthy weight by balancing energy intake and energy expenditure

TABLE 12.7 **Daily Guide to Food Choices**

| Dietary Component | Source of | DAILY RECOMMENDED SERVINGS | | |
|---|---|---|---|---|
| | | **1600 kcal** | **2200 kcal** | **2800 kcal** |
| Water | Fluids to maintain water balance and hydration | 64 oz | 64 oz | 64 oz |
| Grains* | Riboflavin, thiamin, niacin, iron, selenium, protein, fiber, magnesium | 5 oz* (2.5oz from whole grains) | 7 oz* (3.5 oz from whole grains) | 10 oz* (5 oz from whole grains) |
| Vegetables | Vitamins A and C, folate, potassium, magnesium, iron, fiber | 2 cups | 3 cups | 3.5 cups |
| Fruits | Vitamins A and C, folate, potassium, iron fiber | 1.5 cups | 2 cups | 2.5 cups |
| Dairy | Calcium, potassium, protein, riboflavin, niacin, vitamins A and D, B12, phosphorus | 3 cups | 3 cups | 3 cups |
| Protein Foods | Zinc, iron, vitamin $B_{12}$, vitamin $B_6$, niacin, thiamin, riboflavin, vitamin A, vitamin E, folate, magnesium, phosphorus, | 5 oz | 6 oz | 7 oz |
| Fats and oils | Mix of saturated and unsaturated fatty acids, energy | 5 teaspoon (tsp) | 6 tsp | 8 tsp |
| Added sugar | Energy | Women:6 tsp<br>Men: 9 tsp | Women: 6 tsp<br>Men: 9 tsp | Women: 6 tsp<br>Men: 9 tsp |
| Alcohol** | Not a good source of energy; converted into fatty acids | **Women: up to 1 drink/day.<br>**Men: 2 drinks/day | **Women: up to 1 drink/day<br>**Men: 2 drinks/day | **Women: up to 1 drink/day<br>**Men: 2 drinks/day |

*It is recommended that half of grains consumed are whole grains.
**If alcohol is consumed, USDGA recommends moderate consumption.
Courtesy of Connie Mobley, RD, PhD, University of Nevada Las Vegas, School of Dental Medicine, Las Vegas, Nevada.
Data from USDA Healthy US-Style Pattern—Recommended Intake Amounts, https://health.gov/our-work/food-nutrition/2015-2020-dietary-guidelines/guidelines/appendix-3/#table-a3-1-healthy-us-style-eating-pattern-recommended-amounts-o, Accessed August 19, 2020; and Johnson RK, Appel LJ, Brands M, et al: Dietary sugars intake and cardiovascular health: a scientific statement from the American Heart Association, *Circulation* 120:1011–1020, 2009. Appendix 9. Alcohol. U.S. Department of Health and Human Services and U.S. Department of Agriculture. *2015 – 2020 Dietary Guidelines for Americans*. 8th Edition. December 2015. Available from: https://health.gov/dietaryguidelines/2015/guidelines/appendix-9/ (Accessed April 13, 2019)

b. If the requirement for energy is low (e.g., weight-reducing diet), reduce the consumption of foods such as alcohol, sugars, fats, and oils that provide calories but few other essential nutrients
c. Use salt in moderation; recommended intake is no more than 2300 mg (1 teaspoon) per day; 1500 mg/day for those with hypertension
d. Select a nutritionally adequate diet from the foods available by each day consuming appropriate servings of low-fat dairy products, lean meats or legumes, vegetables, fruits, cereals, grains, and breads (Table 12.7)
e. Select as wide a variety of foods in each of the major food groups as practical to ensure a high probability of adequate quantities of all essential nutrients

5. The USDA MyPlate (see Fig. 12.3)
   a. Graphic design is similar to a pie chart; organizes foods into four colorful sections with a side portion for dairy
      (1) Red represents fruits; green is for vegetables; orange is for grains; purple is for protein (a separate blue section for dairy is on the side of the plate)
      (2) Encourages healthier eating habits and the consumption of a more plant-based diet
      (3) Promotes balanced proportions of each food group to be consumed at meals
         (a) Half of your plate should be fruits and vegetables
         (b) At least half of your grains should be whole grains
         (c) Make the switch to fat-free or low-fat milk
         (d) Balance calories
         (e) Avoid oversized portions
      (4) Recommends reduced intake of those foods high in sodium; read labels to compare
      (5) Supports the consumption of water over sugary drinks

B. Methods for collecting data on food intakes
   1. Nutritional Screening and Assessment of Dietary Intake Questionnaire (Fig. 12.4)
      a. Description—interviewer collects data from the patient about all food consumed in the previous 24-hour period; additional questions help determine frequency of sugar and food group intake
      b. Nutrition tools used to guide recommendations
         (1) USDA MyPlate
         (2) Dietary guidelines
         (3) DRI based on life stage
      c. Advantages
         (1) Can be filled out by the patient while waiting in the oral health care setting
         (2) Requires only 15 to 20 minutes to complete
         (3) Allows analysis of food group consumption
         (4) Allows evaluation of sugar intake
      d. Limitations
         (1) No nutrient analysis
         (2) Relies on the patient's memory
   2. The 24-hour dietary recall

**Nutritional Screening and Assessment of Dietary Intake Questionnaire**

Client's Name______________________________________ Gender: M F Age: _______

Height _____ Weight _____ # IBW _____ Occupation/Activity Level ____________________

FOR THE EDENTULOUS CLIENT, COMPLETE ONLY THOSE ITEMS WITH AN ASTERISK (*).

*_________ Complete Oral Health Evaluation CRA Score†: low moderate high very high

*Review client chart and Oral Health Evaluation Form for the following:

____ Does client have a chronic disease (diabetes, hypertension, etc.)?
____ Is client taking medication or a dietary supplement with nutritional implications?
____ Does client have periodontal disease or xerostomia?
____ Does client have a dietary screening score greater than 3?

*Obtain typical dietary intake information: (record 24-hour recall of dietary intake)
*Use nutritional tools as a guide to making recommendations (USDA MyPlate, Dietary Guidelines, DRIs/RDIs)

| **Determine if diet is caries promoting, using the following criteria:** | | **If YES, circle:** |
|---|---|---|
| a. | Do the total number of servings from the combined sugars and sweet beverages group exceed the number of servings from the grains group? | **4 points** |
| b. | Are food and beverage sources of sugars consumed alone? | **2 points** |
| c. | Are foods from the grains group consumed alone? Are foods from the grains group consumed in combination with foods that are sources of sugars? Are these combined foods eaten alone? | **2 points** |
| d. | Is diet lacking foods and/or adequate servings of foods from 1 or more food groups? Do number of servings for food groups exceed recommendations? | **2 points** |
| e. | Does the client have an unusual meal pattern?<br>–Eating snacks or drinking beverages in place of meals<br>–Spacing meals/snacks more than 6 hours apart<br>–Eating or drinking every 1–2 hours | **1 point** |
| f. | Does the client eat or drink late in the evening or immediately prior to bedtime? | **1 point** |
| g. | Does the client report chewing gum that is not sugar free? | **1 point** |
| | **Total Score (6=caries promoting diet)** | |

*Chart findings using SOAP format.

*Educate client, using appropriate nutrition education handouts and models. Refer client to other healthcare professionals, as appropriate.

**Fig. 12.4** Nutritional Screening and Assessment of Dietary Intake Questionnaire.The caries risk assessment (CRA) score is determined from an oral health evaluation tool that is used to determine the level of caries risk on an individual basis. (Modified from Connie Mobley, RD, PhD, University of Nevada Las Vegas, School of Dental Medicine, Las Vegas, Nevada.)

a. Description—interviewer collects data from the patient about all food consumed in the previous 24-hour period
b. Advantages
   (1) Requires 20 minutes or less for the interview
   (2) Allows nutrient analysis
   (3) Allows analysis of food group consumption
   (4) Allows evaluation of sugar intake
c. Limitations
   (1) Requires a trained interviewer
   (2) Relies on the patient's memory
   (3) Represents only 1 day of food consumption

(4) Requires a nutrient data file on foods to effectively analyze nutrients

3. A 3- to 7-day food record or diary
   a. Description—patient keeps a record of food and eating patterns for 3 to 7 days
   b. Advantages
      (1) No interviewer required except to give directions on how to fill out the record
      (2) Allows for analyses of both nutrients and food groups
      (3) Allows for evaluation of sugar intake
      (4) An average intake of several days may be more representative of patient's food intake than that of just 1 day
   c. Limitations
      (1) Represents the food consumption of only the days included in the record
      (2) Relies on the cooperation and ability of the patient to keep the record
      (3) Requires a nutrient data file for more comprehensive nutrient analysis

B. Methods for evaluating food intake
1. USDA MyPlate
   a. Nutrient contributions (see Table 12.7)
      (1) Role in general health
      (2) Role in oral health
   b. Advantages for use in counseling
      (1) Patient participation
      (2) Simple
      (3) Inexpensive
      (4) Fairly accurate
      (5) Detailed nutrient analysis
   c. Limitations
      (1) No provisions made for combination foods (e.g., pizza, casseroles); need to break down into ingredients that correspond to the six groups
      (2) Website can be difficult to navigate
2. Computerized analysis of diet
   a. Definition—food nutrient data are individually entered into a computer program, and the specific amounts of each nutrient for each food consumed are calculated
   b. Nutrient data file (software)—comprehensive analysis of foods and their nutrients; Nutritionist Pro analysis software and ESHA Research are examples of companies that provide software.[6,7] NutritionCalc Plus 5.0 and ESHATrak online nutrition and fitness app also by ESHA Research can be used by the novice learner. These data programs can be used to analyze and monitor personal diet and health goals or patient diet and health goals.[6,7] More detailed applications for these programs and advanced dietary counseling should be used and performed by a registered dietitian who is specifically trained in this area.
   c. DRI and RDA values—used as a standard for comparison with the patient's daily nutrient intake
   d. Advantages
      (1) Accurate
      (2) Specific
      (3) Cost-efficient when technology is available
         (a) Computers in oral health care settings with Internet access
         (b) Services available for a fee outside the oral health care setting
   e. Limitations
      (1) Limited patient participation and home use
      (2) Hardware and software availability
      (3) Expense
      (4) Requires training for accurate interpretation of output
3. Sugar analysis and evaluation
   a. Dental caries and periodontal disease are multifactorial infectious diseases that result from the interaction of the resistance of oral tissues (host factor) with the destructive effects of bacterial biofilm and acids (agent factor) produced from the metabolism of dietary sugars (diet or environment factor); dental disease occurs when all three factors exist simultaneously; often called the "triad" of dental disease; nutritional assessment of exposure to sugar is an essential part of nutritional counseling in disease prevention programs and can be conducted by using precise or simplified methods
      (1) Precise analysis—computer analysis of the diet for carbohydrate content: total carbohydrate in grams, monosaccharides and disaccharides in grams (e.g., grams of sucrose), and fiber in grams; percentage of the total daily calorie intake from simple and complex carbohydrates can be calculated and compared with the recommendations; added sugars should contain no more than 10% of total calories consumed; fiber needs range from 21 to 38 g, depending on age and gender[2]
      (2) Simplified analysis—dietary sugars (sweets and foods processed with sugars; see Table 12.3) are circled on the food record or recall; cariogenicity of the diet is assessed on the basis of frequency and form of sugar exposure; frequent exposure to retentive solid sugars, especially between meals, is harmful; acid production potential of the diet can be calculated by using the following formula:
   a. The formula is based on research that shows glucose-rich food products (either liquid or sugar) result in a decrease of oral pH below the critical level (pH 5.5, the point at which acids decalcify enamel) and that it takes 20 minutes after consumption of liquid sugars for healthy saliva to neutralize acids and raise the pH to a safe level; solid sugars adhere to teeth and have approximately double the potential for acid production.
   b. Caries activity tests—often involve counting the number of acidogenic bacteria or measuring the acids produced by these bacteria; provide information about the current oral environment and help to detect dental caries risk; are valuable adjuncts in biofilm control programs and can be used to monitor a patient's progress in oral home care and diet modifications

## Nutritional Counseling Techniques

A. Direct approach—counseling technique that focuses on the dietary problem
   1. Role of the patient—the patient provides information about his or her diet; is passive and listens to the counselor
   2. Role of the counselor—the counselor controls the session; analyzes and evaluates the patient's diet and makes recommendations for improvement
   3. Advantages—easier for the counselor and often requires less time than a more patient-oriented approach
   4. Limitations—fosters patient dependence; little chance of success if the patient is not committed to dietary changes; patient is not involved in decision making
B. Nondirect or behavior modification approach—counseling technique that focuses on the patient
   1. Role of the patient—the patient actively participates in the diet analysis, evaluation, and modification program
   2. Role of the counselor—the counselor provides information on the causes of dental disease, the role of the diet, and the use of dietary assessment tools
   3. Method
      a. Assumption—dietary habits are learned behaviors and can be "unlearned" and replaced with new behaviors
      b. Collection of baseline data
      c. Patient takes ownership of his or her dietary problems and is committed to change
      d. Patient determines his or her behavioral changes and goals; develops own reward system to use when goals are met
      e. Changes are gradually made in small steps; appropriate changes are rewarded and failures ignored
      f. Close monitoring of progress until new behaviors become self-reinforcing
   4. Advantages—fosters patient independence; success is more likely because the patient is in control of the change process
   5. Limitations—more time and effort needed to arrive at appropriate solutions to dietary problems and rewards for behavior modification
C. Factors that influence the patient's food intake—any combination of the following influences affects food choices and needs to be addressed in a modification program:
   1. Environmental influences—economics, lifestyle, geography, seasons, markets
   2. Social influences—family, culture, religion, social pressures, marketing strategies
   3. Psychological influences—self-image, emotions, stresses, values, priorities
D. Determinants for dental patient selection
   1. High-risk patients—those with conditions that would benefit most from nutritional counseling
      a. Pregnancy—nutrient needs are high; hormonal changes may lead to exaggerated responses to biofilm and bacterial toxins; maternal diet affects the formation of fetal oral tissues
      b. Adolescence—nutrient needs are high; vulnerable to nutritional problems from "fad" diets for weight loss and muscle building; frequent snacking on empty-calorie foods; problems of anorexia and bulimia can lead to enamel erosion, irritation of oral mucosa, and infected or enlarged salivary glands, with possible xerostomia
      c. Rampant caries—high bacterial biofilm and calculus and a positive caries activity test may indicate a problem of frequent exposure to sugar
      d. Periodontal disease or NUG—frequent exposure to sugar and nutritional deficiencies can contribute to the development and progression of these conditions
      e. Oral and maxillofacial surgery—nutritional counseling before and after surgery is important for optimal surgical recovery; postsurgical nutrient needs are high because of blood loss, tissue repair, and host defense activities; modifications in food texture (e.g., soft foods) are made according to the patient's ability to masticate
      f. Edentulism—inability to masticate can result in nutrient deficiencies because of the limited nutrient content in soft and liquid foods
         (1) Food choices are altered because of difficulties with chewing or fear of choking; reduced intake of meats, fresh fruits, and vegetables; softer foods are usually eaten
         (2) Lowered intake of magnesium, folic acid, fluoride, zinc, and calcium
      g. Oral cancer—nutrient needs are high because of host defense activities and tissue repair from cancer and its treatment; cancer or treatment may result in inadequate food intake because of decreased appetite, altered taste perceptions, irritated oral tissues, and xerostomia
   2. Dental office resources—availability of trained personnel, time, and facilities to conduct nutrition counseling services
   3. Patient factors—level of patient motivation to use and benefit from nutritional counseling and financial and intellectual capabilities for using nutritional counseling services

## Dietary Modifications for Specific Dental Conditions

A. Dental caries (see Tables 12.4 and 12.5)
   1. Role of nutrients in tooth formation
      a. Preeruptive effects—nutrients are used systemically for enamel, dentin, and pulp formation; tooth bud formation begins at 6 weeks in utero, and calcification is completed at 13 years
      b. Posteruptive effects—fluoride aids in the remineralization of small enamel lesions; evidence indicates that specific minerals or combinations of minerals and fats have local cariostatic properties
   2. Local effect of dietary carbohydrates on bacteria growth and biofilm formation

3. Role of diet and nutrients in salivary gland function
    a. Nutrients are used systemically for the normal development and secretory function of salivary glands
    b. Foods of firm texture (e.g., raw vegetables) enhance mastication, stimulate the salivary flow rate, and modify the concentration of constituents in saliva, possibly improving antibacterial properties and the buffering capacity to neutralize decalcifying acids

B. Periodontal disease (see Table 12.5)
1. Role of nutrients in the formation of periodontal tissues
    a. Nutrients are used systemically for the normal development of the gingiva, periodontal ligament, cementum, and alveolus
    b. Periodontal tissues are metabolically active throughout a person's life, and nutrients are constantly needed for maintenance (e.g., the cell population of the sulcal epithelium completely renews itself within 3 to 6 days)
2. Local effect of dietary carbohydrates on bacteria growth and biofilm formation
3. Role of nutrients in the host defense system
    a. During the initial stages of periodontitis, the nutritional status of the patient is important in cellular immunocompetence for combating bacterial insults to the periodontium
    b. After periodontal surgery, cellular immunocompetence is important for optimal healing and prevention of infection

C. Oral and maxillofacial surgery
1. Presurgical nutritional counseling
    a. Adequate nutrient intake is needed to build up nutrient reserves in tissues to cope with postsurgical nutrient demands and complications
    b. Counseling is helpful for advising the patient to plan and purchase appropriate foods before surgery in anticipation of convalescence
    c. Need for referral to registered dietitian prior to surgery should be evaluated
2. Postsurgical nutritional counseling
    a. Nutrient requirements are high because of blood loss, increased catabolism, tissue repair, and host defense activities
    b. Dietary intake is influenced by surgical complications of anorexia, dysphagia, and oral discomfort; a liquid diet should be used initially for the first few days, followed by a soft diet until the patient can eat normally; during convalescence, high-protein liquid products fortified with vitamins and minerals (e.g., Ensure, Sustacal, Instant Breakfast) are helpful but contain cariogenic sweeteners; safe levels of vitamin and mineral supplements (100% to 200% of DRI or RDA values) may be recommended

D. Prosthodontics
1. Nutritional counseling in the preparation of the mouth for a prosthesis
    a. Nutrients—systemically important for the health of oral soft tissues and the alveolar ridge
        (1) Surgery—if surgery is necessary, nutrient requirements will be higher for postsurgical healing
        (2) Tissue state—if any inflamed or soft tissue injuries and bone resorption conditions exist, nutrient requirements will be higher for repair and host defense activities
    b. Dietary sugars—condition of the remaining dentition is important for maintaining the use of a new prosthesis; cariogenic sugars need to be restricted to control bacterial growth, acid production, and bacterial biofilm formation
    c. Texture of foods—partial or fully edentulous patients will often need to eat chopped, soft foods; if nutrient intake is compromised, fortified liquid products or nutrient supplements are helpful
2. Nutritional counseling after prosthesis insertion
    a. Food texture—liquid foods for the first 24 hours, followed by soft foods and chopped or cut-up foods; this minimizes biting and chewing and allows time for the muscles and tongue to adjust to the new prosthesis
    b. Counter-dislodgement forces—for every bite of food, food should be evenly divided in the right and left sides of the mouth before chewing to equalize occlusal forces
    c. Nutrients—AI for the integrity of the oral mucosa and alveolar ridge
    d. Dietary sugars—should be restricted to prevent bacterial growth, acid production, and bacterial biofilm formation on the remaining dentition and prosthesis
    e. Food flavors—initially, flavors of foods will be altered because of the new prosthesis, but this side effect will eventually disappear with continued denture use

E. Orthodontics
1. Role of nutrients—systemically important for the integrity of periodontal tissues; requirements are higher as stresses of tooth movement result in more bone apposition and the synthesis of a new periodontal ligament; nutrients are needed for the healing and repair of gingival injuries and irritations from orthodontic bands
2. Role of sugars—to prevent enamel erosion and decay, dietary sugars (especially retentive sweets) must be restricted during the wearing of appliances
3. Role of food textures—when appliances or bands are tightened, chewing hard-textured foods may be painful, and liquid and soft foods should be eaten temporarily; retentive and sticky foods should be avoided because they become trapped in the appliance and are difficult to remove

## Dietary Considerations for Immunocompromised Patients and Those With Special Needs

A. Oral cancer
1. Nutritional support for healing and cellular immunocompetence
    a. Compromised nutritional status—weight loss and nutrient deficiencies increase the risk of not withstanding the physiologic stresses of cancer and anticancer therapies

b. Surgical treatment—primary method in treating cancer; nutrient requirements are higher as a result of the increased catabolic activities, tissue repair, and host defense activities
c. Chemotherapy and radiation treatment—nutrient needs are higher because of the destruction of healthy cells and tissues that occurs during these types of treatments
d. Possible need for referral to registered dietitian to monitor patient's dietary intake during the compromised state
2. Diet modifications useful in treating complications from cancer or cancer treatments
a. Patient unable to ingest or digest food
(1) Home enteral feedings can provide nutrients (e.g., nasogastric tube feedings)
(2) Home parenteral feedings can provide nutrients (e.g., intravenous feedings)
b. Eating problems arising from complications or side effects of anticancer therapies
(1) Nausea and vomiting—patient should suck on ice chips; eat frequently; eat dry, bland foods; eat and drink slowly; avoid highly spiced and fatty foods; new antinausea medications are effective
(2) Loss of appetite—patient should eat foods that are appealing; make up nutrient requirements at times when the appetite is good; eat foods with a high nutrient density
(3) Food aversions and alterations in taste and smell—patient should eliminate offending foods; include highly spiced and distinctive textures to improve taste perceptions; cook and serve food with plastic utensils rather than metal utensils
(4) Dry mouth (xerostomia)—patient should use xylitol-containing gum, mints, and sprays; suck on ice chips or use synthetic saliva; drink liquids with meals; eat cold-temperature foods rather than hot-temperature foods; concentrate on highly nutritious liquids
(5) Radiation-induced caries—patient should restrict cariogenic foods; because of changes in both the quality and the quantity of saliva after cancer treatment, rapid demineralization of the tooth surface can occur
(6) Glossitis and stomatitis—patient should eat a variety of soft, easy-to-chew foods; eat stewed foods rather than broiled and fried foods; avoid highly spiced or acidic foods; eat moderate-temperature foods; use straws if swallowing is difficult

B. Human immunodeficiency virus (HIV)
1. Causes of malnutrition in HIV-infected persons
a. Reduced food intake
(1) Drug treatments cause vomiting, nausea, and food aversions
(2) Fatigue, depression, and fear cause anorexia
(3) Oral infections alter taste, cause pain, and reduce saliva flow
(4) Esophageal infections and respiratory complications hamper swallowing
b. Increased nutrient loss
(1) Cancers of the GI tract cause malabsorption
(2) Drugs cause diarrhea and malabsorption
(3) PEM leads to malabsorption
c. Altered metabolism
(1) Cancer, infections, and fevers increase BMR
(2) Drug therapy alters nutrient utilization
2. Nutrient support
a. Any subclinical nutrient deficiencies and weight loss should be corrected at the time of a positive HIV test
b. At least 100% of the DRI or RDA values of all vitamins and minerals must be provided
c. Patient must avoid all foodborne illnesses
d. The nutrition plan should be designed on the basis of individual complications, with emphasis on controlling weight loss by eating nutrient-dense foods throughout the day
e. Dietary recommendations should be regulated only by a medical physician (MD) or a registered dietitian (RD), or both

C. Patients with special needs (see Chapter 19)
1. Dental problems—unmet oral health care needs in this population significantly exceed those in the general population
a. The oral caries rate may be higher than that of the general population because of poor oral hygiene and cariogenic food habits
b. Increased periodontal disease compared with the general population because of:
(1) Poor oral hygiene; limited self-care
(2) Diets consisting of soft-textured foods
(3) Frequent exposures to fermentable carbohydrates
(4) Metabolic disturbances affecting disease resistance and the reparative process
(5) Nutritional deficiencies associated with diet or metabolic disturbance
(6) Malocclusion and developmental defects
c. Barriers to health care
2. Nutritional problems—slow growth, excessive weight loss or gain, and nutrient deficiencies can occur in the following situations:
a. Inability to consume an adequate diet
(1) Absence or weak sucking response (e.g., cleft lip and palate)
(2) Poor control of arm and head (e.g., cerebral palsy)
(3) Inadequate control of jaw, lip, and tongue (e.g., tongue thrust and tonic bite)
(4) Attention deficit (e.g., intellectual disability and hyperactivity)
b. Impaired nutrient use
(1) Malabsorption conditions (e.g., cystic fibrosis)
(2) Inborn errors of metabolism (e.g., phenylketonuria)
(3) Drug-nutrient interactions (e.g., anticonvulsant medications can interfere with calcium and phosphorus use)
(4) Poor muscle control (e.g., constipation)

c. Excessive intake of foods, calories, and sweets
   (1) Food, especially sweets, often used to reinforce good behavior
   (2) Overfeeding because of parental guilt
   (3) Overemphasis on feeding because mealtime is perceived as the most important time for parent-child interaction
   (4) Excessive calorie intake resulting from inactivity and the pleasurable aspects of eating

## WEBSITE INFORMATION AND RESOURCES

| Source | Website Address | Description |
|---|---|---|
| Food and Nutrition Center: US Department of Agriculture National Agricultural Library | https://www.nal.usda.gov/fnic | Resource for *Dietary Guidelines for Americans,* and *DRI Calculator* that determines daily nutrient needs by age and gender. |
| *Healthy People 2030* | http://www.healthypeople.gov | Information on development of *Healthy People 2030.* Oral health objectives provide a valuable resource for community-based activities. |
| American Dental Association | http://www.mouthhealthy.org/en/nutrition | Provides a nutrition link for food tips, nutrition concerns, and nutrition during pregnancy |
| Choose My Plate | http://www.choosemyplate.gov | Provides guidance on balance, moderation, and adequate consumption of essential food groups; interactive resource for individual groups. Provides specific dietary requirement based on age, gender, and level of physical activity. |
| National Information of Health, Office of Dietary Supplements | https://ods.od.nih.gov/Health_Information/Dietary_Reference_Intakes.aspx | Information available on dietary reference intakes of macronutrients and micronutrients. |

## CHAPTER 12 REVIEW QUESTIONS

Answers and rationales to the review questions are available on this text's accompanying Evolve site. See inside front cover for details.

1. All the following are disaccharides EXCEPT one. Which one is the EXCEPTION?
   a. Glucose
   b. Sucrose
   c. Lactose
   d. Maltose
2. Oligosaccharides are composed of how many monosaccharide units?
   a. More than six identical monosaccharide units
   b. Two to six monosaccharide units
   c. Two monosaccharide units
   d. One monosaccharide unit
3. In the mouth, salivary amylase initiates the enzymatic hydrolysis of starch. Salivary amylase also activates pepsin and denatures proteins in the mouth.
   a. Both statements are TRUE
   b. Both statements are FALSE
   c. The first statement is TRUE; the second statement is FALSE
   d. The first statement is FALSE; the second statement is TRUE
4. Which of the following emulsifies fat during the digestive process?
   a. Pancreatic enzymes
   b. Bile salts
   c. Brush-border enzymes
   d. Salivary enzymes
5. All the following are monosaccharides EXCEPT one. Which one is the EXCEPTION?
   a. Galactose
   b. Sucrose
   c. Glucose
   d. Fructose
6. Quantity of sucrose or carbohydrate eaten is less cariogenic than the frequency consumed. Sucrose eaten with a meal is less cariogenic than when consumed in between meals.
   a. The first statement is TRUE; the second statement is FALSE
   b. The first statement is FALSE; the second statement is TRUE
   c. Both statements are TRUE
   d. Both statements are FALSE
7. One of the end products of glycolysis is
   a. Carbon dioxide
   b. Adenosine triphosphate
   c. Lactic acid
   d. Water
8. What is the process called in which glycogen is the short-term storage form of glucose in the liver and muscle?
   a. Glycogenolysis
   b. Gluconeogenesis
   c. Glycogenesis
   d. Glyconeogenesis

9. Anabolic hormones raise the blood glucose levels. Catabolic hormones lower the blood glucose level.
   a. Both statements are TRUE
   b. Both statements are FALSE
   c. The first statement is TRUE; the second statement is FALSE
   d. The first statement is FALSE; the second statement is TRUE
10. Anabolic hormones are metabolic regulators of all the following EXCEPT one. Which one is the EXCEPTION?
   a. Lower blood glucose level
   b. Stimulate gluconeogenesis
   c. Increase glycogenesis
   d. Increase lipogenesis
11. Which of the following is an example of a soluble fiber?
   a. Oat bran
   b. Cellulose
   c. Hemicellulose
   d. Lignin
12. All the following are biologic roles of carbohydrates EXCEPT one. Which one is the EXCEPTION?
   a. Provides an energy source of 4 kcal/g
   b. Protein sparing
   c. Structural component of cell membrane
   d. Precursors of structural and functional molecules
13. The congenital absence of lactase enzyme is considered a primary lactose intolerance. Temporary or permanent loss of lactase enzyme activity as a result of injury or illness is considered a secondary lactose intolerance.
   a. Both statements are TRUE
   b. Both statements are FALSE
   c. The first statement is TRUE; the second statement is FALSE
   d. The first statement is FALSE; the second statement is TRUE
14. Which of the following nonnutritive sweeteners should be avoided by patients who have phenylketonuria?
   a. Saccharin
   b. Acesulfame-K
   c. Sucralose
   d. Aspartame

## CASE A

Cecilia recently reported to the dentist for her 6-month recall appointment. During the dental exam, four new areas of interproximal decay were noted. The hygienist questioned Cecilia about changes in her oral hygiene or dietary patterns. Cecilia told the hygienist that she was a full-time student at the local community college. She also commented that she had taken a part-time job to help her parents with college expenses. Due to her busy academic and work schedule, she doesn't have time to eat regular meals so she packs snacks such as baked chips, pretzels, and trail mix to eat during the day. She also consumes energy drinks frequently throughout the day to keep her going.

***Use Case A to answer questions 15 to 17.***

15. Which of the following dietary factors could contribute to Cecilia's new areas of decay?
   a. Frequency of intake
   b. Form and consistency
   c. Timing
   d. A and C only
   e. A, B, and C
16. What dietary advice would be helpful for Cecilia in regard to the consumption of her energy drinks?
   a. Encourage her to switch to caffeinated soft drinks for energy
   b. Encourage her to sip on the energy drink rather than consuming a large amount at once
   c. Encourage her to pair with a starchy food to decrease risk of demineralization
   d. Encourage her to consume the energy drink all at once within 30 minutes
   e. Encourage her to avoid energy drinks and consume carbonated water
17. All of the following are factors that may influence Cecilia's food choices and may need to be addressed during nutrition counseling by the dental hygienist EXCEPT one. Which is the EXCEPTION?
   a. Environmental influences
   b. Social influences
   c. Physiological influences
   d. Psychological influences

## CASE B

Mr. Farmer is a single, semiretired 76-year-old Caucasian male with carious lesions on tooth #s 8-M, #9-M, #3-MO, and #19-D. He has moderate supragingival calculus and slight to moderate subgingival calculus. He has generalized bleeding with more than 20 periodontal pocket sites that measure 4 mm. He has a 5 mm periodontal pocket on four distal surfaces of posterior teeth. He is currently taking clonazepam and Vitamin D. He says his mouth feels dry so he frequently keeps cinnamon hard candies in his mouth to stimulate his saliva. Throughout the day, he sips on Dr. Pepper or coffee containing 2 T sugar and Almond Joy creamer to keep his mouth moist. Mr. Farmer lives alone and his cooking skills are minimal. He snacks frequently throughout the day on granola bars, pretzels, and trail mix with raisins, nuts, and banana chips. Breakfast usually consists of a cinnamon raisin bagel, instant brown sugar oatmeal, or a store-bought muffin. Lunch is typically a sandwich of some sort with a bowl of soup. When arriving home at the end of his workday, he drinks one glass of red wine to unwind from his long commute home in traffic. He admits he often skips the evening meal because he doesn't have the energy or desire to cook. If he does eat dinner, he eats a microwavable frozen dinner. To take the edge off his hunger before he goes to bed, Mr. Farmer often snacks on peanut butter crackers or his personal favorite—a bowl of chunky monkey chocolate banana ice cream.

***Use Case B to answer questions 18 to 20.***

18. The forms of foods that Mr. Farmer consumes does not put him at increased risk for dental caries; however the frequency and timing of his snacks and beverages are risk factors.
   a. Both statements are TRUE
   b. Both statements are FALSE
   c. The first statement is TRUE; the second statement is FALSE
   d. The first statement is FALSE; the second statement is TRUE

19. Which of the following dietary factors put Mr. Farmer at the greatest risk for caries?
   a. Banana chips
   b. Cinnamon candy
   c. Cinnamon raisin bagel
   d. Peanut butter crackers
   e. Chocolate banana ice cream
20. Which of the following methods would be the best choice to further assess and provide a more accurate account of Mr. Farmer's dietary intake?
   a. 24 hour dietary recall
   b. 3-to 7-day food record or diary
   c. Dietary Intake Questionnaire
   d. 24 hour dietary recall combined with 3- to 7-day food record.
   e. 24 hour dietary recall and Dietary Intake Questionnaire
21. What is the recommended daily allowance (RDA) for digestible carbohydrate for adults and children?
   a. 50 g
   b. 65 g
   c. 100 g
   d. 130 g
22. All the following are TRUE about patients with type 2 diabetes EXCEPT one. Which one is the EXCEPTION?
   a. A specialized diet is recommended to maintain blood glucose control
   b. Daily injections of insulin are needed
   c. Routine blood testing to monitor blood sugar levels is recommended
   d. Medication is often prescribed to facilitate glucose metabolism
23. All the following signs and symptoms of diabetes mellitus EXCEPT one. Which one is the EXCEPTION?
   a. Recurring gingival infections
   b. Excessive thirst
   c. Poor appetite
   d. Frequent urination
24. Alcoholism can cause B-vitamin depletion. It can also depress antidiuretic hormone, resulting in a loss of magnesium, potassium, and zinc in urine.
   a. Both statements are TRUE
   b. Both statements are FALSE
   c. The first statement is TRUE; the second statement is FALSE
   d. The first statement is FALSE; the second statement is TRUE
25. Essential amino acids can be synthesized by the body and do not need to be provided by the diet. Nonessential amino acids are found in food of animal origin.
   a. Both statements are TRUE
   b. Both statements are FALSE
   c. The first statement is TRUE; the second statement is FALSE
   d. The first statement is FALSE; the second statement is TRUE
26. Although an ovolactovegetarian diet can provide essential amino acids that are inadequate in incomplete plant proteins, which of the following nutrients might an ovolactovegetarian be deficient?
   a. Iron
   b. Vitamin $B_{12}$
   c. Calcium
   d. Zinc
27. The linear sequence of the components of amino acids is referred to as which type of structure?
   a. Primary
   b. Secondary
   c. Tertiary
   d. Quaternary
28. Absorption of proteins occurs at the brush border of the microvilli of the small intestine. Absorption occurs only by active transport at specific amino acid sites.
   a. Both statements are TRUE
   b. Both statements are FALSE
   c. The first statement is TRUE; the second statement is FALSE
   d. The first statement is FALSE; the second statement is TRUE
29. All the following are used for de novo synthesis of proteins EXCEPT one. Which one is the EXEPTION?
   a. Deoxyribonucleic acid
   b. Alpha keto acid
   c. Messenger ribonucleic acid
   d. Ribosomal ribonucleic acid
30. Positive nitrogen balance is the normal situation for building protein-containing tissue. Negative nitrogen balance indicates net protein breakdown.
   a. Both statements are TRUE
   b. Both statements are FALSE
   c. The first statement is TRUE; the second statement is FALSE
   d. The first statement is FALSE; the second statement is TRUE
31. All the following are examples of anabolic hormones EXCEPT one. Which one is the EXCEPTION?
   a. Growth hormone
   b. Adrenocortical hormones
   c. Insulin
   d. Thyroid hormone
32. The cariogenic potential of foods:
   a. Can be affected by the amount of sugar in food
   b. Is related to the retentive quality of the food
   c. Is related to the time foods are beverages are in the mouth
   d. All the above
   e. Both b and c
33. Which of the following anthropometric measures is sensitive indicator of muscle mass reflective of protein stores?
   a. Bioelectrical impedance
   b. Arm muscle circumference
   c. Skinfold thickness measurement
   d. Dual energy x-ray absorptiometry (DEXA)
34. Nutrients needs are often lower for patients undergoing treatment for oral cancer; diet modifications are often

necessary due to complications from cancer or cancer treatments.
a. Both statements are TRUE
b. Both statements are FALSE
c. The first statement is TRUE; the second statement is FALSE
d. The first statement is FALSE; the second statement is TRUE

35. Which of the following eating disorders is most often found in middle income and upper income adolescent females?
a. Obesity
b. Anorexia
c. Bulimia
d. Other Specified Eating or Feeding Disorder

36. Which of the following can occur as a result of nutritional deficiencies that affect the papilla and/or tongue?
a. Stomatitis
b. Cheilosis
c. Glossitis
d. Necrotizing ulcerative gingivitis

37. All the following are TRUE about water-soluble vitamins EXCEPT one. Which one is the EXCEPTION?
a. They are sensitive to heat, light, and oxygen
b. They are absorbed into the blood by both active and passive transport
c. Deficiency symptoms are slow to develop
d. They are transported free and unbound

38. Vitamins are inorganic substrates that are essential to life. Minerals are organic substrates that are essential to life.
a. Both statements are TRUE
b. Both statements are FALSE
c. The first statement is TRUE; the second statement is FALSE
d. The first statement is FALSE; the second statement is TRUE

39. Which of the following have cariostatic properties, providing a coating on the tooth's surface and forming a protective pellicle on the tooth?
a. Proteins
b. Carbohydrates
c. Lipids (fats)
d. Vitamins

40. All the following are examples of fat-soluble vitamins EXCEPT one. Which one is the EXCEPTION?
a. Vitamin A
b. Vitamin C
c. Vitamin D
d. Vitamin K

41. The energy required to digest, absorb, and metabolize food is known as which of the following?
a. Basal metabolic rate
b. Kilocalories
c. Thermic effect of food
d. Adenosine triphosphate

42. What is a more accurate method of determining central or abdominal obesity?
a. Body mass index
b. Ideal body weight
c. Waist circumference
d. Weighing on a scale

43. Which of the following statements is TRUE regarding the diet of individuals who are edentulous or who have limited mastication due to loss of teeth?
a. There is a reduced intake of dairy products
b. There is a reduced intake of grain products
c. There is reduced intake of meats
d. More fruits and vegetables are consumed

44. All the following are important posteruptive effects of carbohydrate on the teeth EXCEPT one. Which one is the EXCEPTION?
a. *Streptococcus mutans* synthesizes polysaccharides from sucrose, which enhances bacterial biofilm formation
b. Carbohydrates provide an energy source for oral bacteria
c. Lactic acid, pyruvic acid, or acetyl–coenzyme A are the end products of glycolysis for acidogenic bacteria
d. Carbohydrates contribute to enamel remineralization

45. Increased caries rate is attributed to a deficiency of vitamin D. Pulp calcification can occur if there is an excess of vitamin D.
a. The first statement is TRUE; the second statement is FALSE
b. The first statement is FALSE; the second statement is TRUE
c. Both statements are TRUE
d. Both statements are FALSE

## CASE C

Margaret is a 56-year-old patient who presents to the dental clinic for her 4-month recare appointment. As a divorced mother, she has been struggling to support her three children in college. She is currently self-employed and cleans homes and babysits for a living. Her chief complaint is sensitivity to hot and cold when eating. She also complains of dry mouth and states she sips on citrus-flavored water throughout the day.

Margaret's medical history reveals she is currently being treated by a physician for type 2 diabetes, hyperlipidemia, hypertension, and gastroesophageal reflux disease (GERD). Her medications include 1000 mg of metformin, 15 mg of atorvastatin, 30 mg of atenolol, 20 mg of Prilosec, 81-mg aspirin tablet, 600 mg of calcium twice daily, and a multivitamin. Her height is 5 feet, 2 inches, and she weighs 150 pounds. Her BMI is 27.43 and her waist circumference is 37. She reports brushing her teeth morning and night, and she tries to floss but is not very compliant. Her biofilm score is 43%. She has several "watches" that were noted on previous dental charting. New bitewing radiographs were taken at this appointment. Secondary decay was identified on the distal of tooth #19 and mesial of tooth #30. Her periodontal assessment reveals isolated probing depths of 4 to 5 mm on the maxillary and mandibular posterior teeth.

The dental hygienist questions Margaret about her diet. She reports she eats small meals throughout the day and states that she "would rather snack than eat full meals." She is also lactose intolerant, so she avoids dairy products. She likes fruits and vegetables but thinks it is time-intensive to have to prepare them, so she has developed a new habit of juicing fruits and vegetables and having a morning "smoothie" with fresh fruit and kale or spinach. Margaret states she also consumes energy drinks each day because she believes they give her "an extra boost" to get through her day. Additionally, she likes to snack on Baked Cheetos and Wheat Thins throughout the day.

***Use Case C to answer questions 46 to 50.***

46. The secondary decay is most likely caused by all the following EXCEPT:
    a. GERD
    b. Lactose intolerance
    c. Energy drink consumption
    d. Flavored-water consumption
    e. Juicing with fresh fruits and vegetables
47. Based on her calculated body mass index (BMI) of 27.43, Margaret would be classified in which of the following categories?
    a. Obesity
    b. Overweight
    c. Underweight
    d. Normal weight
    e. Extreme obesity
48. The direct-approach counseling technique would be best used to address Margaret's dietary concerns in relation to her oral disease risk. The counselor (dental hygienist) should provide information on the causes of the dental disease, the role of the diet, and the use of dietary assessment tools, with the patient (Margaret) as an active participant.
    a. Both statements are TRUE
    b. Both statements are FALSE
    c. The first statement is TRUE; the second statement is FALSE
    d. The first statement is FALSE; the second statement is TRUE
49. During nutrition counseling with Margaret, it is important for the dental hygienist to:
    a. Assess patient knowledge of information provided
    b. Tell the patient which diet to follow
    c. Include the patient in the diet planning
    d. All the above
    e. Both a and c
50. Margaret has a 43% biofilm score. Supragingival biofilm formation is influenced by frequent intake of which of the following in the diet?
    a. Dietary monosaccharides and disaccharides
    b. Fiber-rich foods
    c. Protein-rich foods
    d. Fat-rich foods

## REFERENCES


1. Johnson RD, Lawrence LJ, Brands M, et al. Dietary sugars intake and cardiovascular health scientific statement from the American Heart Association. *Circulation*. 2009;120:1011–1020.
2. Institute of Medicine (IOM). *National Academy of Sciences, Food and Nutrition Board: Dietary Reference Intakes for Energy, Carbohydrates, Fiber, Fat, Fatty Acids, Cholesterol, Protein, and Amino Acids*. Washington, DC: The National Academy Press; 2010. http://www.nap.edu/openbook.php?record_id=10490. Accessed April 11, 2019.
3. Varela-Lopez A, Giampieri F, Bullon P, et al. Role of lips in the onset, progression and treatment of periodontal disease. A systematic review of studies in humans. *Int J Mol Sci*. 2016;17(8):1202. https://doi.org/10.3390/ijms17081202.
4. Hales CM, Carroll MD, Fryar CD, Ogden CL. *Prevalence of Obesity Among Adults and Youth: United States, 2015–2016. NCHS Data Brief, No 288*. Hyattsville, MD: National Center for Health Statistics; 2017. https://www.cdc.gov/nchs/data/databriefs/db288.pdf. Accessed April 11, 2019.
5. US Department of Health and Human Services and US Department of Agriculture. *2015 – 2020 Dietary Guidelines for Americans*. 8th ed. ; December 2015. Available at: https://health.gov/dietaryguidelines/2015/guidelines/.
6. Axxya Systems: Nutritionist Pro Diet Analysis Software, 16932 Woodinville Redmond Rd NE, Suite A201, Woodeinville, WA 98072. https://www.nutritionistpro.com/. Accessed April 10 2019.
7. ESHA Research. Nutrition software, Databases and Consulting services. 4747 Skyline R. S, suite 100, Salem, OR 97306. http://www.esha.com. Accessed April 11, 2019.


## SUGGESTED READINGS


Harper Mallonee L, Boyd L, Stegeman C. Practice paper of the Academy of nutrition and Dietetics (AND). Oral health and nutrition. *J Acad Nutr Diet*. 2014;114:958. Full article available for purchase to the public at http://www.sciencedirect.com/science/article/pii/S2212267214003670. Accessed April 8, 2019.

Lamster IB. Preface. Primary health care in the dental office. *Dent Clin North Am*. 2012;56(4):ix–xi.

Mallonee LF. Diet and Dietary Analysis. In: Boyd LD, Mallonee LF, Wyche CJ. Wilkins' Clinical Practice of the Dental Hygienist. 13th ed. Burlington, MA: Jones&Bartlett Learning; 2021.

Palmer CA, Boyd LD. *Diet and Nutrition in Oral Health*. 3rd ed. Upper Saddle River, NJ: Pearson; 2017.

Stegeman CA, Davis JR. *The Dental Hygienist's Guide to Nutritional Care*. 5th ed. St. Louis, MO: Elsevier Saunders; 2019.

Touger Decker R, Mobley C. Position Paper of the Academy of Nutrition and Dietetics (AND). Oral health and nutrition. *J Acad Nutr Diet*. 2013;113(5):693–701.

Touger -Decker R, Mobley C, Epstein JB. *Nutrition and Oral Medicine*. 2nd ed. Morristown, NJ: Springer; 2014.

13

# Biomaterials

*John M. Powers, Stephen C. Bayne*

Biomaterials, restorative materials, and tissue engineering are fundamental to dental hygiene practice and are used in a variety of dental hygiene roles. This chapter provides an overview of general applications, terminology, and classification for specific biomaterials, including preventive and restorative materials. Structure and the properties of materials, including physical, chemical, mechanical, and biologic characteristics, are also reviewed.

Direct applications of materials include dental amalgams; dental composites; pit-and-fissure sealants; infiltrants and silver diamine fluoride analogs for lesions; bonding agents; cement liners and bases and luting cements; fluoride-releasing restorative materials, topical fluorides and fluoride varnishes; dentifrices and prophylactic pastes; and bleaching agents. Indirect applications include impression materials, provisional materials, models, casts, dies, waxes, investment materials, casting alloys, dental solders, chromium alloys for partial dentures, porcelain-fused-to-metal (PFM) alloys, dental ceramics, crown-and-bridge cements, acrylic appliances, acrylic denture bases, denture teeth, denture liners, denture cleansers, mouth protectors, veneers, digital scanning, computer-assisted design and computer-assisted machining (CAD/CAM), three-dimensional (3-D) printing, and dental implants. Indirect applications continue to move toward digital workflow in which all fabrication operations use computer operations to replace all traditional fabrication stages. Originally, these depended on subtractive processes (e.g., CAD/CAM machining from blocks of ceramic or composite), but many newer applications (e.g., stereolithography, inkjet printing, selective layer sintering) are additive processes.

## INTRODUCTION

### General Considerations

A. Applications for dental biomaterials
  1. Direct preventive and restorative dental procedures
  2. Indirect preventive and restorative dental procedures
B. Definitions and terminology
  1. Materials science terminology
  2. Biomaterials terminology for classification
C. Classification of materials for applications by:
  1. Key parts of composition-influencing properties
  2. Extent of cavity preparation

### Structure

A. Composition
  1. Generally, two components in a specific ratio
    a. Powder and liquid (P/L)
    b. Powder and powder (P/P)
    c. Water and powder (W/P)
    d. Paste and paste (p/p)
    e. Paste and light
  2. Generally, the liquid part is the major reactant
B. Reaction during use
  1. Physical reaction—solidification by drying or cooling with no chemical reaction
  2. Chemical reaction—solidification by creating new primary bonds within the composition
C. Manipulation
  1. Proportioning variables
    a. Ratio of parts
    b. Temperature
    c. Relative humidity
  2. Mixing variables
    a. Manual mixing
      (1) Method of combining components (e.g., stirring and stropping)
      (2) Rate of mixing (e.g., fast and slow)
    b. Auto-mixing and machine mixing
  3. Stages of manipulation
    a. Definitions of times
      (1) Mixing time—time elapsed from onset to completion of mixing
      (2) Working time—time elapsed from onset of mixing to onset of initial setting time
      (3) Initial setting time—time at which sufficient reaction has occurred to cause the materials to be resistant to further manipulation
      (4) Final setting time—time at which the material is practically set, as defined by its resistance to indentation
    b. Definitions of intervals
      (1) Mixing interval—length of time of mixing stage
      (2) Working interval—length of time of working stage
      (3) Setting interval—length of time of setting stage
    c. All water-based materials lose their gloss at the time of setting

### Properties

A. Physical properties—events that do not involve changes in composition or primary bonds
  1. Descriptive properties
    a. Weight—gravitational force that attracts a body

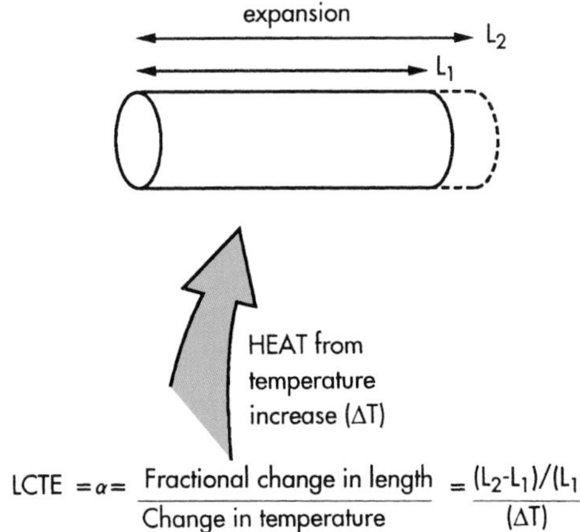

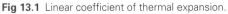

**Fig 13.1** Linear coefficient of thermal expansion.

b. Mass—resistance of a body to acceleration (or being moved)
c. Volume—a defined region in three-dimensional space
d. Density—a body's weight per unit of volume

2. Thermal properties
   a. Linear coefficient of thermal expansion (LCTE, α)
      (1) Rate of expansion or contraction of one dimension of a material with temperature change (Fig. 13.1)
      (2) LCTE values—tooth, 9 to 11 ppm/°C; amalgam, 25 ppm/°C; composite, 35 to 45 ppm/°C; inlay wax, 300 ppm/°C
      (3) When the thermal expansion of restorative material does not match the tooth structure, percolation of fluids occurs at the margins during cyclic heating and cooling
   b. Thermal conductivity
      (1) Insulators transmit heat poorly (e.g., dental enamel, dental cements, acrylic polymers, dental porcelain, ceramic restorations)
      (2) Conductors transmit heat easily (e.g., dental amalgam, cast-gold alloys)
      (3) Teeth with metal restorations may be sensitive to hot and cold foods because of their good thermal conduction
      (4) Individuals wearing dentures may not sense normal temperature differences attributable to the thermal insulation by the acrylic denture base
      (5) To be an effective insulator, the material must be at least 0.5 mm thick
3. Electrical properties—electrical conductivity
   a. Conductors transmit electrons easily (e.g., metals)
   b. Semiconductors transmit electrons sometimes, including ceramics and often composites
   c. Insulators transmit electrons poorly (e.g., ceramics, polymers)
4. Surface properties
   a. Contact angle—internal angle of liquid droplet with solid surface
      (1) Good wetting (angle = 0 degrees)
      (2) Spreading (angle < 90 degrees)
      (3) Poor wetting (angle ≥ 90 degrees)
   b. Reflection—degree of surface backscattering
5. Color properties
   a. Perception—physiologic response to physical stimulus by the eye, which can distinguish three parameters
      (1) Dominant wavelength—blue, green, yellow, orange, and red
      (2) Luminance—lightness of color from black to white
      (3) Excitation purity—saturation of light
   b. Measurement
      (1) Munsell Color System (e.g., 5R 6/4)
         (a) Hue—color family (R, YR, Y, GY, G, BG, B, PB, P, RP)
         (b) Value—lightness from black to white (0/ to 10/)
         (c) Chroma—saturation from gray upward (/0 to /18)
      (2) Instrumentation techniques—record the spectral reflectance versus wavelength curves (405 to 700 nm for visible light)
      (3) L*a*b* color system
         (a) L* is value
         (b) a* is red, – a* is green
         (c) b* is yellow, – b* is blue
      (4) Dental manufacturer shade guides
         (a) Custom product shades guides
         (b) VITA Classical
         (c) VITA Linearguide 3D-Master
         (d) VITA Bleachguide 3D-Master
   c. Definitions
      (1) Metamerism—colors with different spectral energy distributions that look the same under certain lighting conditions but look different with different light sources
      (2) Fluorescence—emission of light by a material when a beam of light is shined on it
      (3) Opacity—degree of light absorption by a material
      (4) Translucency—degree of internal light reflection
      (5) Transparency—degree of light transmission through a material

B. Chemical properties
1. Primary chemical bonding types
   a. Types
      (1) Metallic (e.g., metals)
      (2) Ionic (e.g., ceramics)
      (3) Covalent (e.g., polymers)
   b. Events related to changes in primary chemical bonding
      (1) Contraction attributable to chemical reaction
         (a) Rate of contraction of size of material during chemical reaction or phase change at constant temperature
         (b) Values reported as percentage changes
      (2) Corrosion of surfaces
2. Secondary chemical bonds
   a. Types
      (1) Hydrogen bonding—where hydrogen is attracted to an electronegative atom or molecule section; found in most water-based liquids
      (2) Van der Waals forces—dispersion forces caused by fluctuating dipoles; found in dental composites and acrylics

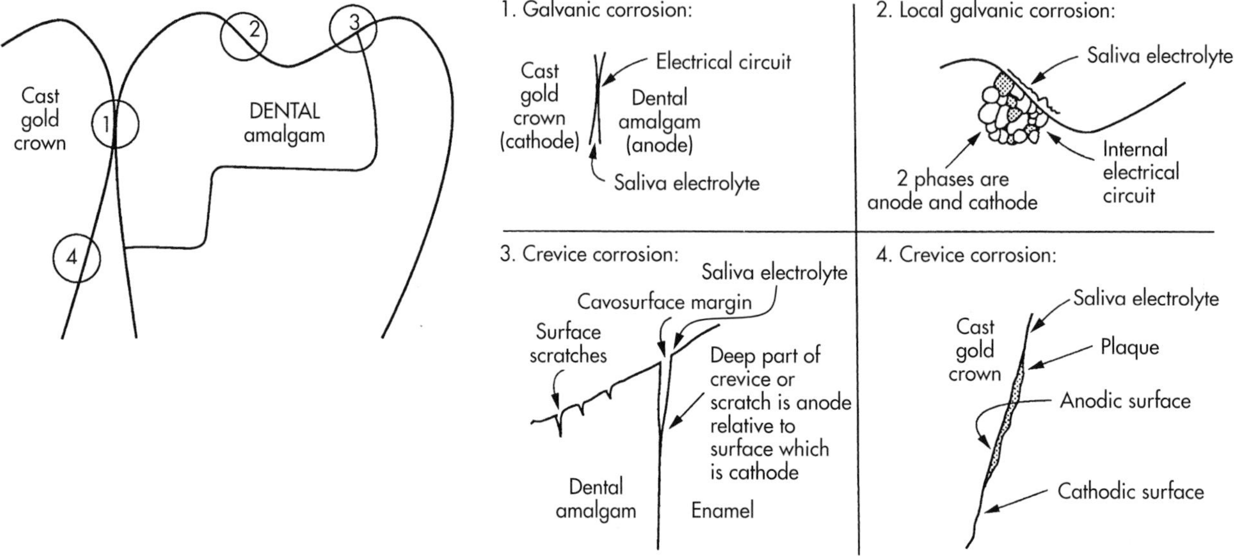


**Fig 13.2** Electrochemical corrosion.

b. Events related to changes in secondary chemical bonding
   (1) Adsorption—uptake "onto" the surface of the solid
   (2) Absorption—uptake "into" the solid
      (a) Example—water absorbed by denture
      (b) Example—moisture absorbed by alginate (imbibition)
   (3) Desorption—fluid lost from the solid; for example, water lost from alginate (syneresis)
   (4) Solubility—material loss by dissolution of surface
   (5) Disintegration—material loss by disruption of solid, usually by absorbed water
3. Corrosion
   a. Chemical corrosion—chemical reaction at surface
      (1) Products may be soluble
      (2) Products may be insoluble and form layers (tarnish)
   b. Electrochemical corrosion—chemical reaction that requires an anode (e.g., dental amalgam), a cathode (e.g., gold crown), an electrolyte (e.g., saliva), and an electrical circuit (e.g., contact) for electron flow (Fig. 13.2)
      (1) Galvanic corrosion—dissimilar metals in contact (previous examples)
      (2) Local galvanic corrosion (structure selective corrosion)—dissimilar phases in the same metal in contact
      (3) Crevice corrosion—corrosion in the crack under plaque, between a restoration and the tooth structure, or in the scratch on the surface of a restoration, where the metals may be the same but the electrolytes are different locally
   c. Corrosion potential
      (1) Immune—does not corrode (i.e., cathodic)
      (2) Active—corrodes readily (i.e., anodic)
      (3) Passive—corrosion produces protective film, for example, chromium oxide film on stainless steel

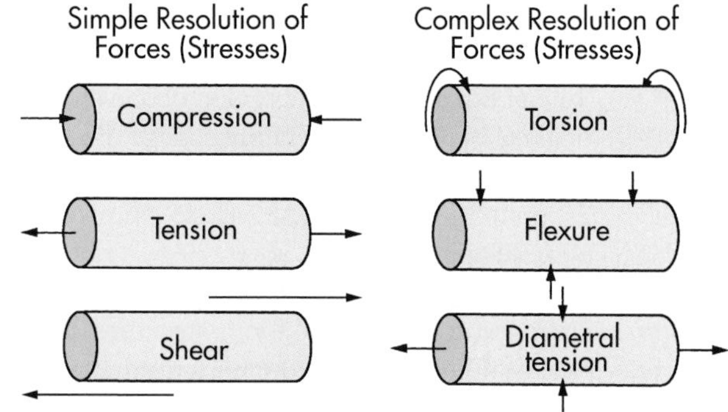


**Fig 13.3** Resolution of forces.

C. Mechanical properties
1. Resolution of forces (Fig. 13.3)
   a. Uniaxial (one-dimensional) forces—compression, tension, and shear
   b. Complex forces—torsion, flexure, and diametral tension or compression
2. Normalization of forces and deformations
   a. Stress
      (1) Applied force (or material's resistance to force) per unit area
      (2) Stress = force/area
   b. Strain (Fig. 13.4)
      (1) Change in length per unit of length because of force
3. Stress-strain diagrams
   a. Plot of stress (vertical) versus strain (horizontal)
      (1) Allows convenient comparison of materials
      (2) Different curves for compression, tension, and shear
      (3) Curves depend on rate of testing and temperature
   b. Analysis of curves (see Fig. 13.4)
      (1) Elastic behavior
         (a) Elastic strain—initial response to stress (*elastic*—when the stress is removed, the strain returns to zero and the material returns to its original length)

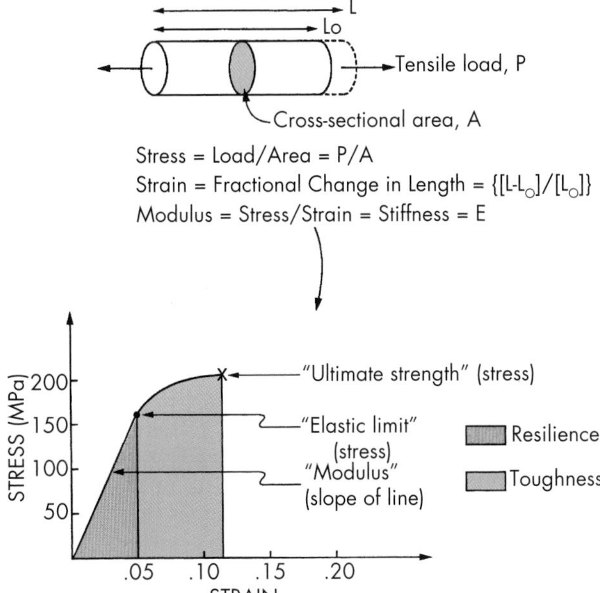


**Fig 13.4** Stress-strain curve.

(b) Elastic modulus—slope of first part of curve; represents the stiffness of the material, or the resistance to elastic deformation under force

(c) Elastic limit (proportional limit)—stress above which the material no longer behaves totally elastically

(d) Yield strength—stress that is an estimate of the elastic limit at 0.002 permanent strain

(e) Hardness—value on a relative scale that estimates the elastic limit in terms of a material's resistance to indentation

Examples—Knoop hardness scale, Diamond pyramid hardness scale, Brinnell hardness scale, Rockwell hardness scale, Barcol scale, Shore A hardness scale, Mohs hardness scale (Table 13.1)

Hardness values are used to determine the ability of abrasives to alter the substrates they contact

(f) Resilience—area under the stress-strain curve up to the elastic limit; estimates the total elastic energy that can be absorbed before the onset of plastic deformation

(2) Elastic and plastic behavior

(a) Beyond the stress level of the elastic limit, a combination of both elastic and plastic strain exists

(b) Ultimate strength—highest stress reached before fracture; the ultimate compressive strength is greater than the ultimate shear strength and the ultimate tensile strength

(c) Elongation (percent elongation)—percent change in length up to the point of fracture = strain × 100%

**TABLE 13.1 Mohs' Scale for Hardness***

| Number | Hardness |
|---|---|
| 10 | Diamond |
| 9 | Corundum |
| 8 | Topaz |
| 7 | Quartz |
| 6 | Orthoclase |
| 5 | Apatite |
| 4 | Fluorite |
| 3 | Calcite |
| 2 | Gypsum |
| 1 | Talc |

*Standard for checking hardness of abrasives and substrates.

(d) Brittle materials—less than 10% elongation at fracture

(e) Ductile materials—greater than 10% elongation at fracture

(f) Toughness—area under the stress-strain curve up to the point of fracture (it estimates the total energy absorbed up to fracture)

(3) Time-dependent behavior

(a) Strain rate sensitivity—the faster a stress is applied, the more likely a material is to store the energy elastically and not plastically

(b) Creep—strain relaxation with time in response to a constant stress, such as dental wax deforming because of built-in stresses created during cooling

(c) Stress relaxation—with time in response to a constant strain

(d) Fatigue—failure caused by cyclic loading

4. Tooth biomechanics

a. Enamel—strong in compression; weaker in flexion or tension

b. DEJ—strong boundary layer between enamel and dentin

c. Dentin—key tissue for absorbing and dissipating energy during tooth loading

d. CEJ—weak boundary between enamel and cementum covered dentin

(1) Sharp cervical notches

(a) Caused by abrasive dentifrices and sawing action of tooth brushing

(b) Involve several adjacent teeth simultaneously

(2) Abfractions

(a) Sauder-shaped or notch-shaped cervical lesions on surfaces

(b) Caused by tooth flexure during excessive loading forces

(c) May be accompanied by wear facets on occlusal surfaces

(d) May occur on individual teeth without adjacent teeth effects

(e) Forces fracture enamel and dentin at CEJ and lead to material losses

**TABLE 13.2 Hardness Values for Dental Substrates***

| Hardness Value | Number |
|---|---|
| CAD/CAM ceramic | 6-7 |
| Porcelain | 6-7 |
| Composite | 5-7 |
| Glass | 5-6 |
| Dental enamel | 5-6 |
| Dental amalgam | 4-5 |
| Dentin | 3-4 |
| Hard gold alloys | 3-4 |
| Pure gold | 2-3 |
| Acrylic | 2-3 |
| Cementum | 2-3 |

*Based on Mohs' hardness scale: diamond = 10; talc = 1 (see Table 13.1).

(f) Self-cleaning areas that do not require restorations except for esthetics
(g) Usually restored with composite or glass ionomer
(e) Cementum

5. Principles of cutting, polishing, and surface cleaning
   a. Terminology
      (1) Cutting—gross removal of excess material from the surfaces of restorations or teeth
      (2) Finishing—fine removal of surface material in an effort to produce finer surface scratches
      (3) Polishing—smoothing of surfaces by removal of fine scratches
      (4) Debriding—removal of unwanted material attached to surfaces
      (5) Air abrasion (air polishing)—removal or polishing of hard tissue by the kinetic energy from particles sprayed against the surface
      (6) Microabrasion—removal of stains by a mixture of an abrasive and hydrochloric acid
   b. Surface mechanics for materials (Table 13.2)
      (1) Cutting—requires materials with the highest possible hardness to produce the cuts
      (2) Finishing—requires materials with the highest possible hardness for the best effect, except at the margins of restorations, where the tooth structure may be inadvertently affected
      (3) Polishing—requires materials with small particles and with a Mohs hardness that is only 1 to 2 units above that of the substrate
      (4) Debriding—requires materials with a Mohs hardness that is less than or equal to that of the substrate to prevent scratching
   c. Factors affecting cutting, polishing, and surface cleaning
      (1) Applied pressure
      (2) Particle size of abrasive
      (3) Hardness of abrasive
      (4) Hardness of substrate
      (5) Speed of rotary instrument
   d. Factors affecting air abrasion
      (1) Abrasive particle size: 27-μm or 50-μm aluminum oxide
      (2) Air pressure—higher air pressure cuts faster but may cause discomfort
   e. Precautions
      (1) During cutting, heat will build up and change the mechanical behavior of the substrate from brittle to ductile and with formation of a smear layer interfering with cutting
      (2) Instruments may transfer debris onto the cut surface from their own surfaces during cutting, polishing, or cleaning operations (this has important implications in cleaning dental implant surfaces)

D. Biologic properties
1. Definitions of biohazards
   a. Toxicity—cell or tissue death attributable to material concentration
   b. Sensitivity—systemic reaction to a substance
      (1) Allergy—reaction to relatively small amounts of a material
      (2) Hypersensitivity—reaction to minute amounts of a material
2. Definitions of local tissue interactions with biomaterials
   a. Fibrous tissue capsule formation (tissue encapsulation)
   b. Integration at the interface (osseo-integration)
      (1) Bone ingrowth
      (2) Bone ongrowth
   c. Biodegradation (desorption or resorption)
3. Classification of biologic materials—tissue interfaces
   a. Intraoral and supragingival—in enamel or dentin
   b. Intraoral, pulpal, or periapical
   c. Transcutaneous
   d. Subcutaneous
   e. Intraosseous
4. Clinical analysis of biocompatibility
   a. Risk versus benefits
   b. Safety and efficacy
5. Agencies that oversee materials, devices, and therapeutics
   a. Regulatory agencies—U.S. Food and Drug Administration (FDA)
   b. Standards development for manufacturing practices (for physical, chemical, mechanical, and biologic properties and for clinical testing)
      (1) American Dental Association (ADA)—Council on Scientific Affairs and Standards Committee on Dental Products (SCDP)
      (2) American National Standards Institute (ANSI)
      (3) Fédération Dentaire Internationale (FDI; International Dental Association)
      (4) International Standards Organization (ISO)

## DIRECT PREVENTIVE AND RESTORATIVE MATERIALS

### Dental Amalgam

A. General considerations
   1. Applications
      a. Load-bearing restorations for posterior teeth (class I, class II)
      b. Pin-retained restorations
      c. Buildups (foundations) or cores for cast restorations
      d. Retrograde root canal filling material
   2. Terminology
      a. Amalgam alloy—powder particles of silver-tin-copper-(zinc), or Ag-Sn-Cu-(Zn) (minor elements are indicated in parentheses)
      b. Amalgam—reaction product of any material with mercury
      c. Dental amalgam—reaction product of amalgam alloy (Ag-Sn or Ag-Sn-Cu) with mercury
   3. Classification of dental amalgam by:
      a. Powder particle shape
         (1) Irregular (comminuted, filing, or lathe-cut)
         (2) Spherical (spherodized)
         (3) Blends, including irregular-irregular, irregular-spherical, or spherical spherical
      b. Total amount of copper
         (1) Low-copper alloys (conventional, traditional); less than 5% copper (Ag-Sn-Cu)
         (2) High-copper alloys (corrosion-resistant); 12% to 28% copper (Ag-Sn-Cu)
      c. Presence of zinc
      d. Other modifications
   4. Examples
      a. Low-copper, irregular-particle alloy (e.g., 70Ag-26Sn-4Cu)
      b. High-copper, blended-particle alloy with irregular particles (e.g., 70Ag-26Ag-4Cu) and spherical particles (e.g., 72Ag-28Cu)
      c. High-copper, spherical-particle alloy (e.g., 60Ag-27Sn-13Cu)

B. Structure
   1. Components
      a. Mercury (Hg) mixed with amalgam alloy
      b. Mercury reacts with periphery of alloy particle to produce crystalline silver-mercury, tin-mercury, and copper-tin phases
   2. Reaction (Fig. 13.5)

$$Hg + Ag - Sn \rightarrow Ag - Sn + Ag - Hg + Sn - Hg$$
$$Hg + Ag - Sn - Cu \rightarrow Ag - Sn - Cu + Ag - Hg + Cu - Sn$$
$$Hg + Ag - Sn + Ag - Cu \rightarrow$$
$$Ag - Sn + Ag - Cu + Ag - Hg + Cu - Sn$$

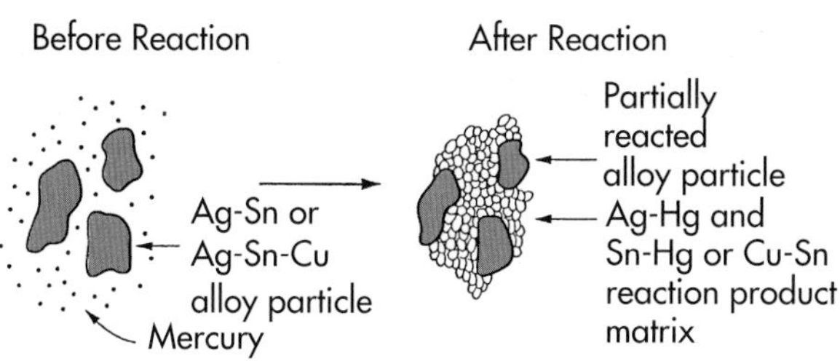

**Fig 13.5** Amalgam reaction.

   3 Manipulation
      a. Selection—based on clinical requirements for strength
      b. Packaging
         (1) Powder or pressed tablets; mercury
         (2) Precapsulated powder and mercury
      c. Mixing
         (1) Mercury alloy—specific to each product but generally less than 1:1 so that amalgam contains 41% to 50% mercury
         (2) Mechanical amalgamators—variable time, speed (frequency and amplitude), and amalgamator motion for different equipment; variables affect the mixing process
         (3) Each amalgamator has specific settings for each different amalgam alloy (e.g., high-copper amalgams require 5 to 10 seconds)
         (4) Amalgamator capsules are recyclable
         (5) Pestle may be included in the capsule for mixing efficiency
         (6) Overmixed mass is difficult to remove from capsule
         (7) Undermixed mass is crumbly
      d. Condensation
         (1) Adaptation of amalgam to cavity walls
         (2) Removal of excess mercury-rich matrix produces a stronger and more corrosion-resistant amalgam because it minimizes the formation of the matrix phases of amalgam, which are the least desirable parts of the set material
         (3) Amalgams with spherical alloys are more fluid and require larger-tipped condensers
         (4) It is important to condense in small increments, overpack restoration, avoid delays, and avoid saliva contamination
      e. Finishing
         (1) The anatomy should be carved within a few minutes after condensing
         (2) The surface should be burnished or the final finish performed at least 24 hours later

C. Properties
   1. Physical
      a. Coefficient of thermal expansion = 25 ppm/°C
      b. Thermal conductivity—high (therefore the amalgam may need an insulating liner or base in very deep cavity preparations)
   2. Chemical
      a. Dimensional change on setting, should be less than ± 20 μm (excessive expansion can produce postoperative pain)
      b. The cavity varnish or the bonding agent electrically insulates a dental amalgam restoration, but it does not prevent corrosion
      c. Chemical corrosion produces a black or green tarnish on the surface that is aesthetically unacceptable but is not detrimental to oral health

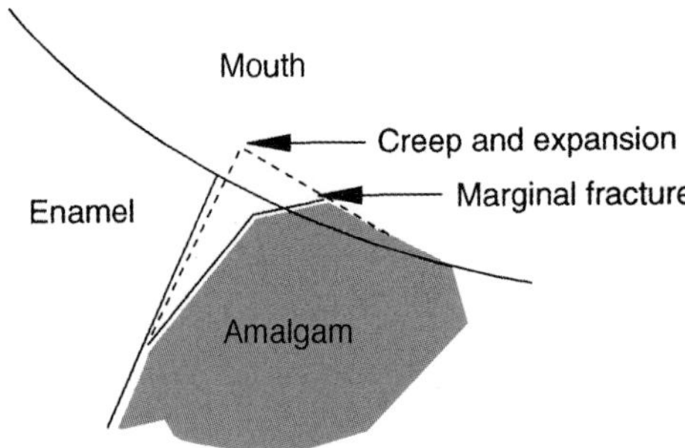


**Fig 13.6** Marginal ditching in an amalgam restoration is produced by creep and expansion, which elevate the margins of the amalgam, and functional stresses produce marginal fracture.

d. Electrochemical corrosion produces penetrating corrosion of low-copper amalgams but produces only superficial corrosion of high-copper amalgams
e. Long-term reaction continues, resulting in slow expansion that is worn away on occlusal surfaces but extrudes the restoration on other surfaces

3. Mechanical
   a. Compressive strength—ranges from 310 to 480 MPa, comparable with enamel (410 MPa) but is not significant in preventing marginal fracture
   b. Because of low tensile strength, enamel support is needed at the margins
   c. Spherical high-copper alloys develop high tensile strength quickly and can be polished sooner than other alloys
   d. Excessive creep occurs during the Ag-Hg phase of incorrectly mixed amalgams and contributes to early marginal fracture
   e. Marginal fracture is correlated with creep and electrochemical corrosion in low-copper amalgams (Fig. 13.6)
   f. Bulk fracture (isthmus fracture) occurs across the thinnest portions of amalgam restorations because of high stresses during traumatic occlusion, the accumulated effects of fatigue, or both
   g. Dental amalgam is relatively resistant to abrasion, that is, wear; similar to human enamel
   h. Amalgam undergoes very slow expansion over years and is worn away occlusally but causes slight expansion on non-wearing surfaces
4. Biologic
   a. Mercury hygiene
      (1) All personnel must be trained; all personnel must be made aware of mercury sources in the oral care setting
      (2) A proper work-area design is important; personnel must work in well-ventilated spaces; the treatment area atmosphere must be periodically checked for mercury vapor
      (3) Precapsulated products should be stored in tight containers
      (4) Mercury should not come into contact with the skin
      (5) Spills should be cleaned up immediately to minimize mercury vaporization
      (6) Amalgamators should be used with covers enclosing the mixing arm
      (7) High-vacuum suction should be used during amalgam alloy placement, setting, polishing, or removal when mercury may be vaporized
      (8) All scrap amalgam should be salvaged and stored in tightly closed containers and recycled in accordance with applicable laws
      (9) Mercury-contaminated items must be disposed of in sealed bags and not in medical waste containers
      (10) The dental office personnel must be aware of aerosols created by vacuuming mercury spilled on the floor or the carpet
      (11) Floor coverings should be replaced every 5 years to eliminate spilled mercury that might have accumulated in carpet pores
      (12) Professional clothing must be removed before leaving the workplace
   b. Mercury bioactivity
      (1) Depends on whether the form is metallic, inorganic, or organic mercury
      (2) Metallic mercury is the least toxic form and is absorbed primarily through the lungs rather than through the gastrointestinal (GI) tract or skin
      (3) Mercury accumulated in the body may come from air, water, food, dental sources (a low amount), or medical sources
      (4) Average half-life for mercury elimination from the body is 55 days
      (5) The U.S. Occupational Safety and Health Administration (OSHA) has set the average level for mercury toxicity by exposure as less than 50 $\mu g/m^3$ per 40-hour workweek
      (6) Incidence of mercury hypersensitivity is estimated to be less than 1 per 100 million persons
   c. Environment issues-important to:
      (1) Use best management practices (BMPs)
      (2) Use precapsulated alloys
      (3) Manage mercury through recycling—recycle used disposable amalgam capsules; salvage, store, and recycle noncontact amalgam; salvage amalgam pieces from restorations after removal, and recycle amalgam waste
         (a) Use chairside traps to retain amalgam and recycle contents
         (b) Recycle contents retained by vacuum pump filter or other amalgam-collecting devices
         (c) Disinfect extracted teeth that contain amalgam restorations using bleach, and recycle them with chairside trap wastes
         (d) Mercury regulation
            (1) Minamota Convention (2013)—adopted pledge to reduce use of mercury everywhere

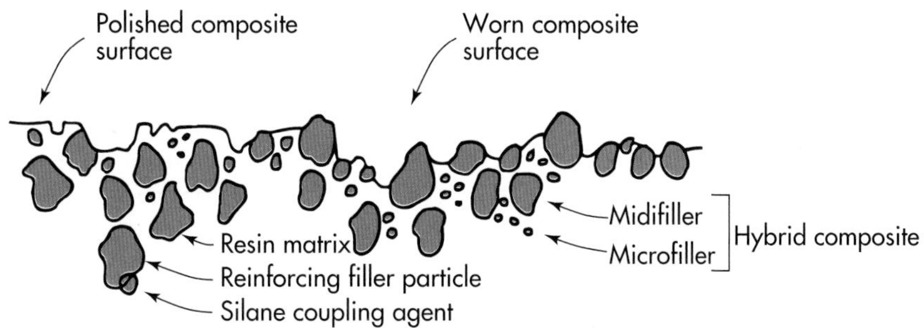

**Fig 13.7** Hybrid dental composite.

D. Amalgam alternatives
   1. Direct esthetic filling materials (composites, compomers)
   2. Indirect filling materials (cast gold, PFM, all-ceramic materials)

## Dental Composites

A. General considerations
   1. Applications
      a. Anterior restorations created for aesthetic purposes (class III, IV, and V cervical erosion, or abrasion lesions)
      b. Low-stress posterior restorations (small class I and II)
      c. High-stress posterior restorations with certain formulations
      d. Veneers
      e. Cores for cast restorations
      f. Cements for ceramic restorations
      g. Cements for resin-bonded bridges
      h. Repair systems for composites or ceramic restorations
   2. Terminology (Fig. 13.7)
      a. Composite—physical mixture of materials to average the properties of the materials involved
      b. Dental composite—restorative material resulting from the mixture of ceramic reinforcing filler particles in a monomer matrix that is converted to polymer on setting
      c. Polymerization—reaction of small molecules (monomers) into very large molecules (polymers)
      d. Cross-linking—tying together of polymer molecules by chemical reaction between the molecules to produce a continuous 3-D network
   3. Classification by:
      a. Amount of filler—25% to 85% by volume, 45% to 90% by weight
         (1) Very high—bulk-fill; packable or condensable composite
         (2) High—universal composite (packable and flowable)
         (3) Moderate—flowable composite
         (4) Low—microfill
      b. Filler particle size
         (1) Average sizes—minifill = 0.1 to 1.0 μm; microfill = 0.01 to 0.1 μm; nanofill = 0.001 to 0.01 μm
         (2) Mixture of sizes—hybrid (microhybrid = mini + micro)
         (3) Presence of pre-cured composite (heterogeneous)
      c. Polymerization method
         (1) Auto-cured (also self-cured, SC)
         (2) Visible light–cured (VLC)
         (3) Dual-cured (VLC + SC)
      d. Matrix chemistry
         (1) Bisphenol A–glycidylmethacrylate (Bis-GMA) or Bis-GMA–like monomers
         (2) Urethane dimethacrylate (UDM or UDMA) monomers
         (3) Tetraethylene glycol dimethacrylate (TEGDMA)—diluent monomer to reduce viscosity
         (4) Expanding monomers—to control overall polymerization shrinkage

B. Structure
   1. Components
      a. Filler particles—colloidal silica or silicate glasses (noncrystalline) of various particle sizes (containing Ba, Li, Al, Zn, Yr, and others)
      b. Matrix—Bis-GMA (or UDMA) with lower-molecular-weight diluents (e.g., TEGDMA) that co-react during polymerization; ring-opening monomers
      c. Coupling agent—silane, which chemically bonds the surfaces of the filler particles to the polymer matrix
   2. Reaction
      a. Free-radical polymerization—monomers + initiator + accelerators → polymer molecules
      b. Initiators—start polymerization by decomposing and reacting with monomer
         (1) Benzoyl peroxide typically used in SC systems
         (2) Camphorquinone typically used in VLC systems
      c. Accelerators—speed up initiator decomposition; different amines used for accelerating initiators in SC and VLC systems
      d. Retarders or inhibitors—prevent premature polymerization
   3. Manipulation
      a. Selection
         (1) Microfill composites or microhybrids for anterior class III, IV, and V restorations
         (2) Microhybrids for class I, II, III, IV, and V restorations
      b. Conditioning of enamel and dentin (see section on "Bonding Agents")
         (1) Total-etch technique:
            (a) Acid-etch with 15% to 38% phosphoric acid

(b) Rinse for 5 to 10 seconds with water
(c) Air-dry enamel for 5 to 10 seconds, but do not desiccate or dehydrate
(d) Apply bonding agent and polymerize
(2) Self-etch technique (apply bonding system)

c. Mixing (if required)—two pastes are mixed for 20 to 30 seconds
(1) Self-cured composite—working time is 60 to 120 seconds after mixing
(2) Light-cured composite—working time is nearly unlimited; used for most anterior and some posterior composite restorations; natural light and dental chair lights may slowly start the reaction
(3) Dual-cured composite—working time is 5 to 8 minutes

d. Placement—a plastic instrument or syringe or a unidose (compule) should be used

e. Light curing—it is important to:
(1) Check the output of the light-curing unit
(2) Use high-intensity quartz-tungsten-halogen (QTH) or light-emitting-diode (LED) or polywave light
(3) Cure incrementally in 1.5 to 2.0 mm–thick layers; use a matrix strip, where possible, to produce a smooth surface and to contour the composite

f. Finishing and polishing—it is important to:
(1) Remove the oxygen-inhibited layer (with alcohol swab)
(2) Use stones, carbide burs, or diamonds for gross reduction
(3) Use multi-fluted carbide burs or special diamonds for fine reduction
(4) Use aluminum oxide strips or discs for finishing or rubber points, cups, and discs
(5) Use fine aluminum oxide or diamond finishing pastes
(6) Microfill and nanofill composites develop smoothest finish because of small size of filler particles
(7) Keep in mind that liquid polishes provide short-term smooth-surface coatings

C. Properties—generally improve with filler content

1. Physical
   a. Radiopacity depends on the ions in silicate glass
   b. Coefficient of thermal expansion is 35 to 45 ppm/°C and decreases with increasing filler content
   c. Thermal and electrical insulators
2. Chemical
   a. Water absorption is 0.5% to 2.5% and increases with polymer content
   b. Acidulated topical fluorides (e.g., acidulated phosphate fluoride [APF]) tend to dissolve glass particles, and thus composites should be protected with a non–petroleum-based jelly during these procedures, or a different topical fluoride (e.g., neutral sodium fluoride) should be used
   c. In the past, major color changes occurred in resin matrix with time because of oxidation, which produces colored by-products, but the modern composites are highly color stable; some composites experience a slight shade shift when light-cured
3. Mechanical
   a. The compressive strength is 310 to 410 MPa, which is adequate
   b. Wear resistance—improves with higher filler content, higher percentage of conversion in curing, use of microfiller, and closer interparticle spacing of fillers
   c. Surfaces that are rough from wear retain plaque biofilm and stain more readily
   d. Apical margins are more susceptible to staining
   e. Stained margins should not be aggressively cleaned with prophy paste because of potential damage
4. Biologic—the components may be cytotoxic, but the cured composite is biocompatible as restorative filling material

## Pit-and-Fissure Sealants

A. General considerations—see the section on "Dental Sealants" in Chapter 16.

1. Applications
   a. Occlusal surfaces of newly erupted posterior teeth
   b. Lingual surfaces of anterior teeth with fissures
   c. Occlusal surfaces of teeth in older persons with reduced flow of saliva (because low levels of saliva increase susceptibility to dental caries)
2. Classification by:
   a. Polymerization method
      (1) Self-curing
      (2) Light-curing—90% of current products
   b. Filler content
      (1) Unfilled—many systems are unfilled because filler tends to interfere with and wear away from self-cleaning occlusal areas; sealants are designed to wear away, except where no self-cleaning action occurs; a common misconception is that sealants should be wear resistant
      (2) Lightly filled—10% to 30% by weight

B. Structure

1. Components
   a. Monomer—Bis-GMA–like or UDMA monomers with TEGDMA, a diluent monomer, to facilitate flow into pits and fissures before cure
   b. Initiator—benzoyl peroxide (in self-cured) and camphorquinone (in light-cured)
   c. Accelerator—amine
   d. Opaque filler—1% titanium dioxide or other colorant to make the material detectable on tooth surfaces
   e. Reinforcing filler—silicate glass (generally not added because wear resistance is not required within pits and fissures)
   f. Fluoride—may be added for slow release
2. Reaction—free-radical reaction (see the previous section on "Dental Composites")

3. Manipulation
   a. Preparation—this involves:
      (1) Cleaning the pits and fissures of organic debris
      (2) Etching the occlusal surfaces, pits, and fissures with 37% phosphoric acid
      (3) Washing the occlusal surfaces for 5 to 10 seconds
      (4) Drying the etched area for 5 to 10 seconds with clean air spray
      (5) Applying the sealant and polymerizing
   b. Mixing or dispensing
      (1) Self-cured—equal amounts of liquids are mixed in a Dappen dish for 5 seconds with a brush applicator
      (2) Light-cured—syringes or unidose tips are used for dispensing
   c. Placement—pits, fissures, and occlusal surfaces; this involves:
      (1) 60 seconds for self-cured materials to set
      (2) Light-curing according to manufacturer's instructions
   d. Finishing
      (1) Unpolymerized (air-inhibited layer) and excess materials should be removed
      (2) The hardness and marginal adaptation of the sealant should be examined
      (3) Occlusal adjustments should be made, where necessary, in the sealant; most unfilled sealant materials are self-adjusting

C. Properties
1. Physical—wetting: low-viscosity sealants wet acid-etched tooth structure the best
2. Mechanical
   a. Wear resistance should not be too great because the sealant should be able to wear off from the self-cleaning areas of tooth
   b. To prevent loss, sealants should be protected during polishing procedures with air-abrading units
3. Biologic—no apparent biologic problems
4. Clinical efficacy
   a. Effectiveness is 100% if retained in pits and fissures
   b. Requires routine clinical evaluation (every 1.5 to 2 years) to check the integrity and resealing of defective areas if sealant loss is attributable to poor retention
   c. Sealants resist attack from topical fluorides (also applied for prevention of dental caries)

## Infiltrants

A. General considerations
1. Applications—approximal and smooth-surface uncavitated lesions where sealing would not be a permanent solution to stop lesion growth and to create good esthetics
2. Definition—a resin system capable of penetrating through slightly porous enamel, embedding into an existing decalcified region of dentin, stopping lesion activity by preventing the diffusion of organic acids below plaque and restoring the esthetics of the tooth structure
3. Classification—this is a new and novel approach to minimally invasive dentistry for interproximal, uncavitated lesion repair; currently, only one system is available on the market
   a. Approximal application kit
   b. Smooth-surface application kit

B. Structure
1. Components—acrylic monomer infiltrant after use of a hydrochloric acid (HCl; hydrogen chloride, hydrochloride) etchant to create micropores in the enamel overlying the lesion and to allow resin penetration
2. Reaction—the resin is light-cured
3. Manipulation (approximal repair)
   a. Wedging of teeth to separate interproximal contacts
   b. Application of acid etchant (more than 90 seconds with 15% aqueous HCl) to create micropores through the overlying enamel by using a unique holder and a film packet to deliver materials
   c. VLC materials

C. Properties
1. Physical—the tooth structure appears to have normal color and opacity after infiltration
2. Chemical—no evidence of dentin decalcification after infiltration
3. Mechanical—previously decalcified dentin is restored to approximately the same hardness
4. Biologic—no evidence of any threat to the pulp before setting
5. No special maintenance required

## Silver Diamine Fluoride (SDF) and Analog Products

A. General considerations
1. Applications – approximal, smooth surface, and occlusal caries to prevent further disease progression

B. Structure
1. Aqueous solution of SDF or analog procedure
2. Reacts with the surface of tooth structure to produce a superficial caries resistant zone

C. Properties
1. Silver diamine fluoride—when painted on enamel or dentin stops dental caries and prevents future progression but it stains tooth structure black
2. Silver diamine fluoride analog—after SDF application, a potassium iodide solution is applied over top to prevent black staining— and teeth are restored with. glass ionomer as needed.

## Bonding Agents

A. General considerations
1. Applications—composites, resin-modified glass ionomers, compomers, bonded ceramic restorations, veneers, orthodontic brackets, desensitizing dentin by covering exposed tubules, resin-bonded bridges, composite-repair and ceramic-repair systems, and amalgams
2. Definitions
   a. Smear layer—thin layer (0.5 to 5.0 µm) of compacted debris on enamel and dentin resulting from the cavity-

preparation process (Fig. 13.8) that is weakly held to the surface (5 to 6 MPa) and that limits bonding agent strength if not removed

b. Etching (or conditioning)—smear layer removal and production of microspaces for micromechanical bonding by dissolving minor amounts of surface hydroxyapatite crystals
   (1) Total-etch (or etch-and-rinse) system—phosphoric acid should be used
   (2) Self-etch system—reliance on acidic monomer to dissolve smear layer, etch surface of intertubular dentin, and embed collagen fibers; no rinsing
c. Priming—micromechanical (and possibly chemical) bonding to the microspaces created by the conditioning step
d. Conditioning and priming agent (self-etching primer)—agent that accomplishes both actions
e. Bonding—formation of resin layer that connects the primed surface to the overlying restoration (e.g., composite)

3. Classification
   a. Major substrate
      (1) Enamel and dentin bonding system—for bonding to enamel and dentin composite or other restorative materials

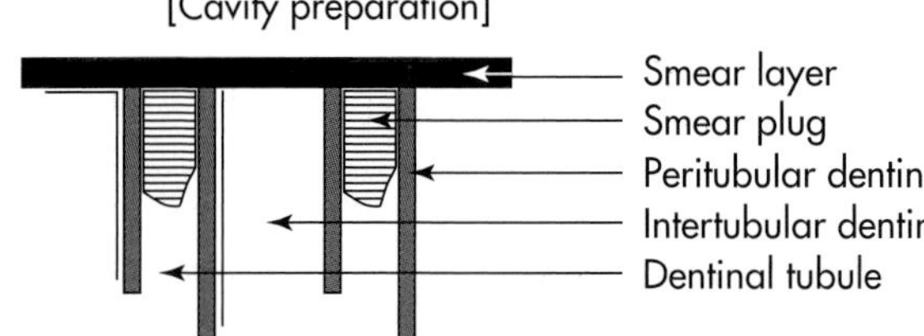


**Fig 13.8** The surface of cut dentin, with a smear layer and smear plugs occluding the dentinal tubules.

      (2) Amalgam bonding system—for bonding amalgam to enamel and dentin to amalgam
      (3) Universal bonding system—for bonding an appliance to enamel, dentin, amalgam, ceramic, metallic alloy, or any other substrate that may be necessary for a restorative procedure using the same set of procedures and materials
   b. Number of components and type of etching (Fig. 13.9)
      (1) Three-component total-etch system—etching + priming + bonding (E + P + B) (also called *fourth-generation*; involves two layers of material)
      (2) Two-component total-etch system—etching + priming/bonding (E + PB) (also called *fifth-generation*; involves one layer of material)
      (3) Two-component self-etch system—etching/priming + bonding (EP + B) (also called *sixth-generation type 1*; involves two layers of material)
      (4) One-component self-etch system—etching/priming/bonding) (EPB)—materials are mixed (if necessary) and scrubbed onto the surface to be bonded using the applicator tip [also called *sixth-generation type 2* or *seventh-generation* (no mixing), involves one layer of material]
      (5) Universal system—etching/priming/bonding (EPB) system—self-etching but also compatible with etching with phosphoric acid, system may contain components that prime zirconia-based ceramics, silica-based ceramics, and metals

B. Structure
   1. Components of bonding systems
      a. Conditioning agent—mineral (e.g., 10% to 40% phosphoric acid), organic acid (e.g., polyacrylic acid), or acidic acrylic monomer (e.g., phosphonate)

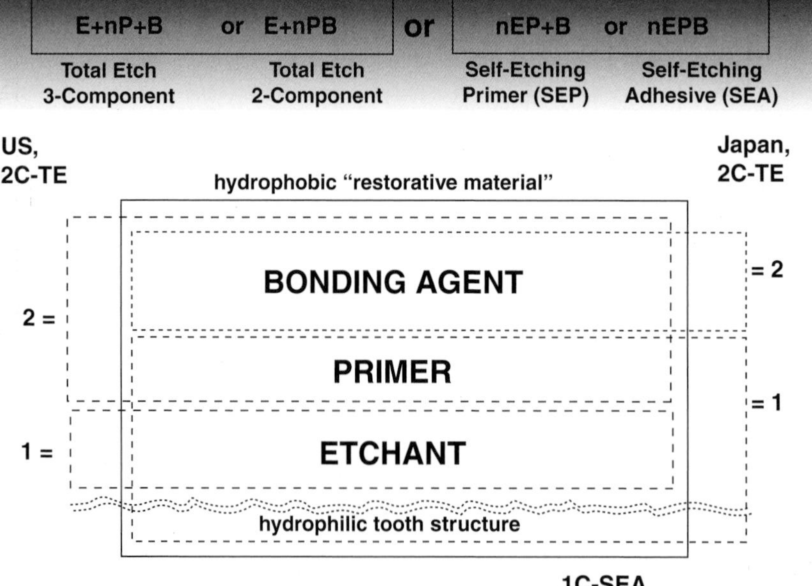


**Fig 13.9** Evolution of bonding system types with fewer components.

b. Priming agent—resin and monomer (e.g., HEMA) in alcohol, acetone, or water
c. Bonding agent—Bis-GMA or UDMA monomers
2. Reaction
a. Bonding occurs primarily by intimate micromechanical retention, with the relief created by the conditioning step
b. Chemical bonding is possible but is not recognized as contributing significantly to the overall bond strength
3. Manipulation (manufacturer's instructions should be followed)
a. Conditioning
(1) Total-etch technique—this involves:
(a) Applying phosphoric acid solution or equivalent
(b) Rinsing and drying without desiccation (dentin should be kept moist with "glistening" appearance)
(c) In case of overdried dentin, remoistening surface with water or a rewetting solution for 10 to 15 seconds
(2) Self-etch technique—this involves applying an acidic primer or a bonding agent, no rinsing
b. Priming—this involves:
(1) Applying a priming agent, and gently drying to remove excess solvent (but air-thinning must not be done unless recommended by manufacturer)
(2) Applying several layers until dentin is fully impregnated to surface
c. Bonding—this involves:
(1) Applying one to two coats of bonding agent when bonding composites
(2) Applying multiple coats of the bonding agent or mixing it with a thickening agent in preparation for bonding with amalgam restorations

C. Properties
1. Physical—thermal expansion and contraction may create fatigue stresses that debond the interface and permit microleakage
2. Chemical—water absorption into the bonding agent may chemically alter the bonding
3. Mechanical—mechanical stresses may produce fatigue that can debond the interface and permit microleakage
a. Enamel bonding—adhesion occurs by macrotags (between enamel prisms) and microtags (into enamel prisms) to produce micromechanical retention
b. Dentin bonding—adhesion occurs by removal of smear layer and formation of microtags within intertubular dentin to produce a hybrid zone (interpenetration or diffusion zone) that microscopically intertwines collagen bundles and bonding agent polymer; macrotags within tubules do not add much to retention because they are poorly polymerized and poorly adapted
4. Biologic
a. Conditioning agents may be locally irritating if they come into contact with soft tissue
b. Uncured priming agents, particularly those based on hydroxyethyl methacrylate (HEMA), may become skin sensitizers for dental personnel after several contacts
(1) Hands and face must be protected from inadvertent contact with unset materials and their vapors
(2) HEMA and other priming monomers may penetrate through rubber gloves in relatively short times (60 to 90 seconds)

## Cement Liners (Calcium Hydroxide; Zinc Oxide–Eugenol; Bioceramic)

A. General considerations—applications (if remaining dentin thickness is less than 0.5 mm)
1. Thermal insulation where the cavity preparation is close to the pulp or pulpal bridging
2. Delivering medications to the pulp
a. Calcium hydroxide (CH) liners—in self-cured and light-cured versions that stimulate reparative dentin
b. Zinc oxide–eugenol (ZOE) relieves pain by desensitizing nerves
c. Bioceramic promotes remineralization
d. Mineral trioxide aggregate (MTA)

B. CH structure (for ZOE types; see the section on "Dental Cements")
1. Components
a. Paste of CH reactant powder, ethyl toluene sulfonamide dispersant, zinc oxide filler, and zinc stearate radiopacifier
b. Paste of glycol salicylate reactant liquid, titanium dioxide filler powder, and calcium tungstenate radiopacifier
2. Reaction
a. Chemical reaction of calcium ions with salicylate to form methylsalicylate salts
b. Moisture absorbed to allow CH to dissociate into ions to react with salicylate
c. Mixture sets from outside surface to inside as water diffuses
3. Manipulation
a. Dentin should not be dehydrated, or material will not set
b. A drop each of the pastes should be mixed together for 5 seconds
c. The material should be applied to dentin; 1 to 2 minutes should be allowed for the material to set

C. CH properties
1. Physical—good thermal and electrical insulator
2. Chemical—poor resistance to water solubility, so may dissolve
3. Mechanical—low compressive strength (0.7 to 3.4 MPa)
4. Biologic—releases constituents, which diffuse toward the pulp and stimulate reparative dentin formation

## Cement Bases

A. General considerations (limited use)
1. Applications
a. Thermal insulation below a restoration (Fig. 13.10)
b. Mechanical protection where dentin is inadequate to support amalgam condensation pressures

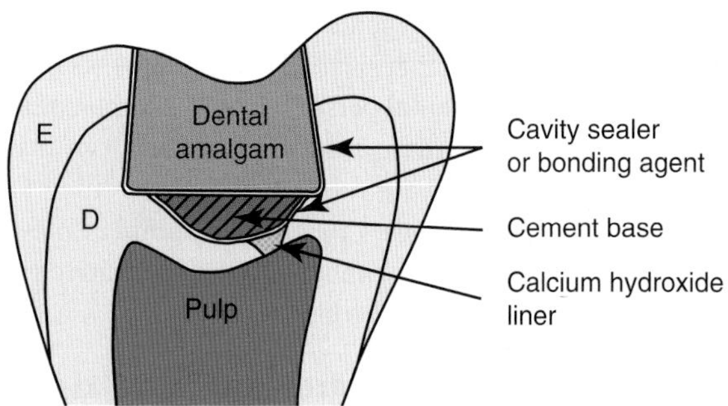


**Fig 13.10** Sealer, liner, and base applications for use with dental amalgam. E, Enamel; D, dentin.

2. Classification (many materials have been used in the past)
   a. Glass ionomer (GI) cement bases
   b. Resin-modified glass ionomer (RMGI)—light-curing compositions

B. Structure (see the section on "Crown-and-Bridge Cements")
1. Components
   a. Self-curing cements (ZP, PC, GI)—reactive powder (chemically basic) and reactive liquid (chemically acidic)
   b. Light-curing cements (RMGI)—paste
   c. Bioceramic—paste containing calcium silicate or bioactive filler and resin
   d. MTA—aqueous calcium silicate components
2. Reaction
   a. Self-curing cement—acid–base reaction that forms salts or cross-linked matrix; reaction may be exothermic
   b. Light-curing cements—monomer polymerization is exothermic
3. Manipulation—consistency for basing includes more powder, which improves all of the cement properties

C. Properties
1. Physical—excellent thermal and electrical insulation
2. Chemical—much more resistant to dissolution than cement liners
   a. Polycarboxylate (PC) and GI cements are chemically adhesive to tooth structure
   b. Solubility of all cement bases is lower than that of cement liners if they are mixed at higher powder-to-liquid ratios
3. Mechanical—much higher compressive strengths (80 to 210 MPa) than those of luting cements
   a. Light-cured RMGI cements are the strongest
   b. ZOE cements are the weakest
4. Biologic (see the section on "Crown-and-Bridge Cements" for details)—PC, GI, and RMGI cements, properly handled, provide good biocompatibility with pulp

## Other Cement Applications

A. Root canal sealers
1. Applications
   a. Cementing of silver cone or gutta percha point
   b. Paste filling material
2. Classification
   a. Zinc oxide–eugenol cement types
   b. Noneugenol cement types
   c. Therapeutic cement types
   d. Flowable composite types
3. Important properties
   a. Physical—radiopacity
   b. Chemical—insolubility
   c. Mechanical—flow; tensile strength
   d. Biologic—inert

B. Gingival tissue packs
1. Application—provide temporary displacement of gingival tissues
2. Composition—slow-setting ZOE cement mixed with cotton twills for texture and strength

C. Surgical dressings
1. Application—gingival covering after periodontal surgery
2. Composition—modified ZOE cement (containing tannic acid, rosin, and various oils)

D. Orthodontic cements
1. Application—cementing of orthodontic bands
2. Composition—composite (see the sections on "Crown-and-Bridge Cements" and "Bonding Agents")
3. Manipulation
   a. Resin (composite) cements use total-etch or self-etch bonding systems for improved bonding
   b. Band, bracket, or cement removal requires special care

## Fluoride-Releasing Restorative Materials

A. General considerations
1. Applications for glass ionomers (GIs), resin-modified glass ionomers (RMGIs), compomers, and atraumatic restorative technique (ART) materials
   a. Class V restorations—GIs and RMGIs for geriatric dentistry
   b. Class I and II restorations—RMGIs and compomers in pediatric dentistry; and ART temporary restorations in people living in the underserved regions of the world
   c. Class III restorations—RMGIs and compomers
2. Classification by composition (Fig. 13.11)
   a. Conventional GIs—limited use
   b. Metal-modified GIs—limited use
   c. RMGIs (hybrid ionomers)—popular use for temporaries, ART, and permanent restorations in pediatric dentistry applications (representing the largest use of GI restorative material)
   d. Compomers—limited use
   e. Giomers—limited use

B. Structure
1. Components
   a. Conventional glass ionomers—aluminosilicate glass powder and liquid water solution of co-polymers (or acrylic acid with maleic, tartaric, or itaconic acid)
   b. Metal-modified glass ionomers—glass ionomer admixed with amalgam alloy particles-used for cores

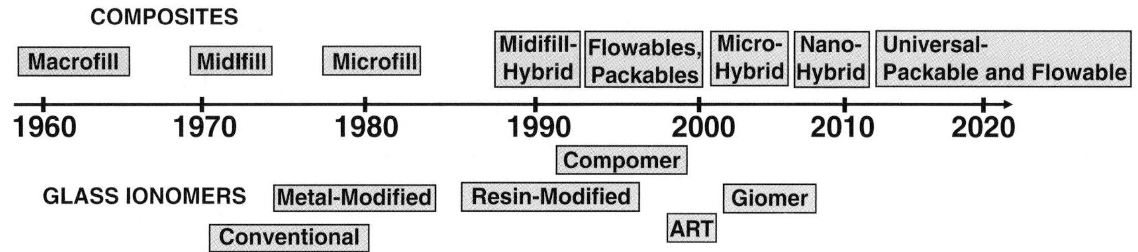


**Fig 13.11** Evolution of glass ionomers and composites over 60 years.

   c. Resin-modified glass ionomers—aluminosilicate glass powder and liquid with water solution of co-polymers (or acrylic acid with maleic, tartaric, or itaconic acids) and water-soluble monomers, for example, HEMA
   d. Compomers—hybrid of RMGI and composite
   e. Giomers—compomers with precured GI particles blended into a mixture
   f. Resin-reinforced (ART materials)—high fluoride-releasing conventional GI that may have small amounts of resin added for increased tackiness
2. Reactions (may involve several reactions and stages of setting)
   a. Glass ionomer reaction (acid-base reaction of polyacid and ions released from aluminosilicate glass particles)
      (1) Calcium, aluminum, fluoride, and other ions released by the outside of the powder particle dissolving in acidic liquid
      (2) Calcium ions initially cross-link acid-functional co-polymer molecules
      (3) Calcium cross-links are replaced in 24 to 48 hours by aluminum ion cross-links, with increased hardening of system
      (4) If no other reactants are present in the cement (e.g., resin modification), protection from saliva is required during the first 24 hours, unless otherwise indicated by manufacturer's instructions
   b. Polymerization reaction (polymerization of double bonds from water-soluble monomers or pendant groups on the co-polymer to form cross-linked matrix)
      (1) Polymerization reaction can be initiated with chemical (self-curing) or light-curing steps
      (2) Cross-linked polymer matrix ultimately interpenetrates the GI matrix
      (3) Occurs in resin-modified GI materials and compomers
3. Manipulation
   a. Self-curing materials—powder and liquid components may be manually mixed or may be precapsulated for mechanical mixing; light-curing materials—directly placed from a syringe or a unidose tip
   b. Placement—mixture is normally placed by using a syringe
   c. Finishing—can be immediate if the system is resin modified or is a compomer system (but otherwise must be delayed 24 to 72 hours until aluminum ion replacement reaction is complete)
   d. Sealing—the resin sealer is applied to smooth the surface (and to protect against moisture affecting the GI reaction)

C. Properties
   1. Physical
      a. Good thermal and electrical insulation
      b. Better radiopacity than with most composites
      c. Linear coefficient of thermal expansion and contraction is closer to that of the tooth structure than that of composites (but is less well matched for resin-modified and compomer systems)
      d. The esthetics of resin-modified and compomer systems is not quite as good as those of most composites
   2. Chemical
      a. Reactive acid side groups of co-polymer molecules produce chemical bonding to the tooth structure
      b. Fluoride ions are released
         (1) Rapid release at first because of excess fluoride ions in the matrix
         (2) Slow release after 7 to 30 days because of slow diffusion of fluoride ions out of aluminosilicate particles (Fig. 13.12)
         (3) Presence of fluoride in topical fluorides and fluoride-containing toothpastes may recharge the fluoride content in the cement matrix temporarily for 2 to 3 days
      c. The solubility resistance of resin-modified systems is close to that of composites
   3. Mechanical
      a. Compressive strength of resin-modified systems and compomers is much better than that of conventional glass ionomers but not quite as strong as that of composites
      b. Glass ionomers are more brittle than are composites
   4. Biologic
      a. Ingredients are biologically compatible with pulp
      b. Fluoride ion release may reduce the incidence and severity of secondary caries (Fig. 13.12), but no definitive clinical research studies exist

## Topical Fluorides and Fluoride Varnishes

A. General considerations (see the section on "Fluoride Agents for Professional Application" in Chapter 16)
   1. Applications—used to prevent smooth-surface caries
   2. Classification
      a. Acidulated phosphate fluoride (APF) gels (acid pH)
      b. Neutral fluoride gels (sodium fluoride at neutral pH)
      c. Fluoride varnishes (5% sodium fluoride, 2.26% fluoride, 22,600 ppm fluoride)

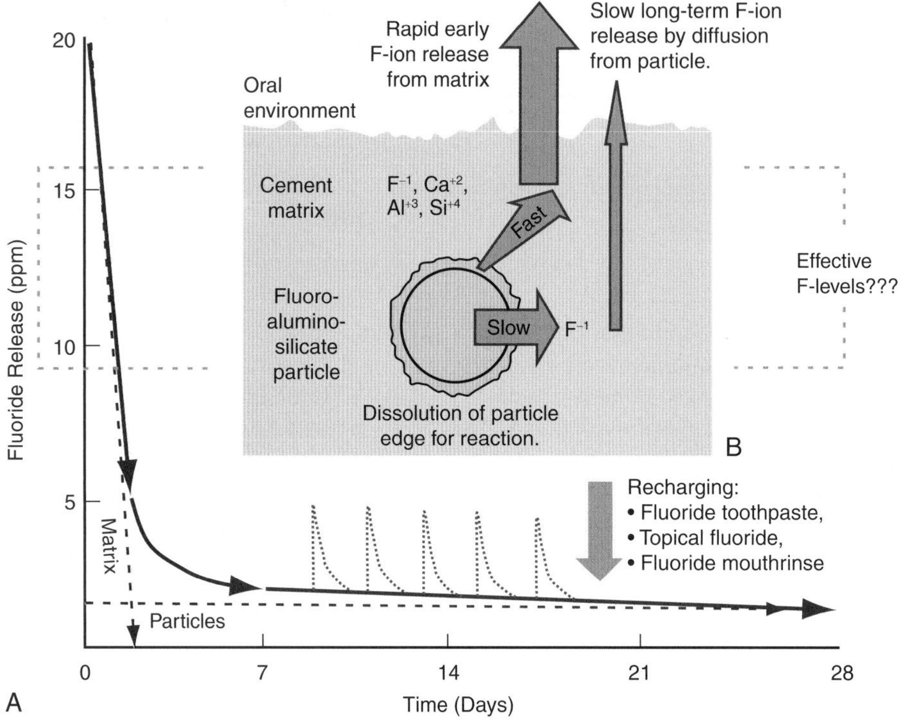


**Fig 13.12** A, Fluoride ion release from glass ionomer. Diffusion from cement. B, Fluoride concentration released over time. (From Bayne SC, Thompson JY: Biomaterials. In Roberson TM, Heymann HO, Swift EJ, editors: *Sturdevant's Art and Science of Operative Dentistry,* 5th ed. St Louis: Mosby; 2006)

B. Structure for APF
   1. Composition
      a. Acidulated phosphate fluoride
         (1) Fluoride ion concentration ranges from 1.22% to 1.32%
         (2) Ingredients—2% sodium fluoride, 0.34% hydrogen fluoride, 0.98% orthophosphoric acid, thickening agent, flavoring agent, coloring agent, and aqueous gel
         (3) pH ranges from 3 to 4; may dissolve glass in restorations, thus those surfaces must be protected
      b. Neutral fluoride gels
      c. Fluoride varnishes—fluoride source mixed with urethane or other resin and dissolved in solvent
   2. Reactions
      a. APF—acid demineralization of the outer layer of enamel; fluoride accelerates the remineralization of demineralized enamel; fluoride ions are incorporated to produce fluoride-substituted hydroxyapatite
      b. Neutral fluoride gels—form fluoride salts on surfaces of teeth
      c. Fluoride varnishes—provide temporary film to allow longer-term fluoride diffusion from varnish into enamel
   3. Manipulation
      a. Gels are applied in a soft, spongy tray after extrinsic stain removal; teeth should be free from saliva; maxillary and mandibular trays are loaded, placed in position, and squeezed to mold the trays tightly around teeth; the tray is held in position for 4 minutes (shorter applications are not effective); the client is told not to eat, smoke, or drink for 30 minutes
      b. Varnishes are painted onto all tooth surfaces; wear away after several hours

C. Properties
   1. Chemical—enamel solubility is decreased by fluoride ion incorporation
   2. Biologic—enamel is more resistant to carious dissolution

## Dentifrices and Prophylactic Pastes

A. General considerations
   1. Cleansing—removal of exogenous stains, pellicle, materia alba, and other oral debris without causing undue abrasion to tooth structure
   2. Polishing—smoothing surfaces (without significant abrasion) of amalgam, composites, glass ionomers, ceramic, and other restorative materials
   3. Factors influencing cleaning and polishing
      a. Hardness of abrasive particles versus that of the substrate (see Tables 13.1 and 13.2)
      b. Particle size of abrasive particles
      c. Pressure applied during procedure
      d. Temperature of abrasive materials
      e. Speed of the rotating instrument used (easiest factor to control)

B. Structure
   1. Composition—contain abrasives, such as kaolinite, silicon dioxide, calcined magnesium silicate, diatomaceous silicon dioxide, pumice, sodium-potassium–aluminum silicate, and zirconium silicate; some pastes also may contain sodium fluoride or stannous fluoride, but they have not been shown to produce therapeutic effects

2. Reactions—abrasion for cleansing and polishing
3. Manipulation (see the earlier section on "Properties," B. Mechanical properties)

C. Properties
1. Mechanical
   a. Products with pumice and quartz enable more efficient cleansing but also generate greater abrasion of enamel and dentin
   b. Coarse pumice is the most abrasive
   c. Dentin is abraded five to six times faster than enamel, regardless of the product used, and cementum is abraded even more quickly than is dentin
   d. Polymeric restorative materials such as denture bases, denture teeth, composites, and composite veneers can easily be scratched during polishing
   e. Ceramic restorations that are externally characterized should not be polished, or the surface color will be lost
2. Biologic—no known problems

## Whitening Agents

A. General considerations
1. Lighten discolored teeth
2. Classification by:
   a. Site of application
      (1) External—applied to the tooth surface
      (2) Internal—applied inside the pulpless (endodontically treated) tooth
   b. Method of application
      (1) In-office—applied professionally
      (2) At-home—dispensed by the dentist or obtained over the counter (OTC) and applied by the client

B. Structure
1. In-office systems use light, heat, or both to "activate" a high concentration (up to 30% to 39%) hydrogen peroxide gel or paste, but little evidence that light or heat provides any benefit
2. At-home systems typically use a 10% carbamide peroxide (equivalent to 3.4% hydrogen peroxide) or higher (15% to 20% carbamide peroxide) concentration that is applied in a custom-fitted, mouthguard-type, soft-plastic tray
3. New systems use thin polyethylene strips impregnated with 5.3% hydrogen peroxide (OTC) and 14% hydrogen peroxide (office dispensed)

C. Properties
1. The effectiveness of whitening depends on application time and dose
2. In-office whitening can provide faster results but is more expensive than at-home bleaching
3. Yellow-colored teeth bleach more rapidly than do gray-colored teeth
4. Tetracycline-stained teeth whiten very slowly (several months of daily at-home treatment needed) or not at all
5. Most common side effects are tooth sensitivity and gingival irritation; both are transient

# INDIRECT PREVENTIVE AND RESTORATIVE MATERIALS

## Impression Materials

A. General considerations
1. Applications
   a. Dentulous impressions
      (1) For casts in prosthodontics
      (2) For pediatric and orthodontic appliances
      (3) For study models in orthodontics
   b. Edentulous impressions for casts in denture construction
2. Terminology
   a. Rigid—inflexible and cannot be removed from undercut area
   b. Flexible—can be removed from undercut area
   c. Hydrocolloid—gel produced by interconnection of small particles (colloid, less than 1 μm) dispersed in water
   d. Elastomeric—based on flexible polymeric material
3. Classification
   a. Rigid impression materials (very limited use)
      (1) Plaster
      (2) Compound
      (3) Zinc oxide–eugenol
   b. Flexible hydrocolloid impression materials
      (1) Agar-agar (reversible hydrocolloid [limited use])
      (2) Alginate (irreversible hydrocolloid)
   c. Flexible, elastomeric, general-purpose impression materials
      (1) Polysulfide elastomer (mercaptan rubber [limited use])
      (2) Silicone elastomer (condensation silicone [laboratory use])
      (3) Polyether (PE) elastomer
      (4) Polyvinyl siloxane (VPS) (addition silicone)
   d. Precision impression materials used for prosthodontics
      (1) Addition silicones—contain surfactants to make surface wetting easier
      (2) Polyethers—more hydrophilic

B. Structure
1. Components (Table 13.3)
   a. Most contain fillers to control shrinkage
   b. Matrix
2. Reaction (Table 13.3)
   a. Physical reaction—cooling causes reversible hardening
   b. Chemical reaction—irreversible reaction during setting
3. Manipulation
   a. Mixing
      (1) Powder-liquid (P/L) types mixed in bowl (plaster and alginate)
      (2) Thermoplastic materials not mixed (compound and agar-agar)
      (3) Hand-mix—paste-paste (p/p) types are hand-mixed on a pad (ZOE, polysulfide rubber, silicone rubber, PE rubber, and VPS)

**TABLE 13.3 Impression Materials**

| Materials | Type | Reaction | Composition | Manipulation | Initial Setting Time |
|---|---|---|---|---|---|
| Plaster (limited use) | Rigid | Chemical | Calcium sulfate hemihydrate, water | Mix powder and liquid (P/L) in bowl | 3-5 min |
| Compound (limited use) | Rigid | Physical | Resins, wax, stearic acid, and fillers | Soften by heating | Variable (sets on cooling) |
| Zinc oxide–eugenol (limited use) | Rigid | Chemical | Zinc oxide powder, oils, eugenol, and resin | Mix pastes on pad | 3-5 min |
| Agar-agar (limited use) | Flexible | Physical | 12%-15% agar, borax, potassium sulfate, and 85% water | Conditioned in heated bath | Variable (sets on cooling) |
| Alginate | Flexible | Chemical | Sodium alginate, calcium sulfate, retarders, and 85% water | Mix P/L in bowl | 4-5 min |
| Polysulfide (limited use) | Flexible | Chemical | Low-molecular-weight (LMW) mercaptan polymer, fillers, lead dioxide, copper hydroxide, or peroxides | Mix pastes on pad | 5-7 min |
| Silicone (limited use) | Flexible | Chemical | Hydroxyl functional dimethyl siloxane, fillers, tin octoate, and orthoethyl silicate | Mix pastes on pad | 4-5 min |
| Polyether | Flexible | Chemical | Aromatic sulfonic acid ester and polyether with ethylene imine groups | Mixing gun or mixing machine | 4-6 min |
| Vinyl polysiloxane (addition silicone) | Flexible | Chemical | Vinyl silicone, filler, chloroplatinic acid, LMW silicone, and filler | Mixing gun or mixing machine | 4-5 min |

(4) Auto-mix—p/p types are mixed through a disposable nozzle on an auto-mixing gun (VPS, PE)
(5) Machine-mix—components mixed and extruded through a disposable nozzle using small machine (e.g., Dynamix speed, Pentamix 3)

b. Placement
(1) Mixed material—carried in a tray to the mouth (full arch, quadrant, or triple tray)
(2) The material sets in the mouth more quickly because of higher temperature

c. Removal—rapid removal of the impression encourages deformation to take place elastically rather than permanently (elastic recovery requires approximately 20 minutes)

d. Cleaning and disinfection of impressions (see the section on "Maintaining the Treatment Area During Client Care" in Chapter 10)

e. Problems—VPS may be inhibited from bonding at the surface of the preparation wall by the bonding agent and also may be dissolved by subsequent infection control solutions; components from latex gloves can contaminate the impression

## Provisional Materials

A. General considerations
1. Applications
a. While waiting for laboratory fabrication of cast restoration
b. While observing the reaction of pulp tissue
2. Terminology
a. Temporary—provisional or nonpermanent; range of use is 2 to 52 weeks
b. Short-term use—2 to 6 weeks
c. Longer-term use—6 to 52 weeks
d. Provisional materials—usually include both provisional restoration and provisional cement
e. Direct—set intraorally (in situ)
f. Indirect—set out of the mouth
3. Objectives
a. Physiologic objectives—protection of hard and soft tissues, pulpal protection, delivery of medication, stabilization of tooth, provision of function for chewing, patient comfort
b. Esthetic objectives—short-term resistance to staining
c. Clinical objectives—ease of use, low cost, ease of repair, low polymerization exotherm, minimal surface reactions on curing, absence of sensitivity reactions
d. Material performance objectives—fracture resistance, wear resistance
4. Classification
a. Provisional resins
b. Temporary or provisional cements

B. Structure
1. Components
a. Provisional restorations
(1) ZOE cement, with cotton fibers
(2) Acrylic P/L products
(3) Bis-acryl and bis-methacryl resin products
b. Provisional cements
(1) ZOE-based cements
(2) Calcium hydroxide cements
(3) Admix cements (cements mixed with petroleum jelly)
(4) Composite cements (without bonding systems)
2. Reaction (see the sections on "Dental Composites" and "Cement Liners")
3. Manipulation (see "Dental Composites" and "Cement Liners")

**TABLE 13.4 Gypsum Products**

| Characteristics | Plaster | Stone | Diestone |
|---|---|---|---|
| Chemical name | β-Calcium sulfate hemihydrates | α-Calcium sulfate hemihydrate | α-Calcium sulfate hemihydrate |
| Formula | $CaSO_4 \cdot \times ½ H_2O$ | $CaSO_4 \cdot \times ½ H_2O$ | $CaSO_4 \cdot \times ½ H_2O$ |
| Uses | Plaster models, impression plaster | Cast stone, investments | Improved stone, diestone |
| Water (W) | | | |
| Reaction water | 18 mL | 18 mL | 18 mL |
| Extra water | 32 mL | 12 mL | 6 mL |
| Total water | 50 mL | 30 mL | 24 mL |
| Powder (P) | 100 g | 100 g | 100 g |
| W/P ratio | 0.50 | 0.30 | 0.24 |

C. Properties
1. Physical
   a. Excellent thermal and electrical insulation
   b. Percolation resistance is good for cements but poor for resins
2. Chemical—generally good resistance to dissolution
3. Mechanical
   a. Good short-term resistance to fracture
   b. Poor resistance to abrasion
   c. Limited color stability and stain resistance
4. Biologic—cements are biocompatible, but resins with low-molecular-weight monomers may cause pulpal inflammation if cured in situ without caution

## Model, Cast, and Die Materials

A. General considerations
1. Applications
   a. Gold casting, ceramic, and porcelain-fused-to-metal veneer fabrication procedures
   b. Orthodontic and pediatric appliance construction
   c. Study models for occlusal records
2. Terminology
   a. Models—replicas of hard and soft tissues for study of dental symmetry
   b. Casts—working replicas of hard and soft tissues for use in the fabrication of appliances or restorations
   c. Dies—working replicas of one tooth (or a few teeth) used for the fabrication of a restoration
   d. Duplicates—second casts prepared from original casts
3. Classification by materials
   a. Models (model plaster, orthodontic stone, or 3D printed resin)
   b. Casts (regular stone or printed resin)
   c. Dies—may be electroplated (very limited use)
      (1) Diestone—gypsum product
      (2) Epoxy dies—epoxy polymer; abrasion-resistant dies
      (3) Printed resin—produced from digital files using 3D printer

B. Structure of gypsum products
1. Components (Table 13.4)
   a. Powder (calcium sulfate hemihydrate = β-$CaSO_4 \times ½ H_2O$)
   b. Water (for mixing and reacting with powder)
2. Reaction
   a. Calcium sulfate hemihydrate (one-half mole of water) crystals dissolve and react with water
   b. Calcium sulfate dihydrate (two moles of water) form and precipitate new crystals
   c. Unreacted (excess) water is left between crystals and slowly evaporates
3. Manipulation of gypsum products
   a. Selection—based on strength for models, casts, or dies
   b. Manual mixing
      (1) Appropriate proportions of water and powder are dispensed (Table 13.4)
      (2) The powder is sifted into the water in a rubber mixing bowl
      (3) A stiff-bladed spatula is used to mix the mass on the side of the bowl
      (4) The mixing is completed in 60 seconds
   c. Auto dispenser
   d. Placement
      (1) Vibration is used to remove air bubbles created through mixing
      (2) Vibration is used to keep the mixture wet and help it flow into the impression

C. Properties of gypsum products
1. Physical
   a. Excellent thermal and electrical insulator
   b. Dense
   c. Excellent dimensional accuracy (setting expansion)
      (1) Plaster: 0.20%
      (2) Stone: 0.10%
      (3) Diestone: 0.05%
      (4) High-expansion diestone: 0.20% (for all-ceramic restoration fabrication)
   d. Good reproduction of fine detail of hard and soft tissues
2. Chemical
   a. Heating will reverse the reaction, that is, decompose the material into calcium sulfate hemihydrate, the original dry component
   b. Models, casts, and dies should be wet during the grinding or cutting to prevent heating
3. Mechanical

a. Better powder packing and lower water content at mixing lead to higher compressive strengths (plaster < stone < diestone)
b. Poor resistance to abrasion (polymer added to improve resistance)
4. Biologic
a. Materials are safe for contact with external epithelial tissues
b. Masks should be worn during grinding or polishing operations, which are likely to produce gypsum dust
D. 3D printed resin—produced from digital files using 3D printer

## Waxes

A. General considerations
1. Applications
a. Making impressions
b. Registering of tooth or soft tissue position
c. Creating restorative patterns for laboratory fabrication
d. Aiding in laboratory procedures
2. Terminology
a. Inlay wax—used to create a pattern for inlay, onlay, or crown for subsequent investing and casting in a metal alloy
b. Casting wax—used to create a pattern for metallic framework for removable partial dentures
c. Baseplate wax—used to establish the vertical dimension, plane of occlusion, and initial arch form of a complete denture
d. Corrective impression wax—used to form a registration pattern of soft tissues on an impression
e. Bite registration wax—used to form a registration pattern for the occlusion of opposing models or casts
f. Boxing wax—used to form a box around an impression before pouring a model or cast
g. Utility wax—soft, pliable adhesive wax for modifying appliances, such as alginate impression trays
h. Sticky wax—sticky when melted and used to temporarily adhere pieces of metal or resin in laboratory procedures
i. Printed wax—produced from digital files using 3-D printer
3. Classification
a. Pattern waxes—inlay, casting, and baseplate waxes
b. Impression waxes—corrective and bite registration waxes
c. Processing waxes—boxing, utility, and sticky waxes
B. Structure
1. Components
a. Base waxes—hydrocarbon (paraffin) or ester waxes
b. Modifier waxes—carnauba, ceresin, beeswax, rosin, gum dammar, or microcrystalline waxes
c. Additives—colorants
2. Reaction—waxes are thermoplastic (soften on heating, harden on cooling)
C. Properties
1. Physical
a. High coefficients of thermal expansion and contraction
b. Insulators (cool unevenly); should be placed in increments to allow heat dissipation
2. Chemical
a. Degrade prematurely if overheated
b. Designed to degrade into $CO_2$ and $H_2O$ during burnout for inlay waxes
3. Mechanical—stiffness, hardness, and strength depend on modifier waxes used and on temperature

## Investment Materials

A. General considerations
1. Applications
a. Mold-making materials for casting alloys or castable ceramics to facilitate the creation of oversize mold space to compensate for shrinkage during cooling of casting alloy
b. Mold-making materials for denture production
2. Terminology—*investment* refers to the mold-making material
3. Classification
a. Gypsum-bonded investment (GBI)—based on gypsum products for matrix
b. Phosphate-bonded investment (PBI)
c. Silicate-bonded investment (SBI)
d. Specialty investments—for glass ceramics, titanium alloys, and other specialized fabrication procedures
B. Structure—66% filler, 33% binder (matrix forms on setting), 1% modifiers
1. Components
a. Liquid—water or other reactant starts the formation of the matrix binder by reacting with the powder
b. Powder—reactant powder, filler, or modifiers
2. Reactions and mold expansion
a. Setting expansion while material reacts, forming crystals that push on each other
b. Hygroscopic expansion while setting mold placed under water
c. Thermal expansion during heating of mold to casting temperature
d. Filler expansion caused by the inversion of crystalline lattice during heating
3. Manipulation
a. P/L is mixed and placed in a container around the wax pattern
b. After setting, the investment is heated to eliminate the wax pattern in preparation for casting

## Casting Alloys

A. General considerations
1. Applications—inlays, onlays, crowns, and bridges
2. Terminology
a. Precious (metals)—based primarily on valuable elements (Au, Pt, Pd, Ag, Ir, Rh, Rd)

b. Noble or immune—corrosion-resistant element or alloy
c. Base or active—corrosion-prone alloy
d. Passive—corrosion resistant because of surface oxide film (*passivation* is prevention of corrosion by formation of a thin, adherent oxide film on metal surface, which acts as a barrier to further oxidation)
e. Purity by weight (99.99% = "4 nines pure")
f. Karat (24 karat is 100% gold; 18 karat is 75% gold)
g. Fineness (1000 fineness is 100% gold; 500 fineness is 50% gold)

3. Classification
   a. High-gold alloys are greater than 75% wt gold or other noble metals (= 50% atoms that are immune)
      (1) ADA type I alloys are 83% wt noble metals (e.g., in simple inlays)
      (2) ADA type II are ≥ 78% wt noble metals (e.g., in inlays and onlays)
      (3) ADA type III are ≥ 75% wt noble metals (e.g., in crowns and bridges)
      (4) ADA type IV are ≥ 75% wt noble metals (e.g., in partial dentures)
   b. Medium-gold alloys are 25% wt to 75% wt gold or other noble metals
   c. Low-gold alloys are less than 25% wt gold or other noble metals
   d. Gold-substitute alloys do not contain gold
      (1) Palladium-silver alloys—passive because of mixed oxide film
      (2) Cobalt-chromium or nickel-chromium alloys—passive because of $Cr_2O_3$ oxide film
   e. Titanium alloys are based on 90% to 100% titanium; passive because of $TiO_2$ oxide film

B. Structure
1. Components of gold alloys
   a. Gold contributes to corrosion resistance
   b. Copper contributes to hardness and strength
   c. Silver counteracts orange color of copper
   d. Palladium increases melting point and hardness
   e. Platinum increases melting point
   f. Zinc acts as oxygen scavenger during casting
2. Manipulation
   a. Heated to just beyond melting temperature for casting
   b. Cooling shrinkage causes substantial contraction

C. Properties
1. Physical
   a. Electrical and thermal conductors
   b. Relatively low coefficient of thermal expansion
2. Chemical
   a. Silver content affects susceptibility to tarnish
   b. Corrosion resistance is attributed to high noble metal content or passivation
3. Mechanical
   a. High tensile and compressive strengths but relatively weak in thin sections such as margins; can be deformed relatively easily
   b. Good wear resistance except in contact with ceramic

## Dental Solders

A. General considerations
1. Applications—fabrication of cast bridges and metallic orthodontic appliances
2. Terminology
   a. Soldering—joining using filler metal that melts below 500°C
   b. Brazing—joining using filler metal that melts above 500°C
   c. Welding—melting and alloying of pieces to be joined
   d. Fluxing
      (1) Oxidative cleaning of area to be soldered
      (2) Oxygen scavenging to prevent oxidation of alloy being soldered
   e. Numerical terminology: 16 to 650 = 650 fineness solder to be used with 16-karat alloys; *fineness* refers to the gold or other precious metal content
3. Classification
   a. Gold solders—bridges
   b. Silver solders—gold-substitute bridges and orthodontic alloys

B. Structure of gold solders
1. Composition—lower gold content than of alloys being soldered
2. Manipulation—solder must melt below melting temperature of alloy

C. Properties
1. Physical—similar to alloys being joined
2. Chemical—more prone to chemical and electrochemical corrosion
3. Mechanical—similar to alloys being joined but weaker
4. Biologic—similar to alloys being joined

## Chromium Alloys for Partial Dentures

A. General considerations
1. Applications—casting partial denture metal frameworks
2. Classification
   a. Cobalt-chromium
   b. Nickel-chromium

B. Structure
1. Composition
   a. Chromium—produces a passivating oxide film for corrosion resistance
   b. Cobalt—increases the rigidity of the alloy
   c. Other elements—increase strength and castability
2. Manipulation
   a. Require higher temperature investment materials (PBI or SBI)
   b. More difficult to cast because less dense than gold alloys; usually require special casting equipment
   c. Much more difficult to finish and polish because of higher strength and hardness

C. Properties
1. Physical—less dense than gold alloys
2. Chemical—passivating corrosion behavior
3. Mechanical—stronger, stiffer, and harder than gold alloys
4. Biologic

a. Nickel may cause sensitivity in some individuals (approximately 6% of men, and 11% to 24% of women)
b. Beryllium in some alloys forms oxide that is toxic, which is a significant problem for dental laboratory technicians if grinding dust is inhaled

## Porcelain-Fused-to-Metal Alloys

A. General considerations
1. Applications—substructures for porcelain-fused-to-metal (PFM) crowns and bridges
2. Classification
a. High-gold alloys
b. Palladium-silver alloys
c. Cobalt-chromium alloys

B. Structure
1. Composition
a. High-gold alloys are 98% gold, platinum, palladium, or both
b. Palladium-silver alloys are 50% to 60% palladium and 30% to 40% silver
c. Chromium-cobalt alloys are 60% to 65% chromium and 25% to 30% cobalt, with other metals
2. Manipulation
a. Must have melting temperatures above that of porcelains (low-fusing porcelains) that will be fabricated onto their surfaces
b. More difficult to cast (see the previous section on "Chromium Alloys for Partial Dentures")

C. Properties
1. Physical
a. Except for high-gold alloys; others are less dense alloys
b. Alloys are designed to have low thermal expansion coefficients that must be matched to the veneering porcelain
2. Chemical—high-gold alloys are immune to corrosion; others passivate
3. Mechanical—high modulus and hardness
4. Biologic—biologically acceptable if they do not corrode

## Dental Ceramics

A. General considerations
1. Applications
a. Veneering material for PFM crowns and bridges
b. All-ceramic, high-strength inlays, onlays, crowns, and bridges
c. Denture teeth
2. Terminology
a. Ceramic—any inorganic material containing metallic and nonmetallic elements, generally formed at a high temperature
b. Porcelain—ceramic composition based primarily on silica, alumina, and potassium oxide; created by mixing clay, feldspar, and quartz, and then heating
c. PFM restoration—metal-based coping (substructure) coated with a porcelain veneer
d. All-ceramic—inlay, onlay, crown, bridge, or veneer made entirely of ceramic
e. Fusing—coalescence of packed layer of particles into a single porcelain mass
f. High-strength ceramics—ceramics that include one or more crystalline phases or strengthening mechanisms to make the composition mechanically more crack resistant than conventional porcelains
g. Glass-ceramics—initially noncrystalline (glassy) ceramics from which some crystalline phase is precipitated for strengthening
h. Glass-infiltrated ceramic—partially sintered ceramic particles that are infused with a glassy matrix (e.g., InCeram)
3. Classification
a. Feldspathic porcelains—produced by traditional laboratory fabrication with porcelain particles painted into position as a water slurry (condensed) and then heated for particle coalescence (sintered)
(1) High-fusing porcelains—for denture teeth
(2) Medium-fusing porcelains—for jacket crowns; not commonly used
(3) Low-fusing porcelains—veneering material for PFM restorations
b. High-strength ceramics—produced by specialized laboratory fabrication technique
(1) Lucite-reinforced porcelains—pressure molded
(2) Alumina-reinforced porcelains
(3) High-density alumina core materials
(4) Infiltrated materials—glass or resin infiltrated
(5) Hydroxyapatite-based materials
c. Glass-ceramics
(1) Mica-based glass-ceramics—used as starting blocks for CAD/CAM restorations
(2) High-strength glass-ceramic core materials, such as lithium disilicate or lithium silicate glass-ceramic
d. High-strength crystalline single-phase materials
(1) Zirconia (yttria-stabilized tetragonal zirconia)

B. Porcelain structure
1. Components
a. Large number of oxides—principally silicon oxide (silica), aluminum oxide (alumina), and potassium oxide, created by combining clay, feldspar, and quartz raw materials
b. Minor oxides contribute properties of opacity, translucency, and color
2. Manipulation
a. Traditional porcelain fabrication
(1) Porcelain powder mixed with water, padded onto substrate, compacted, and heated to produce coalescence with shrinkage
(2) Shrinkage is approximately 30% on firing (sintering); thus porcelain layer must be made oversized and built up by several stages of application
b. Special ceramic laboratory fabrication procedures—require specialized equipment and furnaces
c. Milling—requires specialized equipment

C. Properties
  1. Physical
    a. Excellent electrical and thermal insulation
    b. Low coefficient of thermal expansion and contraction
    c. Good color and translucency; excellent esthetics (superior to all other materials)
  2. Chemical
    a. Porcelain not resistant to fluorine-containing acids and can be dissolved by contact with APF topical fluoride treatments
    b. Porcelain can be acid-etched with hydrofluoric acid or other strong acids for providing micromechanical retention for cements
  3. Mechanical
    a. Harder than tooth structure and will cause opponent wear, although some glass-ceramics are comparable in hardness to enamel
    b. Can be polished with diamond pastes
    c. Poor fatigue behavior of glasses when compared with metal alloys
  4. Biologic—relatively inert

## Crown-and-Bridge Cements

A. General considerations (Table 13.5)
  1. Applications
    a. Luting inlays, onlays, crowns, and bridges
    b. Luting orthodontic bands and brackets
  2. Terminology—luting: attachment by gross mechanical interdigitation with crown and tooth surfaces
  3. Classification
    a. Traditional cements (typically P + L) (rarely used)—zinc oxide–eugenol (ZOE) and zinc phosphate (ZP)
    b. Polymeric cements (typically precapsulated or paste-paste)—polycarboxylate (PC), glass ionomer (GI), resin-modified glass ionomer (RMGI), resin or composite (CC), and universal cement (UC)

B. Structure
  1. Components (see Table 13.5)
    a. Traditional cements—powder (reactant; chemically basic); liquid (reactant; chemically acidic)
    b. Polymeric cements—polymer cross-linking reaction (PC, GI), polymerization reaction (RMGI, CC, UC), or both
  2. Reaction
    a. Traditional cements—acid-base reaction that forms salt; great excess of powder leaves residual powder as filler
    b. Polymeric cements—setting produced by cross-linking reactions similar to GI or composite setting reactions
  3. Manipulation
    a. Traditional cements—all reactions are exothermic; reaction controlled by chilling components, chilling mixing slab, or incrementally adding powder to the liquid
    b. Polymeric cements—powder is added to liquid as quickly as possible to complete mixing in 30 seconds or mixed in triturators and used quickly; may include preplacement of bonding system as well; paste-paste systems are dispensed using auto-mix syringes

C. Properties
  1. Physical properties
    a. All luting cements are electrical and thermal insulators
    b. All luting cements have low coefficients of thermal expansion and contraction
    c. Ideally 50–100 μm film thickness
  2. Chemical properties
    a. In acidic environments, cements tend to disintegrate
    b. PC and GI cements will adhere chemically to calcium ions on the surface of tooth structure and to oxides contained within the set cements
    c. PC and GI are most resistant to microleakage
    d. GI cements release fluoride ions (and most PC cements initially release fluoride because of small $CaF_2$ contents included as mixing aids)
  3. Mechanical properties—compressive strength; composite has the highest compressive strength, and ZOE has the lowest
  4. Biologic properties

**TABLE 13.5 Luting Cements**

| Cement | Abbreviation | Powder or Filler Components | Liquid or Matrix Components |
|---|---|---|---|
| **Traditional (or Conventional) Types** | | | |
| Zinc oxide–eugenol (ZOE), unmodified (limited use) | ZOE | Zinc oxide | Eugenol |
| Zinc phosphate (ZP) (limited use) | ZP | Zinc oxide | Phosphoric acid in water |
| **Polymeric (or Resin) Types** | | | |
| Polycarboxylate | PC | Zinc oxide | Polyacrylic acid in water |
| Glass ionomer, conventional | GI* | Fluoro-aluminosilicate glass | Polyacrylic acid in water |
| Resin-modified glass ionomer | RMGI* | Fluoro-aluminosilicate glass | Copolymer acid in water; water-soluble monomers |
| Compomer | CM* | Fluoro-aluminosilicate glass; silicate glass | Bis-GMA–like monomers |
| Universal cement (esthetic resin cement, adhesive resin cement, self-adhesive resin cement, RC) | UC or RC* | Fluoro-aluminosilicate glass | Bis-GMA–like monomers |

*Principal cements in use today.

a. Eugenol-based cements produce obtundent (pain-soothing) effects
b. PC and GI cements are most gentle to the dental pulp (when manipulated correctly)

## Acrylic Appliances

A. General considerations
1. Application—space maintenance and tooth movement for orthodontics and pediatric dentistry
2. Classification—none

B. Structure
1. Components
a. Powder—PMMA (polymethylmethacrylate) powder, peroxide initiator, and pigments
b. Liquid—MMA (methylmethacrylate) monomer, hydroquinone inhibitor, cross-linking agents, and chemical accelerators (*N, N*-dimethyl-*p*-toluidine)
2. Reaction
a. The PMMA powder makes mixture viscous for manipulation before curing
b. Chemical accelerators cause the decomposition of benzoyl peroxide into free radicals that initiate the polymerization of the monomer
c. New PMMA is formed as a matrix that surrounds the PMMA powder
d. Linear shrinkage of 5% to 7% during setting, but dimensions of appliances are not critical
3. Manipulation
a. The mixture of powder and liquid is painted onto the working cast to create the shape for the acrylic appliance
b. Orthodontic wires may be part of the appliance
c. After curing the mixture, the shape and fit are adjusted by grinding with burrs and stones, with a slow-speed handpiece
(1) Caution—acrylic dust is irritating to epithelial tissues of nasopharynx and skin and may produce allergic dermatitis or other reactions
(2) Grinding may heat the polymer to temperatures that depolymerize and release monomer vapor, which may be an irritant

C. Properties (see "Acrylic Denture Bases")
1. Physical
2. Chemical—may contain 2% to 3% unreacted monomer that can cause soft tissue irritation in approximately 4% of the population
3. Mechanical
4. Biologic

## Acrylic Denture Bases

A. General considerations
1. Application—used to support artificial teeth
2. Classification
a. PMMA/MMA dough systems
b. PMMA/MMA injected-resin systems
c. PMMA/MMA pour resins
d. UDMA VLC resins

B. Structure of PMMA/MMA types
1. Components
a. Powder—PMMA polymer, peroxide initiator, and pigments
b. Liquid—MMA monomer, hydroquinone inhibitor, and cross-linking agents
2. Reaction
a. Heat (or chemicals) used as an accelerator to decompose peroxide into free radicals
b. Free radicals initiate polymerization of MMA into PMMA
c. New PMMA is formed as a matrix around residual PMMA powder particles
d. Linear shrinkage—5% to 7% of monomer on polymerization; reduced by processing procedures
3. Manipulation
a. P/L mixed to form dough or fluid resin to fill mold
b. Mold heated to start and control reaction

C. Properties
1. Physical
a. Thermal insulator—prevents the patient's sensations of food temperature
b. High coefficient of thermal expansion and contraction
c. Poor distortion resistance at higher temperatures; therefore, dentures should not be cleaned in hot water
d. Good resistance to color change
2. Chemical
a. Stored in water before delivery to reach equilibrium absorption level
b. Absorbs water and must be kept hydrated
c. Not resistant to strong oxidizing agents
3. Mechanical
a. Low strength, but flexible; good fatigue resistance
b. Poor scratch resistance; clean tissue-bearing surfaces of denture with soft brush, and do not use abrasive cleaners
4. Biologic—occasional allergic reactions to minute residual monomer have been reported in newly processed dentures

## Denture Teeth

A. General considerations
1. Applications—complete or partial dentures
2. Classification
a. Porcelain teeth
b. Acrylic resin teeth—95% of all denture teeth
c. Abrasion-resistant teeth—composite veneered and interpenetrating network (IPN) teeth

B. Structure and properties
1. Porcelain teeth (high-fusing porcelain)
a. Bonded into denture base mechanically
b. Harder than natural teeth or other restorations and are capable of abrading those surfaces
c. Good esthetic appearance
d. Used when clients have good ridge support and sufficient room between the arches

2. Acrylic resin teeth—PMMA
    a. Bonded pseudo-chemically into the denture base; teeth are wetted with monomer before forming denture base
    b. Soft and easily worn by abrasive foods
    c. Good initial esthetics
    d. Used for clients with poor ridges and those who are opposed to natural teeth
3. Abrasion-resistant teeth (composite veneered)
    a. Bonded pseudo-chemically into the denture base
    b. Much better abrasion resistance than acrylic resin teeth but poorer bonding

## Denture Soft Liners

A. General considerations
1. Applications—for clients with soft tissue irritation
2. Classification
    a. Long-term liners (soft liners)—used over months for patients with severe undercuts or continually sore residual ridges
    b. Short-term liners (tissue conditioners)—used to facilitate tissue healing over several days

B. Structure
1. Soft liners—plasticized acrylic co-polymers or silicone rubber
2. Tissue conditioners—PEMA (polyethylmethacrylate) plasticized with ethanol and aromatic esters

C. Properties
1. Liners flow under low pressure, allowing adaptation to soft tissues, but are elastic during chewing forces
2. Low initial hardness, but the liner becomes harder as plasticizers are leached out during intraoral use
3. Some silicone rubber liners support the growth of yeasts

## Denture Cleansers

A. General considerations
1. Applications—for removal of soft debris, use light brushing and then rinsing of denture; hard deposits require professional repolishing
2. Classification
    a. Alkaline perborates—do not remove bad stains; may harm liners
    b. Alkaline hypochlorites—may cause bleaching, corrode base-metal alloys, and leave residual taste on appliance
    c. Dilute acids—may corrode base-metal alloys
    d. Abrasive powders and creams—can abrade denture surfaces
3. Techniques recommended for denture cleaning
    a. Full dentures without soft liners—immerse denture in solution of one part 5% sodium hypochlorite (Clorox) and three parts water
    b. Full or partial dentures without soft liners—immerse denture in solution of 1 tsp of sodium hypochlorite (Clorox) and 2 tsp of glassy phosphate (Calgon) in a half glass of water
    c. Lined dentures—clean any soft liner with a cotton swab and cold water; clean the denture with a soft brush

B. Properties
1. Chemical—cleansers can swell plastic surfaces or corrode metal frameworks
2. Mechanical—cleansers can scratch the surfaces of denture bases or denture teeth

## Mouth Protectors (Athletic Mouthguards)

A. General considerations
1. Applications—to protect against blows to the chin, the top of the head, and the face or to prevent grinding of teeth; typically used by football, basketball, soccer, and hockey players (contact sports)
2. Terminology—mouth protectors, teeth protectors, or athletic mouthguards
3. Classification
    a. Stock protectors—least desirable because of poor fit
    b. Mouth-formed protectors ("boil-and-bite")—made by client; improved fit compared with stock type
    c. Custom-made protectors—fabrication by dentist is preferred because of durability, low levels of speech impairment, and comfort

B. Structure
1. Components
    a. Stock protectors—thermoplastic co-polymer of polyvinyl acetate–polyethylene (PVA-PE)
    b. Mouth-formed protectors—thermoplastic co-polymer
    c. Custom-made protectors—thermoplastic co-polymer or polyurethane
2. Reaction—hardening during cooling
3. Fabrication
    a. Alginate impression made of maxillary arch
    b. High-strength stone cast poured immediately
    c. Thermoplastic material is heated in hot water and vacuum-molded to cast
    d. Mouth protector trimmed to within 2 mm of labial fold, clearance provided at the buccal and labial frena, and edges smoothed by flaming
    e. Gagging, taste, irritation, and impairment of speech are minimized with properly fabricated mouth protector
4. Instructions for use—client must:
    a. Rinse before and after use with cold water
    b. Clean protector occasionally with soap and cool water
    c. Store the protector in a rigid container
    d. Protect the protector from heat and pressure during storage
    e. Evaluate the protector routinely for evidence of deterioration

C. Properties
1. Physical—thermal insulators
2. Chemical—absorbs water and stains during use
3. Mechanical— after water absorption, tensile strength, modulus, and hardness decrease, but elongation, tear strength, and resilience increase
4. Biologic—nontoxic as long as no bacterial, fungal, or viral growth occurs on surfaces between uses

## Veneers

A. General considerations
   1. Applications—generally anterior maxillary teeth
   2. Terminology
      a. Extracoronal—bonded over existing enamel, that is, no tooth preparation
      b. Intracoronal—bonded into an intraenamel cavity preparation
   3. Classification by materials
      a. Direct composite veneer
      b. Indirect composite veneer (laboratory processed)
      c. Ceramic veneer (stacked or pressed ceramic)
      d. CAD/CAM ceramic veneer
B. Structure
   1. Components—composite, porcelain, or ceramic
   2. Manipulation
      a. Bonding—enamel etching and bonding
      b. Finishing and polishing must be done with care to avoid scratching the surfaces
   3. Maintenance
      a. Polishing with abrasive materials or scaling with metal instruments must be avoided
      b. The protector must be protected with petroleum jelly during topical acidulated phosphate fluoride (APF) treatments, or neutral sodium fluoride must be used
C. Properties
   1. Physical—good esthetic appearance; but some coloring may occur because of the composite resin cement used for bonding the veneer
   2. Chemical
      a. Composite veneers have good acid resistance
      b. Ceramic and CAD/CAM veneers should be protected from APF or other acids
   3. Mechanical
      a. Composite veneers are subject to scratching
      b. Ceramic and CAD/CAM veneers have good abrasion resistance
   4. Biologic—no known problems

## CAD/CAM Restorations

A. General considerations
   1. Applications—inlays, onlays, veneers, crowns, bridges, implants, and implant prostheses
   2. Stages of fabrication of CAD/CAM restorations
      a. Scanning—computerized surface digitization; acquisition of surface contours and geometry, can be intraoral or scanning of impressions
      b. CAD—computer-aided (assisted) design; digital design of restoration
      c. CAM—computer-aided (assisted) machining; fabrication of restoration from block of material
   3. Classification
      a. Chairside or in-office CAD/CAM systems
      b. Laboratory CAD/CAM systems
      c. Examples of CAD/CAM systems in dentistry
         (1) CEREC (DENTSPLY Sirona)
         (2) Planmeca Fit (Planmeca)
B. Structure
   1. Materials
      a. Feldspathic porcelains
      b. Machinable leucite-reinforced ceramic
      c. Machinable lithium disilicate and lithium silicate
      d. Machinable high-strength zirconia ceramics
      e. Metal alloys (limited use)
      f. Composites
   2. Milling
      a. Hard machining—milling solid shape
      b. Soft machining—milling partially sintered shape and final sintering to shape
   3. Cementing
      a. Etching enamel and dentin for micromechanical retention—use of phosphoric acid or self-etching primer
      b. Bonding agent for retention to etched surface
      c. Composite as a luting cement for reacting chemically with bonding agent and with silanated surfaces of restoration
      d. Silane for wetting and chemical bonding to etched ceramic (or metal) restorations and for co-reaction with luting composite cement
      e. Hydrofluoric acid for gel etching of silica-based ceramics or sandblasting of zirconia to create spaces for micromechanical retention on surface of restoration
      f. Ceramic primer for zirconia
C. Properties
   1. Physical properties
      a. Thermal expansion coefficient well-matched to tooth structure
      b. Good resistance to plaque biofilm adsorption or retention
      c. Good esthetics (for shade matching)
   2. Chemical properties—silica-based ceramics are not resistant to hydrofluoric acid and should be protected from APF
   3. Mechanical properties
      a. Excellent wear resistance (but may abrade opposing teeth)
      b. Some wear of luting cements but self-limiting
      c. Excellent toothbrush abrasion resistance
      d. Limited fatigue resistance caused by brittleness (low-fracture toughness of some glass ceramics) and initiation and propagation of cracks
   4. Biologic properties—excellent compatibility with natural tissues

## Dental Implants

See the sections on "Dental Implants" in Chapter 14 and "Advanced Instrumentation Techniques" in Chapter 17

A. General considerations
   1. Applications
      a. Single-tooth implants
      b. Abutments for bridges (freestanding, attached to natural teeth)
      c. Abutments for overdentures

2. Terminology
   a. Endosseous—into the bone; represents more than 90% of all current types
   b. Subperiosteal—below the periosteum but above the bone; second most frequently used type
   c. Transosteal—through the bone
   d. Endodontic—through the root canal space and into the periapical bone
   e. Intramucosal—within the mucosa
3. Classification by geometric form
   a. Endosteal root forms
      (1) Screws
      (2) Cylinders
   b. Other endosteal forms
      (1) Blades
      (2) Staples
   c. Circumferential
4. Classification by materials type
   a. Metallic—titanium (majority of types; uncoated and coated), stainless steel, and chromium-cobalt
   b. Polymeric—PMMA
   c. Ceramic—hydroxyapatite, zirconia
5. Classification by attachment design
   a. Bioactive surface retention by osseo-integration—integration of bone with implant; most favored type of attachment
   b. Nonactive porous surfaces for micromechanical retention by osseo-integration
   c. Nonactive, nonporous surface for ankylosis by osseo-integration
   d. Gross mechanical retention designs (e.g., threads, screws, channels, or transverse holes)
   e. Fibro-integration by formation of fibrous tissue capsule
   f. Combinations of the above designs

B. Structure
1. Components
   a. Root (for osseo-integration)
   b. Neck (for epithelial attachment and percutaneous sealing)
   c. Intramobile elements (for shock absorption)
   d. Prosthesis (for dental form and function)
2. Manipulation
   a. Selection—based on remaining bone architecture and dimensions
   b. Sterilization—RF glow discharge leaves the biomaterial surface uncontaminated and sterile; autoclaving or chemical sterilization contraindicated for some designs
   c. Handling—must be handled with an instrument of like composition; that is, titanium instruments used to handle titanium implants to avoid metallic contamination and localized electrochemical corrosion

C. Properties
1. Physical—should have low thermal and electrical conductivity
2. Chemical
   a. Should be resistant to electrochemical corrosion
   b. Do not expose surfaces to acids (e.g., APFs)
   c. The effects of adjunctive therapies, for example, 0.12% chlorhexidine gluconate mouth rinse must be kept in mind
3. Mechanical
   a. Should be abrasion resistant and have a high modulus
   b. During scaling operations, care must be taken to avoid abrading (e.g., with metal scalers or air-abrasive systems); see the sections on "Advanced Instrumentation Techniques" and "Selective Stain Removal" in Chapter 17.
4. Biologic—depend on osseo-integration and epithelial attachment

## Tissue Engineering

A General considerations
1. Applications—replacement of any orofacial tissues, particularly intraoral tissues
2. Terminology
   a. Tissue engineering—attempt to regenerate tissue for the body, either in the laboratory or in the patient, through manipulation of cellular material, biologic mediators, and natural or synthetic matrices
   b. Cells (in tissue engineering)—living cells that are either precursors of more differentiated cells or disorganized collections of cells that grow, divide, and organize into physiologically functioning tissue
   c. Signals—any physical, chemical, or biologic mediators (extracellular or intracellular) that initiate, propagate, or otherwise stimulate cellular development into fully organized tissue
   d. Scaffolds—any extracellular matrix structure (natural or synthetic, temporary or permanent, hard or soft) that provides a foundation for cells to become attached, organized, and proliferate to generate the tissue of interest
3. Classification by materials by tissue replacement therapies
   a. Autografts—from one's own body
      (1) Best chance of clinical success
      (2) Genetic match (no immunity problems)
   b. Allografts (or homografts)—from same species (usually from cadavers)
      (1) Can be antigenic (sensitize the patient)
      (2) Concerns about transmitted diseases
   c. Xenografts—from different species
      (1) Limited range of use (e.g., porcine heart valve)
      (2) Heavily treated before use
   d. Synthetics—entirely man-made
      (1) Can be metals, ceramics, polymers, or composites
      (2) Prone to long-term mechanical breakdown
      (3) Can produce a toxic response
   e. Tissue-engineered replacement—rebuilding tissues in the laboratory to be implanted, or causing the body to "rebuild the tissue" artificially in situ
      (1) Use of mixture of natural and synthetic materials
      (2) Offers the possibility of a "near-perfect" replacement
      (3) Can potentially solve transplant availability problems

B. Structure
1. Components
a. Cells (cellular material)
(1) Stem cells (undifferentiated)
(2) Specific cells (e.g., osteoblasts, fibroblasts)
b. Signals (biologic mediators)
(1) Growth factors, such as bone morphogenic proteins (BMPs)
(2) Genetic material
c. Scaffolds (matrices)
(1) Polymers—native (e.g., collagen) or synthetic (e.g., PLA/PGA)
(2) Ceramics—native (e.g., bone chips) or synthetic (e.g., Bioglass)
(3) Composites—combination of native and synthetic (e.g., hydroxyapatite-coated collagen fibers)
2. Manipulation
a. Design and grown human tissues outside the body for later implantation to repair or replace diseased tissues
(1) Not necessarily patient specific
(2) Ideal for large-volume need such as skin grafts
b. Implantation of cell-containing or cell-free devices (with appropriate signal molecules) that induce the regeneration of functional human tissues; guided tissue regeneration, for example, use of Perioglass combined with appropriate growth factors in treatment of severe periodontal disease
c. Development of external or internal devices containing human tissues designed to replace the function of diseased internal tissues
(1) Involve use of stem cells or specific differentiated cells from the patient
(2) Ideal for load-bearing tissues (e.g., bone, tendon)
C. Properties—physical, chemical, and mechanical properties should be similar to those of natural tissues

## WEBSITE INFORMATION AND RESOURCES

| Source | Website Address | Description |
|---|---|---|
| Clinicians Reports | http://www.cliniciansreport.org | Updates on dental materials and devices |
| International Association for Dental Research (IADR) Dental Materials Group | http://www.dentalresearch.org/DMG/ | List of all dental materials sites and dental materials manufacturer websites |
| MEDLINE/PubMed | http://www.ncbi.nlm.nih.gov/pubmed | Public access to National Library of Medicine (NLM) abstract index that includes all dental research abstracts for published articles in dental journals |
| Dental Advisor | http://www.dentaladvisor.com | Evaluation of current dental products |

## CHAPTER 13 REVIEW QUESTIONS

Answers and rationales to chapter review questions are available on this text's accompanying Evolve site. See inside front cover for details.

1. Which mixing method is used for some VPS impression materials?
a. Capsule in triturator
b. Mixing pad
c. Agitation using vibration
d. Spatula and a mixing bowl
e. Mixing nozzle
2. What is the final setting time?
a. Elapsed time from the start of mixing until the start of setting
b. Elapsed time from the start of the working interval until the end of the setting interval
c. The setting interval
d. Elapsed time from the start of mixing until the end of setting
e. The time available by the operator to handle and place a dental material
3. Which material does NOT set by polymerization?
a. Flowable dental composite
b. Hybrid glass ionomer cement
c. Gypsum-bonded investment
d. Polyether impression material
e. Pit-and-fissure sealant
4. Which material involves imbibition problems?
a. Pit-and-fissure sealant
b. Flowable composite
c. Glass ionomer luting cement
d. Alginate impression material
e. Zirconia
5. Which restoration is a good thermal conductor?
a. Glass ionomer cement
b. Dental amalgam
c. Packable composite
d. Zirconia all-ceramic inlays
e. Ceramic veneers
6. Which material may undergo crevice corrosion under plaque?
a. Polycarboxylate cement
b. Cast gold restoration
c. Ceramic orthodontic bracket
d. Zirconia
e. None of the above
7. Which one of the following is best for pulp protection?

a. Surface sealant over restoration
b. 1 mm of calcium hydroxide liner
c. 1 mm of remaining dentin thickness
d. 3 mm of composite restoration
e. 5 mm of dental amalgam restoration

8. Which term is not related to color?
a. Chelation
b. Munsel
c. L*a*b*
d. VITA
e. Metamerism

9. Which one of the following is not associated with electrochemical corrosion?
a. Crevices
b. Plaque
c. Stress
d. Passivation
e. Radiopacity

10. What is a material's strength?
a. Highest stress supported before failure
b. Maximum deformation before failure
c. Maximum elastic behavior before failure
d. Toughness
e. Resilience

11. Engineering stress is computed as:
a. Modulus multiplied by the plastic deformation
b. Difference between the total strain and plastic strain
c. Deformation divided by the original length
d. Applied load divided by original cross-sectional area
e. Deformation divided by the volume of the object

12. Engineering strain is computed as:
a. Load at yield divided by elastic deformation
b. Applied load divided by the total elastic deformation
c. Deformation divided by the original length of the object
d. Change between the initial and final strain divided by the time
e. Area under the stress-strain curve

13. What is another name for a material's stiffness?
a. Fracture strength
b. Modulus
c. Fatigue resistance
d. Brittleness
e. Toughness

14. What is the definition of an abfraction?
a. Fracture of amalgam margins resulting from creep and occlusal loading
b. Wear of occlusal surfaces of posterior teeth
c. Fractures oriented parallel to the long dimension of a tooth
d. Saucer or notch-shaped cervical tooth loss due to tooth flexure
e. Loss of a posterior tooth cusp due to cracks coming from an amalgam restoration

15. What primarily contributes to abfraction formation?
a. Toothbrush abrasion when brushing
b. Tooth flexure
c. Improper tooth development
d. Cervical caries
e. Excessive consumption of acidic foods

16. What property is being compared on the Mohs scale ranking?
a. Toughness
b. Resilience
c. Ultimate strength
d. Hardness
e. Fatigue

17. What is the Mohs' hardness value for enamel?
a. 2
b. 3–4
c. 5–6
d. 7
e. 9

18. Which phase in dental amalgam is strongest?
a. Ag-Sn
b. Ag-Cu
c. Cu-Sn
d. Ag-Hg
e. Sn-Hg

19. Which method of amalgam mixing minimizes mercury vapor escape?
a. Precapsulated alloy and mercury
b. Covered mixing arm on the triturator
c. Mortar and pestle
d. Friction-fit capsule
e. More rapid trituration

20. High-copper dental amalgam alloys involve what range of copper in their composition?
a. 12%–30%
b. 6%–12%
c. 1%–5%
d. 0.5%–1%
e. 0.1%–0.5%

21. What is the major advantage of high-copper over low-copper dental amalgam restorations?
a. Lower corrosion tendency
b. Greater polishability
c. Lower coefficient of thermal expansion
d. Lower thermal conductivity
e. Better compressive strength

22. What agency regulates exposure to mercury vapor in air during a 40-hour work week?
a. OSHA
b. EPA
c. CDC
d. ADA
e. FDI

23. What is the melting temperature of the Ag-Hg matrix phase in a set dental amalgam restoration?
a. 127° C
b. 137° C
c. 147° C
d. 157° C
e. 167° C

24. What is a major problem associated with polishing a dental amalgam?
    a. Burnishing of surface corrosion products into the amalgam
    b. Localized surface melting of the amalgam with mercury smearing
    c. Production of grayish color
    d. Smearing amalgam onto enamel to cause staining
    e. Creation of marginal ditching
25. Which guidelines advise on dental amalgam handling in the office and include polishing?
    a. EPA water quality standards
    b. EPA air quality standards
    c. ADA standards for recapture devices
    d. Best management practices
    e. Recycling of amalgam capsules
26. What is the principal reason for the shift away from dental amalgam use?
    a. Composite cost is much lower
    b. Patients prefer tooth-colored restorations
    c. Minamata agreement commits to reduce worldwide Hg use
    d. Patients desire all-ceramic restorations
    e. Improved dentin bonding techniques
27. What is the mechanical reason for failure of a high-copper dental amalgam restoration?
    a. Occlusal marginal ditching
    b. Creep
    c. Wear facets
    d. Bulk fracture
    e. Black or green tarnish
28. Which restorative material may be substituted for dental amalgam in posterior restoration applications in permanent teeth?
    a. Composite
    b. Glass ionomer cement
    c. Direct gold
    d. Porcelain restoration
    e. ART restoration
29. What is the reason an older Class V amalgam may have surfaces slightly elevated above surrounding tooth structure?
    a. Amalgams very slowly expand and without abrasion become extruded
    b. Amalgams are often poorly placed in Class V sites
    c. Excessive corrosion causes amalgam creep on facial surfaces
    d. Secondary caries may help extrude the amalgam surface
    e. Reaction of F ions with amalgam produces excessive surface expansion
30. Which one of the following is true about pit-and-fissure sealants?
    a. Sealants should be filled to improve their mechanical properties
    b. Tinted sealants are more useful than colorless ones
    c. Sealant inspection is unnecessary after 2 years
    d. Partial sealing of pits and fissures is better than no sealing at all
    e. Uncured sealant along air-exposed surfaces will finish curing in 24 hours
31. Which event does not alter an existing composite restoration?
    a. Extensive tea exposure
    b. APF application
    c. Tobacco use
    d. Gum chewing
    e. Whitening techniques
32. Which of the following is most likely observed with Class V composite or glass ionomer restorations over time?
    a. Ditching of the coronal margin
    b. Staining of the apical margin
    c. Surface roughness over a few years
    d. Resin discoloration over a few years
    e. Fracture of the restoration
33. What is the best management for a stained occlusal margin of a composite?
    a. Use of whitening toothpaste by the patient
    b. Swabbing of the margin area with a peroxide soaked cotton
    c. Heavy pressure during prophy procedures
    d. Brushing with abrasive toothpaste
    e. No treatment other than normal prophy procedures
34. Which one of the following is likely to be deceptive in appearance in a radiograph?
    a. Infiltrant
    b. Dental composite restoration
    c. Dental sealant
    d. Temporary restoration
    e. Glass ionomer restoration
35. Which one of the following is the primary use for infiltrant?
    a. Infiltration of non-cavitated proximal lesion
    b. Repair of secondary caries at the margin of a composite
    c. An alternative pit-and-fissure sealant
    d. Repair of deep proximal restoration leakage
    e. Sealer over lesions treated with sodium diamine fluoride
36. What is the most appropriate way to manage long-term wear or discoloration of posterior dental composite surfaces?
    a. Replace the composite with a dental amalgam
    b. Repair the worn areas with resin-modified glass ionomer
    c. Resurface the old composite with new composite
    d. Adjust the occlusion of the opponent tooth
    e. Replace the restoration with a new high-strength ceramic
37. Which procedure does NOT require phosphoric acid etching?
    a. Dental sealant
    b. Ceramic orthodontic bracket attachment
    c. Total-etch dentin bonding procedure

d. Self-etch dentin bonding procedure
e. Amalgam bonding procedure

38. What is required to produce good bond strength to dentin?
a. Drying of dentin
b. Pre-application of chlorhexidine
c. Post-curing with visible light
d. Hybrid layer formation
e. Long conditioning (etching) times

39. How do self-etching bonding systems work?
a. Wetting agent helps adaptation and replaces need for micromechanical bonding
b. New monomers chemically adhere to hydroxyapatite
c. Phosphoric acid is mixed with other components of the bonding system
d. Chemical bonding to collagen replaces need for micromechanical bonding
e. Acidic monomers replace need for phosphoric acid etching

40. Which one of the following is true?
a. Bonding agent films are very thin (1–5 μm) and not disturbed by polishing
b. Bonding agents may react with components of prophy materials
c. Regular bonding agents are close to the same thickness as dental cements (50–100 μm)
d. Bonding agents are very susceptible to discoloration
e. Bonding agents help to provide thermal protection to restorations

41. What product most likely contains water-miscible acrylic monomers?
a. APF
b. Pit-and-fissure sealant
c. Dentin primer
d. Resin surface sealer
e. Polishing paste

42. Which component of a dentin bonding system is most likely to cause skin sensitization in dental personnel?
a. Ethanol
b. HEMA
c. UDMA
d. BIS-GMA
e. Camphorquinone

43. What is the shorthand representation for a three-component total-etch adhesive?
a. E
b. EP+B
c. E+P+B
d. E+PB
e. EPB

44. Which material requires surface protection with petroleum jelly during APF application?
a. Amalgam
b. Porcelain ceramic
c. Cast gold
d. Orthodontic wire
e. Dental sealant

45. What is the primary purpose of fluoride in APF surface treatments?
a. Precipitate $CaF_2$ on tooth surface
b. Incorporate F ion into hydroxyapatite to increase acid resistance
c. Kill bacteria in the biofilm
d. Increase the resistance of teeth to discoloration
e. Repair leakage problems of pit and fissure sealant

46. Which constituent may have a palliative action on the dental pulp?
a. HEMA
b. Eugenol
c. UDMA
d. BIS-GMA
e. Calcium hydroxide

47. What is the primary component of most composite fillers?
a. Zirconium oxide
b. Aluminum oxide
c. Zinc oxide
d. Calcium oxide
e. Silica (silicon oxide or silicon dioxide)

48. Which one of the following dental cements does not include polymer as part of the matrix?
a. Polycarboxylate cement
b. Glass ionomer cement
c. Resin-modified glass ionomer cement
d. Composite cement
e. Zinc phosphate cement

49. Which material does not release fluoride?
a. Resin-modified glass ionomer
b. Compomer
c. Provisional composite restoration
d. ART restoration
e. Traditional glass ionomer

50. Fluoride-release from glass ionomer follows what pattern?
a. Rapid decrease to low level after 24 hours
b. Rapid decrease over 7 to 14 days
c. Some decrease after 3 months
d. Some decrease after 6 months
e. Some decrease after 12 months

51. What is the effectiveness of a recharging glass ionomer restoration?
a. Does not work
b. Increases F release for a few days
c. Increases F release for a few months
d. Increases F release for 1-2 years
e. Permanently re-establishes F release from the material

52. Which of the following applications typically involves an ART material?
a. Class I and II restorations
b. Class III and IV restorations in permanent teeth
c. Liner under composite restorations
d. Temporary crowns
e. Class V esthetic restorations

53. Which one of the following materials is a potent anticaries agent?
   a. Fluoride-releasing glass ionomer
   b. Tin oxide
   c. Ultraviolet light
   d. Silver diamine fluoride
   e. Zirconium dioxide
54. What is a new strategy to restore primary teeth with rampant caries?
   a. Extraction of all teeth
   b. Caries removal and restoration with fluoride-releasing resin-modified glass ionomer
   c. Caries removal, SDF or analog treatment, and/or GI restoration
   d. Infiltration of the lesions
   e. Caries removal and repair with calcium phosphate cement
55. Which impression material is a hydrogel?
   a. Alginate
   b. Polysulfide
   c. Polyether
   d. Vinyl polysiloxane
   e. ZOE
56. What happens to water phase in a set alginate impression?
   a. Stable over time
   b. Quickly lost from impression surfaces
   c. Quickly absorbs additional water from air
   d. Quickly contaminated by things in air
   e. Tends to move toward the bottom of the impression
57. Which statement about vinyl polysiloxane impression material is FALSE?
   a. Low shrinkage on setting
   b. Dimensionally stable
   c. Should be poured immediately
   d. Contains filler
   e. Accurate
58. Which application typically requires the strongest gypsum material?
   a. Denture fabrication
   b. Repairing casts
   c. Master cast
   d. Removable die
   e. Orthodontic model
59. What is the chemical composition of set gypsum product?
   a. Calcium sulfate trihydrate
   b. Calcium sulfate dihydrate
   c. Calcium sulfate monohydrate
   d. Calcium sulfate unhydrated
60. What is the chemical composition of gypsum powder mixed with water to form models?
   a. Calcium chloride
   b. Calcium phosphate
   c. Calcium carbonate
   d. Calcium fluoride
   e. Calcium sulfate hemihydrate
61. How much “water of reaction” is required for the actual setting of 100 g of calcium sulfate hemihydrate powder?
   a. 12 mL
   b. 18 mL
   c. 24 mL
   d. 32 mL
   e. 50 mL
62. Why is more water than the reaction amount required to mix plaster or stone?
   a. Water helps to absorb the heat from the setting reaction
   b. Additional water is used to control the reaction rate
   c. Excess water is needed for hygroscopic expansion
   d. Excess water fills spaces between powder particles for mixing
   e. Excess water stabilizes the dihydrate reaction product
63. What is the major difference between plaster and stone powders?
   a. Sterilization technique
   b. Powder particle packing
   c. Hydration state
   d. Color
   e. Crystal structure
64. Why does plaster require more water for mixing than diestone?
   a. Diestone undergoes a different reaction than stone
   b. Diestone powder particles are less porous and imbibe less water
   c. Diestone chemical reaction generates more heat and requires more cooling
   d. Diestone contains fillers
   e. Diestone powder particles pack more efficiently
65. Why should molten wax be applied slowly in thin layers onto dies?
   a. Promote wetting onto dies
   b. Minimize porosity
   c. Avoid distortion from thermal contraction during wax cooling
   d. Avoid sag due to the low weight of wax
   e. Avoid water absorption
66. What is the major component in most dental waxes?
   a. Paraffin
   b. Beeswax
   c. Ceresin
   d. Carnuba
   e. Microcrystalline wax
67. What is the main goal in the design of dental inlay waxes?
   a. Low hardness
   b. Low coefficient of thermal expansion
   c. Complete pyrolysis on heating to $CO_2$ and $H_2O$
   d. Low melting temperature
   e. High cost
68. Which statement best describes an investment material?
   a. Two fillers
   b. Two liquid binders
   c. Matrix, filler, and modifier
   d. Two filled pastes that are mixed
   e. Binder and accelerator

69. What is the principal advantage of phosphate-bonded investment (PBI) over gypsum- bonded investment (GBI)?
    a. Stronger
    b. Less setting expansion
    c. Faster reacting
    d. Lower cost
    e. More stable at higher temperatures
70. What is the karat designation for a 75% by weight Au alloy?
    a. 10 karat
    b. 12 karat
    c. 15 karat
    d. 18 karat
    e. 20 karat
71. In high-gold casting alloys, which element is primarily responsible for hardness?
    a. Ag
    b. Zn
    c. Au
    d. Pd
    e. Cu
72. What element is responsible for producing the corrosion resistance of stainless steel instruments?
    a. Cr
    b. C
    c. Co
    d. Ni
    e. Fe
73. What level of chromium is required in steel alloys to produce effective passivation?
    a. 10%–14%
    b. 14%–18%
    c. 18%–28%
    d. 28%–40%
    e. >40%
74. Which statement is false for a solder joint?
    a. More corrosion-resistant than parent metals being joined
    b. Not as strong as the parent metals being joined
    c. Categorized using a fineness scale
    d. Different from brazed or welded joints
    e. Typically gold or silver color
75. Which application does not use gold alloys?
    a. Cast alloy bridge
    b. Cast alloy crown
    c. Cast post and core
    d. Implant
    e. Partial denture framework
76. Which dental materials cannot cause nickel sensitivity?
    a. Stainless steel crowns
    b. Dental amalgams
    c. Some partial denture framework alloys
    d. Some PFM alloys
    e. Some orthodontic wires
77. What is the approximate incidence of nickel sensitivity for men?
    a. ~ 6%
    b. ~12%
    c. ~18%
    d. ~24%
    e. ~30%
78. Which event contributes to a relatively high nickel sensitivity level in women?
    a. Genetic differences
    b. Less protective skin and hair during metal contact
    c. Contact dermatitis from nickel-based jewelry
    d. Greater contact with stainless steel
    e. Greater contact with metal coinage
79. Which of the following is a practical definition of a ceramic?
    a. Glassy or crystalline brittle material
    b. Material with a Mohs hardness value of 5-10
    c. Any insulating material
    d. Material typically used as an abrasive
    e. Composition with primarily metallic and non-metallic elements
80. What are the three principal components of dental porcelains?
    a. Silica, calcium oxide, and alumina
    b. Alumina, potassium oxide, and calcium oxide
    c. Calcium oxide, magnesium oxide, and chromium oxide
    d. Silica, alumina, and potassium oxide
    e. Alumina, zinc oxide, and calcium fluoride
81. What component of dental porcelain contributes primarily to esthetics?
    a. Silica
    b. Potassium oxide
    c. Chromium oxide
    d. Titanium oxide
    e. Aluminum oxide
82. What is the main component of very-high-strength ceramic restorations?
    a. Silicon carbide
    b. Potassium oxide
    c. Chromium oxide
    d. Zirconia
    e. Silica
83. Which statement is true about feldspathic porcelain?
    a. Used to veneer metal castings
    b. Used for all-ceramic restorations
    c. Very high strength
    d. Poor translucency
    e. Difficult to color
84. Which one of the following dental materials is not a ceramic?
    a. Silicon dioxide (silica)
    b. Corundum
    c. Hydroxyapatite
    d. Zirconia
    e. Titanium dioxide
85. Which of the following is false for feldspathic porcelain?
    a. Brittle
    b. General category of ceramic
    c. Often used to veneer metal
    d. Based on silica, alumina, and potassium oxide
    e. Strength rivals zirconia

86. What is an ideal film thickness range for dental cements for luting restorations?
    a. 1–5 μm
    b. 5–10 μm
    c. <25 μm
    d. 25–50 μm
    e. 50–100 μm
87. Which dental cement composition requires staged addition of powder to the liquid during mixing on a chilled glass slab to control the reaction?
    a. Polycarboxylate cement
    b. Resin-modified glass ionomer cement
    c. Compomer cement
    d. Universal resin cement
    e. Zinc phosphate cement
88. What is the primary monomer involved in denture base fabrication?
    a. HEMA
    b. BIS-GMA
    c. EMA
    d. UDM
    e. MMA
89. Why are acrylic resin teeth popular for denture fabrication?
    a. Ease of cleaning
    b. Excellent wear resistance
    c. Easily bonded to denture base
    d. Light weight
    e. Best esthetics
90. What is the major problem for tissue conditioners during the first few days?
    a. Increased hardness
    b. Bad taste
    c. Loss of bonding
    d. Discoloration
    e. Fungal growth
91. How should mouth protectors be cleaned?
    a. Dilute chlorhexidine solution
    b. Cool soap-and-water solution
    c. Denture-cleaning solution
    d. Dilute chlorine bleach in water
    e. Ultrasonic agitation in baking soda solution
92. Mouth protectors are typically fabricated from what material?
    a. Impression material
    b. Gutta percha
    c. Composite
    d. Denture base resin
    e. Thermoplastic polymer
93. What does the "A" represent in "CAD/CAM?
    a. Augmented (or additional)
    b. Automated (or automatic)
    c. Assisted (or aided)
    d. Aged
    e. Aligned
94. What is the term for partial sintering, milling, and then final sintering of ceramic?
    a. High-temperature vitrification
    b. Soft machining
    c. Milling during vitrification
    d. Laser milling
    e. Hard machining
95. Which process does not harm the protective titanium dioxide surface on dental implants?
    a. Use of polishing agents
    b. Abrasive dentifrices
    c. Scaling with metal instruments
    d. Dental floss
    e. APF application
96. Which material is now being used for dental implants in addition to titanium?
    a. Zirconia
    b. Alumina
    c. Aluminosilicate
    d. Silicon carbide
    e. Porcelain
97. Which dental fabrication process is classified as additive?
    a. Inkjet printing
    b. CAD/CAM machining of composite
    c. CAD/CAM machining of zirconia
    d. Casting
    e. None of the above
98. What are the major requirements for tissue engineering?
    a. Collagen, hydroxyapatite, and signals
    b. Cells and collagen
    c. Cells and bone
    d. Cells and scaffolds
    e. Cells, signals, and scaffolds
99. Which biomaterial utilizes tissue from a cadaver?
    a. Xenograft
    b. Allograft
    c. Synthetic tissue
    d. Engineered tissue
    e. Autograft
100. Which of the following is not a scaffold material for tissue engineering?
    a. Gold wire mesh
    b. Polylactic acid (PLA)
    c. Bioglass
    d. Collagen
    e. Bone chips

## SUGGESTED READINGS

Powers JM, Wataha JC. *Dental Materials: Foundations and Applications.* 11th ed. St Louis: Elsevier; 2017.

Sakaguchi R, Ferracane J, Powers J. *Craig's Restorative Dental Materials.* 14th ed. St Louis: Elsevier; 2019.

# 14

# Periodontics

*Janet Kinney*

The vast majority of periodontal needs are related to the treatment of gingivitis and early periodontitis, the prevention of periodontal disease, and the maintenance of periodontal health after therapy. The demand for these services, provided by dental hygienists, continues to grow. An understanding of periodontics is critical to the process of dental hygiene care.

## BASIC FEATURES OF THE PERIODONTIUM

A. The periodontium is composed of gingiva, periodontal ligament, cementum, and alveolar bone (Fig. 14.1)
B. The function of the periodontium is to attach the teeth to the alveolar bone tissues of the mandible and the maxilla

### Gingiva

#### Definition

A. Part of the oral masticatory mucosa that surrounds the cervical portions of the teeth and covers the alveolar process of the jaws
B. Components
   1. Marginal gingiva (unattached or free gingiva)
      a. Unattached cuff-like tissue that surrounds all surfaces of the teeth
      b. Parts of marginal gingiva
         (1) Gingival margin—most coronal portion; located at or approximately 0.5 mm coronal to the cemento-enamel junction (CEJ)
         (2) Gingival groove—when present, it is located 1 to 1.5 mm apical to the gingival margin at the base of the gingival sulcus
         (3) Gingival sulcus—space formed by the tooth and the sulcular epithelium laterally and by the coronal end of the junctional epithelium (base of the sulcus) apically; a sulcular measurement of 1 to 2 mm facially and lingually and 1 to 3 mm interproximally is considered normal
         (4) Interdental gingiva—occupies the interdental space coronal to the alveolar crest (clinically, it fills the embrasure space beneath the area of tooth contact)
            (a) Interdental gingiva—consists of two interdental papillae (one facial and one lingual) that are connected by the concave interdental *col*
            (b) Col is absent when teeth are not in contact
   2. Attached gingiva
      a. Portion of the gingiva that is attached to the underlying periosteum of the alveolar bone and to the cementum by connective tissue fibers and the epithelial attachment
      b. Boundaries
         (1) Apically demarcated from the alveolar mucosa by the mucogingival junction
         (2) Coronally demarcated by the base of the gingival sulcus
      c. Width varies from 1.8 to 4.5 mm
         (1) Generally widest in the facial anterior maxillary areas and narrowest in the mandibular premolar facial areas
         (2) The width is not measured on the palate because it cannot be clinically distinguished from the palatal mucosa
   3. Changes in the width of attached gingiva result from changes at the coronal end

#### Histologic Features[1]

See the sections on "Oral Histology," "Oral Mucosa," and "Dento-Gingival Junction" in Chapter 2.

A. Epithelium
   1. Sulcular (crevicular) epithelium—stratified squamous, nonkeratinized epithelium that is continuous with the oral epithelium; lines the peripheral surface of the sulcus, extending to the coronal border of the junctional epithelium
   2. Junctional epithelium—stratified squamous, nonkeratinized epithelium that surrounds and attaches to the tooth on one side and attaches on the other side to the gingival connective tissue; new cells originate from the cells in the apical portion adjacent to the tooth and from the cells in contact with the connective tissue; epithelial cells are shed at the coronal end of the junctional epithelium, at the base of the gingival sulcus
      a. The junctional epithelium is more permeable than the oral epithelium
      b. The junctional epithelium serves as the route for the passage of fluid and cells from the connective tissue into the sulcus and for the passage of bacteria and bacterial products from the sulcus into the connective tissue
      c. The junctional epithelium is easily penetrated by the periodontal probe; penetration is increased in inflamed gingiva
      d. The length of the junctional epithelium ranges from 0.25 to 1.35 mm

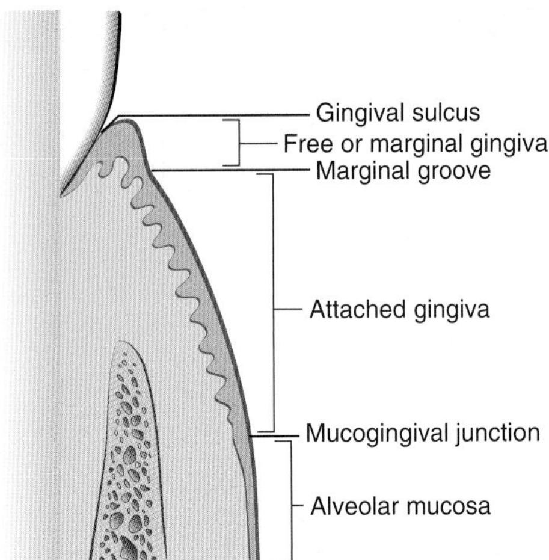


**Fig. 14.1** Anatomy of the periodontium.

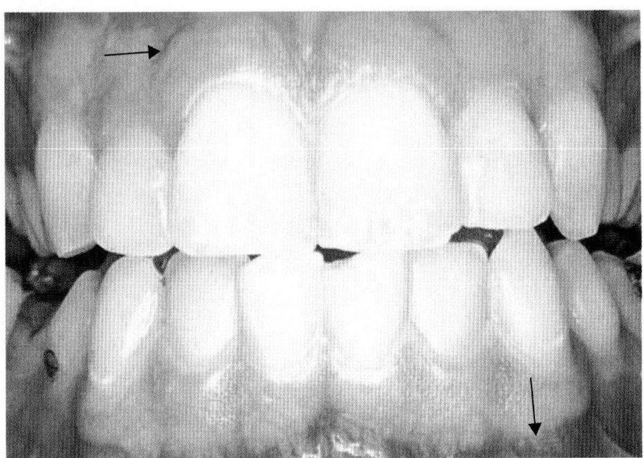

**Fig. 14.2** Normal/healthy gingiva in a young adult. Note the demarcation, referred to as the mucogingival line *(arrows)*, between the attached gingival and the darker alveolar mucosa. (From Newman MG, et al. *Carranza's Clinical Periodontology.* 12th ed. St. Louis: Elsevier; 2015.)

3. Epithelial attachment—basal lamina, hemidesmosomes, adhesion proteins (laminins), and anchoring fibrils that connect the junctional epithelium to the tooth surface at or slightly coronal to the CEJ

B. Connective tissue (or lamina propria)—composed of gingival fibers (connective tissue fibers), intercellular ground substance, cells, and vessels and nerves (see Chapter 2, Figs. 2.20 and 2.27)
   1. Gingival fibers—composed of collagen fibers (60% of connective tissue volume) and an elastic fiber system composed of oxytalan, elaunin, and elastin fibers; fiber bundle groups provide support for marginal gingiva, including the interdental papilla (see Chapter 2; Fig. 2.28B and the section on "Periodontal Ligament" for gingival fiber groups)
   2. Intercellular ground substance (or matrix)—similar to connective tissue in the periodontal ligament
   3. Cells
      a. Fibroblasts (predominant cells)
         (1) Produce various types of fibers found in connective tissue
         (2) Instrumental in synthesis of intercellular ground substanceWound healing or healing after therapy is regulated by fibroblasts (see the section on "Regeneration and Wound Healing" in Chapter 7)
      b. Other connective tissue cellular components—host defense cells
   4. Vessels and nerves (see the section on "Blood Supply, Lymph, and Innervation of the Periodontium")

### Normal/Healthy Clinical Features (Fig. 14.2)

A. Color—in light-skinned individuals, pale or coral pink; in dark-skinned individuals, coral pink to brown; color varies, depending on (1) the degree of vascularity, (2) amount of melanin, (3) epithelial keratinization, and (4) thickness of epithelium

B. Texture
   1. Gingival margin—dull, smooth surface
   2. Attached—stippled, "orange peel" surface present on facial surfaces; may not always be present in health

C. Consistency
   1. Gingival margin—firm and resilient; resists displacement
   2. Attached gingiva—firmly bound to the underlying alveolar bone and cementum

D. Contour and shape
   1. Papillary contour—pointed; papilla fills proximal embrasure space to the contact point
   2. Marginal contour—most coronal edge should form a knife-like edge with a scalloped configuration mesiodistally (follows the CEJ)
   3. The contour varies with the shape and alignment of teeth and with the size and position of contacts

## Periodontal Ligament

See the section on "Periodontal Ligament" and Fig. 2.27 in Chapter 2.

### Functions

A. Physical—attachment of the tooth to the bone, transmission of occlusal forces to the bone, absorption of the impact of occlusal forces, and maintenance of the proper relationship of gingival tissues to teeth

B. Formative—participation in formation of cementum and bone and remodeling of the periodontal ligament by activities of connective tissue cells (cementoblasts, fibroblasts, osteoblasts)

C. Resorptive—by the activity of connective tissue cells (primarily osteoclasts)

D. Nutritive—nutrients carried through blood vessels to cementum, bone, and gingiva

E. Sensory—proprioceptive and tactile sensitivity provided by innervation to the ligament

### Clinical Considerations

A. Thickness varies from 0.05 to 0.25 mm (mean, 0.2 mm), depending on the stage of eruption, the person's age, and the function of a tooth; the ligament is thickest in the apical area and is thicker in functioning than in nonfunctioning teeth and thicker in areas of tension than in areas of compression

B. Periodontal ligament cells that form collagen in ligament bundles can also remodel the ligament through secretion of new collagen (fibroblasts) and resorption of older collagen (fibroclasts), as well as lateral resorption of adjacent bone (osteoclasts) when altered forces are applied (e.g., orthodontics)
C. Accidentally exfoliated teeth can be reimplanted if handling of torn ligament is minimized before reimplantation; heal by reattachment

## Cementum

See the section on "Cementum" in Chapter 2.

### Clinical Considerations

A. Compensates for occlusal wear and continuous eruption by apical deposition of cementum throughout life
B. Protects the root surface from resorption during tooth movement
C. Has a reparative function, which permits reestablishment of new connective tissue attachment after certain types of periodontal therapies
D. When enamel and cementum do not meet, cervical hypersensitivity and caries are more likely

## Alveolar Process

See the section on "Alveolar Bone" and in Chapter 2.

### Shape, Thickness, and Location

A. The contour of the alveolar bone follows the contour of the CEJ and the arrangement of the dentition
B. The shape of the alveolar crest is generally parallel to the CEJ of adjacent teeth; is approximately 1.5 to 2 mm apical to the CEJ
C. Cortical plates generally are thicker in the mandible than in the maxilla
D. Posterior areas—bone generally is thick, and cancellous bone separates the cortical plate from the alveolar bone proper
E. Anterior areas—bone is thin, with little or no cancellous bone separating the cortical plate from the alveolar bone proper
F. Dehiscence—situation in which the marginal alveolar bone is denuded, forming a defect extending apical to the normal level, exposing an abnormal amount of root surface
G. Fenestration—situation in which the margin of alveolar bone is intact; an isolated lack of alveolar bone on the root surface leaves it covered only by the periosteum and gingiva

### Radiographic Features of the Normal Periodontium (Fig. 14.3)

A. Alveolar crest—thin, radiopaque line continuous with the lamina dura; the shape depends on the proximity of adjacent teeth and roots and level of adjacent CEJs
B. Interdental septum—proximal alveolar bone bordered by the alveolar crest

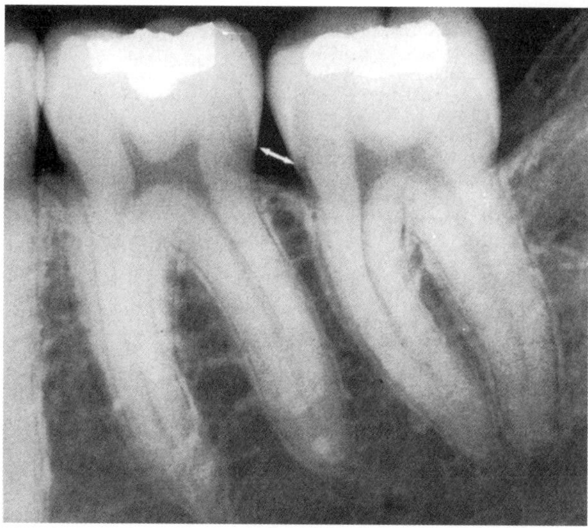

**Fig. 14.3** Crest of interdental septum, which is normally parallel to a line drawn between the cemento-enamel junction of adjacent teeth *(arrow)*. Note the radiopaque lamina dura around the roots. (From Newman MG, et al. *Carranza's Clinical Periodontology.* 12th ed. St. Louis: Elsevier; 2015.)

C. Lamina dura—radiographic image of the alveolar bone proper; may or may not be present as a thin radiopaque line surrounding the bone adjacent to the periodontal ligament
D. Periodontal ligament space—thin radiolucent line surrounding each tooth between the root and adjacent alveolar bone
E. Supporting bone—radiopacity of the trabecular pattern varies, depending on the amount, pattern, and presence of cancellous and cortical bone
F. Limitations of radiographs—radiographs:
   1. Do not show the relationships between soft and hard tissues
   2. Do not show the initial signs of early bone loss
   3. Do not show bone changes on facial or lingual surfaces; these bony plates are obscured by teeth roots
   4. Do not reveal current cellular activity; only reflect past events
   5. Have their diagnostic value affected by variations in technique

### Blood Supply, Lymph, and Innervation of the Periodontium[1]

See the sections on "Blood and Lymph" and "Nerve Tissue" in Chapter 2.

A. Blood supply originates from the inferior and superior alveolar arteries
B. Lymph drains into larger lymph nodes and veins
C. The nerve supply is derived from the branches of the trigeminal nerve and thus is sensory in nature; nerve branches terminate in the periodontal ligament, on the surface of alveolar bone, and within gingival connective tissue; receives stimuli for pain (nociceptors) and for position and pressure (mechanoreceptors and proprioceptors)

## DISEASES OF THE PERIODONTIUM

See the section on "Periodontal Diseases" in Chapter 9.

A. Importance of disease classification

1. Useful for dental hygiene diagnosis, prognosis, care plans, and legal documentation
B. Current classifications of periodontal diseases and conditions[2–12]
1. Periodontal health, gingival diseases and conditions
a. Periodontal health and gingival health
b. Gingivitis: dental biofilm-induced
c. Gingival diseases: nondental biofilm-induced
2. Periodontitis
a. Necrotizing periodontal diseases
b. Periodontitis
c. Periodontitis as a manifestation of system disease
3. Other conditions affecting the periodontium
a. Systemic diseases or conditions affecting the periodontal supporting tissues
b. Periodontal abscesses and endodontic–periodontal lesions
c. Mucogingival deformities and conditions
d. Traumatic occlusal forces
e. Tooth and prosthesis-related factors

(Table 14.1)

## Disease Classification: Periodontal Health, Gingival Diseases and Conditions[5–7] (Table 14.1)

A. Periodontal Health and Gingival Health[5]
1. Four levels: (1) pristine periodontal health (total absence of clinical inflammation); (2) clinical periodontal health (absence or minimal levels of clinical inflammation with normal support); (3) periodontal disease stability (reduced periodontium); and (4) periodontal disease remission/control (reduced periodontium)
2. Levels 3 and 4 are differentiated based upon ability to control modifying factors and therapeutic response

B. Gingivitis: dental biofilm–induced[6]
1. Associated with biofilm alone
a. Inflammation of the gingiva resulting from biofilm at the gingival margin
b. Most common form of periodontal disease; prevalent in all age groups
c. Change in gingival color and contour (redness, swelling, enlargement); increased sulcular temperature and gingival exudate; bleeding on provocation; reversible with biofilm removal
d. Sensitivity or tenderness can occur, although not present in all patients
e. Absence of attachment loss and bone loss is characteristic; after active periodontal treatment and resolution of inflammation in periodontitis, tissue becomes healthy, but attachment loss remains; dental plaque–induced (biofilm-induced) gingivitis on a reduced periodontium can occur in these patients if gingival inflammation arises without evidence of progressive attachment loss
2. Mediated by systemic or local factors
a. Sex hormones such as androgens, estrogens, and progestin modulate the periodontal tissues and in the presence of biofilm produce gingival inflammation
b. Puberty—occurs in adolescents during puberty in both genders when the dramatic rise in hormone levels has a transient effect on gingival inflammation; signs of gingivitis exist in the presence of relatively sparse deposits
c. Menstrual cycle—significant and observable inflammatory changes occur most frequently during ovulation but often not present
d. Pregnancy—some of the most remarkable endocrine changes occur during pregnancy because of increased plasma hormone levels; features are similar to biofilm-induced gingivitis, but little biofilm may be present; increased prevalence and severity have been reported. Pregnancy-associated pyogenic granuloma (pregnancy tumor) is a pronounced response of gingiva to dental biofilm at gingival margin in the form of a sessile or pedunculated protuberant mass; most common interproximally; regresses after parturition
e. Oral contraceptives—current low-dose contraceptives do not induce the clinical changes in the gingival tissues once reported
f. Hyperglycemia—commonly found in children with poorly controlled type 1 diabetes
g. Leukemia—primarily found in patients with acute leukemia; pronounced inflammatory response to biofilm with noted changes in gingival color and contour; increased bleeding on provocation
h. Smoking—a major lifestyle risk factor for periodontal disease; local and systemic effects observed; microvasculature and gingival fibrosis clinically observed; increase level of biofilm and rate of disease progression; reduced clinical signs of gingival inflammation
i. Malnutrition—vitamin C deficiency (i.e., scurvy) has been shown to have detrimental effects on the periodontium; more research is needed to determine the ill effects of other nutritional deficiencies on the periodontal structures
3. Modified by oral factors
a. Subgingival restoration margins—convex nature of subgingivally placed margins increase local accumulations of biofilm
b. Hyposalivation/xerostomia—can be a cause of diseases such as Sjögren's syndrome, anxiety, and poorly controlled diabetes; side effect of medications such as antihistamines, decongestants, antidepressants, and antihypertensives can also cause xerostomia; patient at increased risk of dental caries, taste disorders, halitosis, and inflammation
4. Drug-influenced gingival enlargements
a. Most often associated with:
(1) Antiepileptic agents (e.g., phenytoin and sodium valproate)
(2) Calcium channel blockers (e.g., nifedipine, verapamil, diltiazem, amlodipine, felodipine)
(3) High-dose oral contraceptives

TABLE 14.1 **Classification of Periodontal and Peri-Implant Diseases and Conditions 2017**

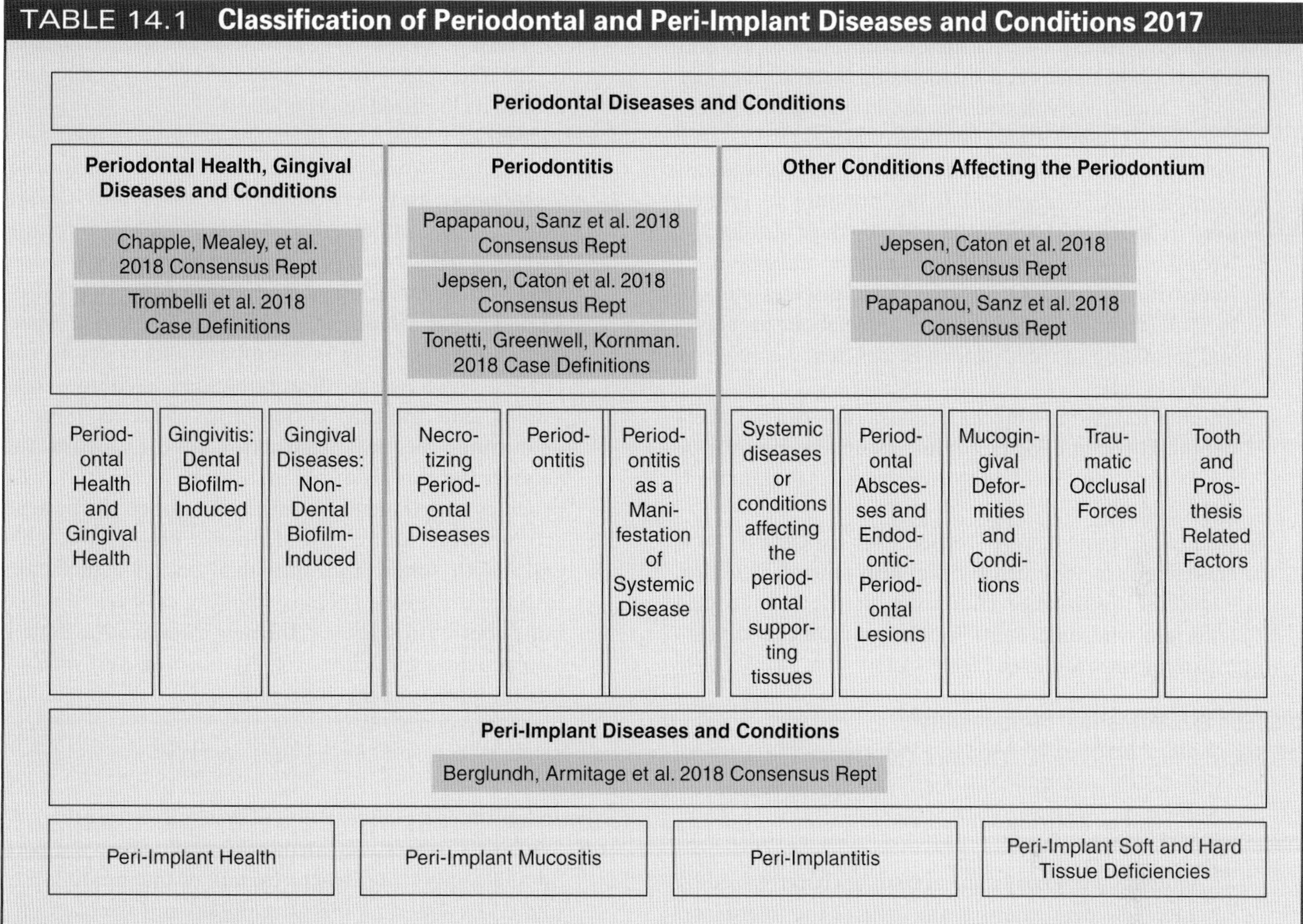


Caton JG, Armitage G, Berglundh T, et al. A new classification scheme for periodontal and peri-implant diseases and conditions - introduction and key changes from the 1999 classification. *J Clin Periodontol.* 2018;45 Suppl 20:S1–S8. https://doi.org/10.1111/jcpe.12935

b. Occurs most frequently in the anterior gingiva, especially in younger populations; onset within 3 months of drug regimen
c. Changes in gingival contour, size, and color because of enlargement; increased gingival exudate and bleeding on provocation can coexist; first occurs interproximally
d. Found in the gingiva, with or without bone loss; not associated with attachment loss

C. Gingival diseases: nondental biofilm-induced[7]
1. Genetic/developmental abnormalities—hereditary gingival fibromatosis (HGF) is a rare disease presenting as generalized fibrous gingival enlargement of tuberosities, anterior free/attached gingival and retro-molar pads; genetic mutation in *Son of Sevenless* gene
2. Specific infections
   a. Bacterial origin—necrotizing gingivitis (NG), necrotizing periodontitis (NP), and necrotizing stomatitis (NS) are severe infections in patients with underlying risk factors (poor oral hygiene, smoking, stress, poor nutrition, compromised immune status); the term "necrotizing periodontal disease" (NPD) is used to describe all three conditions; bacteria associated with NPD are *Treponema* spp., *Selenomonas* spp., *Fusobacterium* spp., and *Prevotella intermedia*
   b. Other bacterial infections—uncommon; arise when homeostasis between nonplaque-related pathogens and innate host resistance is lost
   c. Viral origin—most common are Coxsackie viruses, herpes simplex virus types 1 and 2 and varicella-zoster virus; primary infection usually occurs in childhood but may be observed in adults
   d. Fungal origin—most common is candidiasis; occur in immunocompromised patients
3. Inflammatory and immune conditions
   a. Allergic reactions in the oral mucosa are uncommon but can be caused by dental restorations, dentifrices, mouthwashes, and food allergens; signs and symptoms do not resolve when oral hygiene is instituted
   b. Autoimmune diseases of skin and mucous membranes—dermatologic diseases, including lichen planus, pemphigoid, pemphigus vulgaris, and lupus erythematosus, also may present with gingival manifestations; the diagnosis depends on clinical findings and biopsy specimens (see the sections on "Major Aphthous Ulcers," "Skin Diseases," and "White Lesions" in Chapter 8)

c. Granulomatous inflammatory conditions (orofacial granulomatosis) —persistent enlargement of the oral cavity soft tissues and surrounding facial region; can be concurrent with systemic conditions such as tuberculosis, Crohn's disease and sarcoidosis

4. Reactive processes—nonneoplastic proliferations; asymptomatic; exaggerated tissue response to limited local irritations or trauma; classified by their histology
5. Neoplasms—classified as premalignant or malignant
6. Endocrine, nutritional, and metabolic diseases—ascorbic acid (vitamin C) instrumental in metabolic processes and formation of catecholamines; deficiency is referred to as scurvy)
7. Traumatic lesions—mechanical trauma can be accidental, iatrogenic, or factitious; results in gingival or tooth abrasion, recession, ulceration, inflammation, or laceration
8. Gingival pigmentation—related to exogenous and endogenous factors such as drugs heavy metals, genetics, endocrine disturbance (Addison's disease), syndromes (Albright syndrome, Peutz-Jeghers syndrome) and post-inflammatory reactions. (Table 14.1)

## Disease Classification: Periodontitis[5-7]

A. Necrotizing Periodontal Diseases (NPD)[4]—term used to describe necrotizing gingivitis (NG), necrotizing periodontitis (NP), and necrotizing stomatitis (NS)
   1. NG
      a. Acute inflammatory clinical finding characterized by crater-like depressions at the crest of the interdental papilla that progress into the marginal gingiva
      b. Surface of the lesion(s) is covered by a gray, necrotized slough surrounded by an obvious erythematous (red) zone; interproximal necrosis
      c. Bleeding may be spontaneous and will occur even when necrotic tissue is removed gently
      d. Initially, moderate pain increases as the disease advances
      e. Strong, fetid odor and increased salivation
      f. Swelling and tenderness of regional lymph nodes (especially submandibular nodes)
      g. Fever and malaise may be present
   2. Necrotizing ulcerative periodontitis
      a. Inflammatory condition of the periodontium characterized by necrosis/ulcer of the interdental papillae
      b. Gingival bleeding, halitosis, and pain
      c. Rapid destruction of periodontal attachment and bone loss
      d. Pseudomembrane formation, lymphadenopathy, and fever can be common
   3. NS
      a. Severe inflammatory condition of the periodontium and oral cavity
      b. Occurs in persons who have human immunodeficiency virus (HIV) infection or acquired immunodeficiency syndrome (AIDS), other immunocompromising diseases, or severe malnutrition
      c. May lead to exposure of the alveolar bone and sequestration
      d. Chief complaint may be "jaw pain" or "deep aching pain"
      e. Can be localized or generalized

B. Periodontitis[2,3]
   1. At the 2017 World Workshop on the Classification of Periodontal and Peri-implant Diseases and Conditions, a new framework for identifying periodontitis was accepted. Changes made to the former system were based upon emerging new evidence from population studies, basic science investigations, and the prospective studies assessing environment and systemic risk factors. The new classification system is composed of staging and grading periodontitis patients. Staging determines the past destruction of the disease and assesses the complexity of managing the case. Grading provides supplemental information about the patient, estimates the future risk of disease progression, general health status, and individual patient risk factors into the diagnosis, such as smoking or level of metabolic control in diabetes. The new classification system also provides guidelines for establishing peri-implant health, peri-implant mucositis, and peri-implantitis (see Chapter 14).

(Table 14.2)

(Table 14.3)

C. Periodontitis as a manifestation of systemic diseases[8,9]
   1. Systemic diseases and medications can affect the periodontal supporting structures; rare or uncommon; profound loss of periodontal attachments and alveolar bone; periodontal destruction is often the first sign of disease
   2. Example is Papillon Lefévre syndrome
   3. Categories are based on the magnitude of impact (major, moderate, and destruction independent of plaque-induced disease) on the periodontal apparatus as well as the mechanisms by which they affect the periodontium
   4. Systemic disorders that have a major impact on the loss of periodontal tissue by influencing periodontal inflammation include genetic disorders, diseases affecting the oral mucosa and gingival tissue, diseases affecting connective tissues, metabolic and endocrine disorders, AIDS, and inflammatory diseases
   5. Systemic disorders which have an impact on the loss of periodontal structures by influencing the pathogenesis of periodontal diseases include emotional stress and depression, smoking, and medications such as cytotoxic chemotherapeutics
   6. Systemic conditions affecting the periodontal structures independent of periodontitis often mimic clinical characteristics of periodontitis and can only be differentiated from periodontitis by biopsy and histopathologic examination

## Disease Classification: Other Conditions Affecting the Periodontium

A. Systemic diseases or conditions affecting the periodontal supporting tissues[8,9]

## TABLE 14.2 Periodontitis Staging

| PERIODONTITIS STAGE | | Stage I | Stage II | Stage III | Stage IV |
|---|---|---|---|---|---|
| **Severity** | **Interdental CAL site of greatest loss** | 1 to 2 mm | 3 to 4 mm | ≥5 mm | ≥5 mm |
| | **Radiographic bone loss** | Coronal third (<15%) | Coronal third (15% to 33%) | Extending to mid-third of root and beyond | Extending to mid-third of root and beyond |
| | **Tooth loss** | No tooth loss due to periodontitis | | Tooth loss due to periodontitis of ≤4 teeth | Tooth loss due to periodontitis of ≥5 teeth |
| **Complexity** | **Local** | Maximum probing depth ≤4 mm<br>Mostly horizontal bone loss | Maximum probing depth ≤5 mm<br>Mostly horizontal bone loss | In addition to stage II complexity: probing depth ≥ 6 mm<br>Vertical bone loss ≥3 mm<br>Furcation involvement Class II or III<br>Moderate ridge defect | In addition to stage III complexity: need for complex rehabilitation due to: masticatory dysfunction<br>Secondary occlusal trauma (tooth mobility degree ≥2)<br>Severe ridge defect<br>Bite collapse, drifting, flaring<br>Less than 20 remaining teeth (10 opposing pairs) |
| **Extent and Distribution** | **Add to stage as descriptor** | For each stage, describe extent as localized (<30% of teeth involved), generalized, or molar/incisor pattern | | | |

The initial stage should be determined using CAL; if not available then RBL should be used. Information on tooth loss that can be attributed primarily to periodontitis, if available, may modify stage definition. This is the case even in the absence of complexity factors. Complexity factors may shift the stage to a higher level, for example furcation II or III would shift to either stage III or IV irrespective of CAL. The distinction between stage III and stage IV is primarily based on complexity factors. For example, a high level of tooth mobility and/or posterior bite collapse would indicate a stage IV diagnosis. For any given case only some, not all, complexity factors may be present; however, in general it only takes one complexity factor to shift the diagnosis to a higher stage. It should be emphasized that these case definitions are guidelines that should be applied using sound clinical judgment to arrive at the most appropriate clinical diagnosis. For posttreatment patients CAL and RBL are still the primary stage determinants. If a stage-shifting complexity factor(s) is eliminated by treatment, the stage should not retrogress to a lower stage since the original stage complexity factor should always be considered in maintenance phase management.
*CAL*, clinical attachment loss; *RBL*, radiographic bone loss.
(From Tonetti MS, Greenwell H, Kornman KS. *J Periodontol.* 2018;89(Suppl 1):S159–S172.)

## TABLE 14.3 Periodontitis Grading

| PERIODONTITIS GRADE | | | Grade A: slow rate of progression | Grade B: moderate rate of progression | Grade C: rapid rate of progression |
|---|---|---|---|---|---|
| **Primary criteria** | Direct evidence of progression | Longitudinal data (radiographic bone loss or CAL) | Evidence of no loss over 5 years | <2 mm over 5 years | ≥2 mm over 5 years |
| | Indirect evidence of progression | % bone loss/age | <0.25 | 0.25 to 1.0 | >1.0 |
| | | Case phenotype | Heavy biofilm deposits with low levels of destruction | Destruction commensurate with biofilm deposits | Destruction exceeds expectation given biofilm deposits; specific clinical patterns suggestive of periods of rapid progression and/or early onset disease (e.g., molar/incisor pattern; lack of expected response to standard bacterial control therapies) |
| **Grade modifiers** | Risk Factors | Smoking | Nonsmoker | Smoker <10 cigarettes/day | Smoker ≥10 cigarettes/day |
| | | Diabetes | Normoglycemic/ no diagnosis of diabetes | HbA1c <7.0% in patients with diabetes | HbA1c ≥7.0% in patients with diabetes |
| **Risk of systemic impact of periodontitis (a)** | Inflammatory burden | High sensitivity CRP (hsCRP) | <1 mg/L | 1 to 3 mg/L | >3 mg/L |
| **Biomarkers** | Indicators of CAL/ bone loss | Saliva, gingival crevicular fluid, serum | ? | ? | ? |

Grade should be used as an indicator of the rate of periodontitis progression. The primary criteria are either direct or indirect evidence of progression. Whenever available, direct evidence is used; in its absence indirect estimation is made using bone loss as a function of age at the most affected tooth or case presentation (radiographic bone loss expressed as percentage of root length divided by the age of the subject, RBL/age). Clinicians should initially assume grade B disease and seek specific evidence to shift towards grade A or C, if available. Once grade is established based on evidence of progression, it can be modified based on the presence of risk factors. (a) Refers to increased risk that periodontitis may be an inflammatory comorbidity for the specific patient. CRP values represent a summation of the patient's overall systemic inflammation, which may be in part influenced by periodontitis, but otherwise is an he specific patient. CRP values represebe valuable to assess in collaboration with the patient's physicians. The grey color of the table cells refers to the need to substantiate with specific evidence. This element is placed in the table to draw attention to this dimension of the biology of periodontitis. It is envisaged that in the future it will be possible to integrate the information into periodontitis grade to highlight the potential of systemic impact of the disease in the specific case. Question marks in the last row indicate that specific biomarkers and their thresholds may be incorporated in the table as evidence will become available.
*HbA1c*, Glycated hemoglobin; hsCRP, high sensitivity C-reactive protein; PA, periapical; CAL, clinical attachment loss.
(From Tonetti MS, Greenwell H, Kornman KS, *J Periodontol.* 2018;89(Suppl 1):S159–S172.)

1. A new classification of periodontal diseases
2. Affect the periodontal structure independent of biofilm-induced periodontitis

B. Periodontal abscesses and endodontic–periodontal lesions
1. Most frequently occur in existing periodontal pockets; presentation of localized accumulation of exudate in the pocket; patient at risk for systemic effects of the infection; classified according to the etiology of the abscess
2. Microbiology—*Streptococcus viridans* is the most common isolate; similar to microbiota found in deep periodontal pockets
3. Factors associated with abscess formation
   a. Occlusion of pocket orifices or incomplete calculus removal during treatment
   b. Periodontal pocket
   c. Furcation involvement
   d. Systemic antibiotic treatment
   e. Diabetes mellitus
4. Periodontal abscesses
   a. Gingival abscess—a localized purulent infection involving the marginal gingiva or interdental papilla; may have bluish hue; does not involve the underlying periodontium
   b. Periodontal (or lateral) abscess[1]—localized, purulent area of inflammation within periodontal tissue
      (1) Clinical findings—the abscess may be:
         (a) In the supporting periodontal tissues lateral to the root; may result in a sinus (fistula) opening through the bone extending out to the external surface
         (b) In the soft tissue wall of a deep periodontal pocket, adjacent to a periapical lesion, or after deep scaling or periodontal debridement if incomplete
         (c) Acute or chronic
            [1] Acute—extreme pain, sensitivity, mobility, enlarged lymph nodes; the gingival area is edematous, red, and smooth with a shiny surface; exudate may be expressed from the gingival margin on pressure
            [2] Chronic—usually asymptomatic or episodes of dull pain; elevation of the tooth; desire to grind on the tooth (may have acute episodes)
      (2) Radiographic findings (many variations according to the location, stage, and extent of the lesion)—typical appearance is that of a discrete radiolucent area along the lateral aspect of the root
      (3) Treatment—debridement with 0.12% chlorhexidine or povidone–iodine irrigation; antibiotics if fever, swelling, or lymph node involvement is present; combined periodontic–endodontic therapy if related to periapical abscess
   c. Pericoronal abscess—inflammation of the tissue flap (operculum) surrounding the crown of a partially erupted tooth; also called *pericoronitis*; most common in third-molar areas; may be acute, subacute, or chronic
      (1) Clinical findings if acute
         (a) An extremely red, swollen lesion with exudate is present
         (b) The area is painful; may radiate to the ear, throat, and floor of the mouth
         (c) A foul taste is present in the mouth
         (d) Inflammation may progress so that swelling, inability to close the jaw, fever, and malaise occur; the symptoms are less obvious when chronic
      (2) Cause—accumulation of food debris and bacterial growth between the soft tissue flap and the tooth; inflammation may be compounded by trauma from the opposing tooth
      (3) Treatment
         (a) Antibiotics if fever, swelling, or lymphadenopathy is present
         (b) Cleansing of the area (lavage, debridement) and creation of access for the drainage of the exudate
         (c) Frequent rinsing with warm water and return for follow-up care after 24 hours
         (d) Extraction of the involved tooth or removal (excision) of the soft tissue flap after the pain subsides and the infection is controlled
5. Endodontic–periodontal lesions
   a. Pathologic communication between the pulpal and periodontal tissues; pulpal lesion can subsequently affect the periodontium, periodontal destruction can affect the root canal or cause concomitant occurrence of both pathologies; can be acute or chronic; classified by etiology
      (1) Endo-periodontal lesion with root damage—further broken down by root fracture or cracking; root canal or pulp chamber perforation; or external root resorption
      (2) Endo-periodontal lesion without root damage—further broken down to lesion in periodontitis patient or in nonperiodontitis patient

C. Mucogingival deformities and conditions[10]
1. Highly prevalent; lack of keratinized tissue and gingival recession are most common
2. Gingival recession—apical migration of the gingival margin in relation to the CEJ; associated with attachment loss; frequently observed in adults; increases with age; observed in patients with adequate and inadequate home care; impact includes negative esthetic outcomes, dentin hypersensitivity, and carious and noncarious cervical lesions
   a. Etiology—unclear but predisposing factors have been identified:

(1) Thin periodontal biotype, absence of attached gingiva, and reduced thickness of the alveolar bone due to abnormal tooth position
(2) Improper toothbrushing—duration of toothbrushing, brushing force, frequency of changing the toothbrush, bristle hardness, and brushing technique
(3) Cervical restoration margins—low level of evidence supporting the placement of intra-sulcular restoration margins on gingival recession
(4) Orthodontics—during or after treatment; direction of tooth movement and the bucco-lingual thickness of the gingival may affect occurrence of gingival recession
(5) Other conditions—low level of evidence supporting chronic gingival inflammation results in gingival recession

b. Clinical significance
(1) Exposed roots are susceptible to dental caries and abrasion
(2) Wearing away of cementum on the exposed surface exposes dentin, which may be sensitive to mechanical, chemical, or thermal stimuli
(3) Interproximal recession creates space for the accumulation of biofilm and debris

c. Treatment—nonsurgical or surgical
(1) Removal of causative or risk factors
(2) Daily thorough oral self-care practices and periodontal maintenance
(3) Root desensitization, if needed
(4) Gingival graft, regenerative, or periodontal flap surgery may be performed

D. Traumatic occlusal forces[11]
1. Occlusal trauma and excessive occlusal forces remains a controversial subject; do not initiate periodontitis or loss of connective tissue; when occlusal trauma and plaque-induced periodontitis

E. Tooth- and prosthesis-related factors[12]
6 Multiple tooth- and prosthetic-related factors have the potential to increase the likelihood for plaque retention and lead to gingival inflammation, loss of attachment, and hypersensitivity reactions
a. Tooth-related factors include cervical enamel projections and enamel pearls, developmental grooves, fractures (tooth and root), root resorption, tooth position, root proximity, and open contacts
b. Fixed dental restorations and prostheses include class II restorations and overhang margins
c. Dental materials include the surface characteristics and the location in relation to the gingiva; metal ions and particles have been found in plaque, the periodontium and several organs and tissues; hypersensitivity reactions can appear as gingivitis
d. Removable dental prostheses—in the presence of effective plaque control have not been shown to cause gingivitis, periodontitis, or mobility

## Epidemiology of Periodontal Diseases and Related Risks[1,13]

A. Basic terminology
1. Incidence—number of new cases in an identified population during a specific period
2. Prevalence—percentage of affected people in an identified population
3. Extent—number or percentage of teeth or sites affected by a disease or condition
4. Severity—degree of severity or advancement of a given disease or condition
5. Risk factor—environmental, behavioral, or systemic characteristic or exposure that is associated strongly with a disease, without causality established; usually confirmed through longitudinal studies
6. Risk indicator—a probable or putative risk factor that has been associated with a given condition or disease through cross-sectional studies; not confirmed in longitudinal studies
7. Risk predictor or marker—a factor that has been associated with future development of a given disease or condition; considered potentially predictive without established causality
8. Odds ratio—odds represent the ratio of the probability that an event will occur to the probability that the event will not occur; an odds ratio of 1.0 means that people exposed to a particular event or factor are no more likely than a normal, healthy individual to develop that disease or condition; greater than 1.0 is more likely

B. Natural history of periodontal disease
1. Landmark studies of the natural history of periodontal disease by Löe and colleagues[14] established important features of the disease
a. Severe disease tends to cluster in a small percentage of the population
b. Pronounced differences in susceptibility to periodontal destruction can be independent of the environment
2. These studies examined the course of periodontal disease during a 20-year period in two cohorts: Sri Lankan tea workers who were generally healthy, but had never received dental care and did not know of toothbrushing, and students and academicians from Norway who had lifelong dental care and oral self-care education
3. Plaque, calculus, and gingivitis, which were common conditions in both groups, led to a slow loss of periodontal attachment with increasing age
4. Periodontal attachment loss progressed at a rate of 0.3 mm per year in Sri Lanka and 0.1 mm per year in Norway; professional care and self-care prevented or slowed the progression of disease
5. In the Sri Lankan group with no periodontal therapy, the disease patterns identified were:
a. No progression beyond gingivitis (11%)
b. Moderate progression of 4-mm attachment loss (81%)

c. Rapid progression of 9-mm attachment loss (8%)
6. Periodontal diseases are most often slowly progressive; however, whereas some individuals show no progression even without care, others show rapid progression
7. Plaque, calculus, and gingival inflammation were present in both cohorts; thus, studies have identified other risk factors associated with periodontal disease

C. Current model of pathogenicity
1. All individuals are not equally susceptible to periodontal disease
2. Only a low percentage of sites with gingivitis will develop into periodontitis
3. Periodontal disease is a highly complex disease, and variations in its epidemiology can be attributed to both local (environmental) factors and host susceptibility

D. Epidemiology of periodontal diseases[1,13]
(see also the section on "Epidemiology of Oral Diseases and Conditions" in Chapter 20)
1. Gingivitis
a. Prevalence—large-scale national studies in the United States have estimated that 50% of adults have gingivitis; this may be an underestimation because of study designs
(1) Gingival bleeding in at least one site was seen in 63% of adults
(2) Gingivitis is more prevalent, severe, and extensive in groups of participants with extensive dental deposits, low socioeconomic status, limited access to health education and dental care, less education, and low health literacy, as well as in adolescents, underserved minorities, and cognitively and developmentally challenged persons
b. Risk factors—may be environmental or systemic
(1) Systemic conditions that produce vascular changes, including acute leukemia, hemophilia, Sturge-Weber syndrome, and Wegener's granulomatosis
(2) Systemic conditions that affect host response, including diabetes mellitus, Addison's disease, thrombocytopenia, combined immunodeficiency diseases, and HIV infection
(3) Systemic conditions related to hormonal changes, such as pregnancy and puberty
(4) Environmental factors or local factors such as plaque-retentive factors (calculus, poorly fitting restorations), tooth malalignment or crowding, and smoking
c. Causative factors—cause-and-effect studied
(1) Dental biofilm is causative in gingivitis—plaque-retentive factors such as calculus, incorrect restorative margins, prostheses, and orthodontics increase risk of gingival inflammation; gingivitis is preventable in most people with frequent and effective personal and professional plaque control measures
(2) Prescription drugs can cause drug-influenced gingival enlargement, resulting, in whole or in part, from systemic drug use; these drugs can cause drug-influenced gingival enlargement, or their effects can be exacerbated by bacterial plaque
d. Possible influence of diet and nutrition
(1) No direct link has been established between nutrition and periodontal disease except in the case of scurvy and severe ascorbic acid (vitamin C) deficiency
(2) The relationship of diet and nutrition to disease susceptibility, tissue integrity, and defense mechanisms cannot be ignored

## CHANGES IN THE PERIODONTIUM ASSOCIATED WITH DISEASE

See the section on "Inflammation" in Chapter 7.

A. Pathogenesis and stages of the periodontal lesion[1]
1. Pathogenesis—mode of origin or development of a disease; bacterial virulence factors, constituents, or metabolites that are capable of disrupting protective host mechanisms or causing disease initiation, progression, or both are required for the occurrence of periodontal disease
2. Stage I gingivitis, or initial lesion—2 to 4 days after biofilm accumulation
a. Changes are not clinically visible; subclinical lesion
b. Histologic changes
(1) Brief vasoconstriction followed by "widening" of small capillaries (vasodilation), margination, emigration, and migration of polymorphonuclear neutrophils (PMNs)
(2) Increase in leukocytes, particularly PMNs (neutrophils) and macrophages, in the connective tissue, junctional epithelium, and gingival sulcus; neutrophils are the earliest responders, or the first line of defense, in inflammation
(3) Host systems (e.g., complement and kinin systems and arachidonic pathways)
(4) Increase in the flow of gingival crevicular fluid (GCF) into the sulcus
(5) Inflammatory infiltrate occupies 5% to 10% of the gingival connective tissue where collagen has been lost
3. Stage II gingivitis or early lesion—begins 4 to 7 days after bacterial plaque accumulation; may persist for 21 days or longer
a. Clinical signs of gingivitis appear (erythema, edema, and bleeding on stimulation)
b. Histologic changes
(1) Persistence of inflammation from initial lesion
(2) The sulcular lining is ulcerated (allowing bleeding)
(3) Inflammatory infiltrate in the connective tissue dominated by lymphocytes (75%); primarily T cells, with some macrophages, plasma cells, and mast cells

(4) The junctional epithelium becomes densely infiltrated with inflammatory cells and begins to proliferate into connective tissue
(5) Destruction of collagen fibers (especially circular and dento-gingival) in the infiltrated area; fibroblasts are altered
(6) Migration of leukocytes, macrophages, dendritic cells, and lymphocytes into the junctional epithelium and the gingival sulcus
(7) GCF peaks 6 to 12 days after clinical signs of gingivitis

4. Stage III gingivitis or established (chronic) lesion—the period varies; may persist for months or years without progressing to stage IV (periodontitis)
   a. Clinical changes
      (1) Erythema (redness) of the gingiva resulting from proliferation of capillaries, or a bluish hue superimposed over the reddened gingiva as a result of congested blood vessels, sluggish blood flow, or both
      (2) Bleeding may occur on probing because of thinning of the sulcular epithelium, ulceration of the sulcular epithelium, or both
      (3) Color changes begin in the gingival margin and papilla, then spread to the attached gingiva
      (4) Consistency may be soft and spongy or firm; depends on whether destructive changes or reparative changes within the gingiva are dominant
      (5) Texture may be smooth and shiny (inflammation) or stippled and nodular (reparative, fibrotic)
      (6) Increase in size of gingiva (enlargement)
      (7) Increase in depth of the gingival sulcus—may be caused by enlargement of the gingival tissue only; creates a gingival pocket or pseudopocket
         (a) Begins with papillary enlargement
         (b) Extends into margins, producing rounded and bulbous gingival margins
      (8) Progression of inflammation orchestrated by the progression of cytokines
         (a) May remain only within gingival tissue (gingivitis)
         (b) May extend into supporting periodontal tissue in stage IV (periodontitis) *Note:* Periodontitis must be preceded by gingivitis, but gingivitis does not always progress to periodontitis
   b. Histologic changes
      (1) Vascular proliferation and increase in number of B cells and plasma cells (produced by B lymphocytes) invade the connective tissue; blood vessels are congested, and blood flow is impaired
      (2) Widened intercellular spaces in the junctional epithelium contain lysosomes, lymphocytes, and monocytes; pathogens such as *Aggregatibacter actinomycetemcomitans* and *Porphyromonas gingivalis* invade host tissues
      (3) Periodontal pathogens found in plaque biofilm, such as *A. actinomycetemcomitans, P. gingivalis,* and *Tannerella forsythia,* produce collagenase and elastinase, enzymes that destroy connective tissue; *A. actinomycetemcomitans, P. gingivalis,* and *Treponema denticola* also produce a trypsin enzyme that kills lymphocytes; *Prevotella intermedia, Capnocytophaga,* and *P. gingivalis* degrade antibodies
      (4) The junctional epithelium continues to protrude into the connective tissue; sulcular lining is ulcerated
      (5) Collagenase and other enzymes actively break down connective tissue, resulting in continued loss of collagen
      (6) Simultaneous proliferation of collagen fibers and epithelium (enlargement) occurs
      (7) Bone loss has not occurred

5. Stage IV—pathway of inflammation from the gingiva to supporting periodontal tissue (transition from gingivitis to periodontitis), or advanced lesion
   a. Characterized by loss of connective tissue attachment to teeth, including gingival and periodontal ligament fibers and their attachment to cementum, concurrent gingival inflammation, resorption of alveolar bone, and apical migration of the epithelial attachment along the root surface (i.e., clinical attachment level [CAL])
   b. Generally follows the course of blood vessels through soft tissues and into alveolar bone; the pattern of inflammatory pathway affects the pattern of bone destruction
   c. Initially, the inflammation penetrates and destroys gingival fibers near the gingival fiber attachment to cementum and then spreads
      (1) Interproximally—into bone and the periodontal ligament
      (2) Facially and lingually—from bone to the periodontal ligament, from the gingiva to the periosteum and periodontal ligament, and from the periosteum into bone

B. Formation of the periodontal pocket[1]
   1. Persistent, chronic gingivitis may progress to periodontitis, which results in loss of connective tissue attachment, bone destruction, and periodontal pocket formation
   2. Periodontal pocket—pathologic deepening of the gingival sulcus produced by the destruction of supporting tissue and apical migration of the junctional epithelium
   3. Classification (Fig. 14.4)
      a. Suprabony pocket—base of the pocket is coronal to the alveolar crest; also called *supracrestal* or *supraalveolar pocket*
      b. Infrabony pocket—base of the pocket is apical to the alveolar crest; also called *intrabony, intraalveolar,* or *subcrestal pocket*
   4. Histopathology
      a. The gingival epithelium may show evidence of inflammatory changes

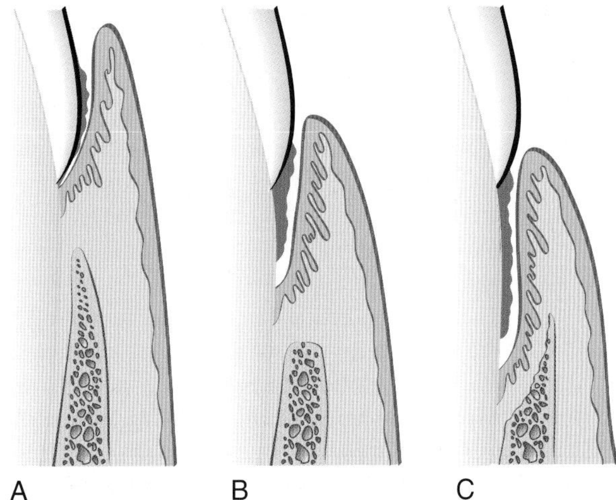


**Fig. 14.4** Different types of periodontal pockets. (A) Gingival pocket. No destruction of the supporting periodontal tissues is seen. (B) Suprabony pocket. The base of the pocket is coronal to the level of the underlying bone. Bone loss occurs horizontally. (C) Infrabony pocket. The base of the pocket is apical to the level of the adjacent bone. Bone loss occurs vertically. (From Newman MG, et al. *Carranza's Clinical Periodontology.* 12th ed. St. Louis: Elsevier; 2015.)

b. Connective tissue changes
   (1) Inflammatory cells infiltrate the connective tissue and proceed through it
   (2) Degeneration of gingival connective tissue fibers; gingival cells release inflammatory mediators or chemicals that destroy bone
   (3) Tissue invasion by periodontal pathogens
c. Changes within supporting bone as inflammatory process progresses
   (1) Cytokines and effector molecules (e.g., interleukins, prostaglandin $E_2$ [$PGE_2$], matrix metalloproteinase) have proinflammatory effects and stimulate osteoclasts that degenerate mineral content of bone; PMNs, macrophages, and mononuclear cells degenerate organic matrix of bone by producing collagenase
   (2) Bone marrow component (fatty tissue) is replaced by inflammatory cell infiltrate, fibroblastic proliferation, and deposition of collagen fibers
   (3) The cortical plate of the interdental septum (crest) is the first area to be involved
   (4) Once this central breakthrough has occurred, supporting bone is destroyed in a lateral direction; bone loss is accompanied by both resorption and formation
   (5) Periodontal pockets are constantly undergoing repair

C. Common clinical changes associated with periodontitis
   1. Similar changes in the gingiva as seen in gingivitis, but usually more chronic
   2. Areas of gingival recession
   3. Bleeding on probing
   4. Periodontal attachment loss
   5. True periodontal pockets
   6. Loose, extruded, or migrated teeth; diastemas may develop
   7. Exudate from the gingival margin in response to pressure; suppuration (pus) is a sign of secondary infection
   8. Symptoms—generally painless; patient may complain of itching gums, loose teeth, food impaction, and bad taste; relief is felt with pressure applied to the gums
   9. Furcation involvement

D. Radiographic changes associated with periodontitis (usually follow this sequence)
   1. Fuzziness and discontinuity off the crest of the interdental septum in the proximal area
   2. Wedge-shaped radiolucent area formed between the mesial or distal aspects of the alveolar crest and the root surface of the involved tooth; also called *triangulation*
   3. Center of the crestal portion of the interdental septum also becomes fuzzy, and faint cup-shaped areas of alveolar crest bone loss appear; bony crater
   4. Bone destruction patterns in periodontitis (Fig. 14.5 and 14.6)
      a. Horizontal bone loss is most common; bone is reduced in height but remains parallel to the CEJ of adjacent tooth surfaces
      b. Osseous defects or bone deformities
         (1) Vertical or angular defects occur in an oblique direction; most frequently, infrabony pockets accompany vertical defects
         (2) Classified by number of remaining walls; may have one, two, or three walls
      c. Osseous craters are concavities in the crest of interdental bone, common in posterior segments
      d. Bulbous bone or bony enlargements occur as adaptations to excess function
      e. Craters result from complete loss of interdental bone without loss of radicular bone
   5. Limitations of radiographs in the diagnosis of periodontitis
      a. The radiograph does not reveal minor destructive changes in bone
      b. The involvement of facial and lingual surfaces cannot be seen
      c. Angulation errors can affect radiographic image of alveolar bone
      d. The internal morphology of infrabony craters or defects cannot be seen
      e. As a general rule, bone loss is always greater than that revealed by the radiograph

E. Periodontal disease activity
   1. Refers to the stage(s) of periodontal disease characterized by loss of alveolar bone and connective tissue attachment
   2. Implies that the natural history of periodontal disease has periods of active destruction and periods of relative inactivity, although chronic inflammation persists

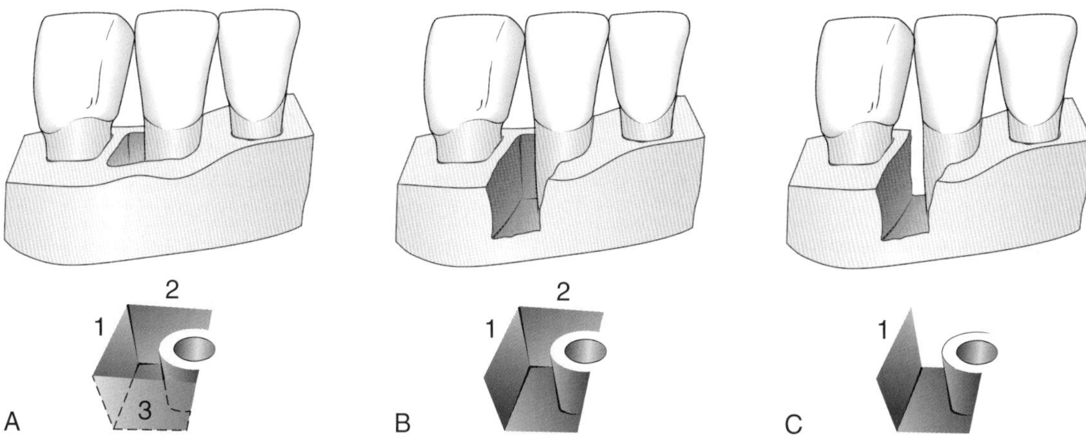


**Fig. 14.5** One-, two-, and three-wall vertical defects on the right lateral incisor. (A) Three bony walls: *1,* distal; *2,* lingual; and *3,* facial. (B) Two-wall defect: *1,* distal, and *2,* lingual. (C) One-wall defect: *1,* distal only. (From Newman MG, et al. *Carranza's Clinical Periodontology.* 12th ed. St. Louis: Elsevier; 2015.)

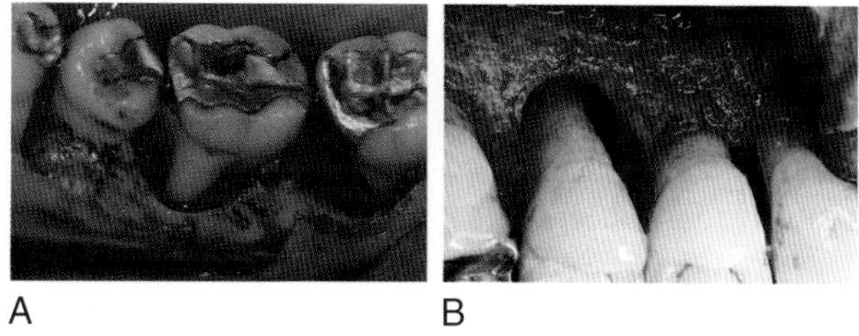


**Fig. 14.6** Angular defects. (A) Infrabony pockets around the molars. (B) Circumferential vertical defect in relation to the maxillary canine and premolars. (From Newman MG, et al. *Carranza's Clinical Periodontology.* 12 ed. St. Louis: Elsevier; 2015.)

## BACTERIAL DENTAL BIOFILM[1]

See the sections on "Microbiology of the Oral Cavity" and "Bacterial Plaque" in Chapter 9.

A. Definition—complex community of bacteria that forms on any surface that is exposed to the fluids in the mouth; communication of bacteria within the biofilm allows for production of byproducts; dense, noncalcified, highly organized; firmly adherent to teeth or other hard materials within the mouth; cannot be washed off by salivary or water flow
   1. Biofilms protect bacteria housed within them (sessile), offering greater potential than freestanding (planktonic) bacteria
   2. Microorganisms produce a matrix called *glycocalyx* and extracellular proteins that encase and coat bacteria in the biofilm, providing protection from the oral environment, retentive qualities essential to being adherent to the tooth surfaces, and pathogenic byproducts (e.g., dextrans and levans, uronic acid, and others); referred to as the slime layer
   3. The matrix, or slime layer, of a biofilm provides a barrier from antimicrobial and antibiotic agents, making the biofilm resistant to chemotherapy
   4. The matrix or slime layer provides structure for the biofilm, nutritional advantages required for growth and maturation of bacteria within the biofilm, and strength against forces that attempt to detach bacteria from tooth surfaces
B. Two categories of bacterial plaque—supragingival and subgingival
C. Stages in plaque formation
   1. Acquired pellicle
   2. Bacterial plaque biofilm
      a. Complex microbial community forms, allowing for communication of bacteria within the biofilm and providing firm adherence to the tooth and other such surfaces
      b. Rate of formation varies from person to person, from tooth to tooth, and between areas on the same tooth; seen on teeth after 24 to 48 hours without oral hygiene
      c. Growth of microcolonies within the matrix and co-aggregation and adhesion of bacteria allow for increased thickness of the biofilm; shifts in the types of microorganisms occur; bacteria deep within the biofilm are more metabolically active and better protected than those on the surface that can be more easily dislodged
D. Supragingival versus subgingival plaque biofilms
   1. Supragingival plaque
      a. As plaque ages, the percentage of gram-positive organisms decreases
      b. As plaque ages, aerobic bacteria decrease and anaerobic bacteria increase
   2. Subgingival plaque
      a. Inflammatory changes in the gingival sulcus or periodontal pocket resulting from supragingival plaque modify the relationship between the gingival margin and the tooth surface, creating a protected subgingival area
      b. This environment allows subgingival bacteria to colonize and adhere to other bacteria, the tooth, or the epithelial tissue surrounding the sulcus or the pocket

c. Pathogenic anaerobic bacteria and spirochetes become well established in the subgingival plaque biofilm
d. Subgingival plaque may be attached or loosely adherent (epithelium associated)
   (1) Attached subgingival plaque (also called tooth-associated subgingival plaque)
      (a) Similar to supragingival bacterial plaque; inner layers are dominated by gram-positive rods and cocci and facultative bacteria; species of the genera *Streptococcus, Veillonella, Prevotella, Neisseria, Gemella,* and *Actinomyces*
      (b) Apical portions are dominated by gram-negative rods, with some filaments present; secondary colonizers such as *P. intermedia, Capnocytophaga* spp., *Fusobacterium nucleatum,* and *P. gingivalis* coaggregate
   (2) Loosely adherent or unattached subgingival plaque
      (a) Extends from the gingival margin apical to the junctional epithelium, adjacent to the gingival epithelium or the pocket lumen
      (b) Primarily gram-negative rods as well as motile organisms, filaments, and spirochetes that are not highly organized; predominance of species such as *P. gingivalis, A. actinomycetemcomitans, T. denticola, P. intermedia, T. forsythia* (formerly *Bacteroides forsythus*) (pathogenic), and *Capnocytophaga ochracea* (beneficial)
e. Bacterial invasion of periodontal tissues
   (1) Bacteria have been found within diseased periodontal tissue
   (2) Widened intercellular spaces in the gingival epithelium or the pocket lining may allow for the penetration of organisms from subgingival bacterial plaque
   (3) Bacterial invasion may occur, or the presence of bacteria within the tissue may be a result of displacement or manipulation rather than actual invasion
   (4) *Aggregatibacter actinomycetemcomitans* and *Porphyromonas gingivalis* are believed to be tissue-invading organisms

E. Bacterial specificity
   1. Specific plaque hypothesis—suggests that specific combinations of bacteria communicating with the biofilm cause various forms of periodontal disease; only certain microorganisms are pathogenic
   2. Research is further defining the bacterial causes and host response effects of destructive periodontal disease

F. Dental calculus—bacterial plaque that has mineralized
   1. Calculus plays a secondary role in the etiology of periodontal diseases by serving as a plaque-retentive factor; not all plaque necessarily calcifies; all calculus in humans is covered by bacterial plaque
   2. Earliest mineralization occurs along the inner surface of the plaque or in attached subgingival plaque; calcium and phosphorus come from the saliva for the mineralization of supragingival calculus and from the GCF for the mineralization of subgingival calculus
   3. Its porosity serves as a reservoir for bacteria and endotoxins that are destructive to the periodontium; impossible for the patient to remove
   4. Modes of attachment to teeth
      a. By acquired pellicle
      b. By direct attachment of the calculus to the tooth surface; penetrates cementum
      c. By mechanically locking into tooth surface irregularities
   5. Effect on the periodontium—because bacterial plaque always covers calculus, it is primarily a bacterial irritant (not mechanical); calculus plays a significant role as a secondary, contributing factor in the pathogenesis of periodontal disease; a plaque-retentive factor

G. Pathogenic effect on periodontium (see the sections on "Acute Inflammation" and "Chronic Inflammation" in Chapter 7)
   1. Bacterial plaque biofilm contributes to periodontal breakdown by direct injury to tissue and by stimulating host-mediated responses that result in tissue injury
   2. Direct injury is caused by toxins and enzymes produced by bacteria and proinflammatory metabolic byproducts of bacterial metabolism; most significant pathologic effects during the early stages of disease
      a. Exotoxins are proteins and other metabolic byproducts such as hydrogen sulfide, uric acid, and fatty acids released by organisms that cause direct injury to tissue
      b. Endotoxins called *lipopolysaccharides* (LPS) or cytotoxic agents are cellular components of gram-negative bacteria that are toxic to surrounding cells, contribute to the inflammatory process, and induce bone resorption; endotoxins are released from the cell wall on the death of gram-negative bacteria, initiating inflammation and tissue destruction
      c. Enzymes—mainly proteases, collagenase, hyaluronidase, chondroitin sulfatase, fibrinolysin, and phospholipase A—directly degrade surrounding tissue and penetrate by breaking down structural barriers
   3. Indirect toxicity results when subgingival bacteria act as antigens and a resultant local immune reaction occurs; the host response attempts to control the bacterial attack, and some destruction of tissue results by a variety of immunopathologic reactions

H. Host response—protective (see Figs. 7.1 to 7.4 in Chapter 7); host-mediated destructive processes play a role in the cause of inflammatory periodontal infections once the protective elements of the periodontium are overwhelmed

I. Host response—destructive
   1. Cytokines, including interleukins and $PGE_2$, participate in periodontal pathologic changes; these low-molecular-weight (LMW) proteins are produced by fibroblasts and inflammatory cells (e.g., monocytes, lymphocytes); LPS stimulates cytokines
   2. Collagenase and lysosomal enzymes destroy connective tissue

3. Aspartate transaminase (AST, aspartate aminotransferase)—an intracellular enzyme that indicates cell death or tissue destruction when present extracellularly
4. Elevated levels of host-derived enzymes (e.g., collagenase, AST, β-glucuronidase, elastase) in GCF can be used as markers for periodontitis
5. Tumor necrosis factor alpha (TNF-α)—an inflammatory mediator that contributes to bone resorption; shares properties with interleukins
6. Matrix metalloproteinase (MMP)—produces collagenase contributing to CAL

## CLINICAL ASSESSMENT OF THE PERIODONTIUM[1,15]

A. Indices—system for documenting clinical observations to help patients become aware of their current status, to demonstrate changes in the patient's health over a certain period, and to survey large populations for current status and trends in health (see Chapter 20)
B. Periodontal documentation
   1. Used to document existing periodontal status; baseline for future reference
   2. Updated periodically to determine changes in periodontal health or disease progression
   3. Necessary for care planning
   4. Serves as a guide for the clinician during treatment and evaluation
   5. Serves as a legal document; a risk management technique to reduce risks associated with failure to diagnose and treat periodontal disease
C. Periodontal assessment—complete periodontal documentation should be based on a thorough periodontal assessment, which includes the following:
   1. A description of gingival tissue—includes visual signs of inflammation
   2. Findings from examination of the periodontium with a periodontal probe (see the section on "Probe" in Chapter 17), which include the following:
      a. Presence of bleeding—widely accepted as an indicator of gingival inflammation; more sensitive than visual signs; however, inflamed sites do not always bleed, and bleeding is a poor predictor of attachment loss (only 30%), unless multiple sites are found in conjunction with deep pockets, attachment loss, or both; these combined conditions help make important risk prediction for attachment loss
      b. Probing depth (also called *sulcus* or *pocket depth*)—gives a historical record of past periodontal disease activity; useful in monitoring the success of periodontal therapy; important in determining patient's ability to maintain health through plaque biofilm control; the periodontal probe remains the best diagnostic aid for detecting periodontal pockets and CAL
      c. Clinical attachment loss (CAL)—measures from the CEJ to the attachment; determines the amount of apical migration of the junctional epithelium or the amount of lost periodontal connective tissue attachment to the tooth; most accurate measure of severity of periodontal disease because the measurement is not influenced by the position of the gingival margin influenced by inflammation and recession, and because CEJ is a static reference point when measuring CAL
         (1) Because the gingival attachment is located slightly apical to the CEJ in a fully erupted tooth, and the gingival margin is slightly coronal to the CEJ in normal gingival contour, probing depth will be slightly greater than CAL
         (2) When gingival recession is present and the gingival margin is apical to the CEJ, the probing depth will be less than CAL; therefore, a normal sulcus depth can be present in an area of connective tissue and bone loss
         (3) If the gingival margin meets the CEJ, the probing depth and CAL are equal
      d. Recession—measured from the CEJ to the gingival margin; indicates apical migration of the gingiva
      e. Presence of purulent exudate (suppuration)—in response to lateral digital pressure on the gingival margin or probing; suggests advanced lesion of periodontitis and secondary infection at site
      f. Adequacy of width of attached gingiva—measured from attachment to mucogingival junction; the amount varies, depending on location; adequate zone necessary to withstand stresses from mastication; if none is present, the gingival margin will move with alveolar mucosa; if inadequate, a mucogingival problem or defect exists
   3. Alternatives to use of standard periodontal probe for periodontal examination[1] (see the section on "Periodontal Assessment" in Chapter 15)
      a. Periodontal screening and recording system (PSR)—provides thorough screening and recording for all patients while saving time in recording aspect of initial examination
      b. Electronic periodontal probes—increase accuracy by reducing the margin of error, standardizing pressure, or both; reduce time required for probing and recording
   4. Presence and distribution of bacterial plaque and calculus (may use indices)
   5. Condition of tooth proximal contacts—loose or open contacts permit food impaction
   6. Degree of pathologic tooth mobility (see "Periodontal Assessment" in Chapter 15 for a specific classification system)
      a. Pathologic tooth mobility is caused by loss of periodontal support (bone loss), trauma from occlusion, inflammation extending into the periodontal ligament from the gingiva or the apex (abscesses), periodontal surgery (temporarily), hormonal changes associated with pregnancy and sometimes menstruation or use of hormonal contraceptives, and pathologic processes of the jaws that destroy the bone or roots of teeth (e.g., osteomyelitis, tumors)
      b. Tooth mobility is usually assessed by using the blunt ends of the handles of two dental instruments (single-ended); can be measured electronically

7. Presence of furcation involvement (see "Periodontal Assessment" in Chapter 15 for a specific classification system)
8. Presence of malocclusion or malposition of teeth
9. Presence and condition of dental restorations and prosthetic appliances; missing teeth; dental implants
10. Presence of overhanging restorations (overhangs)—contributing causative factor in periodontal disease from accumulation of bacterial plaque and food impaction
11. Assessment of disease progression by longitudinal comparison of probing depths, attachment levels, and interproximal bone height (radiographic)
12. Interpretation of a satisfactory number of bitewing and periapical radiographs of diagnostic quality (see the section on "Radiographic Interpretation" in Chapter 6). Evidence of periodontal destruction is referred to a "radiographic bone loss"
    a. Level of alveolar crest in relation to the CEJ and interdental bone
    b. Furcation areas
    c. Width of periodontal ligament space
    d. Existing dental restorations and caries
    e. Periapical disease
    f. Length, shape, and position of roots

D. Documentation of oral habits
1. Bruxing (grinding) or clenching of teeth
2. Chewing on fingernails or foreign objects
3. Smoking or drinking (alcohol) habits
4. Temporomandibular joint (TMJ) trauma (evidenced by crepitus, tenderness, or deviations)

E. Assessment of occlusion—includes:
1. Classification and anterior relationships
2. Excessive wear patterns (facets)
3. Defective prematurities—isolated occlusal contacts that cause deflection in the pathway of physiologic mandibular movement
4. Teeth, restorations, or prosthetic appliances that may interfere with the normal movements of the mandible
5. TMJ discomfort
6. Fremitus—tooth movement when teeth occlude and grind in all functional positions
7. Tooth sensitivity to pressure and to hot and cold substances

F. Classification of occlusal trauma[1]
1. Primary occlusal trauma—trauma results from excessive occlusal forces when periodontal support is normal; result could be mobility, excessive wear of a tooth or teeth, sensitivity of involved teeth, or fremitus
2. Secondary occlusal trauma—the supporting periodontium is not normal (some loss of supporting structures because of periodontitis); one or more teeth are not able to withstand even normal occlusal forces, and particularly excessive occlusal forces; could result in mobility or sensitivity

G. Additional information obtained through patient interview
1. Complete documentation of the patient's past and current health status, including pharmacologic history and risk factors
2. Complete documentation of the patient's dental, fluoride, social, and cultural histories
3. Patient's daily oral hygiene routine
4. Patient's knowledge level and attitude toward oral health

H. Supplemental diagnostic tests[1]
1. Traditional approach to periodontal diagnosis measures only the results of periodontal inflammation and destruction; the goals for developing newer diagnostic approaches include the ability to detect the presence of disease early to predict destruction before it occurs; prognostic devices or tests also are able to assess the risk of disease
2. Validity of a diagnostic test is determined by calculating its sensitivity and specificity
    a. Sensitivity—the probability of a test being positive when a disease truly is present
    b. Specificity—the probability of a test being negative when a disease truly is not present
    c. Predictive value—refers to the probability that a disease will be present when the test is positive or not present when the test is negative; influenced by the prevalence of disease in a particular population
3. Prognostic device or test—predicts the likelihood that a disease will occur in the future
4. Supplemental diagnostic tests can be used for screening (to separate the diseased from healthy individuals) or to detect sites or individuals at high risk for progressive disease
5. General categories of supplemental diagnostic tests (microbiologic monitoring)
    a. DNA (deoxyribonucleic acid) probes—paper points are inserted into specific site(s) and sent to a laboratory for analysis of presence of eight known pathogens to provide general information useful in antibiotic selection in refractory or aggressive cases
        (1) Culturing—plaque samples from specific sites are placed in a vial containing transport medium and sent to a laboratory for analysis; specific percentages of various bacterial species are identified with specific recommendations for antibiotic
        (2) Enzyme-linked immunosorbent assay (ELISA)—matches sample DNA and bacterial antigens to periodontal pathogens; used in research rather than in clinical practice
    b. Bacterial risk assessment test (BANA)—tests three anaerobes typically associated with periodontal disease risk; based on chairside incubation and testing of samples of subgingival biofilm
    c. Local measures of host response;[1] host-derived enzymes in GCF, which are produced by inflamed pocket wall and primarily composed of inflammatory cells and serum proteins as well as inflammatory mediators and tissue breakdown and bacterial byproducts (e.g., collagenase, $PGE_2$, AST)
    d. Genetic testing—determines genotype status through an in-office test for periodontal disease susceptibility (see the section on "Genetics" in Chapter 7)
    e. Automatic calculus detection systems
        (1) Fiberoptic probe—lights up and sounds when subgingival calculus is detected
        (2) Periodontal endoscope—a specific type of endoscopy used to explore and visualize the root surface, periodontal pocket, and furcation areas

f. Risk assessment tool—internet-based periodontal risk calculator that assesses a person's risk for periodontal disease on the basis of nine weighted risk factors

## SYSTEMIC EFFECTS OF PERIODONTAL DISEASE[1]

A. Periodontal disease is a chronic inflammatory response to a given stimulus (virulent bacteria in biofilm) that has been associated with increased risk for conditions such as myocardial infarction, stroke, cardiovascular disease, peripheral vascular disease, adverse pregnancy outcomes, and pneumonia; a relationship between periodontal disease and these diseases has been documented, although a cause-and-effect connection has not been established
   1. Periodontal infection presents a chronic inflammatory burden at the systemic level
   2. Bacterial pathogens released from biofilm in the periodontal pocket enter tissues through ulcerations in the pocket epithelium and colonize other body parts; systemic exposures to these gram-negative pathogens and LPS trigger inflammatory mediator expression in the affected tissues (i.e., release of proinflammatory mediators and acute-phase proteins), contributing to systemic inflammation, atherogenesis, and other pathology
   3. Patient-based clinical outcomes such as disease morbidity and mortality and surrogate markers (e.g., serum inflammatory markers such as cross-reactive protein) are used instead of traditional markers or outcomes (e.g., bleeding, pocket depth)

B. Research into the associations between periodontal diseases and the occurrence and severity of systemic diseases and conditions is ongoing.

## TREATMENT[1,14]

### Initial Care Plan

See the section on "Planning" in Chapter 15.

A. Collection of data to assess the status of the periodontium (see the previous section on "Clinical Assessment of the Periodontium")

B. Formulation of initial care plan based on data collection and assessment
   1. Determination of all causative and contributing factors (risk factors and risk indicators)
   2. Removal or control of etiologic and risk factors in an organized, logical sequence
      a. Plaque removal and control and removal of any plaque-retentive factors
      b. Reduction, control, or elimination of risk factors
      c. Elimination of inflammation; pocket reduction or elimination
   3. Order of treatment will depend on:
      a. Severity of the patient's periodontal condition and prognosis
      b. General health status of the patient
      c. Patient's motivation, cooperation, needs, and desires

C. Contributing factors influencing the prognosis
   1. Local factors
      a. Degree of periodontal destruction (amount of attachment loss)
      b. Rate of periodontal destruction (amount of attachment loss per unit of time)
      c. Presence of contributing local factors (e.g., malocclusion, parafunctional habits, position of teeth in alveoli, malalignment, root proximity, missing teeth)
      d. Quality of restorations present
   2. Risk factors—related to the patient's general health (presence or absence of systemic disease), factors affecting host response, and environmental factors (stress, smoking)

### Preventive Therapy or Treatment of Biofilm-Induced Gingivitis

A. Control biofilm—patient coinvolvement in daily self-care; remove biofilm-retentive factors
   1. Address risk factors
   2. Oral prophylaxis (versus nonsurgical periodontal therapy (NSPT) for periodontitis)
      a. The objective is to prevent the initiation of gingivitis and, failing that, to prevent the conversion of gingivitis to periodontitis; therapeutic goal of oral prophylaxis is to establish gingival health through the elimination of causative factors
      b. Performed for patients with healthy periodontium or with gingivitis; NSPT is performed for patients with loss of periodontal support
      c. Oral prophylaxis includes supragingival and subgingival debridement to remove deposits; removal or correction of biofilm-retentive factors; and coronal polishing, if necessary, for stain removal or for patient satisfaction
   3. The term *scaling* refers to supragingival or subgingival calculus removal without intentional removal of tooth surface

B. NSPT; also called *initial therapy* or *phase I therapy*);[1,15] (see the section on "Concepts in Periodontal Instrumentation" in Chapter 17)
   1. Objective—to treat and manage established periodontal disease and to create conditions conducive to health
   2. Principles—elimination or suppression of pathogenic microorganisms through the removal and control of biofilm and its retentive factors (e.g., calculus, overhangs, food impaction, improper contacts); control of the infection and prevention of reinfection; resolution of inflammation
      a. Oral hygiene self-care, including plaque biofilm removal and control
      b. Periodontal instrumentation—scaling, root planing (intentional removal of the cementum), periodontal debridement (gross removal of hard and soft deposits)

c. Adjunctive use of antiplaque and antigingivitis agents, as indicated (Table 14.4)
3. Consider and, if possible, control behavioral, systemic, and environmental host risk factors
4. Restoration or maintenance of comfort, function, and esthetics
5. Decreasing the likelihood of disease progression

C. Components of NSPT
1. Dental biofilm control—patient as cotherapist: self-care, goal setting, long-term commitment; customized oral hygiene instruction, correction of biofilm–retentive factors, and supragingival and subgingival debridement; antimicrobial or antigingival agents or devices may be used as adjuncts to mechanical self-care methods; long-term success of NSPT depends on adequate biofilm control and regular periodontal maintenance visits
2. Adequate periodontal instrumentation for removal and control of biofilm and biofilm–retentive factors
a. Rationale—periodontal instrumentation and biofilm control result in a significant reduction of gram-negative periodontal pathogens and encourage repopulation with the gram-positive microorganisms that are associated with health; a reduction in inflammatory cytokines responsible for tissue damage occurs after the bacterial composition is altered; calculus, overhanging restorations, and other biofilm-retentive factors that harbor bacterial plaque also are removed; all these components of NSPT reduce inflammation, promote tissue

**TABLE 14.4 Local Chemotherapy for Prevention and Control of Oral Diseases or Conditions**

| Agent and Delivery | Mechanism of Action | Alcohol | Directions for Use | Efficacy | Main Side Effects |
|---|---|---|---|---|---|
| Chlorhexidine 0.12% Mouthrinse | Cationic bisbiguanide ruptures bacterial cell wall; highly substantive | 11.6% or 0% formulations | Rinse with 15 mL for 30 seconds 2 × daily; separate from dentifrice or fluoride by 30 minutes | 45%–61% plaque and gingivitis reduction; antihalitosis | Extrinsic stain, altered taste, increase in supragingival calculus |
| Essential oils and phenolic compounds:<br>Tymol 0.06%<br>Eucalyptol 0.09%<br>Methyl salicylate 0.06%<br>Menthol 0.04%<br>Mouthrinse | Antiseptic form interrupts bacterial cell wall and inhibits bacterial enzymes | 21.6%–26.6% in antiseptic formulation; 0% alcohol formulation is not marketed as antigingivitis (only antihalitosis) | Rinse with 20 mL for 30 seconds 2× daily | 30%–35% reduction in plaque and gingivitis; nonalcohol formulation is antihalitosis | Burning sensation and bitter taste during use; caution with xerostomia and recovering alcoholic patients |
| Cetylpyridinium chloride (CPC)<br>0.045%-0.07%<br>Mouthrinse | Solubilizes bacterial cell wall membrane | 0%–18% (0.07% formulation has 10.8%) | Rinse with 20 mL for 30 seconds 2 × daily | Higher % CPC: small but significant reduction (14%–24%) in gingivitis; 29% reduction in plaque versus control<br>Lower % CPC: for antihalitosis benefits | Low % CPCs have light extrinsic staining |
| Stannous fluoride<br>Dentifrice (0.045%)<br>Gel (0.04%)<br>Mouthrinse (0.063%) | Sn (tin ion) is bacteriocidal and bacteriostatic; also desensitizing effect | 0% | Apply small amount to toothbrush and brush thoroughly at least 2× daily | 18%–22% gingivitis<br>7%–23% plaque reductions<br>1100 ppm fluoride for cavity protection | Extrinsic staining light |
| Chlorine dioxide, zinc, or combination | Neutralizes volatile sulfur compounds (VSCs) | 0% available | Available as oral spray, dentifrice, or rinse; follow manufacturer's instructions | Antihalitosis | No adverse effects known |
| Povidone–iodine | An iodophor effective against many bacteria, fungi, and viruses | 0% | Primarily used during treatment for preprocedural rinsing or as irrigant, especially with immunocompromised status | Antimicrobial | Caution about allergy to iodine; contraindicated with allergy, thyroid dysfunction, and pregnant or lactating women |
| Hydrogen peroxide | Oxygenating effect is intended to affect anaerobes linked with periodontal disease | 0% | Short-term use 2× daily diluted with water | | Safety concern if full-strength use – precancerous or cancerous cells; dilute 1:1 with water maximum |

regeneration, and create a biologically acceptable root surface; control, alteration, or elimination of risk factors (e.g., diabetes, smoking, stress, medications) alters the host response to bacterial pathogens and has the potential to slow periodontal disease progression

b. Supragingival and subgingival scaling, periodontal debridement, root planing, (intentional removal of cementum) or a combination of all is performed; all these procedures are technically demanding; definitive treatment procedures are designed to remove cementum or surface dentin that is diseased, embedded with calculus, toxins, or microorganisms; treatment often requires local anesthesia; when performed thoroughly, some soft tissue removal, termed *incidental curettage,* is unavoidable; in the case of root planing, the need for extensive cementum removal to obtain a glassy, smooth surface is debatable because of a lack of clarity about its absolute necessity, the possibility of overtreatment, and resultant hypersensitivity
   (1) Complete removal of calculus from root surfaces is unlikely, especially as pocket depth and inaccessibility increase; complete removal of detectible calculus remains the initial clinical end point because thorough instrumentation remains paramount to the success of therapy, whether nonsurgical or surgical
   (2) The areas most susceptible to residual deposits after treatment include furcations, line angles, root concavities, and the CEJ

c. NSPT most often requires multiple appointments after assessment for treatment (e.g., four appointments 1 week apart for a quadrant therapy approach) to remove or correct all detectible deposits and plaque-retentive factors; some evidence suggests longer appointments within 24-hour and 48-hour periods for complete mouth debridement, termed *full-mouth disinfection,* are necessary to reduce cross-contamination from untreated areas to treated areas

d. Hand-activated or mechanized instruments (sonic, ultrasonic) may be effectively used for root planing and periodontal debridement; ultrasonic instruments are advocated for debridement and associated lavage

e. NSPT has been shown to be successful in treating early to moderate periodontitis, especially for initial pocket depths of 4 to 6 mm; results are less predictable in periodontal pockets more than 6 mm in depth, if tooth movement occurs, or when furcation involvement is present; NSPT is the definitive treatment for early to moderate periodontitis and an initial therapy for those expected to require surgical therapy

f. Root planing in healthy sulcus areas or shallow crevices is contraindicated; has been shown to cause a loss of attachment in crevices less than 3 mm

g. Use of lasers in periodontics appears to be equally effective to traditional instruments for scaling, root planing, and periodontal debridement

3. Initial evaluation of NSPT—occurs during and on completion of instrumentation by careful tactile exploration of tooth and root surfaces; a clear field, adequate illumination, and use of air to facilitate assessment are required
   a. The term *periodontal debridement* refers to treatment of periodontal disease through mechanical removal of tooth and root surface irregularities (including biofilm, clinically detectable calculus, and all biofilm–retentive factors) depending on the health of adjacent soft tissue
   b. The difference between periodontal debridement and root planing, as used in the literature, is in the desired initial end point and the extent of instrumentation; root planing is performed until root smoothness is obtained with reasonable time and effort, whereas debridement attempts to preserve tooth surface by removing only enough deposits and biofilm-retentive factors to achieve periodontal health; "periodontal debridement" is used on national certification examinations for dental hygienists

4. Ultimate evaluation of NSPT—tissue response (i.e., elimination of inflammation and bleeding)
   a. Commonly referred to as periodontal reevaluation
   b. Thorough reevaluation 4 to 6 weeks after scaling, root planing, or periodontal debridement to determine the need for additional therapy (e.g., surgery, physician referrals, antimicrobials, antibiotics) by means of a periodontal examination; it is critical to determine if clinical judgment regarding the extent of root planing and periodontal debridement was adequate to achieve periodontal health; if unsuccessful, retreatment is indicated; 4 to 6 weeks is considered appropriate for the resolution of inflammation and periodontal tissue healing; relevant findings of the reevaluation are documented in the patient's legal treatment record
   c. Reevaluation includes:
      (1) Evaluation and reinforcement of the patient's self-care
      (2) Updated periodontal assessment, including bleeding points, probing depths, and attachment levels
      (3) Reassessment of the clinical health of tissues; if areas still show signs of inflammation, the cause should be determined
   c. Bacterial plaque and calculus self-care should be reviewed; perform scaling, debridement, or root planing as indicated if the condition is localized; the need for rescheduling and retreatment with active therapy should be determined if the condition is generalized
      (1) If no plaque, calculus, or inflammation is noted, the patient's success is reinforced and the importance of periodontal maintenance emphasized

(2) If the pocket depth is still moderate to severe, controlled drug delivery and surgical procedures might be warranted; the patient must be referred for evaluation by a periodontist

(3) If inflammation and bleeding are still severe, unexplained, or generalized, physical examination by a physician should be considered, including differential blood counts and complete physical examination for a possible previously undetected or undiagnosed systemic host condition

D. Use of topical antimicrobial agents as adjuncts (see the section on "Mouthrinses or Chemotherapeutics" in Chapter 16); also referred to as *local chemotherapy*; can be employed in preventive therapy, in initial or nonsurgical therapy, during the healing stage following periodontal surgery, or during continuing care for periodontal health maintenance

1. Indicated for control of supragingival biofilm and gingivitis; effectiveness in periodontitis has not been documented; used to augment oral self-care efforts that are only partially effective; also recommended for extensive restorative cases and dental implants; aids healing after periodontal surgery (see the sections on "Oral Irrigation" and "Dental Implant Maintenance" in Chapter 16)

2. Antiplaque and antigingivitis agents (see Table 14.4)

a. Chlorhexidine gluconate

(1) Most effective antimicrobial agent for reducing plaque and gingivitis in the long term (45% to 61%); the "gold standard" for topical antimicrobial mouthrinses; 0.12% concentration in the United States and 0.2% outside the United States

(2) High substantivity—ability to adhere to soft and hard tissues for a long duration while releasing active ingredient; a cationic bisbiguanide that ruptures bacterial cell membranes

(3) Adverse effects—staining, reversible desquamation, poor taste or alteration of taste, increase in supragingival calculus deposits; especially with long-term use

(4) Alcohol content 11.6%, or alcohol-free form available

(5) Twice-daily use promotes compliance; patient should be instructed to use 15 mL of rinse for 30 seconds; rinse should be separate from fluoride dentifrice by 30 minutes for full effectiveness

(6) Also recommended for wound healing after surgery or as pre-rinse to reduce salivary bacterial load and aerosols during periodontal therapy and mechanized instrumentation

b. Phenolic compounds (essential oils)

(1) Antiseptic form is a safe and effective antimicrobial and antigingivitis agent (e.g., Listerine antiseptic)

(2) Long-term studies indicate approximately 30% to 45% reduction in plaque and gingivitis

(3) Available antiseptic products have variable alcohol content (21.6% to 26.9% alcohol); thymol, menthol, eucalyptol, and methyl salicylate are active ingredients; act by bacterial cell wall disruption and inhibition of bacterial enzymes

(4) Adverse effects—burning sensation and bitter taste; some report soft tissue irritation; caution with significant xerostomia and recovering alcoholic patients; some formulations have high alcohol content; some are now alcohol free; however, they are for reduction of halitosis rather than as an antiseptic antigingivitis agent

(5) Twice-daily use promotes compliance; patient should be instructed to use 15 mL of rinse for 30 seconds after brushing

(6) Also recommended as preprocedural rinse to reduce salivary bacterial load and aerosols during periodontal therapy and mechanized instrumentation

2. Other agents used in periodontal therapy

a. Povidone–iodine

(1) An iodophor with polyvinyl–pyrrolidone added to iodine; effective against many organisms, including bacteria, viruses, and fungi

(2) Primarily used as a preprocedural rinse or during mechanized instrumentation for antiseptic lavage or irrigation; often recommended for use during treatment of immunocompromised patients who might have multiple organisms affecting their oral health; can be effective antimicrobial and antigingivitis agent, but only with short-term use

(3) Adverse effects—concern for iodine toxicity with prolonged use; contraindicated in those with iodine sensitivity or allergy, thyroid dysfunction and pregnant or lactating women; temporary extrinsic tooth staining

b. Stannous fluoride

(1) Antimicrobial mechanism of action appears to be related to the stannous (tin) ion rather than fluoride

(2) Long-term studies have shown significant reductions in gingivitis without concurrent significant reductions in biofilm and gingival inflammation

(3) Available in dentifrice; in gel form; or in rinses containing 0.63% concentrations; however, the dentifrice and gel forms are most effective

(4) Stannous fluoride has low to moderate substantivity, depending on concentration; twice-daily use promotes compliance

(5) Adverse effects may include unpleasant taste in the mouth and tooth staining after prolonged use (2 to 3 months) in some individuals

(6) Stannous fluoride has the American Dental Association (ADA) Seal of Acceptance for anticaries activity; the dentifrice formulation has been approved for plaque-reducing and gingivitis-reducing properties; dentifrice and gels also approved for dentinal hypersensitivity reduction

c. Quaternary ammonium compounds (cetylpyridinium chloride)
   (1) The most common formulation is cetylpyridinium chloride used alone or with domiphen bromide; cationic surface active agents rupture bacterial cell walls; the compound binds to oral tissues but releases rapidly, which may limit its substantivity and therefore effectiveness in the oral cavity
   (2) Six-month studies show 14% to 24% reduction in bacterial biofilm and gingivitis; the therapeutic value of the product is questionable
   (3) Has benefit in reducing halitosis; often alcohol free
   (4) Adverse reactions are minimal; may include possible slight staining

d. Oxygenating agents—hydrogen peroxide: antiinflammatory properties decrease the clinical signs of inflammation, but bacterial pathogens may not be reduced; studies do not support long-term use of 100% hydrogen peroxide as oral rinse; ration with water 1:1 recommended as maximum; safety issues such as tissue injury and cocarcinogenicity have been raised with long-term use of hydrogen peroxide; 2–3% peroxide solution sold over the counter is being diluted to 1%–1.5% and used as a preprocedural mouth rinse prior to dental services as part of a coronavirus disease 2019 (COVID-19) infection prevention and control procedure

e. Oxidizing agents (chlorine dioxide, zinc)—have no therapeutic value but are recommended for breath freshening and to reduce halitosis; reduce volatile sulfur compounds (VSCs) that are believed to be responsible for halitosis

3. Methods for topical delivery of antimicrobial agents
   a. Mouthrinses, dentifrices, and gels deliver agents supragingivally; subgingival penetration is 0 to 1 mm—most common method
   b. Oral irrigation can deliver agent subgingivally; complete plaque removal is not achieved, but periodontal pathogens found in loosely adherent plaque can be removed; recommended as an adjunct to mechanical biofilm control; often used during the maintenance of periodontal health after completion of active periodontal therapy; pulsating oral irrigators may be used as water flossers
   c. Oral irrigation can be accomplished with water or antimicrobial agents; both reduce bleeding and gingivitis, but antimicrobials are more effective in removing bacterial plaque and making it less pathogenic; effect on periodontitis is not well documented
   d. Depth of penetration with oral irrigation is related to type of tip used; standard jet tip is shallow; subgingival tip 6 mm or less; cannula deepest but concern for patient safety
   e. Oral irrigation can have value in conjunction with daily self-care regimen for mechanical plaque biofilm removal in the treatment of gingivitis or in periodontal maintenance therapy
   f. Professionally administered oral irrigation, with and without root planing and periodontal debridement, has been studied; the main benefit is from mechanical debridement; a single application of an antimicrobial irrigant has little value because of low substantivity in the periodontal pocket

E. Sustained-release, local drug delivery systems (also called *controlled drug delivery*)[1]
   1. Systems are available for site-specific, sustained, local delivery of antibiotics or antimicrobials to specific subgingival sites (e.g., gels, chips, collagen film, bioabsorbable materials); the objective is to eliminate periodontal pathogens; these methods of local delivery provide the benefits of antibiotic or antimicrobial therapy with greater safety and compliance; delivery mechanisms allow the antibiotic or antimicrobial agent to be delivered for up to 14 days (varies by product) after placement; controlled delivery releases the material's active ingredient over time, maintaining a constant and sufficient release of the active ingredient
   2. Controlled delivery offers the advantage of sustained release of a high concentration of the active ingredient to the site of periodontal infection without systemic involvement; can be used in conjunction with scaling, debridement, and root planing during initial periodontal therapy in pockets greater than 5 mm with bleeding on probing, at reevaluation for recalcitrant sites, or during continuing care for localized sites needing adjunctive therapy for the maintenance of periodontal health; few use these systems as a monotherapy
   3. Contraindicated in the presence of allergy to the active ingredient or to any component of the delivery system and during pregnancy or lactation; not useful for treatment of generalized diseased sites
   4. Studies have shown that these controlled delivery systems result in improved CALs or probing depths of 2 mm or greater at 30% to 40% of sites treated in multiple-center, randomized clinical trials, a level considered both statistically and clinically significant
   5. Examples of available sustained-release systems for subgingival application used most often in conjunction with scaling and root planing
      a. Chlorhexidine chip—2.5-mg chlorhexidine gluconate in a hydrolyzed gelatin biodegradable film; self-retentive on contact with moisture, placed using cotton pliers

b. Minocycline hydrochloride microspheres (2%)—consist of antibiotic minocycline hydrochloride in a bioabsorbable polymer of poly-D, L-lactide-CO-glycolide; microspheres are dispensed subgingivally from a capsule placed in a syringe; the tip is inserted into the base of the pocket and then withdrawn after the drug has been applied
c. Doxycycline hyclate gel (10%)—solidifying liquid, biodegradable polymer that hardens after exposure to fluid in the periodontal pocket; delivered by injection from a syringe with a blunt cannula inserted into the pocket; common use is with scaling and root planing

F. Use of systemic antibiotics[1]—drugs that target the bacterial load
1. Sometimes used in conjunction with periodontal therapy (surgical or nonsurgical); however, no evidence that antibiotics alone arrest periodontal disease exist; may be prescribed for patients who are nonresponsive to periodontal therapy, acute periodontal infections with systemic manifestations, for prophylaxis in medically compromised patients, and in conjunction with surgical or nonsurgical therapy when systemic health or classification of periodontal disease warrants use after consideration of risks and benefits
   a. Generalized recurrent or refractory periodontal disease despite appropriate treatment—often related to impaired host resistance or persistent, superinfecting microorganisms
   b. Aggressive forms of periodontitis—related to neutrophil defects and tissue-invasive microorganisms (*A. actinomycetemcomitans* and *P. gingivalis*)
   c. Acute, severe infections (e.g., periodontal abscess, necrotizing ulcerative gingivitis)—especially with fever, malaise, lymphadenopathy, or other systemic signs and symptoms
   d. Immunocompromised status—used with extreme caution to avoid development of resistant strains
2. Not recommended for the routine treatment of gingivitis or chronic periodontitis; problems such as adverse drug reactions, drug hypersensitivity, development of antibiotic-resistant strains, interactions with other prescribed medications taken by the patient, and patient nonadherence limit widespread use; the Centers for Disease Control and Prevention (CDC) recommends judicious use of antibiotics because of growing concerns about overuse and consequently the development of drug-resistant strains of bacteria, which has led to a resurgence of diseases previously well controlled by antibiotics (e.g., tuberculosis, staphylococcal infections, diphtheria); particular concerns about use in pregnant or lactating women do exist, and a higher risk of drug interactions is present with long-term use of cardiovascular disease, asthma, seizures, and diabetes medications
   a. Common side effects include nausea, vomiting, diarrhea, rashes, changes in vaginal or intestinal flora, and allergy; prolonged use can be associated with bleeding problems
   b. Specific reactions include the disulfiram (Antabuse) effect of metronidazole taken with alcohol, discoloration or deformed teeth with tetracycline use in children under 8 years of age, and increased risk of pseudomembranous colitis with clindamycin
3. Restricted use and careful selection are indicated on the basis of response to mechanical therapy, medical history analysis, possible drug interactions, and risks; indiscriminate use is prohibited; microbial analysis, antimicrobial sensitivity testing, or a combination of both before prescribing systemic antibiotics for periodontal therapy is recommended
4. Common agents include tetracylcines (doxycycline), nitroimidazoles (metronidazole), lincomycins (clindamycin), quinolones (ciprofloxacin), and macrolides (azithromycin but not erythromycin); combination therapy includes metronidazole and amoxicillin or metronidazole and ciprofloxacin; the combination is synergistic and increases the spectrum of drug activity; penicillins and cephalosporins are not considered drugs of choice

G. Use of host-modulating drugs;[1] host response is the target
1. While studies of nonsteroidal antiinflammatory drugs (NSAIDs), bisphosphonates, and most recently, lipoxims and resovins have shown proof of concept, only low-dose doxycycline has been FDA approval for treatment of periodontal disease
   a. Subantimicrobial-dose doxycycline (SDD)—used systemically in subantimicrobial doses to inhibit proteases and periodontal disease progression; downregulates the activity of matrix metalloproteinases that are active during periods of periodontal tissue breakdown and thus play a major role in inflammation and the destruction of collagen and bone
   b. Has not been shown to substitute for meticulous home care and periodontal maintenance
   c. Administered 20 mg twice daily (instead of the 50-mg or 100-mg dosage used as antibiotic) for 6 to 9 months or up to 12 months concurrent with periodontal therapy; a low dose eliminates most side effects, although SDD is contraindicated when known allergy to tetracyclines is present
   d. Research has shown slight but statistically significant gains in clinical attachment and reductions in probing depths

## Additional Clinical Interventions

A. Gingival curettage[1,15]—a procedure to remove the ulcerated, chronically inflamed tissue lining a periodontal pocket; evidence fails to support the efficacy of this procedure
1. Studies of gingival curettage have almost always combined this technique with root planing; research indicates that gingival curettage is ineffective and that root planing alone can, in most cases, reduce inflammation, shrink tissue, and promote healing

2. In some states, gingival curettage is a legally permissible procedure that can be performed by dental hygienists
3. If new connective tissue attachment is the goal of a particular periodontal treatment plan, curettage has no justifiable application; healing occurs by means of a longer junctional epithelium and tissue shrinkage, as it does with root planing or periodontal debridement; surgical intervention is the therapy of choice when new attachment is the desired end point

B. Lasers—stands for Light Amplification by the Stimulated Emission of Radiation
   1. Many different types of lasers, each using a different type of laser medium
   2. Used for removal of diseased pocket lining epithelium, bactericidal effect on pathogenic microbiota, elimination of calculus, and root surface detoxification
   3. Laser-assisted new attachment procedure (LANAP) using a free running pulsed Nd:YAG laser has demonstrated regeneration of the cementum mediated attachment apparatus

C. Treatment of occlusal trauma[1]
   1. Definitions
      a. Occlusal trauma—injury to the periodontal attachment apparatus resulting from occlusal forces when those forces exceed the reparative and adaptive capacity of the attachment apparatus
      b. Primary occlusal trauma—injury to the periodontium as a result of excessive occlusal forces when the periodontal attachment apparatus and the attachment level are normal
      c. Secondary occlusal trauma—injury to a compromised periodontium with loss of attachment or bone loss resulting from normal or excessive occlusal force
   2. Clinical features and diagnosis
      a. When injury to the periodontal ligament occurs, collagen is destroyed, vascular elements are affected, and osteoclasts are increased on the pressure side, all of which results in a widening of the periodontal ligament space because of the lateral resorption of the bony socket wall, especially in the crestal area when the force is great enough to cause necrosis of the ligament; when a back-and-forth motion, or "jiggling," of the tooth in the socket (fremitus) occurs from occlusal trauma, changes are seen on both the tension and the pressure side, resulting in a funnel-shaped widening of the periodontal ligament and loss of bone; as such, mobility is the hallmark of occlusal trauma, and radiographic findings reveal widening of the ligament space, infrabony defects, or both; parafunctional habits such as bruxism and clenching or iatrogenic factors causing premature contacts (e.g., "high" restorations) most frequently result in occlusal trauma; tissues can regenerate on removal of the occlusal force that is causing destruction; therefore, constant evaluation and reevaluation are indicated
      b. Although necrosis of the ligament and loss of bone can occur from occlusal trauma, it is important to note that attachment loss characterized by apical migration of the periodontal attachment, such as that caused by periodontitis, does not occur solely from occlusal trauma; occlusal trauma can contribute to advancing loss of attachment once attachment loss or bone loss from periodontitis has weakened tooth support
      c. Positive diagnosis is made on the basis of signs and symptoms of injury (e.g., tooth mobility or migration; pain on percussion or chewing; radiographic changes such as widened periodontal ligament, crestal infrabony [angular] defects, and condensing osteitis, or root resorption; TMJ dysfunction, severe wear facets; crown or root fractures; or *fremitus* (a term used when tooth movement or vibration occurs with the teeth occluded and grinded in all functional positions); clinicians correlate clinical findings with radiographic findings; pathologic occlusion shows evidence of disease interfering with comfort, function, or esthetics that can be attributed to occlusal forces
      d. Pulp vitality testing, evaluation of parafunctional habits, clinical assessment of occlusal discrepancies and bone, fremitus and mobility, radiographic assessment of the periodontal ligament and bone, and other adjunctive diagnostic procedures generally are required for differential diagnosis
   3. Once diagnosed, occlusal traumatism may be treated; however, plaque-induced inflammation also must be eliminated

## Surgical Interventions

A. Principles of periodontal surgery
   1. Rationale
      a. Eliminate active infection
      b. Render the periodontium more cleansable by the patient and maintainable by the professional
         (1) Improvement in the contours of hard and soft tissues
         (2) Pocket elimination or reduction
      c. Replace damaged or destroyed periodontium
         (1) Soft tissue replacement (gingival grafts)
         (2) Hard tissue replacement (osseous grafts)
      d. Surgery is rarely performed solely to remove inflammation or infection but, rather, in an attempt to:
         (1) Eliminate both hard and soft defects created by disease
         (2) Restore normal architecture and physiologic function
         (3) Gain regeneration or new attachment of the supporting structures
   2. Case preparation (see the sections on "Implementation" and "Evaluation" in Chapter 15)
      a. Patients need to complete the initial therapy before entering the surgical phase; initial care aims to remove the causative factors, control active disease, and educate the patient in the role as a cotherapist

b. Completion of initial therapy prepares tissue for surgery by reducing marginal inflammation and improving tissue tone, which allows more predictable incisions and suturing and reduces surgical bleeding
c. The prognosis is improved overall after initial preparation or therapy
d. The patient's response to NSPT is assessed in relation to healing response; motivation and supplemental self-care devices may be needed for adequate healing
e. Completion of initial therapy can reduce the number of sites requiring surgery or even eliminate the need for surgery in a given sextant or quadrant

B. Types of surgical intervention
1. Resective periodontal surgery
a. Gingivectomy—surgical procedure for pocket reduction by excision of the soft tissue pocket wall; indicated for gingival pockets composted of fibrotic enlargement or to correct gingival form; only involves the gingiva
b. Gingivoplasty—reshaping of the gingiva to obtain a physiologic form similar to that characteristic of healthy tissue by using a rotary instrument; frequently combined with gingivectomy
c. Periodontal flap procedures—may be used as a method of surgical curettage (e.g., modified Widman flap) or for pocket elimination by apically repositioning the soft tissue; most common form of surgery; provides access for thorough scaling and root planing when access is not possible through NSPT (deep pockets, furcation areas, or other areas of complex anatomy); can access bony deformities or craters
d. Osseous resective surgery or osseous resection
(1) Objectives—removal of alveolar bone to produce a more physiologic architecture or contour; ultimately, pocket reduction in one-walled infrabony or vertical defects; also for lengthening the clinical crown for root restoration; the goal is to remove a minimal amount of bone; may include ostectomy, osteoplasty, or both
e. Root resection or hemisection—the objective is removal of the crown, root, or both to eliminate the involved furcation when osseous resection or regenerative surgery is not feasible; resection is removal of one molar root when two roots are involved to include class II or III furcations; also requires endodontics and restorative dentistry; hemisection is converting a two-rooted tooth into a single-rooted tooth by removing both one root and a portion of the crown
2. Regenerative and reconstructive surgery
a. Bone grafts and regenerative surgery
(1) Objective—to promote regeneration of connective tissue, periodontal ligament, cementum, and alveolar bone
(2) Indications—two-walled and three-walled vertical defects, class II furcation defects, circumferential defects (Figs. 14.5 and 14.6)
b. Options available
(1) Guided tissue regeneration (GTR) and guided bone regeneration (GBR)—involve using a semipermeable membrane between the epithelium and the underlying ligament and bone to prevent rapid downgrowth of the epithelium or connective tissue, which would interfere with connective tissue regrowth after surgical debridement of the defect; nonresorbable membranes most frequently used
(2) Bone grafts—involve placing bone-grafting material into a debrided defect to the level of the uninvolved crest to promote bone healing and regeneration; the graft stimulates new bone formation and thus new attachment; autografts are obtained from the same patient, allografts are transferred from genetically dissimilar individuals within the same species (e.g., processed human cadaver bone that is freeze-dried or demineralized); alloplastic grafts use biologic fillers (e.g., bioactive glass ionomers, biocompatible composite polymers) or organic materials such as coral and bone; xenografts are obtained from another species
(3) Biologic and biomimicry mediators—biologic agents such as enamel matrix derivatives or synthetic biomimicry agents such as platelet-derived growth factors, platelet-rich plasma, and bone morphogenetic proteins are being studied for their potential to enhance periodontal regeneration
3. Periodontal plastic and reconstructive surgery
a. Includes mucogingival surgery to correct defects or deficiencies in the shape, position, or amount of keratinized, attached gingiva surrounding teeth; mucogingival therapy to correct these types of defects in soft tissue and underlying bone; periodontal plastic surgery to create morphology and appearance that is acceptable to the patient and the clinician, including root coverage, crown lengthening, ridge preservation, and augmentation; esthetic surgery around implants; and exposure of teeth for orthodontics
b. Includes gingival augmentation to increase the width of the attached gingiva, establish vestibular depth, arrest progressive gingival recession, and facilitate self-care; frenectomy for the elimination of abnormal frenum often in conjunction with a soft tissue graft; alveolar ridge augmentation resulting from tooth loss; esthetic crown lengthening when anterior teeth are shorter than normal; papillary retention and reconstruction to correct deficient interproximal height of papillary gingiva; or surgical movement of impacted teeth for orthodontics

## Healing Following Periodontal Therapy

See the section on "Regeneration and Wound Healing" in Chapter 7.

A. In health, periodontal tissue constantly undergoes renewal; the oral epithelium maintains thickness by the mitotic activity of epithelial cells, fibroblasts generate and regenerate connective tissue, and cementoblasts form new cementum; periodontal ligament cells and bone are continually remodeled by fibroblasts and osteoblasts
B. Basic healing processes after all forms of periodontal therapy are the same
   1. Regeneration—growth and differentiation of new cells and intercellular substances to form or re-form tissues or parts of the same type as the precursor; primary means of healing after NSPT, creating a longer junctional epithelium
   2. Repair—also referred to as *healing by scar tissue* or *fibrosis*; does not necessarily restore the original architecture or function of the tissue or part
   3. Epithelial adaptation—close adaptation of the marginal gingival epithelium without complete pocket elimination; occurs with shrinkage of the gingiva after therapy; often occurs in conjunction with the regeneration of a longer junctional epithelium
   4. New attachment—embedding of new periodontal ligament fibers into new cementum and formation of a new gingival attachment in an area previously degenerated by disease rather than repair of the periodontal attachment apparatus after an injury (reattachment)
      a. Goal of periodontal surgery—the rapid downgrowth of the epithelium must be prevented to allow the formation of connective tissue and bone; this is the basis of using a barrier in regenerative surgery
      b. Requires adequate removal of local etiologic factors through debridement; immobilization of mobile teeth and elimination of occlusal stress in a weakened periodontium are necessary

### Sutures

A. Objectives
   1. Used to hold soft tissue in place until the healing process has progressed to the point at which tissue placement can be self-maintained
   2. Stabilization of the soft tissue helps:
      a. Maintain blood clotting around the wound
      b. Protect the wound area during the healing process
B. Types of suture materials
   1. Absorbable—surgical gut (from intestines of sheep); polyglactin and polyglecaprone; absorb through proteolysis by enzymes in saliva in 7 to 10 days, thus eliminating the need for removal
   2. Nonabsorbable—surgical silk most common; must be professionally removed after 7 to 10 days
C. Procedure for suture removal
   1. Grasp the knotted end of suture with cotton pliers, and gently pull it away from the tissue
   2. Insert the tip of scissors under the suture, and cut the suture material that had been in the tissue
   3. Gently pull the knotted end so that only the suture material that had previously been incorporated within the tissue will pass through the tissue during the removal process
   4. Count and record the number of sutures removed, and compare this number with the suture placement record
   5. Gently cleanse the wound sites, and check for bleeding; control the bleeding, as needed

### Periodontal Dressings

A. The rationale for the use of periodontal dressing is to protect the tissues after surgery; have no curative properties; wound healing progresses at the same rate with or without dressings; sometimes used for patient comfort or for protection of the wound area
B. Types—dressings using metallic oxide and fatty acids (noneugenol) are most common; clear, translucent light-cured dressings are preferred by some clinicians for esthetics
C. Removal of the periodontal dressing
   1. Remove the dressing within 5 to 7 days; tease the edges of the dressing away from teeth with a curette or cotton pliers; be sure that sutures are not embedded in the dressing
   2. After the pack has been removed, gently cleanse the area with warm water or dampened cotton tips; remove sutures; assess tissue healing, but do not probe sulcular areas

## POSTOPERATIVE CARE

### Patient Instructions and Education

A. Discomfort—the patient should:
   1. Expect some discomfort after the local anesthesia wears off; use the prescribed pain medication
   2. Rest and limit physical activities during the first few days to prevent excessive bleeding and promote healing
   3. Use an ice pack to prevent swelling
   4. Eliminate spicy, hot, cold, hard, or sticky foods and liquids and tobacco use to limit tissue irritants and protect the dressing
B. Home care recommendations—provide the following instructions to the patient:
   1. Do not rinse the mouth on the first day because this may disturb the process of blood clotting that is necessary for wound healing
   2. After the first day, rinse gently with lukewarm water or a small amount of an antimicrobial rinse (e.g., chlorhexidine gluconate) to help control bacterial biofilm; brush and floss nonsurgical areas as usual but gently
   3. Using a soft brush and water, very gently clean the surface of the dressing
   4. Slight seepage of blood during the first few hours is normal; any unusual, persistent bleeding should be reported to the periodontist

### Follow-up Care

A. Patient returns approximately 7 days after surgery
B. Dressing and sutures are removed; new dressing may or may not be applied

C. Dentinal hypersensitivity may be experienced; desensitization is indicated for dentinal hypersensitivity; desensitization methods may be prescribed (see the section on "Assessment of Dentinal Hypersensitivity" in Chapter 16)
D. Home-care instructions are provided for biofilm control
E. Long-term postoperative care requires periodic evaluation (also known as *periodontal maintenance care, continued care,* or *recare*)

## Periodontal Maintenance

A. An extension of periodontal therapy; also called *periodontal maintenance*
   1. Initiated after completion of active periodontal treatment and continued at various intervals for the life of the dentition or its implant replacements
   2. Periodontal maintenance is an extension of active therapy, whether nonsurgical or surgical
B. The objectives of periodontal maintenance care is to:
   1. Minimize any recurrence and progression of periodontal disease in previously treated patients
   2. Reduce tooth loss incidence by monitoring the patient's periodontal status at regular intervals
   3. Reevaluate results after active periodontal therapy (nonsurgical or surgical) over the long term
   4. Reinforce self-care instructions and encourage patient's long-term protective oral health behaviors
   5. Determine the need for additional treatment in a timely manner
C. Components of periodontal maintenance care
   1. Need for the cooperation of patient, dental hygienist, dentist, and periodontist
   2. Emphasis on scaling, root planing, and periodontal debridement; extrinsic stain removal; and reinstruction of patient in self-care to maintain attachment levels
   3. Optimization of protective factors; minimization and elimination of risk factors
D. Periodic reevaluation and assessment
   1. Review and update of patient's health, pharmacologic, and dental histories; review and control of associated risk factors
   2. Radiographic review
   3. Examination of extraoral and intraoral soft tissues
   4. Dental charting of caries, tooth mobility and fremitus, and other tooth-related problems
   5. Periodontal assessment and charting of gingival recession, probing depths, bleeding on probing; levels of plaque and calculus, furcation involvement, exudation, occlusal trauma, tooth mobility; and other signs or symptoms of periodontal disease
   6. Evaluation of patient's oral self-care behavior, attitude, values, and skill
   7. Examination of dental implants and peri-implant tissues
E. Treatment—based on assessment
   1. Always encourage the patient; provide oral self-care reinstruction, and reinforce patient's compliance with recommended maintenance intervals
   2. Healthy periodontium—removal of supragingival deposits; no root planing indicated
   3. Presence of bleeding or inflammation of the gingiva—treatment depends on the cause and pocket depths; removal of deposits and contributing factors, as necessary; possible use of an antimicrobial rinse (e.g., 0.12% chlorhexidine) or sustained-release, locally delivered antibiotic or antimicrobial agent
   4. Presence of periodontal pockets—scaling, periodontal debridement, and root planing followed by reevaluation in 4 to 6 weeks to determine the need for adjunctive therapy or possible periodontal surgery
   5. Determination of frequency of periodontal maintenance must be individualized
      a. The frequency increases when patients have less than optimal oral self-care practices
      b. Longer intervals are acceptable if patients can control bacterial plaque (dental) biofilm, unless systemic disease or advanced periodontitis exists
      c. The goal is to control the clinical signs of inflammation and to stabilize attachment levels
      d. Frequent intervals (3 months or less) are generally necessary for subgingival and supragingival plaque and calculus removal in the presence of periodontitis
      e. Generally, the shorter the interval, the greater the long-term success, particularly during the healing phase (1 year) after surgery
F. Indications for retreatment
   1. Increase in probing depth or attachment loss of 2 mm or more
   2. Bleeding on probing that does not respond to periodontal maintenance procedures
   3. Severity—to be considered in determining treatment regimens (nonsurgical or surgical); retaining questionable teeth is not recommended
   4. Generalized deterioration—systemic complication might be suspected
   5. Dental implants with bone loss or mobility

# DENTAL IMPLANTS

See the sections on "Dental Implants" in Chapter 13 and "Advanced Instrumentation Techniques" in Chapter 17.

A. Definition—artificial replacements of teeth that are permanently affixed into alveolar bone by a biomedical device and usually composed of an inert metal or a metallic alloy
   1. Implants offer an alternative to removable dentures for edentulous or partially edentulous persons; single or multiple teeth can be replaced
   2. Implants provide a permanent anchor for artificial teeth by serving as an abutment for fixed or removable prostheses
      a. Implant—portion surgically placed within the bone
      b. Abutment—metallic post attached to the implant so that a restoration can be placed over it

c. Superstructure—prosthetic replacement (e.g., crown, bridge, denture) that is affixed to the abutment or a removable replacement tooth that the patient can remove and clean
d. Implant-assisted prosthesis—removable tissue dentures (overdentures) supported in the arch by endosseous dental implants

B. Limiting factors
1. Systemic—age is a consideration only if the patient's jaws are still growing because implants are contraindicated until full growth is attained; any condition or disease that affects an individual's ability to fight infection should be carefully considered because implant failure is often caused by infection; greater failure also occurs in poor quality and density of bone, so conditions such as osteoporosis also require careful consideration; cigarette smoking is a documented risk factor for implant failure, so tobacco cessation is essential before implant placement; factors affecting the patient's ability to withstand surgery also are paramount (e.g., malnutrition, recent cardiac arrest, bleeding problems)
2. Local—unfavorable ridge morphology or other bone quality and density changes caused by resorption; sufficient bone and soft tissue for implant positioning must be similar to that of a natural tooth within the tissue and the alveolar ridge—orthodontics and surgical augmentation or correction may be possible; severe malocclusion or parafunctional habits that would cause excessive trauma would contraindicate implants; uncontrolled periodontal disease is also a contraindication; an immobile implant generally is not attached to a natural tooth with periodontal ligament mobility

C. Implant design
1. Systems—either two stage (submerged) or one stage (nonsubmerged)
a. Submerged—designed to protect the implant from occlusal stress and bacterial exposure during the healing phase; the implant is placed in two steps, allowing osseo-integration for 3 to 6 months before exposing the implant to the oral cavity for abutment placement; a prosthetic device is later connected to the implant
b. Nonsubmerged—the implant has a collar that extends through tissue and attaches the prosthesis supragingivally or slightly subgingivally at the time of placement; only one surgery is involved for patient comfort and convenience
c. Shape and size vary in either system; most common are screw-shaped, root-shaped, or cylinder-shaped implants
2. Materials typically used for dental implants—must be biocompatible
a. Titanium—a metallic element; pure, plasma sprayed, or titanium alloy
b. Hydroxyapatite—plasma sprayed

D. Types of implants most frequently used
1. Endosseous implants (inside bone)
a. The implant is placed directly into a socket, which has been prepared through a process called *trephining*; uses a series of specially prepared drills and burs
(1) Osseo-integration refers to the implant being in direct contact with bone without intervening connective tissue (i.e., no periodontal ligament or connective tissue attachment); the implant is in effect "ankylosed" within bone
(2) After initial loss of 1 to 2 mm of alveolar bone during the first year, crestal bone should be stable with no more than 0.1 to 0.2 mm per year thereafter
b. After bone and soft tissue heal, the final bridge or denture is placed
2. Transosteal implants—means "through the bone"; mandibular denture anchors are placed all the way through the mandible from under the border into the oral cavity

E. Implant–tissue interface
1. The implant–tissue interface is the basis of implant success
2. The epithelial attachment to the implant may be similar to the attachment to a natural tooth (i.e., basal lamina and hemidesmosomes); no periodontal ligament; called *perimucosal seal*
3. Perimucosal seal, or biologic seal, is defined as the adaptation of keratinized or nonkeratinized epithelium to the abutment cylinder of an implant; critical to implant retention
4. Osseo-integration—contact established between normal and remodeled bone and the implant surface without the interposition of connective tissue

F. Criteria for successful treatment outcomes
1. Immobility of the implant
2. No peri-implant radiolucency on the radiograph
3. Width of implant
4. Width of attached gingiva
5. Medical conditions
6. Smoking
7. Absence of signs and symptoms such as pain, bleeding, infections, paresthesias, or mandibular canal involvement
8. Minimum success rate of 85% at 5 years and 80% at 10 years of observation

G. Implant management
1. Periodic evaluation of implants, surrounding tissue, and oral hygiene essential to long-term success; considerations in periodic evaluation include:
a. Extent of biofilm and dental calculus
b. Clinical appearance of peri-implant soft tissue
c. Radiographic appearance—no periodontal ligament space or bone loss; no peri-implant radiolucency
d. Absence of occlusal interference or trauma; stability of implant and prostheses—no mobility
e. Probing depths (if other signs of disease present)—gentle, careful technique
f. Absence of bleeding or exudate
g. Adequacy of maintenance interval
h. Patient comfort and function

2. Goals
   a. Maintenance of the health of the implant and supporting tissue
   b. Prevention of loss of perimucosal seal
   c. Prevention of gingivitis and, failing that, prevention of conversion of gingivitis to peri-implantitis, a periodontitis-like disease process that can affect dental implants
      (1) Infectious failure—failing implants with a primarily infectious cause
      (2) Traumatic failure—failing implants with a primarily traumatic cause
   d. Provision of preventive and maintenance therapies with minimal damage, or surface scratching, to implants
   e. Control of bacterial plaque biofilm

H. Preventive instrumentation (see the sections on "Dental Implant Maintenance" in Chapter 16 and "Instrumentation of Dental Implants" in Chapter 17)

I. Peri-implant diseases and conditions[17]
   1. During the 2017 World Workshop on the Classification of Periodontal and Peri-Implant Diseases and Conditions a new classification for peri-implant diseases and conditions was developed. The goal of the classification system was to describe all aspects of the disease and pertinent site conditions and deformities.
      a. Peri-implant diseases and conditions
         (1) Peri-implant health - absence of visual signs of inflammation and bleeding upon probing around implants with normal or reduced bone support
         (2) Peri-implant mucositis - visual signs of inflammation and bleeding upon probing which are reversible with plaque is removed
         (3) Peri-implantitis - plaque-induced irreversible destruction of the supporting structures
         (4) Hard and soft tissue deficiencies - alveolar process/ridge deformities around an implant caused by multiple etiological factors which may compromise survival of the implant and require therapeutic interventions

(Table 14.1)

## WEBSITE INFORMATION AND RESOURCES

| Source | Website Address | Description |
|---|---|---|
| American Academy of Periodontology | http://www.perio.org | Position papers, parameters of care, scientific information, and related links in periodontics as well as related information for consumers |
| Cochrane Collaboration | http://www.cochrane.org | Evidence-based health care databases; site search for "periodontal" provides excellent related systematic reviews |
| European Federation of Periodontology | http://www.efp.org | Publications, news, patient information |
| National Center for Dental Hygiene Research | https://dent-web10.usc.edu/dhnet/ | Current topics in dental hygiene and periodontics with links to related government sites, product companies, and professional associations |
| Centers for Disease Control and Prevention Smoking and Tobacco Use | https://www.cdc.gov/tobacco/index.htm | Wide variety of resources related to tobacco use, quit tips and cessation materials, and state and community programs |

## CHAPTER 14 REVIEW QUESTIONS

1. Recession is noted in the mandibular anterior region, and the attached gingiva measures 0.5 mm, requiring evaluation by a dentist or periodontist. If periodontal surgery is indicated, a mucogingival surgery would be performed to correct this condition.
   **a.** Both statements are TRUE
   **b.** Both statements are FALSE
   **c.** The first statement is TRUE; the second statement is FALSE
   **d.** The first statement is FALSE; the second statement is TRUE
2. Which of the following devices would be MOST effective for plaque biofilm removal in the mandibular anterior region when recession has resulted in open embrasure spaces?
   **a.** Dental floss
   **b.** Dental tape
   **c.** Oral irrigation
   **d.** Interproximal brush
3. According to the new 2017 World Workshop on the Classification of Periodontal and Peri-Implant Diseases and Conditions, all of the following are goals of staging a periodontitis patient EXCEPT one. Which one is the exception?
   **a.** Classify the severity of the disease based on the extent of destroyed and damaged tissue
   **b.** Assess specific factors that might determine the complexity of managing current disease
   **c.** Estimate future risk of periodontitis progression to guide the intensity of the therapy and monitoring the disease activity
   **d.** Determine the percent of radiographic bone loss
4. An oxygenating mouthrinse would be beneficial for a patient with halitosis because these mouthrinses are the most effective in reducing bacterial plaque biofilm.
   **a.** Both the statement and the reason are correct and related
   **b.** Both the statement and the reason are correct but are NOT related
   **c.** The statement is correct, but the reason is NOT correct
   **d.** The statement is NOT correct, but the reason is correct
   **e.** NEITHER the statement NOR the reason is correct

5. Which of the following periodontal therapies would be BEST recommended for a patient who presents with probing depths of 3 to 5 mm, slight bone loss detected on the radiographs, and a history of infrequent dental hygiene care?
   a. Regenerative periodontal surgery
   b. Gingival curettage
   c. Nonsurgical periodontal therapy
   d. Oral prophylaxis
   e. Periodontal maintenance therapy
6. Which of the following would be the BEST indicator of treatment success at the reevaluation appointment 4 to 6 weeks after initial periodontal therapy?
   a. Relatively free of plaque biofilm
   b. Stable periodontal probing depths
   c. Absence of gingival inflammation and bleeding
   d. No re-formed dental calculus deposits
7. What change in alveolar bone on a dental radiograph indicates early loss of bone?
   a. Fuzziness in the crest of the bone
   b. Faint cup-shaped areas interproximally
   c. Vertical or angular defects
   d. Furcation involvement
8. After thorough periodontal debridement is performed, which is the first inflammatory cell to respond to avoidable resultant irritation of the gingiva?
   a. B lymphocytes
   b. Plasma cells
   c. Neutrophils
   d. T lymphocytes
   e. Macrophages
9. Which of the following changes result in a false or pseudo periodontal pocket?
   a. Apical migration of the junctional epithelium
   b. Apical migration of the gingival margin
   c. Resorption of the alveolar bone
   d. Swelling of the gingival margin without bone loss
10. Which of the following diagnostic procedures is MOST accurate for determining severity of periodontal attachment loss?
    a. Full-mouth digital radiographic survey
    b. Microbial testing of plaque biofilm
    c. Detection of pathologic tooth mobility or furcation
    d. Periodontal probing of all sulcular areas
    e. Determining presence or absence of bleeding on probing
11. In patients of periodontitis, what is the first area to be involved in bone resorption?
    a. Facial and lingual aspects of supporting bone
    b. Cribriforme plate or lamina dura
    c. Cancellous portion of supporting bone
    d. Cortical plate of the interdental septum
    e. Bone surrounding the apical area of the tooth
12. Which one of the following bacteria are predominant in supragingival plaque biofilm associated with gingivitis?
    a. Chromogenic bacteria
    b. Gram-negative anaerobic bacteria
    c. Aerobic and facultative bacteria
    d. Gram-positive *Streptococcus* spp.
13. Which of the following types of cells are responsible for resorption of cementum and bone in periodontal destruction?
    a. Cementoblasts
    b. Fibroblasts
    c. Osteoblasts
    d. Cementoclasts
    e. Osteoclasts
14. Which of the following histologic changes in inflamed gingiva results in redness?
    a. Vasodilation within the gingival connective tissue
    b. Ulceration of the sulcular lining
    c. Lymphoid cell accumulation
    d. Collagenase destroying the lamina propria
    e. Alteration of fibroblasts in the connective tissue
15. Tooth mobility and fremitus can be signs of occlusal trauma because trauma can result in lateral resportion of bone.
    a. Both the statement and the reason are correct and related
    b. Both the statement and the reason are correct but are NOT related
    c. The statement is correct, but the reason is NOT correct
    d. The statement is NOT correct, but the reason is correct
    e. NEITHER the statement NOR the reason is correct
16. Which radiographic findings will MOST LIKELY be seen in dental plaque–induced gingivitis? Select all that apply.
    a. A thin periodontal ligament space
    b. Slight changes in the lamina dura
    c. Condensing osteitis
    d. Normal lamina dura and crestal bone
    e. Slight fuzziness at the alveolar crest
17. According to the new 2017 World Workshop on the Classification of Periodontal and Peri-Implant Diseases and Conditions, which of the following are goals of grading a periodontitis patient? Select all that apply.
    a. Classify the severity of the disease based on the extent of destroyed and damaged tissue
    b. Assess specific factors that might determine the complexity of managing current disease
    c. Estimate future risk of periodontitis progression to guide the intensity of the therapy and monitoring the disease activity
    d. Estimate the potential systemic health interactions with periodontitis to allow co-management with medical colleagues
18. Which of the following tissues consist(s) of nonkeratinized epithelium? Select all that apply.
    a. Crevicular epithelium
    b. Attached gingiva
    c. Interdental papilla
    d. Junctional epithelium
    e. Marginal gingiva
19. Which of the following microbes is associated with necrotizing ulcerative gingivitis and periodontitis?
    a. *Actinomyces viscosus*
    b. *Porphyromonas gingivalis*
    c. *Prevotella intermedia*
    d. *Treponema pallidum*
    e. *Capnocytophaga ochracea*

20. Which of the following types of drugs have been associated with fibrotic gingival overgrowth? Select all that apply.
    a. Oral contraceptives
    b. Antidepressants
    c. Calcium channel blockers
    d. Antihistamines
    e. Anticonvulsants
21. Which gingival fiber group runs from the cervical area of one tooth across to an adjacent tooth?
    a. Dentogingival fibers
    b. Circumferential fibers
    c. Transseptal fibers
    d. Alveologingival fibers
22. Which of the following BEST describes the sulcular epithelium?
    a. Keratinized epithelium
    b. Basal cell epithelium
    c. Squamous cell epithelium
    d. Simple cuboidal epithelium
    e. Parakeratinized epithelium
23. Which type of periodontal disease is characterized by gray, sloughing tissue, pain, and spontaneous bleeding with rapid connective tissue loss and exposed alveolar bone?
    a. Pericoronitis
    b. Periodontal abscess
    c. Necrotizing ulcerative gingivitis
    d. Necrotizing stomatitis
24. Which of the following are possible causes of gingival recession? Select all that apply.
    a. Faulty toothbrushing
    b. Bacterial plaque biofilm
    c. Tissue response to medication
    d. Dental caries
    e. Periodontal disease
25. All the following are risk factors associated with periodontal disease EXCEPT one. Which one is the exception?
    a. Genetics
    b. Immunosuppression
    c. Hormonal changes
    d. Frequent fermentable carbohydrates in diet
    e. Poor oral hygiene
26. Which of the following situations would be an indication for a gingivectomy?
    a. Edematous 5-mm pseudopocket
    b. Severe drug-influenced gingival enlargement
    c. Infrabony pocket of 6 mm on the distal aspect of tooth #30
    d. Gingival recession that extends into the alveolar mucosa
    e. Periodontal abscess
27. Which of the following is an objective of periodontal reconstructive surgery?
    a. Improve the esthetics of the patient's face
    b. Create gingival contour and appearance acceptable to the patient
    c. Remove alveolar bone to improve contour and correct defects
    d. Remove enlarged tissue to assist the patient in daily plaque control
    e. Promote regeneration of a new attachment
28. All the following are substances produced by the host response to bacterial plaque biofilm EXCEPT:
    a. Lipopolysaccharide (LPS)
    b. Matrix metalloproteinase (MMP)
    c. Cytokines
    d. Interleukin-1 (IL-1)
    e. Prostaglandin $E_2$ ($PGE_2$)
29. Which of the following are necessary for new attachment after periodontal surgery? *Select all that apply.*
    a. Thorough removal of bacterial irritants
    b. Immobilization of mobile teeth
    c. Shrinkage of the gingival margin
    d. Regeneration or generation of new tissues or parts
    e. Rapid apical growth of epithelium
30. All the following are advantages of controlled (sustained-release) drug delivery over systemic drug administration in periodontal therapy EXCEPT:
    a. Less concern about patient adherence throughout indicated time frame
    b. Site-specific antimicrobial action in periodontal pocket
    c. High concentration delivered to the site of infection
    d. Can be used when periodontal infection is generalized or severe
31. A female patient, age 40, returns for periodontal maintenance therapy every 3 months for 1 year after nonsurgical periodontal treatment for Stage III/Grade A periodontitis. The inflammation has been resolved, and periodontal probing depths have decreased from 5 or 6 mm to 4 mm or less in most treated areas, with the exception of the distal surface of tooth #15, where the probing depth has increased from 4 to 6 mm. Radiographs reveal no change on tooth #15 distal. All the following explain this finding EXCEPT:
    a. Continuing clinical attachment loss
    b. Error in periodontal probing technique
    c. Calculus deposits affecting accuracy of initial reading
    d. Inaccessibility and poor visibility in pocket areas
    e. Increased inflammation of the gingival tissues
32. Which of the following materials could be used in curettes for maintaining dental implants? Select all that apply.
    a. Stainless steel
    b. Carbon steel
    c. Plastic resin
    d. Titanium
33. Which of the following findings would indicate a failed dental implant?
    a. Peri-implant inflammation
    b. Bleeding on provocation
    c. Alveolar bone loss
    d. Loosening of the prosthetic crown
    e. Mobility
34. How is clinical attachment loss measured with a periodontal probe?
    a. From the margin of the gingiva to the epithelial attachment
    b. From the cemento-enamel junction to the base of the pocket
    c. From the margin of the gingiva to the cemento-enamel junction

d. From the cemento-enamel junction to the margin of the bone

35. In which area of the mouth would the width of the attached gingiva be expected to be the narrowest?
a. Mandibular anterior area
b. Mandibular premolar areas
c. Maxillary molar areas
d. Lingual of the maxillary teeth

36. Where is the lamina propria located in the periodontium?
a. In the periodontal ligament
b. In the alveolar bone
c. At the cemento-enamel junction
d. In the gingival mucosa

37. Which of the following changes would result in pocket reduction after periodontal debridement in an edematous pocket? Select all that apply.
a. Reattachment
b. New attachment
c. Longer junctional epithelium
d. Shrinkage of the gingival margin
e. Downward growth of the junctional epithelium

38. Occlusal trauma can result in all the following EXCEPT:
a. Periodontal pockets
b. Attrition of the tooth
c. Temporomandibular joint discomfort
d. Fractured teeth and restorations

39. Restorative margins placed within the supracrestal connective tissue attachment are associated with which of the following?
a. Primary occlusal trauma
b. Secondary occlusal trauma
c. Passive eruption
d. Inflammation and/or loss of periodontal supporting tissues

40. When applying the new 2017 World Workshop on the Classification of Periodontal and Peri-Implant Diseases and Conditions, what is the first step in classifying the patient?
a. Determine the complexity of the periodontal patient
b. Determine the clinical attachment loss (CAL)
c. Assess the patient's smoking status
d. Assess the patient's HbA1c level

41. Gingival recession only occurs during orthodontic therapy. The direction of tooth movement and bucco-lingual thickness of the gingiva play a critical role in the alteration of the gingival tissues.
a. Both statements are TRUE
b. Both statements are FALSE
c. The first statement if TRUE; the second statement is FALSE
d. The first statement is FALSE; the second statement is TRUE

42. All of the following increase the risk of plaque retention EXCEPT one. Which one is the exception?
a. Tooth positioning such as cross-bite and crowding
b. Supra-gingival placed crown margins
c. Developmental grooves
d. Enamel pearls

43. Which area presents the most challenging to perform a thorough scaling and root planing on?
a. Proximal surfaces of the maxillary anterior teeth
b. Trifurcations of maxillary molars
c. Distal of second mandibular molars
d. Mesial surface of maxillary premolar

44. Which type of microorganism is most prevalent in older (day 14–21) plaque biofilm?
a. Cocci
b. Filamentous and slender rods
c. Fusobacteria
d. Vibrios and spirochetes

45. Which of the following are signs and symptoms of an endo-periodontal lesion? Select all that apply.
a. Deep periodontal pocket extending to the root apex
b. Radiographic bone loss in the apical or furcation region
c. Negative or altered pulp vitality test
d. Purulent exudate/suppuration

## CASE A (FIG. 14.7A–14.9B)

The patient is a 55-year-old African American female, 5'5" in height and weighing 150 lbs. Sitting blood pressure is 134/88 mmHg and pulse of 78 BPM at first reading and 136/86 mmHg and pulse of 78 BPM on second reading 10 minutes later. Patient's medical history includes overactive bladder (had an implant placed in 1985), osteoarthritis (diagnosed for 18 years), seasonal allergies (self-reported), and type 2 diabetes (diagnosed 4 years ago). She has been taking Metformin up until 1 month ago when she did not refill her prescription because of finances. She is not aware of her current HbA1c level but states that her HbA1c level was 8.2% 1 month ago. The patient is allergic to penicillin. The patient denies a history of tobacco use, alcohol consumption or drug use. The patient reported moderate sugar consumption.

### Dental History

The patient presents for periodontal evaluation and treatment. Her last dental visit for cleaning was 2 years ago. Patient reports no pain around her teeth or in her mouth. Patient reports #2 fractured over 5 years ago. Dental history: amalgam: #5(DO), #14(O), #20(OD), #29(MO), #30(MO); composite:#8(D,M), #9(D) and extraction of #1, #4, #12, #13, #16, #17, #31, and #32. Patient had #1, #16, #17, and #32 extracted as a teenager. Teeth #4, #12, #13, and #31 extracted because of "gum disease."

### Chief Complaint

"My teeth are shifting and I am having trouble eating. I would like to replace the missing teeth with implants."

***Use Case A to answer questions 46 to 53.***

46. According to the newest American Heart Association and the American College of Cardiology high blood pressure guidelines, what category of blood pressure does this patient have?
a. Normal
b. Elevated
c. Stage 1
d. Stage 2
e. Hypertensive crisis

47. Which of the following would be the BEST ASA category to assign this patient?
a. ASA I
b. ASA II
c. ASA III
d. ASA IV

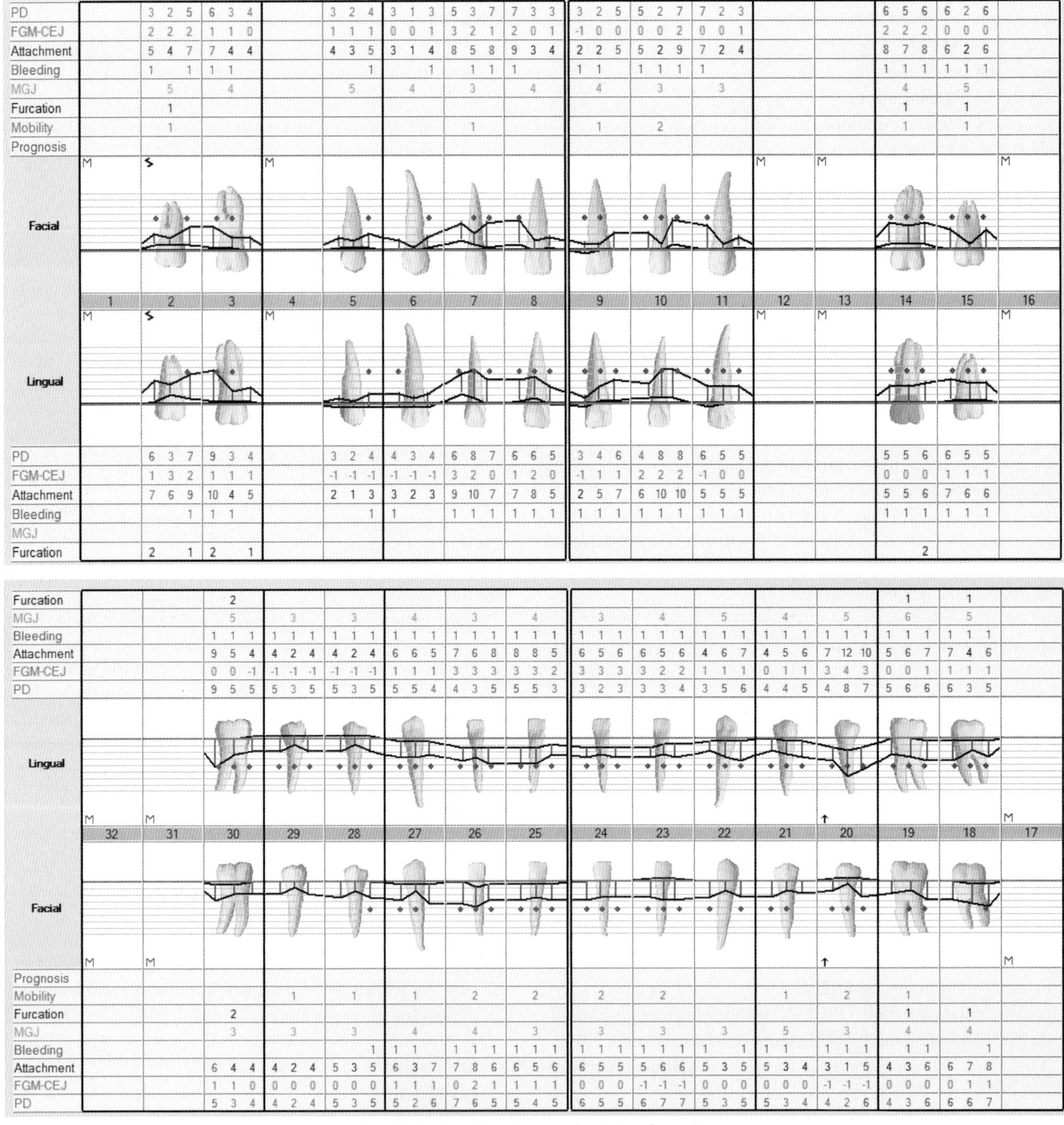

| | 1 | 2 | 3 | 4 | 5 | 6 | 7 | 8 | 9 | 10 | 11 | 12 | 13 | 14 | 15 | 16 |
|---|---|---|---|---|---|---|---|---|---|---|---|---|---|---|---|---|
| **Facial** | | | | | | | | | | | | | | | | |
| PD | | 3 2 5 | 6 3 4 | | 3 2 4 | 3 1 3 | 5 3 7 | 7 3 3 | 3 2 5 | 5 2 7 | 7 2 3 | | | 6 5 6 | 6 2 6 | |
| FGM-CEJ | | 2 2 2 | 1 1 0 | | 1 1 1 | 0 0 1 | 3 2 1 | 2 0 1 | -1 0 0 | 0 0 2 | 0 0 1 | | | 2 2 2 | 0 0 0 | |
| Attachment | | 5 4 7 | 7 4 4 | | 4 3 5 | 3 1 4 | 8 5 8 | 9 3 4 | 2 2 5 | 5 2 9 | 7 2 4 | | | 8 7 8 | 6 2 6 | |
| Bleeding | | 1 1 | 1 1 | | 1 | 1 | 1 1 | 1 | 1 1 | 1 1 1 | 1 | | | 1 1 1 | 1 1 1 | |
| MGJ | | 5 | 4 | | 5 | 4 | 3 | 4 | 4 | 3 | 3 | | | 4 | 5 | |
| Furcation | | 1 | | | | | | | | | | | | 1 | 1 | |
| Mobility | | 1 | | | | | 1 | | 1 | 2 | | | | 1 | 1 | |
| Prognosis | | | | | | | | | | | | | | | | |
| **Lingual** | | | | | | | | | | | | | | | | |
| PD | | 6 3 7 | 9 3 4 | | 3 2 4 | 4 3 4 | 6 8 7 | 6 6 5 | 3 4 6 | 4 8 8 | 6 5 5 | | | 5 5 6 | 6 5 5 | |
| FGM-CEJ | | 1 3 2 | 1 1 1 | | -1 -1 -1 | -1 -1 -1 | 3 2 0 | 1 2 0 | -1 1 1 | 2 2 2 | -1 0 0 | | | 0 0 0 | 1 1 1 | |
| Attachment | | 7 6 9 | 10 4 5 | | 2 1 3 | 3 2 3 | 9 10 7 | 7 8 5 | 2 5 7 | 6 10 10 | 5 5 5 | | | 5 5 6 | 7 6 6 | |
| Bleeding | | 1 | 1 1 | | 1 | 1 | 1 1 1 | 1 1 1 | 1 1 1 | 1 1 1 | 1 1 1 | | | 1 1 1 | 1 1 1 | |
| MGJ | | | | | | | | | | | | | | | | |
| Furcation | | 2 1 | 2 1 | | | | | | | | | | | 2 | | |

| | 32 | 31 | 30 | 29 | 28 | 27 | 26 | 25 | 24 | 23 | 22 | 21 | 20 | 19 | 18 | 17 |
|---|---|---|---|---|---|---|---|---|---|---|---|---|---|---|---|---|
| **Lingual** | | | | | | | | | | | | | | | | |
| Furcation | | | 2 | | | | | | | | | | | 1 | 1 | |
| MGJ | | | 5 | 3 | 3 | 4 | 3 | 4 | 3 | 4 | 5 | 4 | 5 | 6 | 5 | |
| Bleeding | | | 1 1 1 | 1 1 1 | 1 1 1 | 1 1 1 | 1 1 1 | 1 1 1 | 1 1 1 | 1 1 1 | 1 1 1 | 1 1 1 | 1 1 1 | 1 1 1 | 1 1 1 | |
| Attachment | | | 9 5 4 | 4 2 4 | 4 2 4 | 6 6 5 | 7 6 8 | 8 8 5 | 6 5 6 | 6 5 6 | 4 6 7 | 4 5 6 | 7 12 10 | 5 6 7 | 7 4 6 | |
| FGM-CEJ | | | 0 0 -1 | -1 -1 -1 | -1 -1 -1 | 1 1 1 | 3 3 3 | 3 3 2 | 3 3 3 | 3 2 2 | 1 1 1 | 0 1 1 | 3 4 3 | 0 0 1 | 1 1 1 | |
| PD | | | 9 5 5 | 5 3 5 | 5 3 5 | 5 5 4 | 4 3 5 | 5 5 3 | 3 2 3 | 3 3 4 | 3 5 6 | 4 4 5 | 4 8 7 | 5 6 6 | 6 3 5 | |
| **Facial** | | | | | | | | | | | | | | | | |
| Prognosis | | | | | | | | | | | | | | | | |
| Mobility | | | | 1 | 1 | 1 | 2 | 2 | 2 | 2 | | 1 | 2 | 1 | | |
| Furcation | | | 2 | | | | | | | | | | | 1 | 1 | |
| MGJ | | | 3 | 3 | 3 | 4 | 4 | 3 | 3 | 3 | 3 | 5 | 3 | 4 | 4 | |
| Bleeding | | | | | 1 | 1 1 | 1 1 1 | 1 1 1 | 1 1 1 | 1 1 1 | 1 1 | 1 1 | 1 1 1 | 1 1 | 1 | |
| Attachment | | | 6 4 4 | 4 2 4 | 5 3 5 | 6 3 7 | 7 8 6 | 6 5 6 | 6 5 5 | 5 6 6 | 5 3 5 | 5 3 4 | 3 1 5 | 4 3 6 | 6 7 8 | |
| FGM-CEJ | | | 1 1 0 | 0 0 0 | 0 0 0 | 1 1 1 | 0 2 1 | 1 1 1 | 0 0 0 | -1 -1 -1 | 0 0 0 | 0 0 0 | -1 -1 -1 | 0 0 0 | 0 1 1 | |
| PD | | | 5 3 4 | 4 2 4 | 5 3 5 | 5 2 6 | 7 6 5 | 5 4 5 | 6 5 5 | 6 7 7 | 5 3 5 | 5 3 4 | 4 2 6 | 4 3 6 | 6 6 7 | |

**Fig. 14.7** Periodontal chart of patient (Case A).

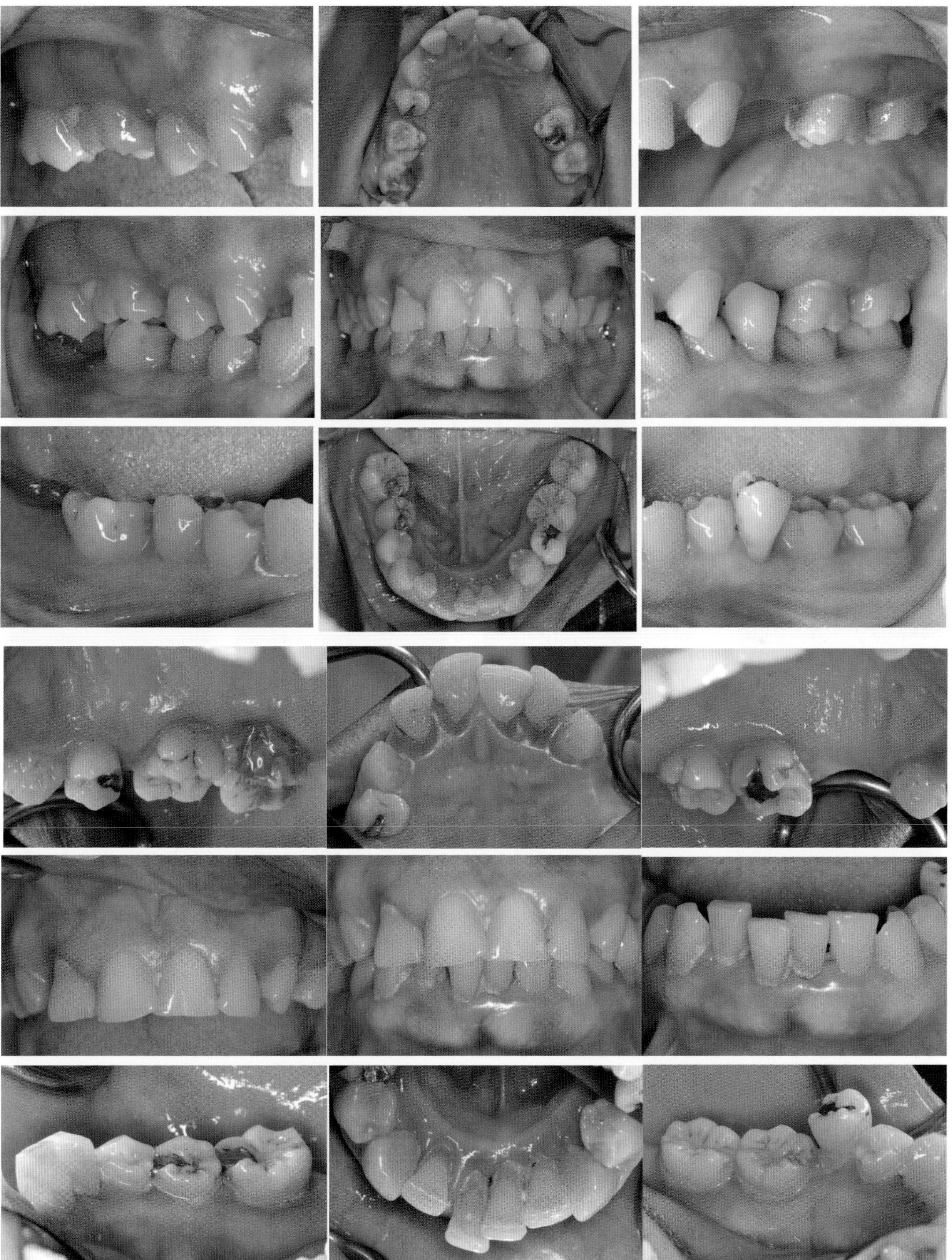

Fig. 14.8 Intraoral photos of patient (Case A).

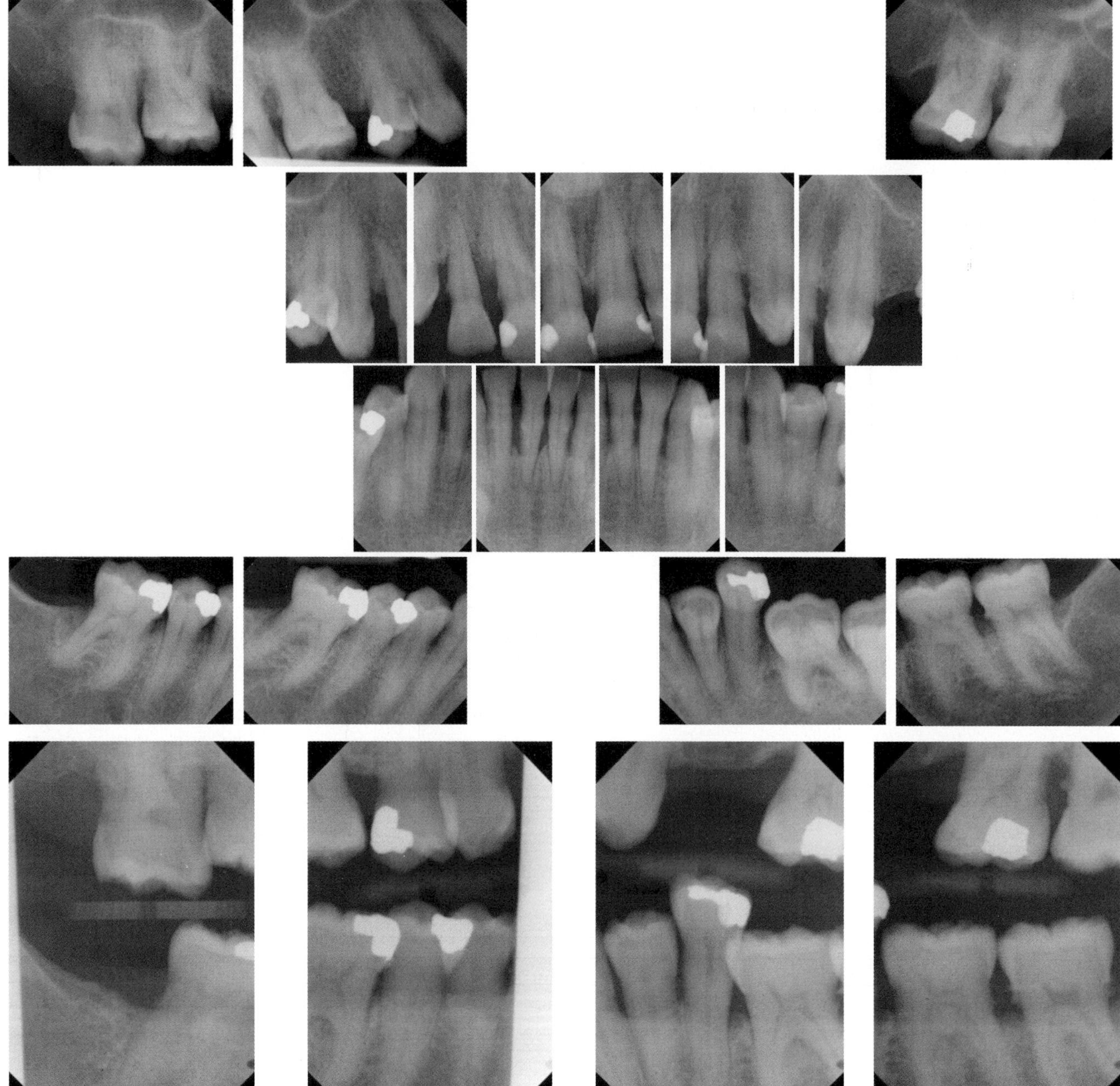

Fig. 14.9 FMX and BW radiographs of patient (Case A).

48. Which of the following is the BEST reason for selecting this ASA category?
    a. The patient's uncontrolled hypertension and diabetes
    b. The patient's uncontrolled diabetes and weight
    c. The patient's history of osteoarthritis and number of missing teeth
    d. The number of missing teeth and uncontrolled hypertension
49. Using the 2017 World Workshop on the Classification of Periodontal and Peri-Implant Diseases and Conditions, which is the BEST stage classification for this patient?
    a. Stage I
    b. Stage II
    c. Stage III
    d. Stage IV
50. Using the 2017 World Workshop on the Classification of Periodontal and Peri-Implant Diseases and Conditions, which is the BEST grade classification for this patient?
    a. Grade A
    b. Grade B
    c. Grade C
    d. Undetermined
51. Which of the following is a grade modifier risk factor associated with this case? Select all that apply.
    a. Smoking status
    b. History of smoking status
    c. Elevated (>7.0%) HbA1c level
    d. Poor plaque control

52. What is the most likely reason why #2 and #20 are hypererupted?
 a. Both have no opposing teeth
 b. Both have periapical lesions
 c. Both have residual calculus
 d. Both have unmet restorative needs
53. Which tooth shows radiographic evidence of vertical bone loss?
 a. #5M
 b. #11D
 c. #18D
 d. #28M

## CASE B (FIG. 14.10A–14.12A)

The patient is a 67-year-old Caucasian male, 6'0" in height and weighing 185 lbs. Sitting blood pressure at initial visit was 118/76 mmHg and pulse was 66 BPM. Patient's medical history included hypertension (diagnosed 8 years ago) and seasonal allergies (self-reported). He was hospitalized in 1994 due to pneumonia and he has recovered since then. The patient is taking Lisinopril for hypertension and monitors his blood pressure on a regular basis at home. The patient reported no allergy to medications or food. The patient quit smoking about 22 years ago and he does not drink alcoholic beverages. The patient reported small sugar consumption.

**Dental History**

The patient reports no pain currently around his teeth or in his mouth. Dental history: amalgam filling at #2(O), #4(O), #12(MOD), #18(O), #28(OD); single crowns at #3, #13, #14, #19, #29, and #30; composite restorations at #5, #6, #7, #8, #9, #10, #11, and #20; extractions of #1, #16, #17, and #32 (extracted as a teenager); RCT of #7, #8, #11, and #29. The patient also reported that his last cleaning was about 6 months ago.

**Chief Complaint**

"I was told that I need treatment for the gum disease."

***Use Case B to answer questions 54 to 60.***

54. According to the newest American Heart Association and the American College of Cardiology high blood pressure guidelines, what category of blood pressure does this patient have?
 a. Normal
 b. Elevated
 c. Stage 1
 d. Stage 2
55. Which of the following would be the BEST ASA category to assign this patient?
 a. ASA I
 b. ASA II
 c. ASA III
 d. ASA IV
56. Which of the following is the BEST reason for selecting this ASA category?
 a. The patient's well-controlled hypertension
 b. The patient's uncontrolled hypertension
 c. The patient's history of pneumonia
 d. The patient's history of smoking
57. Using the 2017 World Workshop on the Classification of Periodontal and Peri-Implant Diseases and Conditions, which is the BEST stage classification for this patient?
 a. Stage I
 b. Stage II
 c. Stage III
 d. Stage IV
58. Using the 2017 World Workshop on the Classification of Periodontal and Peri-Implant Diseases and Conditions, which is the BEST grade classification for this patient?
 a. Grade A
 b. Grade B
 c. Grade C
 d. Undetermined
59. There appears to be an iatrogenic risk factor (amalgam overhang) on which tooth?
 a. Tooth #4
 b. Tooth #12
 c. Tooth #18
 d. Tooth #28
60. What pattern of bone loss does this patient primarily exhibit?
 a. Vertical
 b. Vertical and horizontal
 c. Horizontal
 d. Molar/incisor

## CASE C (FIG. 14.13A–14.15B)

Patient is a 33-year-old Caucasian male, 5'6" in height and weighing 280 lbs (BMI 45). His blood pressure (BP) at initial visit was 156/92 mmHg and pulse was 77 BPM at the first reading. The second BP was 150/92 mmHg and pulse was 75 BPM. Patient's medical history includes chronic obstructive pulmonary disease, skin cancer (excision, cleared), back problems, seasonal allergies, depression, and high cholesterol. He is taking the following medications: ibuprofen and Tylenol #3 for back pain; atorvastatin for high cholesterol level; and trazodone for depression. The patient stated that he started to smoke in his teens and smoked about 1 pack/day over the years. He is currently smoking 1 pack/day. His last dental visit was 12 years ago because he lost his dental insurance.

**Dental History**

Patient reports no pain currently around his teeth or in his mouth. Dental history: extractions at #1, 2, 10, 14, 15, 16, 17, 23, 24, 25, 26, 29, 30, and 32 due to "gum disease"; composite fillings at #3DO, amalgam fillings at #7, #10, #12, #18, and #19; root canal treatment at #9 and #19, single crowns of #8 and #9. Note: radiographs were taken prior to extraction of #10, #15, #23, #24, #25, #26, #29, and #30.

**Chief Complaint**

"I was told that I need treatment for my gum."

***Use Case C to answer questions 61 to 65.***

61. According to the newest American Heart Association and the American College of Cardiology high blood pressure guidelines, what category of blood pressure does this patient have?
 a. Normal
 b. Elevated
 c. Stage 1
 d. Stage 2
 e. Hypertensive crisis
62. Which of the following would be the BEST ASA category to assign this patient?
 a. ASA I
 b. ASA II

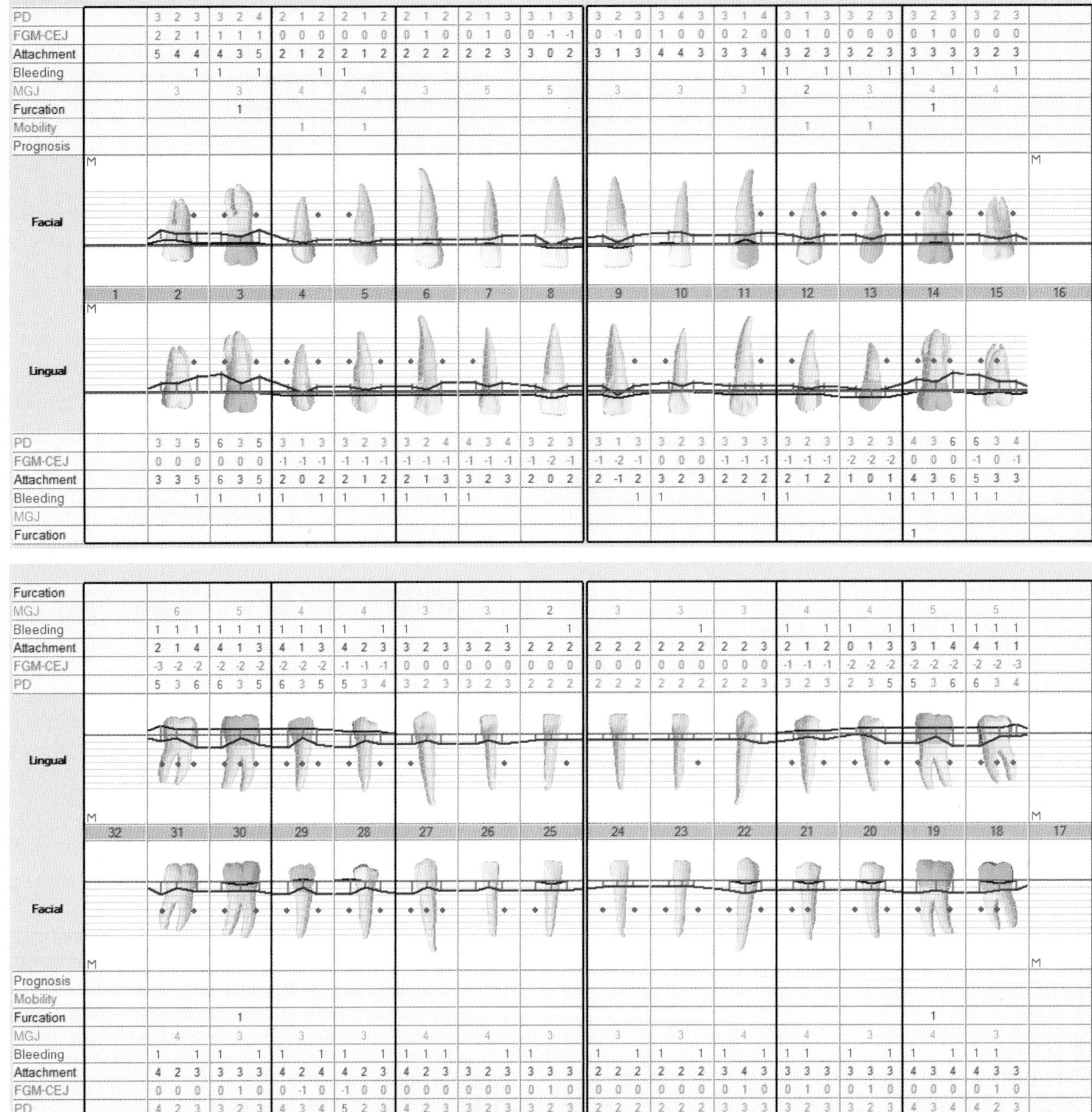


**Fig. 14.10** Periodontal chart of patient (Case B).

c. ASA III
d. ASA IV

63. Using the 2017 World Workshop on the Classification of Periodontal and Peri-Implant Diseases and Conditions, which is the BEST stage classification for this patient?
   a. Stage I
   b. Stage II
   c. Stage III
   d. Stage IV

64. Which of the following are reasons for selecting the stage category EXCEPT one. Which one is the *exception*?
   a. Less than 20 opposing pairs of teeth
   b. Radiographic bone loss between 15%–33%
   c. Drifting of multiple teeth
   d. Greater than five teeth lost due to periodontitis

65. Using the 2017 World Workshop on the Classification of Periodontal and Peri-Implant Diseases and Conditions, which is the BEST grade classification for this patient?
   a. Grade A
   b. Grade B
   c. Grade C
   d. Undetermined

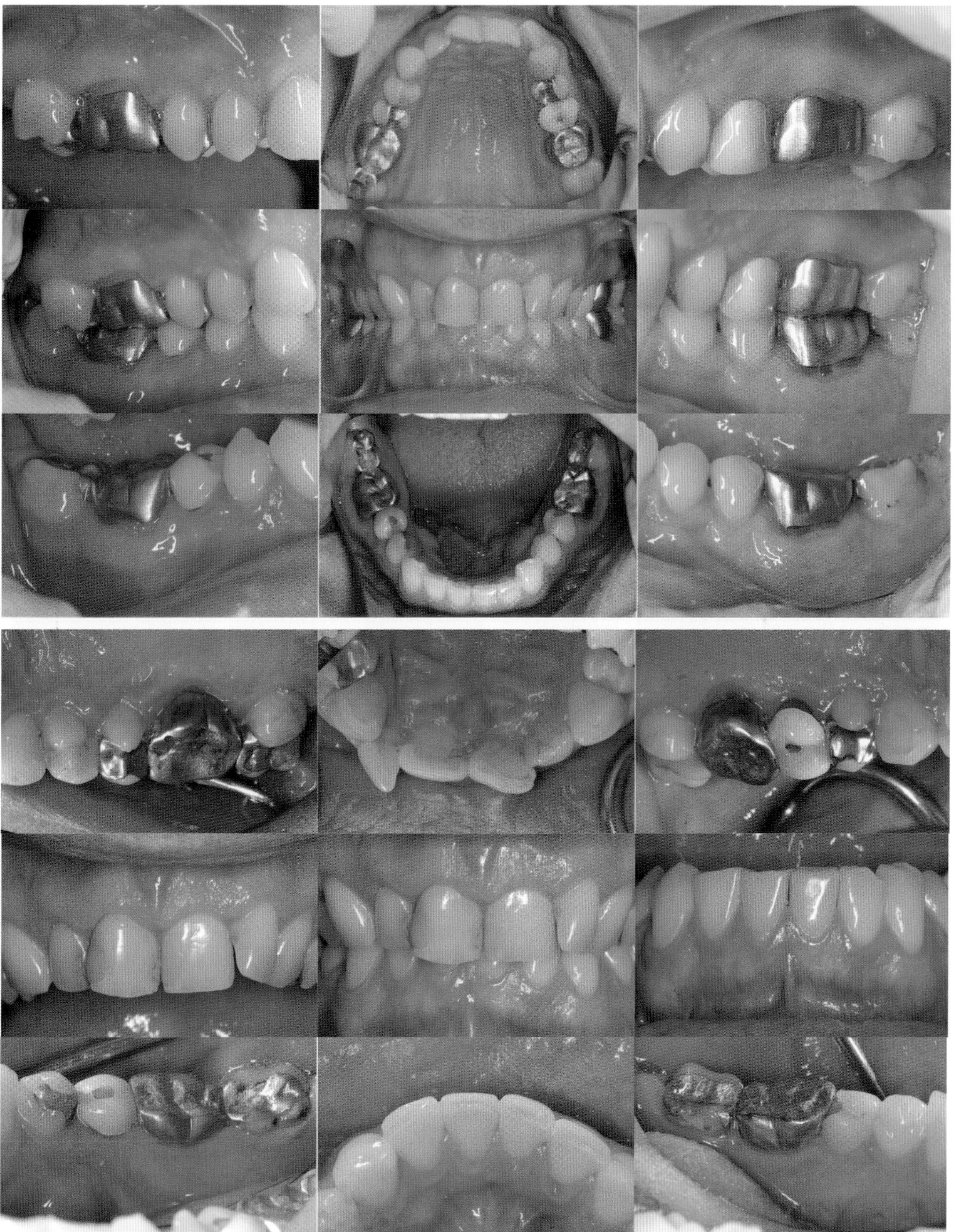

**Fig. 14.11** Intraoral photos of patient (Case B).

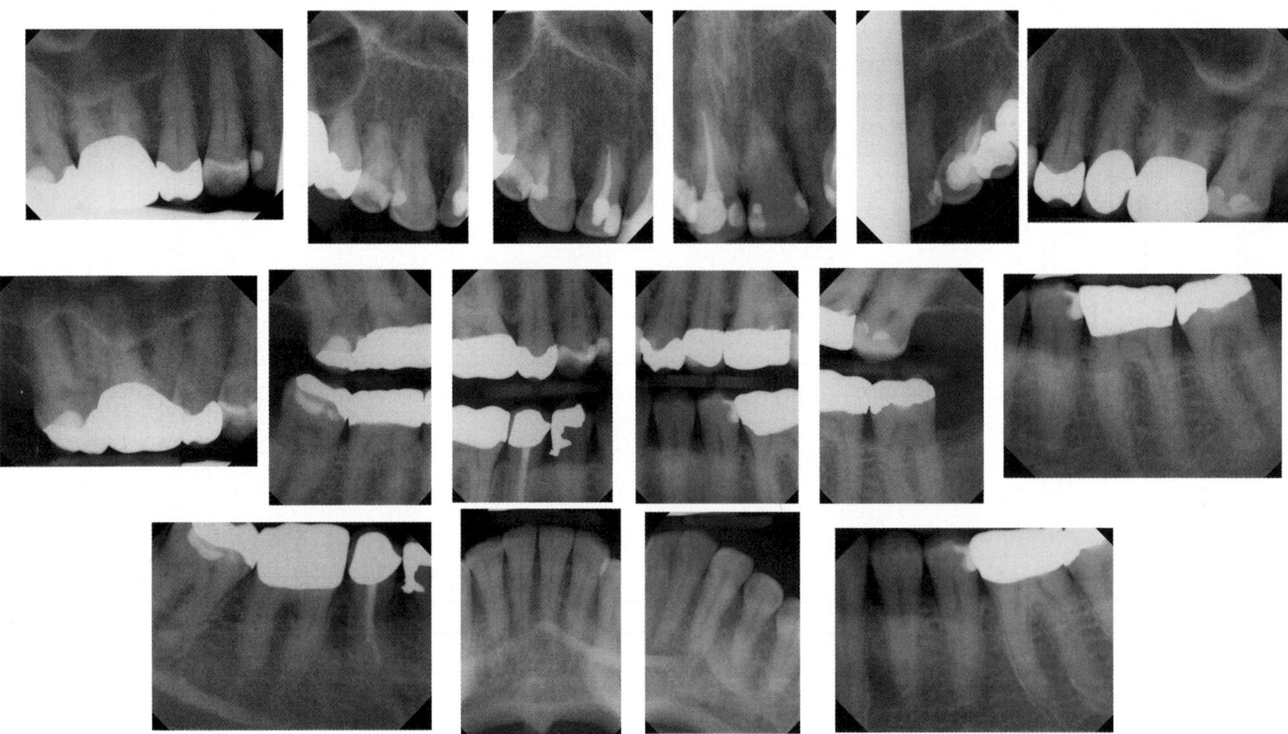

**Fig. 14.12** FMX of patient (Case B).

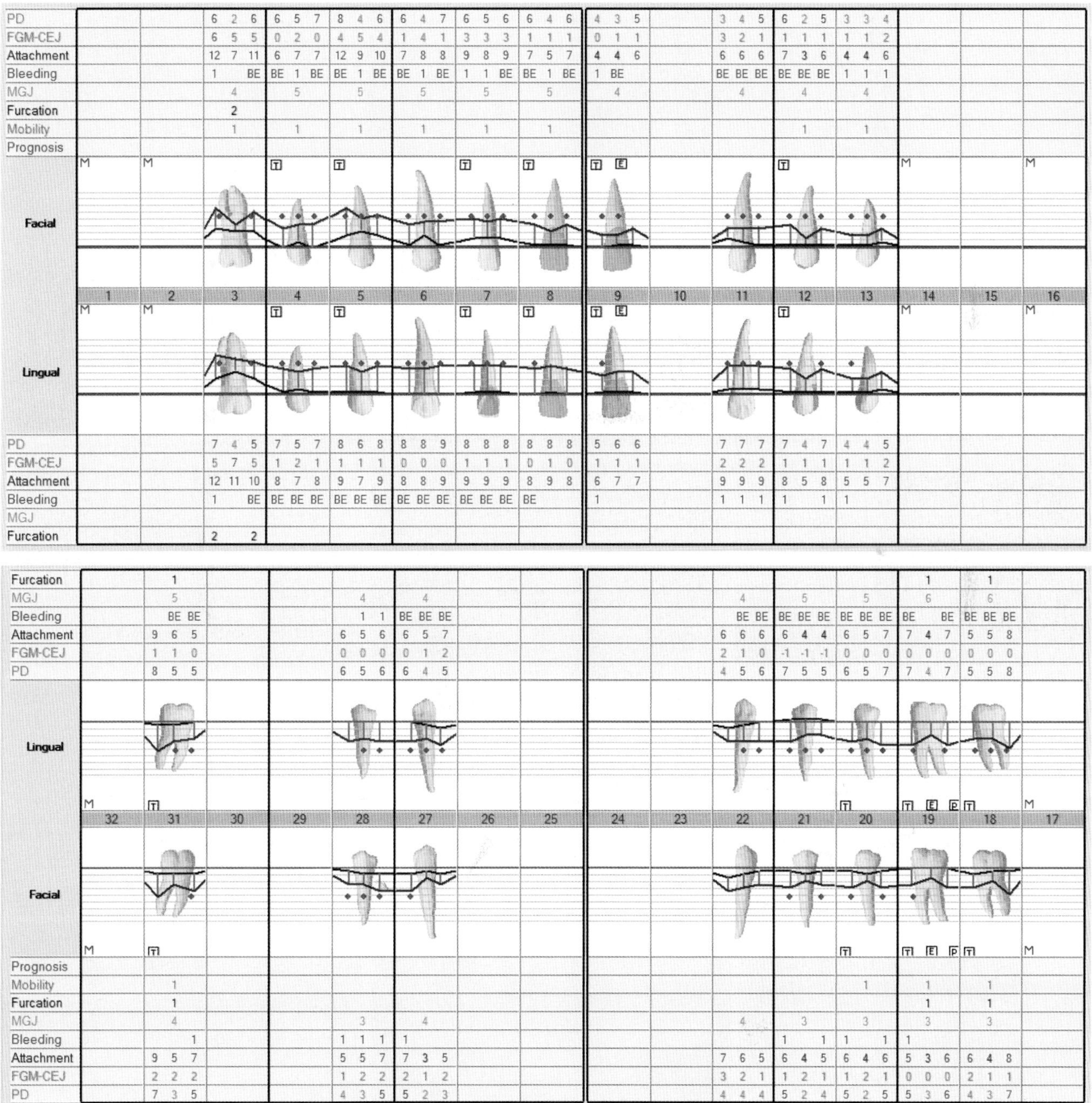

| Facial |  |  |  |  |  |  |  |  |  |  |  |  |  |  |  |  |
|---|---|---|---|---|---|---|---|---|---|---|---|---|---|---|---|---|
| Tooth | 1 | 2 | 3 | 4 | 5 | 6 | 7 | 8 | 9 | 10 | 11 | 12 | 13 | 14 | 15 | 16 |
| PD |  |  | 6 2 6 | 6 5 7 | 8 4 6 | 6 4 7 | 6 5 6 | 6 4 6 | 4 3 5 |  | 3 4 5 | 6 2 5 | 3 3 4 |  |  |  |
| FGM-CEJ |  |  | 6 5 5 | 0 2 0 | 4 5 4 | 1 4 1 | 3 3 3 | 1 1 1 | 0 1 1 |  | 3 2 1 | 1 1 1 | 1 1 2 |  |  |  |
| Attachment |  |  | 12 7 11 | 6 7 7 | 12 9 10 | 7 8 8 | 9 8 9 | 7 5 7 | 4 4 6 |  | 6 6 6 | 7 3 6 | 4 4 6 |  |  |  |
| Bleeding |  |  | 1 BE | BE 1 BE | BE 1 BE | BE 1 BE | 1 1 BE | BE 1 BE | 1 BE |  | BE BE BE | BE BE BE | 1 1 1 |  |  |  |
| MGJ |  |  | 4 | 5 | 5 | 5 | 5 | 5 | 4 |  | 4 | 4 | 4 |  |  |  |
| Furcation |  |  | 2 |  |  |  |  |  |  |  |  |  |  |  |  |  |
| Mobility |  |  | 1 | 1 | 1 | 1 | 1 | 1 |  |  |  | 1 | 1 |  |  |  |
| Prognosis |  |  |  |  |  |  |  |  |  |  |  |  |  |  |  |  |
|  | M | M |  | T | T |  | T | T | T E |  |  | T |  | M |  | M |

| Lingual |  |  |  |  |  |  |  |  |  |  |  |  |  |  |  |  |
|---|---|---|---|---|---|---|---|---|---|---|---|---|---|---|---|---|
| Tooth | 1 | 2 | 3 | 4 | 5 | 6 | 7 | 8 | 9 | 10 | 11 | 12 | 13 | 14 | 15 | 16 |
|  | M | M |  | T | T |  | T | T | T E |  |  | T |  | M |  | M |
| PD |  |  | 7 4 5 | 7 5 7 | 8 6 8 | 8 8 9 | 8 8 8 | 8 8 8 | 5 6 6 |  | 7 7 7 | 7 4 7 | 4 4 5 |  |  |  |
| FGM-CEJ |  |  | 5 7 5 | 1 2 1 | 1 1 1 | 0 0 0 | 1 1 1 | 0 1 0 | 1 1 1 |  | 2 2 2 | 1 1 1 | 1 1 2 |  |  |  |
| Attachment |  |  | 12 11 10 | 8 7 8 | 9 7 9 | 8 8 9 | 9 9 9 | 8 9 8 | 6 7 7 |  | 9 9 9 | 8 5 8 | 5 5 7 |  |  |  |
| Bleeding |  |  | 1 BE | BE BE BE | BE BE BE | BE BE BE | BE BE BE | BE | 1 |  | 1 1 1 | 1 1 | 1 |  |  |  |
| MGJ |  |  |  |  |  |  |  |  |  |  |  |  |  |  |  |  |
| Furcation |  |  | 2 2 |  |  |  |  |  |  |  |  |  |  |  |  |  |

| Lingual |  |  |  |  |  |  |  |  |  |  |  |  |  |  |  |  |
|---|---|---|---|---|---|---|---|---|---|---|---|---|---|---|---|---|
| Furcation |  | 1 |  |  |  |  |  |  |  |  |  |  |  | 1 | 1 |  |
| MGJ |  | 5 |  |  | 4 | 4 |  |  |  |  | 4 | 5 | 5 | 6 | 6 |  |
| Bleeding |  | BE BE |  |  | 1 1 | BE BE BE |  |  |  |  | BE BE | BE BE BE | BE BE BE | BE BE | BE BE BE |  |
| Attachment |  | 9 6 5 |  |  | 6 5 6 | 6 5 7 |  |  |  |  | 6 6 6 | 6 4 4 | 6 5 7 | 7 4 7 | 5 5 8 |  |
| FGM-CEJ |  | 1 1 0 |  |  | 0 0 0 | 0 1 2 |  |  |  |  | 2 1 0 | -1 -1 -1 | 0 0 0 | 0 0 0 | 0 0 0 |  |
| PD |  | 8 5 5 |  |  | 6 5 6 | 6 4 5 |  |  |  |  | 4 5 6 | 7 5 5 | 6 5 7 | 7 4 7 | 5 5 8 |  |
|  | M | T |  |  |  |  |  |  |  |  |  |  | T | T E P | T | M |
| Tooth | 32 | 31 | 30 | 29 | 28 | 27 | 26 | 25 | 24 | 23 | 22 | 21 | 20 | 19 | 18 | 17 |

| Facial |  |  |  |  |  |  |  |  |  |  |  |  |  |  |  |  |
|---|---|---|---|---|---|---|---|---|---|---|---|---|---|---|---|---|
| Tooth | 32 | 31 | 30 | 29 | 28 | 27 | 26 | 25 | 24 | 23 | 22 | 21 | 20 | 19 | 18 | 17 |
|  | M | T |  |  |  |  |  |  |  |  |  |  | T | T E P | T | M |
| Prognosis |  |  |  |  |  |  |  |  |  |  |  |  |  |  |  |  |
| Mobility |  | 1 |  |  |  |  |  |  |  |  |  |  | 1 | 1 | 1 |  |
| Furcation |  | 1 |  |  |  |  |  |  |  |  |  |  |  | 1 | 1 |  |
| MGJ |  | 4 |  |  | 3 | 4 |  |  |  |  | 4 | 3 | 3 | 3 | 3 |  |
| Bleeding |  | 1 |  |  | 1 1 1 | 1 |  |  |  |  |  | 1 1 | 1 1 | 1 |  |  |
| Attachment |  | 9 5 7 |  |  | 5 5 7 | 7 3 5 |  |  |  |  | 7 6 5 | 6 4 5 | 6 4 6 | 5 3 6 | 6 4 8 |  |
| FGM-CEJ |  | 2 2 2 |  |  | 1 2 2 | 2 1 2 |  |  |  |  | 3 2 1 | 1 2 1 | 1 2 1 | 0 0 0 | 2 1 1 |  |
| PD |  | 7 3 5 |  |  | 4 3 5 | 5 2 3 |  |  |  |  | 4 4 4 | 5 2 4 | 5 2 5 | 5 3 6 | 4 3 7 |  |

**Fig. 14.13** Periodontal chart of patient (Case C).

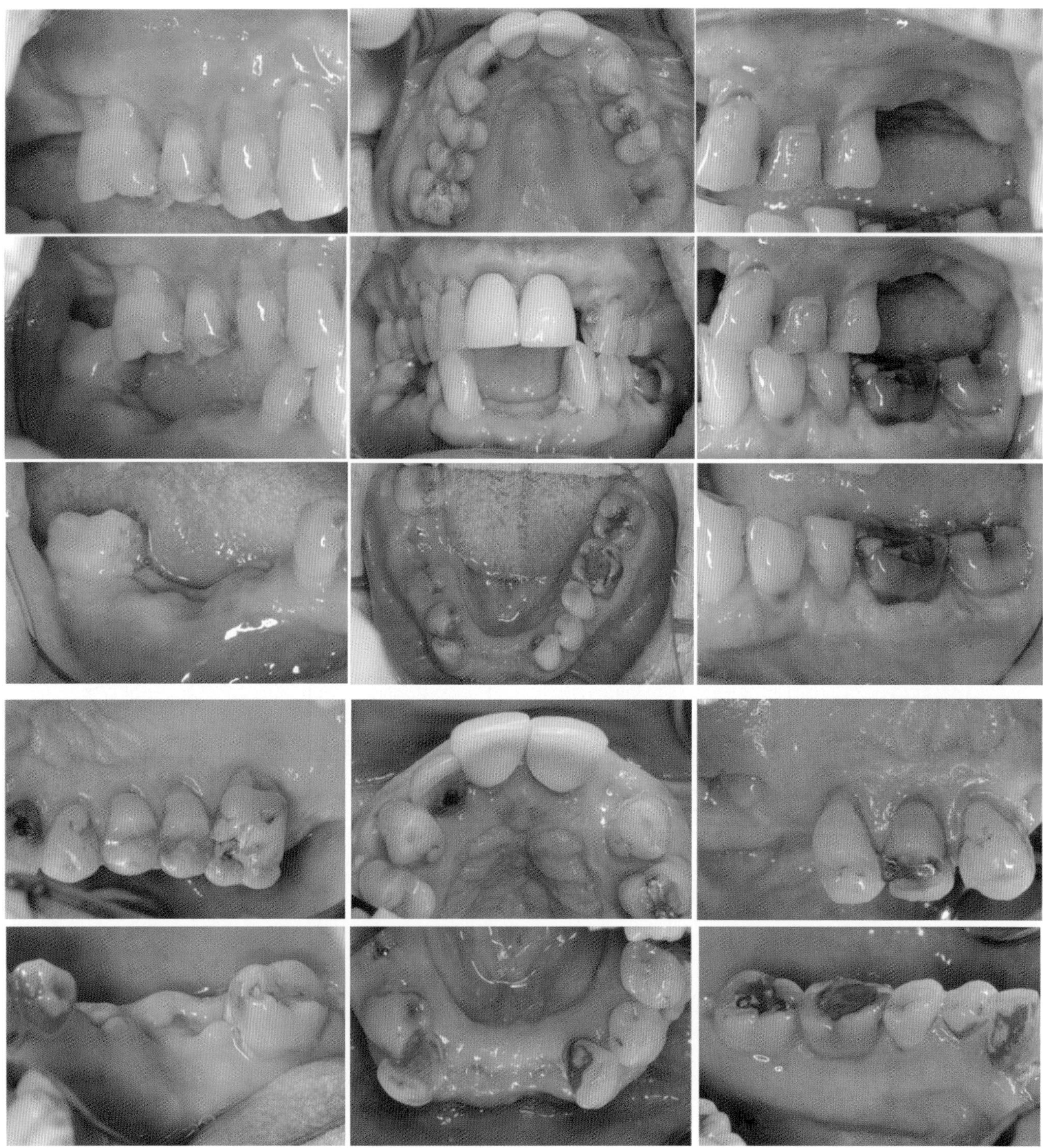

**Fig. 14.14** Intraoral photos of patient (Case C).

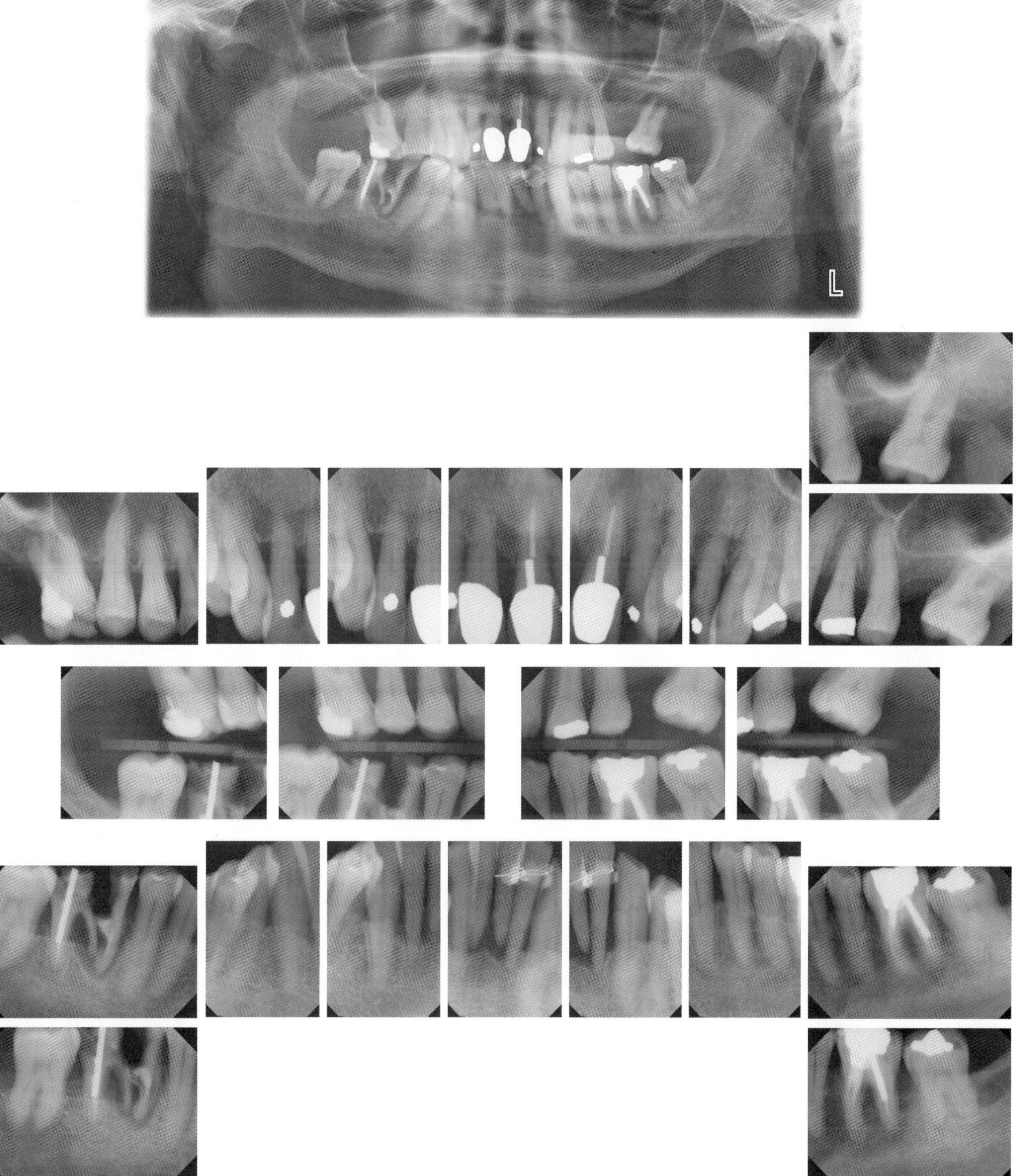


Fig. 14.15 Panoramic and FMX radiographs of patient (Case C).

## REFERENCES


1. Newman MG, Takei HH, Klokkevold P, et al. *Carranza's Clinical Periodontology*. 12th ed. St. Louis: Saunders; 2015.
2. Tonetti MS, Greenwell H, Kornman KS. Staging and grading of periodontitis: framework and proposal of a new classification and case definition. *J Periodontol.* 2018;89(suppl 1):S159–S172.
3. Caton JG, Armitage G, Berglundh, et al. A new classification scheme for periodontal and peri-implant diseases and conditions – introduction and key changes from the 1999 classification. *J Periodontol.* 2018;89(suppl 1):S1–S8.
4. Papapanou PN, Sanz M, Buduneli N, et al. Periodontitis: consensus report of workgroup 2 of the 2017 World Workshop on the classification of periodontal and peri-implant diseases and conditions. *J Periodontol.* 2018;89(suppl 1):S173–S182.
5. Lang NP, Bartold PM. Periodontal health. *J Periodontol.* 2018;89(suppl 1):S9–S16.
6. Murakami S, Mealey BL, Mariotti A, et al. Dental plaque-induced gingival conditions. *J Periodontol.* 2018;89(suppl 1):S17–S27.
7. Holmstrup P, Plemons J, Meyle J. Non-plaque-induced gingival diseases. *J Periodontol.* 2018;89(S 1):S28–S45.
8. Jepsen S, Caton JG, Albandar JM, et al. Periodontal manifestations of systemic diseases and development and acquired conditions: consensus report of workgroup 3 of the 2017 World Workshop on the Classification of Periodontal and Peri-Implant Diseases and Conditions. *J Periodontol.* 2018;89(suppl 1):S237–S248.
9. Albandar JM, Susin C, Hughes FJ. Manifestations of system diseases and conditions that affect the periodontal attachment apparatus: case definitions and diagnostic considerations. *J Periodontol.* 2018;89(suppl 1):S183–S203.
10. Cortellini P, Bissada NF. Mucogingival conditions in the natural dentition: narrative review, case definitions, and diagnostic considerations. *J Periodontol.* 2018;45(suppl 20):S190–S198.
11. Fan J, Caton JG. Occlusal trauma and excessive occlusal forces: narrative review, case definitions, and diagnostic considerations. *J Clin Periodontol.* 2018;45(suppl 20):S199–S206.
12. Crcoli C, Caton JG. Dental prostheses and tooth-related factors. *J Periodontol.* 2018;89(suppl 1):S223–S236.
13. Eke PI, Thornton-Evans G, Dye BA, et al. Advances in surveillance of periodontitis: the Centers for Disease Control and Prevention periodontal disease surveillance project. *J Periodontol.* 2012;83:1337–1342.
14. Löe H, Anerud A, Boysen H, et al. Natural history of periodontal disease in man: the rate of periodontal destruction after 40 years of age. *J Periodontol.* 1978;49:607–620.
15. Bowen DM, Pieren JA. *Darby and Walsh Dental Hygiene Theory and Practice*. 5th ed. St. Louis: Elsevier; 2020.
16. Jha A, Gupta V, Adinarayan R, LANAP, periodontics and beyond: a review. *J Lasers Med Sci.* 2018;9(2):76–81.
17. Berglundh T, Armitage G, Araujo MG, et al. Peri-implant diseases and conditions: consensus report of workgroup 4 of the 2017 World Workshop on the classification of periodontal and peri-implant diseases and conditions. *J Periodontol.* 2018;89(suppl 1):S313–S318.

15

# Dental Hygiene Process of Care

*Laura Mueller-Joseph, Cristina Casa-Levine*

The dental hygiene process of care is a systematic, problem-solving approach to the provision of quality oral health care. This process provides a framework for evidence-based decision making and sound clinical judgment while identifying and resolving patient needs within dental hygiene practice.[1] The dental hygiene process is a standard of practice recognized by the American Dental Hygienists Association (ADHA) and is an educational standard of the American Dental Association (ADA) and Commission on Dental Accreditation.[2,3] This chapter reviews components of the dental hygiene process of care: assessment, diagnosis, planning, implementation, evaluation, and documentation, including prognosis and legal-ethical considerations.

## BASIC CONCEPTS

### Dental Hygiene Paradigm[1]

A. A *paradigm* is composed of major concepts selected for study by a discipline
B. The paradigm for the discipline of dental hygiene includes four concepts[4]:
   1. Patients—recipients of dental hygiene care; include individuals, families, groups, and communities from all age, cultural, gender, and economic groups
   2. Environment—external factors that affect the patient's optimal oral health; includes economic, psychological, cultural, physical, legal, educational, ethical, and geographic dimensions
   3. Health and oral health—status of the overall health and the oral wellness or illness of the patient
   4. Dental hygiene actions—interventions that a dental hygienist initiates to promote wellness, prevent and control oral disease, and encourage active patient participation and collaboration
C. Dental hygiene practice—based on a systematic process of care that involves assessment, diagnosis, planning, implementation, evaluation, and documentation (Fig. 15.1)
D. The dental hygiene process of care provides a logical system for determining the health and disease status of a patient and for selecting appropriate interventions and measuring treatment outcomes
E. The dental hygiene process of care is integrated with a patient's comprehensive dental hygiene diagnosis and care plan

### Human Needs Theory and Assessment[1,5]

A. Most widely known model in the discipline of dental hygiene—human needs conceptual model; requires assessment of each patient's human needs as the framework for providing care
B. Based on the theory that human activity is dominated by behaviors aimed at need fulfillment; an internal drive exists in all humans to satisfy unmet needs; unmet needs motivate specific behaviors to eliminate the perceived deficit; the model encourages establishing an environment that is more patient-oriented than task-oriented
C. The human needs model uses eight needs relevant to oral health that should be considered in the implementation of the dental hygiene process of care (Fig. 15.2)
D. During baseline assessment, deficits in eight human needs are identified, and a dental hygiene diagnosis is made; planning, implementation, and evaluation of dental hygiene care are carried out to address the patient's unmet needs
E. Human needs assessment form—an instrument to assist in the summation and organization of gathered assessment data; used to provide a written record of unmet needs, dental hygiene diagnoses, patient goals, treatment and preventive care plans, and outcome evaluation of dental hygiene care (Fig. 15.3)

### Assessment

A. Definition—comprehensive and systematic collection of data used to identify a patient's needs, oral health status, and general health and well-being
B. Assessment—first phase of dental hygiene process of care
C. Data collection—continuous process of collecting and documenting subjective and objective patient information
D. Data are continuously updated and documented during the dental hygiene process of care
E. Data are collected by interview, questionnaire, observation, measurement, and examination
F. Data recordings are discussed with the patient and other health care professionals responsible for the patient's care
G. Data collection and documentation—includes comprehensive personal, health, and dental histories; pharmacologic history; identification of a patient's chief concerns and human needs; clinical examination; periodontal examination and risk status; analysis of diagnostic radiographs; microbiologic or other tests for assessing periodontal status and risk levels related to dental caries

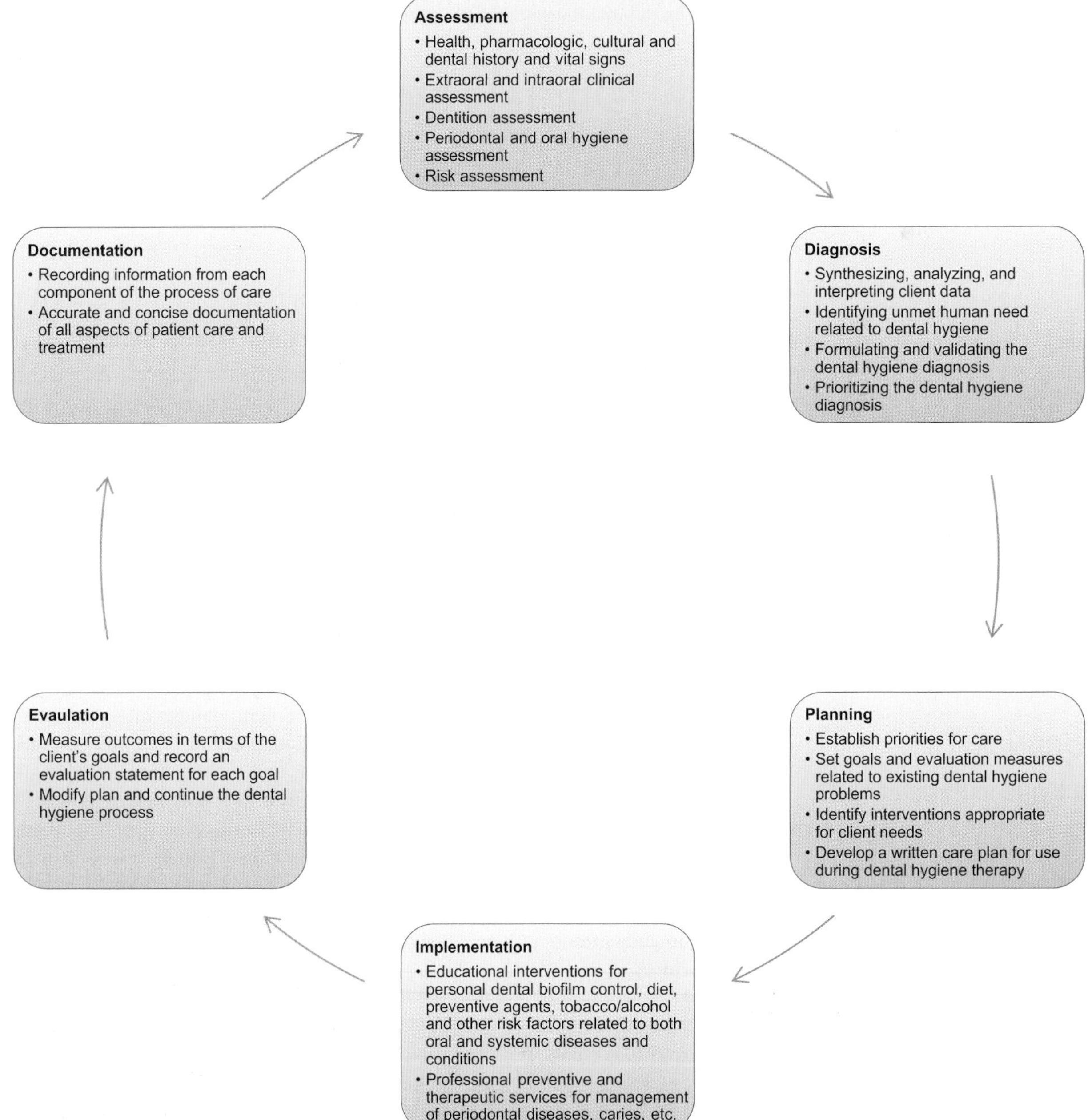

Assessment
• Health, pharmacologic, cultural and dental history and vital signs
• Extraoral and intraoral clinical assessment
• Dentition assessment
• Periodontal and oral hygiene assessment
• Risk assessment
Diagnosis
• Synthesizing, analyzing, and interpreting client data
• Identifying unmet human need related to dental hygiene
• Formulating and validating the dental hygiene diagnosis
• Prioritizing the dental hygiene diagnosis
Planning
• Establish priorities for care
• Set goals and evaluation measures related to existing dental hygiene problems
• Identify interventions appropriate for client needs
• Develop a written care plan for use during dental hygiene therapy
Implementation
• Educational interventions for personal dental biofilm control, diet, preventive agents, tobacco/alcohol and other risk factors related to both oral and systemic diseases and conditions
• Professional preventive and therapeutic services for management of periodontal diseases, caries, etc.
Evaulation
• Measure outcomes in terms of the client's goals and record an evaluation statement for each goal
• Modify plan and continue the dental hygiene process
Documentation
• Recording information from each component of the process of care
• Accurate and concise documentation of all aspects of patient care and treatment


**Fig. 15.1** Dental hygiene process-of-care algorithm.

## HEALTH HISTORY EVALUATION

A. Health history—taken to identify and evaluate predisposing conditions and risk factors that may affect dental hygiene interventions, patient management, potential for an emergency, and oral and general health outcomes; such conditions and factors include, but are not limited to, allergies, chronic diseases, human immunodeficiency virus (HIV) infection, coronavirus COVID-19, pregnancy, tobacco use, substance abuse, and medications
B. Health history form—legal document containing past and present information about a patient's health
   1. Provides baseline information about a patient's health status and assists in medical and dental diagnoses
   2. Information used to assess the overall physical and emotional health of a patient and allow identification of:
      a. Needed precautions to ensure a patient's need for safety
      b. Potential medical emergencies
      c. Needed referrals to a physician or other health care provider
      d. Diseases, conditions, or medications that contraindicate dental or dental hygiene care
      e. Previous history of reactions to medications or drugs
      f. Infectious diseases that could endanger other individuals
      g. Physiologic state of a patient, including pregnancy, puberty, menopause, and use of hormones
   3. Health history questionnaire should be completed in ink, and comprehensive information should be recorded on a questionnaire form or a summary sheet; this may be a component of an electronic patient record

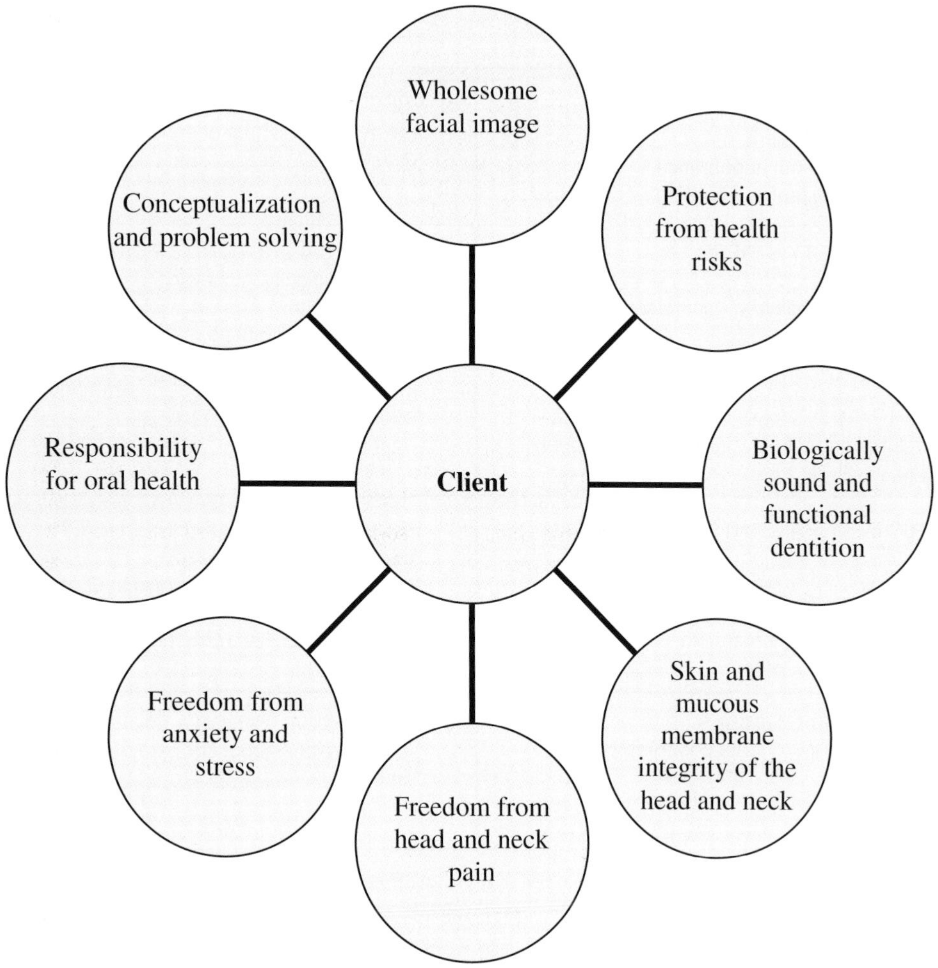


**Fig. 15.2** Eight human needs related to oral health and disease. (Modified from Walsh MM, Darby ML. Human needs theory and dental hygiene care. In Darby ML, Walsh MM, eds. *Dental Hygiene Theory and Practice*. 4th ed. St. Louis: Saunders; 2015.)

4. The health history should be reviewed by the patient and dental hygienist and updated at each dental hygiene appointment
5. The patient should sign the written health history form at each appointment to confirm its accuracy; if the patient is a minor, a parent or legal guardian must sign and date the health history form; electronic signatures are used in the electronic health record
6. The dental hygienist should sign the health history form at each appointment indicating medical and pharmacologic updates were obtained and verified; electronic signatures are used in the electronic health record
7. The health history form should be thorough and concise and legible, using simple language to facilitate understanding

## Health History Questions

A. Personal, social, and cultural histories related to health and disease
1. Information should include social determinants of health (e.g., age, living environment, workplace) that affect health status and quality of life

B. Dental history information should include:
   1. Main concern—why the patient is seeking dental or dental hygiene care
   2. In the case of new patients, the date of the last dental or dental hygiene visit
   3. Areas of pain or discomfort identified during the health history interview, but not associated with the patient's main concern
   4. Nervousness or anxiety about treatment; history of an upsetting experience; the patient's need for freedom from anxiety and stress should be addressed
   5. Pain, swelling, or gingival bleeding
   6. The patient's satisfaction with his or her teeth and oral health
   7. Past or current orthodontics, periodontal surgery, extractions, temporomandibular joint (TMJ) problems, occlusal equilibration, fixed and removable dentures
   8. Oral habits such as clenching or grinding, biting lips or cheeks, mouth breathing, and holding foreign objects between teeth

C. Radiographic history information (see Chapter 6)
   1. Purpose—the radiation exposure history of the patient should be obtained to make safe decisions for radiographic prescriptions
   2. Information should include:
      a. Whether the patient is regularly exposed to radiation in his or her work environment

| **ASSESSMENT** (circle signs and symptoms present)<br>1) WHOLESOME FACIAL IMAGE<br>*expresses dissatisfaction with appearance<br>–teeth –gingiva –facial profile –breath *other _____ | 5) FREEDOM FROM HEAD AND NECK PAIN<br>*extra-/intra-oral pain or sensitivity<br>*other _____ |
|---|---|
| 2) FREEDOM FROM ANXIETY/STRESS<br>*reports or displays:<br>–anxiety about proximity of clinician, confidentiality, or previous dental experience<br>–oral habits –substance abuse<br>*concern about:<br>–infection control, fluoride therapy, fluoridation, mercury toxicity | 6) BIOLOGICALLY SOUND & FUNCTIONAL DENTITION<br>*reports difficulty in chewing<br>*presents with:<br>–defective restorations –ill-fitting dentures, appliances<br>–teeth with signs of disease –abrasion erosion<br>–missing teeth –rampant caries<br>*other _____ |
| 3) SKIN & MUCOUS MEMBRANE INTEGRITY OF HEAD AND NECK<br>–extra-/intra-oral lesion –pockets ≥4 mm<br>–swelling –attachment loss ≥4 mm<br>–gingival inflammation –xerostomia<br>–bleeding on probing –other _____ | 7) RESPONSIBILITY FOR ORAL HEALTH<br>*plaque & calculus present<br>*inadequate parental supervision of oral health care<br>*no dental exam within the last 2 years<br>*other _____ |
| 4) PROTECTION FROM HEALTH RISKS<br>*BP outside of normal limits *need for prophylactic antibiotics<br>*potential for injury *risk factors<br>*other _____ | 8) CONCEPTUALIZATION & UNDERSTANDING<br>*has questions about DH care and/or oral disease<br>*other _____ |

**DENTAL HYGIENE DIAGNOSIS** (List the human need not met, then be specific about the etiology and signs & symptoms evidencing a deficit)

(Unmet Human Need) DUE TO (Etiology) EVIDENCED BY (Signs & Symptoms)

| **CLIENT GOALS** | **INTERVENTIONS** (Target etiologies) | **EVALUATION** (goal met, partially met, or unmet) |
|---|---|---|
| | | |

**Appointment Schedule:** _____

**Continued-care recommendations:**

**Fig. 15.3** Assessment form. (Adapted from Darby ML, Walsh MM: Application of the human needs conceptual model to dental hygiene practice, J Dent Hyg 74:230, 2000.)

**TABLE 15.1 Health History Screening Questions**

| Risk Factor Category | Sample Questions | Significance of Finding |
|---|---|---|
| Overall health | How do you rate your general health?<br>Has there been any change in your general health within the past year?<br>Have you been under the care of a medical doctor during the past 2 years?<br>What is the date of your last physical examination?<br>Have you ever been hospitalized or had a serious illness? | Hospitalization history can provide a good record of past serious illnesses that may be significant to dental hygiene care<br>Knowledge of why a patient was hospitalized is used to evaluate the patient's ability to tolerate stress involved during treatment<br>Knowledge of any problems for which the patient required medical intervention can increase the ability to evaluate the patient's condition before treatment |
| Weight fluctuation history | Have you unintentionally lost or gained more than 10 pounds in the past year?<br>Are you on a medically recommended diet? | Unexpected weight changes may indicate heart failure, hypothyroidism, hyperthyroidism, or uncontrolled diabetes<br>Information may identify an underlying systemic problem, such as diabetes, hyperthyroidism, or cancer |
| Cardiovascular disease | When you walk up stairs or take a walk, do you ever have to stop because of pain in your chest or shortness of breath or because you are very tired?<br>Do your ankles swell during the day?<br>Do you require more than two pillows to sleep, or do you have an elevated bed? | Patients with cardiovascular disease are more susceptible to physical or emotional challenges during dental hygiene care<br>These signs may indicate possible valvular disease, arrhythmia, or congestive heart failure |
| Diabetes | Are you on a medically recommended diet?<br>Do you have to urinate more than six times a day?<br>Are you frequently thirsty?<br>Does your mouth frequently become dry?<br>If yes, what is the probable cause? | Determine family history or potential for diabetes; consultation with a physician may be indicated<br>Complications of diabetes include blindness, hypertension, kidney failure, and delayed healing |
| Tuberculosis or other respiratory diseases | Do you have a nonproductive persistent cough?<br>Do you have a productive persistent cough?<br>Do you have night sweats?<br>Do you have difficulty breathing? | May indicate current or past history of tuberculosis<br>History of the disease must be defined, and medical consultation may be indicated |
| Hematologic disorder | Do you bruise easily?<br>Do you have a tendency to bleed longer than normal?<br>Have you ever had a blood transfusion? | Need to determine whether a blood disorder is present; medical consultation may be indicated<br>Concerns about delayed healing, prolonged bleeding, and infection |
| Latex allergy | Have you experienced a skin reaction (redness, rash, hives, or itching) to adhesive tape, adhesive strips, kitchen gloves, or rubber or latex products?<br>Have you experienced swelling of the lips, tongue, or skin after dental treatment, after blowing up a balloon, or after contact with rubber or latex products?<br>Have you experienced a runny nose, itchy eyes, scratchy throat, or difficulty breathing after contact with rubber or latex products?<br>Do you have an allergy to bananas, kiwis, potatoes, tomatoes, avocados, chestnuts, or other foods? | Need to assess risk for reaction<br>May need medical consultation to determine risk of anaphylaxis<br>Provide a latex-reduced environment |
| COVID-19 | Have you ever tested positive for COVID-19? If yes, when?<br>In the past two weeks have you had contact with someone who has been diagnosed with COVID-19?<br>Have you or anyone you live with had a fever in the past two weeks?<br>Are you experiencing any of the following: shortness of breath, difficulty breathing, pain or pressure in chest, fever or chills, cough, fatigue, muscle or body aches, headache, loss of taste or smell, sore throat, congestion, runny nose, nausea, vomiting, diarrhea, new confusion, inability to wake or stay awake, bluish lips or face? | Will indicate current or past history of COVID-19<br>Symptoms experienced may indicate an undiagnosed case of COVID-19, which will impact patient management |

b. The dates and total number of dental and medical films exposed during a 5-year period

## Health History Information

See Chapters 7, 8, and 19 for more detailed discussions of health conditions.

A. Screening questions are designed to assess risk factors or undiagnosed diseases to enable a clinician to determine the need for a physician consultation or referral before dental hygiene care (Table 15.1)

B. Detailed questions are designed to identify diseases or conditions that a patient previously had or currently has and to determine the need for precautionary measures, physician consultation before dental hygiene care, or need for antibiotic prophylaxis (Table 15.2)
   1. When practitioner questions the patient regarding his or her disease status, specific information should include:
      a. Type and onset of disease
      b. Treatment received in the past
      c. Severity of disease or extent of damage

**TABLE 15.2 American Dental Association (ADA) and American Association of Orthopedic Surgeons (AAOS) Antibiotic Premedication Guidelines for Professional Oral Health Care**

| Dental Procedures That Require Premedication in Highest-Risk Patients[a] | ADA Recommendations for Cardiac Conditions | ADA and AAOS Recommendations for Orthopedic Conditions | Other Conditions That May Necessitate Antibiotic Premedication Based on Physician Consultation |
|---|---|---|---|
| | Highest-risk category: only people at greatest risk of negative outcomes from infective endocarditis (IE) should receive short-term preventive antibiotics before identified dental (and medical) procedures<br>Patients at the greatest danger of adverse outcomes from IE and for whom preventive antibiotics are worth the risks include those with:<br>- Artificial heart valves, including transcatheter-implanted prostheses and homografts<br>- Artificial material for heart valve repair<br>- History of having had IE<br>- Heart transplant with valve regurgitation<br>- Certain specific, serious congenital heart conditions, including:<br>- Unrepaired cyanotic congenital heart disease, including those with palliative shunts and conduits<br>- Any repaired congenital heart defect with residual shunts or valvular regurgitation at the site or adjacent to the site of a prosthetic patch or prosthetic device<br>- Pediatric patients with incompletely repaired cyanotic congenital heart disease<br>- Pediatric patients with a congenital heart condition repaired with artificial materials or a device, during the first 6 months after procedure<br>- Pediatric patients with repaired congenital heart defects with residual defects | Antibiotic premedication is generally not recommended for patients with prosthetic joint replacements<br>Treatment decisions should be made in light of all circumstances; appropriate use criteria should be considered to assist with decision making; consulting the patient and orthopedic surgeon in the presence of significant medical risk may be required[b]<br>Immunocompromised or immunosuppressed patients<br>Inflammatory arthropathies (e.g., rheumatoid arthritis, systemic lupus erythematosus)<br>Drug-induced immunosuppression<br>Radiation-induced immunosuppression<br>Patients with comorbidities (e.g., diabetes, human immunodeficiency virus [HIV])<br>Previous prosthetic joint infections<br>Previous complications associated with joint-replacement surgery<br>Malnourishment<br>Hemophilia<br>HIV infection<br>Insulin-dependent (type 1) diabetes<br>Malignancy<br>Megaprostheses | Prophylaxis consultation recommended<br>Renal transplants or dialysis<br>Immunosuppressive therapy (e.g., cyclosporine)<br>Uncontrolled diabetes<br>Sickle cell anemia<br>Spina bifida (ventriculoatrial shunt) |

[a]Every attempt should be made to complete procedures and services in as few appointments as possible; follow-up appointments should be scheduled at least 9 days apart if patient is premedicated.

[b]Clinical judgment may indicate antibiotic use in selected circumstances that may cause significant bleeding.

Modified from American Dental Association Antibiotic Prophylaxis Prior to Dental Procedures, June 25, 2018, https://www.ada.org/en/member-center/oral-health-topics/antibiotic-prophylaxis; from Sollecito TP, Abt E, Lockhart PB, Truelove E, Paumier TM, Tracy SL, Tampi M, Beltrán-Aguilar ED, Frantsve-Hawley J. The use of prophylactic antibiotics prior to dental procedures in patients with prosthetic joints: Evidence-based clinical practice guideline for dental practitioners — a report of the American Dental Association Council on Scientific Affairs, *JADA*. 146(1), 11–16, https://jada.ada.org/article/S0002-8177(14)00019-1/pdf; and from American Academy of Orthopedic Surgeons, American Association of Orthopedic Surgeons: Prevention of orthopedic implant infection in patients undergoing dental procedures: evidence-based guidelines and evidence report, https://www.aaos.org/globalassets/quality-and-practice-resources/dental/pudp_guideline.pdf. Accessed January 31, 2019.

   d. Type of current medical care
   e. Results of follow-up testing
   f. Classification of the patient's risk for a medical emergency using the American Society of Anesthesiologists (ASA) Physical Status Classification System (Table 15.3)
2. Questions regarding cardiovascular disease (CVD) are significant because patients with various forms of CVD are especially vulnerable to physical or emotional challenges that may be encountered during dental hygiene care; for most CVDs, implementing a stress reduction protocol, based on the ASA system, is necessary (see the sections on "Vasoconstrictors" in Chapter 18; "Congenital Heart Disease," "Cardiac Arrhythmias and Dysrhythmias," "Hypertensive Disease," "Ischemic Heart Disease," "Cerebrovascular Accident," and "Congestive Heart Failure" in Chapter 19; and "Vital Signs" in Chapter 21)
   a. Hypertension can result in myocardial infarction (MI) and stroke (cerebrovascular accident, CVA) and contribute to arteriosclerosis, impaired kidney function, and cardiac enlargement; hypertension guidelines must be followed during professional care to reduce the risk of a medical emergency (Table 15.4)
   b. When CVD is identified, it is important for the clinician to conduct a thorough interview to assess the severity and level of control of disease and to determine alterations in care (e.g., physician consultation, antibiotic prophylaxis, stress reduction protocol)
   c. Patients undergoing corrective surgery for congenital heart disease and who have prosthetic material or a prosthetic device are susceptible to transient bacteremia for up to 6 months and must receive antibiotic prophylaxis; at 6 months after surgery, antibiotic prophylaxis is not usually recommended (see Table 15.2)

**TABLE 15.3 American Society of Anesthesiologists (ASA) Physical Status Classification System[a] and Stress Reduction Protocols**

| ASA Classification | Patient Risk Description | Examples of Medical Conditions | Precautionary Measures for Stress Reduction |
|---|---|---|---|
| Physical status 1 | Normal healthy patient without systemic disease<br>Little or no anxiety<br>Elective dental hygiene care can be implemented | Healthy, nonsmoking, no or minimal alcohol use | Determine patient's level of anxiety<br>Schedule morning appointment<br>Minimize waiting time<br>Consider shorter appointments for anxious patients<br>Optimize adequate pain control during therapy |
| Physical status 2 | Patient with mild systemic disease<br>Healthy patient with extreme anxiety<br>Elective dental hygiene care can be implemented with minimal risk, but measures for stress reduction should be taken | Mild diseases only without substantive functional limitations; examples include current smoker, social alcohol drinker, pregnancy, obesity (30 < BMI < 40), well-controlled diabetes or hypertension, mild lung disease | Identify the patient's medical risk potential<br>Complete a physician consultation before starting dental hygiene care, as indicated<br>Schedule a morning appointment time<br>Take and record vital signs at each appointment |
| Physical status 3 | Patient with severe systemic disease that limits activity but is not incapacitating<br>Elective dental hygiene care is not contraindicated, but risk is increased and precautionary measures for stress reduction should be taken | Substantive functional limitations; one or more moderate to severe diseases; examples include poorly controlled diabetes or hypertension, COPD, morbid obesity (BMI > 40), active hepatitis, alcohol dependence or abuse, implanted pacemaker, moderate reduction of ejection fraction, ESRD patient undergoing regularly scheduled dialysis, premature infant PCA 60 weeks, history (> 3 months) of MI, CVA, TIA, or CAD/stents | Optimize adequate pain control during therapy<br>Shorter appointments, not to exceed 90 minutes<br>Arrange appointments during the beginning of the week (Monday to Wednesday) |
| Physical status 4 | Patient with incapacitating systemic disease that is a constant threat to life<br>Elective dental hygiene care is contraindicated until the medical condition has improved to at least ASA physical status 3 | Examples include recent (within 3 months) MI, CVA, TIA, or CAD/stents; ongoing cardiac ischemia or severe valve dysfunction; severe reduction of ejection fraction; sepsis; DIC; ARD; ESRD patient not undergoing regularly scheduled dialysis | Immediate medical consultation |

*ARD,* Acute renal disease; *BMI,* body mass index; *CAD,* coronary artery disease; *COPD,* chronic obstructive pulmonary disease; *CVA,* cerebrovascular accident; *DIC,* disseminated intravascular coagulation; *ESRD,* end-stage renal disease; *MI,* myocardial infarction; *PCA,* postconceptual age; *TIA,* transient ischemic attack.

[a]*Note:* Physical status 5 and 6 are used primarily in medical practice.

Modified from American Society of Anesthesiologists: ASA Physical Status Classification System, https://www.asahq.org/standards-and-guidelines/asa-physical-status-classification-system; accessed January 27, 2019; and Malamed SF. Knowing your patients, *J Am Dent Assoc.* 2010:141;3S–7S.

d. When antibiotic prophylaxis is necessary, 9 to 10 days should be scheduled between appointments to allow oral bacteria to return to the original state; patients currently following an antibiotic regimen must use an alternative regimen of antibiotic therapy; if antibiotic medication is inadvertently missed, administer within 2 hours after the procedure

3. Questions regarding diseases of the immune system and blood disorders assess a patient's potential risk for infection in dental hygiene care and his or her ability to handle stress through the appointment; primary concerns include prolonged bleeding, delayed healing, and secondary infections; physician consultation may be required for more chronic or involved conditions
   a. For patients with diabetes, concerns exist about a hypoglycemic incident, susceptibility to oral infections (abscesses, periodontal diseases), impaired wound healing, and impaired glycemic control because of the presence of periodontal disease; consultation with a physician is indicated in most cases, and referral is based on health history, dialogue, and oral conditions. A sugar source must be available in the oral care facility in case of an episode of hypoglycemia or hyperinsulinism
   b. Oral assessment should be initiated to determine the presence of infections and the extent of periodontal disease before consultation with a patient's physician; glycated hemoglobin values ($A_{1c}$) and blood glucose levels are requested from the physician; the patient should be asked to bring his or her glucometer, or a glucometer should be available in the oral care facility (Box 15.1)
   c. For patients with well-controlled diabetes, no alteration of the care plan is indicated unless complications of diabetes such as hypertension, congestive heart failure (CHF), MI, angina, or renal failure are present. Patients who are managed with medication should take their medication and eat before their scheduled appointment

**TABLE 15.4 Classification of Adult Blood Pressure (BP) and Precautionary Measures**

| Category | Systolic (mm Hg) | | Diastolic (mm Hg) | Dental Management Considerations |
|---|---|---|---|---|
| Normal | < 120 | and | < 80 | Routine dental management<br>Recheck at continued-care (recare) visit |
| Elevated | 120–129 | and | <80 | Routine dental management<br>Advise patient of status, recommend follow-up with physician, and recommend lifestyle management<br>Recheck at recare visit |
| Hypertension: Stage 1 | 130–139 | or | 80–89 | Routine dental management<br>Advise patient of status, recommend follow up with physician, and recommend lifestyle management<br>Recheck at recare visit |
| Hypertension: Stage 2 | ≥ 140 | or | ≥ 90 | **140–159 (systolic) or 90–99 (diastolic):** Monitor BP at consecutive appointments<br>If all exceed these guidelines, seek medical consultation<br>Stress reduction protocol<br>Recheck at recare visit<br>**160–179 (systolic) or 100–110 (diastolic):** Recheck BP in 5 minutes<br>If BP still elevated within this range, seek and receive medical consultation before dental hygiene therapy<br>Noninvasive care only<br>Definitive emergency care only if BP is less than 180/110 mm Hg<br>Stress reduction protocol<br>Continue to monitor BP at consecutive appointments<br>Recheck at each visit |
| Hypertensive crisis | > 180 | and/or | > 120 | Recheck BP in 5 minutes<br>If BP still elevated, immediate medical consultation is indicated<br>No dental or dental hygiene care, elective or emergent, until BP is decreased<br>Noninvasive emergency care with drugs: analgesics or antibiotics are indicated<br>Refer to hospital for immediate invasive dental care |

Modified from Little JW, Miller C, Rhodus NL, Falace D. *Dental Management of the Medically Compromised Patient.* St. Louis: Evolve; 2018; Whelton PK, Carey RM, Aronow WS, et al. 2017 ACC/AHA/AAPA/ABC/ACPM/AGS/APhA/ASH/ASPC/NMA/PCNA guideline for the prevention, detection, evaluation, and management of high blood pressure in adults: a report of the American College of Cardiology/American Heart Association Task Force on Clinical Practice Guidelines. *Hypertension.* 2018; *71*:e13–e115; and US Department of Health and Human Services, National Institutes of Health, National Heart, Lung, and Blood Institute, National High Blood Pressure Education Program: JNC 7 Express, Seventh Report of the Joint National Commission on Prevention, Detection, Evaluation, and Treatment of High Blood Pressure, Bethesda, MD: NIH Pub No 03-5233, 2004, http://www.nhlbi.nih.gov/guidelines/hypertension/jnc7full.htm; Accessed January 27, 2019.

4. Metabolic syndrome (MetS) is closely associated with insulin resistance, in which the body cannot use insulin efficiently; patients with MetS are at increased risk of coronary heart disease, stroke, peripheral vascular disease, and type 2 diabetes
   a. MetS is identified by the presence of three or more components: obesity measured by waist circumference (men >40 inches and women >35 inches), fasting blood triglycerides (>150 mg/dL), blood high-density lipoprotein (HDL) cholesterol (men <40 mg/dL and women <50 mg/dL), blood pressure (BP) (>130/ 85 mm Hg), and fasting glucose (>100 mg/dL)
   b. Physician referral, medical consultation, or both may be required for patients who do not have regular medical care, to determine the presence of associated conditions or the level of control of existing conditions
5. Questions regarding respiratory disease, chronic obstructive pulmonary disease (COPD), or COVID-19 assess the level of compromised respiratory function; clinicians should use precautionary measures to avoid further depression of respiration (see the section on "Chronic Obstructive Pulmonary Disease" in Chapter 19); delayed treatment is required for patients suspected to have COVID-19.
6. Musculoskeletal system disorders may be associated with chronic use of salicylates or nonsteroidal antiinflammatory drugs (NSAIDs), which can alter blood clotting and corticosteroid therapy and increase the risk of acute adrenal insufficiency
7. Neurologic and psychological disorders must be identified and the degree of control determined; medications used to control seizures can cause drug-influenced gingival enlargement, and psychiatric drugs have the potential to interact adversely with the vasoconstrictors in local anesthetic agents
8. Other disorders, such as glaucoma, sexually transmitted infections (STIs), herpes, chemical dependency, and tobacco use, have significant implications for treatment; for patients with glaucoma, anticholinergics are contraindicated because these agents increase intraocular pressure; chemical dependency and tobacco use are risk factors for infectious

**BOX 15.1 Glycemic Management for Adults (Nonpregnant) With Diabetes**

| Blood Glucose Level (mg/dL) | |
|---|---|
| < 70 | Tendency toward hypoglycemia; give 15 g[a] of carbohydrate, and wait 15 minutes; monitor again to assess whether the treatment should continue; notify patient's physician |
| 70–130 (Preprandial)<br>< 180 (Peak postprandial)[b] | Acceptable |
| 180–239 | Risk for infection |
| > 240 | Unacceptable for treatment; refer to a physician, and reschedule or postpone treatment until the patient reports control and acceptability of treatment |
| Glycosylated hemoglobin | Level periodically determined to assess plasma glucose control during the preceding 1 to 3 months |
| Hemoglobin $A_{1c}$ ($HbA_{1c}$) | Prediabetes 5.7–6.4%<br>Diabetes ≥ 6.5% |

[a]15 g = 3 glucose tablets, a tube of glucose gel, or 4 ounces of fruit juice.
[b]Postprandial glucose measurements should be made 1 to 2 hours after the beginning of the meal.
Modified from American Diabetes Association. Standards of medical care in diabetes 2019 abridged for primary care providers. *Clin Diabetes.* 2019;37(1):11–34.

diseases, malignancies, CVD, pulmonary diseases, and periodontal diseases; dental hygiene care for patients with active herpes, STIs, or active transmissible diseases should be postponed until the disease is no longer active

9. The physiologic state of women identifies their status related to pregnancy and endocrine changes
10. The identification of the risk of latex allergy is essential to reduce the chances of an allergic reaction; types of reactions include irritant contact dermatitis, allergic contact dermatitis (delayed hypersensitivity), and latex allergy
    a. Irritant contact dermatitis—the most common reaction; causes dry, itchy areas of irritation on the skin
    b. Allergic contact dermatitis (type IV hypersensitivity reaction)—results from exposure to chemicals added to latex during harvesting of rubber, processing, or manufacturing
    c. Latex allergy, or immediate allergic urticaria (type I hypersensitivity reaction)—results from certain proteins in latex rubber; symptoms range from skin redness, rash, hives, or itching to runny nose, itchy eyes, asthma, and anaphylaxis
    d. Patients at risk for latex reaction should be treated in a latex-reduced environment; physician consultation is indicated for patients with risk of an anaphylactic reaction
11. Listing of current medications—used to determine medications taken by the patient and possible interactions with other medications; these medications may be the only clue to the patient's existing condition (*Physicians' Desk Reference* or *Mosby's Dental Drug Reference* can help with the identification of adverse reactions, precautions, contraindications, and dental considerations)
12. Identification of medication allergies informs health care professionals of the patient's previous adverse reactions to medications
13. Vital signs (see the section on "Vital Signs" in Chapter 21)
    a. Vital signs are values given to measurements of BP, respiration, pulse, and temperature; serve as a baseline in a medical emergency; a temperature ≥100.0°F may indicate COVID-19
    b. Abnormal or elevated BP values should be brought to the patient's immediate attention; on the basis of the BP values, monitoring of BP at every appointment or a physician consultation may be required before initiation of dental hygiene care (see Table 15.4)
    c. BP, respirations, and pulse are measured and recorded before the administration of local anesthetic agents or nitrous oxide–oxygen ($N_2O$-$O_2$) analgesia
14. Conditions being treated with medications—may influence or contraindicate certain procedures; for example, anticoagulant therapy may require a lower dose; antihypertensive drugs may alter the choice of local anesthetic; antipsychotic medications may alter the choice of $N_2O$-$O_2$ analgesia (see the sections on "Anticoagulants" in Chapter 11; "Toxicity," "Vasoconstrictors," and "Conscious Sedation with Nitrous Oxide–Oxygen" in Chapter 18; and Chapter 21)
15. Physician consultations—may be necessary, depending on the information obtained from health history or physical examination; written documentation from the physician is necessary (see Fig. 15.4)
    a. Written informed consent is obtained from the patient before submitting the request for physician consultation
    b. Medical consultation can be faxed or mailed to the physician's office

C. Health history information is gathered through interviews, written questionnaires, or a combination of both
    1. The interview method allows the dental hygienist to develop patient rapport and ensures that the patient understands the questions
    2. The self-administered written questionnaire is the most common format used to gather information pertaining to the patient's health status
    3. Use of both the interview and the written questionnaire is the best approach to collect accurate and comprehensive health information

## EXTRAORAL AND INTRAORAL ASSESSMENT

A. Purpose—to assess and recognize deviations from normal conditions significant to a patient's health
B. Establishment of an assessment sequence that is followed systematically—skills used in performing extraoral and intraoral examination include direct observation, palpation, auscultation, and olfaction
    1. Direct observation—visual inspection techniques used to examine a patient's movement, body symmetry, color, texture, contour, consistency, and form of skin and mucous membrane

**REQUEST FOR MEDICAL CONSULTATION**

Date: ____________________

TO: **CLIENT INFORMATION**

RE: ____________________

____________________ Physician's Name — Client's name

____________________ Address — ____________________ Address

____________________ Address — Gender:_____ Birthdate:______

**Request:** It is anticipated that dental hygiene treatment will extend for (# of appointments) over (time period) (weekly/monthly) for (appointment length) hour durations. Your Client reported (or we observed) the following:

_____Cardiac arrhythmia, diagnosed ___________
_____High blood pressure (readings(s)/date) _________
_____Congential heart disease (CHD)_______________
_____ Anticoagulant therapy, (medication dose/name)
_____Diabetes, Type 1, glucose level ________
_____Diabetes, Type 2, glucose level_________
_____Total joint replacement (type & date replaced)
_____Other:______________________________

The treatment planned for ________________ includes:

_______Deep scaling and root planing/debridement (hemorrhage will occur)
_______Use of local anesthetic agent
_______Use of nitrous oxide-oxygen analgesia
_______Other:______________________________

Our concerns for ______________________ include the need for:

______Antibiotic prophylactic according to the AHA guidelines (2007)
______Evaluation of high blood pressure prior to dental hygiene care
______Evaluation of prothrombin time prior to dental hygiene care; INR score___
______ Evaluation of glucose level of control. Please provide most recent diabetes laboratory test results ____ $H1A_{1c}$
______Other:______________________________.

____________________ Dentist — ____________________ Registered Dental Hygienist

**RECOMMENDATIONS: Please indicate the definitive diagnosis and/or level of control. Also provide applicable laboratory test results in the space provided:**

____________________ Physician Signature — ____________________ Date

Adapted with permission from Idaho State University, Department of Dental Hygiene

**Fig. 15.4** Request for medical consultation.

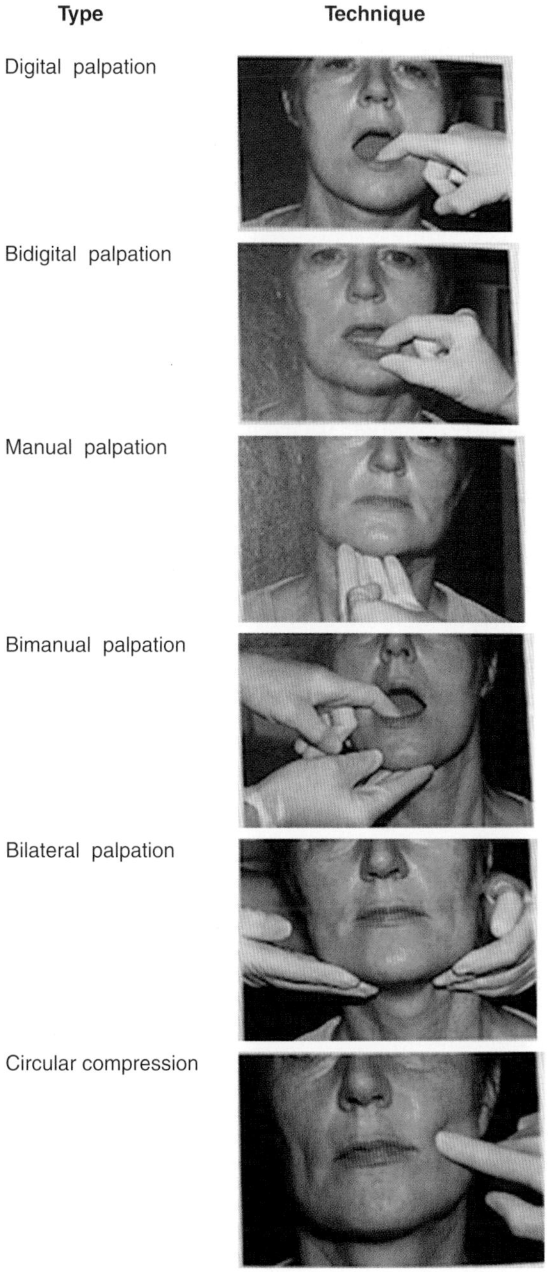

| Type | Technique |
|---|---|
| Digital palpation | |
| Bidigital palpation | |
| Manual palpation | |
| Bimanual palpation | |
| Bilateral palpation | |
| Circular compression | |

**Fig, 15.5** Palpation techniques. (Modified from Walsh MM, Darby ML. Palpation methods for assessing the oral cavity. In Darby ML, Walsh MM, eds. *Dental Hygiene Theory and Practice.* 4th ed. St. Louis: Saunders; 2015:216.)

2. Palpation—sense of touch used to examine for tenderness, texture, masses, and variations in structure and temperature within the head and neck region (see Fig. 15.5)
   a. Digital palpation—use of single (index) finger to move or press against the tissue of the floor of the mouth or hard palate
   b. Bidigital palpation—use of two or more fingers and thumb to move or compress the tissue of lips, tongue, cheeks, and vestibule
   c. Bimanual palpation—simultaneous use of the index finger of one hand and the fingers and thumb of the other hand to move or compress the tissue of the floor of the mouth
   d. Manual palpation—use of all the fingers of one hand to move and compress tissue to assess cervical lymph nodes
   e. Bilateral palpation—use of both hands simultaneously to move or press the tissue on the contralateral sides of the head to assess the submandibular nodes, TMJ, inferior border of mandible, and temporalis and masseter muscles
   f. Circular compression—use of fingers that move in a rotating, circular motion while slight pressure is applied
3. Auscultation—listening to and detecting sounds made by the body, such as clicking (crepitation) of the TMJ; speech disorders; and vocal hoarseness
4. Olfaction—use of the olfactory sense to detect variations in breath odors, such as alcohol breath, fruity ketosis (diabetic acidosis), and halitosis associated with dental caries, periodontitis, and necrotizing ulcerative gingivitis

## Extraoral Examination Procedure

See also Chapter 4.

A. Head, neck, and face—the overall appearance of patient should be assessed via visual inspection
B. The symmetry of skin, eyes, nose, and ears should be observed; areas of unusual discoloration should be inspected
   1. Skin (see the section on "Skin Diseases" in Chapter 8)
      a. Normal texture is continuous, firm, and pigmented in relation to normal variations associated with race and ethnicity
      b. Abnormal textures or pigmentations should be recorded (e.g., scarring, swelling, moles, freckles, pallor, redness, severe acne, tumors, jaundice)
      c. Abnormal lesions should be measured and documented in writing, with details about color, size, shape, and surface texture
   2. Face
      a. Face and head should be symmetrical and have normal function
      b. Asymmetry or lack of function may be associated with injury, Bell's palsy, tumor, abnormal growth and development, difficulty swallowing, Parkinson's disease, Tourette syndrome, and abuse
      c. Facial expression can indicate the patient's general frame of mind (e.g., anxious, happy, sad, angry)
   3. Eyes (see the section on "Visual Impairment" in Chapter 19)
      a. Clarity of the sclera should be noted; a yellowing color may indicate the presence of jaundice
      b. Pupil size and response to light should be reported; pupil abnormalities can indicate nerve damage, a medical condition, or be a side effect of medication
      c. Excessively dry or irritated eyes may be a result of medication side effects
   4. Nose
      a. Breathing should be assessed; flared nostrils or ragged breath could indicate difficulty breathing
      b. An enlarged, bulbous, and red nose may be associated with an overgrowth of sebaceous and sweat glands from alcohol abuse (rhinophyma)

5. Ears (see the section on "Hearing Impairment" in Chapter 19)

C. The symmetry of bones, muscles, lymph nodes, and salivary glands should be observed
   1. The inferior border of the mandible should be assessed for asymmetry by using bimanual palpation from the midline to the posterior angle
   2. The TMJ and the muscles of mastication should be inspected
      a. The TMJ should be assessed for deviation, pain, crepitus, grinding, and reduced range in opening or closing; evaluated through patient interview and bilateral palpation with index fingers anterior to outer meatus; patient is asked to open and close the mouth slowly several times; any deviation or symptomatology is recorded
      b. Masseter and temporalis muscles are assessed for overdevelopment, pain, swelling, and unusual hardness by using bilateral circular compression; patient is asked to clench the teeth together while the muscles are palpated
   3. The mentalis muscle is assessed for overdevelopment and smoothness of contraction during the swallowing movement; evaluated by digital palpation; tissue is moved over the mandible, and patient is asked to swallow
   4. The larynx is assessed for unrestricted movement by bimanual palpation; the larynx is gently moved from side to side to check movement
   5. Lymph node chains are assessed (Fig. 15.6)
      a. Occipital lymph nodes are assessed for pain, swelling, enlargement, unusual hardness, or fixed position by using bilateral palpation
      b. Auricular and parotid lymph nodes are examined for pain, swelling, enlargement, unusual hardness, or fixed position by using bilateral palpation
      c. Superficial cervical lymph nodes are assessed for pain, enlargement, unusual hardness, and fixed position by placing patient's head to one side with the chin slightly lowered and by palpating with fingers along the sternocleidomastoid muscle
      d. Deep cervical lymph nodes are examined for pain, enlargement, unusual hardness, and fixed position by placing patient's head upright and by palpating deep tissues along the sternocleidomastoid muscles with the thumb and fingers
   6. Submental and submandibular glands are examined for asymmetry, noncontinuous borders, pain, tenderness, swelling, enlargement, unusual hardness, or difficulty in swallowing by bilateral digital palpation
   7. The thyroid gland is assessed for asymmetry and enlargement by a combination of bidigital palpation and circular compression; patient is asked to sit upright and to swallow
   8. Parotid glands are examined for pain, swelling, enlargement, and hardness by using bilateral circular compression; salivary flow can be observed at the opening of Stensen's duct when the gland is compressed

## Intraoral Examination Procedure

A. Screen the patient to detect lesions that may be pathologic, particularly lesions that may be cancerous

B. Prevent the development of advanced, irreversible, or untreatable oral disease through early recognition of initial lesions

C. Oral piercing and tongue splitting are forms of body art. Tongue splitting is considered a body modification
   1. Inspect the tongue, lips, cheeks, frenum, and uvula for piercings and modifications
   2. Barbells and rings are the most common types of jewelry
   3. Complications from piercing include excessive hemorrhage; transmission of communicable diseases; nerve damage; infection; bacteremia; Ludwig's angina; cracked, fractured, or abraded teeth; recession; dehiscence; speech and mastication issues; and aspiration or ingestion of jewelry[6]
   4. Jewelry should be removed during the radiography procedure
   5. Complications from tongue splitting include nerve damage; infection; and excessive bleeding[6]

D. The oral mucosa, lips, floor of the mouth, tongue, salivary ducts, hard and soft palates, and oropharynx should be examined and evaluated (see Chapter 5 Table 5.1)
   1. The lips are examined by visual inspection and palpation for:
      a. Changes in size—may be caused by swelling or allergic reaction
      b. Chapping—may be caused by mouth breathing or nutritional deficiency
      c. Blistering—may be associated with herpetic lesions
      d. Cracking—may be associated with angular cheilosis, candidiasis, or vitamin B deficiency (see the section on "Vitamins" and Table 12.4 in Chapter 12)
      e. Scar tissue or irritations—may be associated with habitual lip biting or trauma; bruising at commissures may indicate binding or gagging associated with physical abuse
      f. Abnormal texture, lack of moistness or firmness—may be associated with dehydration and excessive sun exposure
      g. Limitations of opening; muscle elasticity, and muscle tone—may be associated with stroke or TMJ dysfunction
   2. Labial and alveolar mucosa and the gingiva are examined by using bilateral and bidigital palpation
      a. Signs of tissue trauma from biting, toothbrush abrasion, burns, or physical abuse; lacerated or torn frenum (tissue tags) may indicate binding, gagging, or forced feeding
      b. Ulcerated lesions such as herpetic lesions or aphthous ulcers
      c. Tight or low frenum attachments, which can cause gingival defects such as recession and loss of attached gingiva
      d. "Spit tobacco" lesion (leukoplakia), hyperkeratinized tissue; white, sometimes corrugated in appearance; patient should be taught self-assessment techniques

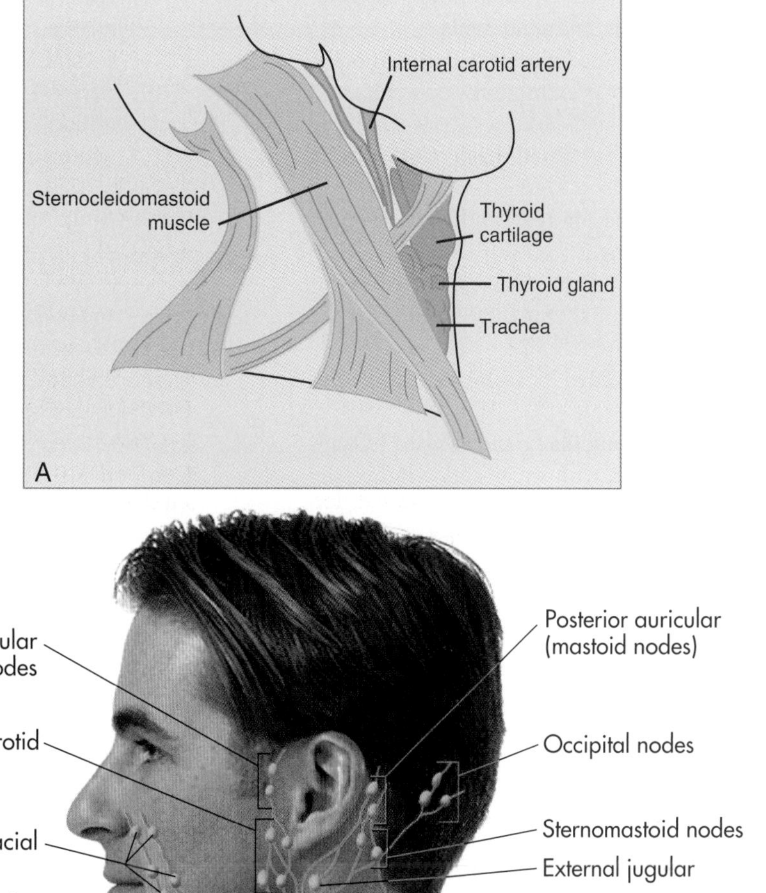

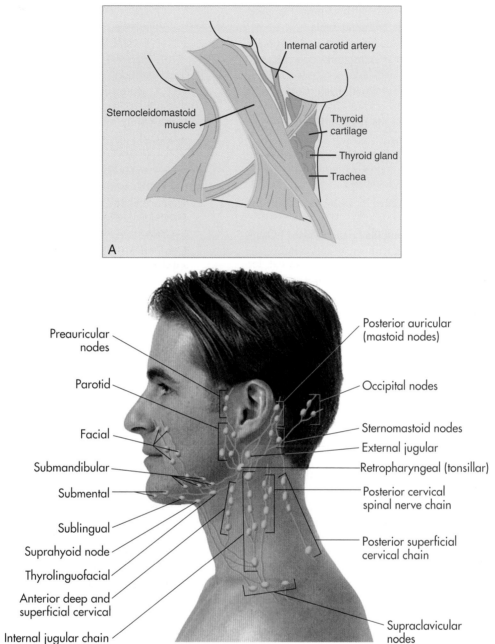


**Fig. 15.6** (A) Location of the thyroid gland and major muscle groups. (B) Lymph nodes of the head and neck region. (Modified from Ball JW, et al. *Seidel's Guide to Physical Examination.* 8th ed. St. Louis: Elsevier; 2015.)

e. Amalgam tattoo, blue-and-black coloration, size variations—can be found on any area of soft tissue (see section on "Amalgam Tattoo" in Chapter 8)
f. Fordyce granules—ectopic sebaceous glands

3. The buccal mucosa is assessed by using bidigital palpation; the mouth mirror is used to reflect light and to inspect the buccal mucosa
   a. The buccal mucosa is examined for color and texture
   b. The parotid papilla and duct (Stensen's duct) are evaluated; the duct is palpated to assess salivary function
   c. Atypical findings include traumatic lesions related to cheek biting, linea alba adjacent to occlusal plane, ectopic sebaceous glands (Fordyce granules)
4. Hard and soft palates and alveolar ridges are examined by visual inspection; the mouth mirror is used to reflect light; digital palpation is used on the hard palate and alveolar ridges; palpation is not recommended for soft palate to avoid triggering the gag reflex
   a. The hard palate, including the incisive papilla, rugae, and palatine fovea, is examined and assessed for:
      (1) Shape of the palate—low, high, narrow vault; alterations in shape may require alteration in oral radiographic techniques
      (2) Petechiae, torus palatinus, trauma (food burns, denture irritation), stomatitis (nicotine, ulcerative, necrotizing, and denture), fistulas from draining abscesses, denture-related candidiasis

b. The soft palate is assessed for inflammation, petechiae, trauma, stomatitis, and bifid uvula
c. Alveolar ridges are assessed for impacted third molars, scarring from third-molar extractions, opercula, and exostosis
5. Oropharynx is assessed by visual inspection with a mouth mirror
a. Patient is asked to say "ah" to relax and lower the posterior portion of the tongue
b. Anterior and posterior pillars are assessed for inflammation, petechiae, trauma, stomatitis, and enlarged tonsillar tissues
6. Floor of the mouth is examined by visual inspection and bimanual palpation
a. Function of the submandibular gland is tested by wiping each Wharton's duct with gauze and compressing it with a gloved finger to observe salivary flow
b. Entire floor of the mouth is palpated; the finger of one hand and the finger and thumb of the other hand are placed under patient's chin to palpate
c. Enlargement or masses, Wharton's duct, sublingual caruncle, and lingual frenum are assessed
d. Varicosities, tight frenum attachment (ankyloglossia), and blocked salivary duct are inspected
e. Exostosis along lingual surface of mandible and mandibular tori—significant if interfering with prosthetic appliances
7. The tongue is examined by visual inspection and digital palpation
a. The dorsal surface is inspected; the entire tongue is palpated, and the lateral borders of the tongue are examined by using gauze to gently hold the tongue
b. The ventral surface is examined by having patient touch the palate with the tongue
c. The tongue is assessed for:
(1) Coating on the dorsal surface and the condition of papillae; the extent is assessed
(2) Size; macroglossia associated with Down syndrome or cretinism (see the section on "Down Syndrome" in Chapter 19)
(3) Lingual frenum; tight frenum restricting movement (ankyloglossia)
(4) Fissured tongue; deep grooves and crevices along the lateral borders and the dorsal surface; the lateral borders are common sites of oral cancer
(5) Geographic tongue—benign condition in which a sporadic migration of dorsal papilla occurs; tenderness is assessed
(6) Nutritional deficiencies; burning or glossy tongue (see the section on "Abnormalities Affecting the Tongue" in Chapter 8)
(7) Black hairy tongue related to proliferation of filiform papillae; caused by irritants such as smoking, alcohol, and rinsing with hydrogen peroxide (see the section on "Abnormalities Affecting the Tongue" in Chapter 8)
(8) Hairy leukoplakia caused by extensions of keratin on the lateral borders of the tongue; associated with HIV infection
(9) Atypical lesions, including aphthous ulcerations, trauma-associated fibroma, hemangiomas, and white plaque

## ASSESSMENT OF DENTITION

A. Purpose—to assess and document the position and condition of teeth, restorations, and dental caries, noting normal and abnormal findings on a detailed dentition chart
1. Used for care planning, communication with patient, legal documentation, forensic use, and financial audits
2. Components include study models, occlusion assessment, dentition charting, pulp vitality testing, and strain assessment
B. Study models—impressions for study models taken to obtain visual reproduction of teeth, gingiva, and adjacent intraoral structures and to assist with dentition and periodontal charting
C. Occlusion assessment—presence of malocclusion or tooth position determined; signs of parafunctional habits resulting in occlusal traumatism noted (see the sections on "Intra-arch and Interarch Relationships" in Chapter 5 and "Clinical Assessment of the Periodontium" in Chapter 14)
D. Dentition charting—graphic representation of a patient's teeth at assessment (see Fig. 15.7)
1. Includes developmental anomalies and defects, condition of teeth, dental caries activity, restorative history, and other problems; a combination of radiographs and direct visual inspection is used to assist with accurate recording of tooth assessment (Box 15.2)
2. Office guides and professional organizations' dentition charting symbols may be adopted for use; the ADA's National Board Dental Examination (NBDE) provides a dental charting symbol key in each patient case used
3. Universal Numbering System—most widely used notation system; permanent teeth numbered from 1 to 32 and primary teeth lettered from A to T; 1 to 16 or A to J are located on the maxillary arch, moving right to left; 17 to 32 or K to T are located on the mandibular arch, moving left to right (from patient's perspective)
4. Developmental anomalies that affect enamel and dentin, developmental defects that affect tooth shape, number of teeth, and tooth size are noted (see Chapter 8)
5. Tooth positions, eruption patterns, and missing teeth are recorded (see the sections on "Eruption" and "Intra-arch and Interarch Relationships" in Chapter 5)
6. Tooth damage that results in loss of integrity of tooth surface is recorded; common forms of damage include attrition, abrasion, erosion, fracture, and dental caries (see Chapter 8)
7. Dental caries is an infectious, transmittable, and multifactorial disease of bacterial origin; carious lesions are

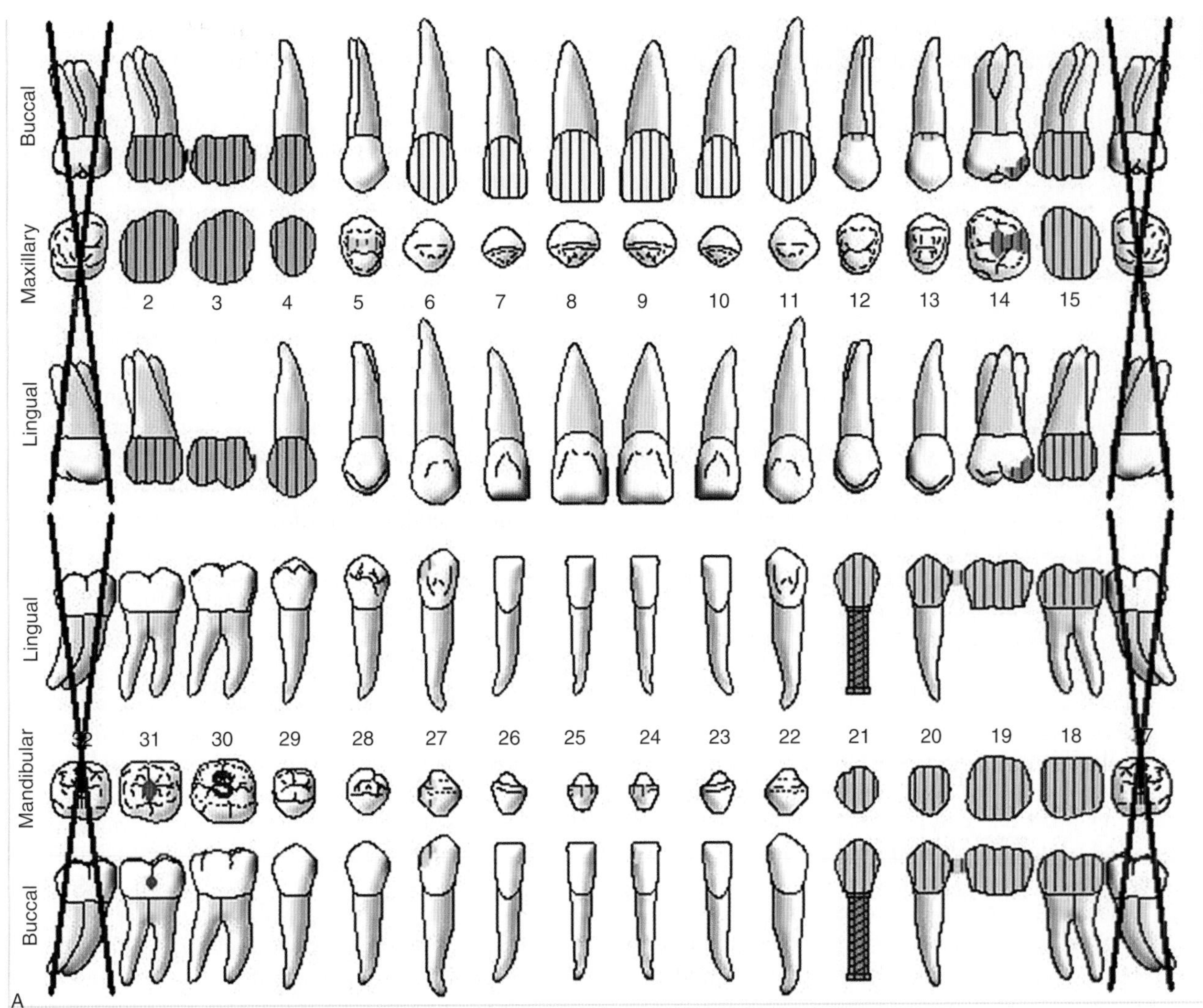


B

| Tooth/Teeth # | Restoration/Condition |
|---|---|
| **1, 16, 17, 18** | Extracted |
| **2, 3, 4** | High noble metal bridge (2 and 4 abutment ; 3 pontic) |
| **5** | Class I composite |
| **6, 7, 8, 9, 10, 11** | Porcelain veneer |
| **12, 13** | Class V composite |
| **14** | Class II amalgam |
| **15** | Porcelain fused to metal crown |
| **18, 19, 20** | Porcelain fused to metal bridge (18 and 20 abutment; 19 pontic) |
| **21** | Implant and porcelain fused to metal crown |
| **24** | Class IV composite |
| **25** | Class VI composite |
| **27** | Class III composite |
| **30** | Occlusal sealant |
| **31** | Decay on occlusal surface and buccal pit |

**Fig. 15.7** (A) Restorative charting. (B) Restorative chart key. (Courtesy Eagle Soft. With permission from Patterson Dental Supply Inc.)

classified by the type and location of the lesion by using visual inspection with magnification, laser fluorescence, light fluorescence, digital imaging, fiberoptic transillumination, gentle probing, and radiographic examination with standard bitewing or digitized view

a. Classification for carious lesions includes rate, direction, and type of disease progression; used to determine level of priority for restorative therapy
   (1) Rampant caries—a rapidly progressive decay process that affects the smooth surfaces of numerous teeth and requires urgent intervention; frequently found with early-childhood caries (formerly called *nursing bottle syndrome*)
   (2) Chronic caries—slow progressive decay process
   (3) Arrested caries—carious lesion that has been reversed because of the remineralization process

## BOX 15.2 Systematic Approach for Dentition Charting Sequence

Complete a general appraisal of teeth, and note developmental anomalies and defects affecting tooth shape, number of teeth, tooth size, and presence of partial or complete dentures (e.g., generalized moderate fluorosis, amelogenesis imperfecta, peg laterals, number of teeth present, mandibular partial denture)
Chart all missing or erupted supernumerary teeth before recording specific tooth-by-tooth information
Using radiographs, chart all unerupted or impacted teeth
Chart teeth indicated for extraction
Chart existing restorations (amalgam, tooth-colored, and temporary restorations; inlays, onlays, and gold foils; crowns, veneers, and bridges)
Chart signs of tooth damage (dental caries, risk areas, attrition)
Chart areas of plaque-retentive factors and defective restorations needing replacement (overhangs, deficient margins, unpolished amalgam restorations, fractured restorations, improper anatomical contour, occlusal surfaces indicated for pit-and-fissure sealants)
When treatment has been completed on teeth indicated for restorative or supportive care, update the chart using a different color to quickly identify teeth that were restored after original baseline charting
Update the dentition charting at each recare visit, and record any areas of change

(4) Backward caries—lateral spread of decay at the dentino-enamel junction through an undermining process; the surface lesion appears small, but destruction is extensive underneath
(5) Recurrent or secondary caries— new decay located around existing restorations

b. Carious lesions described by specific location on tooth surface (see the section on "Dental Caries" in Chapter 9)
(1) Pit-and-fissure caries—develop in the pits and grooves of the occlusal surfaces of premolars and molars, lingual pits of maxillary incisors, buccal grooves of mandibular molars, and lingual grooves of maxillary molars; pit-and-fissure sealants are an effective preventive strategy to protect tooth surfaces (see "Dental Sealants" in Chapter 16)
(2) Smooth surface caries—found on the facial, lingual, mesial, and distal surfaces of teeth
(3) Root caries—found on exposed root surfaces

c. G.V. Black's classification of dental caries and restorations provides a precise description of the types and location of caries and restorations
(1) Class I—pits and fissures on the occlusal, buccal, and lingual surfaces of posterior teeth and the lingual surfaces of anterior teeth
(2) Class II—proximal surface of posterior teeth, usually involving the occlusal surfaces
(3) Class III—proximal surfaces of incisors and canines, not including the incisal edge
(4) Class IV—proximal surfaces of incisors and canines, including the incisal edge
(5) Class V—gingival third of facial or lingual surfaces of any tooth
(6) Class VI—cusp tips of posterior teeth and the incisal edge of anterior teeth

8. Charting of existing restorations, treatment procedures (endodontics, apicoectomy), and tooth replacement methods (implants, crown, bridge) completed by using accepted dental symbols
a. Restorations should be charted with G.V. Black's classification system and should reflect the actual restoration
b. The restoration morphology, margin quality and location, and biocompatibility of restorative material with soft tissue are evaluated
(1) The restoration and the surrounding tooth structure are assessed for new or recurrent dental caries
(2) The marginal and structural integrity assessed for open margins or signs of restorative material fatigue or fractures; the appropriate margin is smooth to tactile evaluation and does not show any overhang
(3) The interproximal and occlusal contours and the proximal contact are assessed; the appropriateness of faciolingual and occlusocervical dimensions are determined; indication for amalgam polishing or recontouring to improve restoration is assessed
(4) Surface finish is assessed to determine whether it meets the functional and esthetic requirements of the patient; indication for amalgam polishing or finishing is assessed
c. Faulty restorations are usually in need of replacement because of the presence of recurrent dental caries, fractures, or factors that encourage microbial plaque biofilm retention and may contribute to the development of secondary caries, periodontal disease, and dentinal hypersensitivity
d. Overhangs on class II restorations should be assessed for removal (margination procedures) to correct defective margins and to provide a smooth surface that will not harbor bacterial plaque biofilm
(1) Type I overhang—less than one-third of the interproximal space; treated with margination procedure and repolishing of restoration; may be detected radiographically
(2) Type II overhang—one-third to one-half of the interproximal embrasure space; treated with margination procedure if the predicted final result is good (prognosis for the tooth, complexity, and cost of replacement are considered); usually radiographically and clinically detectable
(3) Type III overhang—more than half of the interproximal embrasure space; treated with replacement of restoration; clinically and radiographically detectable

9. Implant identification (see the sections on "Dental Implants" in Chapter 14)—to assess for peri-implantitis and the stability of the implant

10. Prosthetic appliances—assessed for stability and functionality

E. Pulpal vitality testing—when applicable (see the section on "Pulpal Vitality and Testing Devices" in Chapter 16)

F. Stain assessment (see the section on "Selective Stain Removal" in Chapter 17)—to determine the extent and type of stain present
   1. Stains are primarily factors related to esthetics; result from deposits of chromogenic bacteria, foods, and chemicals
   2. Heavy tobacco stains encourage bacterial plaque biofilm retention

## PERIODONTAL ASSESSMENT

See the section on "Clinical Assessment of the Periodontium" in Chapter 14.

A. Recognition of oral health, gingivitis, or periodontitis must occur through systematic and comprehensive periodontal examination to determine whether oral prophylaxis, nonsurgical periodontal therapy (NSPT), periodontal maintenance (PM), or other periodontal therapy is indicated and to what extent (Fig. 15.8)

B. During general periodontal examination, anatomical features such as position, size, and shape of gingiva and interdental papillae and position of frena must be recorded
   1. The presence, location, and severity of gingival inflammation are assessed—soft tissue description (color, texture, consistency, marginal and papillary shape)
   2. Mucogingival relationships are evaluated to identify the deficiencies of keratinized tissue, abnormal frenum insertions, and other tissue abnormalities, such as clinically significant gingival recession (e.g., recession, loss of attachment/clinical attachment level, attached gingiva)

C. Periodontal probing is done to assess the probing depth and to provide information on the health of subgingival areas, including the presence of bleeding on probing (see the section on "Using Periodontal Probes" in Chapter 17)
   1. Probing depths are measured on six tooth sites (distofacial, facial, mesiofacial, distolingual, lingual, mesiolingual) and recorded on the periodontal chart
   2. Clinical pocket depth measurements and loss of attachment readings are used to determine the presence of pseudopockets (false or gingival pockets) or periodontal pockets

D. Periodontal soft tissues, including peri-implant tissues, should be examined

E. The presence of purulent exudates and gingival crevicular fluid (GCF) should be determined; increased GCF and purulent exudate indicate inflammatory changes within the pocket wall; these are considered risk factors for disease progression and require further assessment to determine cause and to plan interventions

F. The presence and amount of bleeding on probing is noted to assist in the determination of disease severity

G. The presence and distribution of bacterial plaque biofilm and calculus—location, extent, and tenacity of deposits are identified to assist with appropriate care planning and instrument selection (see the section on "Dental Explorers" in Chapter 17)

H. Degree of mobility of teeth and dental implants
   1. Mobility—risk factor for periodontal disease progression; should be measured when moderate to advanced disease is present
   2. Measured by bidigital evaluation with two instrument handles when teeth are not occluded and by direct observation (fremitus) when teeth are occluded; classified by degree of movement
      a. Class 1 or I—slight mobility, greater than normal
      b. Class 2 or II—moderate mobility, greater than 1 mm
      c. Class 3 or III—severe mobility, tooth can move in all directions and can be depressed into the socket
   3. Contributing factors—trauma from occlusion, inflammation in periodontal ligament, periodontal surgery, physiochemical changes (pregnancy or hormonal changes) in periodontal tissues, and pathologic conditions (tumors)

I. The presence, location, and degree of clinical furcation involvement are determined
   1. Occurs when loss of attachment extends into bifurcation or trifurcation of multi-rooted teeth; classified by degree of involvement
      a. Class I—exposure of furcation; but bone remains between roots
      b. Class II—loss of some bone between roots; but not complete communication from one surface to another
      c. Class III—through-and-through involvement with complete loss of bone between roots; opening covered by gingiva
      d. Class IV—through-and-through involvement with complete loss of bone between roots; entrance clearly visible
   2. Furcation involvement—risk factor in predicting periodontal breakdown; compromises the prognosis of a tooth; detection and thorough periodontal debridement essential at the earliest point

J. Bacterial culturing, genetic testing, deoxyribonucleic acid (DNA) or ribonucleic acid (RNA) probes, antibody and enzyme markers should be used, when indicated (see the section on "Clinical Assessment of the Periodontium" in Chapter 14)
   1. Microbial assessments are not recommended routinely because tests fail to identify specific diseases or predict disease progression; however, microbiologic monitoring may be used in patients who continue to experience disease progression despite regular NSPT, surgical intervention, and effective oral self-care; those at high risk for disease progression or medically compromised patients with aggressive periodontitis may benefit from microbiologic monitoring
   2. Commercially available genetic tests assess susceptibility to chronic periodontitis and assist in risk assessment
   3. Salivary diagnostic advances allow for identification of periodontal bacteria and genetic testing; although use in clinical practice is limited[7]

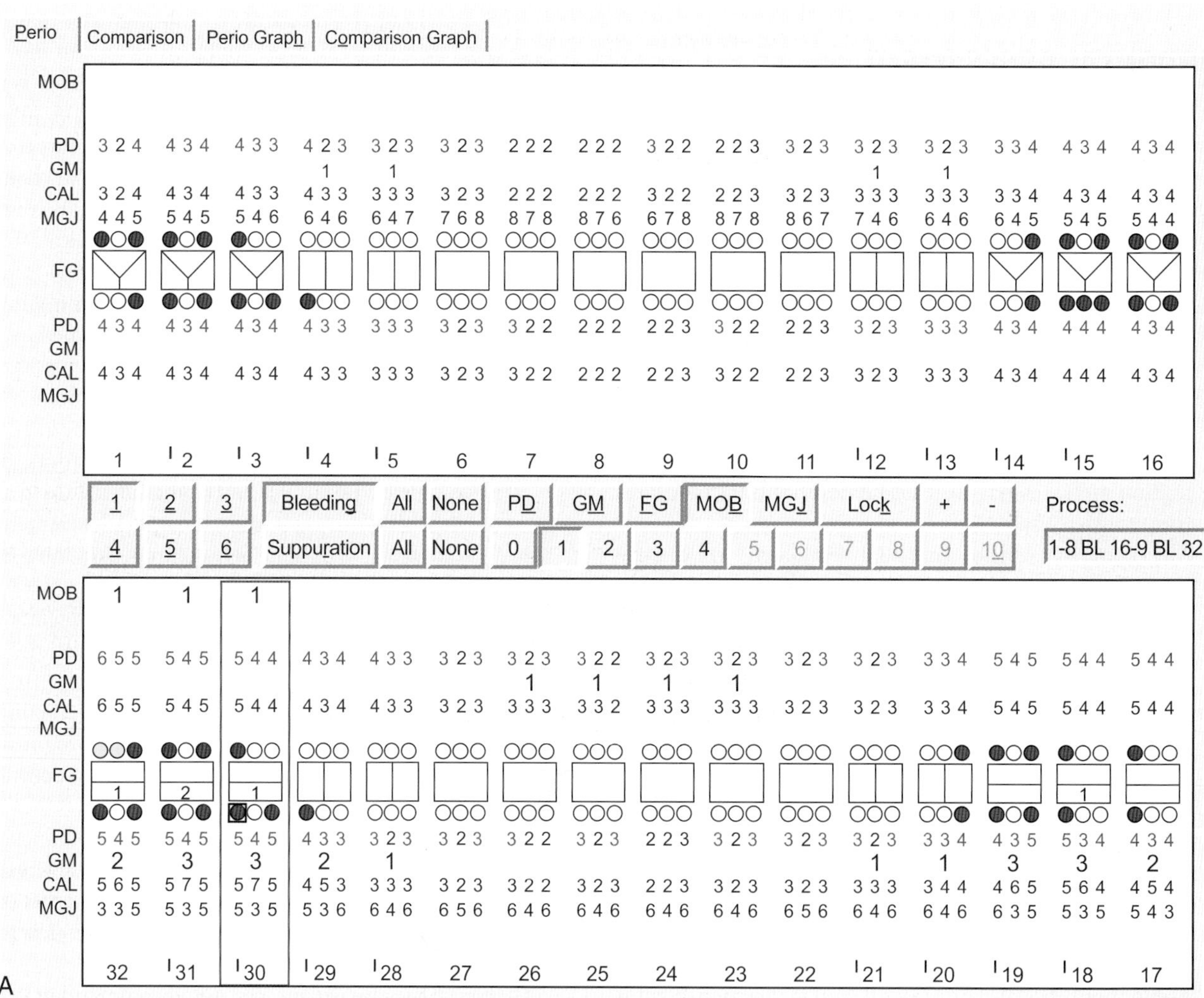
Perio | Comparison | Perio Graph | Comparison Graph
MOB
PD 324 434 433 423 323 323 222 222 322 223 323 323 323 334 434 434
GM 1 1 1 1
CAL 324 434 433 433 333 323 222 222 322 223 323 333 333 334 434 434
MGJ 445 545 546 646 647 768 878 876 678 878 867 746 646 645 545 544
FG
PD 434 434 434 433 333 323 322 222 223 322 223 323 333 434 444 434
GM
CAL 434 434 434 433 333 323 322 222 223 322 223 323 333 434 444 434
MGJ
1 2 3 4 5 6 7 8 9 10 11 12 13 14 15 16
1 2 3 Bleeding All None PD GM FG MOB MGJ Lock + - Process:
4 5 6 Suppuration All None 0 1 2 3 4 5 6 7 8 9 10 1-8 BL 16-9 BL 32
MOB 1 1 1
PD 655 545 544 434 433 323 323 322 323 323 323 323 334 545 544 544
GM 1 1 1 1
CAL 655 545 544 434 433 323 333 332 333 333 323 323 334 545 544 544
MGJ
FG 1 2 1 1
PD 545 545 545 433 323 323 322 323 223 323 323 323 334 435 534 434
GM 2 3 3 2 1 1 1 3 3 2
CAL 565 575 575 453 333 323 322 323 223 323 323 333 344 465 564 454
MGJ 335 535 535 536 646 656 646 646 646 646 656 646 646 635 535 543
32 31 30 29 28 27 26 25 24 23 22 21 20 19 18 17
A

**Fig. 15.8** (A) Periodontal chart.

**TABLE 15.6 Asking the Clinical Question: PICO Mnemonic**

| Element (PICO) | Descriptive Question(s) to Ask | Example |
|---|---|---|
| **P**atient, or problem | How would I describe a group of patients similar to mine? What are the most important characteristics for this patient? | A patient with generalized marginal biofilm and inflammation |
| **I**ntervention, cause, or prognosis | Which main intervention or prognostic factor am I considering for this patient? | A powered toothbrush |
| **C**omparison, or control | What is the main alternative to compare with the intervention? | Compared with a manual toothbrush |
| **O**utcome, or outcomes | What can I hope to accomplish, measure, or improve? | Decrease marginal biofilm and inflammation |

Modified from Forest JL, Miller SA. Translating evidence-based decision making into practice: EBDM concepts and finding the evidence, *J Evid Based Dent Pract*. 2009;9:(2):59–72.

2. A computerized literature search is conducted to gather information that may be used to answer the PICO question—randomized controlled clinical trials (RCTs), systematic reviews, or meta-analysis studies provide the best evidence for answering the question
3. Evidence obtained from the literature search is critically evaluated to determine validity and clinical applicability—studies are reviewed to identify the results and determine whether they are valid and whether they apply to the patient
4. Evidence gathered from the literature appraisal is applied to clinical practice by discussing the findings with the patient and offering recommendations for treatment
5. The process and the clinician's performance are evaluated

## PLANNING

A. Definition—identification and prioritization of current and potential dental and dental hygiene care needs, establishment of patient goals, and determination of interventions and outcomes to meet these needs

B. Patients are more likely to express their wants, needs, and desires and to commit to a care plan if they are actively involved in the development of goals, priorities, interventions, and appointment planning

C. Assessment data and diagnosis should be used to develop a logical plan of therapy to eliminate disease, slow disease progression, and maintain and promote health

D. Four components to consider when completing written care plan:
1. Establish priorities for care that require a collaborative approach among the patient, the dental hygienist, and the dentist; address the following:
   a. Needs of the patient based on conditions that pose the greatest threat to comfort, life, health, and safety
   b. Main concerns or preferences of the patient (chief complaint)
   c. Motivational level of the patient
2. Set patient-oriented goals and evaluation measures that reflect the expected and desired outcomes of dental hygiene care
   a. For each dental hygiene diagnosis, at least one goal and intervention should be established; some diagnoses may require multiple interventions
   b. Goals should focus on the cognitive, affective, or psychomotor domain and contain a subject, verb, measurement criteria, and specific time element:
      (1) Cognitive goals focus on increasing knowledge level
      (2) Affective goals focus on changes in beliefs, attitudes, and values
      (3) Psychomotor goals focus on skill development when skill deficiencies are present
   c. Expected outcomes and evaluation measures are used to determine whether goals are being met during care or after completion of therapy; when indicated, modify the diagnosis or care plan if goals are not being met; two forms of evaluation should be considered when planning care:
      (1) Evaluation that occurs throughout the implementation phase of care (formative evaluation)
      (2) Evaluation or reevaluation that occurs after the completion of initial therapy (summative evaluation)
3. Identify interventions as part of care planning that specifically address the dental hygiene diagnosis (Table 15.7)
   a. Traditional phases of dental care planning include[14]:
      (1) Preliminary phase—focuses on treating periodontal or dental emergency needs
      (2) Phase I therapy—focuses on controlling the risk factors responsible for disease; includes self-care education, diet control, removal or correction of biofilm-retentive factors, antimicrobial therapy, and dental caries management
      (3) Phase II therapy—focuses on surgical care; includes periodontal surgery, placement of implants, and endodontic therapy
      (4) Phase III therapy—focuses on prosthetic treatment and final management of dental caries, along with periodontal examination to reevaluate response to restorative procedures
      (5) Phase IV therapy—focuses on long-term PM therapy; includes assessment, self-care education, deposit removal, and evaluation of continued-care (recare) interval
   b. Common system of periodontal disease classification; there are three major forms of periodontitis[15,16] (see the section on "Diseases of the Periodontium" in Chapter 14)
      (1) Necrotizing periodontitis
         (a) Necrotizing gingivitis
         (b) Necrotizing periodontitis
         (c) Necrotizing stomatitis
      (2) Periodontitis as a manifestation of systemic diseases
         (a) Classified according to International Statistical Classification of Diseases and Related Health Problems (ICD) codes

**TABLE 15.7 Components of Dental Hygiene Care**

| Component | Elements |
|---|---|
| General assessment | Medical and dental history |
| | Chief concern |
| | Clinical examination |
| | Radiographic analysis |
| | Microbiologic, genetic, and biochemical diagnostic tests |
| | Extraoral and intraoral examinations |
| Periodontal and restorative assessment | Risk assessment |
| | Plaque or biofilm, calculus |
| | Dental restorations |
| | Caries assessment |
| | Dental implants |
| | Probing depth (bleeding and suppuration) |
| | Clinical attachment level and gingival recession |
| | Furcation status |
| | Prosthetic appliances |
| | Occlusion (mobility, occlusal discrepancy, fremitus) |
| | Proximal contact relationships |
| | Periodontal–systemic interrelationships |
| Self-care education | Risk factors |
| | Disease theory education |
| | Skill enhancement |
| | Behavior interventions (nutrition counseling, tobacco cessation, medical referral) |
| Instrumentation and supportive therapy | Pain and anxiety control methods |
| | Plaque biofilm and calculus removal |
| | Restoration overhang removal |
| | Desensitization for dentinal hypersensitivity |
| | Fluoride therapy |
| | Sealant application |
| | Local or systemic chemotherapeutic agents |
| | Implant maintenance |
| | Mouthguard fabrication |
| Selection of polishing procedures | Selective stain removal (polishing) |
| | Restoration enhancement (finishing, polishing) |
| Referrals | Medical consultation |
| | Restorative therapy |
| | Periodontal surgery |
| | Orthodontics |
| | Endodontics |
| | Oral surgery |
| | Oral pathology diagnosis |

Modified from American Academy of Periodontology: Statement on comprehensive periodontal therapy. 2011. https://onlinelibrary.wiley.com/doi/pdf/10.1902/jop.2011.117001. Accessed January 27, 2019.

(3) Periodontitis; characterized by stage and grade
  (a) Stage (based on severity and complexity of management)
    [1] Stage I: Initial periodontitis
      i. Severity:
        1. Interdental clinical attachment loss (CAL) of 1–2 mm at site of greatest loss
        2. Radiographic bone loss extending to the coronal third of the root with less than 15% of teeth involved
        3. No tooth loss due to periodontitis
      ii. Complexity:
        1. Maximum probing depth ≤ 4 mm
        2. Mostly horizontal bone loss
    [2] Stage II: moderate periodontitis
      i. Severity:
        1. Interdental CAL of 3–4 mm at site of greatest loss
        2. Radiographic bone loss extending to the coronal third of the root with 15%–33% of teeth involved
      ii. Complexity:
        1. Maximum probing depth ≤ 5 mm
        2. Mostly horizontal bone loss
    [3] Stage III: severe periodontitis with potential for additional tooth loss
      i. Severity:
        1. Interdental CAL of ≥ 5 mm at site of greatest loss
        2. Radiographic bone loss extending to the middle third of the root and beyond
        3. Four or less teeth lost due to periodontitis
      ii. Complexity (in addition to Stage II complexity):
        1. Probing depths ≥6 mm
        2. Vertical bone loss ≥3 mm
        3. Class II or III furcation involvement
        4. Moderate ridge defects
    [4] Stage IV: Severe periodontitis with potential for loss of the dentition
      i. Severity:
        1. Interdental CAL of ≥5 mm at site of greatest loss
        2. Radiographic bone loss extending to the middle third of the root and beyond
        3. Five or more teeth lost due to periodontitis
      ii. Complexity (in addition to Stage III complexity); need for complex rehabilitation due to:
        1. Masticatory dysfunction
        2. Secondary occlusal trauma
        3. Bite collapse, drifting, flaring
        4. <20 remaining teeth (10 opposing pairs)
  (b) Extent and distribution (localized, generalized, molar-incisor distribution); added to stage descriptor
  (c) Grade (evidence or risk of rapid progression, anticipated treatment response). Grade modifiers are risk factors that can affect the rate of progression.
    [1] Grade A: slow rate of progression
      i. Grade modifiers:
        1. Nonsmoker
        2. No diagnosis of diabetes

[2] Grade B: moderate rate of progression
i. Grade modifiers:
1. Smoking less than 10 cigarettes daily
2. Diabetic patients with A1c less than 7.0%

[3] Grade C: Rapid rate of progression
i. Grade modifiers:
1. Smoking 10 or more cigarettes daily
2. Diabetic patients with A1c greater or equal to 7.0%

c. Interventions for common forms of periodontal disease include:
(1) Therapy for gingivitis—includes oral self-care education, supragingival and subgingival debridement, antimicrobial agents, and correction of plaque biofilm–retentive factors completed during a 1-hour appointment; may include reevaluation at another appointment if extensive bleeding occurs on probing or pseudopockets are present
(2) Therapy for initial periodontitis (stage I)—includes elimination, modification, or control of systemic diseases and other risk factors; oral self-care education; and supragingival and subgingival debridement, including scaling and root planing with a quadrant approach, during four 60- to 90-minute appointments, and reevaluation
(3) Therapy for moderate periodontitis (stage II)—includes elimination, alteration, or control of systemic diseases and other risk factors; oral self-care education; and supragingival and subgingival debridement, including scaling and root planing with a sextant or quadrant approach, during four to six 60- to 90-minute appointments, and reevaluation for surgery
(4) Therapy for severe periodontitis with potential for additional tooth loss (stage III) or loss of the dentition (stage IV) includes elimination, modification, or control of systemic diseases and risk factors; oral self-care education; debridement, including scaling and root planing with a sextant approach during six 60- to 90-minute appointments; subgingival microbial sampling; and extraction of teeth that have a poor prognosis. Reevaluation for surgery, possible stabilization or restoration of masticatory function,[17] and the potential for referral are options to consider following treatment

4. Written care plan provides permanent documentation and becomes a contract between the dental hygienist and a patient; elements of care plan include:
a. Procedure—course of action or procedures to be rendered; associated risks and benefits
b. Alternative treatment options
c. Appointment sequence—order in which therapy will be given
d. Approximate time for each procedure and total time for each appointment
e. Expected outcomes and limitations of care

## CASE PRESENTATION

A. Definition—presentation of assessment data to include dental and dental hygiene diagnosis and proposed care plan
B. Purpose—to satisfy legal and ethical responsibilities for care, reach agreement for therapy, and obtain informed consent
C. A collaborative approach between patient and clinician should be encouraged
D. Case presentation should be accurate, direct, and concise; should describe:
1. Existing oral conditions and related causative and contributing factors presented in terms that are understandable to the patient
2. Treatment procedures and how therapy may differ from previous appointments (e.g., number of appointments, length, purpose of each appointment, services to be incorporated, description of services)
3. Desired outcomes of treatment and provisional prognosis
4. Risks and benefits of all treatment options involved
5. Consequences of rejecting treatment or not proceeding with all components of care
6. Alternative approaches to care, if any exist (e.g., mechanized vs. hand-activated instrumentation; NSPT vs. surgery when advanced disease is present)
7. Patient's responsibility as a cotherapist (e.g., commitment to self-care and continued-care recommendations)
8. Patient's right to decline care by providing an opportunity to initially consent for care and to withdraw from treatment at any time
9. Time and cost involved in professional care

## INFORMED CONSENT

A. Definition—legal process by which a patient agrees to a proposed treatment after a complete case presentation (see Chapter 22)
B. Informed consent provides the patient with the necessary information to make a decision regarding their treatment; includes:
1. A description of the patient's condition
2. A description of proposed treatment
3. Alternative treatment options
4. A description of risks and benefits for all treatment (proposed and alternative)
5. Outcomes expected for each treatment option presented
6. Referral information, if necessary
C. The patient must understand all information provided to make an informed decision; an opportunity for questions and answers are provided
D. Includes use of a written informed consent form (stating elements listed above), signed by the patient or guardian, the clinician, and a witness as documentation of consent; should be completed before implementation of care plan
E. An *informed refusal form* is completed when a patient declines some or all of the care plan; includes:
1. Proposed dental and dental hygiene care planned
2. Risks involved without treatment

3. List of procedures being refused
4. Date the informed refusal form was signed
5. Signature of the patient, the dental hygienist or the dentist, and a witness

## IMPLEMENTATION

See the section on "Preventive Therapy or Treatment of Biofilm-Induced Gingivitis" in Chapter 14.

A. Definition—delivery of preventive and therapeutic procedures identified in an individualized care plan to meet a patient's human needs (see Table 15.7)
   1. Activities—reduction or elimination of risk factors for disease, health promotion, self-care education, mechanical and mechanized instrumentation, pharmacotherapeutic interventions, pain control strategies, selective polishing; supporting interventions include overhang removal, desensitization, dietary assessment and counseling, dental caries management, and occlusal therapy
   2. Modifications to the initial care plan are made as new assessment criteria become available during the implementation of care (i.e., improved self-care, increase in healing response time)
B. Self-care discussion—presenting information about disease control, health maintenance, behavior change and health promotion strategies aimed at improving oral health; should occur at each appointment before instrumentation procedures; strategies are those implemented by the patient at home (see Chapter 16)
C. Pain and anxiety control should be used when indicated to prevent or manage apprehension and pain and promote the patient's cooperation and compliance; includes local anesthetic agents, $N_2O$-$O_2$ analgesia, topical anesthetic agents, and psychosomatic methods (see Chapter 18)
D. Instrument selection—based on intraoral conditions discovered in the assessment phase of care: periodontal pocket depth, furcation involvement, root concavities, deposit size, configuration, mode of attachment, and location (see Chapter 17)
   1. Hand-activated instrumentation—use of sharp curets and files, with fundamental instrumentation principles during scaling and debridement
   2. Mechanized instrumentation—ultrasonic and sonic scaling equipment and techniques for scaling and debridement
E. Polishing procedures—use of abrasive agents, prophy angle, low-speed handpiece, toothbrush, or air abrasion unit to remove bacterial plaque biofilm and stain and to produce a smooth, lustrous tooth surface
   1. Selective polishing—esthetic procedure accomplished with a rubber cup and paste or air-polishing unit (air abrasion) to remove extrinsic stain remaining after periodontal instrumentation (see the section on "Selective Stain Removal" in Chapter 17)
   2. Therapeutic polishing—prophylaxis pastes may include supplemental ingredients for added benefits, including fluoride, xylitol, and calcium phosphate compounds
   3. Polishing and finishing restorations prevent recurrent caries and deterioration of restorations, maintain periodontal health, and prevent occlusal problems
F. Maintenance therapy (formerly known as *supportive therapy*)—a term used for interventions directed at sustaining oral health and controlling disease progression (e.g., debridement for control of periodontal diseases and maintenance of periodontal health, fluoride therapy, sealant application, occlusal appliance fabrication, oral irrigation, desensitization, local or systemic antibiotics, implant maintenance) (see the section on "Periodontal Maintenance" in Chapter 14 and "Oral Irrigation," "Fluorides," "Mouthrinses or Chemotherapeutics," "Dental Sealants," "Care of Fixed and Removable Prostheses," "Dental Implant Maintenance," "Tobacco Use Interventions," and "Assessment of Dentinal Hypersensitivity" in Chapter 16.)
G. *Ergonomics* focuses on the prevention of exposure to injury within the work environment; involves clinician and patient positioning, tasks and procedures performed, equipment design and use, and impact of these actions on musculoskeletal health
   1. Cumulative trauma disorders (also known as *repetitive strain disorders*)—musculoskeletal and nerve impairments caused by repetitive work activities, especially when performed aggressively, in awkward positions, or both
   2. Prevention of ergonomic hazards—involves daily application of ergonomic principles while providing dental hygiene care (e.g., posture, grasp, properly fitted gloves, instrument and equipment design, exercise for hand and body, positioning of equipment and materials in the environment)

## PATIENT MANAGEMENT WITH EFFECTIVE COMMUNICATION

A. Communication—giving or exchanging information, signals, or messages through facial expression, behavior, talking, gestures, and writing; effective communication is essential in creating an environment conducive to modifying a patient's psychomotor skills, level of knowledge, values, attitudes, and lifestyle
B. Intrapersonal communication—processing a message within oneself; often affected by one's personal life experiences, culture, beliefs, and values
C. Interpersonal communication—messages between two or more people; focuses on the interaction and interpretation of a conversation with nonverbal behaviors and spoken words; effective interpersonal communication may reduce the incidence of miscommunication and patient management problems and increase the patient's commitment to care
   1. Nonverbal behaviors—nonspoken messages, including body orientation, posture, facial expressions, gestures, touch, distance, voice tone, and hesitation in speech
   2. Verbal behaviors—spoken messages, including language, active listening, paraphrasing, and reflective responding
      a. The language used in communication should be carefully selected based on the patient's characteristics and presented in a straightforward and nonthreatening manner
      b. Active listening requires maintaining eye contact and concentration and focusing on what the patient is communicating

   c. Paraphrasing is restatement or summary of what the patient said; provides the opportunity to correct any misunderstandings
   d. Reflective responding addresses the actual feelings of the patient; response is presented in manner that restates, rewords, or reflects what the patient said
D. Enhancement of patient–dental hygienist relationship through confidence and trust requires:
   1. Acceptance—accepting the patient without judgment
   2. Comfort—ability to deal with embarrassing or emotionally painful topics related to an individual's health
   3. Concreteness—communicating in a clear and precise manner with terms understandable to a patient
   4. Empathy—listening and understanding the emotions and feelings of an individual
   5. Genuineness—communicating in an open and honest manner
   6. Respect—ability to convey honor and esteem for an individual
   7. Responsiveness—ability to reply to messages at the very moment they are sent
   8. Self-disclosure—sharing personal experiences with a patient
   9. Warmth—displaying personal feelings and empathy

## EVALUATION

See the sections on "Treatment" and "Periodontal Maintenance" in Chapter 14.

A. Definition—measurement of extent to which patient has achieved specified goals in care plan and determination of success of interventions; ensures that high-quality care has been provided
B. Indicates the achievement of goals or the need for treatment or referral
C. The quality of dental hygiene care is assessed by certain criteria and standards
   1. Criteria—qualities or characteristics by which the knowledge, skill, or oral health status of a patient is measured through descriptions of acceptable levels of performance of patient or dental hygienist (e.g., probing attachment levels are reduced by 1 to 2 mm and no sites with bleeding on probing)
   2. Standards—acceptable and expected levels of performance by the dental hygienist or other health care professionals, established through national consensus[2]
C. Measurement of outcomes of dental hygiene interventions involves collecting evaluation data to determine whether the patient's goals established during the planning phase of care have been met, partially met, or not met
D. *Supervised neglect* occurs when the patient needs further professional care to achieve higher levels of oral wellness or to prevent or control oral disease process, but has been discharged from care under the false assumption that a healthy state was achieved
E. Two forms of evaluation:
   1. Evaluation—occurs continually throughout implementation phase of care; provides the mechanism for modifying the care plan as new assessment criteria become available during treatment (e.g., improved patient self-care, increase in healing response time)
   2. Reevaluation—occurs 4 to 6 weeks after therapy is completed to evaluate response to initial care and to recommend additional therapy as needed (e.g., decrease in probing depths, elimination of bleeding points)
F. Elements of reevaluation appointment include components of the dental hygiene process of care: assessment, diagnosis, planning, and implementation
   1. Assessment
      a. Reassessment of initial assessment data and periodontal status to evaluate improvement, such as effective self-care methods, reduction of 1 to 2 mm in probing measurements, no bleeding on probing, and healthy-appearing gingival tissue
      b. Determination of the presence of residual deposits, newly accumulated deposits, or unresponsive areas indicated by bleeding on probing or gingival inflammation
      c. Reevaluation of the patient's self-care practices
   2. Diagnosis—reevaluation of dental or dental hygiene diagnosis, if indicated, based on assessment data
   3. Planning—care plan developed on the basis of assessment findings; includes, when indicated, modification to self-care practices, localized debridement, chemotherapy, appropriate referrals, and establishment of continued-care schedule or PM therapy
   4. Implementation—provision of self-care education; removal of residual deposits and plaque biofilm–retentive factors; debridement of nonresponsive areas; provision of indicated therapy, and reassessment of continued-care schedule
G. The continued-care (recare) schedule is determined on the basis of individual patient needs, degree of risk for oral disease, and disease progression; patient is informed of the rationale for and the importance of continued care[14]
   1. Continued-care schedules with intervals of 1 to 3 months are recommended to patients who display poor results after therapy, have significant risk factors, have advanced or aggressive disease, have poor self-care, have furcation involvement, or have complicated prostheses
   2. Intervals of 3 months are recommended to patients who complete routine NSPT with uneventful healing and demonstrate moderate to high risk for oral diseases and disease progression
   3. Intervals of 3 to 4 months are recommended to patients who have maintained generally good results for 1 year or longer after therapy but display significant risk factors (e.g., inconsistent or poor oral hygiene, heavy calculus formation, systemic disease or condition, tobacco use, localized pockets, occlusal problems, complicated prostheses, ongoing orthodontic therapy, dental caries activity, localized teeth with less than 50% of alveolar bone support)
   4. Intervals of 6 months to 1 year are recommended to patients who maintain excellent results for 1 year or longer and have been able to eliminate or control risk factors for oral disease (e.g., good oral hygiene, minimal calculus, no occlusal problems, no complicated prosthesis, no remaining pockets, no teeth with less than 50% of alveolar bone remaining, low risk for dental caries)

H. Documenting the outcomes of dental hygiene care aids in preventing possible legal charges related to inadequate documentation and patient feeling inadequately informed about his or her oral health status; should include:
   1. Status and prognosis for the case, sites at risk for disease progression, and sites with disease progression
   2. Sites with plaque biofilm and calculus, bleeding, and areas of inflammation
   3. Need for restorative and periodontal treatment and for referral to a specialist
   4. Discussion that took place with the patient regarding his or her health or disease status
   5. Past commitment of the patient and recommendations suggested by the clinician
   6. Time interval required for the next appointment (continued-care interval)
   7. Acceptance or rejection of any further needed therapy

## DOCUMENTATION

A. Definition—the process of accurately recording all aspects of the process of care, including assessment data, diagnosis, care plan, treatment rendered, patient education, and evaluation findings, for the purpose of establishing the patient's health record
B. Accurate documentation of all assessment findings is the legal responsibility of all clinicians (see Table 15.7)
C. Assessment findings should be clearly recorded and dated using ink on appropriate data collection forms: health history forms, extraoral and intraoral examination forms, dentition and periodontal charting forms, and radiographic interpretation forms
   1. Documentation and monitoring of abnormal lesions must be followed; if after 1 week to 10 days the lesion or abnormality remains, procedures should be implemented to diagnose the condition (e.g., excisional or incisional biopsy, brush biopsy) (see the section on "Diagnostic Tools for Oral Cancer Detection" in Chapter 16)
   2. Active disease or any deviations from normal should be documented and monitored
D. Additional information that was assessed (e.g., risk factors) and discussed with the patient, but not charted, should be recorded on a record-of-services form
E. Diagnostic report documentation includes clearly written statements that connect assessment findings with possible causes that can be prevented, reduced, or resolved by dental hygiene interventions
F. Care-planning documentation, as previously mentioned, should outline all interventions needed to address patient needs, including the estimated number of appointments
G. Implementation documentation is the recording of all treatments and educational interventions administered to the patient, with the appropriate date of service; must include the signature of the provider of care
H. Documentation of evaluation includes the resulting outcomes of the interventions provided as well as any updated information found during the reassessment process; next steps are communicated to the patient and detailed in the patient's permanent record

## ETHICAL, LEGAL, AND SAFETY ISSUES

Provision of comprehensive, quality care by licensed dental hygienists includes legal, ethical, regulatory, and safety issues that require consideration (see Fig. 15.10)

### Ethical, legal, regulatory, and safety issues that place the hygienist at risk

**Ethical issues**

- Failure to refer to a medical professional or other dental specialist when indicated
- Failure to maintain client confidentiality
- Failure to perform a thorough case presentation so that a client can make an informed decision about the dental hygiene care
- Failure to perform comprehensive assessment to detect oral diseases, abnormalities, and degree of client risk for disease or disease progression

**Legal and regulatory issues**

- Failure to comply with the Health Insurance Portability and Accountability Act (HIPAA); the clinician must verify that clients have read the HIPAA policy and obtain a written Acknowledgment of Receipt of the Notice from the client
- Failure to assess, diagnose, treat, or refer for disease; even when under the supervision of a dentist, a licensed dental hygienist is accountable and responsible for client care
- Failure to obtain written informed consent before initiating care
- Failure to provide necessary care on the basis of assessment findings; constitutes "supervised neglect"
- Failure to provide evidence-based care
- Failure to document assessment, care plan, informed consent, services rendered, and client response to care

**Safety issues**

- Failure to protect a client from harm during care
- Failure to assess accurately the client's health and pharmacologic history and to make necessary physician referrals
- Failure to allow time during appointment for the provision of adequate care
- Failure to evaluate therapy after completion of care or to recommend an appropriate continued-care interval
- Failure to follow established protocol that protects the clinician and the client during therapy (e.g., standard precautions; see Chapter 10)
- Failure to use instrumentation in effective and responsible manner (e.g., not using sharp instruments, not selecting appropriate instruments based on conditions present, and causing tissue trauma)
- Failure to follow the manufacturer's instructions in the use of equipment, devices, and dental materials

**Fig. 15.10** Ethical, legal, regulatory, and safety issues that place the hygienist at risk.

## WEBSITE INFORMATION AND RESOURCES

| Source | Website Address | Description |
|---|---|---|
| Medline and PubMed | http://www.ncbi.nlm.nih.gov/pubmed/ | Used for evidence-based decision making |
| National Center for Dental Hygiene Research & Practice | https://dent-web10.usc.edu/dhnet/default.asp?section=1 | Focus for many dental hygiene research-related topics and links |
| National Institutes of Health | http://www.nih.gov | Health topics, funding, news, events |
| American Academy of Periodontology | http://www.perio.org | Association website; parameters of practice and position papers related to the treatment of periodontal diseases |
| National Institute of Dental and Craniofacial Research | http://www.nidcr.nih.gov | Oral health information, educational resources and research |

## CHAPTER 15 REVIEW QUESTIONS

1. The dental hygiene process of care provides a logical system for:
   - **a.** Determining the health and disease of a patient
   - **b.** Selecting appropriate interventions to address patient needs
   - **c.** Measuring treatment outcomes and modifying the treatment plan accordingly
   - **d.** Determining the health and disease of a patient, selecting appropriate interventions, and measuring treatment outcomes
2. The health history form provides information about a patient's health used for establishing medical and dental diagnoses. Completion and review of a patient's health history falls under the assessment phase of the process of care.
   - **a.** Both statements are TRUE
   - **b.** Both statements are FALSE
   - **c.** The first statement is TRUE. The second statement is FALSE
   - **d.** The first statement is FALSE. The second statement is TRUE
3. What blood pressure category is represented by the reading 135/85 mm Hg?
   - **a.** Normal
   - **b.** Elevated
   - **c.** Stage I
   - **d.** Stage II
4. When performing the intraoral assessment, all of the following structures are assessed using palpation techniques along with visual inspection EXCEPT one. Which is the EXCEPTION?
   - **a.** The tongue
   - **b.** The soft palate
   - **c.** The floor of the mouth
   - **d.** The hard palate
5. All of the following relate to proper management of the adult patient with diabetes EXCEPT one. Which is the EXCEPTION?
   - **a.** Requesting A1c levels
   - **b.** Treating the patient with a blood glucose level of 245
   - **c.** Scheduling appointments after the patient has taken medication and eaten
   - **d.** Requesting blood glucose levels
6. Formulating the dental hygiene diagnosis statement involves:
   - **a.** Identification of the condition/problem, contributing factors, and signs/symptoms
   - **b.** Identification of the condition/problem and contributing factors
   - **c.** Identification of the factors contributing to a problem and signs/symptoms
   - **d.** Identification of the signs/symptoms of a condition/problem
7. In patients with a blood pressure reading that is categorized as elevated hypertension, dental hygiene care should not be performed. In patients presenting with a blood pressure reading that is categorized as hypertensive crisis, dental hygiene care should be performed.
   - **a.** Both statements are TRUE
   - **b.** Both statements are FALSE
   - **c.** The first statement is TRUE. The second statement is FALSE
   - **d.** The first statement is FALSE. The second statement is TRUE.
8. Tooth #2 is severely mobile, can be moved in all directions, and can be depressed into the socket. Which mobility class does this represent?
   - **a.** Class 0
   - **b.** Class I
   - **c.** Class II
   - **d.** Class III
9. All of the following are classic symptoms of diabetes EXCEPT one. Which one is the EXCEPTION?
   - **a.** Excessive hunger
   - **b.** Excessive thirst
   - **c.** Excessive urination
   - **d.** Excessive joint pain
10. The comprehensive and systematic collection of data used to identify a patient's needs, oral health status, and general health and well-being defines:
    - **a.** The assessment phase of the dental hygiene process of care
    - **b.** The diagnosis phase of the dental hygiene process of care
    - **c.** The planning phase of the dental hygiene process of care
    - **d.** The implementation phase of the dental hygiene process of care

11. The informed consent form is to be completed and signed before implementation of the care plan. The informed consent form is to be signed by the clinician only.
    a. Both statements are TRUE
    b. Both statements are FALSE
    c. The first statement is TRUE. The second statement is FALSE
    d. The first statement is FALSE. The second statement is TRUE
12. The preliminary phase of dental care planning focuses on which of the following?
    a. Controlling risk factors
    b. Surgical care
    c. Treating periodontal or dental emergency needs
    d. Long-term periodontal maintenance therapy
13. All of the following are included on an informed refusal form EXCEPT one. Which one is the EXCEPTION?
    a. Planned dental hygiene care
    b. The patient's vital signs
    c. Risks involved without treatment
    d. Signature of the patient, dental hygienist, and a witness
14. A risk factor for caries development is:
    a. Optimal fluoride exposure
    b. Frequent exposure to sugary and starchy foods
    c. Adequate salivary flow
    d. Well coalesced pits and fissures
15. Dental hygienists should use current best evidence when providing care. Evidence-based decision making integrates clinical expertise, patient values and circumstances, and best evidence.
    a. Both statements are TRUE
    b. Both statements are FALSE
    c. The first statement is TRUE. The second statement is FALSE
    d. The first statement is FALSE. The second statement is TRUE
16. According to G.V. Black's classification of dental restorations, what type of restoration is an amalgam filling located on the occlusal surface of tooth #15?
    a. Class I
    b. Class II
    c. Class III
    d. Class IV
17. All of the following are elements of an evidence-based question EXCEPT one. Which one is the EXCEPTION?
    a. Patient, or problem
    b. Intervention, cause, or prognosis
    c. Caries risk
    d. Outcome, or outcomes
18. Prediction of duration, course, and termination of disease and response to treatment is defined as:
    a. Diagnosis
    b. Prognosis
    c. Evaluation
    d. Documentation
19. A systematic and comprehensive periodontal examination should be performed on every patient. Performing a systematic and comprehensive periodontal examination allows the clinician to determine the type of periodontal therapy/treatment indicated.
    a. Both statements are TRUE
    b. Both statements are FALSE
    c. The first statement is TRUE. The second statement is FALSE
    d. The first statement is FALSE. The second statement is TRUE
20. Using the American Society of Anesthesiologists (ASA) physical status classification system, what is the classification for a healthy patient with extreme dental anxiety?
    a. ASA P1
    b. ASA P2
    c. ASA P3
    d. ASA P4
21. What phase of the dental hygiene process of care comes immediately before implementation?
    a. Assessment
    b. Diagnosis
    c. Planning
    d. Evaluation
22. Dental hygiene treatment should be postponed when a patient presents with all of the following conditions EXCEPT one. Which one is the EXCEPTION?
    a. Controlled diabetes, an A1c level of 6.5, a blood glucose level of 160 taken one hour after breakfast, and no other medical conditions
    b. An active herpetic lesion
    c. Active tuberculosis
    d. A blood pressure reading of 165/100 mm Hg
23. Presentation of assessment data that includes the dental diagnosis, dental hygiene diagnosis, and proposed care plan is called:
    a. The case presentation
    b. Informed consent
    c. Informed refusal
    d. Documentation
24. Maintenance therapy is a term used for interventions directed at sustaining oral health and controlling disease progression. The application of occlusal sealants is an example of maintenance therapy.
    a. Both statements are TRUE
    b. Both statements are FALSE
    c. The first statement is TRUE. The second statement is FALSE
    d. The first statement is FALSE. The second statement is TRUE
25. The continued-care (recare) schedule is determined by:
    a. Patient preferences
    b. The electronic health record software
    c. Patient needs, degree of risk for oral disease, and disease progression
    d. Degree of risk for oral disease
26. All of the following are components to consider when completing the written care plan EXCEPT one. Which one is the EXCEPTION?
    a. Goals and evaluation measures
    b. The priorities for care established by the patient, dental hygienist, and dentist
    c. Interventions that address the dental hygiene diagnosis

d. Collecting information about the patient's social determinants of health

27. Communicating the care plan to the patient is necessary prior to the implementation phase of the process of care. As long as the care plan is explained to the patient, the dental hygienist can proceed with all preventive and therapeutic procedures identified regardless of the patient accepting the planned care.
   a. Both statements are TRUE
   b. Both statements are FALSE
   c. The first statement is TRUE. The second statement is FALSE
   d. The first statement is FALSE. The second statement is TRUE
28. Antibiotic premedication is indicated for which of the following?
   a. Mitral valve prolapse
   b. History of infective endocarditis
   c. Heart murmur
   d. Rheumatic heart disease
29. The delivery of preventive and therapeutic procedures specified in the care plan to meet a patient's needs defines:
   a. The diagnosis phase of the dental hygiene process of care
   b. The planning phase of the dental hygiene process of care
   c. The implementation phase of the dental hygiene process of care
   d. The evaluation phase of the dental hygiene process of care
30. Dental procedures that require antibiotic premedication are those that involve the manipulation of gingival tissues or the periapical region of teeth, or perforation of the oral mucosa. The extraoral and intraoral examination is an example of a procedure that requires antibiotic premedication.
   a. Both statements are TRUE
   b. Both statements are FALSE
   c. The first statement is TRUE. The second statement is FALSE
   d. The first statement is FALSE. The second statement is TRUE

## CASE A

A 30-year-old female presents for her 6-month recare dental hygiene appointment. The updated health history reveals that the patient is 5 months pregnant.

Her dental records indicate that she has a history of slight generalized marginal inflammation, minimal bleeding on probing, light generalized plaque biofilm, and 1 to 2 mm of gingival recession in the posterior sextants. Existing restorations include amalgams on #18MO and #30O. Slight bone loss localized to the molar regions in addition to a restoration overhang on #18M are evident on the radiographs. Good home care practices were documented.

During the current recare appointment, the patient complains that her "gums" bleed when she brushes. Since being pregnant she has frequently been eating cookies and drinking apple juice. She has only been brushing once a day and has not been flossing because she is tired. During the periodontal assessment, the dental hygienist records moderate generalized gingival inflammation, moderate generalized plaque biofilm and subgingival calculus deposits, generalized bleed on probing, 2 to 4 mm probing depths, and a 5 mm probing depth on the mesiolingual of #18. A protrusive, red, soft, circular, 6 mm mass is found on the labial gingiva between tooth #9 and tooth #10.

*Use Case A to answer questions 31 to 40.*

31. What is the patient's ASA physical status classification?
   a. ASA P1
   b. ASA P2
   c. ASA P3
   d. ASA P4
32. The overhang on tooth #18 allows for accumulation of bacterial plaque biofilm. The harboring of bacterial plaque biofilm around the overhang is most likely the cause of the 5 mm probing depth on mesiolingual of tooth #18.
   a. Both statements are TRUE
   b. Both statements are FALSE
   c. The first statement is TRUE. The second statement is FALSE
   d. The first statement is FALSE. The second statement is TRUE
33. According to G.V. Black's classification of dental restorations, the amalgam on tooth #18 is:
   a. A class I restoration
   b. A class II restoration
   c. A class III restoration
   d. A class IV restoration
34. All of the following are factors that can contribute to the patient's increased gingival inflammation EXCEPT one. Which one is the EXCEPTION?
   a. Pregnancy
   b. Inadequate brushing and flossing
   c. The presence of biofilm
   d. Evidence of radiographic bone loss
35. Which best defines the protrusive, red, soft, circular, 6mm mass found on the labial gingiva between teeth #9 and #10?
   a. Pyogenic granuloma
   b. Verruca vulgaris
   c. Primary herpetic gingivostomatitis
   d. Mucocele
36. Which answer choice best explains the prognosis for the mass found on the labial gingiva between teeth #9 and #10?
   a. The mass may resolve when the hormone levels return to normal
   b. The mass may resolve after using 0.12% chlorhexidine rinse for a week
   c. The mass may resolve after brushing twice a day for two weeks
   d. The mass may resolve after using an interproximal brush for 5 days
37. Reviewing the health history as well as examining the dentition, periodontal conditions, and home care practices of the patient are all components of the assessment phase of the dental hygiene process of care. Interpretation of the data collected during the assessment phase is not needed to develop a dental hygiene diagnosis.
   a. Both statements are TRUE
   b. Both statements are FALSE
   c. The first statement is TRUE. The second statement is FALSE
   d. The first statement is FALSE. The second statement is TRUE

38. All of the following are factors that place the patient at risk for developing caries EXCEPT one. Which one is the EXCEPTION?
    a. Visible plaque biofilm
    b. Having a dental home
    c. Plaque retentive factors
    d. Frequent exposure to sugary foods and beverages
39. The patient inquires about tooth whitening. Tooth whitening is contraindicated because:
    a. The patient has amalgam restorations that will not lighten
    b. The patient has not been flossing
    c. The patient is pregnant
    d. The patient has slight localized bone loss
40. All of the following are patient education topics and home care instructions to be discussed with the patient EXCEPT one. Which one is the EXCEPTION?
    a. The connection between pregnancy and periodontal disease
    b. Dietary risk factors for dental caries
    c. Daily use of an interproximal cleaning aid
    d. Brushing twice a day using the Fones method

## CASE B

**Patient Information**
Age: 55
Sex: M
Height: 5′9″
Weight: 185 lbs

**Medical History**
Patient has a history of myocardial infarction and is under the care of his cardiologist.

**Social History**
Patient is an attorney at an extremely busy law firm; patient has a stressful position.
Patient smokes approximately 5 cigarettes a day.

**Dental History**
History of nonsurgical periodontal therapy. Since nonsurgical periodontal therapy has been completed, the patient visits the office once every 4 months.

**Current Medications**
Plavix 75 mg once daily

**Vital Signs**
Blood pressure: 125/75 mm Hg
Pulse rate: 70 bpm
Respiration: 18 rpm

**Chief Complaints**
Sensitivity to cold on upper left
Discomfort around temporomandibular joint
Food gets caught between last two teeth on lower right

**Oral Assessment**
Bilateral crepitus of TMJ

**Dental and Restorative Assessment**
3rd molars were extracted due to impaction; all other teeth are present
Attrition on posterior teeth
Open contact between teeth #30 and #31
Existing restorations include #31MO and #30DO

**Periodontal Assessment**
Gingival recession of 2 mm on direct buccal surfaces of teeth #12 and #13
Interdental CAL of 1–2 mm
Probing depths 4 mm or less
Radiographic bone loss extending to the coronal third of root on less than 15% of teeth
Mostly horizontal bone loss
No evidence of attachment loss in over 5 years
Light generalized inflammation

**Deposit Present**
Light generalized plaque biofilm

***Use Case B to answer questions 41 to 50.***

41. Smoking is a risk factor for all of the following EXCEPT one. Which one is the EXCEPTION?
    a. Oral cancer
    b. Cardiovascular disease
    c. Periodontal disease
    d. TMJ disorders
42. The patient is taking Plavix to prevent blood clots from forming. Since the patient is taking Plavix, bleeding should be closely monitored while providing dental hygiene care.
    a. Both statements are TRUE
    b. Both statements are FALSE
    c. The first statement is TRUE. The second statement is FALSE
    d. The first statement is FALSE. The second statement is TRUE
43. What is the patient's periodontal classification?
    a. Stage I Grade A
    b. Stage I Grade B
    c. Stage II Grade B
    d. Stage III Grade C
44. Given the blood pressure reading, what does appropriate patient management consist of?
    a. Advise patient of blood pressure status, recommend follow-up with physician and lifestyle management, and recheck at recare visit
    b. Seek medical consultation prior to dental hygiene treatment
    c. Recheck blood pressure in 5 minutes, if reading remains the same continue with noninvasive care only
    d. Recheck blood pressure in 5 minutes, if reading remains the same refer to hospital for immediate evaluation
45. All of the following are interventions included in the dental hygiene care plan EXCEPT one. Which one is the EXCEPTION?
    a. Implementation of tobacco cessation strategies
    b. Application of desensitizing agent
    c. Educate the patient about the benefits of using a night guard
    d. Record probing depths on periodontal chart

46. Which of the following is most likely the cause of sensitivity?
    a. Plaque biofilm
    b. Gingival recession
    c. 4 mm probing depths
    d. The existing restorations
47. The attrition present on the posterior teeth is most likely caused by:
    a. Aggressive toothbrushing habits
    b. Bruxism
    c. Bone loss
    d. Food impaction
48. All of the following are appropriate diagnostic statements for this case EXCEPT one. Which one is the EXCEPTION?
    a. Potential for increased pocket depth related to food accumulation in open contact between teeth #30 and #31.
    b. Potential for root exposure related gingival recession
    c. Sensitivity related to exposed root surfaces
    d. TMJ discomfort related to bruxism
49. Some cardiac conditions call for antibiotic premedication to be taken prior to invasive dental hygiene procedures. The patient in this case needs to take antibiotic premedication because of his history of myocardial infarction.
    a. Both statements are TRUE
    b. Both statements are FALSE
    c. The first statement is TRUE. The second statement is FALSE
    d. The first statement is FALSE. The second statement is TRUE
50. Today's 3-month appointment is best defined as:
    a. Surgical therapy
    b. Periodontal maintenance
    c. Restorative therapy
    d. Preliminary therapy

## REFERENCES


1. Darby ML, Walsh MM, eds. *Dental Hygiene Theory and Practice.* 5th ed. St. Louis: Saunders; 2019.
2. American Dental Hygienists Association. *Standards for Clinical Dental Hygiene Practice.* Chicago: ADHA; 2016.
3. Commission on Dental Accreditation. *Accreditation Standards for Dental Hygiene Education Programs.* Chicago: American Dental Association; 2018.
4. American Dental Hygienists Association. *Policy Manual: ADHA Framework for Theory Development.* Chicago: ADHA; 2018.
5. Darby ML, Walsh MM. Application of the human needs conceptual model to dental hygiene practice. *J Dent Hyg.* 2000;74(3):230–237.
6. American Dental Association. *Intraoral/perioral Piercing and Tongue Splitting*; 2018. https://www.ada.org/en/member-center/oral-health-topics/oral-piercing. Accessed January 27, 2019.
7. Ghallab NA. Diagnostic potential and future directions of biomarkers in gingival crevicular fluid and saliva of periodontal diseases: review of the current evidence. *Arch Oral Biol.* 2018;87:115–124.
8. American Academy of Periodontology. Parameter on systemic conditions affected by periodontal diseases. *J Periodontol.* 2000;71:880–883.
9. Fiore MC, Jaén CR, Baker TB, et al. Treating Tobacco Use and Dependence: 2008 Update. Clinical Practice Guideline. Rockville, MD: US Department of Health and Human Services, Public Health Service; 2008. https://www.ncbi.nlm.nih.gov/books/NBK63952/?report=printable.
10. Bershaw K, Davis C, CAMBRA. From research to practice. *J Calif Dent Hyg Assoc.* 2016;33(2):9–16.
11. Novak KF, Goodman SF, Takei HH. Determination of prognosis. In: Takei HH, Klokkevold PR, Carranza FA, eds. *Newman MG.* 12th ed. Clinical Periodontology; St. Louis: Saunders; 2015:10–14.
12. Bowen DM, Forrest JL. Translating research for evidence-based practice. *Access.* 2017;89:10–14.
13. Franstve-Hawley J, Clarkson JE, Slot DE. Using the best evidence to enhance dental hygiene decision making. *J Dent Hyg.* 2015;89(suppl 1):39–42.
14. Merin RL. Supportive periodontal treatment. In: Takei HH, Klokkevold PR, Carranza FA, eds. *Newman MG.* 12th ed. Clinical Periodontology; St. Louis: Saunders; 2015.
15. Papapanou PN, Sanz M, et al. Periodontitis: consensus report of Workgroup 2 of the 2017 world workshop on the classification of periodontal and peri-implant diseases and conditions. *J Periodontol.* 2018;89(suppl 1):S173–S182.
16. Caton J, Armitage G, Berglundh T, et al. A new classification scheme for periodontal and peri-implant diseases and conditions – Introduction and key changes from the 1999 classification. *J Periodontol.* 2018;89(suppl 1):S1–S8.
17. Tonetti MS, Greenwell H, Kornman KS. Staging and grading of periodontitis: framework and proposal of a new classification and case definition. *J Periodontol.* 2018;89(suppl 1):S159–S172.


## SUGGESTED READINGS


Albandar JM, Susin C, Hughes FJ. Manifestations of systemic diseases and conditions that affect the periodontal attachment apparatus: case definitions and diagnostic considerations. *J Clin Periodontol.* 2018;45(suppl 20):S171–S189.

Beemsterboer PL. *Ethics and Law in Dental Hygiene.* 3rd ed. St. Louis: Elsevier; 2017.

Bronstein D, Suzuki JB. Periodontal disease management. *Dimens Dent Hyg.* 2018;16(7):42–45. https://dimensionsofdentalhygiene.com/article/periodontal-disease-management/.

Dalonges DA, Fried JL. Creating immediacy using verbal and nonverbal methods. *J Dent Hyg.* 2016;90(4):221–225.

Gurenlian JR, Swigart DJ. Dental hygiene diagnosis. *Dimens Dent Hyg.* 2018;16(12):36–39. https://dimensionsofdentalhygiene.com/article/dhdx-dental-hygiene-diagnosis/.

Little JW, Miller C, Rhodus NL. *Dental Management of the Medically Compromised Patient.* 9th ed. St. Louis: Elsevier; 2018.

Malamed SF. *Medical Emergencies in the Dental Office.* 7th ed. St. Louis: Elsevier Mosby; 2015.

16

# Strategies for Oral Health Promotion and Disease Prevention and Control

Michelle C. Arnett

The role of the dental hygienist is oral health promotion and disease prevention. As valued members of the health care team, the application of evidence-based strategies and interventions that support prevention-oriented health care is fundamental to the practice of dental hygiene. The complex relationship between an individual's behaviors, environment, and lifestyle contribute to the prevalence of oral diseases. The success of a preventive oral health program depends on an individual's self-care behaviors. Therefore, a dental hygienist must be knowledgeable in behavior change theories and concepts to support and motivate positive lifestyle behaviors and individual adherence to self-care regimens. This chapter focuses on the dental hygienist's role in health promotion at the individual level.

## PREVENTIVE CARE PLANNING

### Basic Concepts

The discipline of dental hygiene includes concepts of the patient, the environment, health/oral health, and dental hygiene actions, with a perspective that includes a focus on disease prevention and oral health promotion. Scientific evidence informs decision-making within the dental hygiene care process. Person-centered care provides the framework for delivery of dental hygiene treatment and encompasses patient desires, values, family situations, social circumstances and lifestyles; seeing the person as an individual, and working together to develop appropriate solutions.

A. Initiation and progression of oral diseases depend on the interaction of host, agent, and environmental factors. Therefore, prevention and control of oral diseases require attention to all primary and contributing factors in each category.
B. Dental caries and inflammatory periodontal diseases are complex disease states that involve colonization by specific pathogenic bacteria in dental plaque biofilm; thus the control of plaque biofilm is essential in any oral disease prevention program.
C. Effective preventive programs assess disease risk and identify active disease; individuals at high risk for dental caries, periodontal disease, and oral lesions require multiple preventive strategies applied frequently and aggressively (see the sections on "Epidemiology of Periodontal Diseases and Related Risks" in Chapter 14 and "Risk Factor Assessments" and Table 15.6 in Chapter 15).
D. The prevention of oral disease requires the participation of individuals who understand oral disease processes and personal level of risk and adopt effective oral care practices.
E. Patients must possess skills in implementing oral self-care, and the motivation to practice preventive behaviors. Therefore, understanding concepts related to behavioral theory is necessary to support behavior change.

### Human Behavior Principles

A. Values
   1. Values form the basis for behaviors
   2. Individuals come to the dental hygienist with existing values
   3. Conflicts between individuals' existing values and those values that support and enable preventive oral health care practices must be recognized and resolved
   4. Individuals who have value systems that support preventive health behaviors will adopt new behaviors that fit readily into their existing value system
B. Motivation
   1. Definition—a desire to fulfill an unmet human need (deficit); an inner force that causes a person to act; motivation may be internally or externally generated
      a. Intrinsic— motivation focuses on one's own perceived needs; generally longer lasting
      b. Extrinsic— motivation is based on offers of reward or avoid punishment; generally of shorter duration

### Maslow's Hierarchy of Needs

A. Theory about human nature that is used to explain the motivational process; Maslow suggested that inner forces (needs) drive a person to action and classified four levels of human basic needs in a pyramid according to their importance to the individual, his or her ability to motivate themselves, and the importance placed on the needs being satisfied. Only when an individual's lower needs are met will an individual become concerned about higher-level needs; once those needs have been met, they no longer function as motivators (Fig. 16.1).
B. Hierarchy of needs
   1. Physiologic—survival needs are the most powerful and must be met before any others; include the components necessary for body homeostasis, such as food, water, oxygen, sleep, temperature regulation, and sex

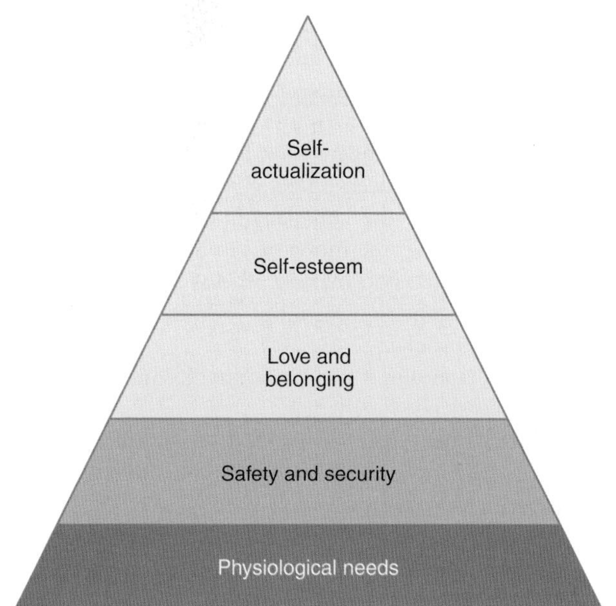


**Fig. 16.1** Maslow's hierarchy of needs. (From Darby ML, Walsh MM. *Dental Hygiene Theory and Practice*. 5th ed. Philadelphia: Saunders; 2019. Modified from Potter PA, Perry AG. *Fundamentals of Nursing*. 9th ed. St. Louis: Mosby; 2017.)

2. Security and safety—these needs are required for protection against physical or psychological damage and are more cognitive than physiologic in nature; include shelter, a job for economic self-sufficiency, and a well-organized and stable environment
3. Social—once physiologic and security needs have been met, the need for love and social belonging become prime motivators, including belonging to a group and having the chance to give and receive friendship and love
4. Esteem or ego—of the two categories of needs that exist at this level, one involves feelings of worth, such as competence, achievement, mastery, and independence; the other involves gaining the esteem of others and triggers learning and the desire to acquire status, power, and higher-level skills
5. Self-actualization or self-realization—these needs drive the individual to reach the very top of his or her field; based on positive actions toward development, growth, and self-enhancement

C. Application—assessment of an individual's level of needs may aid in the identification of motivational factors that can be targeted for enhancing behavior change

## Health Belief Model[3]

A. Based on the concept that one's beliefs direct behavior; the model is used to explain and predict health behaviors and acceptance of health recommendations; the emphasis is on the perceived world of an individual, which may differ from objective reality.

B. Components
1. Susceptibility—individuals must believe that they are susceptible to a particular disease or condition

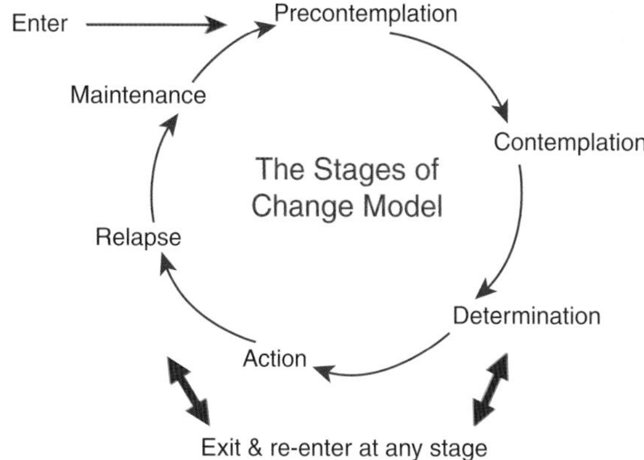


**Fig. 16.2** The Stages of Change Model. (From Gobat N, Bogle V, Lane C. The challenge of behavior change. In: Ramseier CA, Suvan JE. *Health Behavior Change in the Dental Practice*. Ames (IA): Wiley-Blackwell; 2010. 13–34.)

2. Severity—individuals must believe that if they contract the particular disease or condition, the consequences will be serious
3. Asymptomatic nature of disease—individuals must believe that a disease can be present without their being fully aware of it
4. Benefit of behavior change—individuals must believe that effective means of preventing or controlling the potential or current problem exist, and that action on their part will produce positive results

C. Cues to action—once these beliefs have been accepted, the individual will act on them when necessary; the stronger the beliefs, the greater the potential that appropriate action will occur

## Transtheoretical Model[3,4,5]

A. Conceptualizes behavior change through a series of steps; progression through these steps depends on the balance of the advantages and disadvantages of the decision

B. Provides a framework to determine and select appropriate interventions to assist individuals in improving their health behaviors

C. Stages of change (Fig. 16.2):
1. Precontemplation—the individual has not acknowledged there is a problem with a behavior
2. Contemplation—the individual acknowledges there is a problem; unsure if intends to make a change
3. Preparation—the individual is determined to make a change and has taken some behavioral steps in this direction
4. Action—the individual has practiced changed behaviors
5. Maintenance—the individual has maintained the changed behavior
6. Relapse—the individual abandoned the changed behavior

## Psychological Concepts

### Locus of Control

1. Internal locus of control—individuals believe that they have control over their own outcomes and that their behavior will make a difference; they are most likely to adopt preventive health behaviors

2. External locus of control—individuals believe that the outcomes are out of their control and that whatever they do will not affect the outcomes; they are less likely to change behaviors and rely more on the dental professional to take care of their problems

## Motivational Interviewing: Evidenced-Based Approach (Fig. 16.3)[6-9]

A. Motivational interviewing (MI)—is a patient-centered counseling approach to support an individual's intrinsic motivation toward a positive behavior change
   1. Patient-centered counseling supports an individual to become responsible for their own health and enhances development of autonomy for their decisions
   2. Designed to strengthen an individual's motivation for and movement toward a specific goal by eliciting and exploring ambivalence
   3. Allows the provider to demonstrate partnership, acceptance, empathy, and compassion (spirit of MI) to evoke a positive change from within the individual.
   4. Shown to have positive effects on health behavior change related to smoking, exercise and weight reduction, diabetes management, medication adherence, condom use, and oral health

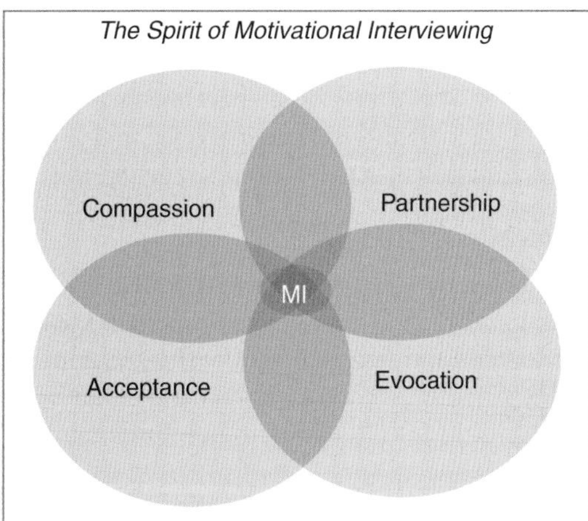


**Fig. 16.3** The Spirit of Motivational Interviewing. (From Miller WR, Rollnick S. Motivational interviewing helping people change. 3rd ed. New York: The Guilford Press; 2013. *Chapter 2, The spirit of motivational interviewing*; p.25-37.)

B. The four principles of MI (empathy, discrepancy, rolling with resistance, and supporting self-efficacy) allow individuals to maintain their autonomy during the behavior change process. Guiding strategies of open-ended questions, affirmations, reflective listening, and summaries (OARS) can assist and support an individual to achieve a behavior change. The dental hygienist may utilize OARS to elicit an individual's desire, ability, reasons, and need for change ("change talk")
   1. Open-ended question—those that cannot be answered with a "yes" or "no" statement
   2. Affirmations—provides encouragement and acknowledgment for the individual's strength
   3. Reflective listening—encompasses the provider listening without judgement to understand the individual's perception and ambivalence
   4. Summaries —utilized to close the MI session and confirm that the clinician understands the individual's perception
   5. Ultimately, the decision to change resides within the individual, not the clinician; in this sense, the dental hygienist allows the individual to have complete autonomy in the decision-making process
      a. Resisting the righting reflex (refraining from trying to fix the problem)
      b. Understanding the individual's motivation and ambivalence for change

C. Brief motivational interviewing (BMI)[10]—is a derivate of MI and is useful for clinicians that have limited time (5–10 minutes) to discuss a positive behavior change with an individual. BMI encompasses the MI principles and guiding strategies to assess the individual's motives, awareness, and support change

## Concepts of Patient-Centered Education

See Table 19.14 for dental management considerations for individuals who have special needs.

A. Effective education involves the facilitation of learning to help make positive changes in an individual's behaviors.
B. To maximize learning, these four principles apply to the design of an educational plan:
   1. Small step size—present only what person can assimilate in one session; provide conceptual or factual information when the "need to know" is evident
   2. Active participation—provide time and opportunity for the person to ask questions; offer suggestions and monitor the practicing of new skills to enhance learning and retention
   3. Immediate feedback—provide the learner with early and frequent information regarding progress; make suggestions for improvement, and use positive reinforcement to support and encourage learning
   4. Self-pacing—recognize that each person will progress at a different pace; recognize the learner's needs, and establish an instructional pace tailored to each individual
C. Visual aids enhance verbal instructions:
   1. Use of visual aids available in print or on the Internet can enhance individual comprehension of oral hygiene instructions
   2. Demonstration of dental plaque biofilm control techniques on models before intraoral demonstration may be helpful
   3. Written instructions and illustrated pamphlets reinforce in-office instructions
   4. Use of an intraoral camera that projects images on a monitor enables individuals to see the conditions in their mouth

## Factors Influencing Individual Adherence to Preventive Regimen

A. Individual–clinician relationship
   1. The quality of communication and the relationship between the individual and the hygienist is critical to achieving individual adherence

2. Individuals must be encouraged to share the responsibility for their oral health
3. Authoritarian or autocratic verbal and nonverbal messages from the dental hygienist will be less effective than messages that allow for genuine individual involvement and assumption of responsibility
4. The dental hygienist must recognize that established behaviors are difficult to change because they generally satisfy needs; new behaviors are adopted slowly

B. Health literacy[11]
1. The ability to comprehend health, medical, dental, and overall health information
2. Individuals who exhibit greater understanding of information provided in the health care setting are more likely to be compliant in home care instructions
3. Low dental health literacy is considered a barrier to good oral health outcomes
4. Clinicians need to explain health related information in an easily understandable vocabulary
5. Screening instruments are available to evaluate an individual's health literacy

C. Individual's support systems
1. Individual's lifestyle and significant others influence the individual's willingness and ability to carry out self-care regimens
2. Support systems are important, especially with children and individuals with disabilities, who must depend on caregivers to carry out home care practices

D. Complexity of therapy
1. Individuals must agree that time and effort required to practice preventive behaviors are reasonable
2. Changes in basic lifestyle are more difficult to achieve than modest modifications to existing behaviors
3. Product cost and availability affect adherence to oral self-care regimens

### Prevention Principles for Children[12]

A. Proactive counseling of parents about anticipated developmental changes in their children
B. Information provided to parents or caregivers in appropriate-sized "bites" on the basis of the developmental milestone anticipated in their children
C. Guidance is based on the rationale that people are ready to apply information that is most relevant to them and their children
D. Box 16.1 provides suggestions for obtaining compliance from pediatric individuals

> **BOX 16.1 Tips for Dental Hygienists Working With Children**
>
> Modified from American Dental Hygienists' Association: Tips for dental hygienists working with kids [members-only section, requires registration and password].
>
> When a child visits your practice, your priority is to create a positive dental experience. The child is more important than his or her teeth. Incorporating the ideas from this fact sheet as you interact with children will help them to become both comfortable and compliant.
>
> - Make the reception area a friendly, colorful place. Include toys, games, and videos. Books about visiting a dental office and a doll dressed as an oral health care provider will help children discuss any fears they may have.
> - Each staff member should greet the child by name in a friendly and welcoming manner. Bend down or squat so that you are at the level of the child's head, and listen to what the child has to say.
> - The treatment room should be decorated in a way that is visually accessible and appealing to children. Show the child the instruments you will be using, and explain how they are used. Make everything that looks unfamiliar look friendly. For example, you might draw friendly faces on masks used for demonstration, and some practitioners like to call the suction "Mr. Thirsty." Demonstrate the buttons on the chair and how it moves up and down, but do not put the chair back if doing so makes the child nervous.
> - Allow the parent into the treatment area if the child desires, especially for the first visit. Both you and the room will look less frightening with a familiar face present.
> - Explain exactly what you are going to do during the appointment. Use age-appropriate terms to explain why it is so important that teeth be kept healthy.
> - Turn the appointment into a game. For example, count eyes, ears, and fingers before moving on to counting teeth. Always give the child a choice of flavors. Write down preferences so that you will have all the child's favorites ready for the next visit. If the light shines in the child's eyes, produce a pair of sunglasses and say how cool he or she looks.
> - Use a new toothbrush presented during the brushing lesson. Apply fluoride varnish. Let the child know that you are in control, with a fast solution to every problem.
> - Praise the good, but don't criticize the bad. A child may take "these teeth don't look so good" very personally and feel he or she has done something wrong. Concentrate on teaching the proper way to take care of teeth.
> - Don't use tricks or lie; keep your promises. If you say, "Just let me do one more thing," do it and let the child go. If a child will not cooperate, try again another day.
> - When the visit is over, let the child pick a treat from a "treasure box." Praise good behavior, and let the child give the parent the "good news" about the child's teeth.
> - Snap a picture of the child's sparkling smile and create a gallery of photos in the office. Seeing his or her own picture is something a child can look forward to at the next appointment.

## DENTAL PLAQUE BIOFILM VISUALIZATION

### General Considerations

A. Dental plaque biofilm is relatively invisible and tooth surfaces are not easily accessed, teaching individuals dental disease–control skills can be challenging
B. Agents that make biofilm visible supragingivally can enhance the teaching–learning process by:
1. Demonstrating a relationship between the presence of plaque biofilm and the clinical signs of disease
2. Guiding the development of skills that are applied before biofilm removal
3. Allowing evaluation of the effectiveness of skills that are applied after biofilm removal
4. Promoting self-evaluation of skills that are applied by the individual at home

C. The presence of subgingival plaque biofilm cannot be demonstrated by using disclosing agents
D. The plan for disease control education should include establishing the associations among the presence of plaque, clinical signs of disease such as bleeding, the presence of risk factors, and possible links to systemic disease

E. Subgingival biofilm detection by the individual is best managed when the individual has an understanding of the gingival sulcus (or pocket) and of the clinical changes that occur with ineffective plaque biofilm removal

### Disclosing Agents

A. Erythrosine (FD&C Red No. 3 or No. 28)
   1. A red dye available in tablet or solution form; most widely used agent
   2. Can be dissolved into a solution or chewed to dissolve in mouth
   3. Tends to stain soft tissues, making post application evaluation of gingiva difficult
B. Fluorescein dye (FD&C Yellow No. 8)
   1. Plaque biofilm stained with sodium fluorescein; visible only with use of an ultraviolet light source
   2. More expensive to use but has the advantage of not interfering with gingival assessment or leaving a visible stain on oral tissues
C. Two-tone dyes (FD&C Red No. 3 and Green No. 3)
   1. Combination solution; has the advantage of differentiating mature plaque biofilm (stains blue) from new plaque biofilm (stains red)
   2. Discloses plaque biofilm but not gingival tissues
D. Precautions
   1. Avoid staining restorative materials that may be susceptible to permanent discoloration
   2. Dispense the solution into a disposable cup; do not contaminate the solution by introducing applicators into the storage container bottle
   3. To avoid staining the lips, apply a light coat of nonpetroleum or water-based lubricant (e.g., K-Y jelly)
   4. Avoid using the agent before application of a dental sealant
   5. Avoid any risk of staining clothing, that is, provide appropriate protective drapes to the individual, and use small amounts of the solution

### Plaque and Gingival Indices

Recording a plaque score at consecutive appointments enables the individual to see progress (see Table 20.13 for information on indices and computing indices).

## MECHANICAL PLAQUE BIOFILM CONTROL ON FACIAL, LINGUAL, AND OCCLUSAL TOOTH SURFACES

### Basic Concepts

A. Microbial population of dental plaque biofilm contributes to the initiation of dental caries and periodontal diseases
B. Mechanical disruption of organized plaque biofilm colonies, both supragingivally and subgingivally, is effective and widely used to prevent and control dental diseases
C. Toothbrushing—most widely used and effective means of controlling plaque biofilm
D. Toothbrushes are available in many shapes, sizes, and textures
E. The selection of the type of toothbrush should be based on the individual's needs, oral characteristics, and preferences
F. Special attention to subgingival plaque biofilm control in areas greater than 3 mm is essential; toothbrushes are generally ineffective in depths greater than 3 mm and in furcations; additional tools must be selected
G. Toothbrushes should be replaced after 2 to 3 months of use and when filaments become bent or splayed
H. Individuals who are immunosuppressed, debilitated, or diagnosed with a known infection and those about to undergo surgery should disinfect their toothbrushes or use disposable ones

### Manual Toothbrushes

A. Description
   1. Parts include the handle, head, and shank; the head, or the working end, holds clusters of bristles (tufts) in a pattern
   2. Design variables
   3. Bristle characteristics:
      a. Handle can be in the same plane with the head or offset at an angle
      b. The length varies, with adult brushes being longer than those recommended for children
      c. Tuft placement can be in two to four rows, with 5 to 12 tufts per row; bristles may be of varying lengths
      d. The brushing planes can be even, flat, or uneven
      e. Many brushes have contoured or thick handles, angled shanks, and flexible heads
      f. Nylon bristles, or filaments, are manufactured for uniformity in texture, shape, and size; nonabsorbent nylon bristles are easily cleaned, dry quickly, and are durable
      g. Relative stiffness—the diameter and length of filaments determine whether the brush will be ranked hard, medium, soft, or extra-soft; variations exist among products from different manufacturers
B. Desirable characteristics of toothbrushes:
   1. Conform to individual requirements in size, shape, and texture
   2. Easily and efficiently manipulated
   3. Readily cleaned and aerated
   4. Impervious to moisture
   5. Durable and inexpensive
   6. Flexible and soft
   7. Contain rounded-end filaments
C. Factors in toothbrush selection and recommendations:
   1. Oral health status
   2. Recommended method of brushing
   3. Periodontal status
   4. Individual's age, dexterity, and ability to use the brush in an effective, nontraumatic manner
   5. Individual's preference and motivation
   6. Unique, special needs of the individual (e.g., arthritis, Parkinson's disease; see Chapter 19)

D. Soft brush head design is important for effective plaque removal and minimal likelihood of trauma to soft and hard tissues
E. Both angled and standard toothbrush designs have little impact on plaque removal capacity; both designs prevent gingival recession as long as soft-bristled toothbrush is used

## Manual Toothbrushing Methods[1]

Although the Bass (sulcular) method is widely recognized as being the most effective and most often recommended, it is helpful to know all the major toothbrushing methods. The method selected should disrupt both supragingival and subgingival plaque biofilm to the extent possible. Although a horizontal scrub technique is often used, it is not recommended because of potential trauma to hard and soft tissues.

In all the following methods, the handle is placed parallel to the occlusal plane for posterior (facial and lingual) and anterior facial surfaces and parallel to the long axis of the tooth (using the toe of the brush) for anterior lingual surfaces. Occlusal surfaces are cleaned with a scrubbing motion.

A. Bass or sulcular brushing method
   1. Technique—direct the bristles into the sulcus at a 45-degree angle to the long axis of the tooth; vibrate the bristles in a short, back-and-forth motion
   2. Indications—plaque biofilm disruption at and under the gingival margin; good gingival stimulation; widely recognized as an effective control technique
B. Stillman's method
   1. Technique—position the bristles on the attached gingiva, and direct them apically at a 45-degree angle to the long axis of the tooth; use firm, gentle vibration, holding the bristles stationary
   2. Indication—gingival stimulation
C. Roll method
   1. Technique—place the sides of the bristles on the attached gingiva and direct them apically; turn the wrist to roll or sweep the bristles over the gingiva and the tooth
   2. Indications—facial and lingual tooth surfaces; often combined with the Bass, Charters', or Stillman's method
D. Charters' method
   1. Technique—position the bristle tips toward the occlusal surfaces at a 45-degree angle to the long axis of the tooth; move the bristles in a short, back-and-forth motion
   2. Indications—cleaning orthodontic appliances, fixed appliances; after periodontal surgery when sulcular brushing must be avoided to allow wound healing
E. Fones (circular) method
   1. Technique—with upper and lower teeth together, place the bristles perpendicular to the buccal tooth surfaces; use a wide circular motion to cover the gingiva and tooth surfaces of both arches; on the lingual surfaces, use smaller circles to brush each arch separately
   2. Indications—when technique must be easy to learn and execute; can be mastered by children
F. Combination methods
   1. Modified-Bass method—combination of Bass and roll methods
   2. Modified-Stillman's method—combination of Stillman's and roll methods

## Power Toothbrushes

A. General description
   1. Brush heads contain bundles of bristles arranged on a variety of brush head shapes; toothbrushes with different brush head shapes are available on the market
   2. The bristles can have flat, bilevel, or multilevel trims; designed for occlusal and smooth surfaces or interdental proximal surface cleaning
   3. The handles are larger than those of manual brushes
   4. Power toothbrushes move in directions and at speeds unattainable by manual toothbrushes
   5. Power toothbrushes have timers to ensure adequate brushing duration and a pressure sensor to monitor the force applied on the toothbrushes
B. Power source—electric rechargeable handle-base; replaceable, rechargeable, and nonreplaceable batteries
C. Motion—distinctly different stroke movement from the motion of manual toothbrushes; motions occur in one of the following directions:
   1. Side-to-side, arcuate, or back-and-forth
   2. Oscillating or rotating
   3. Rotating or counter-rotating
   4. High-frequency pulsating, combined with an oscillating or rotating movement
   5. Sonic vibratory motion from low-frequency acoustic energy
D. Indications for use—recommended for all individuals because of the superiority of power toothbrushes with regard to removing plaque biofilm and reducing gingivitis. Especially valuable to those who:
   1. Lack the manual dexterity, discipline, or motivation to master an effective manual toothbrushing technique, especially children and adolescents who are physically and mentally challenged (recommended to the caregivers who may be doing the toothbrushing for these children and adolescents)
   2. Have orthodontic appliances or implants
   3. Are prone to dental stain
   4. Are aggressive brushers, or exhibit abrasion, erosion, abfraction, or gingival recession
   5. Have periodontal disease or are undergoing periodontal maintenance therapy
E. Power toothbrushes, especially those with oscillating-rotating brushes reduce gingival bleeding and inflammation[13,14]
F. Power toothbrushes reduce plaque biofilm and gingivitis better than the manual toothbrush can, with or without floss[14,15]

## Single-Tufted Brushes

A. Design—flat or tapered
B. Suggested use—to remove plaque biofilm from surfaces not accessible with larger brushes, including areas of crowded

or malpositioned teeth, distal surfaces of terminal molars, around pontics, in furcations, and on lingual surfaces of molars; also used on type II or III embrasure (depending on design) and fixed dental prosthesis[1]

C. Technique—tufts are positioned at or just under the gingival margin, and a sulcular brushing stroke is used; placement of the tapered angled side against teeth allows for the insertion of the bristles several millimeters subgingivally

### Factors in Toothbrushing Effectiveness

A. Sequence
   1. A methodical, systematic approach enhances effectiveness
   2. Suggested sequence—begin systematic, overlapping strokes at the facial aspect of the maxillary right or left terminal tooth; continue around the arch to the terminal tooth on the opposite side; switch to the lingual aspect, and begin working back toward the starting side; use the same pattern for the mandible, and then brush the occlusal surfaces of teeth. Individuals need to be informed to brush the ginigival margin and tongue as well

B. Duration
   1. Monitor the brushing time in an area by counting strokes or seconds after each time the brush is moved
   2. The total manual brushing time of 2 minutes is often recommended; the average brushing time is 1 minute or less

C. Frequency
   1. Thorough removal of plaque biofilm every day is the goal of individual self-care and for maintenance of oral health
   2. Toothbrushing should be performed twice daily; however, the frequency should be increased when gingival or periodontal conditions warrant it or when caries risk is high
   3. Thoroughness in daily brushing is more important than frequency
   4. Emphasis should be placed on effective oral cleaning, not just toothbrushing

D. Skill level
   1. Careful attention should be given to evaluating skill development in all components of toothbrush manipulation, including grasp, placement, activation, wrist movement, and amount of pressure applied
   2. Control of toothbrush placement and motion is essential for effectiveness

### Improper Toothbrushing

A. Need to assess
   1. Improper toothbrushing—may result from lack of education in proper technique, incorrect application following instruction, or long-established habits
   2. The dental hygienist should evaluate the individual's toothbrushing technique and monitor the conditions of hard and soft tissues at each continued-care visit
   3. Faulty placement, overly vigorous motion or pressure, and use of a brush with frayed, splayed, or broken bristles can lead to unwanted consequences

B. Acute consequences—soft tissue injuries such as denuded attached gingiva, lesions that appear "punched out" and red, and clusters of small ulcerations at the gingival margin

C. Chronic consequences
   1. Soft tissue—loss of gingival tissue or change in contour; malpositioned or prominent teeth and an inadequate band of attached gingiva are predisposing factors
   2. Hard tissue—loss of tooth structure and creation of a wedge-shaped defect at the cervical third of tooth (noncarious cervical lesion)

### Toothbrush Maintenance

A. Toothbrushes should be rinsed clean after each use and allowed to air-dry in the upright position

B. Toothbrushes should be replaced when the bristles splay or lose resiliency; generally, they should not be used longer than 2 to 3 months

C. Some toothbrushes have color-indicator bristles to alert the user about replacement time

D. After an acute illness and an oral infection, toothbrushes should be replaced or disinfected with 0.12% chlorhexidine gluconate; power toothbrushes with a built-in sanitizer unit help control toothbrush contamination[1]

## INTERDENTAL PLAQUE BIOFILM CONTROL

### Basic Concepts

A. Toothbrushes—are relatively ineffective on proximal surfaces

B. Interdental cleaning devices—designed for access to interproximal surfaces; essential for effective control of plaque biofilm

C. Interdental col area—protected area that harbors microorganisms that can initiate disease

D. Anatomy of the interdental area—significant factor in both disease initiation and disease control

### Factors to Consider When Selecting Interdental Cleaning Methods

A. The level of oral health or disease, teeth positioning, and condition of the gingiva and attachment should be considered when recommending interdental aids (Fig. 16.5); three types of embrasures:[1]
   1. Type I embrasures are occupied by interdental papillae
   2. Type II embrasures have slight to moderate recession of interdental papillae
   3. Type III embrasures have extensive recession or complete loss of interdental papillae

B. Individual manual dexterity, adherence, skill development, and personal preferences must be considered

### Dental Floss

A. Dental floss—most frequently recommended device for interdental cleaning of type I embrasures[1] (Fig. 16.5)

B. Flossing may precede or follow brushing in a home care regimen

C. As gingival recession increases, as in type II and type III embrasures, the effectiveness of flossing decreases; other interdental plaque control aids should be selected

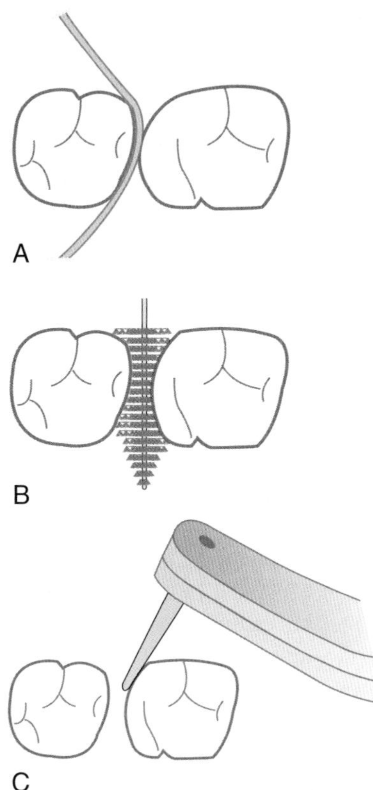


**Fig. 16.4** Use of interdental plaque biofilm control devices. (A) Dental floss. (B) Interdental brush. (C) Toothpick in holder. (From Darby ML, Walsh MM. *Dental Hygiene Theory and Practice.* 5th ed. St. Louis: Saunders; 2019)

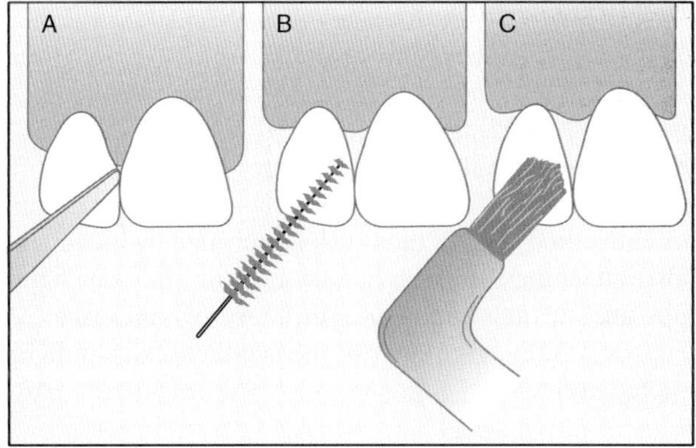


**Fig. 16.5** Interproximal embrasure types and corresponding interdental cleansers. (A) Type I—no gingival recession: dental floss. (B) Type II—moderate papillary recession: interdental brush. (C) Type III—complete loss of papillae: uni-tufted brush. (From Darby ML, Walsh MM. *Dental Hygiene Theory and Practice.* 5th ed. St. Louis: Saunders; 2019. Modified from Newman MG, et al. *Carranza's Clinical Periodontology.* 12th ed. St. Louis: Elsevier; 2015.)

D. Agents to enhance color, taste, and therapeutic value have been incorporated into the dental floss; evidence to confirm the effectiveness of the addition of fluoride and whitening agents is limited
E. Floss type
   1. Unwaxed—unbound filaments are spread on the tooth and have more friction for cleaning; filaments hold plaque and debris for easier removal; the floss slips through contacts more easily
   2. Waxed—resists tearing and shredding on faulty restorations or when moved through very tight contacts
   3. Polytetrafluoroethylene (PTFE) floss—slides through contacts easily; does not fray

## Flossing Technique

A. Floss length—varies with holding technique; 10 to 15 inches when forming a loop; 12 to 24 inches when wrapping around fingers
B. Holding technique
   1. Ends may be tied together to form a loop, wrapped around middle fingers, or tucked into the palm of the hand
   2. With equal tension in both hands, grasp with both thumbs or with the thumb and the forefinger for use on the maxilla or with both forefingers for use on the mandible; leave 1-inch to 2-inch length between fingers
C. Insertion
   1. Approach the embrasure space obliquely, and ease the floss past the contact with a back-and-forth motion
D. Adaptation and stroke
   1. Position fingers such that the floss wraps securely against the proximal surface and forms a "C" shape against the tooth
   2. Slide beneath the gingival margin, and move in an apicocoronal direction several times

## Improper Flossing

A. Acute consequences—snapping through contacts, failure to curve the floss against the proximal surfaces, and application of excessive pressure can result in floss cuts of interdental papillae
B. Chronic consequences
   1. Soft tissue—excessive pressure applied submarginally can be destructive to soft tissue
   2. Hard tissue—repeated heavy sawing movements in a faciolingual direction can abrade proximal tooth structure

## Flossing Aids

A. Types of aids
   1. Floss holders
      a. General description—the floss is threaded through and held on a double-pronged plastic device, forming a span between the prongs
      b. Technique—the prepared holder is positioned for insertion, then adapted and activated in much the same manner as handheld floss; special care should be taken not to snap the floss through the contacts
      c. Indications for use—individual's lack of dexterity to floss properly and individual preference
   2. Floss threaders
      a. General description—firm, flexible, blunt-ended devices for moving the floss through closed contacts or under pontics or orthodontic wires; a variety of designs are available

b. Technique—position the floss in the threader with even lengths on each side; pass the threader through the embrasure from the buccal aspect to the lingual aspect, leaving sufficient length on the buccal aspect; remove the threader and use the floss in the normal manner; slide through the space to remove it

## Interdental Brushes

A. General description
   1. Soft nylon filaments are twisted onto a stainless steel wire to form a tapered or a nontapered small brush; the wire may be plastic coated for use around dental implants and for individual comfort
   2. Interdental brushes must be used with a special handle; some have small handles, and some have contra-angled handles
   3. Interdental brushes provide excellent access to root concavities, furcation areas, and proximal surfaces where papillae do not fill the interdental spaces, as in type II and type III embrasures (see Fig. 16.3)
   4. Interdental brushes come in a variety of sizes, with thin wires and a tapered brush to remove interproximal plaque biofilm from all types of embrasures
B. Technique
   1. Choose a brush of appropriate size, insert interproximally, and use an in-and-out motion from the buccal aspect to the lingual aspect, and vice versa
   2. Brushes may be used in furcation areas in a similar manner
   3. Access into the interproximal pockets may be achieved with careful vertical placement and movement
C. Precautions
   1. Avoid forcing through tight, tissue-filled areas to prevent trauma
   2. Do not aim the wire into tissue
   3. Discard the tip when the filaments lose their original shape
   4. Do not use a brush with a stainless steel wire on an dental implant; the brush must have a plastic-coated wire to prevent damage to the dental implant

### Toothpicks[1]

A. Suggested use—for proximal surfaces and concavities and in exposed furcation areas
B. Technique—round toothpicks can be used alone or inserted into special holders; moisten the tip with saliva, and adapt it to the surface to be cleaned; subgingivally, use a 45-degree angle to the tooth; move the toothpick in and out several times for cleaning the interproximal surfaces, and follow the tooth contour on the facial or lingual surfaces
C. Precautions—rigid pointed tips can cause injury if forced into tight tissue areas; over time, papillae will abrade if toothpicks are used improperly

### Interdental Wedges[1]

A. Suggested use—for cleaning the proximal surfaces or just under the gingival margin; triangular in cross section; should be used interproximally only when adequate space for insertion is available (e.g., type II and III embrasures)
B. Technique—moisten the tip, position the flat base of the triangle at the gingival border, insert with the tip angled slightly toward the occlusal surface, and move the wedge in and out, with moderate pressure against the surface
C. Precautions—discard tip as soon as splaying occurs; repeated insertion with the tip perpendicular to the long axis of the tooth may cause blunting of interdental papillae

### Interdental Tip

A. Suggested uses—for proximal surfaces, in exposed furcations, and under gingival margins; conical or pyramidal, flexible rubber or plastic tip; may be used to maintain interproximal gingival contours or to recontour papillae following periodontal surgery; rubber tips are also used for massaging the gingiva to improve blood circulation, increase keratinization, and provide epithelial thickening[1]
B. Technique
   1. Dental plaque biofilm removal—trace the gingival margin with the tip aimed into the sulcus; move the tip in and out in a buccolingual direction along the proximal tooth surface apical to contact areas
   2. Contouring gingiva—place the tip, without forcing it, into the interdental contour, being careful to follow the gingival form; press the side of the tip against the gingiva, and use a firm rotary motion to apply intermittent pressure
C. Precaution—avoid flattening interdental papillae; use of interdental tips made from rubber should be avoided in individuals with latex sensitivity

## Power Interdental Cleaning Devices

A. Power flossing devices are available to make interdental cleaning easier; include flossers, interdental brushes, dental water jets, and dental air flossers.
B. Technique—usually the unit comes with an attachment (similar to a floss holder, interdental brush, or single-tufted or end-tufted brush); the brush is activated by turning it on after attaching the brush handle; requires only one hand to operate; the tip is aimed into the interproximal space
C. Suggested use—alternative to the handheld floss; individual preference

### Dental Water Jet and Air Flosser[1,15-17]

A. General description—motor-driven pulsating device with a reservoir and specially designed tips to deliver the irrigant to the gingival pocket. Depending on the size of the tip selected, this device has the ability to reach deep periodontal pockets; dental water jets produce a steady stream of fluid; air flosser delivers a combination of air and microdroplets
B. Technique—the reservoir is filled with water or an antimicrobial agent; after inserting the appropriate tip into the handle, the pressure gauge is adjusted to the individual's comfort setting. Starting with posterior teeth, the tip is placed at a 90-degree angle to the long axis of the tooth, following each tooth along the gingival margin
C. Indications for use—individuals with fixed orthodontics, dental implants, crowns, and bridges; those with gingivitis; and persons in periodontal maintenance program

D. Precaution—each manufacturer's product differs; follow each model's instructions for use

## DENTIFRICES

### Basic Concepts

A. Definition—toothpaste used with a toothbrush
B. Purposes
  1. Cosmetic—tooth surfaces are cleaned and polished; breath is freshened
  2. Cosmetic and therapeutic—certain nontherapeutic substances augment the efficiency of brushing in the removal of plaque biofilm, debris, and stain
  3. Therapeutic—vehicle for transporting biologically active ingredients such as fluoride, which inhibits tooth demineralization and promotes remineralization, to the tooth and its environment
C. Basic ingredients[1]
  1. Detergents—lower surface tension to loosen debris and stain; provide foaming characteristic; sodium lauryl sulfate, a common foaming agent, has been implicated in causing aphthous ulcers in susceptible individuals
  2. Cleaning and polishing agents—abrasives that help remove stain, plaque biofilm, and debris from tooth surfaces and give a luster to the tooth surface; should provide maximal cleaning benefit with minimal abrasion; examples include calcium carbonate, silica, calcium pyrophosphate, aluminum oxide, insoluble calcium metaphosphate, magnesium carbonate, and bicarbonate
  3. Humectants—retain moisture to ensure a chemically and physically stable product; for example, glycerin, mannitol, sorbitol, synthetic cellulose, vegetable oils, and propylene glycol
  4. Binding agents—prevent separation by increasing the consistency of a mixture of liquid and solid ingredients; for example, mineral colloids, natural gums, and seaweed colloids
  5. Flavoring and sweetening agents—provide a pleasant and refreshing flavor and aftertaste, and cover unpleasant flavors; for example, peppermint, cinnamon, wintergreen, and noncariogenic artificial sweeteners such as glycerin, sorbitol, menthol, and xylitol
  6. Coloring agents—contribute to the product's attractiveness and desirability; vegetable dyes and titanium dioxide
  7. Preservatives—prevent bacterial growth and prolong shelf life of the product; for example, alcohol, benzoates, and dichlorinated phenols

### Therapeutic and Active Ingredients

A. Definition—biologically active ingredients that produce a beneficial effect on hard or soft tissue; dentifrices claiming therapeutic effects are eligible for acceptance by the American Dental Association (ADA) Council on Scientific Affairs; all products with the ADA Seal of Acceptance are listed at http://www.ada.org
B. Remineralizing agents
  1. Fluoride—substantial data exist to show that approved fluoride dentifrices reduce the incidence of dental caries; fluorides currently used in dentifrices are sodium fluoride (NaF), stannous fluoride ($SnF_2$), $SnF_2$–sodium hexametaphosphate, and sodium monofluorophosphate ($Na_2$-$PO_3F$)[1]
  2. Amorphous calcium phosphate (ACP)—calcium and phosphate were traditionally added to dentifrices as abrasives and lubricants and now for caries control
  3. Xylitol—a sugar alcohol, which has anticaries and antiplaque properties; *Streptococcus mutans* cannot metabolize xylitol, which allows a less acidic environment for tooth demineralization[18]
C. Antimicrobial agents—triclosan is the primary agent used in the United States; its antigingivitis and antiplaque efficacy has been demonstrated
D. Desensitizing agents— desensitization agents work in one of two ways; they either block dentinal tubules (high concentration of fluoride, calcium phosphates, and oxalate salts) or block nerve repolarization (potassium salts, including potassium nitrate and potassium citrate); potassium nitrate is the primary agent used in desensitizing dentifrices[1]
E. Anticalculus agents—function by interfering with the calcium phosphate bond in the calculus matrix; effective only against the formation of supragingival calculus on enamel surfaces
  1. Pyrophosphate system—pyrophosphate has a negative charge, attracts positively charged calcium ions, and interferes with calculus formation
  2. Zinc system—zinc has a positive charge, attracts negatively charged phosphate ions, and interferes with calculus formation
F. Whitening agents—several dentifrices are marketed for their ability to remove or bleach stains; several whitening dentifrices have low abrasive levels; may be effective for the maintenance of cosmetic restorations; whitening agents include papain (Citroxain), silica, hydrogen peroxide, and carbamide peroxide

### Guidelines for Dentifrice Selection

A. Products selected should carry the ADA Seal of Acceptance or the Canadian Dental Association (CDA) Seal of Recognition; this ensures that adequate evidence of safety and efficacy has been demonstrated in controlled clinical trials, that advertising claims comply with ADA and CDA standards for accuracy and truthfulness, and that the therapeutic ingredient will be bioavailable when the dentifrice is used
B. All ADA-accepted and CDA-recognized dentifrices have safe levels of abrasiveness
C. Dentifrices containing fluoride are granted acceptance on the basis of their caries-reducing properties
D. Desensitizing dentifrices that carry ADA and CDA seals have gained acceptance for their proven efficacy in the control of dentinal hypersensitivity

### Guidelines for Dentifrice Use

A. Daily use of fluoride dentifrice should be recommended to all individuals, regardless of caries risk, because these products promote tooth remineralization

B. It is recommended young children should be supervised when using a fluoride dentifrice because children under 6 years of age will most likely swallow the dentifrice. A smear of fluoride dentifrice or the size of a grain of rice is suggested for children 3 years old or younger and a small, pea-sized amount for children 4–6 years old

## CONTROLLING ORAL MALODOR[19]

A. Identifying malodor
   1. Oral malodor (bad breath, or halitosis)— prevalence is 32% of the general population and originates approximately 80%–90% of the time from the mouth/oropharynx region (tongue coating, gingivitis, periodontitis, pharyngitis, and tonsillitis) in addition to systemic causes
   2. Malodors are produced by microorganisms on the tongue and teeth; proteolytic activity results in foul-smelling compounds or volatile sulfur compounds (VSCs)
   3. Oral dryness (xerostomia) exacerbates malodor; smoking, medications, alcohol, and caffeine increase oral dehydration
   4. Bad breath caused by high levels of VSCs is often associated with periodontal infections and overnight denture wearing
   5. Malodor can be measured by sensory or organoleptic (smell) instruments such as gas chromatography (GC) that monitor VCSs (hydrogen sulfide, methyl mercaptan, methyl sulfide)

B. Controlling malodor
   1. Improve oral hygiene by including tongue cleaning in the process
   2. Abstain from tobacco and alcohol use
   3. Avoid caffeine
   4. Stimulate salivary flow by chewing sugarless gum with xylitol
   5. Use ADA-accepted or CDA-recognized antimicrobial mouthrinses
   6. Use saline nasal sprays and humidifiers to control dryness of throat and nasal passages
   7. Use sugar-free (with xylitol) breath sprays, breath fresheners, or drops

## ORAL IRRIGATION

### Basic Concepts

Oral irrigation can be a valuable adjunct to maintaining oral cleanliness and health. Oral irrigating devices force a steady or pulsating stream of water over gingival tissue and teeth, with the goals of removing unattached debris and reducing the concentration of microorganisms and cellular end products that may be present; irrigators also are used to deliver antimicrobial agents supragingivally and subgingivally.

### Home Irrigation

A. Home uses
   1. Before toothbrushing and flossing to remove debris or retained food particles, or after toothbrushing to deliver antimicrobial agents
   2. Debridement of recessed areas of fixed prosthetic or orthodontic appliances; around dental implants
   3. Flushing of periodontal pockets with a controlled, low-intensity, pulsating stream of water

B. Types of irrigators
   1. Hand syringes—blunt tip, side-port cannula; requires high level of dexterity and motivation; not recommended for most individuals
   2. Power-driven device—unit with a water reservoir; plugs into an electrical outlet or battery operated to create a pulsating jet of water; water pressure is regulated by an adjustable dial or sliding switch
   3. Water pressure–driven device—attaches directly to a faucet to deliver a constant stream of water; pressure is controlled by regulating water flow from the faucet
   4. Tips—standard jet tip or flexible subgingival tip; tips with a side-port design or an end-port design show similar effectiveness

C. Use with antimicrobial agents[1,20]
   1. Some studies have documented greater benefits with the addition of antimicrobial agents
   2. Since standard irrigation tips are unable to access periodontal pockets completely, no significant benefits in treating periodontitis is found; demonstrated benefits are limited to parameters such as plaque and bleeding indices, gingivitis, and reduction of bleeding on probing
   3. The use of water alone is as effective as the use of chemotherapeutic agents

D. Precautions—contraindications to use
   1. Individuals should be trained in the proper use of irrigating devices and be monitored for adverse effects
   2. Transient bacteremias may occur following oral irrigation, particularly when untreated disease is present; persons at highest risk for infective endocarditis should not use irrigation as part of their oral self-care
   3. Use of low pressure prevents gingival tissue trauma and allows better access to the base of the pocket

E. Antimicrobial agents
   1. Stannous fluoride—1.64% $SnF_2$; dispense equal parts of 3.28% $SnF_2$ concentrated gel and distilled water; use a fresh mixture for each individual
   2. Chlorhexidine gluconate—0.12% in the United States and 2% in Europe; may be diluted to 0.06% concentration; may become less effective in the presence of sodium laurel sulfate, fluoride, blood, and protein
   3. Essential oils mouthrinse; may be diluted with equal parts water for use in a power irrigator, but most studies use it at full strength

## CARE OF FIXED AND REMOVABLE PROSTHESES

Dental prostheses are replacements for one or more teeth or other oral structures, ranging from a single tooth to a complete denture. Individuals wearing fixed or removable dental prostheses have unique needs that require specific procedures for maintaining the prosthesis as well as retained natural teeth.

## Relevant Terminology[1]

A. Appliance—in dentistry, a general term referring to a device used to provide a functional or therapeutic effect
B. Abutment—tooth, root, or dental implant used for the support and retention of a fixed or removable dental prosthesis
C. Clasp—retains and stabilizes the denture by attaching it to the abutment teeth
D. Denture—artificial substitute for missing natural teeth and adjacent tissues
E. Pontic—artificial tooth on a fixed, partial denture or isolated tooth on a removable, partial denture that replaces lost natural tooth, restores its function, and usually occupies space previously occupied by a natural crown
F. Fixed prosthesis—dental prosthesis firmly attached to natural teeth, roots, or dental implants usually by a cementing agent; cannot be removed by individual
G. Obturator—maxillofacial prosthesis that includes an intraoral structure that replaces all or part of the palate or the maxilla; it may also have a palatal lift that aids in speech or swallowing
H. Overdentures—dentures with retained natural teeth or dental implants
I. Removable prosthesis—dental prosthesis that can readily be placed in the mouth and removed by the individual
J. Orthodontic bracket—a small metal attachment fixed to a band that serves as a means of fastening the archwire to the band
K. Orthodontic band—a thin metal ring that secures orthodontic attachments to a tooth
I. Orthodontic wire—a slender, pliable rod or thread of metal used as a source of force to direct teeth to move in desired directions
M. Implant, or dental implant—a device surgically inserted into the jawbone to be used as a prosthodontic abutment; may be used to support complete dentures
N. Grills ("grillz," fronts)—a decorative, jewel-encrusted encasement for teeth; usually made of precious metals (e.g., gold, platinum)

## Fixed-Prosthesis Maintenance

A. Fixed prostheses such as fixed bridges and orthodontic bands and wires increase the potential for plaque biofilm and debris retention and make access to the proximal surfaces more difficult
B. Home care armamentarium
   1. Floss threaders—allow the floss to move beneath pontics and between pontics and abutments
   2. Interdental brushes—access interdental spaces apical to closed contacts
   3. Special brushes and toothpicks
      a. Orthodontic bilevel toothbrushes—three rows wide, with shorter middle row; moves into and around orthodontic appliances; adapts to areas between the orthodontic appliance and the gingival margin
      b. Two-row brushes—for cleaning of sulci; adapt to narrow areas between brackets and gingivae
      c. Toothpick holders—for cleaning type II embrasures, furcations, and margins of appliances, brackets, and sulci
      d. Single-tuft or end-tuft brushes—for use in type III embrasure areas, furcations, margins of appliances and brackets, and single-teeth abutments
      e. Oral irrigators—flushing action removes loose debris and food material

## Removable-Prosthesis Maintenance

A. Individuals with removable appliances, including orthodontic appliances, must be taught about the importance of conscientious home care
B. Debris, stain, plaque biofilm, and calculus will collect on removable appliances, if the appliances are not cleaned regularly
C. Inadequate cleaning may contribute to the development of soft tissue lesions underlying the appliance or of carious lesions on abutting tooth surfaces; chronic *Candida albicans* infection also may result
D. Removable prostheses can be maintained by:
   1. Brushing with dentifrice after each meal and before retiring to bed at night
   2. Immersion in a solvent that chemically loosens or removes stains and deposits is recommended; the appliance should be brushed after soaking it to remove residual debris and chemicals
   3. Antifungal denture solutions help prevent candidiasis
      a. Special denture brushes have two different arrangements of filaments to access both the inner curved surface and the outer and occlusal surfaces
      b. Special clasp brushes have a narrow, tapered cylindrical design that can adapt to the inner clasp surface, a prime site for plaque biofilm formation and retention
E. Removable appliances should be taken out at night and stored in a covered container with one of the solvents or denture solutions listed above
F. Cleansing procedures
   1. Hold the appliance securely to avoid dropping and/or breaking
   2. When brushing, hold the appliance over a sink partly filled with water or lined with a cushioning material
   3. Avoid overzealous brushing and use of strong abrasives; the plastic resin material can be scratched or abraded to the extent of compromising denture fit
   4. If any denture adhesive material is used, it should be removed from the appliance and the underlying mucosa several times a day
   5. Brush the underlying mucosa at least once daily with a soft toothbrush
   6. Solutions used for cleansing or soaking a denture should be renewed for each use
G. All removable appliances and prostheses, including fluoride carriers, night guards, mouthguards, and bleaching trays should be cleaned on a regular basis and appropriately stored after use[1]

### Dental Implant Maintenance

See the sections on "Dental Implants" in Chapters 13 and 14 and "Instrumentation of Dental Implants" in Chapter 17.

A. Osteo-integrated implants and superstructures require special home maintenance, products, and techniques; individuals must learn the techniques for plaque biofilm control that prevent peri-implant diseases, damage to the implant material, and superstructure
B. The home care armamentarium may include:
   1. Soft-bristled, multitufted nylon toothbrushes
   2. Interdental brushes with nylon coating over metal wire cores; coating prevents scratching of the implant material (usually titanium)
   3. Flat and tapered end-tuft brushes
   4. Dental floss
   5. Implant flossing aids—braided nylon filaments with a hook leader for insertion is recommended; flat cotton floss; or floss containing a soft filament brush component
   6. Rubber tip stimulator; wood sticks
   7. Disclosing tablets or liquid; may be most useful during initial education on plaque biofilm control
   8. Antimicrobial mouthrinse; chlorhexidine used twice daily is the rinse of choice after treatment; other antimicrobial mouthrinses may be used for long-term treatment
   9. Small amount of ADA-approved or CDA-recognized gel or fine-abrasive, fluoridated toothpaste; abrasive toothpastes must be avoided; anticalculus formulas are acceptable
   10. Oral irrigators may be used on the lowest setting, with the tip directed perpendicular to the long axis of the tooth or implant; water, chlorhexidine 0.12%, phenol-based, or plant alkaloid mouthrinses may be used
C. Skill development in plaque biofilm control
   1. Individuals must be shown how to control plaque biofilm on all areas of the implant and the superstructure
   2. Sufficient supervised practice will ensure adequate skill development
   3. Plaque biofilm control must be monitored at each continued-care appointment and techniques modified, as indicated
   4. Research indicates poor plaque control, prior history of periodontal disease, and tobacco use increases dental implant failure[21,22]

## CARIES MANAGEMENT

### Caries Management by Risk Assessment[23]

Caries management by risk assessment (CAMBRA) is an evidence-based approach to the prevention or treatment of dental caries in the earliest stages. The dental hygienist identifies an individual's level of risk by determining the balance between pathologic and protective risk factors. Once the clinician identifies an individual's caries risk (low, moderate, high, or extreme), a therapeutic and/or preventive plan is implemented (see Table 15.5 in Chapter 15).

A. Caries disease indicators—uses acronym WREC to describe:
   1. White spots lesions
   2. Restorations placed within the past 3 years as a result of caries
   3. Enamel proximal lesions
   4. Cavitation of carious lesions penetrating into dentin
B. Pathologic factors
   1. Medium or high level of streptococci and lactobacilli counts
   2. Presence of heavy biofilm on teeth
   3. Frequent snacking between meals
   4. Deep pits and fissures
   5. Recreational drug use
   6. Inadequate salivary flow caused by medication, radiation, or systemic diseases
   7. Exposed roots
   8. Orthodontic appliance
C. Protective factors—biologic or therapeutic factors related to the individual's practice of oral hygiene that can counterbalance the challenge presented by caries risk factors
   1. Drinks fluoridated water on a regular basis
   2. Uses a fluoride toothpaste once or more daily
   3. Uses fluoride-containing mouthrinse daily
   4. Has had fluoride varnish applied in the past 6 months
   5. Has received an in-office topical fluoride treatment in the past 6 months
   6. Has used prescription chlorhexidine daily for 1 week in each of the past 6 months
   7. Has used xylitol gum or lozenges four to five times daily in the past 6 months
   8. Has used calcium and phosphate supplement during the past 6 month
   9. Has adequate salivary flow

## ADJUNCT CARIES DETECTION DEVICES[24,25]

### DIAGNOdent

A. Definition —A caries assessment device with a probe tip that emits laser fluorescence light to be used as an adjunct to radiographs for pits and fissures and interproximal caries
   1. This device uses infra-red signals to display a scale value to indicate caries; healthy enamel will have no to little florescence and a scale reading of 0–14; scale readings of 15–30 may indicate monitoring or operative treatment; potential caries will emit fluorescence and appear as a high scale reading >30
B. Procedure
   1. Requires calibration of placing the probe tip on a calibration disc; a two digit number and audible tone will confirm calibration was successful; calibration needs to be checked frequently
   2. Portable handpiece needs to be disinfected before use and the probe tip needs to be sterilized

### DEXIS CarieVu

A. Definition—A nonionizing caries assessment device that uses near-infrared transillumination technology to support radiographs for occlusal, interproximal, and recurrent caries

1. This tool can be used as an adjunct to radiographs to confirm diagnosis of caries; near-infrared transillumination appears transparent on healthy enamel surfaces and dark in areas with potential caries due to the absorption of light
2. Beneficial for individuals that radiographs are contraindicated (pregnant women or children); individuals who cannot have radiographs due to behavioral, mental, or refusal of radiographs; useful for high caries risk individuals or monitoring of incipient lesion more frequently compared to traditional radiographs

B. Procedure
1. Handpiece with a removal insert tip; removable insert tip has two rubber sides that hug the buccal and lingual surface of the teeth; the insert tip covers the teeth and part of the gingiva
2. The oral health care provider slowly glides the handpiece over the occlusal surface; the near-infrared transillumination light passes through the enamel and is viewable on a computer monitor; images can be viewed as a live video or capture a still image by pressing the button on the side of the handpiece
3. Portable handpiece needs to be disinfected before use and the removal insert needs to be sterilized
4. Studies indicate the DEXIS CarieVu may be utilized as an adjunct tool to radiographs for interproximal caries diagnosis for caries

## Other Caries Adjunct Devices

A. Other adjunct caries devices include Aire Techniques CamX, ACTEON SoproCARE Caries, and SPECTRA (Air Techniques)

B. Radiographs are still the "gold standard" for caries diagnosis

## Fluorides[26,27]

See the section on "Topical Fluorides and Fluoride Varnishes" in Chapter 13 and "Preventing and Controlling Oral Diseases and Conditions" in Chapter 20.

### General Considerations

A. Most effective agent for the prevention and control of dental caries, especially on smooth surfaces

B. A multitherapeutic approach is most effective; three categories of administration:
1. Systemic—community water supplies, institutional water supplies, and dietary supplementation
2. Professional application—gels and varnishes
3. Self-applied—dentifrices, rinses, and gels

C. Safe when used in recommended amounts and concentrations; dental hygienists must be alert to the potential for acute and chronic adverse effects
1. Large quantities of fluoride products should not be stored in the home
2. Institutions that have fluoride programs must handle and store fluoride products safely
3. Parents and caregivers must be educated about supervising home use of products containing fluoride by young children to prevent acute toxic reactions or long-term effects (e.g., dental fluorosis)
4. Products intended for topical application should not be swallowed
5. If excessive amounts have been ingested, vomiting should be induced immediately with ipecac or manually; calcium solution or milk should be administered to slow the absorption rate; emergency medical care should be obtained (see the section on "Drug-Related Emergencies and Poisoning" in Chapter 21)
6. Fluoride therapy is based on the individual's risk assessment

### Ingested Fluorides

A. Drinking optimally fluoridated water (0.7 ppm), especially during tooth formation and professional application of a topical fluoride provides a significant decrease in the overall percentage of dental caries in both children and adults

B. Maximum benefits are obtained when fluoride is provided from the onset of tooth development until tooth eruption is complete and then fluoridated water is used continuously for drinking

C. Fluoride works primarily and most effectively via topical (surface) mechanisms (whether delivered in the drinking water, foods, beverages, or products) to inhibit demineralization, enhance remineralization, and inhibit plaque bacteria

D. The dental hygienist has a key role in educating parents, caregivers, and children about the value of fluoride and its preventive benefits.

### Fluoride Agents for Professional Application

A. Neutral sodium fluoride (NaF)
1. Characteristics—first fluoride used for topical application; available in 2% concentration foam or gel and 5% concentration varnish
2. Advantages—safe for use in dentition with porcelain crowns and composite restorations; varnish is easily applied on the teeth of young children; research highly supports the efficacy of fluoride varnish for caries prevention compared with other professional fluoride methods
   a. Applications of 2% NaF at 6-month intervals; 4-minute application
   b. Fluoride varnish—contains a 5% NaF concentration, approved by the US Food and Drug Administration (FDA) for use as a desensitizing agent and cavity liner; the varnish is used as a topical fluoride treatment; painted on teeth; the varnish is retained on the tooth surface for 3 to 4 hours

B. Acidulated phosphate fluoride (APF)
1. Characteristics—available as foam, gels, and thixotropic gels; 1.23% NaF with 1 molar (M) orthophosphoric acid concentration
2. Application intervals—every 6 months, or more frequently when caries risk is high; 4-minute application
3. Advantages—high level of individual acceptance; nonirritating to soft tissues; does not discolor tooth structure;

highest documented efficacy; most common in-office treatment; 1-minute application not supported by the research literature
4. Disadvantages and precautions—low pH of 3.5 for enhanced fluoride uptake may cause etching of dental sealants and porcelain and some composite restorations; sealants, porcelains, and composites should be protected with a water-based lubricant, or use NaF as an alternative

C. Silver Diamine Fluoride (SDF)[28,29]
1. Characteristics—a liquid containing silver particles and 38% fluoride ion; utilized outside of the United States; FDA approved in 2014 as a desensitizing agent; ongoing clinical trials for caries arrest; used off-label in United States for caries arrest
2. Indications—individuals unable to access or tolerate dental care; early childhood caries, challenging carious lesions for treatment due to behavioral or medical conditions, disability, and/or age of the individual; (children, special needs, and/or the elderly/frail populations)
3. Application—apply to active, asymptomatic caries lesions; isolate tooth from adjacent teeth; apply petroleum jelly to lips and surrounding skin to prevent staining; dry carious lesion; apply liquid 38% SDF with micro brush for 2–3 minutes and wait 1 minute
4. Advantages—arrests caries; prevents progression of carious lesion
5. Disadvantages—esthetic concern because caries turns dark/black in color

## Indications for Professional Application

A. Topical fluoride therapy is an accepted part of the prevention-oriented care plan

B. Assessment of individual's risk for dental caries will determine an individual's fluoride therapy plan

C. Therapy regimen may include both professionally applied (varnish) and self-applied agents

D. Inclusion of topical fluoride in individual's care plan should be based on the following criteria:
1. For children and adults at moderate, high, or highest risk for dental caries—fluoride varnish or fluoride gel is the treatment of choice at continued-care intervals
2. Less than optimally fluoridated drinking water available
3. Fair or poor oral hygiene
4. Decalcification, white spots, or incipient lesions are present; secondary or recurrent caries; active caries
5. Following root instrumentation, dentin can be exposed and dentinal tubules opened; hypersensitive root surfaces that often result can be controlled by fluoride application
6. Fluoride application reduces incidence of root caries and dentinal hypersensitivity associated with exposed root surfaces resulting from gingival recession
7. Irregular professional dental visits
8. Inappropriate dietary practices (e.g., frequent sugar intake)
9. When xerostomia is present as a result of irradiation to the head and neck, certain medications, or salivary gland dysfunction, caries destruction occurs rapidly and is generalized when salivary production is minimal. Multiple fluoride treatments are used to control high risk for dental caries associated with xerostomia
10. Individuals wearing orthodontic, prosthodontic, or any other oral appliances

## Application Principles—General Guidelines for Individual Preparation

A. Explain the indication(s), the steps involved, and the time required for the procedure, the need to control salivary flow and to avoid ingestion, and post application instructions

B. Position the individual to facilitate salivary control and reduce potential for gagging

C. Calculus, extrinsic stains, materia alba, and heavy plaque biofilm should be removed before the application of fluoride

## Application Methods

### *Tray Systems*

A. Designed for use with fluoride gels; trays cover all teeth in an arch, come in a variety of materials, shapes, and sizes; tray systems are not appropriate for solutions because they cannot be adequately retained within tray boundaries

B. Tray examples—most frequently used
1. Disposable polystyrene (Styrofoam)—used for professional fluoride application; ADA and CDA do *not* recommend the use of fluoride foam because of lack of sufficient scientific evidence for its efficacy in caries prevention; ADA and CDA recommend only 4-minute fluoride gel application
2. Custom-fitted polyvinyl—used by the individual for self-application of fluoride gel; provides excellent coverage; must be remade as the dentition matures; relatively expensive

### *Self-Applied Fluorides*

A. Frequent, low doses of fluoride exposure to tooth surfaces are important for enamel remineralization and prevention of demineralization

B. Rinses—available by prescription, except as noted
1. Daily use—low potency, high frequency
2. Weekly use—high potency, low frequency
3. Many commercially prepared fluoride rinses contain alcohol and should *not* be recommended for persons with a history of alcoholism or xerostomia; use alcohol-free rinses with children and individuals who need to avoid exposure to alcohol
4. Fluoride rinses are not recommended for children under 6 years old; swallowing small doses of fluoride over a period may lead to dental fluorosis
   a. 0.044% APF rinse supplement
   b. 0.05% NaF (available over the counter [OTC])
   c. 0.1% $SnF_2$ rinse (0.63% plus water)
   d. 0.2% NaF
   e. Most common concentration used for school-based fluoride rinse programs

C. Gels—available OTC and by prescription
1. 0.4% $SnF_2$ (brush-on or tray application)

2. 1.1% NaF (brush-on or tray application, also available in paste)
3. 0.05% APF (tray application)

D. Some studies indicate that $SnF_2$ may have antiplaque, antihypersensitivity, and anticaries effects

### *Amorphous Calcium Phosphate*[30]

A. ACP contains the same minerals as the hydroxyapatite crystals of tooth enamel
B. Casein phosphopeptide–amorphous calcium phosphate (CPP-ACP), a milk protein peptide, is usually added to stabilize and localize the calcium and phosphate ions on the tooth surface, promoting remineralization of enamel
C. Products that contain ACP should *not* be substituted for fluoride therapy; ACP should be used in conjunction with fluoride to enhance fluoride uptake
D. Several professionally applied and OTC self-applied products, including dentifrices, tooth-whitening agents, prophylaxis paste, and fluoride varnish, contain ACP

### *Xylitol for Dental Caries Prevention*[18,31]

A. Xylitol is a noncariogenic sugar alcohol; *Streptococcus mutans* cannot metabolize xylitol, which causes a decrease in *S. mutans* infections
B. Xylitol inhibits the attachment and transmission of *S. mutans,* reduces plaque biofilm formation, and stimulates salivary secretion.
C. Research on the effectiveness of xylitol in preventing dental caries is inconclusive.
D. Xylitol-containing salivary stimulants can be beneficial for people with xerostomia and diabetes
E. Several products contain xylitol (e.g., chewing gum, lozenges, mints); when used for therapeutic purposes, products must contain 1.55 g of xylitol and must be used at least four or five times daily.

### *Mouthrinses or Chemotherapeutics*[20,32]

A. May have cosmetic and therapeutic value
B. Effectiveness of many mouthrinses is limited to dislodging gross debris, temporarily reducing microorganisms, and providing a feeling of freshness.
C. One category of commercial mouthrinses is approved by the ADA Council on Scientific Affairs: phenol-related essential oils compounds gained acceptance for control of both plaque biofilm and gingivitis and carry the ADA Seal of Acceptance
   1. Chlorhexidine gluconate (Peridex, PerioGard, Pro Dentx, PerioRx)
      a. Available by prescription only
      b. 0.12% concentration in an aqueous solution containing 11.6% alcohol, pH 5.5; also made without alcohol for persons who cannot use alcohol (ask the pharmacist)
      c. Clinical effects are comparable with 0.2% mouthrinse used for many years outside the United States; extensive clinical research has documented its efficacy
      d. Review of numerous studies has established chlorhexidine's safety, stability, and substantivity, which make it effective in preventing and controlling plaque biofilm and reducing and inhibiting gingivitis
      e. May cause brownish yellow stain and supragingival calculus
      f. Unpleasant taste may hinder individual acceptance
      g. Recommended for short-term use only; one 2-ounce, 30-second rinse, twice daily for 6 months
   2. Phenol-related essential oils (Listerine and many equivalent generic store brands)
      a. Available in alcohol-free formulation
      b. Available without a prescription
      c. Contains thymol, menthol, eucalyptol, and methyl salicylate in a hydroalcohol solution, 21.6% to 26.9% alcohol, pH 5.0
      d. Low substantivity
      e. Listerine's efficacy in inhibiting bacterial plaque biofilm and gingivitis has been documented
      f. Various flavors available to enhance individual acceptance and adherence to manufacturer's recommendation for a 30-second rinse twice daily
      g. Essential oils mouthrinses, using basically the same formula as Listerine, are marketed under many store brand names and are also accepted by the ADA Council on Scientific Affairs as having antiplaque and antigingivitis effects
      h. Can be used as preprocedural mouthrinses before aerosol-producing procedures; or as a preprocedural subgingival irrigant
      i. Anticalculus formulation of Listerine containing zinc chloride; inhibits supragingival calculus accumulation; has the ADA Seal of Acceptance
      j. Available in alcohol-free formulation

D. Mouthrinses are recommended as adjuncts to, not replacements for, mechanical plaque biofilm control.
E. Effective on supragingival biofilm only, unless delivered subgingivally with irrigators
F. Approved mouthrinses should be considered for individuals with the following conditions:
   1. Inability to achieve acceptable mechanical plaque biofilm control
   2. Fixed splinting, prostheses, dental implants, and overdentures
   3. Orthodontic appliances
   4. Post periodontal or other oral surgery
   5. Individuals at high risk for dental caries
   6. Medication-induced gingival enlargement
   7. Immunosuppression
   8. Preprocedural application to minimize bacteremia and disease transmission

G. Commercially prepared mouthrinses may contain alcohol or may be alcohol free; other ingredients are water, flavoring, coloring, sweetening agents, and a variety of active ingredients such as:
   1. Antimicrobials to reduce or inhibit biofilm activity (cetylpyridinium chloride, chlorhexidine, sanguinarine, phenolic compounds, triclosan)
   2. Oxygenating agents to debride and release oxygen (hydrogen peroxide)
   3. Astringents to shrink tissue (citric acid, zinc chloride)

4. Anodynes to alleviate pain
5. Buffering agents to reduce acidity, dissolve mucinous films, and relieve soft tissue pain
6. Deodorizing (sodium bicarbonate) and oxidizing (chlorine dioxide) agents to neutralize odors and eliminate VSCs
7. Fluorides to decrease dental caries risk (see the previous section on "Self-Applied Fluorides")
8. Whitening agent such as hydrogen peroxide to reduce intrinsic stains

H. Inexpensive mouthrinses may be prepared by the individual (not recommended for individuals on a low-salt or sodium-free diet) and used following thorough periodontal debridement
   1. Isotonic (normal) saline solution: 1/2 teaspoon salt in 8 ounces of water
   2. Hypertonic saline solution: 1/2 tsp salt in 4 oz water
   3. Sodium bicarbonate solution: 1/2 tsp sodium bicarbonate (baking soda) in 8 oz warm water

I. Mouthrinse use should be monitored by both the individual and the dental hygienist; any adverse effects indicate that use should be evaluated and possibly discontinued

J. The dental hygienist should teach individuals how to be wise consumers of mouthrinses, helping individuals to recognize the benefits, limitations, and appropriate therapeutic regimens for mouthrinses

## DENTAL SEALANTS

### General Considerations

See the section on "Pit-and-Fissure Sealants" in Chapter 13.

A. Pit-and-fissure surfaces of the tooth compared to smooth surfaces do not have the same benefit from systemic and topical fluoride

B. Sealants are a thin resin or glass ionomer coating placed in the pits and fissures of teeth to act as a physical barrier to oral bacteria
   1. Preventive sealant—placed in caries-free pits and fissures
   2. Therapeutic sealant—placed in pits and fissures with incipient carious lesions to halt caries process

C. Pits and fissures allow for the accumulation and stagnation of fermentable substrates and serve as accumulation sites for acidogenic microorganisms capable of demineralizing tooth tissue

D. The effectiveness of dental sealants in the prevention of pit-and-fissure caries has been clearly demonstrated in research settings

E. Protection from caries approaches 100% when pits and fissures remain completely sealed; numerous clinical trials have documented the efficacy of sealants

F. Comprehensive prevention programs incorporate the complementary use of sealants and fluorides

G. Sealants classified by method of polymerization
   1. Auto-polymerizing—chemically cured or self-curing
   2. Photo-polymerizing—cured by visible light

H. Sealants classified by filler content
   1. Filled sealant—composite resin sealant containing particles of glass and quartz
   2. Unfilled sealants—composite resin sealant without particles; less resistant to long-term wear
   3. Glass ionomer—salivary control not a critical factor; ideal for teeth when moisture control is an issue
   4. Fluoride releasing—promotes remineralization
   5. Calcium phosphate—promotes remineralization

I. Sealants classified by color—available in clear, tinted, and opaque color; the color aids in detection and in monitoring retention

### Indications for Application

A. Factors to consider:
   1. Dental caries activity, risk, and pattern
   2. Depth of pits and fissures
   3. Dietary patterns
   4. Current and past fluoride exposure
   5. Eruption status
   6. Frequency of preventive services
   7. Individuals or guardians should be informed about sealants as a primary preventive measure

B. Benefits of sealant placement[1]
   1. Individuals who can benefit from sealant application:
      a. Children with newly erupted teeth with pits and fissures; adults with deep pits and fissures
      b. Persons whose lifestyle, behavior patterns, physical or emotional development, or lack of fluoride exposure put them at high risk for dental caries
      c. People with xerostomia or persons with orthodontic appliances
      d. Other persons who desire sealants as a preventive measure to protect pits and fissures
      e. Teeth with noncavitated lesions should be sealed.[33]

### Contraindications to Sealant Application

A. Presence of frank carious lesion on occlusal surface
B. Presence of carious lesion on proximal surface that necessitates preparation of occlusal surface
C. Previously restored tooth
D. Life expectancy of the primary tooth predicted to be short

### Application Guidelines[1]

A. Read the manufactures instructions and follow the guidelines for sealant placement

B. Mechanical cleansing of enamel
   1. Debride the pit-and-fissure surface of plaque biofilm and surface debris
   2. Cleansing agents include:
      a. Toothbrush
      b. Air polishing, rubber cup polishing
      c. Dental explorer

C. Isolating
   1. Salivary contamination of etched enamel surfaces is a major reason for resin sealant failure
   2. Isolation—using a rubber dam or cotton rolls and bibulous (absorbent) pads is essential for consistent success

D. Drying
 1. Dry isolated tooth thoroughly in preparation for the application of conditioner or etchant
 2. Avoid water contamination if using air/water syringe
E. Conditioning or etching
 1. Acid conditioning etches enamel surface before the application of resin or glass ionomer (sealant) material; etching removes a layer of enamel and increases the total surface area by rendering the deeper enamel regions porous; the sealant's resin material fills the enamel micropores, producing a mechanical "lock" when polymerized
 2. Acid conditioning agents (30% to 50% phosphoric acid)—available in solution or gel form
  a. Apply the solution by gently dabbing the enamel surface with a saturated cotton pellet or brush; avoid rubbing the surface because it causes a breakdown of lattice-like micropores
  b. Gels are applied with a special applicator, brush, cotton tip, or cotton pellet
  c. Whether using gel or solution, cover all susceptible surfaces and cuspal inclines with the etchant
  d. Contact between the etching agent and soft tissues should be avoided
  e. Etch the tooth surface for 10 to 20 seconds; check the manufacturer's instructions for etching time
F. Rinsing the conditioned tooth
 1. Thoroughly rinse the etched enamel surfaces by using a water syringe and a high-speed evacuation system; do not allow the individual to swish; rinsing time may need to be increased to ensure complete removal
 2. Salivary contamination at this point results in substantial reduction in resin sealant bond strength
  a. Do not allow individual to close the mouth, rinse, or touch the conditioned surface with the tongue
  b. When using cotton rolls or bibulous (absorbent) pads, change them as needed, being careful to avoid salivary contamination
G. Drying the conditioned tooth
 1. Prepare the tooth for resin sealant application by drying it thoroughly with compressed air for at least 10 seconds; a completely dry tooth surface is essential for effective application of the resin sealant; it is not as critical when using glass ionomer sealants
 2. Examine the conditioned surface; properly etched surfaces will appear dull and chalky; reetch the tooth surface when these changes are not seen or salivary contamination occurs
H. Applying the sealant material—all susceptible pits and fissures, including the buccal pits of mandibular molars and the lingual grooves of maxillary molars, should be sealed, when possible
 1. Visible light-cured sealants—the resin sealant is applied to the etched surface; the tip of the light source is placed 2 mm from the sealant (see the manufacturer's instructions)
 2. Chemical or self-curing sealants—the catalyst and the sealant are mixed and then placed immediately onto the prepared tooth surface with a brush or a custom dispenser; working time from mixing to setting is 1 to 3 minutes; it is important not to disturb the layer of applied sealant during polymerization
 3. The sealant material should be allowed to flow into all areas to minimize entrapment of air bubbles
 4. Applying excess sealant to the occlusal surface should be avoided because this could alter the individual's occlusion
  a. Light must be delivered for polymerization to occur and for the prevention of sealant failure
  b. Once polymerization is complete, the sealant should be wiped with a wet cotton roll or pellet to remove any air-inhibited layer of nonpolymerized resin; failure to remove this layer will result in an unpleasant taste
  c. The sealant material is delivered in a variety of ways; unit dose dispensers contain enough sealant for one quadrant; this method reduces the risk of cross-contamination, when used properly
I. Evaluating the results
 1. Examine the sealant to determine the adequacy of bond strength and the absence of voids, underextensions, overextensions, or undercuring
 2. The sealed surface should feel completely smooth
 3. Floss teeth to ensure that the sealant has not flowed into interproximal spaces
 4. For the filled-type sealant material, occlusion should be checked with articulating paper; frank high spots should be reduced with a finishing bur or fine stone; in the case of unfilled-type sealant materials, high spots self-adjust after a few days
 5. Evaluate sealant retention at each appointment; replace the material, as needed
 6. Most sealant failures result from "operator error," for example, oil, debris, or moisture contamination, or from not following manufacturer's instructions
J. Document on individual's chart the type of sealant used and the teeth sealed

## TOBACCO USE INTERVENTIONS

### General Considerations[34–36]

A. Types of tobacco are smoked tobacco and unsmoked tobacco
 1. Examples of smoked tobacco include *bidis,* cigars, pipes, cigarettes, water pipe *(hookah),* vaping (vape pens), electronic cigarettes (ECIGS), and clove cigarettes
 2. Unsmoked tobacco is also known as *spit tobacco, snuff, dip, pinch,* or *smokeless tobacco*
B. Tobacco cessation is considered to have occurred when an individual permanently discontinues the use of tobacco
C. Smoking is a primary risk factor for:
 1. Lung cancer
 2. Chronic obstructive lung disease
 3. Heart disease
 4. Head and neck, oropharyngeal, and other cancers
 5. Periodontal disease

D. Oral effects of tobacco use: oral and pharyngeal cancer, failure of periodontal therapy, failure of dental implants, dental caries, tobacco abrasion, extrinsic stain, halitosis, attrition, delayed wound healing, nicotine stomatitis, oral leukoplakia, and tooth loss
E. From a host response perspective, smoking has been found to interfere with the normal function of helper lymphocytes critical to antibody production, impair revascularization in both soft and hard tissues, inhibit collagen production, and increase collagenase activity
F. Spit tobacco use is associated with oral, laryngeal, and pharyngeal cancers
   1. Oral mucosal lesions and gingival recession are mostly observed in individuals using spit tobacco
   2. Oral mucosal lesions often disappear after spit tobacco use is discontinued
G. Dental hygienists must assume the responsibility for supporting individuals from abstaining tobacco use and encouraging nonusers
H. Nicotine itself is not a carcinogen, but it is physiologically addictive; individuals trying to quit may experience withdrawal symptoms (e.g., insomnia, irritability, weight gain); embedded social and psychological factors also contribute to the challenge
I. Dental hygienists should take an active role in the community and in legislative efforts to reduce all tobacco use

### Tobacco Cessation Interventions

A. Oral care and all other health care facilities should be tobacco free
B. Oral health care professionals should strive to quit all tobacco-related habits and serve as positive role models
C. Tobacco use by all individuals should be addressed, assessed, and documented in individuals' permanent records
D. The Agency for Healthcare Research and Quality's Clinical Practice Guideline on Treating Tobacco Use and Dependence recommends a combination of tobacco dependence counseling and medication treatments[37]
   1. Combination of counseling and medication is more effect than counseling or medication alone; health professionals should be trained in effective strategies to assist tobacco users to quit and/or motivate those unwilling to quit; MI techniques have been effective to evoke an individual's intrinsic motivation to quit
      a. Pregnant smokers should be offered one-on-one psychosocial innervations that is *more than* minimal advice to quit because of serious harm to the fetus
      b. Dental hygienists should ask children and adolescents about tobacco use and deliver a powerful message to refrain from usage; question the type of tobacco used (e.g., cigarettes, ECIGS, water pipes [hookahs], vape pens, chewing tobacco, snuff); educate about the health risks of tobacco, negative effects of tobacco on their physical appearance and athletic prowess; encourage to resist peer pressure, pop culture, and social media messages to start using tobacco
   2. Successful individual-provider interactions:[6–9,37]
      a. Ask—at every appointment, identify tobacco use and type, and document
      b. Assess—individual readiness for cessation
      c. Assist—if individual is willing to make an attempt to quit, provide counseling, and pharmacotherapeutic agents
      d. Arrange—a follow-up contact; scheduled within the first week following the quit date
   3. FDA-approved pharmacotherapeutic agents include:
      a. Nicotine reduction therapy—nicotine transdermal patch, gum, lozenge, nasal spray, and oral inhaler
      b. Nonnicotine agents for managing nicotine addiction—sustained-release bupropion hydrochloride (Zyban) tablets and varenicline (Chantix)
G. Tobacco-use assessment should be part of history taking; assessment should include:
   1. Form of tobacco used
   2. Amount used
   3. Duration of habit
   4. Previous quit attempts
   5. Reasons for quitting or abstaining from tobacco use
H. Refer—if individual is motivated to quit, refer to QUITLINES, websites, and local cessation programs; find programs and assistance at http://www.smokefree.gov, or call 1-800-44U-QUIT (1-800-448-7848); these websites and telephone numbers provide resources to use at the chairside
   1. Typically, smokers try to stop multiple times before they succeed

## PERIODONTAL DISEASE RISK ASSESSMENT[22,34,38]

A. Periodontal risk assessment
   1. Involves the identification of individuals and populations at risk of developing periodontal disease
   2. Purpose of risk assessment
      a. Reduce the need for complex periodontal therapy
      b. Improve individual outcome
      c. Reduce risk of chronic systemic diseases
   3. Identification of risk factors and taking steps that can reduce the risk will help prevent periodontal disease; identification of risk factors does not imply cause and effect
B. Common risk factors for periodontal disease
   1. Tobacco use
      a. Heat from smoking enhances attachment loss and increases calculus formation, which in turn creates favorable environment for plaque biofilm retention
      b. Nicotine negatively affects collagen synthesis, protein secretion, and bone formation, leading to impaired bone healing
      c. Use of tobacco products increases production of cytokines because of lower oxygen levels, which cause breakdown periodontal tissues
      d. Tobacco history is assessed during health and social histories
   2. Systemic diseases

a. Have been associated with oral diseases (e.g., periodontal disease, dental caries, salivary gland dysfunction and xerostomia, burning mouth syndrome) and increased susceptibility to oral infections
b. Evidence shows a high chronic systemic inflammatory response in individuals with metabolic syndrome
3. Genetic factors
a. Interleukin-1 (IL-1) polymorphism studies have indicated that IL-1 genotype–positive individuals have greater chance of periodontal disease than IL-1 genotype–negative individuals
b. Oral disease and tooth loss in the family are assessed during the health history.
4. Poor oral hygiene—lack of plaque biofilm removal encourages an environment conducive to the survival of periodontal disease pathogens
5. Metabolic syndrome
a. Group of disorders that increase the risk of heart disease, stroke, and diabetes, including high blood pressure, elevated plasma glucose, excess body fat around the waist and abdominal area, and high cholesterol level
b. Studies on the relationship between periodontal disease and metabolic syndrome are inconclusive

## ORAL CANCER RISK ASSESSMENT

Many oral cancers, unfortunately, are not detected until they have invaded deep tissues and require radical surgery, extensive chemotherapy, irradiation, or all three interventions. Early detection and early treatment are the best ways to manage oral cancer; self-examination can supplement a thorough in-office head and neck, extraoral, and intraoral examination. Individuals can potentially benefit from self-examination skills. It is especially important to educate high-risk persons.

A. Individuals need to be informed about modifiable and nonmodifiable risk factors for oral cancer
1. Modifiable risk factor—can be changed or eliminated (e.g., smoking, sun exposure, or drinking behavior)
2. Nonmodifiable risk factor—cannot be changed or eliminated (e.g., genetic makeup, biological sex)
B. Strategies for reducing risk factors should be part of the dental hygiene care plan

### High-Risk Factors[34–36]

A. Tobacco use
1. Individuals who smoke are estimated to be at greater risk than nonsmokers
2. Individuals who use snuff and spit tobacco are prone to squamous cell carcinomas at or near the site where the tobacco is held
B. Alcohol use—the combination of smoking and alcohol use is responsible for the majority of head and neck cancers[1]
C. Virus—certain viruses, such as human immunodeficiency virus (HIV) and human papillomavirus (HPV), are linked to the development of cancers of the nasopharynx, cervix, and lymphatic system
D. Sun exposure—individuals who work outdoors, especially those with a fair complexion, are at higher risk for basal cell tumors of the skin (predominating around the face and lips).

### Examination Technique

#### Materials Needed

A. Large mirror and adequate light source are essential for self-examination procedures
B. A flashlight, mouth-sized mirror, and gauze or tissue squares help to access and visualize intraoral structures

#### Systematic Approach

A. Face and neck
1. Symmetry—one-sided irregularities should be further investigated; right and left sides should have the same outline and shape; lesions that fail to heal within 2 weeks should be suspect
2. Skin—have the individual remove eyeglasses; check for sores, bumps, and discoloration
3. Neck—palpate lymph chains for lumps or tender areas
B. Visually examine and palpate lips and gums
1. Have the individual remove full or partial dentures
2. Retract the lips; look for sores or color changes
C. Cheek
1. Retract the right side and then the left side to visualize the inner surface; look for red, white, brown, or speckled patches
2. Palpate for lumps or tenderness
3. Run a finger over the inside surface to check for rough or raised places
D. Roof of mouth
1. Tilt the head back and use a flashlight for better visualization
2. Look for sores or color changes; feel for lumps or areas of tenderness
E. Tongue
1. Have the individual extend the tongue, and look at the dorsum
2. Grasp the tongue with a gauze square; pull and roll the tongue to the right side and then to the left side
3. Look for sores, color changes, and irregularities
4. Feel for lumps, areas of tenderness, or roughened surfaces
F. Floor of mouth
1. Have the individual place the tip of the tongue against the roof of the mouth
2. Look for any asymmetry, sores, or color changes
3. Place the fingers of one hand under the individual's jaw, and use the index finger of the other hand to compress structures
4. Check for lumps, tenderness, or irregularities
G. Provide the individual with an assessment of his or her modifiable and non-modifiable risk factors; help the individual to reduce the risks for oral cancer
H. Provide the criteria for determining significant deviations from normal
1. Sores that fail to heal within 2 weeks
2. Appearance of white, red, or dark-colored patches
3. Presence of swellings, lumps, bumps, or growths

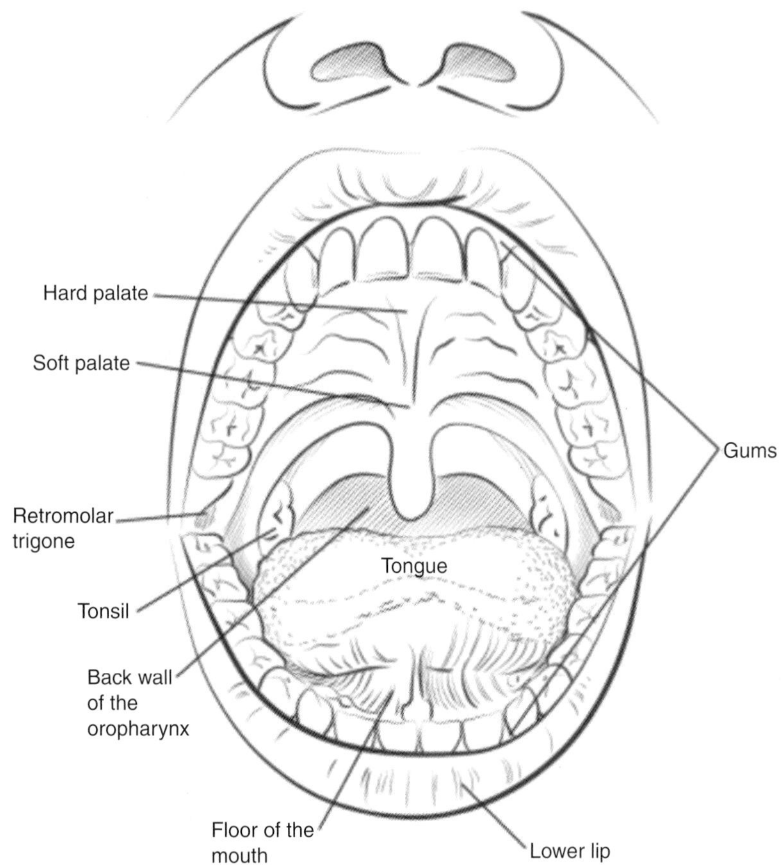


**Fig. 16.6** Intraoral Cancer Screening (©American Cancer Society 2011. Used with permission.

I. Define the oral health professional's role in interpreting findings; the individual should report unusual findings, but should not self-diagnose
J. Establish the concept that self-examination is not meant to be a substitute for periodic regular professional evaluation

## DIAGNOSTIC TOOLS FOR ORAL CANCER DETECTION

### General Considerations

A. The combination of visual examination and palpation is the main approach to detecting epithelial changes in the oral mucosa
B. Routine examination for the detection of oral cancer should be completed for each individual (see the section on "Extraoral and Intraoral Assessment" in Chapter 15)
C. Routine oral cancer screenings can reduce oral cancer incidence and mortality rate[39]
D. The diagnosis of a suspicious lesion is established by traditional biopsy

### Brush Biopsy

#### Definition

A. Transepithelial oral biopsy—samples the superficial, intermediate and basal epithelial layers to detect oral cancer at its earliest stages; indicated for small, innocuous-appearing lesions
B. The dental hygienist's role is to identify red, white, or mixed lesions as well as ulcerated, thickened, traumatized, or irritated oral epithelium to be evaluated using brush biopsy
C. Dental hygienists should consult their state regulatory board or state statutes to determine whether they are legally permitted to perform brush biopsies
D. Accurate detection of precancerous or cancerous areas requires scalpel biopsy

#### Advantages

A. Easy, chairside test to evaluate epithelial changes and lesions that may have received only a clinical follow-up before this test became available
B. Rapid results, generally within 3 days to detect dysplasia or carcinoma
C. Minimally invasive
D. Each specimen is evaluated by both computer-assisted analysis and a pathologist

#### Disadvantages

A. Costs for both obtaining and analyzing the specimen are incurred by the individual
B. As with any biopsy method, false-negative results are possible
C. Brush biopsies with negative results require careful follow-up

### Procedure

A. Armamentarium (see http://www.oralcdx.com)
   1. Sterile brush instrument for biopsy
   2. Microscope specimen slide
   3. Fixative
   4. Laboratory forms
B. Obtaining and preparing the sample
   1. Using the individual's saliva, moisten the biopsy brush
   2. Firmly press the biopsy brush against the lesion
   3. While pressing, rotate the brush over the surface of the lesion until pink tissue or pinpoint areas of bleeding occur; number of rotations will vary, depending on the thickness of the lesion
   4. Use of topical anesthesia is contraindicated because it may distort the sample
   5. To prepare the glass slide, transfer as much of the cellular sample as possible by rotating and dragging brush lengthwise on the slide
   6. Apply the fixative to cover the slide thoroughly; allow drying for 15 minutes
   7. Package the sample and send it to the laboratory for evaluation

## Laboratory Findings for Brush Biopsy

A. Classification categories
   1. Unsatisfactory—specimen is not adequate for diagnosis
   2. Class I: normal—only normal cells are present
   3. Class II: atypical—some cellular changes may be present; no suggestion of malignancy is present
   4. Class III: intermediate—changes may suggest malignancy, but findings are not clear; biopsy is recommended
   5. Class IV: suggestive of cancer—cells with malignant characteristics are present; biopsy is mandatory
   6. Class V: positive for cancer—cells are obviously malignant; scalpel biopsy is mandatory
B. Follow-up needs
   1. Unsatisfactory—the individual should be scheduled for another smear or brush biopsy
   2. Class I or II findings—the individual should be monitored for healing of lesion or reevaluated if the lesion fails to resolve; as with all biopsy methods, false-negative reports are possible; a healed lesion is the best reassurance for reports in categories I and II
   3. Class III, IV, or V findings—the individual should be referred for scalpel biopsy

### Adjunct Oral Cancer Screening Devices[40]

Routine oral cancer visual and tactile examination is the "gold standard" for identification of oral cancer lesions[37] the following adjunct technologies may aid in visual and tactile examination.

### ViziLite

A. Definition—an FDA-approved technology that screens for oral abnormalities potentially indicative of oral cancer
   1. This tool helps oral health care professionals identify lesions before they appear on oral tissue surfaces
   2. ViziLite illumination cannot distinguish keratotic, inflammatory, malignant, or possibly malignant lesions; clinical judgment and scalpel biopsy are essential for proper patient care
B. Procedure
   1. The individual rinses with a solution
   2. The oral health care professional activates a patented light stick intraorally
   3. The light stick illuminates any suboral lesions during the oral cancer screening examination
C. Studies have shown inconsistent results with the use of ViziLite

### VELscope

A. Definition—an FDA-approved handheld device that uses oral fluorescence technology to screen for precancerous and cancerous lesions in the oral cavity
   1. The fluorescence technology shows healthy tissue as green and atypical areas (potentially cancerous lesions) as dark magenta, brown, or black
   2. Changes in tissue can be detected while the change is still subepithelial and otherwise not visualized during conventional oral examination
   3. Tissue margins can be determined, which will help guide complete removal of oral cancers in the operatory
B. This device should be used as an adjunct to clinical screening; clinical judgment and scalpel biopsy are essential for the diagnosis of oral cancer lesions
C. There is higher risk of false-positive results; VELscope does not provide a definitive diagnosis

### Other Devices and Oral Examination

A. Other oral cancer screening devices are available, such as Identafi; however, these devices are unable to provide definitive diagnosis

## ASSESSMENT OF DENTINAL HYPERSENSITIVITY

A. Definition—abnormal condition that occurs when vital dentin is exposed to the environment of the oral cavity; the result is painful stimuli that can reach the pulp and cause pain
   1. Thermal, evaporative, tactile, osmotic, or chemical stimuli can cause fluid movement within the dentinal tubule, exciting the nerve and signaling the pulp to respond
   2. Gingival recession and loss of enamel should be minimized to avoid dentinal hypersensitivity
   3. Treatment of dentinal hypersensitivity is a valuable individual service; symptoms cause considerable discomfort to the individual and may interfere with both control of plaque biofilm and professional treatment
B. Characteristics
   1. Rapid onset
   2. Sharp pain
   3. Short duration
   4. Response to stimuli

## ETIOLOGY

A. Primary causes of hypersensitivity are exposed dentin and open dentinal tubules
B. Dentin exposure occurs:
   1. In 10% of all teeth; during development, enamel and cementum do not join
   2. When enamel or cementum is lost through abrasion, erosion, abfraction, dental caries, or over instrumentation
   3. When soft tissue is lost because of gingival recession, periodontal surgery, or an aggressive toothbrushing technique
   4. When diet exposes the dentin to foods and beverages with a low pH; soft drinks, sport drinks, coffee, and fruit juices/drinks; citrus fruits; yogurt; and some alcoholic beverages; plaque biofilm acids
C. Loss of hard and soft tissues is believed to be accelerated from the combined use of mechanical brushing and a dentifrice applied immediately after exposure to acidic food or drink

### Pain Mechanism

A. Hydrodynamic theory—the most widely accepted
B. Explains the following:
   1. Dentinal tubules are exposed
   2. Pain-producing stimuli are present
   3. Pain-producing stimuli initiate the flow of lymphatic fluid within dental tubules
   4. Odontoblasts and their processes act as receptors and transmitters of sensory stimuli
   5. The movement of tubular fluids causes nerve endings at the pulpal wall to be stimulated and produce pain

### Pain Stimuli

A. Thermal or evaporative stimuli—foods and liquids at extreme temperatures, cold air, and too rapid drying of a tooth surface; cause a concurrent rapid drop in tooth temperature; are more problematic than hot-air changes
B. Mechanical stimuli—instrumentation, home care devices, eating utensils, and friction from removable prosthetic or orthodontic devices
C. Chemical stimuli—foods high in acid or sugars; some topical medications; plaque acids

### Desensitizing Agents

A. Modes of action—desensitizers:
   1. Seal dentinal tubules by surface precipitation of ions, subsurface incorporation of ions, or stimulation of secondary dentin
   2. Decrease the excitability of sensory nerves, thereby making the nerve less sensitive to stimuli
B. Optimal characteristics—professionally applied desensitizing agents should act rapidly and should be nontoxic, easy to apply, and have consistent outcomes and long-term effects

### Types of Desensitizing Treatments

A. No single desensitizing agent or form of treatment is effective for all persons
B. Numerous agents have varying degrees of success, including:
   1. Solutions, gels, or pastes of fluoride in varying compounds and percentages, stannous fluoride, calcium hydroxide, strontium chloride, potassium nitrate, sodium citrate, formaldehyde, glutaraldehyde, arginine and insoluble calcium, casein phosphopeptide–amorphous calcium phosphate complex, or potassium or ferric oxalate
   2. Adhesive, varnish, or bonding materials
   3. Polymerizing agents[1]
   4. Iontophoretic devices—technique sensitive
   5. Laser therapy—one-time treatment that reduces or eliminates dentin sensitivity by sealing dentinal tubules; sensitive dentin treated with laser is found to be harder than untreated dentin
   6. Restorations—restoration may be placed on the surface where dentin is exposed to help reduce sensitivity
      a. Glass ionomer cements (GICs)—used in cervical abrasion and abfraction; the sensitive area is etched with 50% citric acid, rinsed with water, and dried before application of GIC
      b. Adhesive resin primers—reduces dentin permeability by occluding open tubules; the material is rubbed on the sensitive area for approximately 30 seconds and air-dried
      c. Iontophoresis is the application of an electrical current to impregnate tissues with ions from dissolved salts
      d. Fluoride iontophoresis is thought to result in the increased uptake and penetration of fluoride ions into dentin

### Desensitization Methods

A. Self-care regimens
   1. Effective plaque biofilm control strategies are important in gaining and maintaining control of hypersensitivity and modifications to minimize aggressive brushing are critical
   2. Specially formulated toothpastes containing 5% potassium nitrate to desensitize the nerve are often combined with fluoride to promotes remineralization
   3. Daily use of a fluoride gel or rinse is advisable when the problem is generalized or recurrent
B. Professionally delivered regimens should support and enable self-care regimens
   1. Procedure

Pastes are usually burnished in with a wooden point, whereas solutions, gels, or varnishes are painted or bathed on.

      a. Remove all deposits; involved surfaces must be free of barriers to the agent
      b. Local anesthesia is appropriate when instrumentation procedure or application of the agent is too painful
      c. Isolate the sensitive tooth and control saliva
      d. Dry the affected tooth with cotton pellets or gauze; avoid using an air syringe
      e. Apply the agent according to the manufacturer's instructions for method and time required
      f. Remove any excess agent to avoid ingestion by the individual. Some agents have very high concentrations

of fluoride. To prevent nausea, use proper application and techniques to control salivary flow

g. Test for change in pain reaction; this will not be possible with anesthetized areas. Some individuals may experience an acute pain reaction to the agent; immediately remove the agent, wait a few minutes, and then attempt reapplication
h. Plan for future reapplication if desensitization was not successful

## PULPAL VITALITY AND TESTING DEVICES[41]

### Basic Concepts

A. Teeth may become nonvital from bacterial invasion of the pulp associated with caries or periodontal disease or from injuries such as mechanical or thermal trauma
B. Any tooth suspected of being nonvital should be tested for pulpal vitality
C. The preferred method of testing provides a *qualitative* assessment
D. Tests should correlate with or mimic the individual's chief complaint
E. Palpation, percussion, and radiographic findings (e.g., widened periodontal ligament) are other sources of data for pulpal assessment

### Laser Doppler Flowmetry

A. Noninvasive, painless, semiquantitative method; measures pulpal blood flow through assessment of the vascular supply by the passage of light through a tooth; monitors blood flow in response to pressure changes and administration of local anesthesia
B. Useful in young children whose responses are usually unreliable
C. Studies have shown that blood circulation is the most accurate determinant in assessing pulp vitality
D. Laser Doppler flowmetry is more reliable at identifying vital and nonvital teeth earlier than other pulp vitality tests

### Traditional Electrical Testing Devices

A. The electrical pulp tester (also known as a *vitalometer*) and the digital pulp tester use gradations of electrical current to excite a response in pulpal tissue and thus assess response to stimulus
   1. Pulp testers have either a portable battery or a plug-in electrical power source
   2. All testers have rheostats, with a scale (e.g., 1 to 10 or 1 to 50) that indicates the relative amount of current being applied; digital pulp testers provide a digital reading
   3. Electrical pulp testers can be used safely on individuals with implanted cardiac devices
B. Procedure
   1. Armamentarium
   2. Individual preparation
   3. Obtaining a reading
   4. Documentation
      a. Testing device
      b. Cotton rolls
      c. Toothpaste or other conducting medium
      d. Explain the procedure to the individual; use the minimal stimulation necessary to evoke a response
      e. Instruct the individual to raise a hand when the slightest warmth or tingling sensation is felt
      f. Isolate and dry the teeth to be tested; this prevents the conduction of current into the soft tissue
      g. Apply a small amount of toothpaste, or an alternative conductor, to the tester tip
      h. Place the tip on sound tooth structure, within the middle third of the crown for a single-rooted tooth and within the middle third of each cusp for a multirooted tooth; a clip resting on the individual's lip and attached to the handpiece is necessary to create a closed electrical circuit and to activate the tester
      i. Avoid any contact with restorations and soft tissue
      j. Slowly advance the rheostat from zero to increasingly higher numbers until a sensation is felt by the individual; the rheostat should not be moved above that point for that tooth
      k. Two readings should be taken for each tooth tested and the readings averaged
      l. For all teeth tested, record the lowest average reading, the type of testing device and conductor used, and any individual actions or reactions that may have affected the results
C. Variables affecting results
   1. Pulpal conditions may vary from early inflammation to complete necrosis; individual responses vary with each condition; the pulp of the tooth that is tested is considered to be degenerating when, compared with a control, much more current is required to gain a response
   2. Metallic restorations conduct electrical charges more rapidly than tooth structure and can produce false readings
   3. Teeth with splints, bridges, or proximal restorations may produce false-positive reactions because the circuit can be transferred from adjacent vital teeth
   4. Multi-rooted teeth may have some combination of vital and nonvital canals and may give false-positive results
   5. Pain reactions are influenced by the individual's attitude, age, gender, anxiety, emotions, fatigue, culture, and medications

### Thermal Testing

A. Employs a hot or cold stimulus to test for pulpal response
B. The cold test is used most often
C. The heat test is useful when an unidentified tooth is heat sensitive

## ETHICAL, LEGAL, AND SAFETY ISSUES

A. Dental hygienists must have knowledge of evidence-based preventive products and strategies to provide optimal care
B. A combination of frequent review of the literature; focus on information from controlled clinical trials and systematic review articles; the practitioner's knowledge, clinical

experience, and judgment; and individual preferences leads to appropriate evidence-based decision making and best practices

C. Thorough, accurate, and confidential chart documentation is essential; adherence to the regulations of the Health Insurance Portability and Accountability Act (HIPAA) is mandatory
D. The individual's progress with regard to self-care should be documented in the individual record and should include the individual's response, knowledge, adherence, involvement, skills, and measurable oral changes
E. The dental hygienist should discuss all the procedures with individuals on an appropriate level for comprehension, obtain informed consent, and encourage individual participation in the dental hygiene care plan
F. Dental hygiene interventions are offered within the scope of dental hygiene practice and within the legal jurisdiction of the employment setting
G. Individuals have the right to accept or reject the dental hygiene care plan and still retain the respect of the dental hygienist
H. Individuals have the right to receive individualized, cutting-edge, evidence-based recommendations and care

## WEBSITE INFORMATION AND RESOURCES

| Source | Website Address | Description |
|---|---|---|
| National Center for Dental Hygiene Research | https://dent-web10.usc.edu/dhnet/ | Dental hygienists' resources and links |
| American Academy of Periodontology | http://www.perio.org | Periodontics resources and position papers |
| Campaign for Tobacco Free Kids | https://www.tobaccofreekids.org/ | Information and initiatives to keep kids tobacco free |
| American Lung Association—Freedom from Smoking | https://www.lung.org/stop-smoking/join-freedom-from-smoking/ | Information about lung diseases and tobacco cessation |
| American Dental Association | https://www.ada.org/en/science-research/ada-seal-of-acceptance/ada-seal-shopping-list | ADA seal product list |

## CHAPTER 12 REVIEW QUESTIONS

Answers and rationales to chapter review questions are available on this text's accompanying Evolve site. See inside front cover for details.

1. Which of the following focuses on strengthening an individual's motivation for and movement toward a specific goal?
   - **a.** Maslow's hierarchy of needs
   - **b.** Transtheoretical Model
   - **c.** Health Belief Model
   - **d.** Motivational Interviewing
2. A 20-year-old male has completed dental implant therapy. Years ago, during a high school baseball game, he was hit in the face with a ball fracturing #6, #7, and #8. Both #6 and #7 were restored; however, #8 required extraction. Due to his age at the time of injury, he was not a candidate for a dental implant and had a removable prostheses to replace #8. The trauma from the injury and missing #8 impacted his emotional and social well-being. Now at age 20 years old, he has restored #8 with a dental implant and will be attending a major university out of state. Which of Maslow's hierarchy of needs have been met?
   - **a.** Self-actualization
   - **b.** Self esteem
   - **c.** Safety and security
   - **d.** Physiological needs
   - **e.** Love and belonging
3. Which of the following products would you recommend for plaque removal under a of a four-unit bridge #28–#31 (#31 and #28 abutments; #30 and #29 pontics) to an individual with dexterity limitations?
   - **a.** End-tuft brush
   - **b.** Super-floss
   - **c.** Proxy brush
   - **d.** Dental water jet
   - **e.** Both c and d
4. A 45-year-old African American male presents to the clinic for quadrant scaling and root planing. Health history is significant for a 20 year tobacco habit, social alcohol use, type 2 diabetes, hypertension, and high cholesterol. Medications include a calcium channel blocker, metformin, and Lipitor. During the oral cancer screening you notice a 3 mm x 5 mm raised leukoplakia on the left lateral border of his tongue. All the following are risk factors for oral cancer EXCEPT one. Which one is the *exception*?
   - **a.** Medications causing xerostomia
   - **b.** Tobacco and alcohol use
   - **c.** Ethnicity
   - **d.** Periodontitis
   - **e.** Both a and d
5. A 50-year-old Hispanic male presents as a new patient to the dental clinic. His medical, dental, pharmacologic, and social health history are updated. The patient brought a full mouth series of radiographs from his prior dentist that are 18 months old. The dental hygienist records his vitals, full mouth periodontal charting, and the hard and soft tissue evaluation. Collecting this information falls under what step of the dental hygiene process of care?
   - **a.** Assessment
   - **b.** Dental hygiene diagnosis
   - **c.** Planning

d. Implementation
e. Evaluation
f. Documentation

6. Ms. Patel is a 46-year-old female that had quadrant scaling and root planing completed less than two months ago. She presents to the dental clinic for you to review and measure the results of the dental hygiene care plan. What category is this step of the dental hygiene process of care?
   a. Assessment
   b. Dental hygiene diagnosis
   c. Planning
   d. Implementation
   e. Evaluation
   f. Documentation
7. Which of the following viruses are linked to the development of cancers of the nasopharynx, cervix, and lymphatic system?
   a. Human immunodeficiency virus
   b. Epstein-Barr virus
   c. Rhinovirus
   d. Human papillomavirus
   e. Both a and d
   f. Both b and d
8. An individual with plaque-induced periodontal disease can benefit from all of the following EXCEPT:
   a. Patient-centered counseling to support oral hygiene behaviors
   b. Antimicrobial mouthrinse
   c. Power toothbrush
   d. Advice giving or use of fear tactics
   e. Dentifrices with triclosan
9. The following are strategies to maintain a toothbrush except one. Which one is the exception?
   a. Toothbrushes should be changed every three months.
   b. Toothbrushes should be disinfected with 0.12% chlorhexidine gluconate after a cold, the flu, or infection/sore throat or replaced.
   c. Toothbrushes should be rinsed and air-dried after each use.
   d. Tootbrushes can be shared with others after disinfecting with a 11.6% alcohol mouth rinse.
10. A 25-year-old female presents to the dental clinic for her routine six month prophylaxis, bite-wing radiographs, and examination. She recently started a plant-based diet and prefers fruit compared to vegetables. You notice numerous incipient lesions on the bite-wing radiographs. You believe the incipient lesions are a result of her diet change that encompasses high natural sugar and acid found in fruit. The patient wants to maintain a plant-based diet with a high fruit content. However, she is interested in products to arrest the incipient lesions. Which of the following fluoride products is NOT an appropriate recommendation for this patient?
    a. Amorphous calcium phosphate
    b. Casein phosphopeptide–amorphous calcium phosphate
    c. 5% fluoride varnish
    d. Silver diamine fluoride
11. All the following are FALSE statements about silver diamine fluoride (SDF) EXCEPT one. Which one is the exception?
    a. FDA approved as a desensitizing agent and for caries arrest
    b. Should be applied to all individual with caries
    c. The caries lesions will turn black in color after application
    d. Available over the counter for caries prevention
12. All the following can be recommended for plaque control to prevent peri-implant diseases for individuals with a dental implant EXCEPT:
    a. Antimicrobial rinses (i.e., 0.12% chlorhexidine gluconate)
    b. Fluoride products (i.e., topical, varnish, or rinses)
    c. Interdental brushes (i.e., toothpicks, interdental wedges, interdental tips)
    d. Oral irrigation (i.e., dental water jet with or without antimicrobial rinse)
13. A 65-year-old Caucasian male presents to the clinic with the chief complaint of oral malodor. Health history is significant for acid reflux. The individual had a 40-year smoking habit and has been smoke-free for five years. He consumes daily coffee and one glass of red wine every night. During intraoral examination you notice plaque biofilm accumulation on the dorsal surface of the tongue. Which of the following recommendations would NOT be appropriate for this individual?
    a. Oral hygiene education
    b. Tobacco cessation
    c. Dietary counseling
    d. Referral to primary care physician
14. Which of the following is NOT an assessment tools for caries?
    a. Caries management by risk assessment (CAMBRA)
    b. DIAGNOdent
    c. DEXIS CarieVu
    d. Radiographs
15. Which of the following is NOT a therapeutic and active ingredient of dentifrices?
    a. Remineralizing agents
    b. Binding agents
    c. Antimicrobial agents
    d. Desensitizing agents
16. Which of the following are risk factors for peri-implant diseases?
    a. Tobacco use
    b. Plaque biofilm
    c. History of periodontal disease
    d. All of the above
17. A 30-year-old woman recently diagnosed with rheumatoid arthritis presents to the dental clinic. All of the following factors contribute to her caries risk EXCEPT one. Which one is the exception?
    a. Xerostomia associated with medications to manage rheumatoid arthritis
    b. Use of fluoride mouthrinse
    c. Sealants in pits and fissures

d. Poor manual dexterity
e. Both a and d
f. Both b and c

18. Which of the following are contraindications for dental sealants?
a. Individuals with deep pits and fissures
b. Individuals with newly erupted teeth with deep pits and fissures
c. Individuals with carious lesions on the proximal surfaces extending to the occlusal surface
d. Individuals with xerostomia
e. Both a and b
f. Both c and d

19. An oral lesion present more than two weeks should be examined by the following?
a. VELscope
b. Brush biopsy of the lesion
c. ViziLite
d. Biopsy of the lesion
e. Both a and c
f. Both b and d

## CASE A

Ms. Davis is a 42-year-old female with a history of periodontal disease. She presents for her 3-month periodontal maintenance at the dental office. She has been recently diagnosed with stage 2 breast cancer and is scheduled to start chemotherapy. Her oncologist has requested an oral examination and letter documenting she has no oral conditions or diseases before she starts chemotherapy. Health history is significant for hypertension controlled with atenolol and osteoarthritis controlled with nonsteroidal antiinflammatory drugs (NSAIDS). She experiences dry mouth and reports brushing twice daily with an electric toothbrush. She sips juice throughout the day to help relieve her dry mouth. She states she knows sipping juice is not good, but water does not seem to help relieve her dry mouth as much as juice. She has never liked flossing. Ms. Davis has moderate levels of interproximal plaque biofilm and is very concerned her periodontal disease will not be controlled once she starts chemotherapy. She is missing teeth #1, #3, #14, #16, #17, #20, and #32. She has two three-unit bridges (#2–#4 and #13–#15) and one dental implant #20. In addition, she has class II restorations on #5, #21, and #19 placed in the last 3 years. Dental examination indicates no caries, pathology, and her periodontal status is stable and her periodontal status is stable with CAL due to recession and no signs of progression.

***Use Case A to answer questions 20 to 26.***

20. According to the transtheoretical model, what stage of change is Ms. Davis in with regard to sipping juice?
a. Precontemplation
b. Contemplation
c. Preparation
d. Action

21. Which of the following are caries disease indicators for Ms. Davis?
a. History of periodontal disease
b. Restorations placed in the last 3 years
c. Medications
d. Frequent juice consumption
e. Future chemotherapy treatment
f. All of the above

22. Ms. Davis's greatest concern is that her periodontal health will be compromised with chemotherapy. As a dental hygienist, you know the moderate level of plaque contributes to her periodontal status. How can you best support her concern?
a. Provide patient-centered counseling
b. Demonstrate the Spirit of motivational interviewing (MI) (partnership, acceptance, empathy, and compassion)
c. Utilize guiding strategies of open-ended questions, affirmations, reflective listening, and summaries (OARS)
d. Resist the righting reflex
e. All of the above

23. What interdental device would the dental hygienist recommend to Ms. Davis for plaque biofilm removal between #20 and #21?
a. Dental floss
b. Floss threader
c. Interdental brush
d. Oral irrigation
e. Both a and b
f. Both c and d

24. Ms. Davis is at risk for all of the following once she begins chemotherapy EXCEPT one. Which one is the exception?
a. Caries
b. Oral cancer
c. Candida albicans
d. Oral mucositis

25. What information should be included in the letter to Ms. Davis' oncologist?
a. Risk factors for oral conditions and diseases
b. Dietary counseling
c. Request clearance for future periodontal maintenance and dental treatment
d. The letter should include information for a, b, and c
e. A letter should NOT be sent since there was no conditions or diseases found during dental examination

26. Ms. Davis does not like to use dental floss, but she is receptive to suggestions because her periodontal health is important to her. All of the following can be used as an alternative to floss to help maintain periodontal health EXCEPT one. Which one is the exception?
a. Dental water jet
b. Dentifrice with triclosan
c. Fluoride varnish
d. Antimicrobial mouthrinse

## CASE B

Mr. Robinson is a 35-year-old male who presents to the dental clinic as a new patient. His health history reveals he is taking insulin for type 1 diabetes and reports his Alc was 7.5 last month. He smokes one-half of a pack of cigarettes daily. A full mouth radiograph series is completed and reveals generalized 30% bone loss and radiographic calculus. A full mouth periodontal chart is completed with generalized 5–6 mm probing depths, clinical attachment loss of 2–3 mm, and bleeding on probing. There is class II furcation involvement on #19 and #30. Intraoral assessment reveals a coated tongue, bilateral linea alba, and generalized abfraction in the posterior. Mr. Robinson's chief complaint is bad breath and he has not had his teeth cleaned in 7 years.

*Use Case B to answer questions 27 to 37.*

27. Which of the following is contributing to Mr. Robinson's periodontal condition?
    a. Insulin for type 1 diabetes
    b. Plaque biofilm
    c. Smoking
    d. Bruxism
    e. Both a and b
    f. Only b, c, and d
28. The dental hygienist presents the dental hygiene diagnosis of four quadrants of scaling and root planing to treat Mr. Robinson's periodontal disease. Performing scaling and root planing falls under which of the following steps of the dental hygiene process of care?
    a. Assessment
    b. Dental hygiene diagnosis
    c. Planning
    d. Implementation
    e. Evaluation
    f. Documentation
29. All of the following should be included in the care plan for Mr. Robinson EXCEPT one. Which one is the exception?
    a. Tobacco cessation
    b. Oral hygiene education
    c. Occlusal guard
    d. Consult with an endocrinologist
    e. Referral for periodontal surgery
30. What American Society of Anesthesiologists (ASA) Physical Status Classification is applicable to Mr. Robinson?
    a. ASA I
    b. ASA II
    c. ASA III
    d. ASA IV
31. Mr. Robinson returns for the 6 week periodontal reevaluation. Localized areas in the posterior of all four quadrants have not responded to nonsurgical periodontal therapy. The dental hygienist should modify the care plan with the following EXCEPT one. Which one is the exception?
    a. Retreat the areas with nonsurgical periodontal therapy
    b. Place a locally delivered antibiotic
    c. Refer to a periodontist for an evaluation
    d. Schedule for a 2–3 month periodontal maintenance
32. Which of the following dentifrices can Mr. Robinson use to reduce bleeding and inflammation?
    a. Dentifrice containing triclosan
    b. Dentifrice with sodium fluoride
    c. Dentifrice with potassium nitrate
    d. Dentifrice with hydrogen peroxide
33. Mr. Robinson can benefit from all the following to remove plaque biofilm from the furcation of #19 and #30 except for one. Which one is the exception?
    a. Floss
    b. Interdental wedge
    c. Proxy brushes
    d. Daily oral irrigation

## CASE C

Mr. Smith is a 29-year-old Caucasian male who presents for a 6-month prophylaxis. He transferred from another dental office and had his dental records forwarded to the new dental clinic. His medical and dental history is insignificant. His social history revels a prior 10-year tobacco habit. He switched to electronic cigarettes (ECIGS) 2 years ago. In addition, he occasionally uses cannabis in a vape pen. During intraoral and extraoral examination, a 2 mm x 3 mm asymptomatic lesion is noted on the floor of Mr. Smith's mouth. Mr. Smith has no knowledge of the lesion and it was not noted in his prior dental records.

*Use Case C to answer questions 34 to 38.*

34. What is the MOST appropriate next steps for treatment of the white plaque on the floor of the Mr. Smith's mouth?
    a. Smoking cessation
    b. Inform Mr. Smith and document in the patient record
    c. Evaluate the lesion with VELscope or ViziLite
    d. Referral for biopsy
35. What American Society of Anesthesiologists (ASA) Physical Status Classification is applicable to Mr. Robinson?
    a. ASA I
    b. ASA II
    c. ASA III
    d. ASA IV
36. What are Mr. Smith's modifiable risk(s) for developing oral cancer?
    a. Use of ECIGS
    b. Age
    c. Race
    d. Use of cannabis in a vape pen
    e. Both a and d
    f. Only a, b, and d
37. Which of the following should the dental hygienist implement in the care plan for Mr. Smith?
    a. Tobacco cessation
    b. Oral self-examination
    c. Dietary counseling
    d. Caries prevention
    e. Both a and b
    f. All of the above
38. The dental hygienist includes a lesion description in Mr. Smith's patient record. What category is this step of the dental hygiene process of care?
    a. Assessment
    b. Dental hygiene diagnosis
    c. Planning
    d. Implementation
    e. Evaluation
    f. Documentation

## CASE D

Mrs. Lopez is a 48-year-old Hispanic female who had quadrant scaling and root planing (SRP) completed 5 years ago. Mrs. Lopez was on a regular 3-month periodontal maintenance for the first 3 years after the initial SRP. However, she has a new employer, and the new insurance policy only covers periodontal maintenance two times per year. The last 2 years, Mrs. Lopez had a periodontal maintenance on a 6-month recall. Today, she presents with increased probing depths of 1 mm and generalized bleeding on probing. There is moderate plaque and subgingival calculus throughout. Radiographs indicate caries on #2, #3, #14, #20, #28, and #29. During hard tissue examination the dental hygienist finds numerous white spot lesions along the cervical margin of her teeth. Mrs. Lopez states she works in customer service now and would like to whiten her teeth to match the white spots near her gumline. In addition, she started sucking on peppermint candies during the day to keep her breath fresh.

***Use Case D to answer questions 39 to 43.***

39. What is MOST likely the cause of Mrs. Lopez's radiographic caries and cervical white spot lesions?
 a. Plaque biofilm
 b. Bleeding on probing
 c. Insurance policy change
 d. Peppermint candies
 e. Both a and d
40. Which of the following mouthrinses may reduce plaque and caries for Mrs. Lopez?
 a. 0.12% chlorhexidine gluconate
 b. 0.05% sodium fluoride
 c. 0.1% stannous fluoride
 d. Cetylpyridinium chloride
41. Which of the following toothbrushing methods should the dental hygienist suggest for Mrs. Lopez?
 a. Bass method
 b. Charters' method
 c. Stillman's method
 d. Fones method
42. Mrs. Lopez is not interested in changing any behaviors. Which of the following suggestions is MOST appropriate for the dental hygienist to discuss with Mrs. Lopez to reduce her caries risk?
 a. Use a fluoride mouth rinse
 b. Come in for a 3-month periodontal maintenance
 c. Switch to a xylitol mint
 d. Brush and floss more
43. Which of the following is the MOST appropriate chairside intervention for her white spot lesions?
 a. Fluoride varnish
 b. Sliver diamine fluoride
 c. Fluoride gel in tray
 d. Sealants
44. A 19-year-old female college soccer player presents for her 6-month recall. Her chief complaint is sharp pain when she drinks her sports drink during practice. The sharp pain does not occur every time and only lasts a short period of time. Her health history is insignificant. Clinical findings include marginal gingivitis, localized recession on the facials the canines and premolars, and light calculus on the lingual of the mandibular anteriors. What is MOST likely the cause of her sharp pain?
 a. Gingivitis
 b. Dentinal hypersensitivity
 c. Calculus
 d. Caries
45. Dentinal hypersensitivity may be caused by the following stimuli?
 a. Thermal stimuli
 b. Electric stimuli
 c. Mechanical stimuli
 d. Chemical stimuli
 e. Both b and c
 f. Only a, c, and d
46. The dental hygienist placed sealant on the occlusal surface of all first molars on an 8-year-old child. Isolation with a rubber dam was successful on the mandibular arch, but difficult to secure on the maxillary arch. The dental hygienists elected to isolate the maxillary first molars with cotton rolls. The teeth were dried and etched prior to the sealant placement. Six months later the child presents for a routine prophylaxis and examination. The sealants on the maxillary first molars failed. What is MOST likely the cause?
 a. Ineffective etching
 b. Ineffective isolation
 c. Insufficient rinsing of etch material
 d. Insufficient drying of the tooth surface
 e. Both a and c
 f. Both b and d
47. Inadequate homecare of removable oral appliances may result in all of the following oral conditions EXCEPT one. Which one is the EXCEPTION?
 a. Caries lesions
 b. Tissue lesions
 c. Oral cancer
 d. Candid albicans
48. The dental hygienists can use the following for pulpal vitality testing EXCEPT one. Which one is the EXCEPTION?
 a. Periodontal probing
 b. Palpation
 c. Percussion
 d. Radiographs
49. Which of the following are barriers for individuals to obtain information on oral disease prevention?
 a. Access to oral health care
 b. Oral health literacy
 c. Cost or lack of dental insurance
 d. Fear of dental procedures
 e. All of the above
50. Which of the following is the MOST effective method of tobacco cessation intervention?
 a. Tobacco dependency counseling
 b. Professional advice giving
 c. Pharmacotherapeutic agents
 d. Both a and b
 d. Both a and c

## REFERENCES


1. Darby ML, Walsh MM, Bowen DM. *Dental Hygiene Theory and Practice*. 5th ed. St. Louis: Sanders, Elsevier; 2019:1176.
2. Maslow AH. A theory of human motivation. *Psychol Rev*. 1943;50(4):370–396.
3. Skinner CS, Tiro J, Champion VL. The health belief model. In: Glanz K, Rimer BK, Viswanath K, Health *Behavior and Health Education: Theory, Research, and Practice*. 5th ed. San Francisco: Jossey-Bass; 2015:75–93.
4. Prochaska JO, Redding CA, Evans KE. The transtheoretical model and stages of change. In: Glanz K, Rimer BK, Viswanath K, Health *Behavior and Health Education: Theory, Research, and Practice*. 5th ed. San Francisco: Jossey-Bass; 2015:125–148.
5. Wade KJ, Coates DE, Gauld RD, et al. Oral hygiene behaviours and readiness to change using the TransTheoretical Model (TTM). *N Z Dent J*. 2013;109(2):64–68.
6. Miller WR, Rollnick S. *Motivational Interviewing Helping People Change*. 3rd ed. New York: The Guilford Press; 2013:25–37 (Chapter 2), The spirit of motivational interviewing.
7. Cately D, Goggin K, Lynam I. Motivational interviewing (MI) and its basic tools. In: Ramseier CA, Suvan JE, eds. *Health Behavior Change in the Dental Practice*. Ames (IA): Wiley-Blackwell; 2010:59–92.
8. Mills A, Kerschbaum WE, Richards PS, et al. Dental hygiene students' perceptions of importance and confidence in applying motivational interviewing during patient care. *J Dent Hyg*. 2017;91(1):15–23.
9. Bray KK, Catley D, Voelker MA, Liston R, Williams KB. Motivational interviewing in dental hygiene education: curriculum modification and evaluation. *J Dent Educ*. 2013;77(12):1662–1669.
10. Ramseier CA, Suvan JE. *Health Behavior Change in the Dental Practice*. Ames(IA): Wiley-Blackwell; 2010.
11. Macek MD, Atchison KA, Watson MR, et al. Assessing health literacy and oral health: preliminary results of a multi-site investigation. *J Public Health Dent*. 2016;76(4):303–313.
12. Okunseri C, Gonzalez C, Hodgson B. Children's oral health assessment, prevention, and treatment. *PediatrClin North Am*. 2015;62(5):1215–1226.
13. Van der Weijden FA, Slot DE. Efficacy of homecare regimens for mechanical plaque removal in managing gingivitis a meta review. *J Clin Periodontol*. 2015;42(suppl 16):S77–S91.
14. Kurtz B, Reise M, Klukowska M, et al. A randomized clinical trial comparing plaque removal efficacy of an oscillating-rotating power toothbrush to a manual toothbrush by multiple examiners. *Int J Dent Hyg*. 2016;14(4):278–283.
15. Rmaile A, Carugo D, Capretto L, et al. Removal of interproximal dental biofilms by high-velocity water microdrops. *J Dent Res*. 2014;93(1):68–73.
16. Kotsakis GA, Lian Q, Ioannou AL, et al. The effectiveness of interproximal oral hygiene aids. *J Periodontol*. 2018;89:558–570.
17. Goyal CR, Lyle DM, Qaqish JG, et al. Efficacy of two interdental cleaning devices on clinical signs of inflammation: a four-week randomized controlled trial. *J Clin Dent*. 2015;26(2):55–60.
18. Zhan L. Rebalancing the caries microbiome dysbiosis: targeted treatment and sugar alcohols. *Adv Dent Res*. 2018;29(1):110–116.
19. Silva MF, Leite FRM, Ferreira LB, et al. Estimated prevalence of halitosis: a systematic review and meta-regression analysis. *Clin Oral Investig*. 2018;22(1):47–55.
20. Neely AL. Essential oil mouthwash (EOMW) may be equivalent to chlorhexidine (CHX) for long-term control of gingival inflammation but CHX appears to perform better than EOMW in plaque control. *J Evid Based Dent Pract*. 2012;12(3 Suppl):69–72.
21. Lee CT, Huang YW, Zhu L, et al. Prevalences of peri-implantitis and peri-implant mucositis: systematic review and meta-analysis. *J Dent*. 2017;62:1–12.
22. Caton JG, Armitage G, Berglundh T, et al. A new classification scheme for periodontal and peri-implant diseases and conditions—introduction and key changes from the 1999 classification. *J Periodontol*. 2018;89(suppl 1):S1–S8.
23. Fontana M, Gonzalez-Cabezas C. Evidence-based dentistry caries risk assessment and disease management. *Dent Clin North Am*. 2019;63(1):119–128.
24. Makhija SK, Bader JD, Shugars DA, et al. Influence of 2 caries-detecting devices on clinical decision making and lesion depth for suspicious occlusal lesions: a randomized trial from The National Dental Practice-Based Research Network. *J Am Dent Assoc*. 2018;149(4):299–307.
25. Berg SC, Stahl JM, Lien W. A clinical study comparing digital radiography and near-infrared transillumination in caries detection. *J Esthet Restor Dent*. 2018;30(1):39–44.
26. Maguire A. ADA clinical recommendations on topical fluoride for caries prevention. *Evid Based Dent*. 2014;15(2):38–39.
27. Slayton RL, Urquhart O, Araujo MWB, et al. Evidence-based clinical practice guideline on nonrestorative treatments for carious lesions: a report from the American Dental Association. *J Am Dent Assoc*. 2018;149(10):837–849.
28. American Academy of Pediatric Dentistry. Use of silver diamine fluoride for dental caries management in children and adolescents, including those with special health care needs. *Pediatr Dent*. 2017;39(6):146–155.
29. Wright JT, White A. Silver diamine fluoride: changing the caries management paradigm and potential societal impact. *N C Med J*. 2017;78(6):394–397.
30. Sinfiteli PP, Coutinho TCL, Oliveira PRA, et al. Effect of fluoride dentifrice and casein phosphopeptide-amorphous calcium phosphate cream with and without fluoride in preventing enamel demineralization in a pH cyclic study. *J Appl Oral Sci*. 2017;25(6):604–611.
31. Marghalani AA, Guinto E, Phan M, et al. Effectiveness of xylitol in reducing dental caries in children. *Pediatr Dent*. 2017;39(2):103–110.
32. Swango PA. Regular use of antimicrobial mouthrinses can effectively augment the benefits of oral prophylaxis and oral hygiene instructions at 6-month recall intervals in reducing the occurrence of dental plaque and gingivitis. *J Evid Based Dent Pract*. 2012;12(2):87–89.
33. Deery C. Clinical practice guidelines proposed the use of pit and fissure sealants to prevent and arrest noncavitated carious lesions. *J Evid Based Dent Pract*. 2017;17(1):48–50.
34. Eke PI, Thornton-Evans GO, Wei L, et al. Periodontitis in US adults: National Health and Nutrition Examination Survey 2009–2014. *J Am Dent Assoc*. 2018;149(7):576–588.
35. Ramôa CP, Eissenberg T, Sahingur SE. Increasing popularity of waterpipe tobacco smoking and electronic cigarette use: implications for oral healthcare. *J Periodontal Res*. 2017;52(5):813–823.
36. Lortet-Tieulent J, Goding Sauer A, Siegel RL, et al. State-level cancer mortality attributable to cigarette smoking in the United States. *JAMA Intern Med*. 2016;176(12):1792–1798.
37. 2008 PHS Guideline Update Panel, Liaisons, and Staff. Treating tobacco use and dependence: 2008 update US Public Health Service Clinical Practice Guideline executive summary. *Respir Care*. 2008 Sep;53(9):1217–1222.
38. Michaud DS, Fu Z, Shi J, et al. Periodontal disease, tooth loss, and cancer risk. *Epidemiol Rev*. 2017;39(1):49–58.

39. Speight PM, Epstein J, Kujan O, et al. Screening for oral cancer-a perspective from the Global Oral Cancer Forum. *Oral Surg Oral Med Oral Pathol Oral Radiol*. 2017;123(6):680–687.
40. Huber MA. Adjunctive diagnostic techniques for oral and oropharyngeal cancer discovery. *Dent Clin North Am*. 2018;62(1):59–75.
41. Alghaithy RA, Qualtrough AJ. Pulp sensibility and vitality tests for diagnosing pulpal health in permanent teeth: a critical review. *Int Endod J*. 2017;50(2):135–142.

## SUGGESTED READINGS

Harris NO, Garcia-Godoy F. *Primary Preventive Dentistry*. 8th ed. Upper Saddle River, NJ: Pearson Prentice Hall; 2013.

Molina A, García-Gargallo M, Montero E, et al. Clinical efficacy of desensitizing mouthwashes for the control of dentin hypersensitivity and root sensitivity: a systematic review and meta-analysis. *Int J Dent Hyg*. 2017;15(2):84–94.

Naavaal S, Malarcher A, Xu X, et al. Variations in cigarette smoking and quit attempts by health insurance among US adults in 41 states and 2 jurisdictions, 2014. *Public Health Rep*. 2018;133(2):191–199.

Speight PM, Epstein J, Kujan O, et al. Screening for oral cancer-a perspective from the Global Oral Cancer Forum. *Oral Surg Oral Med Oral Pathol Oral Radiol*. 2017;123(6):680–687.

Wilkins EM. *Clinical Practice of the Dental Hygienist*. 12th ed. Philadelphia: Lippincott Williams & Wilkins; 2017.

Papadiochou S, Polyzois G. Hygiene practices in removable prosthodontics: a systematic review. *Int J Dent Hyg*. 2018;16(2):179–201.

17

# Periodontal Instrumentation for Assessment and Care

*Danielle Rulli*

This chapter focuses on the use of periodontal instruments for assessment and nonsurgical periodontal instrumentation. The primary objective of nonsurgical periodontal instrumentation is to restore periodontal tissue to health by removing plaque biofilm, its by-products, and biofilm-retentive factors from tooth surfaces and from within the tooth pocket space. Successful professional care depends on reducing biofilm to a level that is acceptable to the tissue; therefore, instructing and supervising the patient's daily self-care precedes, continues with, and follows instrumentation by the dental hygiene practitioner.

## INSTRUMENT DESIGN

### Parts of an Instrument

A. Handle—the part of a periodontal instrument that the clinician holds; various shapes, weights, sizes, and surface serrations (smooth, ribbed, or knurled) exist
   1. Types
      a. Single-ended—one working end
      b. Double-ended—two working ends; working ends may be unpaired (dissimilar working ends) or paired (mirror-image working ends)
   2. Handle design characteristics
      a. Small-diameter (3/17-inch) handles, with smooth or flat texture, decrease the user's control and increase muscle fatigue
      b. Large-diameter (⅜-inch) handles that are lightweight and have bumpy texturing maximize the user's control and reduce muscle fatigue

B. Shank—connects the working end with the handle; usually bent in one or more places to facilitate placement of the working end against the tooth surface
   1. Functional shank—the part of the shank that allows the working end to be adapted to the tooth surface; begins below the working end and extends to the last bend in the shank nearest the handle
      a. Instruments with short functional shanks are used on teeth crowns
      b. Instruments with long functional shanks are used on both the crown and the root (Fig. 17.1)
   2. Lower (terminal) shank—the bent portion of the functional shank nearest to the working end (Fig. 17.1)
   3. Extended lower shank—3 mm longer than a standard lower shank; provides additional leverage, acting as a fulcrum, and is ideal for working in deep periodontal pockets
   4. Simple shank—bent in one plane (front to back); used primarily on anterior teeth; also called a *straight shank*
   5. Complex shank—bent in two planes (front to back and side to side) to facilitate instrumentation of posterior teeth; this design is necessary to reach around the crown and onto the root surface; also called an *angled shank* or *curved shank*

C. Working end—the part of the dental instrument that contacts the tooth (explorer, curet) or soft tissue (probe) to perform the work of the instrument; begins where the instrument shank ends; an instrument may have one or two working ends
   1. Parts of the working end—identified as the face, back, lateral surfaces, toe, and tip; on a hand-activated periodontal instrument, a cutting edge is formed by the union of a lateral surface and the face of the working end
   2. Application of the working end—the tooth surfaces or areas of the mouth on which an instrument can be used
      a. Anterior use—one single-ended instrument (e.g., anterior sickle scaler, such as a Jacquette 33) can be used to perform procedures on the facial, lingual, mesial, and distal surfaces of anterior teeth
      b. Posterior use—one double-ended instrument (e.g., posterior sickle scaler, such as a Jacquette 34/35) can be used to perform procedures on the facial, lingual, mesial, and distal surfaces of posterior teeth
      c. Universal use—one double-ended instrument (e.g., universal curet, such as a Columbia 13/14) can be used to perform procedures on both anterior and posterior teeth
      d. Area-specific use—an instrument that can be applied only to specific surfaces and areas of the mouth; a set of area-specific instruments (e.g., area-specific curets, such as the Gracey series) is needed for procedures on the entire dentition
   3. Function of the working end
      a. Assessment of teeth, soft tissue, or both
      b. Instrumentation of tooth surfaces (the removal or disruption of calculus deposits and plaque biofilm)

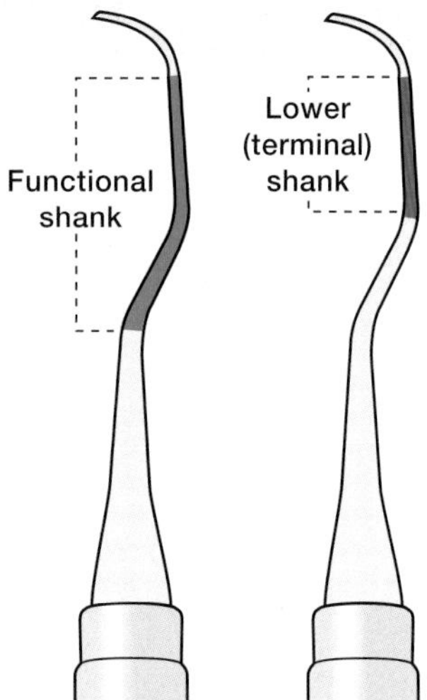


**Fig. 17.1** Functional shank and lower (terminal) shank. (From Nield-Gehrig JS. *Fundamentals of Periodontal Instrumentation and Advanced Root Instrumentation.* 6th ed. Philadelphia: Lippincott Williams & Wilkins; 2013.)

## Design Characteristics

A. Instrument balance—a balanced instrument has working ends that are aligned with the long axis of the handle
   1. During a work stroke—for example, in calculus removal; balance ensures that finger pressure applied against the handle is transferred to the working end, which results in pressure against the tooth
   2. An instrument that is not balanced is more difficult to use and increases stress on the muscles of the user's hand and arm

B. Instrument identification—the unique design name and number that identify each periodontal instrument
   1. Design name—identifies the school or individual responsible for the original design or development of an instrument or group of instruments (e.g., ODU 11/12 periodontal explorer, in which the ODU stands for Old Dominion University; and the TU-17, in which TU stands for Tufts University School of Dental Medicine)
   2. Design number—the number designation of the working end that, when combined with the design name, provides the exact identification of the working end (e.g., Gracey 11, in which Gracey is the design name, and 11 is the design number)
   3. Identification of the working ends of a double-ended instrument—a double-ended instrument will have two design numbers, one number for each working end of the instrument
      a. If the design name and number are stamped along the length of the handle, each working end is identified by the number closest to it
      b. If the design name and number are stamped across the handle, the first number identifies the working end at the top of the handle, and the second number identifies the working end at the bottom

**TABLE 17.1 Use of Hand-Activated Instruments**

| Classification | Purpose |
|---|---|
| Calibrated probe | Measurement of pocket depths, clinical attachment level, width of attached gingiva, gingival recession, and intraoral lesions; evaluation of gingival tissue for consistency and presence of bleeding or exudate |
| Furcation probe | Detection of furcation involvement in multirooted teeth |
| Explorer | Detection of calculus deposits, tooth surface irregularities, defective margins on restorations |
| Sickle scaler | Removal of medium-sized to large-sized calculus deposits from enamel surfaces; provides good access to the proximal surfaces on anterior crowns and the enamel surfaces apical to the contact areas of posterior teeth; should NOT be used on cementum |
| Periodontal file | Used to crush large calculus deposits and prepare burnished calculus before removal with another instrument; should NOT be used directly on cemental surfaces |
| Universal curet | Instrumentation of crown and root surfaces; removal of light to medium-sized supragingival and subgingival calculus deposits; some designs have long functional shanks that allow access to the cervical and middle thirds of root surfaces |
| Area-specific curet | Instrumentation of crown and root surfaces; removal of light supragingival and subgingival calculus deposits; some designs have extended shanks that allow access to the middle and apical thirds of root surfaces |

(From Nield-Gehrig JS. *Fundamentals of Periodontal Instrumentation and Advanced Root Instrumentation.* 6th ed. Philadelphia: Lippincott Williams & Wilkins; 2013.)

# HAND-ACTIVATED INSTRUMENTS

## Classifications

A. Hand-activated nonsurgical periodontal instruments include assessment instruments comprised of periodontal probes, explorers, and mirrors; treatment instruments include sickle scalers, periodontal files, universal curets (or curettes), and area-specific curets (Table 17.1). Hoes and chisels are rarely used because their functions have been largely replaced by ultrasonic and sonic devices

B. Periodontal instruments are divided into classifications based on the specific design characteristics of the working end
   1. Design of the cutting edges, back, lateral surfaces, and shank
   2. Cross section of the working end
   3. Relationship of the face to the lower shank

C. In selecting an instrument for a specific task, one of the most important considerations is the classification of the working end

## Dental Mirror

A. Characteristics
   1. Assessment instrument used to visualize the hard and soft tissues of the oral cavity
   2. The working end has a reflecting (mirrored) surface
   3. Types
      a. Front surface—the reflecting surface is on the front surface of the glass; produces a clear mirror image with no distortion

**TABLE 17.2 Examples of Probe Markings**

| Type | Marking Pattern | Increments (mm) |
|---|---|---|
| UNC15 | All mm marked | 1 to 15 |
| Glickman 26G | No mark at 6 mm | 1–2–3–5–7–8–9–10 |
| Goldman Fox | No mark at 6 mm | 1–2–3–5–7–8–9–10 |
| Merritt | No mark at 6 mm | 1–2–3–5–7–8–9–10 |
| Williams | No mark at 6 mm | 1–2–3–5–7–8–9–10 |
| Maryland Moffitt | No mark at 6 mm; ball-end | 1–2–3–5–7–8–9–10 |
| Michigan "O" | Marks at 3, 6, and 8 mm | 3–6–8 |
| PSR Screening | Colored band from 3.5–5.5; marks at 8.5 and 11.5 mm; ball end | 3.5–5.5–8.5–11.5 |
| CP-18 | Colored bands from 3–5 and 8–10 | 3–5–8–10 |
| CP-11 | Colored bands from 3–6 and 8–11 | 3–6–8–11 |
| CP-12 | Colored bands from 3–6 and 9–12 | 3–6–9–12 |
| Hu-Friedy Novatech | Right-angled probe; available in a wide variety of designs | Available in various increments |

(From Nield-Gehrig JS. *Fundamentals of Periodontal Instrumentation and Advanced Root Instrumentation.* 6th ed. Philadelphia: Lippincott Williams & Wilkins; 2013.)

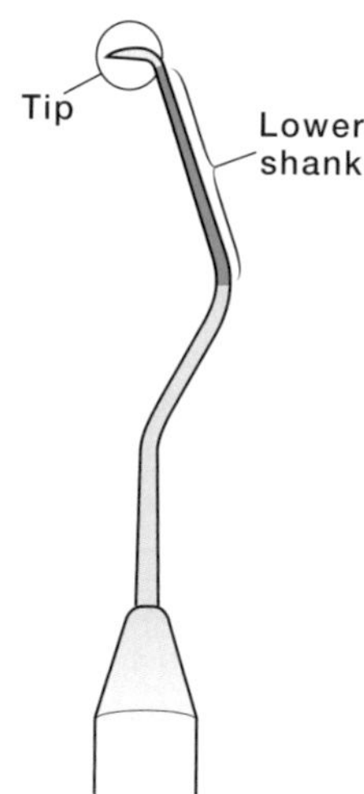


**Fig. 17.2** Design characteristics of a dental explorer. (From Nield-Gehrig JS. *Fundamentals of Periodontal Instrumentation and Advanced Root Instrumentation.* 6th ed. Philadelphia: Lippincott Williams & Wilkins; 2013.)

b. Concave—the reflecting surface is on the front surface of the mirror lens; produces a magnified but slightly distorted image

c. Plane—the reflecting surface is on the back surface of the mirror lens; this type of surface is less easily scratched than a front surface mirror and produces a double or "ghost" image

B. Uses

1. Indirect vision—the mirror's reflecting surface provides a view of the tooth surface or intraoral structure that cannot be seen directly
2. Retraction—using the mirror to hold the patient's cheek or tongue to view tooth surfaces or other structures that are otherwise hidden by the cheeks or tongue
3. Indirect illumination—reflecting light from the mirrored surface into a dark area of the mouth
4. Transillumination—reflecting light from the mirrored surface through anterior teeth

## Probe

A. Characteristics

1. Assessment instrument that is used to evaluate the health of periodontal tissue
2. Two types: calibrated and furcation probes

B. Types

1. Calibrated probe (e.g., Williams, PSR screening probe) has a slender, rod-shaped, blunt working end marked in millimeter increments; can be used as a miniature ruler for making intraoral measurements, such as for measuring sulcus and pocket depths, clinical attachment levels (CALs), width of attached gingiva, or the size of oral lesions; also used to assess for the presence of bleeding or purulent exudate (pus)
2. Furcation probe (e.g., Nabers 1 N) is a curved, blunt-tipped instrument used to detect and assess bone loss in the furcation areas of bifurcated and trifurcated teeth
3. Biotype probe is a flat, plastic, blunt-tipped instrument consisting of three separate tips with different white, green or blue color blocks used to determine thin, medium, or thick tissue, respectively

C. Calibrations—millimeter marks at intervals that are specific for each probe design

1. Calibrated probes
   a. Probe designs may differ in millimeter markings (Table 17.2); only certain millimeter increments may be indicated on the probe (e.g., 1—2—3—5—7—8—9—10 mm), or each millimeter may be indicated (e.g., 1—2—3—4—5—6—7—8—9—10—11—12—13—14—15 mm)
   b. Color-coded probes are marked in bands (often black), with each band being several millimeters in width (e.g., 3 to 5 mm and 8 to 10 mm)
2. Furcation probes
   a. Most furcation probes do not have millimeter markings
   b. Some furcation probes are marked in bands (usually black), with each band being several millimeters in width (e.g., 3 to 6 mm and 6 to 9 mm); these probes usually are used in research investigations to facilitate investigators' calibration

## Explorer

A. Characteristics

1. Assessment instrument with a fine, flexible wire-like working end
2. Provides the best tactile information to the clinician's fingers; used to locate calculus deposits, tooth surface irregularities, and defective margins on restorations

B. Design (Fig. 17.2)

1. The working end is 1 to 2 mm in length and is referred to as the tip; the side of the tip, rather than the actual point, is used for detecting calculus
2. Circular in cross section, the explorer may have paired or unpaired working ends

C. Types—available in a variety of design types; not all design types are well suited to subgingival use; therefore, the clinician must be knowledgeable about the recommended use of each design type
   1. Shepherd hook (e.g., #23 and #54 explorers)—an unpaired explorer with a short, highly curved shank and a sharp point; used for supragingival examinations to detect irregular margins of restorations; not recommended for calculus detection because subgingival use could result in tissue trauma
   2. Straight explorer (e.g., 6, 6A, 6 L, 6XL)—an unpaired explorer with a short lower shank and a sharp point; used for examinations to detect irregular margins of restorations; not recommended for subgingival calculus detection
   3. Curved explorer (e.g., 3, 3A)—an unpaired explorer with a curved shank and a sharp point; limited for use in examining normal sulci or shallow pockets; may be used for calculus detection; however, care must be taken not to injure the junctional epithelium when the working end is used subgingivally
   4. Orban-type explorer (e.g., TU-17, Orban 20)—an unpaired explorer with a straight lower shank that can be used in deep pockets with only slight tissue displacement (stretching of the tissue wall away from the tooth); the explorer tip is bent at a 90-degree angle to the terminal shank, which allows the back of the tip (instead of the point) to be directed toward the junctional epithelium; useful for detecting subgingival calculus on anterior teeth or on the facial and lingual surfaces of posterior teeth; however, the straight lower shank makes it difficult to adapt to the line angles and proximal surfaces of posterior teeth
   5. Pigtail or cowhorn explorer (e.g., 3MI, 3CH, 2A)—a paired universal explorer with a short, broadly curved lower shank and a sharp point; the curved lower shank causes considerable tissue displacement; useful for detecting calculus in normal sulci or shallow pockets extending no deeper than the cervical third of the root
   6. The 11/12-type explorer (e.g., ODU 11/12, 11/12 AF)—a paired universal explorer with an extended lower shank and a tip that is bent at a 90-degree angle to the terminal shank; the tip design allows the back of the tip to be applied to the pocket base without lacerating the junctional epithelium; this effective explorer design adapts well to all surfaces throughout the mouth and is equally useful when exploring a shallow sulcus or a deep periodontal pocket

## Sickle Scaler

A. Characteristics
   1. Calculus removal instrument; limited for use on enamel surfaces
   2. Anterior and posterior designs

B. Design (Fig. 17.3)
   1. Cutting edges—two cutting edges that meet in a point
   2. Back—sharp, pointed back; some types of scalers are made with flattened backs

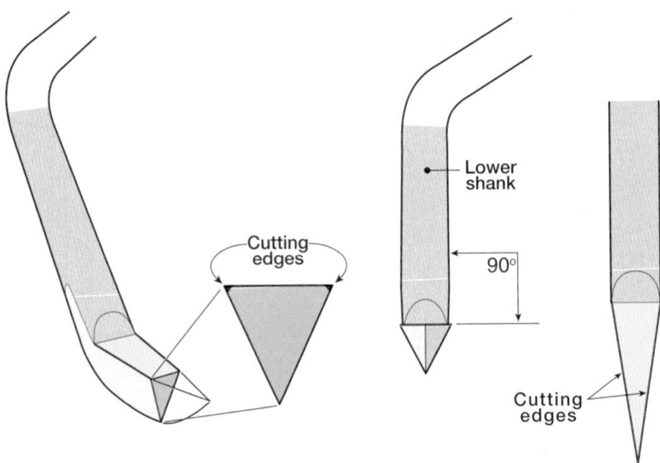


**Fig. 17.3** Design characteristics of a sickle scaler, consisting of two-level cutting edges that meet in a point and an instrument face that is at a 90-degree angle to the lower shank. (From Nield-Gehrig JS. *Fundamentals of Periodontal Instrumentation and Advanced Root Instrumentation*. 6th ed. Philadelphia: Lippincott Williams & Wilkins; 2013.)

   3. Cross section—triangular; lateral surfaces meet the instrument face at an internal angle between 70 and 80 degrees
   4. Face—perpendicular to the lower shank so that the cutting edges are level with each other; level cutting edges require that the lower shank be tilted slightly toward the tooth surface to establish correct angulation
   5. The anterior sickle scaler has an unpaired working end and a simple shank; primarily used on anterior teeth (e.g., Jacquette 33)
   6. The posterior sickle scaler has paired working ends, with complex shanks; primarily used on posterior teeth but may be used on anterior teeth (e.g., Jacquette 34/35)

C. Uses
   1. Removal of medium-sized to large calculus deposits from enamel tooth surfaces
   2. Provides good access to the proximal surfaces on anterior crowns and to the enamel surfaces apical to the contact areas of posterior teeth

D. Limitations
   1. The pointed tip and the straight cutting edges do not adapt well to rounded root surfaces and concavities
   2. The pointed back is not suited to subgingival use (may injure the junctional epithelium)

## Periodontal File

A. Characteristics
   1. Calculus removal instrument used to prepare calculus deposits before removal with another instrument
   2. Anterior and posterior designs

B. Design
   1. Cutting edges—multiple cutting edges at a 90- to 105-degree angle to the lower shank
   2. Working end—thin in width with a large circumference at the base; the base may be round, oval, or rectangular in shape

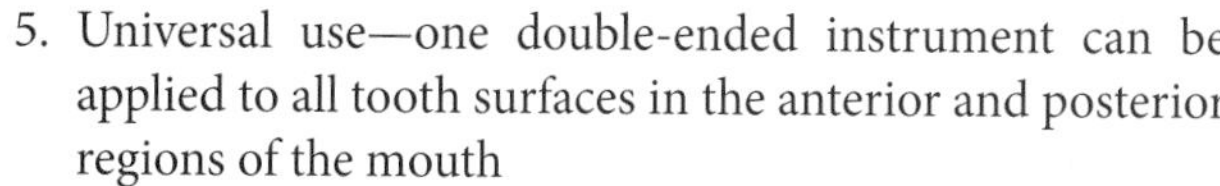

3. Area-specific application—each working end is designed for use on a single surface (four working ends are needed for procedures on all tooth surfaces); files with simple shanks work best on anterior teeth; those with complex shanks work best on posterior teeth

C. Uses
1. Preparation of burnished calculus deposit (a deposit with a smooth outer surface) before definitive removal of the deposit with a curet; a file is used to scratch the surface of a burnished deposit so that it can be removed with another instrument
2. Crushing of a large calculus deposit; once a deposit has been crushed with a file, it is easier to remove with a curet
3. Smoothing overextended or rough amalgam restoration in sites where the file can be effectively adapted

D. Limitations
1. Limited to use on enamel surfaces or to applications on the outer surface of a calculus deposit; gouging could result if a file is used on root surfaces
2. The working ends have straight cutting edges on a flat base; do not adapt well to curved tooth surfaces

## Universal Curet

A. Characteristics
1. One of the most frequently used and versatile of all the instruments for calculus removal
2. Used both supragingivally and subgingivally; two curets usually are paired on a double-ended instrument (the paired working ends are mirror images of each other)

B. Design (Fig. 17.4)
1. Cutting edges—two cutting edges that converge in a rounded toe
2. Back—the rounded back is ideal for subgingival use
3. Cross section—semicircular; lateral surfaces meet the instrument face at an internal angle between 70 and 80 degrees
4. Face—perpendicular to the lower shank so that the cutting edges are level with each other; the level cutting edges require that the lower shank be tilted slightly toward the tooth surface to establish correct angulation

5. Universal use—one double-ended instrument can be applied to all tooth surfaces in the anterior and posterior regions of the mouth

C. Uses
1. Calculus removal from crown and root surfaces
2. Removal of small to medium-sized calculus deposits

D. Limitations
1. The toe is wider than a pointed tip and therefore may be more difficult to adapt for use beneath the contact areas of anterior teeth
2. The level cutting edges require that the lower shank be tilted slightly toward the tooth for correct angulation

## Area-Specific Curet

A. Characteristics
1. Calculus removal instrument with one cutting edge (only one cutting edge per working end is used for procedures); a set of curets is needed to perform procedures throughout the mouth
2. The curet is used supragingivally and subgingivally; especially well-suited for instrumentation of roots within periodontal pockets
3. Designs include area-specific curets with flexible and rigid shanks

B. Design (Fig. 17.5)
1. Cutting edge—one working cutting edge per working end; only the lower, longer cutting edge is used
2. Back—rounded back; ideal for subgingival use
3. Cross section—semicircular; the lateral surfaces meet the instrument face at an internal angle between 70 and 80 degrees
4. Face—tilted at a 60- to 70-degree angle in relation to the lower shank, making one cutting edge (the working cutting edge) lower than the other; this tilted relationship makes the working cutting edge "self-angulated"; that is, when the lower shank is parallel to the tooth surface, the cutting edge is at the correct angulation

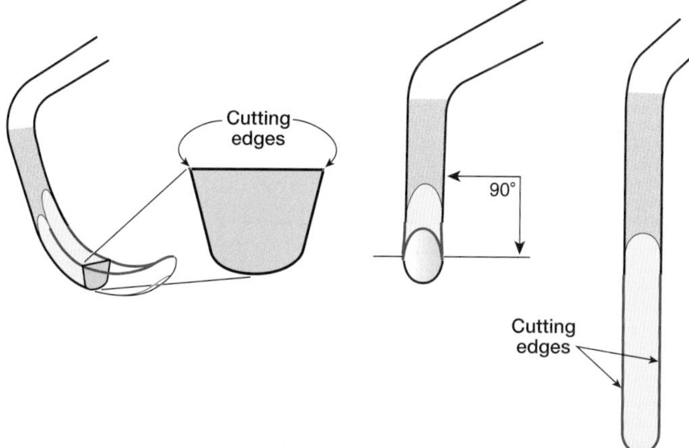


**Fig. 17.4** Design characteristics of a universal curet, consisting of two-level cutting edges and an instrument face that is at a 90-degree angle to the lower shank. (From Nield-Gehrig JS. *Fundamentals of Periodontal Instrumentation and Advanced Root Instrumentation.* 6th ed. Philadelphia: Lippincott Williams & Wilkins; 2013.)

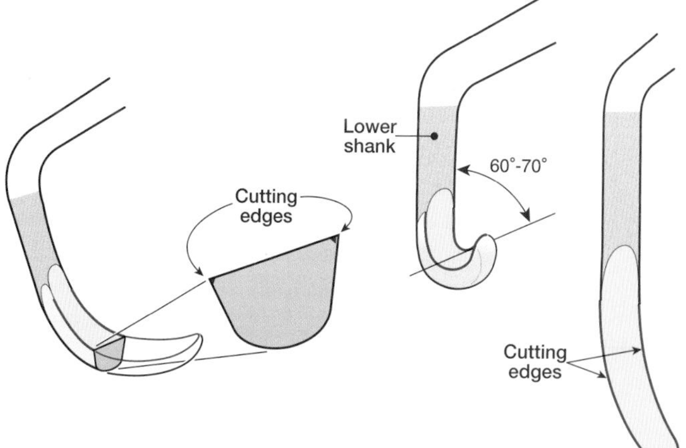


**Fig. 17.5** Design characteristics of an area-specific curet, consisting of one cutting edge, an instrument face at a 70-degree angle to the lower shank, and one cutting edge positioned lower than the other, nonworking cutting edge. (From Nield-Gehrig JS. *Fundamentals of Periodontal Instrumentation and Advanced Root Instrumentation.* 6th ed. Philadelphia: Lippincott Williams & Wilkins; 2013.)

5. Area-specific use—each working end is limited to use only on certain teeth and on certain surfaces

C. Uses
1. Instrumentation of crown and root surfaces
2. Removal of small deposits of calculus and biofilm

D. Limitations
1. The toe is wider than a pointed tip and is therefore more difficult to adapt to the proximal surfaces of anterior crowns
2. A single working cutting edge per working end means exchanging instruments more frequently

### Advanced Root Instrumentation

A. Characteristics
1. The treatment of patients with periodontitis requires specialized instruments with longer shank lengths and miniature working ends for instrumentation of root concavities and furcation areas
2. Designs include area-specific curets with miniature working ends, extended shanks, flexible and rigid shanks, and diamond-coated working ends

B. Examples of advanced periodontal instruments—a variety of periodontal instruments have been developed to increase treatment effectiveness on root surfaces within deep periodontal pockets
1. The 11/12-type periodontal explorer—an 11/12 AF (After Five) explorer has an extended shank and is ideal for use in deep periodontal pockets
2. Advanced curet designs—several curets are ideal for instrumentation within deep periodontal pockets
   a. Vision Curvette curet series—have a working end that is shortened to half the length of a standard Gracey curet, a curved working end, and an extended lower shank, and shank demarcations to identify depth of insertion
   b. Modified Gracey curets
      (1) Several varieties of modified Gracey curets—include modified Gracey curets with extended shanks, miniature Gracey curets, and micro Gracey curets
      (2) Design features for modified Gracey curets—include extended lower shank length, thinner working ends, and working ends that are shorter in length than in a standard Gracey curet
   c. Langer curets—have a 90% angle from the terminal shank to the blade for use on both mesial and distal surfaces
   d. Quétin (kee′-tan) furcation curets—specialized instruments that are used to debride furcation areas and root concavities; each miniature working end has a single, straight cutting edge with rounded corners; the working ends are available in either 0.9-mm or 1.3-mm size
   e. DeMarco furcation curets—specialized instruments that are used to debride furcation areas and root concavities; the working ends are discoid shaped and allow all sides of the blade to debride; available in 0.9 mm or 1.3 mm sizes
   f. O'Hehir debridement curets—area-specific curets that are designed to remove light residual calculus deposits and bacterial contaminants from root surfaces
      (1) The working end of an O'Hehir curet is a tiny circular disc; the entire working end is a cutting edge; the working end curves into the tooth for easy adaptation in furcation areas and developmental grooves
      (2) These curets have extended lower shanks
   g. Instruments with diamond-coated working ends
      (1) The working ends of these instruments do not have cutting edges; instead, they are coated with a very fine diamond grit; for example, a version of the Nabers furcation probe is diamond-coated
      (2) Diamond-coated instruments can be used to remove light, residual calculus deposits
      (3) Because of the abrasive nature of their working ends, these instruments should be used with light, even pressure against the root surface to avoid gouging or grooving

## PRINCIPLES OF INSTRUMENTATION

### Position of the Clinician

A. Neutral, seated position (Fig. 17.6)
1. Head—tilt of 0 to 15 degrees
2. Shoulders—in a horizontal line
3. Back—straight or leaning forward slightly from the waist or hips
4. Thighs—hips slightly higher than the knees

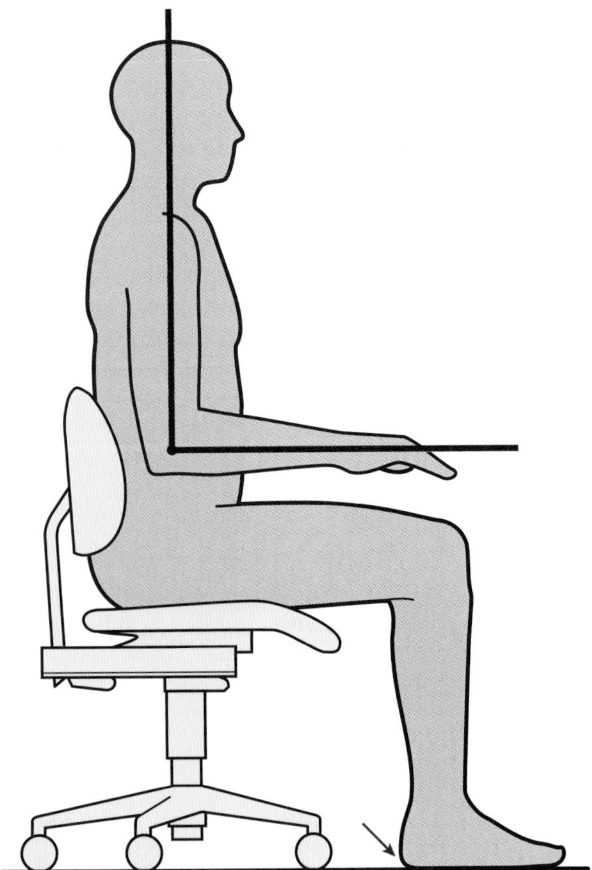

**Fig. 17.6** Neutral seated position for the clinician. (From Nield-Gehrig JS. *Fundamentals of Periodontal Instrumentation and Advanced Root Instrumentation.* 6th ed. Philadelphia: Lippincott Williams & Wilkins; 2013.)

5. Upper arms—parallel to the long axis of the torso
6. Elbows—at waist level; held slightly away from body
7. Forearms—parallel to the floor; raised or lowered, if necessary, by pivoting at the elbow joint rather than by raising the elbows
8. Feet—seat height should be positioned low enough so that the heels of the feet can rest on the floor

B. Relationship to the patient and the dental unit
   1. The patient's chair should be positioned such that the tip of the patient's nose is at a level slightly lower than clinician's elbows; clinician should not have to raise the elbows above his or her waist level to reach the patient's mouth; lower arms should be in a horizontal position or raised slightly so that the angle formed between the lower and upper arm is slightly less than 90 degrees
   2. All instruments and equipment should be positioned within easy reach of the clinician

## Stabilization During Instrumentation

A. Modified pen grasp—the recommended grasp for holding a periodontal instrument that allows precise control of the working end; precise placement of the fingers in the modified pen grasp is important to be successful in instrumentation technique
   1. Finger placement and function (Fig. 17.7)
      a. Index finger and thumb—finger pads hold the instrument handle

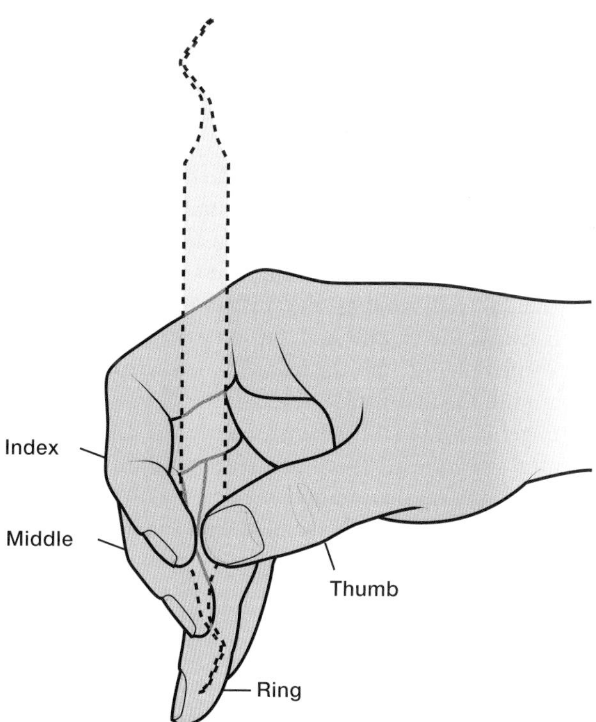


**Fig. 17.7** Finger placement in the modified pen grasp. The index finger and the thumb hold the instrument handle. The middle finger rests on the instrument shank. The ring finger acts as a support for the hand and instrument. (From Nield-Gehrig JS. *Fundamentals of Periodontal Instrumentation and Advanced Root Instrumentation*. 6th ed. Philadelphia: Lippincott Williams & Wilkins; 2013.)

      b. Middle finger—the side of the finger pad rests on the instrument's shank; the clinician's fingers should be able to feel the vibrations in the instrument's shank as the working end encounters roughness on the tooth surface
      c. Ring finger—fingertip rests on a stable surface, usually the occlusal or incisal tooth surface, which stabilizes the hand for control and strength
   2. Technique
      a. A light grasp is needed for increased tactile sensitivity during assessment procedures (e.g., subgingival use of explorer or probe)
      b. A firm grasp is used with hand-activated instruments during calculus removal
   3. Glove fit—proper fit of sterile gloves is important in avoiding muscle strain during instrumentation
      a. Select right-hand and left-hand fitted gloves rather than ambidextrous gloves
      b. Select gloves that come in a range of numbered sizes (e.g., 5½, 6, 6½) rather than those marked in size ranges of small, medium, and large

B. Fulcrum and finger rest
   1. Definitions
      a. Fulcrum—the point of support on which the clinician rests the hand; used to stabilize the clinician's hand during instrumentation; the pad of the ring finger serves as the fulcrum finger during instrumentation to control stroke pressure and length
      b. Finger rest—the place where the fulcrum finger rests during instrumentation
   2. Types of fulcrums
      a. Basic intraoral fulcrum
         (1) The finger rest is placed on a tooth, close to the tooth being worked on; should not be positioned in the line of the instrument's stroke to prevent instrument stick
         (2) The intraoral fulcrum is considered the most desirable because it provides the greatest stability and strength for calculus removal
      b. Basic extraoral fulcrum—placed outside the patient's mouth, usually on the chin or cheek
      c. Advanced fulcrums—variations of the basic fulcrum that may be required for access to posterior teeth or root surfaces within periodontal pockets; advanced fulcrums require greater skill and stroke control than the basic intraoral fulcrum
   3. Advanced fulcrum techniques
      a. Piggybacked—intraoral fulcrum in which the middle finger is stacked on top of the ring finger
      b. Cross-arch—intraoral fulcrum in which the finger rests on the side of the mouth opposite the treatment area (treatment area is mandibular right quadrant, finger rest on mandibular left quadrant)
      c. Opposite arch—intraoral fulcrum in which the finger rests on the arch opposite to the treatment area (treatment area on mandibular arch, finger rest on maxillary arch)

d. Finger-on-finger—intraoral fulcrum in which the finger of the nondominant hand serves as the resting point for the ring finger of the dominant hand
e. Stabilized—intraoral or extraoral fulcrum in which a finger of the nondominant hand is used to concentrate lateral pressure against the tooth surface and to help control the instrument stroke

## Adaptation

A. Definition—positioning the first 1 or 2 mm of the lateral surface of the instrument's working end in contact with the tooth surface
B. Characteristics
 1. Explorer—the first few millimeters of the tip (not the point) are adapted to the tooth surface for calculus detection
 2. Probe—the side of the probe tip is maintained against the tooth surface, with the length of the probe almost parallel to the tooth surface being probed
 3. Sickles and curets—the leading one-third of the cutting edge is positioned to conform to the tooth surface

## Angulation

A. Definition—the relationship between the instrument face and the tooth surface to which the working end is applied
B. Principles
 1. For insertion beneath the gingival margin—the face-to-tooth surface angulation is between 0 and 40 degrees
 2. For calculus removal—the face-to-tooth surface angulation is between 45 and 90 degrees; a 60-degree angulation works well for biofilm removal, whereas a 70- to 80-degree angulation is ideal for calculus removal (Fig. 17.8)

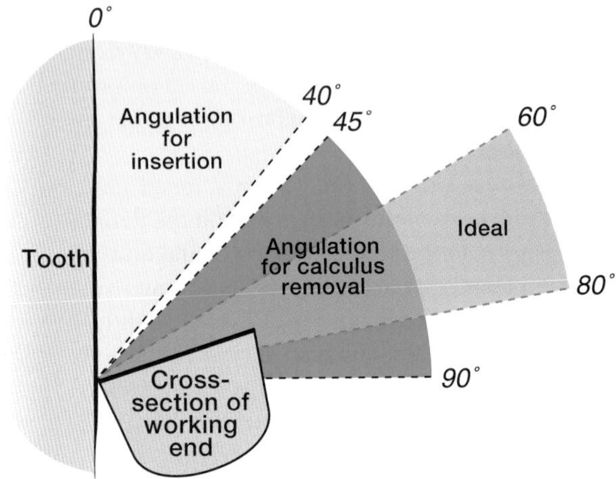


**Fig. 17.8** Angulation for calculus removal should be between 45 and 90 degrees. An angulation between 60 and 80 degrees is ideal for calculus removal. (From Nield-Gehrig JS. *Fundamentals of Periodontal Instrumentation and Advanced Root Instrumentation.* 6th ed. Philadelphia: Lippincott Williams & Wilkins; 2013.)

## Activation

A. Definition—moving an instrument to produce a stroke; it is the action of an instrument in the performance of the task for which it was designed
B. Types
 1. Hand-forearm activation
  a. Made by rotating the hand and forearm as a unit to provide the power for the instrumentation stroke; similar to the action of turning a doorknob
  b. Uses the power of the hand and arm to move the instrument; recommended for calculus removal with hand-activated instruments
 2. Digital (finger) activation
  a. Created by flexing the thumb, index, and middle fingers to move the instrument
  b. Used whenever physical strength is not required during a task, such as when using ultrasonic or sonic instruments, probes, and explorers
C. Stabilization and lateral pressure
 1. Definitions
  a. Stabilization—preparing for an instrument's stroke by locking the joints of the ring finger and pressing the fingertip against the tooth surface to provide control for the stroke
  b. Lateral pressure—applying pressure equally with the index finger and the thumb inward against the instrument's handle to engage the working end apical to a calculus deposit before and throughout a calculus removal or assessment stroke
 2. Stroke pressure
  a. Pressure during stroke activation—stroke pressure is applied in a coronal direction; the pressure ranges from light to firm, depending on the amount of pressure needed for the particular task (e.g., assessment, calculus removal)
  b. Pressure between strokes—finger muscles should be relaxed as the working end is repositioned, using light stroke pressure
D. Maintaining adaptation during stroke production
 1. Hand pivot—turning the hand and arm slightly while resting on the fulcrum to maintain adaptation; used when moving around line angles and onto proximal surfaces
 2. Handle roll—rolling the instrument handle slightly between the thumb and the index finger to maintain adaptation as the instrumentation strokes advance around the tooth surface; either the thumb or the index finger is used to roll the instrument
E. Neutral wrist position—correct wrist position is important to avoid muscle discomfort and injury during the procedure; the wrist should be aligned with the long axis of the forearm; bending the wrist up, down, or to the side should be avoided

## Instrumentation Strokes

A. Types of strokes
 1. Assessment strokes—used to evaluate a subgingival root surface or the health of periodontal tissue
  a. Used with probes, explorers, curets
  b. Angulation—50 to 70 degrees
  c. Lateral pressure—in contact with the tooth surface; light pressure

d. Character—fluid strokes of moderate length
e. Number—many strokes used to cover the entire root surface
2. Work strokes for calculus removal
a. Used with hand-activated sickle scalers, curets, and files
b. Angulation—70 to 80 degrees
c. Lateral pressure—moderate to firm
d. Character—powerful strokes; short in length
e. Number—the number of strokes should be limited to the areas where needed
3. Work strokes for removal of residual calculus deposits and biofilm removal
a. Used with hand-activated curets
b. Angulation—60 to 70 degrees
c. Lateral pressure—light to moderate
d. Character—lighter strokes of moderate length
e. Number—many strokes used to cover the entire root surface

B. Stroke direction
1. Vertical—parallel to the long axis of the tooth; used on facial, lingual, and proximal surfaces of anterior teeth and on the mesial and distal surfaces of posterior teeth
2. Oblique—diagonal to the long axis of the tooth; used most often on facial and lingual surfaces
3. Horizontal—perpendicular to the long axis of the tooth; used at the line angles of posterior teeth, furcation crotch areas, and within pockets that are too narrow to allow vertical or oblique strokes
4. Multidirectional—a combination of vertical, oblique, and horizontal strokes, one by one, used in succession on of a subgingival tooth surface

C. Stroke characteristics
1. Length—short, powerful stroke for calculus removal; longer, lighter stroke for removal of residual calculus deposits and biofilm
2. Overlap—strokes should overlap to ensure complete coverage; long ridges of calculus are treated in sections, in overlapping scaling zones
3. Pattern
a. Large calculus deposits should be removed in sections with a series of short, firm strokes
(1) A calculus deposit should not be removed in layers because removing the outermost layer will leave the deposit with a smooth surface (burnished surface)
(2) A burnished calculus deposit may be indistinguishable (when explored) from the tooth surface
b. For subgingival instrumentation, it is helpful to imagine that the root surface is divided into a series of narrow, diagonal instrumentation zones
(1) Each instrumentation zone is only as wide as the toe-third of the cutting edge
(2) Deposits are removed in each zone, from the junctional epithelium to the gingival margin, before progressing to the next zone

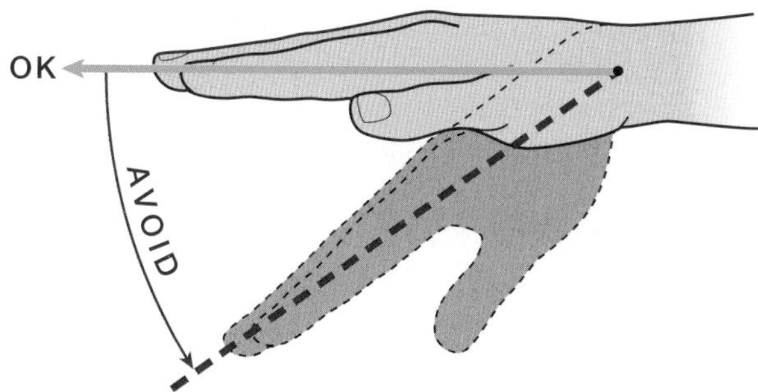


**Fig. 17.9** Neutral wrist position. The wrist should be aligned with the long axis of the forearm. (From Nield-Gehrig JS. *Fundamentals of Periodontal Instrumentation and Advanced Root Instrumentation.* 6th ed. Philadelphia: Lippincott Williams & Wilkins; 2013.)

## STEPS FOR CALCULUS REMOVAL WITH HAND-ACTIVATED INSTRUMENTS

A. Position the dental mirror, and establish a finger rest
B. Grasp the instrument in a modified pen grasp
C. Establish a finger rest
1. Locate the finger rest near the site of instrumentation in the dental arch; precise control of the instrument's stroke becomes more difficult as the finger rest is moved farther away from the site of the procedure
2. Select the correct working end of the instrument

D. Adjust the hand-wrist-forearm as a unit
1. Position the thumb and the index finger across from each other on the instrument handle, near the junction of the handle and shank
2. Lightly rest one side of the middle finger pad on the instrument shank
3. Place the other side of the middle finger pad against the ring finger to allow the hand to function as a unit during the production of the stroke
4. Balance the tip of the ring finger on an occlusal or an incisal surface to support the weight of the hand and instrument
5. Position the wrist in a neutral position so that it is aligned with the long axis of the forearm (Fig. 17.9)

E. Adapt the cutting edge
1. If working subgingivally, close the face of the working end toward the tooth, and slide the working end to the junctional epithelium; use a light grasp while positioning the working end
2. Adapt the toe-third of the cutting edge to the tooth surface just apical to the deposit
3. Establish the instrument face-to-tooth surface angulation of 70 and 80 degrees
4. Fine-tune the grasp and the wrist position

F. Stabilize the grasp, and apply lateral pressure
1. Press down with the ring finger against the finger rest
2. Apply pressure against the instrument handle with the index finger and the thumb

G. Activate a pulling stroke away from the junctional epithelium
1. Use hand-forearm activation for strength and control
2. Activate instrumentation strokes in a coronal direction to prevent particles of calculus from being pushed into soft tissue

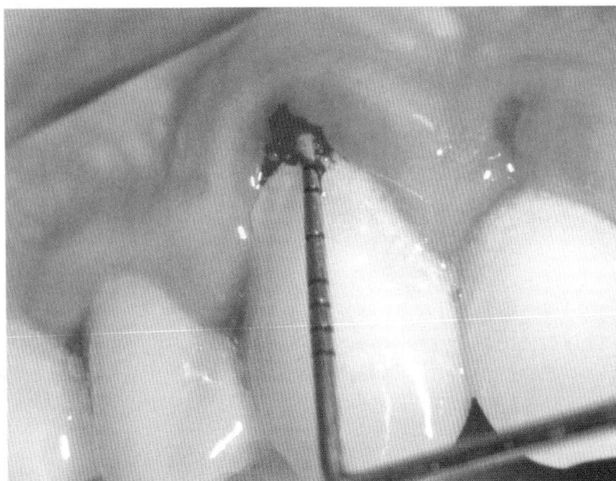

**Fig. 17.10** Assessment for the presence of bleeding. Bleeding on probing is an early clinical sign of inflammation. (From Nield-Gehrig JS. *Fundamentals of Periodontal Instrumentation and Advanced Root Instrumentation*. 6th ed. Philadelphia: Lippincott Williams & Wilkins; 2013.)

3. Use vertical and oblique strokes in most areas; supplement these strokes with horizontal strokes, as needed
4. Use short, powerful strokes for calculus removal and longer, lighter strokes for removal of residual calculus deposits and biofilm
5. Use overlapping strokes to ensure complete coverage of the entire root surface

H. Pause briefly at the end of a stroke
   1. Relax the grasp, the finger rest, and the lateral pressure
   2. Use a relaxed grasp to reposition the working end of the instrument for the next stroke

I. Check the instrumentation area frequently with an explorer to ensure deposit is being removed

## INSTRUMENTATION FOR ASSESSMENT

### Basic Concepts

A. Thorough assessment involves examining all aspects of the periodontium and teeth

B. Patient preparation, based on information from the personal, comprehensive health and dental histories, is essential for safe instrumentation

C. Successful treatment depends on well-developed assessment skills, before instrumentation for dental hygiene care planning and during and after instrumentation for evaluating treatment outcomes

### Assessments With Periodontal Probes

A. Purposes of the periodontal examination
   1. Aid in planning dental hygiene care by determining gingival characteristics, probing depth, level of attachment, and presence of bone loss
   2. Determine the extent of inflammation in conjunction with the probing depth and attachment level; bleeding resulting from probing is an early clinical sign of inflammation (Fig. 17.10)
   3. Evaluation of treatment outcomes according to:
      a. Tissue response to the patient's self-care and nonsurgical periodontal therapy
      b. Evidence of health determined by the probe
         (1) No bleeding on gentle probing
         (2) CALs remain the same or decrease in depth

B. Factors that may affect probing accuracy
   1. Probe design
      a. Calibration—the probe must be clearly and accurately marked and easy to read; the clinician must be knowledgeable about the calibration pattern
      b. Thickness—a thinner probe causes less distention of the sulcus or the pocket wall; use a probe no larger than 0.5 mm in diameter
   2. Influence of tissue health and related factors
      a. Tissue resistance—with light pressure, the probe is inserted until it meets the physical resistance of the base of the sulcus or the periodontal pocket
         (1) Normal tissue—the junctional epithelium offers more resistance; probing is stopped by the coronal portion of the junctional epithelium
         (2) Gingivitis and early periodontitis—the junctional epithelium offers less resistance; the probe tip passes farther into the junctional epithelium
         (3) Advanced periodontitis—the junctional epithelium offers little or no resistance; the probe tip may penetrate the junctional epithelium to reach the attached connective tissue fibers
      b. Dental calculus—large calculus deposits can hinder the placement of the probe
   3. Concepts of probing technique
      a. Adaptation—place the side of the probe tip against the tooth surface, with the length of the probe positioned as parallel as possible to the tooth surface; to assess the col region, tilt the probe so that the tip reaches under the contact area
      b. Stroke technique—strokes must be close to each other as the probe is "walked" along the entire circumference of the junctional epithelium
      c. Pressure—a light pressure of 10 to 20 g should be sufficient

### Probing Technique

A. Parallelism—the probe is positioned as parallel as possible to the tooth surface being probed

B. Adaptation—the side of the probe tip is maintained in contact with the tooth at all times

C. Activation—digital (finger) activation may be used with the probe because only light pressure is used when probing

D. Walking strokes—a series of bobbing strokes made within the sulcus or the pocket while keeping the probe tip against the tooth
   1. The junctional epithelium is continuous around a tooth, and the probing depth may vary considerably on different surfaces; for complete evaluation, the entire circumference of the sulcus or the pocket base should be assessed with a series of probing strokes

2. The probe is gently inserted under the gingival margin, holding the side of the tip against the tooth with a light lateral pressure; the probe tip is moved gently in an apical direction along the tooth surface until it encounters the resistance of the junctional epithelium
3. The tip is moved up and down in short bobbing strokes of 1 to 2 mm while progressing forward in small, 1-mm to 2-mm steps around the circumference of the tooth; with each downward stroke, the probe tip returns to gently touch the junctional epithelium
4. The base of the sulcus or pocket will feel soft and resilient; if the resistance on the probe feels hard, the probe tip has encountered a large calculus deposit before reaching the junctional epithelium
5. The probe should not be removed from the sulcus or the pocket after each instrumentation stroke; repeated insertion and removal is unnecessary and can cause trauma to the free gingival margin

E. Proximal surface probing—the probe is walked across the proximal surface until it touches the contact area; the probe is slanted slightly so that the tip reaches under the contact area; with the probe in this position, it is gently pressed downward to touch the junctional epithelium to take a reading

F. Sequence of steps for probing by quadrants
1. Insert the probe at the distal line angle of the posterior-most tooth in the quadrant; walk the probe in a distal direction, adapting the probe around the line angle and across the distal surface, slightly past the midline of the distal surface (because this is the distal-most tooth in the quadrant, no contact area is present to contend with)
2. Reinsert the probe at the distal line angle, and proceed in a mesial direction, across the distal surface, around the line angle, and across the mesial surface, slanting under the mesial contact area, as needed
3. Remove the probe from the sulcus or the pocket, and reinsert at the distal line angle of the next tooth in the quadrant; assess each tooth in the quadrant in a similar manner, ending with the mesial surface of the central incisor
4. After probing the facial aspect of the quadrant, assess the lingual aspect of the same quadrant

G. Calculus—when a large calculus deposit is encountered, the probe should be moved outward from the tooth and around the deposit and guided back to the tooth, proceeding in an apical direction

H. Recording probing depths—for the purpose of documentation, each tooth is divided into six areas (three on the facial aspect and three on the lingual aspect)
1. The six areas are:
   a. Distofacial line angle to the midline of the distal surface
   b. Facial surface
   c. Mesiofacial line angle to the midline of the mesial surface
   d. Distolingual line angle to the midline of the distal surface
   e. Lingual surface
   f. Mesiolingual line angle to the midline of the mesial surface
2. Only one reading per area is recorded—if the probing depths vary within an area, the deepest reading obtained in that area is recorded (e.g., when readings for an area range from 3 to 6 mm, only the 6-mm reading is entered on the chart for that area)
3. Depths are recorded in millimeters and rounded up (e.g., a reading of 4.5 mm is recorded as a 5-mm reading)

## Clinical Assessment Using Periodontal Probes

A. Bleeding on probing
1. Rationale
   a. Bleeding on probing is a significant clinical indicator of inflammation and is an earlier clinical sign of disease than marginal redness
   b. Bleeding on probing correlates with an increase in motile bacterial organisms, especially spirochetes, in the pocket
   c. Bleeding may indicate an area nonresponsive to nonsurgical periodontal treatment
   d. No bleeding on probing is a criterion for healthy tissue
2. Technique
   a. Insert the probe a few millimeters into the pocket (tip should not be in contact with the junctional epithelium)
   b. Make horizontal sweeping strokes along the pocket wall, using light pressure with the side of the probe
   c. Spongy tissue of a pocket wall will usually bleed near the gingival margin; firm chronic pocket linings usually do not bleed until sweeping strokes are made in the deep part of the pocket (bleeding may not be evident for a few seconds)
   d. Bleeding on probing usually is recorded on the periodontal chart; often indicated by a red dot on the chart

B. Measurement of recession of the gingival margin
1. Definition and rationale
   a. Gingival recession is the movement of the gingival margin from its normal position, slightly coronal to the cemento-enamel junction (CEJ), leading to exposure of a portion of the root surface to the oral cavity
   b. Gingival recession indicates the apical migration of the junctional epithelium
2. Procedure
   a. Position a calibrated probe parallel to the tooth surface with the toe of the probe touching the gingival margin
   b. Measure the extent of recession in millimeters from the CEJ to the gingival margin with a calibrated periodontal probe

C. Measuring probing depths
1. Definition—the distance in millimeters from the gingival margin to the base of the sulcus or the pocket, as measured with a calibrated probe
2. Rationale
   a. Used in mathematically calculating CALs
   b. Useful in prescribing client self-care regimens and in educating clients
3. Limitations—in the presence of gingival recession, probing depth measurements are not an accurate indication of loss of attachment or level of bone support to the tooth

4. Technique
   a. With the probe in a vertical position and in contact with the attached tissue, record the distance from the gingival margin to the base of the sulcus or the pocket
   b. When the gingival margin contacts the probe between the millimeter marks, use the higher number for the final reading

D. Measuring CALs
1. Definition—the position of the attached tissue at the base of the sulcus or the pocket, as measured from a fixed point, usually the CEJ
2. Rationale
   a. Probing depths are not reliable indicators of the position of the junctional epithelium because the measurement is made from the gingival margin; the position of the gingival margin changes with recession and edema
   b. Measurements are taken from a fixed point on the tooth; the CEJ usually is used because it provides a more reliable indication of the level of the attached tissue
   c. When evaluating treatment outcomes, measurements taken from a fixed point provide a better way of monitoring whether the level of the attached tissue has remained the same, decreased, or increased in depth
3. General concepts
   a. Two measurements are made and then used to calculate the clinical attachment; the measurements include:
      (1) The probing depth
      (2) The distance from the CEJ to the gingival margin
   b. Three possible relationships exist between the CEJ and the gingival margin; the clinician must understand how to calculate the CAL for each of these relationships
      (1) Visible gingival recession (gingival margin is apical to the CEJ) (Fig. 17.11)
      (2) Gingival margin is coronal to the CEJ
      (3) Gingival margin is approximately level with the CEJ
4. Calculation technique in areas of visible gingival recession
   a. Measure and record the probing depth (distance from the gingival margin to the base of the pocket)
   b. Measure and record the amount of gingival recession (distance from the CEJ to the gingival margin)
   c. Calculate the CAL by adding the probing depth and the measurement of gingival recession
5. Calculation technique in areas where gingival margin is coronal to the CEJ
   a. Measure and record the probing depth
   b. Apply the probe, and determine the location of the CEJ by tactile sensitivity; measure the distance from the gingival margin to the CEJ
   c. Calculate the CAL by subtracting the distance from the gingival margin to the CEJ from the probing depth
6. Calculation technique in areas where the gingival margin is level with the CEJ—when the gingival margin is within 0.5 mm apical or coronal to the CEJ, the probing depth and the CAL are the same measurement

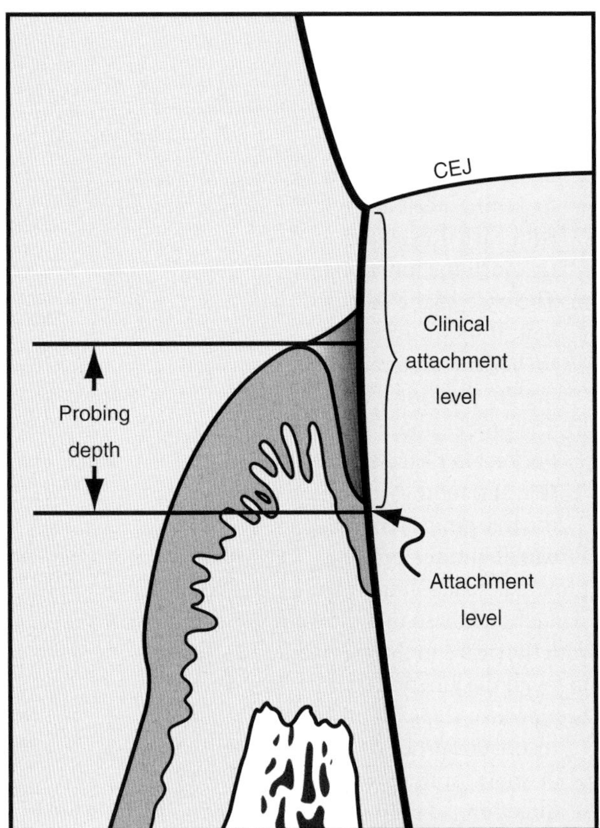


**Fig. 17.11** Comparison of the probing depth and the clinical attachment level (CAL) when the gingival margin is apical to the cemento-enamel junction *(CEJ)*. The CAL provides an accurate estimation of the level of the attached tissues. (From Nield-Gehrig JS. *Fundamentals of Periodontal Instrumentation and Advanced Root Instrumentation*. 6th ed. Philadelphia: Lippincott Williams & Wilkins; 2013.)

E. Mucogingival examination
1. Rationale—to determine the width of the attached gingiva
2. Procedure for determining the amount of attached gingiva
   a. On the external (outer) surface of the gingiva, measure the distance in millimeters from the gingival margin to the mucogingival junction; this is the total width of the gingiva (free and attached gingiva)
   b. Measure the probing depth
   c. Calculate the width of the attached gingiva by subtracting the probing depth from the total width of the gingiva
3. Significance of finding
   a. If the probing depth is equal to or greater than the width of the total gingiva, no attached gingiva (NAG) exists
   b. If the probe tip passes the mucogingival junction, mucogingival involvement exists in this area

F. Furcation involvement
1. Definition—furcation involvement occurs when periodontal infection invades the area between and around the roots of a bifurcated or trifurcated tooth, and the bone level is apical to the furcation crotch area

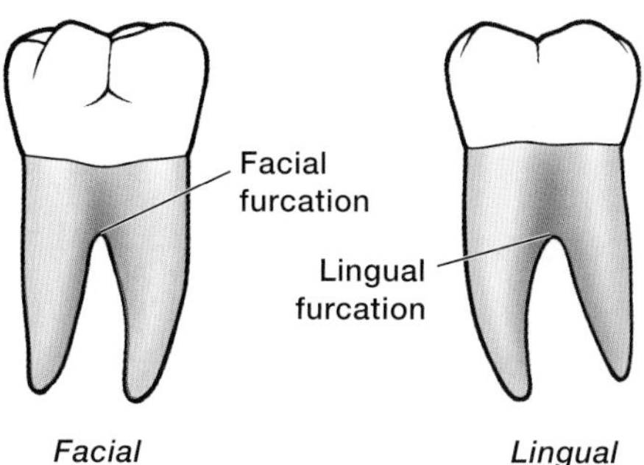


**Fig. 17.12** Furcation morphology on a mandibular molar (mesial and distal roots). The furcation can be examined from the facial and lingual aspects. (From Nield-Gehrig JS. *Fundamentals of Periodontal Instrumentation and Advanced Root Instrumentation.* 6th ed. Philadelphia: Lippincott Williams & Wilkins; 2013.)

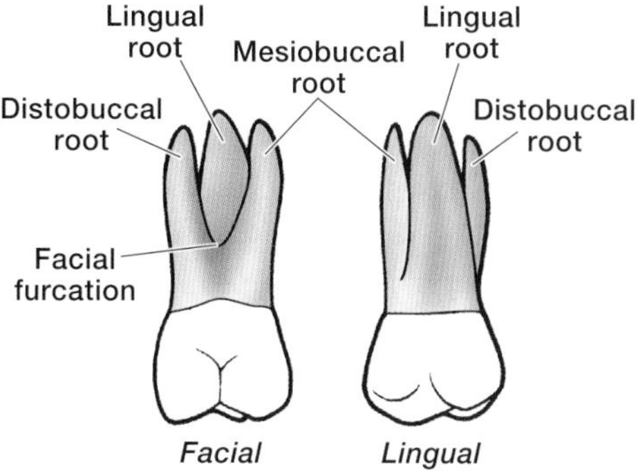


**Fig. 17.13** Furcation morphology on a maxillary molar (mesiobuccal, distobuccal, and palatal roots). The furcation can be examined from the facial, mesial, and distal aspects. (From Nield-Gehrig JS. *Fundamentals of Periodontal Instrumentation and Advanced Root Instrumentation.* 6th ed. Philadelphia: Lippincott Williams & Wilkins; 2013.)

2. Classification—furcation involvement is classified according to the extent of bone loss
   a. Class I—early, or incipient, involvement; the anatomy of the root surfaces can be felt by moving the probe from side to side, passing over the root into the concavity of the furcation area, and up the opposite side to the adjacent root
   b. Class II—moderate involvement; bone has been destroyed to an extent that allows the probe to partially enter the furcation, which extends approximately one-third the width of the tooth between the roots
   c. Class III—severe, or advanced, involvement; in mandibular molars, the probe can pass between the roots, through the entire furcation; in maxillary molars, the probe can pass between the mesiobuccal and distobuccal roots to touch the palatal root
   d. Class IV—same as class III; also, the furca is visible clinically because of the presence of tissue recession
3. Access to furcation area
   a. Bifurcated roots (two roots)
      (1) Mandibular molars—to examine between the mesial and distal roots, probe midfacial and midlingual aspects (Fig. 17.12)
      (2) Maxillary first premolars—to examine between the buccal and palatal roots, probe from the mesial and distal aspects, apical to the contact area
   b. Trifurcated roots (three roots)—maxillary molars; to examine around the palatal root and the two facial roots, probe from the midfacial, mesial, and distal aspects (Fig. 17.13)

G. Evaluation of oral deviations—a calibrated periodontal probe is used to determine the size of an oral lesion or deviation; when documenting measurements, anatomical terminology such as anteroposterior or superoinferior, is used, rather than terms such as length or width

## Clinical Assessment With Dental Explorers

A. Purposes and uses
1. Dental explorers detect, by tactile response, the texture and character of tooth surfaces before, during, and after treatment, to assess the progress and thoroughness of instrumentation
2. Dental explorers examine tooth surfaces for:
   a. Dental calculus
   b. Cemental changes that may have resulted from pocket formation
   c. Anomalies
   d. Anatomical features such as grooves, curvatures, and furcation areas
3. Dental explorers define the extent of instrumentation for treatment procedures of the tooth surface, including:
   a. Removal of calculus deposits and biofilm
   b. Removal of overhanging restorations
   c. Sealant placement

B. Dental calculus (see the sections on "Bacterial Plaque" in Chapter 9 and "Bacterial Dental Biofilm" in Chapter 14)
1. Definition
   a. Calcified or mineralized plaque biofilm is a hard, tenacious mass that forms on tooth surfaces and on dental prostheses
   b. The surface of calculus is rough and is covered by a layer of plaque biofilm
2. Types, distribution, and shape
   a. Supragingival (supramarginal) calculus
      (1) Located coronal to (above) the gingival margin
      (2) Distribution—localized, usually not generalized throughout the mouth
      (3) Most common locations include the lingual surfaces of mandibular anterior teeth, facial surfaces of maxillary molars, teeth out of occlusion, or overlapping teeth
   b. Subgingival (submarginal) calculus
      (1) Located apical to (beneath) the gingival margin
      (2) Distribution—may be localized or generalized; heaviest on proximal surfaces
      (3) Extends along the root surface almost to the base of the pocket; the newest, less calcified calculus is at the most apical area, near the soft tissue attachment

(4) Shape—flattened to conform to pressure from the gingival pocket wall; forms may include combinations of the following:
(a) Nodular deposits (spicules)
(b) Ledge-like or ring-like formations
(c) Thin, smooth veneers
(d) Finger-like and fern-like formations

3. Modes of attachment—calculus is more easily removed from some tooth surfaces than from others; the difficulty in removal usually is related to the manner in which the calculus is attached to the tooth; on any one tooth, more than one mode of attachment can occur
   a. Attachment to acquired pellicle (thin acellular layer on tooth surface)—most common mode of calculus attachment to enamel; calculus may be removed readily because no interlocking of calculus to the tooth exists
   b. Attachment by "locking" into minute irregularities in the tooth surface
   c. Attachment of the calcified calculus matrix to the tooth surface by interlocking of inorganic crystals of the tooth with the mineralizing plaque biofilm

C. Calculus detection
1. Supragingival assessment—unnecessary supragingival exploration should be avoided; adequate light combined with the use of a dental mirror and compressed air will reveal most supragingival deposits
2. Subgingival assessment and adaptation
   a. Instrument grasp and lateral pressure—a relaxed grasp and light lateral pressure are used to enhance tactile sensitivity; pressure with the middle finger against the instrument shank should be avoided, because this reduces tactile sensitivity
   b. Activation—a combination of hand-forearm and digital activation
   c. Strokes—many, overlapping, fluid strokes are used to thoroughly cover the entire root surface

D. Carious lesions
1. Historically, the use of tactile examination of a tooth surface, with firm application of a sharp tip of an explorer into a suspected site of caries, was a common method of carious lesion detection, but this approach is no longer recommended
2. Research has shown this technique to be unreliable for carious lesion detection and to be potentially harmful
3. Firm application of a sharp explorer tip into a carious pit or fissure on a tooth surface may actually cause additional damage to the tooth surface and interfere with subsequent attempts at remineralization of the caries lesion (see Chapter 16)

## CONCEPTS IN PERIODONTAL INSTRUMENTATION

### Instrumentation Terminology

A. Instrumenting—using a periodontal instrument for a task
B. Biofilm management—the disruption or removal of subgingival plaque biofilm and its by-products from cemental surfaces and the pocket spaces
C. Tactile sensitivity—the ability to feel vibrations transferred from the instrument's working end, shank, and handle to the clinician's fingers
D. Assessment—examination of a tooth and periodontium to determine anatomy and detect biofilm-retentive factors, and oral disease status
E. Nonsurgical periodontal instrumentation—removal of hard and soft deposits from the tooth crown, root surfaces, and pocket space to the extent needed to reestablish periodontal health and restore a balance between the bacterial flora and the host's immune responses
F. Overhang removal—recontouring procedures that correct defective margins of restorations to provide a smooth surface that will deter bacterial accumulation
G. Supragingival—located coronal to (above) the gingival margin
H. Subgingival—located apical to (beneath) the gingival margin
I. Biofilm-retentive factors—conditions that foster the establishment and growth of biofilm, such as calculus deposits and overhanging restorations

### Rationale for Nonsurgical Periodontal Instrumentation

A. Arrests the progress of disease
B. Induces positive changes in the subgingival bacterial flora (count and content)
C. Creates an environment that permits the gingival tissue to heal, thereby eliminating inflammation
   1. Converts the pocket from an area experiencing increased loss of attachment to one in which the CAL remains the same or decreases
   2. Eliminates bleeding
   3. Improves integrity of tissue attachment
D. Increases the effectiveness of client self-care
E. Permits reevaluation of periodontal health status; surgery may then be unnecessary, lessened in extent, or confined to specific areas
F. Prevents recurrence of disease through frequent periodontal maintenance therapy

### Rationale for Removal of Overhangs

A. Eliminates irregular surfaces where biofilm can collect
B. Induces positive changes in the microflora of the pocket when the overhang extends subgingivally
C. Encourages resolution of inflammation
D. Facilitates interdental biofilm removal and control by the client

### End Point of Instrumentation

A. The goal of instrumentation is to render the root surface and pocket space acceptable to tissue so that healing occurs
B. Tissue healing occurs slowly, and it is not possible to assess tissue response for at least 1 month after completion of instrumentation

1. The client's appointment for reevaluation should be scheduled 4 to 6 weeks after completion of instrumentation
2. During reevaluation, a periodontal assessment should be completed that includes probing depths, CALs, and bleeding on probing
3. Nonresponsive sites are those that show continued loss of attachment and may exhibit clinical signs of inflammation or bleeding, or both, on probing; nonresponsive sites may require:
   a. Removal of new or residual calculus deposits; or other biofilm–retentive factors
   b. Thorough subgingival biofilm removal, preferably with an ultrasonic instrument or glycine-powder air polishing with a specially designed subgingival nozzle tip
4. Consideration should be given to other risk factors that might be contributing to the disease process (host response, systemic, and local factors)

### Steps for the Preparation for Instrumentation

A. Protect patient safety
   1. Review the patient's personal and health histories for indications of special needs; prepare for a possible emergency
   2. Assess vital signs
   3. Observe the patient for signs of stress
B. Use standard precautions (see Chapter 10)
   1. Postpone treatment for a patient with a communicable disease or an open oral lesion
   2. Provide the means for lowering the bacterial count of the patient's oral surfaces
      a. Provide the patient with a preprocedural antimicrobial mouthrinse or antimicrobial irrigation to lower the count of oral microorganisms
      b. Discuss oral self-care with patient (e.g., plaque control) before any instrumentation

## SHARPENING OF HAND-ACTIVATED INSTRUMENTS

A. Sharp cutting edges are vital to achieve efficient periodontal instrumentation with minimal tissue trauma
B. Sharp cutting edges help provide more efficient treatment because of easier calculus removal, fewer strokes, improved stroke control, increased patient comfort, and reduced clinician fatigue
C. To sharpen instruments correctly, the clinician must understand the design of the working end
   1. A sharp cutting edge is a line without width; a dull cutting edge is a rounded surface
   2. The internal angle formed between the face and lateral surface of a sickle scaler or curet is between 70 and 80 degrees
   3. Most sickle scalers have pointed tips and backs; curets have rounded toes and backs
   4. Sickle scalers and universal curets have two working cutting edges per working end; area-specific curets have one working cutting edge per working end
D. Instruments should be sharpened at the first sign of dullness—the cutting edge of the instrument dulls at various rates because of:
   1. Number of working strokes used
   2. Amount of lateral pressure used
   3. Hardness and tenacity of the deposit
   4. Composition of the metal of the instrument
E. Equipment
   1. A stable, well-lighted work surface
   2. Heat-sterilized rectangular sharpening stone or sharpening tool and plastic sharpening test stick (Table 17.3)
   3. Water or oil to lubricate the stone (depending on the type of stone)
   4. Protective eyewear, facemask, and household gloves (when sharpening contaminated instruments)

## ULTRASONIC AND SONIC INSTRUMENTATION

A. Description
   1. Powered ultrasonic and sonic devices use rapid vibrations of a fluid-cooled instrument tip to fracture and dislodge supragingival and subgingival calculus deposits from the teeth and to cleanse the environment within the periodontal pocket
   2. Ultrasonic devices (magnetostrictive and piezoelectric)
      a. High-frequency electrical energy is converted into mechanical energy in the form of ultrasonic vibrations; instrument tip vibrations range from 25,000 to 50,000 cycles per second (cps, hertz [Hz])
      b. Heat that is produced must be dissipated by a constant flow of water through the handpiece; antimicrobial solutions may be used instead of water in certain units
      c. Ultrasonic instruments provide efficient removal of all types of calculus deposits (old, new, supragingival and subgingival, light and heavy deposits)
   3. Sonic instruments
      a. Air pressure also is used to create rapid mechanical vibrations; sonic instrument tip vibrations range from 3000 to 8000 cycles per second (Hertz)
      b. No heat is generated; although water cooling is not necessary, a water coolant is indicated to obtain the benefits of water lavage
      c. Because of the lower frequency of vibration, sonic instruments are less efficient in removing calculus deposits and have a limited ability to remove tenacious deposits; they function well for the removal of newly formed and light deposits
B. Definitions
   1. Fluid lavage—the fluid stream within the periodontal pocket, produced by the constant flow of fluid through the handpiece, near the instrument's tip; when the fluid strikes the vibrating instrument tip, it creates a spray composed of millions of tiny bubbles
   2. Cavitation—the energy release that occurs when the tiny bubbles in the fluid spray collapse, producing shock waves that may alter or destroy bacteria by tearing the bacterial cell walls
   3. Stroke—the maximum distance the powered instrument tip moves during one cycle of vibration
C. Instrument tip design

**TABLE 17.3 Sharpening Stones and Tools**

| Type | Abrasiveness | Description | Purpose | Lubricant | Sterilization[a] |
|---|---|---|---|---|---|
| Ceramic | Fine | Synthetic stone | Routine sharpening of metal and some plastic implant instruments | Water | All methods |
| Arkansas | Fine | Natural stone | Routine sharpening of metal instruments | Mineral oil | All methods[b] |
| India | Medium | Synthetic stone | Sharpening of metal instruments that are dull | Water or oil | All methods |
| Composition | Coarse | Synthetic stone | Sharpening of metal instruments that are extremely dull or that need reshaping | Water | All methods |
| Nievert Whittler | — | Tungsten carbide steel | Routine sharpening of metal instruments | Water | All methods |
| Reciprocating honing device | — | — | Sharpening of metal instruments | — | — |

[a]Includes autoclave, dry heat, or chemical sterilization.
[b]Natural stones become brittle over time with heat exposure.
Modified with permission.

1. Working ends of ultrasonic/sonic instruments have no cutting edges to cut or tear tissue; less tissue trauma can result in faster healing rates for sites treated with ultrasonic or sonic instruments
2. The entire length of the working end is active; therefore, adaptation is not limited to a single region on the working end
3. Tip selection
    a. Ultrasonic tip selection varies, depending on the manufacturer; the availability of a full range of tip designs is an important criterion when purchasing a mechanized device
    b. Tips may range in size from large, broad tips (standard size), to medium-sized tips to slim-diameter slender tips
    c. Standard tips (ultrasonic and sonic designs)
        (1) Broad, large tips are used to remove heavy, supragingival deposits
        (2) Medium-sized tips are used to remove medium and light deposits; some may be used subgingivally if the tissue permits easy insertion of the tip
    d. Slim-diameter ultrasonic tips
        (1) Similar in diameter to periodontal probes, and significantly smaller in size than the working end of a curet
        (2) Approximately 40% thinner than a standard-sized ultrasonic tip
        (3) Available in straight, right-paired, and left-paired styles
        (4) Used for biofilm and light calculus removal; provide excellent access to deep pockets and furcation areas
4. Energy dispersion—magnetostrictive instrument tips are active on all surfaces while piezoelectric instruments are only active on the lateral sides; by adapting the appropriate tip surface, the clinician can control energy dispersion and patient sensitivity during the procedure
    a. Point—generates the most energy; should not be used directly against the tooth surface
    b. Face (concave surface)—second most powerful surface (generates less energy than the point); usually not recommended for use against the tooth surface

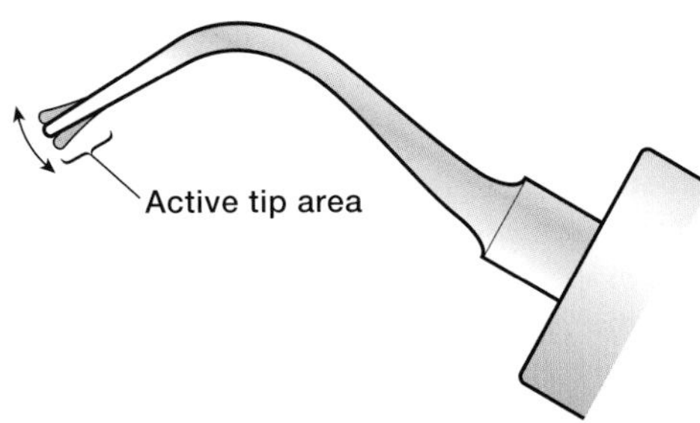


**Fig. 17.14** Active tip area of a mechanized instrument. The active tip area ranges in length from 2 to 3 mm and is the portion of the instrument tip that is capable of doing the work. (From Nield-Gehrig JS. *Fundamentals of Periodontal Instrumentation and Advanced Root Instrumentation.* 6th ed. Philadelphia: Lippincott Williams & Wilkins; 2013.)

    c. Back (convex surface)—generates less energy than the face; follow the manufacturer's recommendations regarding direct use on the tooth surface
    d. Lateral surfaces (sides)—generate the least amount of energy; may be used directly against the tooth surface; adaptation of a lateral surface is recommended for calculus removal and deplaquing
5. Fluid delivery—ultrasonic instruments require a constant stream of fluid running through the handpiece, which disperses in a fine spray at or near the instrument tip to prevent overheating of the vibrating instrument tip
    a. Fluid delivery to the tip
        (1) The external flow tube is adjacent to the instrument's shank
        (2) In the internal fluid flow system, the fluid flows directly through the instrument tip
    b. Water is the most common fluid used; some ultrasonic units have an independent fluid reservoir that can deliver distilled water or other fluid solutions (e.g., sterile saline, stannous fluoride, chemotherapeutic agents) to the instrument tip
6. Tip frequency—the number of times per second that the tip moves back and forth during one cycle
    a. Active tip area—the portion of the tip that is capable of doing work; ranges from 2 to 4 mm in length (Fig. 17.14)

   b. Manual ultrasonic units allow the clinician to adjust the tip frequency by turning an adjustment knob on the unit; automatic ultrasonic units control the tip frequency automatically; sonic instruments have a preset frequency that cannot be controlled by the clinician

D. Several factors influence the force produced by the powered instrument tip
   1. Exposure time—sufficient time must be allowed for the tip to do its work (e.g., ultrasonic instruments are effective, but even they do not instantaneously remove calculus); powered instrument tips work by creating microfractures in a calculus deposit; the tip should be moved back and forth repeatedly over the deposit to allow time for the microfractures to develop
   2. Angle of adaptation—an angle of between 0 and 15 degrees is recommended for direct adaptation to tooth surfaces
   3. Sharp or dull tip—only dull tips are recommended; sharpened tips emit high energy levels that could damage the tooth
   4. Lateral pressure—tips function most effectively with light lateral pressure against the tooth or calculus deposit; moderate or firm lateral pressure decreases or even stops the vibrations of the tip

E. Uses of modern ultrasonic instruments
   1. Removal of attached and unattached plaque biofilm from root surface and pocket space
   2. Removal of supragingival and subgingival calculus
   3. Removal of toxins from root surfaces
   4. Smoothing down overextended or rough amalgam restorations, removing extrinsic stains for esthetic considerations, and removing orthodontic cement (using standard tips)

F. Contraindications
   1. Patient with a communicable disease that can be disseminated by aerosols
   2. Immunocompromised patient with high susceptibility to an infection who could be exposed to microorganisms in contaminated water or aerosols or by other means (e.g., debilitated patient, those with uncontrolled diabetes, immunosuppressed patients)
   3. Patient with respiratory disease or difficulty breathing (e.g., history of emphysema, cystic fibrosis, asthma); the patient is at increased risk of respiratory infection if septic material or oral microorganisms are aspirated
   4. Patient who has difficulty swallowing or is prone to gagging (e.g., multiple sclerosis, amyotrophic lateral sclerosis, muscular dystrophy, paralysis)
   5. Patient with a cardiac pacemaker; the dental clinician should check with the patient's cardiologist if the device is shielded or unshielded for magnetostrictive ultrasonic use
   6. Patient with primary or newly erupted teeth—danger of heat being conducted to large pulp chambers
   7. Direct contact between the instrument tip and porcelain jacket crowns, composite resin restorations that could be damaged by the vibration or the tip, and demineralized enamel surfaces (conservation of demineralized enamel surfaces is indicated) should be avoided
   8. Direct contact with titanium implant surface should be avoided, unless the instrument tip is covered with a specially designed plastic sleeve

G. Precautions
   1. The handpiece and the working end of ultrasonic instruments must be cooled with constant flow of water to dissipate heat
   2. Aerosols produced may be contaminated with pathogens; use of barriers, surface disinfectants, protective clothing, and laminar airflow systems is recommended
   3. The patient may experience sensitivity
   4. Shifts in hearing sensitivity have been reported; the effect of ultrasonic and sonic equipment on the hearing of clinicians who frequently use these instruments has not been studied well

H. Preparation
   1. Employ universal precautions, and ensure that protective attire is worn by the clinician, the assistant, and the patient
   2. Have the patient use a preprocedural antimicrobial mouthrinse, or irrigate the treatment area to reduce the number of airborne microorganisms in aerosols created by water spray
   3. Monitor the condition of the equipment
   4. Replace the instrument tip as soon as it shows signs of wear or damage
      a. Tip wear—1 mm of wear results in approximately 25% loss of efficiency; tips should be discarded at 2 mm of wear; some manufacturers offer wear guides that make it easy to determine tip wear; precision-thin tips must be replaced more frequently than standard tips
      b. Metal stacks of magnetostrictive insert—replace if the stacks are bent or separated, or if the insert does not slide easily into the ultrasonic handpiece
   5. Instrument tips and handpieces should be sterilized according to manufacturer's instructions; use surface disinfectant and barriers on an ultrasonic unit

I. Technique
   1. Biofilm control in water tubing—flush the water tubing of stagnant water for 2 minutes at the start of the day, and for 30 seconds between patients; use units with an independent fluid reservoir or waterline point-of-use filter, or both
   2. Tip selection—select the appropriate instrument tip for the task at hand
      a. Broad, standard tips for removal of heavy and medium-sized supragingival calculus
      b. Medium-sized standard tips for moderate and light supragingival use; also may be used subgingivally if the tissue permits easy insertion of the tip
      c. Slim-diameter tips for removal of light deposits and deplaquing
   3. Power setting—use standard instrument tips at medium-power or low-power setting, and slim-diameter tips at low-power setting; high-power setting is no more effective than medium power and is not recommended
   4. Grasp—use light, relaxed grasp, even during calculus removal
   5. Finger rest—use an intraoral or extraoral rest; advanced fulcrum techniques may be helpful for gaining access to posterior pockets

6. Lateral pressure—use light stroke pressure for effective calculus removal
7. Activation—use digital activation as recommended
8. Fluid adjustment and containment
   a. Adjust the water spray around the instrument tip to create a light mist or halo effect, with no excess dripping of water; insufficient water flow over an ultrasonic tip can result in trauma to the pulp; a warm handpiece is a sign of inadequate fluid flow through the handpiece
   b. Use high-volume suction or a saliva ejector for fluid control; position the suction tip at the corner of the mouth where the fluid will pool; deactivate the instrument tip occasionally to prevent large amounts of fluid accumulation
   c. Use the client's lips and cheeks as barriers to deflect fluid back into the client's mouth
9. Tip adaptation
   a. Adaptation to the tooth surface—position the tip with the point directed toward the junctional epithelium and the length of the tip at a 0- to 15-degree angle to the tooth surface; never apply the point of the tip directly to the tooth surface
   b. Adaptation to a calculus deposit—place the tip directly against the uppermost or outermost edge of the calculus deposit; the lateral surface of a tip may also be adapted to a calculus deposit
10. Instrumentation strokes
   a. Motion—use a tapping motion against large-sized calculus deposits and a sweeping, eraser-like motion against small deposits and for biofilm removal from root surfaces
   b. Pressure—use light pressure; firm pressure decreases effectiveness
   c. Direction—use overlapping vertical, oblique, and horizontal strokes; subgingival strokes should cover the entire root surface for calculus removal and deplaquing
11. Calculus removal
   a. Sequence—work in a coronal-to-apical direction, beginning at the gingival margin and working toward the junctional epithelium (this is the reverse of the sequence for calculus removal with a curet)
   b. Technique for removing stubborn deposits
      (1) Use an adequate number of strokes—move the tip repeatedly over the deposit or tap against the deposit; keep the tip in constant motion
      (2) Select the proper tip for the type of calculus; for example, do not use slim-diameter tips for medium-sized or large deposits
      (3) Approach the deposit from different aspects (e.g., approach an interproximal deposit from both the facial and the lingual aspect)
      (4) Do not apply firm stroke pressure; use of light pressure is most effective
      (5) Increase the frequency on a manually calibrated unit
      (6) Increase the power setting from low to medium

## ADVANCED INSTRUMENTATION TECHNIQUES

### Instrumentation of Dental Implants

A. Definition—dental implant: a nonbiologic device surgically inserted into or onto the jawbone to replace a missing tooth or to provide support for an implant superstructure (e.g., a fixed bridge or denture)
B. General guidelines
   1. Special instruments are recommended for assessment and instrumentation of implants; plastic instruments are used most often because the plastic material is softer than the implant material; titanium instruments are increasing in popularity due to their ability to remove soft and hard deposits safely from the implant surfaces.
   2. Metal instruments (e.g., stainless steel, carbon steel, and metal ultrasonic instruments) may leave scratches on the surface of the implant
      a. Scratches or surface roughness on an implant may promote accumulation of biofilm
      b. Surface coating of an implant may be disturbed, thereby reducing the biocompatibility of the implant with the surrounding tissues
   3. Some plastic instruments may be sterilized by autoclaving; follow the manufacturer's instructions for sterilization and reuse
C. Design of the working end of implant instruments
   1. Wrench-shaped, crescent-shaped, and hoe-shaped working ends on plastic instruments—useful for instrumentation of an implant's superstructure
   2. Working ends that are similar in design to conventional metal probes, sickle scalers, and curets—useful for the assessment and instrumentation of the implant abutment
D. Use of plastic or metal, calibrated probes for assessing peri-implant tissues (soft tissues that surround the dental implant)
   1. Peri-implant probing depths are related to the thickness of the mucosa around the implant; biotype probes for measuring mucosal thickness type are available
   2. Probing depths and CALs are important parameters for the longitudinal monitoring of peri-implant tissue stability; deeper probing depths are found in conjunction with a thicker mucosa
   3. Considerations
      a. Probing may be invasive because the probe may penetrate the weakly adherent biologic seal and could introduce bacteria into peri-implant tissue
      b. Accurate probing depths may be difficult to obtain because of the constricted "cervical" area of some implants
      c. Approach perpendicular to the implant on the buccal or lingual and then stand the probe up; adjust probing to accommodate the shape of the prosthetic for accurate probing
      d. Radiographs are more accurate than probing depths for detecting the absence or presence of bone loss around implants
E. Instrumentation for calculus removal

1. Calculus is removed easily from implants because no interlocking or penetration of the deposit exists within the implant surface
2. Light lateral pressure with a plastic or titanium scaler or curet is recommended; care must be taken not to scratch the surface of the implant
3. Instrumentation should be completed on all areas of the implant accessible if deposit is present

## SELECTIVE STAIN REMOVAL

A. Definitions
   1. Intrinsic—stains that occur within the tooth substance; the process of removal is performed by a dentist using bleaching techniques or prosthetic coverage with a crown
   2. Extrinsic—stains that occur on the external surface of the tooth; removed by patient self-care and professional procedures such as scaling and rubber cup and brush scaling, rubber cup/brush, and conventional air polishing
B. Significance of dental stains
   1. No detrimental effects have been shown to result from the presence of dental stains; research shows that stains do not directly contribute to periodontal disease, dental caries, or any oral disease; however, stains may contribute to biofilm retention
   2. Removal of unsightly dental stains on anterior teeth may benefit the client's appearance and self-esteem
C. Rationale for selective stain removal
   1. Polishing is viewed as a cosmetic procedure with limited application; stain removal provides no therapeutic benefit to the patient and has numerous detrimental effects on teeth and soft tissue
   2. Decision to include stain removal in a patient's care plan can best be made after patient self- care education and after complete periodontal instrumentation because much of the stain may be removed along with calculus deposits
D. Contraindications to polishing
   1. Dental contraindications
      a. Tooth surfaces that have no extrinsic stains or have stains that are not visible when patient smiles or engages in conversation
      b. Areas of dentinal hypersensitivity—application of fluoride is one treatment for tooth sensitivity; protective fluoride must be left undisturbed (see the section on "Assessment of Dentinal Hypersensitivity" in Chapter 16)
      c. Restored tooth surfaces—gold and other restorative materials may be scratched by the abrasive agent
      d. Titanium implants—polishing could scratch the titanium abutment, however, it is critical to remove all deposits and biofilm from implants and their prostheses
      e. Areas of demineralization—conservation of demineralized enamel surfaces is indicated
      f. Gingiva that is enlarged, soft, spongy, or bleeds easily—polishing is not recommended because paste can enter the tissue, and the action of the rotating cup can further traumatize the tissue
   2. Systemic contraindications
      a. Patient with a communicable disease that could be spread by aerosols
      b. Patient with a high susceptibility to infection who could inhale contaminated aerosols (e.g., patient with respiratory or pulmonary disease, debilitated patient)
      c. Patient who has a history of renal insufficiency, Addison's disease, Cushing syndrome, or metabolic alkalosis; is taking mineralocorticosteroids, antidiuretics, or potassium supplements; air polisher use should be avoided
      d. Patient who has a history of hypertension or a sodium-restricted diet; air polishing using a sodium-containing powder is contraindicated; air polishing can be used with one of the newer, sodium-free polishing powder products, such as those composed of aluminum trihydroxide or calcium carbonate
E. Adverse effects of polishing
   1. Aerosol production and spatter from power-driven polisher
      a. Contaminated aerosols present a hazard to the clinician, other dental personnel, and other patients in the oral health care environment; polishing splatter is composed of polishing paste, microorganisms, and saliva
      b. Components of commercial prophylaxis pastes may include various chemicals that can cause a severe inflammatory response in the eye
   2. Iatrogenic damage to tooth surfaces
      a. Enamel surfaces—stain removal with an abrasive agent removes the surface layer of tooth structure where the fluoride content is greatest and most protective; polishing the teeth for 3 minutes with pumice removes 3 to 4 micrometers (μm) of enamel; over time, the loss of enamel can be significant
      b. Cemental surfaces—exposed surface near the CEJ has a thin cementum or dentin surface that can be abraded or removed with an abrasive agent
      c. Heat production—care must be taken to use a wet polishing agent with minimal pressure and low speed to prevent overheating of a tooth, particularly the pulp tissues of small children; primary teeth have large pulp chambers, which make them particularly vulnerable to heat generated by power-driven handpieces
   3. Tissue trauma—during polishing, abrasive paste is forced into the gingival sulcus and even into the tissue itself; some individuals experience a negative tissue response to abrasive particles or chemicals in the paste, which can delay tissue healing
F. Power-driven polisher (rubber cup polishing)
   1. Description
      a. Handpiece—connects to the dental unit's low-speed handpiece line
      b. Prophylaxis angle—attaches to the handpiece; holds polishing cups and bristle brushes
      c. Attachments
         (1) Polishing cups—used for stain removal from tooth surfaces and for polishing restorations

(2) Bristle brushes—used for stain removal from occlusal surfaces; not for use near the gingival margin or on cementum or dentin, where the brush could denude the epithelium or remove cementum

2. Technique considerations
   a. Application of polishing agent—apply agent only to individual teeth requiring stain removal for esthetic purposes
   b. Use the lowest possible handpiece speed
   c. Apply the cup to the tooth with a light, intermittent pressure
      (1) The edges of the cup should just barely flare from the tooth surface
      (2) Use of continuous motion—avoid holding the cup on a single spot for too long to prevent buildup of frictional heat

G. Supragingival and subgingival air polishing
1. Definition—an air-powered device using air and water pressure to deliver a controlled slurry of powder to the tooth surface
2. Technique
   a. Wear protective attire
      (1) Patient—provide a plastic apron, hair cover, eye protection, and lip lubrication
      (2) Clinician and assistant—wear a paper or cloth long-sleeved garment, facemask, hair cover, eye protection, and gloves
   b. Administer a preprocedural mouthrinse to lessen contaminated aerosols; have the patient rinse with an antibacterial mouthrinse
   c. Use lip retractors; these help to provide an unobstructed view, retract the lips and buccal mucosa for instrumentation, and ease of evacuation with a high-volume evacuator
   d. Apply disclosing solution
   e. Direct the powder spray away from the gingival tissue, never direct the spray into the sulcus or pocket space; establish the recommended angulation of the tip to the tooth surface
      (1) Facial and lingual surfaces—position the nozzle tip at a 60- to 80-degree angle to the tooth
      (2) Occlusal surfaces—position the nozzle at a 90-degree angle to the surface of the tooth
   f. Direct the spray in constant motion for only 3 to 5 seconds at any area on the enamel surface
      (3) Subgingival air polishing requires 5-10 seconds on each tooth surface with a constant back-and-forth motion
3. Air Polishing Powders
   a. Polishing powder should be selected based on supra or subgingival polishing, stain, and materials present in the dentition
   b. Sodium bicarbonate, glycine, and erythritol
      (a) Sodium bicarbonate—large, abrasive particle size for supragingival stain and biofilm removal
      (b) Glycine—amino acid salt with very small particle size safe for dentin, cementum, restorative materials including titanium implants, and subgingival air polishing
      (c) Erythritol—sugar alcohol powder similar to xylitol, with the smallest particle size; safe for dentin, cementum, restorative materials including titanium implants, and subgingival air polishing

H. Postoperative procedures for mechanical and air polishing
1. Remove particles of abrasive at the contact areas with dental floss
2. Loosen and remove particles in sulci or pockets by irrigation and aspiration with central suction

## ETHICAL, LEGAL, AND SAFETY ISSUES

A. Provision of quality care by licensed dental hygienists includes ethical, legal, and safety issues
B. A comprehensive review of the patient's medical health and pharmacologic histories is essential to assess the degree of patient risk for dental procedures and to make necessary physician or specialty referrals
C. Adherence to the Health Insurance Portability and Accountability Act (HIPAA) is necessary; thorough, accurate, and confidential chart documentation is essential
D. Comprehensive patient assessment is essential to detect oral diseases and abnormalities and determine the degree of patient risk for caries, periodontal disease, or disease progression
E. Failure to provide necessary care based on assessment findings constitutes supervised neglect; the licensed dental hygienist is accountable and responsible for patient care
F. A thorough case presentation is essential so that the patient can make an informed decision about recommended dental hygiene care; written informed consent should be obtained before beginning care; discussion of all procedures with patients, using everyday language the client can understand, and encouragement of patient participation are essential
G. The dental hygienist has an obligation to provide evidence-based care
H. The dental hygienist has an obligation to protect the client from harm during care
I. The dental hygienist has an obligation to follow established protocol that protects the clinician and the patient during treatment
J. It is essential to allow sufficient time during appointments for provision of adequate care
K. Nonsurgical periodontal instrumentation should be performed in an effective and responsible manner; use of sharp instruments and selection of appropriate instruments for the task are essential
L. It is important to evaluate the success of nonsurgical periodontal instrumentation at appropriate continued-care intervals
M. The dental hygienist has a legal obligation to document thoroughly and accurately the assessment, care plan, informed consent, services provided, and the patient's response to care

## WEBSITE INFORMATION AND RESOURCES

| Source | Website Address | Description |
|---|---|---|
| American Academy of Periodontology | http://www.perio.org | Parameters of care, position papers, scientific information, related links |
| Cochrane Collaboration | http://www.cochrane.org | Evidence-based health care database |
| National Center for Dental Hygiene Research | https://dent-web10.usc.edu/dhnet | Current topics in dental hygiene; links |
| Hu-Friedy | http://www.hu-friedy.com | Online catalogue of periodontal instruments; ultrasonic and air-polishing devices; white papers, material safety data sheets (MSDS), instrument care, articles |
| Premier Dental | http://www.premusa.com | Online catalogue of periodontal instruments; fluoride; continuing education seminar information |
| Deldent Ltd. Air Polishers | http://www.deldent.com | Information about the products marketed by Deldent |
| Dentsply Ultrasonic Units | http://www.dentsply.com | News articles, career and legal information, and information about Dentsply products |
| KaVo America | http://www.kavousa.com | Information about KaVo dental products |
| Parkell Ultrasonic Scalers | http://www.parkell.com | Information about Parkell dental products |

## CHAPTER 17 REVIEW QUESTIONS

Answers and rationales to the review questions are available on this text's accompanying Evolve site. See inside front cover for details.

### CASE A

**Synopsis of Patient History**

Age: 76
Sex: M
Height: 6′1″
Weight: 243 lb

**Vital Signs**

Blood pressure: 122/86
Pulse: 59 bpm
Respiration: 16 rpm

1. Under the care of a physician: x YES ____NO
2. Hospitalized within the last 5 years: x YES ____NO (placement of cardiac stent)
3. Has or had the following conditions:
   Hyperlipidemia
   Hypertension
4. Current medications:
   Simvastatin 20 mg/day, used to treat high cholesterol
   Cardizem 120 mg/day, used to treat angina (chest pain) and hypertension
5. Smokes or uses tobacco products: ____YES x NO

**Medical History**

Sees a physician every 3 months for monitoring of cardiac condition and cholesterol levels
Is compliant in taking medication and monitors fat intake
Patient reports home monitoring of his blood pressure, and that it is typical for his blood pressure to "run a little high"

**Dental History**

Missing all third molars and #3 and #31
Implants #7 and #10 to replace congenitally missing laterals
Gold onlay on #14 and gold inlays on #4 and #29
Large class II amalgams on #30 and #19 with compromised margins and overhangs on the M and D of both teeth
Gingival tissues are inflamed and bleed easily on probing; moderate bleeding interproximally in all posteriors
Tissue in anterior and premolar teeth is hyperplastic

**Social History**

Retired from the US Navy
Had a second career for 20 years as an engineer for an aerospace company

**Chief Complaint**

Has noticed bleeding when brushing and was told by his wife he has "bad breath" and he should have his teeth cleaned
Reports mouth has become very dry

**Current Oral Hygiene Status**

Moderate generalized interproximal calculus
Moderate plaque biofilm at gingival third
Probing depths range 4–7 mm with deepest readings in mandibular left and maxillary right
Clinical attachment levels confirm generalized bone loss

***Use Case A to answer questions 1 to 10.***

1. While checking for subgingival calculus deposits on the mandibular anterior teeth with an ODU 11/12 explorer, the clinician finds it difficult to insert the explorer without unduly distending the tissue. Which of the following techniques might cause less tissue distention?
   a. Switch to an Orban-type explorer
   b. Aim the point of the ODU 11/12 explorer toward the base of the sulcus so that less of the working end is inserted in the sulcus
   c. Switch to a pigtail explorer
   d. Use a calibrated periodontal probe to locate calculus deposits
2. One of the patient's chief complaints is that his medication makes his mouth dry. All the following are useful suggestions for the patient to minimize effects of xerostomia EXCEPT:
   a. Increase intake of caffeine beverages to stimulate saliva production
   b. Use toothpastes and mouthrinses specially designed for individuals with xerostomia
   c. Chew sugarless gum to increase the flow of saliva
   d. Replace lost saliva with saliva substitutes

3. You are using hand instruments to remove the calculus deposits from the patient's teeth. After 30 minutes, your hand muscles are noticeably fatigued. Potentially, all the following can cause hand fatigue EXCEPT:
   a. Glove fit is too big
   b. Instrument handles are of small diameter
   c. Instrument is not balanced
   d. Using finger motion instead of wrist motion activation
4. A large piece of burnished calculus is present on the distal aspect of tooth #2. Which instrument would be MOST effective in preparing the burnished deposit for eventual removal with another periodontal instrument?
   a. Beavertail ultrasonic tip
   b. Rigid Gracey 13/14
   c. Periodontal file
   d. Miniature Gracey 13/14 curet with an extended shank
5. The patient has defective margins (overhangs) on a class II amalgam restoration that abuts a porcelain crown interproximally on each side, reducing his ability to keep the areas clean with floss and resulting in chronic inflammation. What is the BEST choice to help mitigate the circumstance?
   a. Use a standard Gracey to pop off the extra amalgam
   b. Use a sturdy posterior sickle apical to the overhang to try and remove it
   c. Use an ultrasonic tip designed to smooth the defective margin
   d. Use a periodontal file to smooth defective margins
6. After instrumentation on some moderate to heavy calculus deposits, you notice you are burnishing calculus and need to sharpen your instruments. All of the following impact the frequency and need to sharpen EXCEPT?
   a. Amount of lateral pressure used
   b. Design of the instrument
   c. Number of working strokes
   d. Type of metal the instrument is made of
7. The patient has two implants to replace congenitally missing maxillary lateral incisors. All the following statements are TRUE regarding patient treatment EXCEPT:
   a. Use a metal probe around implants #7 and #10
   b. Since calculus does not form on implants or their abutments, there is no need to check the implants for calculus deposits
   c. Avoid using the motor-driven polisher so as not to scratch the restoration
   d. Instrumentation of the implants with titanium instruments is necessary to remove all calculus deposits
8. This patient has several contraindications to rubber-cup polishing. Which of the following is NOT a contraindication for this patient?
   a. Gold onlay tooth #14
   b. Placement of a cardiac stent
   c. Gingival hyperplasia
   d. Implant abutments
9. There is a radiographically visible, large deposit of calculus on the mesial of tooth #14. Before beginning, you decide to take a minute to plan your instrumentation technique. Ensuring all the following steps will help you effectively remove the deposit EXCEPT:
   a. Use of a standard ultrasonic tip to break up the deposit beforehand instrumentation with a curet
   b. The instrument working end angulation is 70 to 80 degrees, and the instrument's lower shank is parallel to the long axis of the tooth
   c. Only the toe-third of the working end is adapted to the tooth
   d. Remove the deposit in a coronal to apical direction
10. The patient has cyanotic, gingival hyperplasia on the facials of the mandibular anterior area. After instrumentation of the lower mandibular anterior teeth, there is evidence of tissue trauma. All the following practices may cause tissue trauma EXCEPT:
   a. Using a standard versus miniature area specific curet
   b. Using a cowhorn explorer instead of an Orban-type explorer
   c. Using an appropriately adapted thin ultrasonic tip
   d. Adapting the anterior third of the working end

## CASE B

**Synopsis of Patient History**
Age: 37
Sex: F
Height: 5′2″
Weight: 130 lb

**Vital Signs**
Blood pressure: 118/74
Pulse: 76 bpm
Respiration: 15 rpm

| | | |
|---|---|---|
| 1. Under the care of a physician: | x YES | ____ NO |
| 2. Hospitalized within the last 5 years: | x YES (car accident) | ____ NO |

3. Has or had the following condition:
Depression and anxiety
4. Current medications:
Prenatal vitamins
Lexapro 5 mg/day used to treat depression
Lorazepam .50 mg/day used to treat anxiety and insomnia

| | | |
|---|---|---|
| 5. Smokes or uses tobacco products: | x YES | ____ NO |
| 6. Is pregnant: | x YES (3 months) | ____ NO |

**Medical History**
Pregnant with first child
Major depression and anxiety

**Dental History**
All third molars have been surgically extracted
Tooth-colored filling on occlusal #20 and mesiolingual of #11
Gingival tissues red and slightly enlarged on maxillary and mandibular anterior teeth

**Social History**
Sociology instructor at a local community college

**Chief Complaint**
Wants teeth cleaned

**Current Oral Hygiene Status**
Light calculus and coffee stains on proximal and lingual surfaces of #6 to #11 and facial surfaces of #22 to #27
Generalized moderate plaque biofilm

*Use Case B to answer questions 11 to 19.*

11. Access to the light subgingival calculus deposits on the proximal surfaces of the anterior teeth is difficult because of papillary enlargement of the gingival tissues. All of the following are correct instrumentation techniques EXCEPT?
    a. Moderate lateral pressure
    b. Selection of a slim-diameter tip
    c. No more than 15-degree angulation
    d. Repeated, back-and-forth strokes
12. Clinical examination shows that the gingival tissues are red and slightly enlarged on maxillary and mandibular anterior teeth. Which of the following should be considered by the hygienist consider as the LEAST likely etiologic factor(s) in the tissue inflammation?
    a. The type of dentifrice the patient is using
    b. The patient is pregnant
    c. The patient suffers from depression and anxiety
    d. Light biofilm at the gingival margin
13. Your patient tells you she has been brushing her teeth with activated charcoal for natural whitening while pregnant, and wants you to use what she's brought to polish her teeth. You know this is not approved by the Food and Drug Administration. Based on ethical and safety obligations as a health care provider, which of the following reasons is the BEST reason for you to educate your patient against its use and refuse?
    a. You must document the conversation in her chart based on HIPAA requirements
    b. You are obligated to provide evidence-based care
    c. You are obligated to protect the patient from harm during care
    d. Both b and c
14. Calculus assessment reveals light, supragingival calculus deposits in sheets on the maxillary and mandibular anterior teeth and maxillary first molars, with generalized plaque biofilm and no pocketing. Of the following instruments, which would you be most likely NOT to use in treating this patient?
    a. Universal curet
    b. Anterior sickle scaler
    c. ODU 11/12 explorer
    d. Beaver tail ultrasonic tip
15. While removing the light calculus on the lingual surfaces of maxillary anterior teeth, you notice a dark semi-circle on the distal lingual of tooth #10, which you suspect to be caries. You noticed this by using your mirror for which of the following mirror techniques?
    a. Retraction
    b. Transillumination
    c. Indirect illumination
    d. Indirect vision
16. You are probing the facial of tooth #4 and note a probing depths of 3mm at the midline of the distal surface, 4 mm at the distofacial line angle, 5 mm on the facial surface, 2 mm on the mesiofacial line angle, and 3 mm at the midline of the mesial surface. Which of the following would be the CORRECT probe depth recording for the facial of tooth #4 from the distal to the mesial?
    a. 4-5-3
    b. 3-2-3
    c. 3-5-2
    d. 4-2-3
17. When removing calculus deposits on interproximal surfaces of the facial aspect of a mandibular anterior sextant, which fulcrum would be the BEST in this situation?
    a. Finger-on-finger
    b. Extra-oral
    c. Opposite arch
    d. Piggyback
18. Which of the following is the correct sequence in steps for executing a subgingival calculus removal stroke?
    a. Open the blade to 70 degrees, adapt the toe-third of the cutting edge on the surface of the deposit, position the mirror, adapt the cutting edge to the tooth, activate pulling stroke coronally with hand-forearm activation
    b. Close the face of the working end and insert, adapt entire working end apical to deposit, adjust and stabilize grasp, activate pushing stroke apically
    c. Close the face of the working end and insert, adapt toe-third apical to deposit, adjust and stabilize grasp, apply lateral pressure, activate pulling stroke coronally with hand-forearm activation
    d. Establish a fulcrum, position the mirror, adapt the cutting edge to the tooth, insert to the junctional epithelium, apply lateral pressure
19. The facial surface of tooth #3 is coated with a large, moderate layer of supragingival calculus that extends subgingivally. All the following stroke patterns should be used to remove this calculus deposit efficiently EXCEPT:
    a. Long, light strokes
    b. Overlapping, strokes in sections
    c. Firm, short strokes
    d. Oblique strokes

## CASE C

**Synopsis of Patient History**

Age: 48
Sex: F
Height: 5′3″
Weight: 165 lb

**Vital Signs**

Blood pressure: 149/92
Pulse: 80 bpm
Respiration: 13 rpm

1. Under the care of a physician: x YES ___ NO
2. Hospitalized within the last 5 years: x YES ___ NO
3. Has or had the following condition:
Hypertension
Type II diabetes
On a physician-directed sodium-restricted diet

4. Current medications:
Lisinopril 10 mg/day
Metformin 500 mg/day
5. Smokes or uses tobacco products: x YES ___ NO
Cigarettes for 18 years

Continued

## CASE C—CONT'D

**Medical History**

History of hypertension diagnosed 5 years ago. Type II diabetes diagnosed 18 months ago. Current HbA1c is 9.0.

**Dental History**

Missing with no replacement: #1, #4, #16, #17, #30, #32
Several large amalgams and tooth-colored anterior restorations
Recurrent caries apical to class V composite on F #9
Pocket depth range 3–6 mm with class III furcation involvement on F #19
6-mm pocket depth on M #3, which has drifted mesially
6-mm pocket depth on D #15
Significant recession on F #19, D and F #14
Moderate tobacco stain
Fibrotic gingival tissues with generalized, light bleeding on probing

**Social History**

Retail store manager
Recently divorced

**Chief Complaint**

Wants teeth to look whiter and wants to replace the "gap" on the lower right

**Current Oral Hygiene Status**

Generalized subgingival calculus deposits in anterior and posterior sextants
Heavy generalized plaque biofilm on gingival thirds of teeth
Radiographs confirm bone loss and furcation involvement in posterior sextants

***Use Case C to answer questions 20 to 29.***

20. Your patient tends to be sensitive, and does not like the ultrasonic to be used. The BEST way to remove supragingival tobacco stain and biofilm for this patient is:
    a. The toe of a universal curet
    b. An air polisher with erythritol
    c. A Nabers diamond-coated file (similar to Nabers furcation probe with diamond coating)
    d. A standard ultrasonic tip
21. Which of the following ultrasonic tips would be the BEST choice to initiate removal of the moderate calculus deposits located subgingivally in a 6mm pocket?
    a. Standard tip with a straight working end
    b. Medium tip with a straight working end
    c. Right and left paired tips
    d. Slim-diameter tip
22. Tooth #19 has class III furcation involvement on the facial aspect. Which of the following instruments would be the BEST choice for light calculus removal and deplaquing the roof of the furcation area?
    a. DeMarco curet
    b. Periodontal file
    c. Mini Gracey curet 1/2
    d. Universal curet with an extended lower shank
23. Your patient has fibrotic tissue, with generalized bleeding on probing. All of the following are likely contributing to her periodontal condition EXCEPT
    a. Poor glycemic control
    b. Smoking
    c. Subgingival hard and soft deposits
    d. The patient's hypertension medication
24. Which instrument would be BEST to detect furcation involvement on multirooted teeth?
    a. Furcation probe, such as a Nabers probe
    b. Periodontal file
    c. A biotype probe
    d. Calibrated periodontal probe
25. All the following statements are TRUE about ultrasonic instrumentation EXCEPT:
    a. The side of the tip should maintain contact with the tooth at all times
    b. Cavitation creates tiny bubbles that collapse and kill bacteria
    c. They are safe to use on composite restorations
    d. There are no cutting edges on the ultrasonic tip
26. You notice that your ultrasonic instrumentation has become less efficient recently. It is taking longer to remove calculus deposits, and even biofilm removal is not as effective. You assess your technique, and find nothing that needs to be adjusted. Which of the following is likely the cause of the decline in your ultrasonic instrumentation?
    a. The water flow needs to be increased
    b. The tips are worn
    c. The power and lateral pressure need to be increased
    d. The time being spent instrumented on each tooth needs to be increased
27. On a tooth with class III furcation involvement, which of the following instruments would you use from the facial aspect to instrument the mesial half of the distal root?
    a. Universal curet
    b. Miniature Gracey 11/12 curet
    c. Miniature Gracey 13/14 curet
    d. ODU 11/12 explorer
28. Tooth #19 has significant recession of the gingival margin. If there were light tobacco stain on the root surface, what would be the BEST way to remove it?
    a. Use a straight, slim-diameter ultrasonic tip with light overlapping strokes
    b. Do not remove the stain, because it is not visible when the patient smiles, and stain does not contribute to periodontal disease or dental caries
    c. Use a rigid Gracey 11/12 curet with light pressure
    d. Use an air polisher with glycine or erythritol
29. Your patient is considering an implant to replace "the gap" where tooth #4 was extracted. Which of the following is NOT likely to be a contraindication for implant placement?
    a. Poor glycemic control
    b. Clinical attachment level
    c. Poor oral hygiene
    d. Smoking

## CASE D

Sophie is a high-achieving, 20-year-old college junior with type 1 diabetes. Her course load, extracurricular volunteering, and studying for the law school admissions test has led to poor diet and decreased oral hygiene. She states she has been drinking multiple cans of energy drinks each day to keep up her pace. She presents with generalized marginal gingivitis, moderate bleeding on probing, light calculus, and heavy plaque biofilm. Dental examination revealed demineralized, white spot lesions on the cervical of #7–#10 facial.

*Use Case D to answer questions 30 to 33.*

30. In addition to controlling local oral factors—biofilm and calculus deposits—the dental team should consider the all the following to assist Sophie in improving her oral health EXCEPT:
    a. Apply fluoride varnish at every visit, and recommend a prescription fluoride dentifrice
    b. Consultation with her primary care provider or endocrinologist
    c. Recommend a gingivectomy to control the marginal gingivitis
    d. Provide nutritional counseling, and explain the connection between poor glycemic control and poor oral health
31. Before beginning instrumentation, you explore to determine the type, amount, and location of calculus deposits. Which of the following explorers is NOT recommended for calculus detection?
    a. ODU 11/12
    b. 6XL straight explorer
    c. Pigtail or cowhorn
    d. Orban type
32. Which of the following patient-positioning suggestions is BEST to ensure an effective and ergonomic instrumentation technique on a dentition with crowded mandibular anterior teeth?
    a. Adjust the chair back to a 45-degree angle, and ask the patient to lower her chin (chin-down position) so that the occlusal plane is parallel to the floor
    b. Wear loupes for better visualization
    c. Ask the patient to keep his chin in an upward position (chin-up position)
    d. Put the chair in an upright position so the clinician can work from a standing position
33. Because the mandibular anterior teeth are crowded and lingoverted, calculus removal on the lingual, interproximal surfaces will be challenging. Which of the following would be the BEST instrument choice?
    a. A Gracey 1/2 curet
    b. A universal curet
    c. An ODU 11/12 explorer since access is narrow
    d. Anterior sickle scaler

## CASE E

Antonio is a healthy 2-year-old toddler whose mother has brought him in for his first dental visit. His mother states she brushes his teeth daily with a nonfluoridated, children's toothpaste, and that they have nonfluoridated well water. On examination, you notice light plaque along the gingival margins that when removed, reveals white-spot lesions.

*Use Case E to answer questions 34 to 36.*

34. Considering the white spot lesions identified, all the following can be used during treatment on this pediatric patient EXCEPT:
    a. Rubber-cup polishing
    b. Toothbrush
    c. Universal curet
    d. Ultrasonic scaler
35. Which of the following approaches is likely to be of MOST benefit to Antonio's ongoing oral health?
    a. Guiding the child as she removes the biofilm herself during the appointment
    b. Using a rubber cup and prophy paste to remove the biofilm
    c. Educating the patient's mother
    d. Fluoride varnish application every six months
36. All the following are acceptable methods of fluoride delivery for this patient EXCEPT:
    a. A smear of fluoridated toothpaste when brushing
    b. 5% NaF varnish
    c. 0.25 mg fluoride supplements daily
    d. 1.23% APF in a tray

## CASE F

Nasim is a new graduate who accepted a position as dental hygienist at a small dental office, replacing a hygienist of 20 years. During his interview, Nasim noticed that the instruments in each hygiene cassette contained a shepherd's hook explorer, one anterior sickle, and one universal curet. The instruments were dull with narrow handles, and there were no ultrasonic units available.

*Use Case F to answer questions 37 and 38.*

37. Dull instruments inhibit efficient patient treatment and causes musculoskeletal fatigue for the operator. All the following statements are TRUE about the importance of using a sharp versus a dull instrument EXCEPT:
    a. Fewer strokes are necessary
    b. More discomfort for the patient
    c. Calculus is more easily removed
    d. Stroke control is much improved
38. Nasim is finding moderate to heavy calculus deposits regularly on a number of patients. He notices that he is regularly having muscle fatigue in his dominant hand at the end of the day. All the following may be contributing to Nasim's muscle fatigue EXCEPT:
    a. Dull instruments are not effective in removing calculus deposits.
    b. Narrow-diameter handles cause the clinician to use more grip pressure, thus causing muscle fatigue.
    c. His instrument selection is limited, forcing him to use an inappropriate instrument, such as using a Gracey 11/12 to remove heavy calculus deposits.
    d. Relaxing the fingers in the grasp after each calculus removal stroke is inefficient and stresses the hand muscles.

## CASE G

George, age 90, is a widower who lives in an assisted living facility and is dropped off at his appointments by the facility's shuttle driver. George presents with generalized posterior recession of the gingival margin and bone loss, heavy biofilm and food impaction in the posteriors with moderate, subgingival calculus. George does not remember his last visit or why he is there, which is a significant decline in his memory since his last visit 6 months ago.

*Use Case G to answer questions 39 to 41.*

39. You decide to use ultrasonic instrumentation for biofilm and food impaction removal. However, you notice that George has trouble swallowing and keeps coughing whenever you apply the ultrasonic. Which of the following would be the BEST alternative?
    a. Continue using the ultrasonic as it will be quicker and more efficient in removing the biofilm and food.
    b. Use a universal curet.

c. Use a toothbrush to remove as much of the biofilm and food as possible before moving to hand instrumentation.
d. Reschedule the appointment.

40. George does not recognize you and does not understand why he is there. You note his blood pressure is more elevated than usual. At what stage of treatment should you assess the patient for signs of anxiety?
    a. After instrumentation of a few teeth
    b. After reviewing the medical history and before beginning instrumentation
    c. While explaining what to expect during ultrasonic instrumentation
    d. Before taking radiographs
41. All the following are ethical and legal concerns when treating this patient EXCEPT:
    a. Obligation to protect the patient from harm or injury during care
    b. Obtaining consent
    c. Assessing for physician or specialty referrals
    d. Sharing information with the assisted living facility regarding George's oral hygiene
42. Which of the following instruments would be BEST to remove moderate to heavy calculus under the contact on the mesial of tooth #15?
    a. Rigid Gracey 13/14 curet
    b. Posterior sickle
    c. Quétin curet
    d. Universal curet

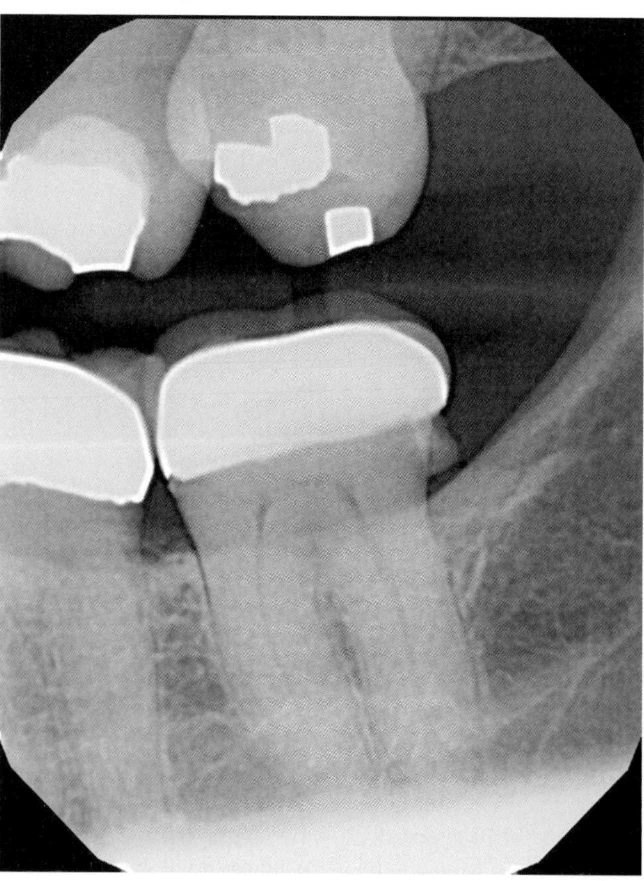

43. Removing subgingival calculus deposits from the distal of terminal molars would be BEST accomplished using:
    a. An area specific curet with a complex, extended shank
    b. Anterior sickle
    c. Standard Gracey ½
    d. Universal curet
44. Tooth #14 has a heavy, tenacious ledge of calculus on the mesiolingual requiring significant lateral pressure for removal. All of the following will ensure effective lateral pressure EXCEPT:
    a. Sharpened instruments
    b. A rigid shank instrument
    c. A miniature-bladed curet
    d. A stabilized fulcrum
45. You realize you have a small area of burnished calculus on the furcation floor of tooth #2. Which of the following hand instruments would be the BEST choice when removing this burnished calculus?
    a. Diamond file
    b. Standard Gracey 13/14
    c. Posterior sickle
    d. Universal curet

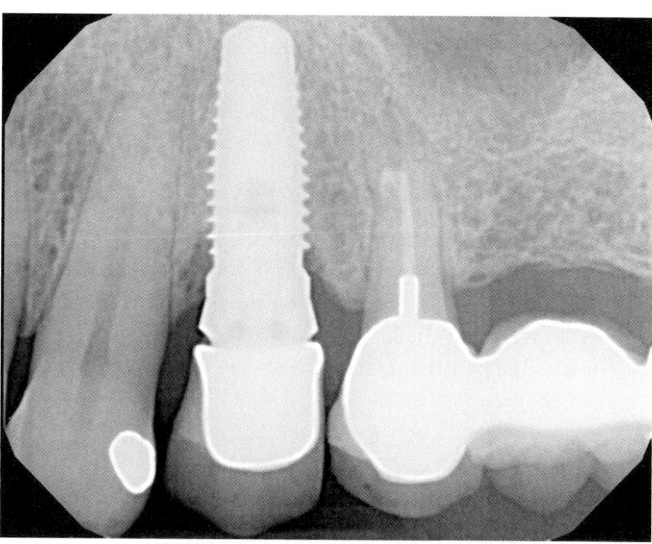

46. Which of the following instruments is BEST for calculus removal from a dental implant?
    a. Titanium curet
    b. Plastic periodontal probe
    c. Standard Gracey curet
    d. An explorer
47. A new patient presents for scaling and root planing. The patient is a smoker of 25 years, and has a diagnosis of chronic generalized periodontitis. All maxillary posterior teeth have moderate, tenacious, subgingival calculus deposits. Which of the following is NOT recommended for removing these calculus deposits?
    a. Subgingival air polishing
    b. Begin with a standard ultrasonic tip, approach the deposits from both the facial and the lingual aspect of the sextant

c. Assess the amount, type, and location of the calculus deposits with a periodontal explorer, such as an ODU 11/12
d. Once the heavy deposits have been removed, use a slim-diameter ultrasonic tip to complete calculus removal

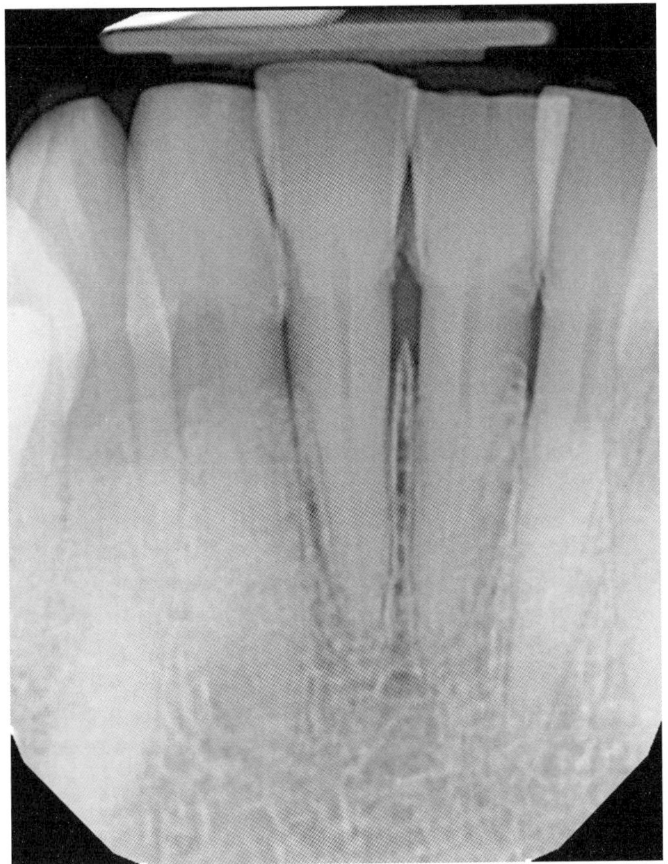

48. Which instrument would be most efficient in removing heavy, supragingival calculus deposits from the linguals of anterior teeth that exhibit crowding?
    a. Universal curet
    b. Beaver tail ultrasonic tip
    c. Gracey miniature 1/2 curet
    d. Anterior sickle scaler
49. The patient has multiple implants and restorations, with generalized, moderate biofilm and bleeding on probing. In addition, the patient has 5–6 mm pocketing in multiple areas but slight to no subginigival calculus. Which would be the BEST option to debride the biofilm?
    a. Subgingival air polisher using glycine powder
    b. Titanium implant instruments
    c. Posterior sickle scaler
    d. A universal curet

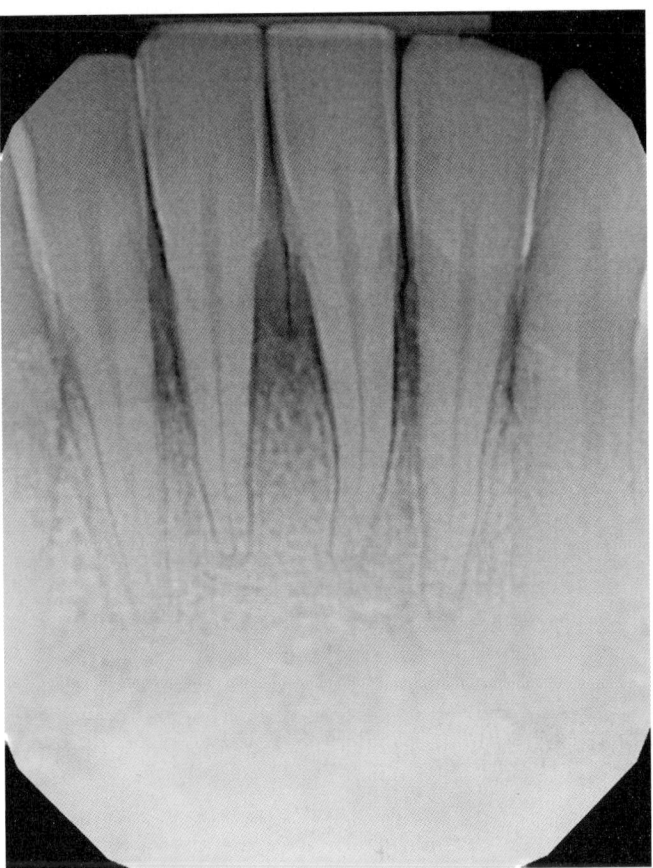

50. The lingual of tooth #26 has a 6 mm pocket with a moderate piece of subgingival near its base. Which would be the BEST hand instrument choice considering the anatomy of the root and pocket depth?
    a. Langer sub zero curvette
    b. Standard Gracey 1/2 curet
    c. Micro-mini Gracey 1/2 curet
    d. Universal curet

## SUGGESTED READINGS

Darby ML, Walsh MM. Instruments and instrumentation theory. In: Darby ML, Walsh MM, eds. *Dental Hygiene Theory and Practice.* 3rd ed. Philadelphia: Saunders; 2010.

Nield-Gehrig JS. *Fundamentals of Periodontal Instrumentation and Advanced Root Instrumentation.* 7th ed. Philadelphia: Lippincott Williams & Wilkins; 2013.

# 18

# Management of Pain and Anxiety

*Margaret J. Fehrenbach, Demetra Daskalos Logothetis*

As clinicians, dental hygienists must be able to manage the patient's pain and anxiety. This requires mastery of head and neck anatomy, physiology, pharmacology, medical emergencies, and clinical technique. This chapter reviews four methods to relieve and manage pain and anxiety: (1) local anesthesia with standard syringe, (2) topical anesthesia, (3) computer-controlled local anesthesia delivery device, and (4) nitrous oxide-oxygen minimal (conscious) sedation.

## DENTAL PAIN

A. Types of dental pain
   1. From disease or trauma (see medical/dental history)
   2. Iatrogenic, meaning from dental treatment
   3. Post dental treatment
B. Pain perception
   1. Physioanatomic process by which pain is received and transmitted by neural structures from end organs and pain receptions and through conductive and perceptive mechanisms
   2. Does not differ much from person to person, same in most healthy individuals, but can be affected by both disease and toxic states
C. Pain reaction
   1. Manifestation of perception of pain that has been perceived by the brain
   2. Determines what patient will do about the unpleasant experience of pain
   3. Differs greatly from person to person because of past dental experiences and various factors such as fatigue, stress, fear, apprehension, age, emotional state, education
D. Pain threshold
   1. Hyporeactive: high pain threshold, tolerates pain well, shows little reaction to pain
   2. Hyperreactive: low pain threshold, does not tolerate pain well, shows more reaction to pain
   3. However, most individuals vary between two types depending on factors (discussed earlier)
E. Responses to pain
   1. Physiologic: increased respiratory rate, increased heart rate (HR), increased blood pressure (BP)
   2. Physical: crying out, tapping feet, cold sweat, altered facial expression, white knuckles, inability to sit still
F. Pain control and dental office
   1. Pain is a major factor that brings patients to the dental office, while fear and anxiety about pain are the most common reasons patients fail to seek dental care; many avoid dental treatment until forced into office with an emergency
   2. Control of pain and anxiety is therefore an essential part of dental practice:
      a. To accomplish this objective, various techniques are used, including psychological approaches, local anesthetics of various types, and combinations of sedative and general anesthetic agents
      b. Choice of most appropriate modality for particular situation is based on training, knowledge, and experience of clinician; nature, severity, duration of procedure; age and physical and psychological status of patient; level of fear and anxiety; previous responses to pain control procedures
   3. Important part of stress reduction protocol, especially in management of cardiovascular disease (CVD) patients

## ANXIETY MANAGEMENT

Anxiety is the feeling of apprehension and fear characterized by physical symptoms such as palpitations, sweating, feelings of stress. Anxiety keeps many people from receiving necessary dental treatment because of fear of pain or discomfort. Fear is excessive apprehension or anxiety. Understanding dental fear can help in selecting appropriate methods for alleviating patient discomfort. Anxiety and fear are common occurrences in the dental office and can be managed by a variety of techniques. Sometimes fear can become excessive and involve a phobia, which promotes inaction (further failure to seek necessary dental treatment).

A. Etiology of dental anxiety and fear:
   1. Anxiety and fear are typically based on past dental experiences
   2. May be based on fearful experiences related by others (friends or family) or portrayed by media
   3. Iatrogenic causes arise from personal experiences with dental situations and personnel (typically during childhood); two greatest dental fears are needles and dental drill
   4. Feeling a loss of control can increase dental anxiety and fear
B. Treatment of dental anxiety, fear, phobias:
   1. Using systemic desensitization (small doses of positive experiences) for highly anxious patients increases tolerance for dental encounters

2. Explaining procedures thoroughly decreases fear of unknown
3. Increasing patient control during each treatment session decreases fear of helplessness and increases sense of trust (allow patient to help with suction by holding patient saliva ejector or pick out favorite flavor of topical)
4. Using relaxation techniques in dental environment, includes headphones or other distracters, calming voice, biofeedback, adhering to time schedule
5. Using pharmacologic control of anxiety:
   a. Moderate sedation with premedication, either orally or IV, with benzodiazepines (BZDs), diazepam (Valium), or alprazolam (Xanax); patient will have less memory of stressful dental procedures (see Chapter 11, Pharmacology)
   b. Topical and/or injected local anesthesia agents can remove pain during dental procedures.
   c. Minimal (conscious) sedation with nitrous oxide can provide more relaxation, increase pain threshold, decrease awareness of time and procedures, increase sense of well-being.
   d. Posttreatment with antiinflammatories (such as ibuprofen) can reduce inflammation and thus pain, helping with healing (see Chapter 11, Pharmacology).

## SENSORY INNERVATION

Peripheral nervous system (PNS) comprises sensory (afferent) nerves that carry sensations of pain to central nervous system (CNS), and motor (efferent) nerves that transmit messages from CNS to muscles and glands. Understanding of sensory nerve anatomy and physiology and action of local anesthetics is essential to pain management.

A. Anatomy of nerve:
   1. Myelinated nerves (comprise most nerves in the body), divided into four zones: (Fig. 18.1)
      a. Input zone: Dendrite (free nerve endings) receives input from other neurons or from sensory stimuli (where majority of input to neuron occurs)
      b. Summation zone: Serves as site where nerve impulses combine and, if total strength exceeds threshold potential, will trigger impulse that will be conducted along axon or conduction zone
      c. Conduction zone: Axon is pipeline that delivers impulses to CNS. Both summation (trigger) zone and conduction zone have many voltage-gated Na+ channels and K+ channels imbedded in plasma membrane
      d. Output zone: (distal end of axon) Where nerve impulse triggers release of neurotransmitters. Output zone includes many voltage-gated Ca++ channels in membrane
   2. Structure of single nerve fiber: myelin sheath covers axon, composed mainly of lipid layers (75%), protein (20%), and carbohydrates (5%)
      a. Lipid layers: act as barriers to some molecules and as binding sites for lipophilic components of local anesthetics
      b. Proteins: act as channels to allow some ions (Na+, K+) to pass through nerve membrane

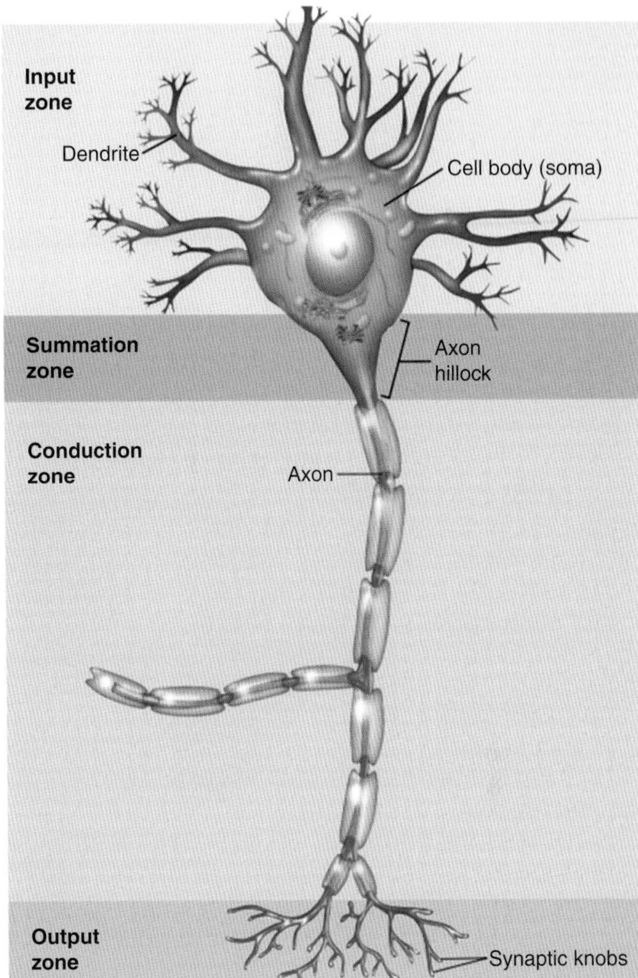


**Fig. 18.1** Functional regions of the neuron's plasma membrane. The input zone receives input from other neurons or from sensory stimuli (stimulus-gated ion channels present). The summation zone serves as the site where the nerve impulses combine and possibly trigger an impulse that will be conducted along the axon, or conduction zone. Both the summation (trigger) zone and conduction zone have many voltage-gated Na+ channels and K+ channels imbedded in the plasma membrane. The output zone (distal end of axon) is where the nerve impulse triggers the release of neurotransmitters. The output zone includes many voltage-gated Ca++ channels in the membrane. (From: Patton K, Thibodeau G. *Anatomy and Physiology*. 9th ed. St Louis: Mosby; 2016.)

   3. Layers of nerve: (Fig. 18.2):
      a. Endoneurium: layer of connective tissue which surrounds each axon within a nerve
      b. Fascicles: nerve bundles that are bundled together in groups
      c. Perineurium: layer of connective tissue that wraps each fasciculi
      d. Epineurium: connective tissue layer that wraps the entire nerve; carries fasciculi, blood vessels, and lymphatic vessels; as anesthetic diffuses through epineural sheath and blood vessels, begins to eliminate anesthetic
   4. Nodes of Ranvier: gaps 0.5 to 3 mm apart; nerve impulses travel from node to node via salutatory conduction (rapid transmission of nerve impulses along myelinated nerve fiber)

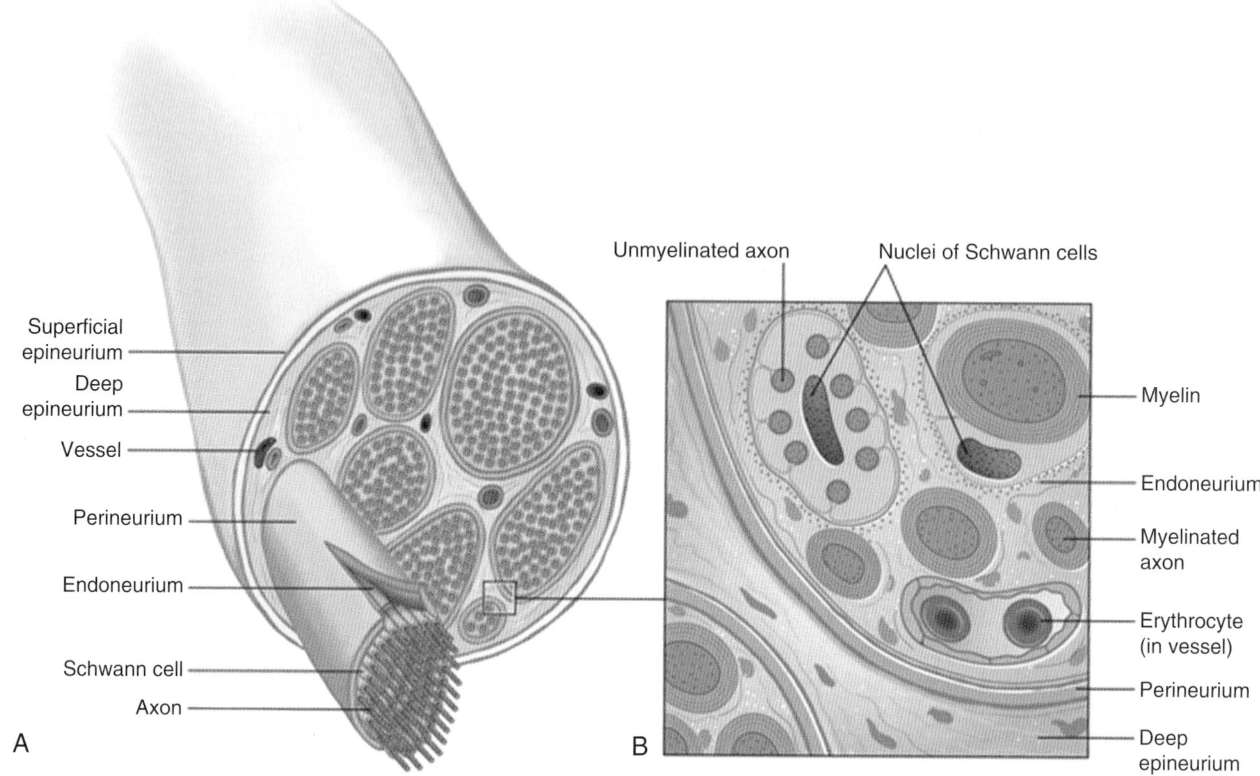


**Fig. 18.2** The nerve. (A) Each nerve contains axons bundled into fascicles. A fibrous endoneurium surrounds each axon and its Schwann cells within a fascicle. A perineurium surrounds each fascicle, forming a blood-nerve barrier. A dense connective tissue epineurium wraps the entire nerve. (B) Inset showing magnified view of individual neurons within a fascicle. (From: Patton K, Thibodeau G. *Anatomy and Physiology*, 21st ed. St Louis: Mosby; 2019.)

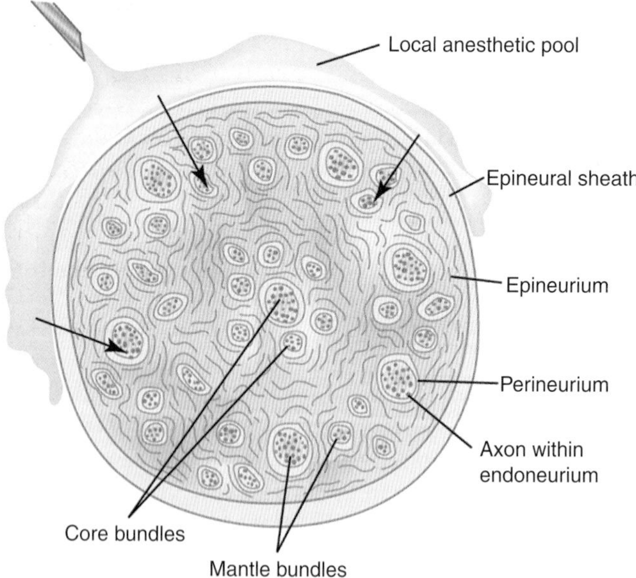


**Fig. 18.3** A schematic cross section of a large peripheral nerve illustrating the composition of nerve fibers and bundles, and how the deposited local anesthetic solution near the nerve sheath must diffuse inward toward the core fibers, reaching the mantle fibers first. (From: Logothetis D.D. *Local Anesthesia for the Dental Hygienist*. 3rd ed. St. Louis; Elsevier; 2021)

B. Structure of nerve bundle: many peripheral nerves have hundreds to thousands of tightly packed axons in the fasciculi bundles (Fig. 18.3)
   1. Mantle bundles: located near the outside of nerve bundle, receive anesthetic first, innervate proximal areas (posteriors), and begin to lose anesthetic properties first, but will be the last fibers to recover completely
   2. Core bundles: located closer to the inside of nerve bundle; receive anesthetic last and in lower concentration because of distance from anesthetic source and presence of more blood vessels; innervate distal areas (anteriors) and lose anesthetic properties by slowly diffusing into mantel bundles and are the first fibers to recover

C. Physiology of nerve:
   1. Resting nerve cell membrane (polarized or nonstimulated):
      a. Nonstimulated nerve has Na+ ions outside membrane, K+ ions and negative ions inside, and resting potential of –70 mV

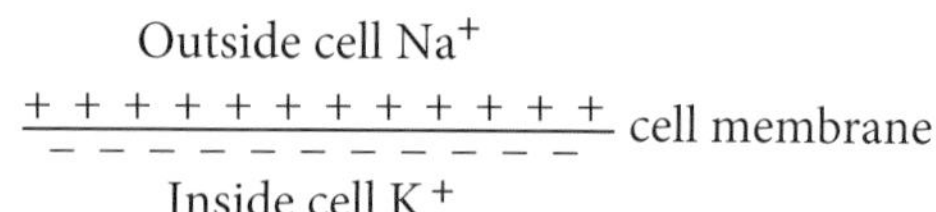


      b. Membrane potential maintained by sodium-potassium pump and permeability of cell membrane
   2. Minimal threshold stimulus:
      a. Stimulus: environmental change that can be chemical, thermal, mechanical, or electrical in nature
      b. Minimal threshold stimulus: magnitude of stimulus required to initiate nerve impulse
      c. "All-or-none" principle: either nerve fires as strongly as possible or it does not fire at all

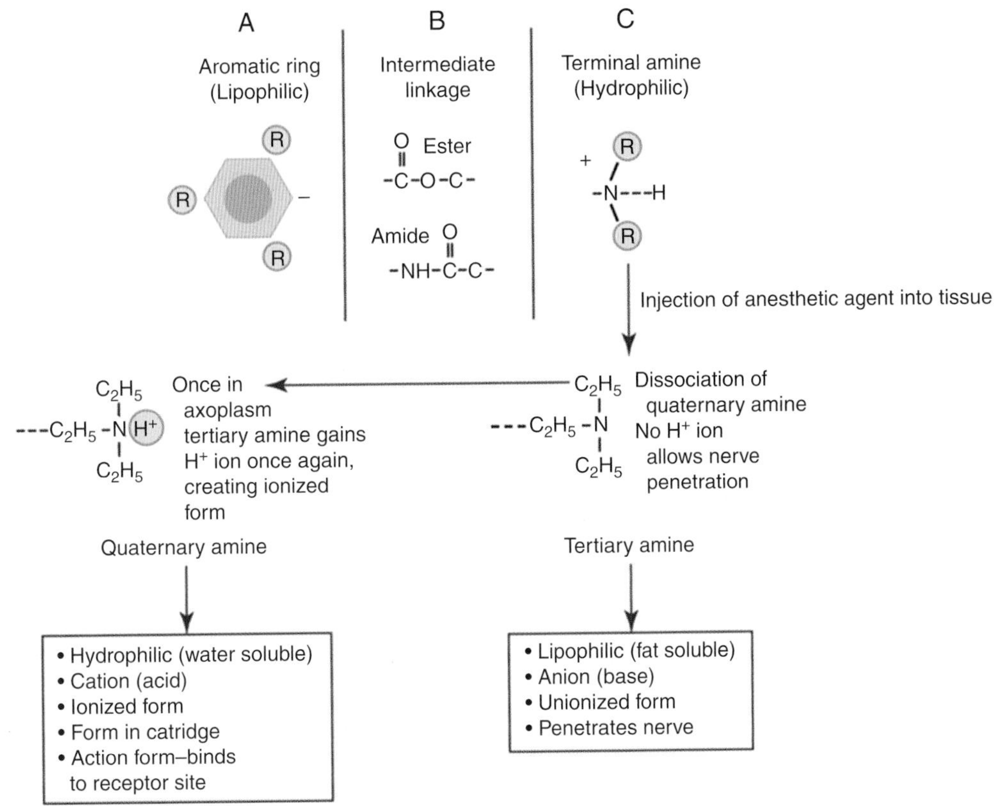


**Fig. 18.4** Chemical formula of a local anesthetic. (From: Logothetis D.D. *Local Anesthesia for the Dental Hygienist*. 3rd ed. St. Louis: Elsevier; 2021)

3. Excitation: When a minimal threshold stimulus excites the nerve:
   a. The permeability of the cell membrane changes:
      (1) Influx: $Na^+$ enters cell
      (2) Efflux: $K^+$ diffuses to outside of cell
   b. Reversed polarity:

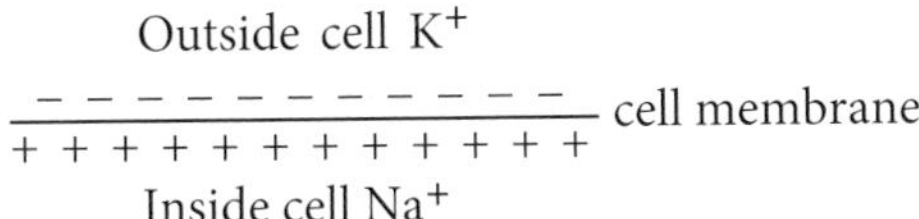


4. Depolarization: time interval that exists while ionic concentrations are reversing
5. Reversed polarity: result of reversal in ionic charges
6. Repolarization: occurs after reversed polarity; membrane becomes hyperpermeable to $K^+$ and impermeable to $Na^+$; polarity is reestablished
7. Action potential: rapid sequence of changes in membrane potential (negative to positive and positive back to negative);
   Stages involved:
   a. Depolarization: resulting in reversed polarity
   b. Repolarization
6. Absolute refractory period: period during depolarization and reversed polarity when cell membrane cannot be reexcited
7. Relative refractory period: during repolarization, nerve cell membrane can be reexcited, but requires greater stimulus than stimulus required for excitation from resting state

## LOCAL ANESTHESIA

Dental patients can benefit from removal of pain during dental procedure with local anesthesia, along with use of topical anesthesia, as well as hemorrhage control from use of a vasoconstrictor. Can be used alone or with a combination of nitrous oxide sedation, the latter which alone does not replace local anesthesia for pain control since it is an analgesic and not an anesthetic. Local anesthetic administration is within the legal scope of dental hygiene practice in most jurisdictions in the United States and may need to be under the supervision of dentist.

A. Mode of action: local anesthetic prevents or blocks depolarization in neurons
   1. Stabilizes nerve membrane so that membrane threshold is elevated to point where depolarization does not occur
   2. Thus Na + channels do not open and Na + ions will not pass through the Na+ channels
   3. Depresses all unmyelinated fibers first and larger myelinated fibers last
   4. General order of loss of function (first to last): pain, temperature, touch, proprioception, motor nerve function
B. Chemical formula of agent (Fig. 18.4):
   1. Aromatic group (lipophilic [hydrophobic] component): affinity for lipid portion of the myelin sheath, which helps local anesthetic agent attach to nerve membrane and block nerve impulse
   2. Intermediate chain: either ester (– COO – R) or amide (NHCO – R) group; determines mode of biotransformation or metabolism (see later discussion)

3. Amino end (hydrophilic component): makes anesthetic agent injectable; amides dissolve poorly in water and are unstable on exposure to air; therefore hydrochloride (HCl) is added to produce a salt that is more soluble and stable

C. Discussion of pH: mathematic measure of acidity and alkalinity, expressed as negative logarithm:
1. Acidic substances have higher concentrations of hydrogen (H+) ions and therefore can give up more H+ ions; alkaline (base) substances have lower concentrations of H + ions and can accept more H+ ions
2. The pH of normal tissue is 7.4; pH of inflamed tissue is lower, between 5 and 6 (more acidic)
3. Decreased extracellular pH does not decrease nerve action; internal pH of nerve is constant; decreased extracellular pH does decrease action of anesthetic
4. The pH of anesthetic without epinephrine (vasoconstrictor) is 5.5; anesthetic with epinephrine is ~ 3.3 pH
   a. Manufacturers acidify anesthetic with sodium bisulfite to inhibit oxidation (breakdown) of epinephrine
   b. Anesthetic may burn slightly on deposition because of difference between pH of anesthetic and pH of tissue
   c. More acidic the anesthetic, slower its onset; using cartridge warmers can break down pH of local anesthetic, increasing burning during deposition

D. Dissociation of local anesthetics: ability of local anesthetic to dissociate, indicated by pKa number
1. The pKa number is a constant that characterizes equilibrium of a particular compound; also measures molecule's affinity for H+ ions:
   a. Equilibrium equation is a pKa equation: RNH+ ⇔ RN + H+
   b. Cation: RNH+ is positively charged molecule that is responsible for binding at receptor site and decreasing the Na+ that enters nerve
   c. Free base: RN is uncharged molecule that is responsible for diffusion of anesthetic through surrounding tissues and the nerve sheath
2. Clinical implications of the pKa number, since each anesthetic has pKa number:
   a. Lower pKa number (below 7.5), more lipophilic free base molecules (creates greater diffusion, quicker onset of action but less cations available to bind anesthetic
   b. When the pH of anesthetic is same as pKa number, equal amounts of base and cation exist
   c. Equilibrium shifts:
      (1) Shifts left (cation state) when there are more hydrogen ions (low pH)
      (2) Shifts right (free base state) when there are fewer hydrogen ions (high pH)
   d. More free base molecules available, greater diffusion of anesthetic through tissue and membrane, and therefore faster onset of action
3. The pH of anesthetic is lowered with addition of epinephrine (pH 3.3):
   a. When more cations exist, more Na + is bound at nerve receptor, which creates greater binding power
   b. Less free base leads to less diffusion and slower onset
   c. Surrounding tissue buffer more acidic solutions
4. The pH of inflamed tissue is low (5 to 6), so more cations exist; therefore Na + is bound at nerve receptor site:
   a. Less diffusion of anesthetic into surrounding tissues causes slower onset and leads to ineffective anesthesia
   b. Surrounding tissues are not able to buffer more acidic solutions because of lower pH
   c. Patient may need more local anesthetic agent because of acidic conditions; nerve block may be more effective than supraperiosteal injection since agent is not near inflamed tissue

## PHARMACOLOGY OF LOCAL ANESTHETICS AND VASOCONSTRICTORS

Understanding the metabolism, action, dosage calculations, and specific functions of topical and local anesthetic agents and vasoconstrictors helps the clinician to request and use these agents more safely and efficiently. Clinician must prevent overdose (OD) situation, which is accidental or intentional use of drug in amount higher than normally used.

A. Types of agents:
1. Ester agents: No longer available as injectables, only with topicals (usually 20% benzocaine):
   a. Biotransformed to paraaminobenzoic acid (PABA) in blood plasma by enzyme pseudocholinesterase
   b. Half-life (rate at which 50% of the anesthetic is eliminated from the blood) is 2 to 8 minutes
   c. Have lower potential for OD (toxicity)
   d. More likely to cause allergic reaction (to PABA)
2. Amide agents
   a. Less likely to cause allergic reaction because methylparaben, which can cause allergic reactions, has been eliminated as preservative
   b. Biotransformed mainly in liver (must have healthy liver tissue)
   c. Have greater potential for OD (when alone and without vasoconstrictor) because higher blood levels occur until agent reaches liver for biotransformation
   d. Half-life is 96 to 162 minutes depending on anesthetic
      (1) Exception: Articaine's half-life is different from other amides
         (a) Falls under amide class, but its associated ester group also allows plasma metabolism via pseudocholinesterase, purportedly increasing rate of breakdown and reducing its toxicity
         (b) Difference in metabolism gives advantage of having 27-minute half life, in contrast to lidocaine, which has 96-minute half-life

B. Distribution and elimination of agents:
1. After entering blood, agents permeate all body tissue
2. Local anesthetics are vasodilators; thus vasoconstrictors are added in most cases to decrease vasodilation
3. Esters and amide agents are both eliminated mostly through kidneys

C. Phentolamine mesylate injection via syringe (Oraverse): accelerates return of normal soft tissue sensation (i.e., sensation of lip and tongue) as well as function following restorative and periodontal procedures. Also helps prevent any self-inflicted oral trauma that may occur with long-lasting injection of local anesthetic containing vasoconstrictor. Contains alpha-adrenergic antagonist that acts as vasodilator, resulting in faster diffusion of anesthetic into cardiovascular system and away from site

## LOCAL ANESTHETIC AGENT ACTION

Local anesthetics are anesthetic drugs that induce local anesthesia by inhibiting nerve excitation or conduction. These agents also have effects on CNS, cardiovascular system (CVS), and respiratory system. See Chapter 21, Medical and Dental Emergencies: local anesthesia emergency protocol in dental setting.

A. CNS effects:
   1. Low levels have no effect but can provide anticonvulsive properties by raising seizure threshold; used to treat epileptic seizures
   2. Preconvulsive levels can cause slurred speech, shivering, twitching, flushed feeling, dream state, lightheadedness, blurred vision, tinnitus
      a. Lidocaine may cause mild sedation or drowsiness, which is indication of possible toxic reaction
      b. Therefore anesthetized patient should never be left alone since onset occurs in 5 to 10 minutes
   3. Convulsive levels cause convulsions, CNS depression, respiratory depression and arrest
B. CVS effects:
   1. Low levels produce no effects
   2. High (non-OD) levels cause mild hypotension (low blood pressure) by relaxing smooth muscles
   3. At OD levels, can produce profound hypotension, which causes decreased myocardial contractions, decreased cardiac output, decreased peripheral resistance
   4. Lethal levels lead to CVS collapse caused by massive peripheral vasodilation, decreased heart contractions, and decreased heart rate (bradycardia)
C. Respiratory system effects:
   1. Non-OD levels relax action of bronchial smooth muscles
   2. OD levels can lead to respiratory arrest as a result of CNS depression

## VASOCONSTRICTOR ACTION WITH LOCAL ANESTHESIA

Vasoconstrictors if used in local areas cause constriction of the arterioles and capillaries. Vasoconstrictors act on alpha (α) and/or beta (β) receptors, depending on the body tissue.

A. Chemical structure of vasoconstrictor:
   1. Benzene ring with two OH groups in third and fourth positions called catechol
   2. Benzene ring with amine group in another position is called catecholamine
   3. Most vasoconstrictors are catecholamines:
      a. Epinephrine, norepinephrine, dopamine: all occur in nature
      b. Levonordefrin and isoproterenol: both synthetics
   4. Do not use cartridge warmers since inactivate vasoconstrictors
B. Adrenergic receptors: present naturally in most body tissue
   1. Includes two types of receptors:
      a. Alpha (α) activation causes contraction of smooth muscles in blood vessels
      b. Beta (β) activation:
         (1) β1 activation in heart and small intestine, responsible for cardiac stimulation and lipolysis
         (2) β2 activation in bronchi, vascular beds, uterus produces bronchodilation and vasodilation
   2. Most vasoconstrictors used in dentistry exert action on adrenergic receptors:
      a. Epinephrine: acts on both α and β receptors, but mainly on β receptors
      b. Norepinephrine: acts on both α and β receptors, but mainly on α receptors
      c. Levonordefrin (synthetic): acts on both α and β receptors, but mainly on α receptors
C. Types of vasoconstrictors:
   1. Epinephrine (adrenalin): one most commonly used in United States:
      a. More potent; found in both natural and synthetic forms
      b. In skeletal muscle and blood vessels, produces both vasodilation (small amounts act on $\beta_2$ sites) and vasoconstriction ( large amounts act on α receptors)
      c. Mainly used at 1:100,000 for nerve blocks and not 1:50,000 concentrations (usually only supraperiosteal/local infiltrations and intraseptal injections); use of additional dosage does not increase duration and/or effectiveness, only hemorrhage control
   2. Norepinephrine (Levarterenol): not used in US but used in other countries:
      a. Less potent than epinephrine (one fourth as potent) and demonstrates less systemic action.
      b. Activation of α receptors in smooth muscles of palatal blood vessels can cause ischemia and then tissue necrosis.
   3. Levonordefrin (Neo-Cobefrin): not as commonly used in US:
      a. Less potent than epinephrine (one sixth as potent); demonstrates less systemic action so used at higher concentration (1:20,000) when used with agents such as 2% mepivacaine; has same onset, depth, duration of anesthesia in both pulpal and soft tissue as lidocaine with epinephrine
      b. Not as strong in hemorrhage control as epinephrine, which is important in dental procedures involving bleeding and need for hemorrhage control, such as dental hygiene procedures
D. Inclusion of vasoconstrictors:
   1. Medical considerations for use of vasoconstrictors:
      a. Absolute contraindications:
         (1) Cardiovascular disease (CVD): acute incident (myocardial infarction [MI, heart attack] or cerebrovascular accident [CVA, stroke]) within

6 months or unable to meet 4 METs (metabolic equivalents); uncontrolled high blood pressure (HBP) ≥140/90 mm Hg; unstable or severe angina pectoris that is relieved by rest
(2) With uncontrolled or undiagnosed hyperthyroidism, may cause thyroid storm
(3) Recreational cocaine (crack) user (within 24 hours); could be fatal
b. Relative contraindications:
(1) Reduced levels needed with most other chronic CVD histories; however, still may need to use limited amount to ensure pain control (reduces endogenous [own] epinephrine of patient with CVD); see next section
(2) Patients taking tricyclic antidepressants (TCAs): neither norepinephrine nor levonordefrin (Neo-Cobefrin) should be used; substitute epinephrine if needed at cardiac dose
2. Consideration for duration of appointment:
a. Addition increases duration of anesthetic effects
b. Concentration and type affect duration of a local anesthetic
3. Consideration for hemostasis during appointment:
a. Epinephrine in large quantities acts as a vasoconstrictor; in smaller quantities becomes vasodilator that has potential to increase bleeding postoperatively
b. Injection should be close to the area of bleeding to be effective; may want to add epinephrine 1:50,000 levels (available with lidocaine agent) as interseptal injection after other injections
c. Epinephrine has better hemostatic control levels than levonordefrin (Neo-Cobefrin), which is important with bleeding that may occur with nonsurgical periodontal maintenance

E. Local anesthetics with vasoconstrictors cause slightly more burning sensation upon injection compared to plain anesthetics because of the preservative (sodium bisulfite), since it is acidic to increase agent's shelf-life

## LOCAL ANESTHETIC AGENTS (SEE TABLE 18.1)

### Potency of Local Anesthesia

A. Definition: lowest concentration of drug needed to consistently produce adequate anesthesia
1. Potency is related directly to lipid solubility
2. If local anesthetic drug is highly potent, lower concentrations are effective in achieving adequate anesthesia
3. However, greater potency also equals greater chance of systemic toxicity (see Table 18.1)

### Toxicity with Local Anesthesia

A. Definition: amount of drug capable of causing adverse systemic reactions in normal persons; adverse reactions occur when rate of drug absorbed is greater than rate of *biotransformation,* which is body's ability to metabolize drug

B. True toxic reactions occur immediately. Most profound effects of toxic reaction are on CNS and cardiovascular system
1. CNS effects
a. CNS stimulation phase: person becomes extremely talkative, restless, and anxious
b. CNS depression phase: convulsions may occur, in extreme cases, unconsciousness may result
2. Cardiovascular effects
a. During stimulation phase: person's blood pressure and pulse rise rapidly
b. During depression phase: person's blood pressure and pulse drop significantly
3. Respiratory failure is primary cause of death
4. Vital functions must be supported until drug is eliminated by biotransformation

### Biotransformation (Metabolism) of Local Anesthesia

A. Definition: process whereby drug is broken down, changed, or combined with other substances to render it physiologically inactive

B. Biotransformation (according to chemical group):
1. Esters: metabolized in plasma through process of hydrolysis; inactivated by plasma cholinesterase (an enzyme)
2. Amides: metabolized in liver; history of cirrhosis, alcoholism, liver disease or liver transplantation, and jaundice may affect the rate of biotransformation
a. Lidocaine, mepivacaine, and bupivacaine are metabolized in liver
b. Prilocaine is metabolized in liver and lungs
c. Articaine is metabolized 95% in plasma and 5% in liver

### Topical Anesthetic

A. Purpose: reduces discomfort associated with initial penetration of needle through mucosa

B. Controversy exists with regard to widespread use
1. Dosage control: impossible to standardize because of variability in factors such as clinician, patient, and area of operation
2. Concentration of topical anesthetic used exceeds that which is administered by injection since mode is less systemic (e.g., 5%, 10%, 20% topical anesthetic vs. 2%, 3%, or 4% local anesthetic)
3. Except for 5% lidocaine (Xylocaine), all other topical anesthetics are esters
4. Lidocaine and prilocaine periodontal gel (Oraqix): amide indicated in adults who require limited pain control during root debridement in periodontal pockets
5. Cetacaine (combination of benzocaine, butamben, and tetracaine hydrochloride): ester indicated in adults who require preinjection, deep scaling, and suture removal anesthesia (available in spray, liquid, or gel form)

C. Esters have greater incidence of allergic reactions and cross-reactivity than amides

D. Topical agents have indications and contraindications; can interact with other medications; clinicians must always assess for potential allergies, side effects, and adverse effects and take appropriate precautions

**TABLE 18-1 Comparison of Frequently Used Local Anesthetic Agents in Dentistry.**

| Generic Name | Lidocaine | | | Mepivacaine | | Prilocaine | | Articaine | | Bupivacaine |
|---|---|---|---|---|---|---|---|---|---|---|
| Available formulations | 2% Plain Light Blue | 2% 1:50,000 Epinephrine Green | 2% 1:100,000 Epinephrine Red | 3% Plain Tan | 2% 1:20,000 Levonordefrin Brown | 4% Plain Black | 4% 1:200,000 Yellow | 4% 1:100,000 Epinephrine Gold | 4% 1:200,000 Epinephrine Silver | 0.5% 1:200,000 Epinephrine Blue |
| ADA color coding band | | | | | | | | | | |
| pKa | 7.7 | 7.7 | 7.7 | 7.6 | 7.6 | 7.7 | 7.9 | 7.8 | 7.8 | 8.1 |
| Onset of action (In minutes) | 2-3 | 2-3 | 2-3 | 2-4 | 1.5–2 | 2–4 | 2-4 | 1-2 (S) 2.0-2.5 (B) | 1-2 (S) 2-3 (B) | 6-10 |
| pH | 6.5 | 3.3-5.5 | 3.3-5.5 | 4.5-6.8 | 3.0-3.5 | 6.0-7.0 | 3.0-4.0 | 4.4-5.2 | 4.6-5.4 | 3.0-4.5 |
| Duration category | Very Short | Intermediate | Intermediate | Short | Intermediate | Short (S) Intermediate (B) | Intermediate | Intermediate | Intermediate | Long |
| Duration pulpal (In minutes) | 5-10 | 60 | 60 | 20 (S) 40 (B) | 60 | 10-15 (S) 40-60 (B) | 60-90 | 60-75 | 45-60 | 90-180 |
| Duration soft tissue (In minutes) | 60-120 | 180–300 | 180-300 | 120-180 | 180-300 | 90-120 (S) 120-240 (B) | 180-480 | 180-360 | 120-300 | 240-540 (Reports up to 720) |
| Half-life (In minutes) | 96 | 96 | 96 | 114 | 114 | 96 | 96 | Approx. 27 | Approx. 27 | 162 |
| MRD (mg/lb) | 3.2 | 3.2 | 3.2 | 3.0 | 3.0 | 3.6 | 3.6 | 3.2 | 3.2 | 0.9* |
| MRD (mg/kg) | 7.0 | 7.0 | 7.0 | 6.6 | 6.6 | 8.0 | 8.0 | 7.0 | 7.0 | 2.0* |
| MRD Absolute mg | 500 | 500 | 500 | 400 | 400 | 600 | 600 | None listed | None Listed | 90 |
| Relative Potency (Reference value = Lidocaine @100%) | 100% | 100% | 100% | 100% | 100% | 100% | 100% | 150% | 150% | 400% |
| Relative toxicity (Reference value = Lidocaine @100%) | 100% | 100% | 100% | 75% | 75% | 60% | 60% | 100% | 100% | Less than 400% |

*Canadian recommendations, No U.S. recommendations available.
*S*, Supraperiosteal; *B*, block
From Logothetis DD: *Local anesthesia for the dental hygienist*, ed 2, St Louis, 2017, Elsevier

### Calculation of Maximum Recommended Dose for Local Anesthetics

A. Maximum recommended dose (MRD): maximum amount of drug administered that does not produce toxic reaction and is based upon mg per pound or mg per kilogram
B. Maximum recommended doses of local anesthetic agents per appointment for healthy patients:
   1. Lidocaine: 3.2 mg/lb, 7.0 mg/kg, 500 mg max
   2. Mepivacaine: 3.0 mg/lb, 6.6 mg/kg, 400 mg max
   3. Prilocaine: 3.6 mg/lb, 8.0 mg/kg, 600 mg max
   4. Articaine: 3.2 mg/lb, 7.0 mg/kg, no max listed
   5. Bupivacaine: 0.9 mg/lb, 2.0 mg/kg, (based on Canadian recommendations, no United States weight based recommendations available), 90 mg max
C. Steps to calculating maximum recommended dose and maximum cartridges:

   **Step 1:** Obtain necessary patient information

   **Step 2:** Calculate number of mg of selected anesthetic in one cartridge;
   - **A.** take percentage of solution and multiply by 10;
   - **B.** take the above answer and multiply by 1.8 (mL in one cartridge) = mg of anesthetic per cartridge

   **Example:** 2% lidocaine: 20 × 1.8 = 36 mg/cartridge

   **Step 3:**
   - **A.** Convert pounds to kilograms if using this unit of measurement lb ÷ 2.2 = kg
   - **B.** Multiply kilograms by mg/kg or pounds by mg/lb

     **Example using kilograms:**

     120 lb patient ÷ 2.2 = 54.5 kg × 7 (mg/kg) = 381.5 mg (MRD) ***or***

     **Example using pounds:**

     120 lb patient × 3.2 (mg/lb) = 384 mg (MRD). This number may be different for each anesthetic and provides MRD in mg for the patient based on weight

   **Step 4:** Convert maximum recommended dose of anesthetic to cartridges
   - **A.** Divide the MRD (Step 3) by number of mg of selected anesthetic per cartridge (Step 2) = maximum number of cartridges

   **Example:** 384 mg ÷ 36 mg (for lidocaine) = 10.6 cartridges
D. Calculating milligrams of anesthetic administered:
   1. Multiply number of cartridges administered by the number of mg of selected anesthetic in one cartridge

   **Example:** administered 2.5 cartridges of 4% articaine:

   2.5 × 72 (mg of articaine in one cartridge) = 180 mL administered

## VASOCONSTRICTORS IN LOCAL ANESTHETIC CARTRIDGE (TABLE 18.2)

A. Vasoconstrictors are combined with local anesthetics to counteract vasodilating properties of local anesthetics
B. Description: all vasoconstrictors can be referred to *adrenergic drugs* or *sympathomimetic amines.*
   1. Adrenergic drug: capable of producing same effects as those of adrenalin
   2. Sympathomimetic amine: mimics sympathetic nervous system and contains amine group within its chemical structure, which is characteristic of vasoconstrictors
   3. All vasoconstrictors can be produced synthetically; two naturally occurring vasoconstrictors, epinephrine and norepinephrine, are produced in adrenal medulla and the sympathetic postganglionic nerve fibers
   4. There are two vasoconstrictors that are added to local anesthetic drugs available in United States: epinephrine and levonordefrin
C. Benefits of vasoconstrictor:
   1. Reduce systemic absorption of local anesthetic agent
   2. Decrease risk of systemic toxicity
   3. Reduce blood flow through the area (hemostasis)
   4. Increase duration of action of anesthetic
   5. Increase in effectiveness of local anesthetic by decrease in diffusion
   6. Lower dose of local anesthetic agents required
D. Mode of action: stimulate α-adrenergic receptors located in walls of arterioles.
   1. α-Adrenergic receptors: responsible for arterial constriction
   2. β-Adrenergic receptors: responsible for bronchial dilation
   3. Each type of vasoconstrictor possesses varying degrees of response of both α- and β-adrenergic activity
E. Termination of action: once absorbed, action of epinephrine is terminated primarily by reuptake action of adrenergic nerves, any epinephrine that escapes reuptake action is inactivated by enzymes catechol-O-methyltransferase (COMT) and monoamine oxidase (MAO) in the blood
F. Pressor potency: ability of a drug to produce vasoconstriction
   1. Epinephrine: most potent vasoconstrictor; pressor potency value = 1
   2. Levonordefrin: another type of adrenergic vasoconstrictor; pressor potency value = ⅙
   3. Concentrations of all vasoconstrictors must be increased to obtain same vasoconstrictive potency as that of epinephrine
G. Vasoconstrictors in solution: unstable; preservative (e.g., sodium bisulfite) is added to prevent oxidation
H. Toxicity: toxicity resulting from vasoconstrictor overdose is caused by constriction of blood vessels, which raises blood pressure and cardiac rate from β-adrenergic receptor stimulation
   1. Symptoms:
      a. Increased blood pressure
      b. Increased heart rate (tachycardia > 150 beats/min)
      c. Talkativeness
      d. Restlessness
      e. Palpitations or irregular heartbeat
      f. Headache
   2. Prevention of cardiac emergencies: strict adherence to MRD in the case of persons with cardiac disease)

**TABLE 18.2 Vasoconstrictors Used in Dental Local Anesthetic Solutions**

| Generic Name | Proprietary Name | Dilutions | Healthy Dose | Cardiac Dose |
|---|---|---|---|---|
| Epinephrine | Adrenalin | 1:50,000<br>1:100,000<br>1:200,000 | 0.2 mg/appt. | 0.04 mg/appt. |
| Levonordefrin | Neo-Cobefrin | 1:20,000 | 1.0 mg/appt. | 0.2 mg/appt. |

From: Logothetis DD. *Local Anesthesia for the Dental Hygienist*. 3rd ed. St Louis: Elsevier; 2021.

I. Maximum recommended dose for vasoconstrictor drugs:
  1. Based on recommendations from the American Heart Association and New York Heart Association
    a. Based on "healthy" or "compromised" individuals, and not weight dependent
    b. Maximum doses of vasoconstrictors are expressed in milligram amounts. Healthy dose for epinephrine is 0.2 mg per appointment, and healthy dose for levonordefrin is 1.0 mg per appointment. Cardiac dose for epinephrine is 0.04 mg per appointment, and cardiac dose for levonordefrin is 0.2 mg per appointment (See Table 18.2)
    c. Vasoconstrictor dilutions are expressed as a ratio
      (1) It is necessary to be able to convert this ratio to the number of milligrams of vasoconstrictor per milliliter of solution
      (2) A 1:1000 dilution means that there is 1g (1000 mg) of vasoconstrictor in 1000 mL of solution or 1 mg of vasoconstrictor in 1 mL of solution
      (3) A 1:10,000 solution contains 1 mg vasoconstrictor in 10 mL of solution or 0.1 mg of vasoconstrictor in 1 mL of solution, and a 1:100,000 solution contains 0.01 mg of vasoconstrictor in 1 mL of solution

J. Steps to calculating vasoconstrictor drug doses:

**Example:** using 1:100,000 epinephrine

**Step 1**: Obtain necessary patient information

**Step 2:** Calculate mg of vasoconstrictor in one cartridge of anesthetic

**Example:** 1:100,000 dilution mean there is 1 gram in 100,000 mL of solution

  A. 1 g = 1000 mg/100,000 mL of solution = 0.01 mg vasoconstrictor/1 mL of solution
  B. To obtain mg in 1 cartridge of 1:100,000 dilution multiply 0.01 mg × 1.8 mL (mL in one cartridge) = 0.018 mg in one cartridge of 1:100,000

**Step 3**: Convert MRD of vasoconstrictor to cartridges

  A. Divide MRD by number of mg of vasoconstrictor per cartridge of anesthetic (from Step 2)
  B. For a healthy patient using MRD for 1:100,000 epinephrine (0.2 mg ÷ 0.018 = 11.1 cartridges); for a cardiac patient using MRD for 1:100,000 epinephrine (0.04 mg ÷ 0.018 = 2.2 cartridges)

K. Limiting drug:
  1. When determining the safety of administering a local anesthetic with a vasoconstrictor, the limiting drug must me determined. To determine which drug limits the amount of solution to be administered, calculate the MRD of both the anesthetic drug and the vasoconstrictor to determine which drug will reach its MRD first; the drug that reaches its MRD first will be the limiting drug
  2. **Example**: 150 pound healthy patient for 2% lidocaine 1:100,000
    a. For local anesthetic (lidocaine) calculation such that 2% = 20 mg/mL × 1.8 mL = 36 mg (in one cartridge of lidocaine) 150 × 3.2 mg/lb = 480 mg MRD such that 480 mg ÷ 36 mg = 13.3 cartridges of lidocaine maximum
    b. For vasoconstrictor (epinephrine) calculation such that 1:100,000 = 1 mg/100 mL = 0.01 mg/1 mL × 1.8 mL = 0.018 mg (in one cartridge of 1:100,000 epinephrine dilution) and 0.2 mg (MRD of vasoconstrictor for healthy patient) ÷ 0.018 mg = 11.1 cartridges maximum
    c. Because 11.1 is lower than 13.3, epinephrine is the limiting drug in this example

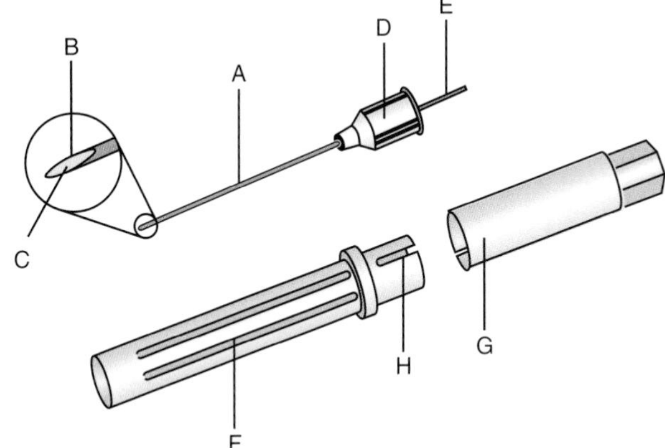


**Fig. 18.5** Components of a hypodermic needle. (A) Shaft or shank, the working end of the needle. (B) Bevel, or angulation, of the tip. (C) Lumen, the hollow interior of the shaft. (D) The hub holds the shaft and is threaded onto the adapter of the syringe. (E) The syringe end enters the anesthetic cartridge. (F), The protective shield sleeve (colored end) covers the needle shaft. (G) The protective shield guard (clear or white) covers the syringe end of the needle. (H) The security seal holds the protective shield sleeve and guard together until the hub is assembled and attached to the syringe.

## LOCAL ANESTHESIA ARMAMENTARIUM

A. Definition: all items essential for administration of a local anesthetic agent

B. Armamentarium categories
  1. Needle:
    a. Components (Fig. 18.5)
    b. Composition: stainless steel

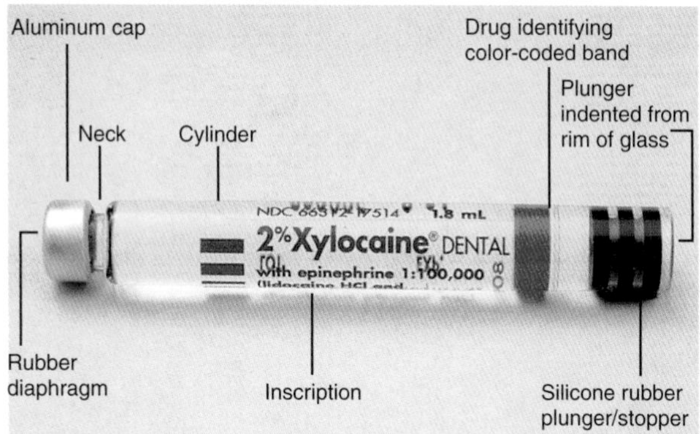


**Fig. 18.6** Components of local anesthetic cartridge. (From: Logothetis D.D. *Local Anesthesia for the Dental Hygienist.* 3rd ed. St. Louis: Elsevier; 2021)

c. Gauge (ga): diameter of lumen is indicated by number
  (1) Larger gauge number, smaller lumen diameter
  (2) The 25-, 27-, and 30-ga needles are most common in dentistry
d. Length: measured from hub to point of bevel
  (1) Short = 1 inch
  (2) Long = 1⅝ inches
e. Method of sterilization: disposable needles come presterilized with security seal

2. Anesthetic cartridge:
  a. Components (Fig. 18.6):
    (1) Aluminum cap: directed toward needle when cartridge is loaded into syringe.
    (2) Round rubber diaphragm: syringe end of needle penetrates diaphragm and enters cartridge
    (3) Cylinder: glass tube containing anesthetic solution
    (4) Inscription: legally required information on cartridge, which includes:
      (a) Volume: 1.8 mL
      (b) Anesthetic agent: generic and brand names
      (c) Percentage of drug
      (d) Vasoconstrictor
      (e) Concentration ratio of vasoconstrictor
      (f) Manufacturer
      (g) Lot number
      (h) Expiration date
    (5) Rubber stopper: seals opposite end of cartridge; it is the movable component of cartridge
  b. Ingredients in anesthetic solution:
    (1) Anesthetic drug
    (2) Vasoconstrictor
    (3) Preservative (sodium bisulfite)
    (4) Sodium chloride: makes solution isotonic
    (5) Distilled water: inert ingredient
  c. Method of storage: away from direct sunlight and ultraviolet light, and maintained at room temperature (68 °F to 77 °F; 20 °C to 25 °C) or slightly cooler

3. Anesthetic syringe (Fig. 18.7):
  a. Components:
    (1) Needle adaptor: hub of needle is threaded onto this part of syringe

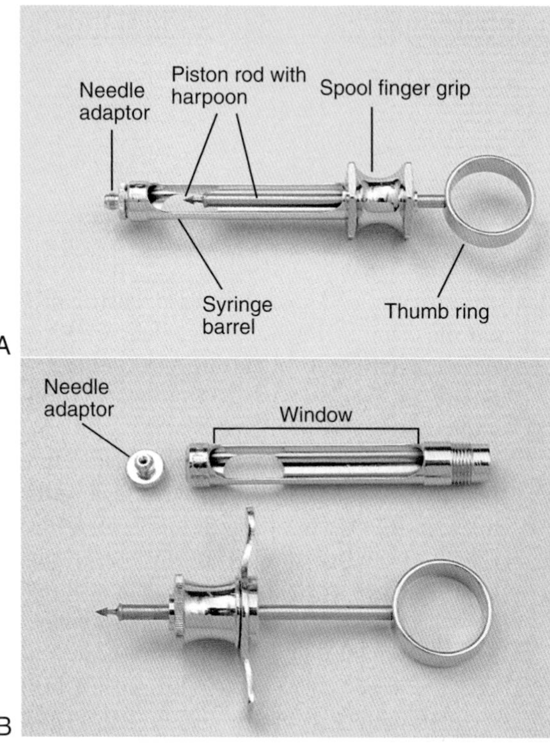


**Fig. 18.7** Components of a standard local anesthetic syringe. (From: Logothetis D.D. *Local Anesthesia for the Dental Hygienist.* 3rd ed. St. Louis: Elsevier; 2021)

    (2) Barrel: holds anesthetic cartridge
    (3) Harpoon: fishhook-shaped tip is forced into rubber stopper
    (4) Piston rod: connects harpoon to thumb ring; can be advanced to expel solution or retracted to aspirate
    (5) Large window: faces clinician during injection; rubber stopper speed, positive aspirations, and volume are observable
    (6) Small window: aids in removing used cartridge
    (7) Spool finger grip: place of rest for index and middle fingers
    (8) Thumb ring: enables clinician to aspirate or express fluid from cartridge
  b. Method of syringe sterilization: bioburden is removed; syringe is dried, packaged, and sterilized
  c. Auxiliary materials: hemostat or cotton pliers; used if needle breaks

C. Record keeping and documentation in patient dental record
  1. Documentation requirements vary by state law
  2. Documentation includes:
    a. Time of administration
    b. Type and percentage of drug administered
    c. Type and ratio of vasoconstrictor
    d. Amount of drug administered in milligrams
    e. Name of injection(s) administered and oral region in which injection(s) administered
    f. Reactions to drug (if any)
    g. Using American Dental Association (ADA) Code D9215 for health insurance reimbursement

TABLE 18.3 **Maxillary Nerve Blocks**

| Injection | Structures Anesthetized | Target Area | Injection Site | Needle Length | Amount Deposited |
|---|---|---|---|---|---|
| ASA | Maxillary anterior teeth<br>Labial periodontium and gingiva of anterior teeth, labial mucosa, and upper lip | ASA nerve superior to apex of maxillary canine approximately 5-6 mm of short needle | Height of mucobuccal fold of maxillary canine and just medial to and parallel to canine eminence | 27-gauge short needle | 0.9 to 1.2 mL or one-half to two-thirds of cartridge<br>Wait 3-5 min |
| MSA | Maxillary premolars and mesiobuccal root of maxillary first molar in 28% of the population<br>Buccal periodontium and gingiva of maxillary premolars and mesiobuccal root of first molar, buccal mucosa and upper lip | MSA nerve superior to apex of maxillary second premolar approximately 5 mm of short needle | Height of maxillary mucobuccal fold of maxillary second premolar | 27-gauge short needle | 0.9 to 1.2 mL or one-half to two-thirds of cartridge<br>Wait 3-5 min |
| IO | Maxillary anterior teeth and premolars as well as the mesiobuccal root of maxillary first molar in approximately 28% of cases<br>Facial periodontium and gingiva of anesthetized teeth; upper lip to midline; medial part of cheek; side of nose; lower eyelid | Infraorbital nerve at IO foramen at approximately 10 mm inferior to midpoint of IO rim with zygomaticomaxillary suture<br>Approximately 16 mm or one-half depth of long needle | Height of maxillary mucobuccal fold of maxillary first premolar | 27-gauge long or 27-gauge short for children (or small adults) | 0.9 to 1.2 mL or one-half to two-thirds of cartridge<br>Wait 3-5 min |
| PSA | Maxillary molars in approximately 72% of cases; however, the mesiobuccal root of maxillary first molar is not anesthetized in approximately 28% of cases due to possible presence of MSA nerve<br>Buccal periodontium and gingiva of anesthetized teeth as well as buccal mucosa and upper lip | PSA nerve at PSA foramina on infratemporal surface of maxilla and posterosuperior on maxillary tuberosity<br>Approximately three-fourths the depth of short needle | Height of maxillary mucobuccal fold of maxillary second molar, distal to zygomatic process of maxilla by inserting needle upward at a 45° angle to maxillary occlusal plane, inward at a 45° angle to maxillary occlusal plane, and backward at 45° angle | 25- or 27-gauge short needle | 0.9 to 1.8 mL or one-half to full cartridge<br>Wait 3-5 min |
| GP | Posterior hard palate and palatal periodontium and gingiva of ipsilateral maxillary posterior teeth<br>Palatal mucosa to midline | GP nerve at GP foramen at junction of the alveolar process of maxilla and hard palate<br>Approximately 4 to 6 mm depth of short needle or until contact with palatine bone | Palatal tissue 1 to 2 mm slightly anterior to greater palatine foramen using pressure anesthesia | 27-gauge extra-short or short with standard syringe or 30-gauge extra-short or short with computer-controlled local anesthetic delivery device | 0.45 to 0.6 mL or one-fourth to one-third of cartridge until blanching of tissue<br>Wait 2-3 min |
| NP | Anterior hard palate and palatal periodontium and gingiva of maxillary anterior teeth<br>Palatal mucosa in anterior hard palate | Nasopalatine nerves at incisive foramen on anterior hard palate approximately 4 to 5 mm depth of short needle or until gentle contact | Palatal tissue lateral to incisive papilla and palatal to maxillary central incisors using pressure anesthesia on opposite side of overlying incisive papilla | 27-gauge extra-short or short with standard syringe or 30-gauge extra-short or short with computer-controlled local anesthetic delivery device | 0.45 mL or one-fourth of cartridge<br>Wait 2-3 min |

*ASA*, Anterior superior alveolar; *MSA*, middle superior alveolar; *IO*, infraorbital; *PSA*, posterior superior alveolar; *GP*, greater palantine; *NP*, nasopalantine.
From: Logothetis DD. *Local Anesthesia for the Dental Hygienist*. 3rd ed. St Louis: Elsevier; 2021.

## LOCAL ANESTHESIA INJECTIONS

A. Injection Types:
1. Supraperiosteal injection (incorrectly called local infiltration): anesthetizes small area, usually one or two teeth and associated structures by injection near apices
   a. Can be administered on any tooth of either dental arch
   b. Increased clinical effectiveness in maxillary arch since bone is less dense than mandibular arch and increased clinical effectiveness of mandibular anterior teeth than mandibular posterior teeth
   c. Target area: superior (or inferior) to apex (apices) near terminal nerve endings
   d. Injection site: needle should be inserted parallel to long axis of tooth usually in height (or depth) of mucobuccal fold or lingual tissue with bevel orientation of needle toward alveolar process
2. Nerve block (see next sections for Maxillary Nerve Blocks and Mandibular Nerve Blocks, see Tables 18.3 and 18.4): usually affects larger area of anesthesia than supraperiosteal injection

TABLE 18.4 **Mandibular Nerve Blocks**

| Injection | Structures Anesthetized | Target Area | Injection Site | Needle | Amount Deposited |
|---|---|---|---|---|---|
| IA | Mandibular teeth to midline<br>Facial periodontium and gingiva of the mandibular anterior teeth and premolars to midline<br>Lingual periodontium and gingiva to midline<br>Lower lip<br>Anterior two-thirds of tongue<br>Floor of the mouth to midline | IA nerve at mandibular foramen on medial surface of mandibular ramus overhung by lingula; lingual nerve by diffusion; at two-thirds to three-fourths distance from coronoid notch to posterior border of mandibular ramus (where pterygomandibular raphe (fold) turns superior towards soft palate)<br>Approximately 20 to 25 mm or two-thirds to three-fourths of a long needle until bone is gently contacted | Center of pterygomandibular space (triangle) at 6-10 mm superior to occlusal plane of mandibular molars | 25-gauge long needle | Approximately 1.8 to 3.6 mL (one to one and a half to two cartridges); save portion for administration of the buccal block, if needed<br>Wait 3-5 min |
| B | Buccal periodontium and gingiva of mandibular molars<br>Skin of cheek | (Long) buccal nerve as it passes over anterior border of mandibular ramus in the area of retromolar pad (triangle)<br>Approximately 2 to 4 mm of needle length until bone is gently contacted | Buccal mucosa distal and buccal to most distal mandibular molar | 25-gauge long (same needle as IA block administered immediately following in most cases) or 27-gauge short (if administered alone in fewer cases) | Approximately 0.3 mL or one-eighth cartridge<br>Wait 1 min |
| M | Facial periodontium and gingiva of mandibular anterior teeth and premolars to midline<br>Lower lip<br>Skin of chin to midline | Mental nerve at mental foramen at depth of mandibular mucobuccal fold inferior to the apices of the mandibular premolars or location determined by radiographs and/or palpation<br>Approximately 5-6 mm of short needle | At mental foramen at depth of mandibular mucobuccal fold inferior to apices of the mandibular premolars or location determined by radiographs and/or palpation | 27-gauge short needle | Approximately 0.6 mL or one-third of cartridge<br>Wait 2-3 min |
| I | Mandibular anterior teeth and premolars to midline<br>Facial periodontium and gingiva of anesthetized mandibular teeth to midline<br>Lower lip<br>Skin of chin to midline | Same as Mental Nerve Block<br>Following injection must massage solution into the mental foramen for 2 minutes | Same as Mental Nerve Block | 27-gauge short needle | Approximately 0.6 mL or one-third of cartridge<br>Wait 2-3 min |
| G-G | Mandibular teeth to midline<br>Lingual periodontium and gingiva of anesthetized mandibular teeth<br>Facial periodontium and gingiva of anesthetized mandibular anterior teeth and premolars to midline and possibly buccal periodontium and gingiva of anesthetized mandibular molars<br>Lower lip, anterior two-thirds of tongue and floor of the mouth to midline<br>Skin over zygomatic bone and posterior part of buccal and temporal regions | IA nerve, lingual nerve, (long) buccal nerve (75% of cases), mental nerve, incisive nerve, mylohyoid nerve, auriculotemporal nerve at anteromedial border of neck of mandibular condyle | Buccal mucosa on medial surface of mandibular ramus, just distal to height of mesiolingual cusp of maxillary second molar using pathway that parallels imaginary extraoral line connecting intertragic notch and ipsilateral corner of the mouth while keeping mouth wide open as well as after for 1 to 2 minutes | 25-gauge long | Approximately 1.8 mL or full cartridge<br>Wait 3-5 minutes |
| V-A | Mandibular teeth to midline<br>Lingual periodontium and gingiva of anesthetized mandibular teeth<br>Facial periodontium and gingiva of anesthetized mandibular anterior teeth and premolars to midline and possibly buccal periodontium and gingiva of anesthetized mandibular molars<br>Lower lip, anterior two-thirds of tongue, and floor of the mouth to midline | IA nerve, lingual nerve, (long) buccal nerve (75% of cases), mental nerve, incisive nerve, mylohyoid nerve at center of pterygomandibular space and at approximately equidistant between the mandibular foramen and neck of mandibular condyle as well as being adjacent to maxillary tuberosity | Medially past coronoid process and then into buccal mucosa on medial surface of mandibular ramus at same height as mucogingival junction of maxillary third or second molar directly across way and with bevel oriented away from the bone of mandibular ramus so it faces toward the midline | 25-gauge long | Approximately 1.8 mL or full cartridge<br>Wait 5 minutes |

*IA*, inferior alveolar nerve block; *B*, buccal nerve block; *M*, mental nerve block; *I*, incisive block; *G-G*, Gow-Gates mandibular block; *V-A*, Vazirani-Akinosi mandibular block.
(From: Logothetis DD. *Local Anesthesia for the Dental Hygienist*. 3rd ed. St Louis: Elsevier; 2021.)

a. Increased level of clinical effectiveness when compared to supraperiosteal injection; can be administered at a distance away from localized inflammation or infection
b. Fewer injections and lesser amounts of agent can be used for anesthesia within a quadrant
c. Target area: near larger nerve trunks

B. Basic injection procedure:
1. Preanesthetic patient assessment and consultation
2. Select anesthetic and dosage based upon preanesthetic patient assessment
3. Confirm dental hygiene care plan
4. Obtain informed consent
5. Select injection(s) based upon areas needing to be anesthetized, presence of infection, and the need for hemostasis
6. Prepare and check equipment
7. Position patient in supine position
8. Apply topical anesthetic
9. Dry tissue and visualize or palpate penetration site to determine any needle access problems
10. Establish fulcrum
11. Make tissue taut
12. Keep syringe out of patient's sight
13. Gently insert needle and slowly move toward target
14. Aspirate, if negative, slowly deposit anesthetic at rate of 1 mL of solution per minute
15. Observe patient; never leave patient
16. Document procedure

## TRIGEMINAL NERVE: MAXILLARY NERVE, SECOND DIVISION ($V_2$)

See the section the "Nervous System" in chapter 4.

### Maxillary Nerve Innervation

A. The $V_2$ branches within pterygopalatine fossa:
1. Zygomatic nerve: fibers for lacrimal gland via lacrimal nerve
   a. Zygomaticofacial nerve
   b. Zygomaticotemporal nerve
2. Pterygopalatine nerves:
   a. Orbital branches
   b. Nasal branches: including nasopalatine (NP) nerve (relevant branch for local anesthesia); both right and left nerves via incisive foramen (with incisive papilla)
   c. Palatine branches: communication between nerves at junctions of distribution:
      (1) Greater palatine (GP) nerve (relevant branch for local anesthesia): via GP foramen
      (2) Lesser palatine nerve: via LP foramen; possible gag reflex by default when soft palate anesthetized with GP nerve
   d. Pharyngeal branch
3. Posterior superior alveolar (PSA) nerve (relevant branch for local anesthesia): via superior dental plexus
   a. External branch: innervation of maxillary molars
   b. Internal branch: via PSA foramina
4. Infraorbital (IO) nerve (relevant branch for local anesthesia): largest contributor via IO foramen; joins PSA nerve or maxillary nerve directly
   a. Anterior superior alveolar (ASA) nerve: via superior dental plexus; possibly involved in crossover-innervation; joins with IO nerve in IO canal
   b. Middle superior alveolar (MSA) nerve: via superior dental plexus in only 28% of cases; joins with IO nerve in IO canal
   c. Lateral nasal nerve
   d. Superior labial nerve
   e. Inferior palpebral nerve

### Maxillary Nerve Blocks (See Table 18.3 and Fig. 18.8)

## TRIGEMINAL NERVE: MANDIBULAR NERVE, THIRD DIVISION ($V_3$)

See the section the "Nervous System" in chapter 4.

### Mandibular Nerve Innervation

A. The $V_3$ branches from undivided main nerve trunk within infratemporal fossa:
1. Meningeal branches (sensory)
2. Medial pterygoid nerve (motor)

B. The $V_3$ branches from divided nerve trunk:
1. Anterior trunk:
   a. Lateral pterygoid nerve (motor)
   b. Masseter nerve (motor)
   c. Anterior deep temporal nerve (motor)
   d. Posterior deep temporal nerve (motor)
   e. (Long) buccal nerve (sensory): relevant branch for local anesthesia; does not serve buccinator muscle
2. Posterior trunk:
   a. Auriculotemporal nerve (sensory) (relevant brand for local anesthesia); can get anesthetized with IA nerve
   b. Lingual nerve (sensory) (relevant branch for local anesthesia); can get damaged with oral surgery and local anesthesia
   c. Inferior alveolar nerve (mixed) (relevant branch for local anesthesia); travels in mandibular canal; via mandibular foramen; can be bifid with two mandibular canals
      (1) Mylohyoid nerve (motor but may provide accessory sensory innervation for mandibular first molar)
      (2) Mental nerve (sensory) (relevant branch for local anesthesia): via mental foramen
      (3) Incisive nerve (sensory) (relevant branch for local anesthesia); travels in mandibular incisive canal; via mental foramen; possibly involved in crossover-innervation

### Mandibular Nerve Blocks (Table 18.4 and Fig. 18.8)

## COMPUTER-CONTROLLED LOCAL ANESTHESIA DELIVERY DEVICE (CCLADD)

A. Three main components (Table 18.5):
1. Drive unit

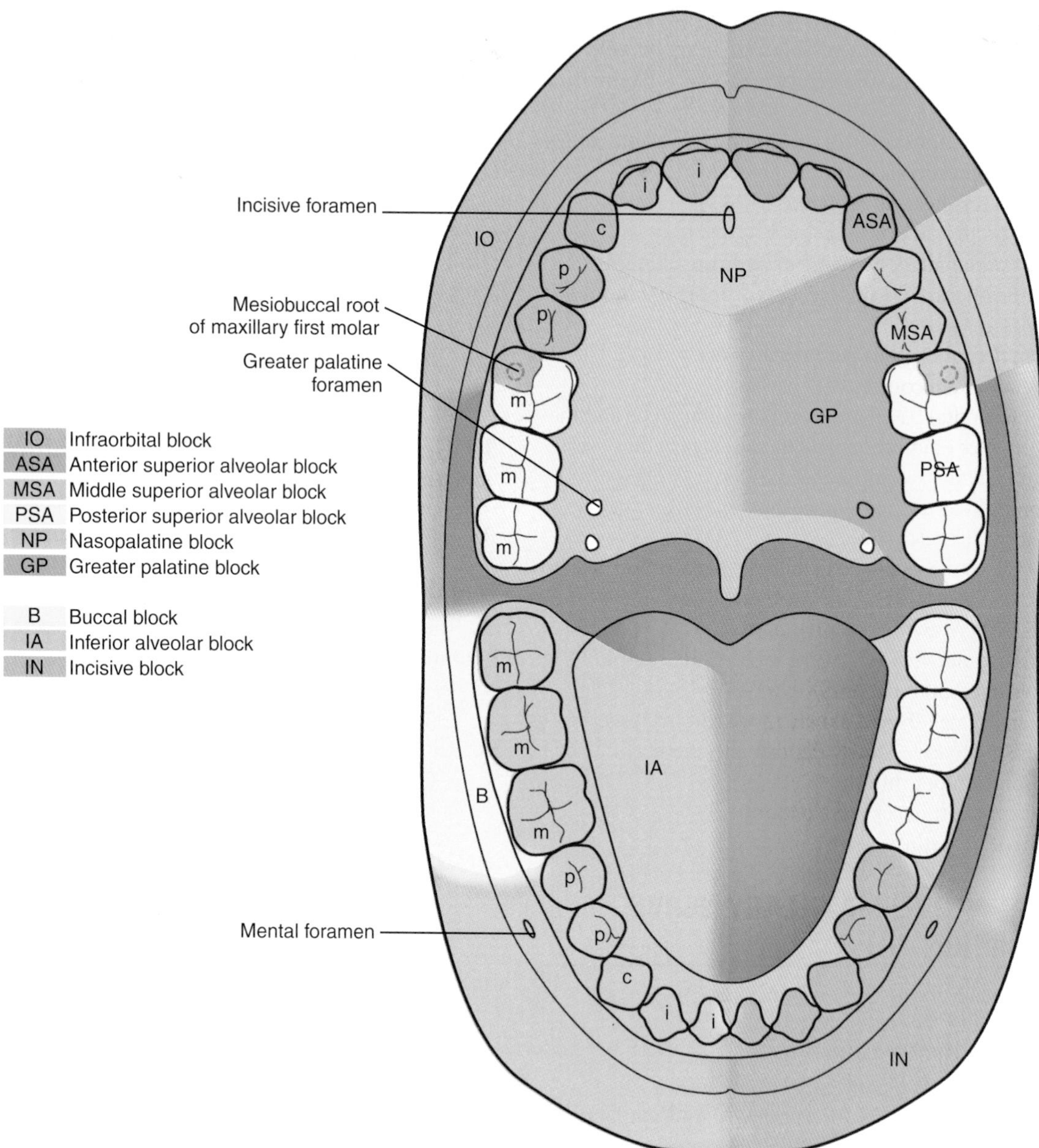


**Fig. 18.8** Local anesthetic nerve blocks with the related structures that are anesthetized. Note that the anterior middle superior alveolar, the mental, and the Gow-Gates or Vazirani-Akinosi mandibular blocks are not included (see also Table 18.3 and Table 18.4). (From: Fehrenbach MJ, Herring SW. *Illustrated Anatomy of the Head and Neck*. 6th ed. St Louis: Elsevier; 2021)

2. Disposable plastic handpiece and tubing
3. Foot control that activates unit and controls two slow/fast flow rates
   a. Slow flow rate:
      (1) Delivers 1 drop every 2 seconds
      (2) 1.8 mL of anesthetic delivered in 2 minutes
   b. Rapid flow rate:
      (1) Delivers steady stream (30-gauge) or rapid drip (27-gauge)
      (2) Takes 1 minute to deliver contents of cartridge

## Basic CCLADD Procedure

A. Decreases main causes of pain associated with dental injections that include:
   1. Initial tissue puncture
   2. Depositing volume of fluid too rapidly into a confined space
B. Advantages of CCLADD (Table 18.5):
   1. Eliminates initial pain from needle penetration by establishing anesthetic pathway
   2. Eliminates pressure pain by constant pressure and controlled volume
C. Anesthetic pathway: anesthetic drip precedes path of needle and can be used for any injection
D. Prepuncture technique used for palatal injections to increase comfort:
   1. Place bevel of needle against the tissue
   2. Use cotton-tipped applicator on top to seal bevel to tissue surface

TABLE 18.5 **Comparison of Standard Syringe to Computer-Controlled Local Anesthesia Delivery Device (CCLADD)**

| | Standard | CCLADD |
|---|---|---|
| Grasp and needle control | Palm grasp<br>Relies on large muscles of wrist, forearm, and shoulder<br>Weighs 80 grams<br>Held 9 inches from insertion site | Pen grasp<br>Control is transferred to small muscles of fingers and thumb<br>Weighs few grams<br>Held within 2 inches of insertion site |
| Fluid delivery | Thumb is used to start and stop flow of agent | Uses a foot control to deliver flow of agent |
| Fluid metering | Pressure and volume cannot be separated; thus is clinician dependent | Maintains constant pressure and controlled volume |
| Aspiration | Relies on clinician control | Automatic (on demand) by releasing foot control |
| Needles | Threaded hub in most cases; luer-lok in fewer cases:<br>25-gauge, long and short<br>27-gauge, long and short | Luer-Lok hub<br>30-gauge, short<br>27-gauge, long |
| Path of insertion | Linear insertion (straight push through tissues, possibly causing needle deflection) | Bi-rotational insertion (180°) between the thumb and index finger to overcome needle deflection |

3. Initiate rate of anesthetic for 2 to 3 seconds to force anesthetic through surface epithelium before actual tissue penetration of palatal tissue

E. Complications: postinjection pain, swelling, necrosis when administered too rapidly and with too much agent

## Computer-Controlled Local Anesthesia Delivery Device (CCLADD) Recommended Injections

A. GP nerve block and NP nerve block, as well as all other nerve blocks

B. Anterior middle superior alveolar (AMSA) nerve block using palatal approach:
1. Teeth anesthetized: maxillary anterior teeth and premolars within one maxillary quadrant; covering area served by ASA, MSA, GP, NP blocks
2. Other structures anesthetized: facial periodontium and gingiva of anesthetized teeth to midline; hard palate and palatal periodontium and gingiva of ipsilateral maxillary posterior teeth and maxillary anterior teeth bilaterally; no regional soft tissue anesthesia of upper lip and face but will need to administer PSA nerve block to complete maxillary quadrant
3. Not as effective anesthesia for nonsurgical periodontal therapy due to multi-tooth and pulpal anesthesia delivered from single injection increased deposition time, variable anesthesia, reduced hemostatic control but with no numbness of lips and of muscles of facial expression so used in cosmetic dentistry
4. Target area: pores in maxilla of hard palate allowing diffusion of agent
5. Injection site: area on palate superior to apices of maxillary premolars and midway between palatal gingival margin and median palatal raphe (suture)
6. Amount: approximately 1.4 to 1.8 mL until blanching of tissue
7. Flow rate: slow flow rate
8. Needle: 30-gauge extra-short or short

C. Palatal-anterior superior alveolar (P-ASA) nerve block:
1. Teeth anesthetized: maxillary central incisors, lateral incisors, and canines (lesser degree) in maxillary anterior sextant; covering area served by bilateral ASA and NP blocks
2. Associated labial as well as palatal periodontium and gingiva bilaterally
3. Not as effective anesthesia for nonsurgical periodontal therapy due to multi-tooth and pulpal anesthesia delivered from single injection with increased deposition time, variable anesthesia, reduced hemostatic control but with no numbness of lips and facial muscles of facial expression so used in cosmetic dentistry
4. Target area: anterior part of superior dental plexus and NP nerve
5. Injection site:
   a. Contralateral to incisive papilla
   b. Needle should be reoriented to gain access to incisive canal (and advance needle to bony wall and aspirate)
6. Amount: 1.4 to 1.8 mL
7. Aspiration: required
8. Duration: 60 to 90 minutes
9. Flow rate: slow flow rate
10. Needle: 30-gauge extra-short or short

D. Periodontal ligament (PDL) injection:
1. Teeth anesthetized: single tooth
2. Other structures anesthetized: associated periodontium and gingiva of selected tooth
3. Pulpal anesthesia for single tooth or supplemental injection to block or supraperiosteal injection (local infiltration)
4. Target area: nearby terminal nerve endings at apex (or apices) so agent can also flow into marrow spaces of alveolar bone proper
5. Injection site: maxillary and mandibular teeth
   a. Long axis of tooth either mesial or distal with single-rooted tooth; mesial or distal to each root for multirooted tooth
   b. Into depth of gingival sulcus and then into alveolar bone proper
6. Aspiration: not necessary
7. Duration: 1 hour
8. Flow rate: slow flow rate
9. Needle:

a. 27-gauge extra-short or short for premolars and molars
b. 30-gauge extra-short or short for incisors

E. Intraseptal injection:
1. Structures anesthetized: interdental periodontium and gingiva of two adjacent teeth
2. Target area: terminal nerve endings within marrow of interdental bone of alveolar process associated with adjacent periodontium and gingiva of two or more teeth
3. Injection site: inject few drops and then use pressure to push needle into interdental bone center of interdental papilla adjacent to selected teeth
4. Aspiration: required
5. Duration: variable
6. Flow rate: slow flow rate
7. Needle: 27-gauge short

## LOCAL ANESTHESIA COMPLICATIONS (SEE TABLE 18.6)

### Minimal (Conscious) Sedation with Nitrous Oxide-Oxygen

Fearful or anxious dental hygiene patients can benefit from the relaxing effects of minimal (conscious) sedation with nitrous oxide ($N_2O$) by inhalation of $N_2O$ through the nose. This sedative can be used alone and in combination with dental local anesthesia. However, $N_2O$ sedation does not replace local anesthesia for pain control, since it is an analgesic and not an anesthetic. Short course can enhance venous distention and visibility if using premedication sedation (see latter note). Nitrous oxide administration by dental hygienists is only allowed in some states within the United States and may only be used under supervision of a dentist.

A. Chemistry, Physiology, and Pharmacology:
1. Colorless, tasteless, sweet-smelling inorganic gas that is not flammable but does support combustion
2. Commercially prepared by heating ammonium nitrate crystals in iron retort at 240 °C, then storing as liquid at 750 pounds pressure per square inch (psi) in blue cylinder and delivered as gas
3. Contents of $N_2O$ cylinder cannot be determined by pressure gauge until it is almost empty. Contrast with $O_2$ that is stored and delivered as gas in green cylinder, and its contents can be determined by reading pressure gauge where full is noted as 2100 psi. Highly recommended to have second tank of each gas immediately available should one be emptied in middle of procedure
4. Inhaled gas does not combine chemically with body tissue but mainly affects CNS
5. Psychosedation provided by $N_2O$ acts on the CNS so pain impulses are not relayed to cerebral cortex or the interpretation of pain impulses is altered
6. Alters mood and increases pain reaction threshold but does not totally block pain sensations
7. Works by stimulating release of inhibitory neurotransmitters at neuropathway junction located within brain. Consequent activation of opioid receptors and descending receptors of Gamma-aminobutyric acid type A (GABA-A) and noradrenergic metabolic sequence occurs which modifies spinal nociceptive process. Anxiolytic effect involves activation of GABA receptors through benzodiazepine binding sites
8. Has no effect on heart rate, blood pressure, and the liver or kidneys, as long as adequate amount of oxygen ($O_2$) is delivered simultaneously
9. Does affect sensations such as touch, pain, warmth, and hearing
10. Reduces gag reflex but does not eliminate it until is exchanged in lungs, beginning with respiratory bronchioles and ending at pulmonary alveolus. Also nonirritating to mucous membranes
11. The $N_2O$ molecule enters bloodstream through lungs, where it displaces nitrogen and is eventually exhaled, unchanged, through lungs
12. Not metabolized in body but is eliminated by diffusion properties from lungs as noted above
13. Toxic reaction associated with too much $N_2O$ is considered hypoxia, which is lack of $O_2$ to tissue and is characterized by headache and nausea (see later notes)
14. Highly soluble in blood plasma, therefore has analgesic properties in concentrations as low as 20%
15. Note that higher altitudes increase demand for higher concentrations of its use because of increased need for $O_2$ in blood
16. Using other sedative plus $N_2O$ and $O_2$ places individual in category of **moderate sedation**, which requires additional monitoring

B. Patient Selection:
1. Effective administration of $N_2O$ sedation involves both correct patient selection and correct management of sedation unit. Very few true contraindications exist. However, its use is not appropriate for everyone
2. Using American Society of Anesthesiologists (ASA) physical classification system for screening:
   a. ASA I and II: considered appropriate candidates with some considerations as noted below
   b. ASA III: greater risk but may be used after medical consult
   c. ASA IV: high risk; must seek medical consult; usually not appropriate to use with this patient
3. Relative contraindications:
   a. Pregnancy must have medical consultation. Regardless, in first trimester, no drugs are recommended. In third trimester, there is concern with low oxygen tension and levels of homocysteine. However, $N_2O$ has no effect on breast milk
   b. Recent eye surgery during which gas was administered to protect eyes after surgery for up to 3 months; can disrupt bubble and cause blindness. Medical consult is advised as to the length of time needed to postpone sedation for both
   c. Cystic fibrosis patients may have bullae, which are bubblelike cavities filled with air in lungs that can become exacerbated; medical consult is advised
   d. Chronic obstructive pulmonary disease, such as emphysema, chronic bronchitis, or lung cancer:
      (1) Depends on lowered blood $O_2$ level to stimulate respiration and with increased $O_2$ saturation may

## TABLE 18.6 Local Complications Associated With the Administration of Local Anesthetics

| Complication | Causes | Prevention | Management |
|---|---|---|---|
| Needle breakage | Sudden, unexpected movement;<br>Poor technique | Patient communication<br>Long, large-gauge needle<br>Do not bend needle<br>Advance needle slowly<br>Never force needle<br>No sudden direction changes<br>Never insert to hub | Remain calm<br>Keep hands in patient's mouth to prevent closure<br>Remove needle fragment if visible<br>Refer to oral surgeon<br>Document incident |
| Pain during injection | Careless technique<br>Dull needle<br>Barbed needle<br>Hitting bone<br>Rapid deposit | Proper technique<br>Sharp needles<br>Topical anesthetic<br>Sterile anesthetics<br>Inject slowly<br>Room temperature solutions | Good communication<br>Reassure patient that pain is only temporary |
| Burning during injection | Contamination of local anesthetics<br>Heated anesthetic<br>Expired solution<br>Rapid deposit | Never store in disinfecting solution<br>Store at room temperature<br>Check expiration date<br>Do not use cartridge warmers<br>Inject slowly<br>Consider buffering local anesthetic | Reassure patient that burning will last only seconds |
| Hematoma | Inadvertent puncturing of a blood vessel<br>Overinsertion of needle during posterior superior alveolar (PSA) block<br>Improper technique<br>Multiple needle penetrations | Short 25-gauge needle for PSA<br>Know dental anatomy<br>Modify injection technique for patient size<br>Minimize number of needle insertions<br>Maintain good technique | Swelling; apply direct pressure<br>Apply ice to region; warm packs the next day<br>Discuss possibility of soreness and limited movement to patient<br>Instruct patient that swelling and discoloration will disappear after 7–14 days<br>Dismiss patient when bleeding has stopped |
| Transient facial paralysis | Inadvertent deposition of local anesthetic in parotid salivary gland during inferior alveolar (IA) block or Vazirani-Akinosi (V-A) block<br>Parotid salivary gland is located on the posterior border of the mandibular ramus and fifth cranial or facial nerve travels through gland<br>Temporary loss of function of muscles of facial expression due to anesthesia of facial nerve | Use proper technique for IA or V-A block<br>Contact bone on the medial surface of the mandibular ramus before depositing agent for the IA or V-A block<br>Redirect barrel of syringe more posteriorly if bone is not contacted | Reassure patient that paralysis is temporary and will last only a few hours<br>Ask patient to remove contact lenses if applicable<br>Close eyelid manually<br>Document |
| Paresthesia | Irritation to nerve following injection of contaminated agent (less nerve fascia)<br>Edema places pressure on nerve<br>Trauma, electrical shock, or even hemorrhage around nerve sheath<br>Higher concentrations of local anesthetic agent may increase risk for paresthesia<br>Controversy on role of articaine | Store dental cartridges properly<br>Avoid placing cartridges in disinfectant solution<br>Use proper technique: do not move needle around in deep tissue, change needle directions when needle is almost completely withdrawn from tissue<br>Use conservative approach by not using articaine for IA block<br>Use alternative blocks to IA block | Reassure patient<br>Arrange examination with dentist<br>Consultation with oral surgeon<br>Record incident<br>Inform insurance carrier of incident |
| Trismus | Trauma to muscles in infratemporal space<br>Multiple needle insertions<br>Using contaminated needles<br>Depositing contaminated agent<br>Depositing large amounts of agent in restricted areas<br>Hemorrhage<br>Low-grade infection | Store anesthetic properly<br>Use sharp, sterile, needles<br>Use appropriate injection technique<br>Use minimal amount of agent<br>Deposit agent slowly | Arrange for exam with dentist<br>Heat therapy<br>Jaw exercises<br>Infection; antibiotic treatment<br>Severe pain; refer to oral surgeon<br>Record incident |
| Infection | Contamination of the anesthetic needle before injection<br>Improper handling of local anesthetic<br>Administration of contaminated agent<br>Improper tissue preparation<br>Administering local anesthetics through areas of dental infection (needle tract) | Sterile needle<br>Sheath needle before and immediately after injection<br>Be aware of the location of the uncovered needle at all times<br>Use appropriate infection protocols<br>Store anesthetic properly<br>Wipe off diaphragm<br>Topical antiseptic<br>Do not administer local anesthetics through areas of dental infection | Treat initially as trismus; if patient does not respond in 3 days, systemic antibiotic therapy may be prescribed by their dentist or physician |

**TABLE 18.6 Local Complications Associated With the Administration of Local Anesthetics—cont'd**

| Complication | Causes | Prevention | Management |
|---|---|---|---|
| Edema | Trauma during injection<br>Administration of contaminated agent<br>Hemorrhage<br>Infection<br>Allergic response; may produce airway obstruction | Appropriate infection control<br>Appropriate technique<br>Adequate preanesthetic assessment | Usually resolves within several days without any required treatment<br>Edema caused by infection may require systemic antibiotics |
| Soft tissue injuries | Lips, tongue, cheeks traumatized by patient while numb<br>Typically seen in children and in special needs patients | Select anesthetic with appropriate duration for treatment<br>Warn patient not to eat, drink hot fluids, or test anesthesia by biting<br>Instruct parent or guardian of danger<br>Place cotton rolls between teeth and soft tissue<br>Warning stickers can be used to remind patient and guardian of dangers associated with being numb<br>Consider administering phentolamine mesylate | Analgesics for pain<br>Antibiotics should be prescribed for infections<br>Recommend warm saline rinses to decrease swelling and discomfort<br>Petrolatum can be used to coat the lips to minimize discomfort |
| Tissue sloughing | Prolonged use of topical anesthetics<br>Sterile abscess may develop after prolonged ischemia, usually on palate caused by vasoconstrictor | Use topical agent for only 2 to 3 minutes and in a small area<br>Avoid high concentrations of vasoconstrictors | Usually requires no treatment |
| Postanesthetic intraoral lesions | Trauma to area of injection | Use appropriate administration techniques | Topical anesthetic agents or pastes for discomfort |

From: Logothetis DD, *Local Anesthesia for the Dental Hygienist*, 3rd ed, St Louis, Elsevier 2021.

go into apnea and stop breathing; match test can be used to check for pulmonary health
   (2) Physician discretion for hypoxic drive; medical consult recommended
  e. Respiratory infection from both viral or bacterial source or active allergies. Active infections must be cleared before use and medications may be of use with allergies. However, asthmatics respond very well and keeps them from getting anxious
  f. Recent pneumoencephaly procedure involving cerebrospinal fluid deplacement with gas for visualization. Medical consult is advised as to the length of time needed to postpone sedation
  g. Claustrophobia since are already not fond of dental professionals in personal space and need to wear traditional nasal hood. However, new nasal hoods are available that are less intrusive and may prove to be more viable option
  h. Language or consent must be considered if unable to give verbal informed consent because of mental capacity reasons or language barriers. Instead discuss with caregiver or arrange for translation services
  i. Drug or alcohol abuse could significantly potentiate any drug already on board in an individual. Practitioners must also be vigilant about security of nitrous oxide supply (see latter discussion)
  j. Bleomycin sulfate treatment for cancer patients; cannot receive hyperoxygenation (100%). Medical consult is advised as to length of time needed to postpone sedation
4. Cautions for use:
  a. Psychiatric patients and patients taking mood altering drugs; care must be exercised, medical consult recommended
  b. Emotional instability that includes history of death, divorce, job loss; care must also be exercised
  c. Vitamin $B_{12}$ (cobalamin) deficiency due to drug abuse (see later discussion) as well as medication use and illnesses that have lowered level. Medical consult and possible premedication with vitamin are indicated or use of general anesthesia instead

C. Administration procedures:
1. For safe administration of $N_2O$ sedation, patient must be screened and monitored for relative contraindications or cautions (see earlier discussion) and sedation unit must be checked for safety; National Institute for Occupational Safety and Health (NIOSH) has shown that controls can allow lower $N_2O$ concentrations in dental operatories
2. Must follow standard precautions for infection control at all times. Any part of tubing that is not corrugated can be sterilized. This can be done after each patient, but it is not necessary. Surface disinfection is adequate
3. Patient considerations:
  a. Take thorough medical history
  b. Monitor during administration of gas to determine consciousness and intolerance. However, pulse oximeter is not necessary since it is used at a minimal sedation level
  c. Instruct patient not to talk to decrease exhalation of gas into room air and keep sedation constant. Music is a welcome addition too because it often promotes relaxation

4. $N_2O$-$O_2$ unit:
   a. Thoroughly check unit for leaks and unsafe equipment. Confirm absence of leaks at pressure connections on unit. Bubbles will appear at leaking locations when soap and water solution is used; inadequate seal will produce audible hissing sound
   b. Monitor main fail-safe features:
      (1) Universal color scheme: used for tanks; blue for $N_2O$; green for $O_2$
      (2) Tanks for two gases are not interchangeable:
         (a) Pin index safety system ensures that $N_2O$ cylinder does not fit into yoke that holds $O_2$ cylinder and vice versa
         (b) Diameter index safety system has diameter of hole at top of cylinder ($O_2$ or $N_2O$) fits only with corresponding cylinder head
      (3) Flowmeter: measures how much of both $O_2$ and $N_2O$ is delivered in liters flow per minute (L/min)
         (a) Minimum flow: the $O_2$ is 2 L/min and $N_2O$ flow is 0.5 L/min; delivers minimum of 30% $O_2$ at all times. Critical to maintain an $O_2$ level of at least that present in ambient air (21%). Minimum of 30% established by the manufacturers allows for a margin of error in calibration. Similarly, equipment is designed to deliver no more than 70% $N_2O$ at any time. For analgesia and sedation purposes, not necessary to administer $N_2O$ concentrations higher than 70%
         (b) Then $N_2O$ shuts off when $O_2$ quits; also, clinician can turn off $N_2O$ at any time; mechanism's function is based on pressure. Then $O_2$ flows into unit at pressure that opens valve to allow flow of $N_2O$. If $O_2$ pressure drops because of depletion of supply, valve closes, thereby preventing flow of $N_2O$
         (c) Alarm systems: used when $O_2$ runs out and automatic turnoff occurs when $O_2$ is depleted
      (4) Scavenger system: removes exhaled gases from face mask (or nasal hood) and room air and reduces environmental $N_2O$ contamination from 900 to 30 parts per million (ppm)
         (a) Scavenging nasal hoods are designed to provide fresh gas to the patient through one-two hoses, while one or two additional hoses evacuate gas being exhaled by patient via vacuum system that exhausts gases out of building
         (b) Maximum allowable contamination in healthcare environments is 50 ppm
      (5) Flush system: available to provide 8 or more liters of 100% $O_2$ to patient if there are signs of intolerance
      (6) Reservoir bag: used to assist or control respiration during procedure and in event of an emergency
      (7) $N_2O$ tank: will show 750 psi until it is mostly empty; meter cannot be used to tell how much is left in tank, unlike tank of $O_2$
5. Preprocedural steps (preparation phase):
   a. Look at chart for last entry involving use and pain control issues for patient
   b. Have patient use restroom and take out contacts since eyes can get dry from air with mask
   c. Obtain preprocedure vital signs
   d. Have patient supine with legs uncrossed to prevent changes in circulation and paresthesia (numbness)
   e. Explain procedure to patient; also explain potential sensations associated with gas
      (1) Percentage noted is only somewhat relevant for current appointment
      (2) Most common mistake is to automatically deliver preset percentage to all patients
      (3) Look for any changes in emotional state and listen for any similar verbal cues
   f. Verbal consent must be obtained before each procedure and written consent is prudent practice
6. Procedural steps (administration and recovery phase):
   a. Turn on unit and push in flush valve to allow air for first breaths
   b. Adjust mask for proper secure fit and turn on scavenger system; piece of gauze may be folded over patient's nose to minimize gas leakage should adjustment be inadequate
   c. Determine and administer to patient correct liter flow using 100% $O_2$; actual percentage of $N_2O$ is calculated by dividing $N_2O$ L/min by total L/min
      (1) Considered minimum flow rate or tidal volume (TV) when patient is breathing comfortably with average adults breathing 4 to 6 L/min, athletes or large adults breathing 7 to 8 L/min, and children or small adults breathing 4 to 5 L/min
      (2) Make sure reservoir bag is not overinflated or underinflated while patient is breathing; should fluctuate as patient breathes
      (3) Certain units automatically determine $O_2$ level when gas level is adjusted
   d. At 1-minute intervals, decrease $O_2$ flow by same amount that $N_2O$ flow is increased until patient acknowledges appropriate effects
      (1) Titration: method of drug administration in which a substance is given in incremental doses until a specific desired clinical endpoint is reached. Process allows $N_2O$ to be titrated, which is current standard of care
      (2) Limits amount of drug that is required; allows for biologic variability and safe performance of prolonged procedure
      (3) Takes 30 to 60 seconds for changes in gas levels to be felt by patient
   e. Once flow is at level where patient is comfortable, start procedure
      (1) If reservoir bag collapses or flattens, fill it again by use of $O_2$ flush valve and increase flow
      (2) If reservoir bag balloons or overinflates, decrease flow until bag is two-thirds full
   f. Increase level of $N_2O$ during painful or stressful portions of treatment by 5% L/min from present levels to ensure pain control

g. Continue to monitor patient for signs of intolerance, including nausea, diaphoresis (or perspiration), unconsciousness, or changes in behavior (see later discussion)
   (1) Patients must never be left unattended; otherwise they may feel that they have been left alone and may panic, become agitated, or remove mask; also oversedation and toxicity could occur
   (2) Once baseline is achieved, level of $N_2O$ should be dropped back 0.5 to 1.0 L/min and $O_2$ turned up by same amount; can also be decreased near end of appointment
h. When $N_2O$ is no longer needed, have patient breathe 100% $O_2$ for at least 5 minutes or as long as necessary until effects of sedation disappear (see later discussion on importance); no titration is needed at this time. Most experts state that although there is no specific time unit, they consider 3 hours as an extended time period

7. Postprocedural steps (postoperative phase):
   a. Always evaluate recovery; verbal should be same as if nothing happened
   b. Obtain postprocedure vital signs. Blood pressure values within 10 mm Hg for both systolic and diastolic from preprocedural readings are considered to be within accepted comparable range; pulse rates within 10 beats/min and respiration rates within 5 breaths/min are acceptable parameters for comparison
   c. Document use in records along with thorough ongoing status (updated medical history, ASA classification, indications for use, and vital signs):
      (1) TV in L/min
      (2) Amount of $N_2O$ in liters or percentage
      (3) Amount of $O_2$ in liters or percentage
      (4) Duration of sedation
      (5) Oxygenation period
      (6) Patient's response
   d. Thank patient for cooperation and reinforce success of appointment
   e. May go to work immediately after use if not concerned about possible tiredness. However, have patient wait 15 minutes before leaving if driving
      (1) Motor skills and attention can be affected for as long as 15 minutes after patient stops breathing gas
      (2) Offense for person to drive while under influence of drugs; dental setting can be held liable

8. Signs and symptoms:
   a. There are basic signs and symptoms associated with $N_2O$ use; however, response varies under sedation. Patients should not be given specific physical signs to expect such as tingling in fingers, toes, cheeks, lips, tongue, head, or chest area
   b. Never liken it to alcohol, since that may upset patient. Patients will remember what procedures were done and with whom they interacted
   c. Since most nonsurgical dental procedures, such as those performed by dental hygienist, use minimal levels of sedation at less than 50% of gas, which is standard of care, patient remains awake and aware while breathing and can participate in treatment

**TABLE 18.7 General Signs and Symptoms in Response to Nitrous Oxide Sedation**

| Concentration of $N_2O$ (%) | Response* |
|---|---|
| 10%-20% | Body warmth, tingling of hands and feet |
| 20%-30% | Numbness of thighs |
| 20%-40% | Numbness of hands, feet, and tongue, droning sounds present, dissociation begins and reaches peak, mild sleepiness, analgesia (minimum at 30%), euphoria |
| 30%-50% | Sweating, nausea, increased sleepiness |
| 40%-60% | Dreaming (possibly sexual), laughing, further increases sleepiness, tending toward unconsciousness, increased nausea and vomiting |
| 50% and over | Loss of consciousness and light general anesthesia |

*Standard of care states that it should be used at <50% for most dental procedures because higher levels increase risk of complicating signs and symptoms as listed.

   d. Patient will still be able to respond to requests and answer questions, but speech may be slightly slurred, and responses may be slower than usual. Will be relaxed and cooperative, probably will not feel any local anesthetic injections or other discomforting parts of dentistry and will lose track of time. Sedated patients may not be able to accurately state how they feel; specific questions are necessary to assess patient. **Example:** "*Are you uncomfortable?*" or "*On a scale of 1 to 10, what is your level of comfort?*"
   e. Effective minimal sedation occurs in most patients; this level of gas keeps from occurring and maintains safety (see Table 18.7). See later discussion of complications
   f. Specific signs:
      (1) Patient awake, drowsy, relaxed appearance
      (2) Eye reaction and pupil size, blood pressure, heart rate, and respiratory normal
      (3) Flushing of skin with slight perspiration and lacrimation
      (4) Little or no gagging or coughing; speech infrequent and slow
      (5) Minimal movement of arms and legs
      (6) Lessened pain reaction
   g. Specific symptoms:
      (1) Feeling of warmth and pleasant floating sensation
      (2) Tingling in hands and feet
      (3) Feeling of heaviness or lightness
      (4) Slight temporary hearing changes

9. Complications:
   a. Procedure is very safe. However, about 15% of patient experience side effects, including headache, nausea, and/or vomiting
   b. Other possible side effects are excessive sweating and shivering
   c. Behavioral problems (such as sexual dreaming) may occur
   d. If patient experiences side effects, gas can be turned off and patient can breathe 100% $O_2$ for up to 5 minutes

e. Most complications result from excessive levels of gas (such as more than 50%) or not monitoring patients while they are under influence of gas
f. Nausea is more common than vomiting
   (1) With prompt recognition, nausea can be eliminated; unrecognized, it can lead to vomiting
   (2) Patient monitoring is most important means of preventing
      (a) Watching face, arms, and body for any unusual expression or movements
      (b) Looking for pained features and other signs such as pallor, sweating, hands over abdomen
   (3) Causes:
      (a) Increased depth or length of sedation; concentration of gas
      (b) Overwrought patient
      (c) If patient has inherent tendency to become nauseated, may be premedicated with prescription or over-the-counter antiemetic drugs (such as dimenhydrinate [Dramamine]); possibly should be avoided during unstable pregnancy symptomology
      (d) Presence or absence of food in stomach; heavy meal (includes fatty, fried foods) is not recommended but does not require empty stomach
      (e) Changes in patient's position; mouth breathing, and prolonged conversation reduce sedation level; once patient is resedated with reminder to nose breathe, may revert to mouth breathing and create situation known as "roller coaster" with sedation going up and down in levels
   (4) Management by decreasing gas concentration by ~ 5% to 10% until patient feels comfortable
g. Vomiting (emesis) prevented by prompt recognition and management of nausea; less common than nausea
   (1) More common in children; may vomit without warning
   (2) Caused by oversedation; higher risk during induction when communication is harder and patient is more likely to mouth breathe
   (3) Vomitus may be aspirated because of position of head in dental chair; potential to produce obstructed airway and its complications
   (4) Warning signs are nausea, pallor, cold sweat, cold and clammy hands, increased salivation, and active swallowing
   (5) Immediately turn off gas flow, permitting patient to breathe 100% $O_2$
      (a) Remove delivery apparatus from face and removable dental equipment from mouth
      (b) Turn head and body to side to allow vomitus to pool in cheek and not in throat (pharynx)
      (c) Use basin and/or high-speed suction (high-volume evacuator) to remove vomitus
   (6) After incident, have patient breathe 100% $O_2$ again to reduce further vomiting
      (a) Patient may not want to have delivery apparatus on again for fear of becoming sick again, so explain need for $O_2$
      (b) Explain that vomiting was unusual occurrence and is unlikely to occur again to avoid discouraging patient from future use
h. Excessive sweating can be a concern
   (1) May become flushed by peripheral vasodilating properties of gas; minor perspiration is usually noted on forehead, arms, or hands
   (2) If severe, concentration of gas is slowly reduced by ~ 5% per in attempt to make patient comfortable
   (3) If unable to stop patient's perspiring, procedure is aborted
   (4) However, if accompanied by pallor, drop in blood pressure, and/or increased heart rate, give patient 100% $O_2$, provide basic life support, and activate emergency medical system
i. Shivering is not uncommon but can be uncomfortable; usually develops at end of procedure
   (1) With flushing and sweating that occur with use, core temperature can be reduced
   (2) Reassure that everything is fine; place blanket over patient to speed warming process
j. May show up in drug screening test since small amount is excreted in urine. However, nitrous oxide is not biotransformed by liver
k. It is possible for patient go to sleep during sedation but this does not occur when using appropriate titration technique. Patient should not be allowed to become drowsy or somnolent

D. Nitrous Oxide Drug abuse:
1. $N_2O$ can be abused by dental personnel for recreational use (with acute) or because of psychologic dependence (with chronic)
2. Short-term effects:
   a. May have slurred speech; difficulty maintaining balance when walking; delay in responding to questions; no response to stimulus such as pain, loud noise, or speech; may lapse into unconsciousness
   b. Person who is rendered unconscious is likely to stop breathing within seconds as result of depressed nervous system; if remains conscious and stops breathing gas, recovery can occur within a few minutes
   c. Person who remains unconscious and continues to inhale pure gas is likely to die
   d. Death also occurs when users, in attempt to reach higher state of euphoria by breathing the gas in confined space, such as a small room, inside automobile, or by placing head in plastic bag
   e. Long-term exposure (within several minutes) is not necessary before death occurs.
3. Effects of chronic use are unusual but can occur; may cause vitamin $B_{12}$ (cobalamin) deficiency
   a. Red blood cell count is lowered, resulting in anemia and nerve degeneration with myelopathy

b. Painful and/or numbing sensations, unsteady walk, or irritated appearance
c. May also result in depression of heart muscular functioning and cardiac disturbances

E. Dental personnel recommendations:
1. Exposures should be minimized to prevent short-term behavioral and long-term reproductive health effects. This includes adopting gas scavenging system in environment with adequate air changes/hour and specific methodologic indications in anesthesia procedure to reduce risk such as correct mask size and adequate pressure of adhesion to patient's face, reduction of time of administration, and dilution of gas concentration
2. Chronic exposure should be avoided by women in first trimester of pregnancy and infertile individuals using in vitro fertilization procedures (linked to spontaneous abortions in surgical nurses in studies); also those with neurologic complaints and immunocompromised persons because of bone marrow suppression. Dental office studies are not conclusive in this regard at this time as are surgical operatories on pregnancy complications

**WEBSITE INFORMATION AND RESOURCES**

| Source | Website Address | Description |
|---|---|---|
| Essential Skeleton 4 | https://itunes.apple.com/us/app/essential-skeleton-4/id623811668?mt=8 | Study bony landmarks, nerves, and muscles pertaining to the administration of local anesthesia |
| Dental—Head and Neck Anatomy | https://play.google.com/store/apps/details?id=com.jass.refapp8 | Same as above |

## CHAPTER 18 REVIEW QUESTIONS

Answers and rationales to review questions are available on this text's accompanying Evolve site. See inside front cover for details.

1. All of the following are desirable properties of local anesthetics EXCEPT one. Which one is the EXCEPTION?
   - **a.** Reversible
   - **b.** Rapid onset
   - **c.** Stability in solution
   - **d.** Slow biotransformation
2. The nerve that supplies the mandibular anterior teeth is a branch of the
   - **a.** Inferior alveolar nerve
   - **b.** Middle superior alveolar nerve
   - **c.** Lingual nerve
   - **d.** Posterior superior alveolar nerve
3. Sodium bisulfite is added to a cartridge of anesthetic to increase the stability of the
   - **a.** Distilled water
   - **b.** Vasoconstrictor
   - **c.** Hydrochloride salt
   - **d.** Plasma cholinesterase
4. Infection and inflammation cause the following effects when administering a local anesthetic?
   - **a.** Make the local anesthetic more effective
   - **b.** Cause the inflamed tissue to have a low pH
   - **c.** Increase the duration of action of the local anesthetic
   - **d.** Cause the inflamed tissue to have a high pH
5. All the following statements are TRUE about lidocaine EXCEPT one. Which one is the EXCEPTION?
   - **a.** It is an amide-linked compound
   - **b.** It is used in 2% concentrations
   - **c.** Is formulated in a 1:50,000 levonordefrin dilution
   - **d.** It has anticonvulsant properties
6. Which of the following gauge numbers indicates the needle with the largest lumen?
   - **a.** 30
   - **b.** 27
   - **c.** 25
   - **d.** 35
7. The maxillary division of the trigeminal nerve is
   - **a.** Sensory only
   - **b.** Motor only
   - **c.** Sensory and motor simultaneously
   - **d.** Mostly sensory and minimally motor
8. In a resting neuron, what negative ion is most abundant inside the plasma membrane?
   - **a.** Potassium
   - **b.** Sodium
   - **c.** Calcium
   - **d.** Chloride
9. Anesthetics decrease or limit the sensation of pain by
   - **a.** Decreasing the firing threshold
   - **b.** Preventing depolarization
   - **c.** Repolarizing the nerve membrane
   - **d.** Causing hyperpolarization
10. Saltatory conduction refers to
    - **a.** Rapid transmission of nerve impulses along a myelinated nerve fiber
    - **b.** Diffusion of sodium into the nerve cell during impulse conduction
    - **c.** Conduction of an impulse along a nonmyelinated nerve fiber at the nodes of Ranvier
    - **d.** Beginning relationship of the nerve to the muscle
11. Chemical synapses use chemical transmitters called:
    - **a.** Neurotransmitters
    - **b.** Chemical transmitters
    - **c.** Synaptic transmitters
    - **d.** Endogenous transmitters
12. The electrical potential of nerve axoplasm in the resting state is approximately:
    - **a.** -70mV

b. -30mV
c. Zero
d. +30 mV
e. +70 mV

13. Signs and symptoms of a vasoconstrictor overdose manifest as:
a. Central nervous system depression
b. Central nervous system stimulations
c. Cardiovascular depression
d. Respiratory depression

14. The mandibular nerve exits the skull via the:
a. Foramen rotundum
b. Foramen ovale
c. Superior orbital fissure
d. Cranial fossa

15. The lipophilic portion of an anesthetic molecule allows the anesthetic solution to
a. diffuse through the nerve tissue
b. diffuse through osseous tissue
c. diffuse through the interstitial tissue
d. be absorbed by the blood supply

16. Which acid is most often combined with a local anesthetic drug making it water soluble?
a. Sodium bisulfite
b. Sodium chloride
c. Acetic acid
d. Hydrochloric acid

17. The patient's medical history indicates past liver damage. Why is the amount of bupivacaine solution a relative contraindication?
a. Bupivacaine increases risk of allergic reaction
b. Bupivacaine undergoes biotransformation in liver
c. Bupivacaine is absorbed much slower at injection site
d. Bupivacaine is long acting anesthetic

18. When is lidocaine 1:50,000 epinephrine most effective?
a. When postoperative pain control is needed
b. When hemostasis is needed
c. When treating a cardiovascularly-involved patient
d. When more profound pain control is needed

19. Where is procaine metabolized?
a. Liver
b. Lungs
c. Plasma
d. Plasma and liver

20. The lipophilic portion of an anesthetic molecule allows the anesthetic solution to diffuse through the interstitial tissues; the hydrophilic portion allows the solution to diffuse through the nerve membrane.
a. Both statements are TRUE
b. Both statements are FALSE
c. The first statement is TRUE; the second statement is FALSE
d. The first statement is FALSE; the second statement is TRUE

21. Vasoconstrictors are added to local anesthetic agents to increase duration and:
a. Reduce toxicity by increasing the efficiency of the heart
b. Reduce toxicity by slowing absorption
c. Extend the half-life of the drug
d. Help biotransformation of the drug

22. Vasoconstrictors are terminated by?
a. Adrenergic nerves
b. Liver
c. Kidneys
d. MAO inhibitors

23. For what purpose is epinephrine added to either prilocaine or mepivacaine local anesthetic agent?
a. To increase the duration of the anesthesia
b. Increase hemorrhage in field of operation
c. To increase the potency of the drug
d. Decrease the onset of action of the anesthetic

24. Which of the following vasoconstrictor agents is used with mepivacaine (Carbocaine) 2%?
a. Neo-Cobefrin
b. Epinephrine
c. Levophed
d. Benzocaine

25. After starting the nonsurgical periodontal therapy, the clinician encounters considerable bleeding from the patient's sulcular tissues. It is decided to administer a local anesthetic for hemostasis. Which dilution of vasoconstrictor will provides the most profound bleeding control?
a. 1:20,000 levonordefrin
b. 1:50,000 epinephrine
c. 1:100,000 epinephrine
d. 1:200,000 epinephrine

26. All of the following are fail-safe components of the nitrous oxide unit EXCEPT one. Which one is the EXCEPTION?
a. Minimum flow of nitrous oxide is 2 L/min
b. Different universal colors are used to label oxygen and nitrous oxide
c. Oxygen and nitrous oxide tanks cannot be interchanged
d. Scavenger system is used to decrease exhaled gases

27. The patient indications for nitrous oxide sedation should ALWAYS include which of the following?
a. Mild anxiety
b. Emotional instability
c. Severe intellectual disability
d. Active respiratory infection

28. Which of the following is a common mistake when using nitrous oxide?
a. Individualizing the amount of nitrous oxide the patient receives
b. Using the oxygen flush button to remove mixture of gases from bag
c. Once baseline is achieved, dropping back the level of nitrous oxide
d. Allowing patients to let the dental staff know how they feel

29. How should the clinician have the reservoir bag while using nitrous oxide?
a. Overinflated
b. Deflated
c. Partially inflated
d. Stored in emergency kit

30. All of the following should be done immediately after the administration of nitrous oxide EXCEPT one. Which one is the EXCEPTION?
    a. Administer 100% oxygen to clear patient
    b. Take blood pressure reading
    c. Allow patient to drive
    d. Thank patient for cooperation
31. Which of the following is the primary site of action for nitrous oxide?
    a. Central nervous system
    b. Urinary system
    c. Respiratory system
    d. Cardiovascular system
32. About how long does it usually take for the patient to feel the changes to the level of the flow of the gases when nitrous oxide is administered?
    a. 5 to 10 seconds
    b. 20 seconds
    c. 30 to 60 seconds
    d. 2 minutes
33. Which of the following signs should be present during general dental treatment levels of sedation with nitrous oxide?
    a. Patient is asleep
    b. Lessened pain reaction
    c. Extra movement of arms and legs
    d. Speech frequent and rapid
34. What should a clinician do immediately if a patient shivers when under nitrous oxide sedation?
    a. Cover patient with blanket
    b. Increase tidal volume
    c. Give the patient 100% oxygen
    d. Abort clinical procedure
35. Which of the following are one of the pharmacologic properties of nitrous oxide?
    a. Sour smelling
    b. Amber colored
    c. Explosive
    D. Inorganic
36. How many cartridges of lidocaine 2% 1:100,000 epinephrine anesthetic agent can be safely administered to a 120-lb patient taking tricyclic antidepressants?
    a. 1.1 cartridges
    b. 2.2 cartridges
    c. 3.3 cartridges
    d. 4.4 cartridges
37. How many cartridges of prilocaine 4% anesthetic agent can a healthy 130-lb patient receive?
    a. 6.5 cartridges
    b. 7.2 cartridges
    c. 7.8 cartridges
    d. 8.3 cartridges
38. What is the target area for the inferior alveolar nerve block?
    a. Mandibular foramen
    b. Lateral surface of mandibular ramus
    c. Anteromedial border of neck of mandibular condyle
    d. Retromolar pad or triangle
39. What is the target area for the posterior superior alveolar nerve block?
    a. Retromolar pad or triangle
    b. Maxillary tuberosity
    c. Posterior superior alveolar foramina
    d. Superior to maxillary canines
40. What is the most common medical emergency observed in the dental office?
    a. Cardiac arrest
    b. Vasodepressor syncope
    c. Seizures
    d. Respiratory failure
41. Which nerve is involved when anesthetizing the palatal gingiva of the maxillary 2nd premolar?
    a. Middle superior alveolar nerve
    b. Nasopalatine nerve
    c. Infraorbital nerve
    d. Greater palatine nerve
42. After administering a posterior superior alveolar nerve block, the maxillary first molar remains sensitive, but the maxillary second and third molars are anesthetized. Which of the following would be the BEST explanation?
    a. Anesthetic agent was deposited too high for the usual landmarks
    b. Not enough anesthetic agent was deposited by the clinician
    c. Mesiobuccal root may not be anesthetized by posterior superior alveolar nerve block
    d. Anesthetic agent was deposited too low for the usual landmarks

## CASE A

| Age | 45 YRS | Scenario |
|---|---|---|
| Sex | ☐ Male ☒ Female | The patient has an appointment for nonsurgical periodontal therapy on her mandibular left quadrant. She is very sensitive to probing and has heavy deposits on her teeth. |
| Height | 5′5″ | |
| Weight | 130 LBS | |
| BP | 102/56 | |
| Chief Complaint | *"My teeth are sensitive and feel dirty!"* | |
| Medical History | Depression | |
| Current Medications | Elavil | |
| Dental History | Has been 5 years since her last appointment | |

***Use Case A to answer questions 43 to 46.***

43. The clinician anesthetizes the mandibular left quadrant using three cartridges of 2% Lidocaine with 1:100,000 epinephrine. Considering the patient's medical history, which of the following statements is TRUE regarding the selection and volume of the anesthetic administered?
    a. The anesthetic selected produces great stress on the heart and is contraindicated
    b. The type and dose of anesthetic are appropriate for the patient

c. The anesthetic selected is acceptable but the volume administered is inappropriate since an overdose was administered
d. The dose is correct but the anesthetic type is inappropriate since a vasoconstrictor is absolutely contraindicated

44. The clinician selected using 2% Lidocaine 1:100,000 over 1:50,000 epinephrine because of the anticipation of a great deal of bleeding. Which of the following is TRUE of the anesthetic choice made by the clinician, considering the patient's medical history?
a. It was inappropriate as more epinephrine is needed to control bleeding
b. It was appropriate as both concentrations of epinephrine will produce bleeding control
c. The change in procedure should never have been considered since neither concentrations has any effect on bleeding
d. Changing procedure due to an anticipation of bleeding is not standard protocol

45. The clinician administers the left inferior alveolar nerve block with the syringe over the contralateral premolars at the height of the coronoid notch. After penetration of almost ½ of the long needle, the needle is met with resistance. What is the best way to proceed?
a. Withdraw the needle completely and reinsert in a different location prior to depositing anesthetic
b. Withdraw the needle slightly and deposit the solution at the area of resistance
c. Withdraw the needle slightly and redirect the syringe by moving it more posteriorly, advance the needle until bone is gently contacted, then deposit the solution
d. Withdraw the needle slightly and redirect the syringe by moving it more anteriorly, advance the needle, reposition over the contralateral premolars, and continue insertion until bone is contacted, then deposit the solution

46. The clinician administers the left inferior alveolar nerve block. During treatment, all teeth on the left are anesthetized except the first molar that remains sensitive. What is the best explanation for this?
a. The clinician administered too little solution
b. The clinician used incorrect needle placement
c. The sensitive tooth is receiving innervation from the mylohyoid nerve
d. The sensitive tooth is receiving innervation from the contralateral side

## CASE B

| Age | 37 YRS | Scenario |
|---|---|---|
| Sex | ☐ Male ☒ Female | The patient has an appointment for nonsurgical periodontal therapy on her maxillary left quadrant. To reduce her fear of needles and her possible gag reflex, the clinician would like to use nitrous oxide sedation during the appointment. Near the end of the appointment, the patient becomes pale, starts to sweat on her forehead, and places her hands on her abdomen. |
| Height | 6′2″ | |
| Weight | 185 LBS | |
| BP | 102/56 | |
| Chief Complaint | *"I am really nervous about the needle!"* | |
| Medical History | Knee replacement surgery twice<br>Back surgery last year | |
| Current Medications | OTC vitamin preparations | |
| Social History | Marathon runner | |

***Use Case B to answer questions 47 to 50.***

47. How does the patient's being an athlete change the treatment using nitrous oxide sedation?
a. Greater volume of air needed for breathing
b. Less volume of air for needed breathing
c. Reduction of exposure to allow for better induction
d. Increased exposure to allow for better stamina

48. How does nitrous oxide sedation help the patient with a possible gag reflex?
a. Increase the reflex for easier diagnosis by the clinician
b. Allow the patient to feel free to vomit if needed
c. Decrease the reflex for effective therapy by the clinician
d. Allow the patient to rinse their oral cavity as needed

49. How will the clinician respond to the patient's fear of needles when using nitrous oxide sedation?
a. Clinician needs to increase nitrous oxide by 10%
b. Clinician needs to decrease oxygen by 20%
c. Clinician needs to increase nitrous oxide by 5%
d. Clinician needs to decrease oxygen by 1%

50. What does it mean when the patient places her hands over her abdomen and becomes pale and sweaty?
a. The patient needs to use the restroom as soon as possible
b. The patient is allowing the nitrous oxide to be removed from her tissue
c. The patient needs basic life support as soon as possible
d. The patient is becoming nauseated due to higher levels of gas

## SUGGESTED READINGS

Bowen DM, Pieren JA. *Darby and Walsh Dental Hygiene Theory and Practice*. 5th ed. Philadelphia: Elsevier; 2020.

Clark MS, Brunick AL. *Handbook of Nitrous Oxide and Oxygen Sedation*. 5th ed. St Louis, Elsevier; 2020.

Fehrenbach MJ, Herring SW. *Illustrated Anatomy of the Head and Neck*. 6th ed. Philadelphia: Saunders/Elsevier; 2021.

Logothetis DD. *Local Anesthesia for the Dental Hygienist*. 3rd ed. St Louis: Elsevier; 2021.

Malamed SF. *Handbook of Local Anesthesia*. 7th ed. St Louis: Mosby; 2019.

# 19

# Dental Hygiene Care for Patients With Special Care Needs

*Susan Lynn Tolle*

Every person has unique abilities and needs. Two of every five patients treated in the oral health care environment may require a modified care plan because of special care needs. These special care needs may be transient, such as pregnancy or a broken foot, or may be lifelong, such as end-stage renal disease or intellectual and developmental disabilities. With ongoing health care reforms, the aging of the population and improved access to care for underserved populations, dental hygienists will be serving increased numbers of persons with special care needs in a variety of settings. The National Institute of Dental and Craniofacial Research describes persons requiring special care as those with genetic or systemic disorders that affect oral, dental, or craniofacial health; whose medical treatments cause oral problems; or whose intellectual or physical disabilities complicate oral hygiene or dental treatment.

## GENERAL CONSIDERATIONS

### Life Span Approach to Care

A. Principles of growth, development, and maturation
   1. Growth includes physical and functional maturation
   2. Growth is generally a continuous and orderly process but can be modified by numerous factors (e.g., nutritional deficiencies)
   3. Different parts of the body grow and mature at different rates
   4. Critical periods exist in growth and development
   5. During growth and maturation, a person's perception of self and of self in relation to others changes
   6. Health status generally progresses from acute illness to chronic illness
   7. Transition from one life stage to another is gradual and not necessarily based on chronologic age
   8. Biologic age is not synonymous with chronologic age
   9. Signs of aging can appear at any age
      a. Immunity and host response

B. The US health care system (see the section on "Provision of Oral Health Care" in Chapter 20). The current system is categorical, with many gaps in services. A continuum of services through people's life stages must ensure:
   1. Universal access
   2. Continuity of care
   3. A comprehensive philosophy of care
   4. A system of planned change
   5. Heterogeneity of persons bearing the same label
   6. Social determinants of health are addressed
   7. Health care providers should consider how social determinants of health affect care

C. Individualized approach to care: oral health needs and approaches to care can differ throughout a person's life cycle (Table 19.1)

### Incidence and Prevalence of Individuals With Special Care Needs

A. National statistics on incidence and prevalence figures are difficult to compile because of:
   1. Unreliable reporting systems
   2. Variable and changing definitions of conditions
   3. Differences between acute conditions versus chronic conditions
   4. Overlap in data when dealing with multiple conditions

B. More than 60 million persons (one in five persons) are considered "disabled" as defined by the Americans with Disabilities Act; of these, approximately 1 million are children younger than 6 years

C. In the United States, 22% of adults have some type of disability

D. Non-Hispanic black (29%) and Hispanic (25.9%) adults are more likely to have a disability than white, non-Hispanic (20.6%) adults

E. Those with lower education levels, lower incomes, and those who are unemployed are more likely to report a disability

Table 19.2 identifies the most common chronic conditions in the older adult population

F. The most common disabilities in the United States are caused by cardiovascular disease, stroke (cerebrovascular accident [CVA]), obesity, arthritis, cancer, and diabetes

G. The prevalence of disability increases with age
   1. Of persons in the United States age 5 to 17, 5.6% are disabled
   2. Of persons in the United States age 18 to 64, 10.6% are disabled
   3. Of persons in the United States age 65 and older, 35.2% are disabled

H. Of individuals with developmental disabilities, 80% live in community-based residences or at home with families

**TABLE 19.1 Life-Span Approach to Oral Health Care**

| Life Stage | General Care Concerns | Usual Oral Concerns |
|---|---|---|
| Early childhood | Teaching parents and caregivers oral care skills<br>Preventing early occurrence of caries or trauma (protecting developing teeth)<br>Controlling risk factors<br>Preventing vertical and horizontal disease transmission | Oral infections<br>Dental caries<br>Dental development |
| Childhood | Developing positive dental attitudes and behaviors<br>Teaching self-care skills<br>Controlling risk factors<br>Preventing vertical and horizontal disease transmission | Dental caries<br>Dental development<br>Gingivitis |
| Adolescence | Motivating toward self-responsibility for seeking and receiving care<br>Controlling risk factors for disease<br>Preventing oral injuries<br>Nicotine use cessation | Dental caries<br>Periodontal diseases<br>Dental development |
| Young adult | Decreasing barriers and integrating oral health care into daily schedule<br>Nicotine use cessation | Periodontal diseases |
| Midlife | Maintaining status and preventing deterioration<br>Controlling risk factors<br>Nicotine use cessation | |
| Older adult | Motivating to continue preventive care and accept new theories and interventions<br>Decreasing barriers to care<br>Controlling risk factors<br>Nicotine use cessation | Periodontal diseases<br>Dental caries<br>Oral cancer |
| Elderly adult | Maintaining status and function and preventing infections and tooth loss<br>Controlling risk factors<br>Nicotine use cessation | Periodontal diseases<br>Dental caries<br>Oral cancer<br>Fractures, tooth loss<br>Oral infections |

**TABLE 19.2 Leading Chronic Conditions in the Older Adult Population**

| Noninstitutionalized Older Adults | Nursing Home Residents |
|---|---|
| Mobility limitations | Arthritis |
| Arthritis | Heart disease |
| Hypertension | Mental illness |
| Hearing impairments | Paralysis |
| Heart disease | |

## The Dental Hygienist and Individuals With Special Care Needs

A. Recognize physical, mental, medical, social, and oral needs
B. Recognize care involves increased awareness, attention, and accommodation by dental team
C. Communicate with patients and caregivers in a positive, appropriate, nondiscriminatory manner
D. Communicate with other professionals and team members to facilitate planning, implementation, and coordination of care
E. Plan, implement, and evaluate community-based and office-based programs
F. Adapt dental hygiene care plans, interventions, and evaluations to meet patients' special needs, considering:
   1. Barriers to care
   2. Resources
   3. Personal skills and abilities
   4. Cultural values and beliefs
   5. Be prepared for medical emergencies
G. Identify and eliminate potential barriers to care
H. Assess one's own attitudes, values, and commitment to provision of oral health services to these patients
I. Evaluate local, state, regional, and national trends for their potential impact on the provision of oral health care
J. Advocate oral health promotion and disease prevention programs, full use of dental hygienists, and development of sound research so that evidenced-based care is provided in oral health care programs
K. Patients may have multiple comorbid medical issues that the dental team needs to be prepared to manage

## General Definitions

These definitions tend to change frequently and often overlap:

A. Labeling—the process of classifying persons for educational, medical, or financial reasons
B. Barrier-free environment—facilities that are physically accessible to everyone
C. Normalization—making available patterns and conditions of everyday life that are as close as possible to the norms and patterns of mainstream society
D. Mainstreaming—integration of persons with special needs into community-based programs and services
E. Access to oral health care—opportunity for each individual to enter into the oral health care system and use needed services

## Goals of Normalization for Persons With Special Care Needs

A. Ensure the same legal and civil rights as others

B. Guarantee appropriate education for continued learning
C. Increase or maintain social skills and problem-solving abilities
D. Increase employment options and decrease employer discrimination
E. Ensure comprehensive network of community resources

## Potential Barriers to Oral Health Care

A. Accessibility
  1. Financial
    a. One-fourth of the older adult population has an inadequate income level; percentages are higher for women, ethnic minorities, and single heads of household
    b. Between 29% to 49% of disabled persons live near the poverty level
    c. Medicaid coverage for oral health care is extremely variable across states and often does not cover adult dental care
    d. Medical and pharmaceutical expenses for many persons with disabilities consume a major portion of their income
    e. Many individuals with special needs who have limited incomes cannot afford standard private practice fees for dental care, have no health insurance, or are underinsured
  2. Transportation and geography
    a. Public transportation is often unreliable, confusing, unaffordable, or nonexistent
    b. Patients with special care needs often rely on others for transportation to dental appointments, which increases their dependence and makes scheduling and compliance difficult. Homebound, hospitalized, or institutionalized patients frequently cannot be transported for care in the community
  3. Physical facilities
    a. Minimum standards for accessibility must be met by dentists according to the Americans with Disabilities Act of 1993
    b. External barriers include parking lots and spaces, walkways, curbs, stairs, narrow doors and entryways, heavy or pressurized doors, and small-print signs
    c. Internal barriers include narrow passageways or doors, cluttered rooms or hallways, loose rugs or heavy shag carpets, abrupt changes in floor textures, and bathrooms without grab-bars or other modifications

B. Psychosocial concerns
  1. Many persons in the United States express positive attitudes toward older adults and persons with disabilities, and yet most really perceive these populations as "different" and "inferior"
  2. Society perceives disabilities, differences, and disease states before recognizing similarities
  3. Feelings of guilt, anxiety, apathy, inadequacy, embarrassment, depression, anger, and resentment about special needs interfere with attempts to seek care
  4. Fear of or inability to comprehend dental procedures, antisocial or atypical behavior, or dependency on oral health care providers interferes with provision of care
  5. Basic daily needs and activities are often overwhelming and can lower the priorities for oral health care
  6. Perception of self-image and worth can affect care planning

C. Provider philosophy and provision of care
  1. The Americans with Disabilities Act requires that public and private dental offices serve persons with disabilities, that treatment is provided on the same basis as for nondisabled persons, and that dentists make reasonable modifications to facilitate access
  2. Despite the Americans with Disabilities Act, surveys indicate some dentists are unwilling to treat persons who are physically or mentally challenged
  3. Reasons given for not treating individuals with special needs include:
    a. Inadequate facilities and equipment
    b. Inadequate training (knowledge and competencies)
    c. Not wanting to expose "normal" patients to "special" patients
    d. Inability to collect adequate fees
    e. Additional effort and time required
    f. Personal discomfort about perceived "differences" of special patients
    g. Treatment of medically complex persons increases insurance premiums

D. Communication and cultural concerns
  1. Sensory impairments (hearing, visual) limit the patient's ability to transmit and receive communications when scheduling or undergoing oral care or participating in oral health care education
  2. The use of technical terminology or inappropriate language level may interfere with understanding
  3. Differences in communication styles (eye contact, physical proximity and contact, formal vs. informal speech, cultural variations, use of nonverbal cues and verbal language) can impair effective communication
  4. Use of condescending voice tones or language levels closes off communication lines
  5. Foreign language barrier may deter a patient from seeking care or reduce effectiveness of care
  6. Inadequate numbers of health care providers possess cross-cultural competence

E. Medical concerns
  1. Situations compromising the provider or patient
    a. Inadequate or inaccurate health histories
    b. Inadequate precautions for potential emergencies
    c. Inadequate knowledge of systemic conditions and their treatments
    d. Treatment barriers and modifications

F. Mobility and stability concerns
  1. Impaired ambulation or use of assistive devices may hinder access to care
  2. Uncontrolled or sudden movements may interfere with home care or dental hygiene interventions
  3. Uncontrolled or aggressive behavior may endanger the care providers and the patient
  4. Spatial disorientation may interfere with patient relaxation in the dental chair or with oral care procedures

## SPECIFIC CONDITIONS

See Chapters 8 and 9.

### Developmental and Cognitive Challenges

A. Definition
   1. Subaverage intellectual functioning originating during the developmental period and associated with impairment in adaptive behavior and significant limitations in daily living skills (formerly known as "mental retardation")
   2. Most common developmental disability
B. Incidence—2.5% to 3% of the US population (57.7 million total), depending on criteria
C. Levels of intellectual disabilities—intelligence quotient (IQ)
   1. Mild—approximate IQ 50 to 70 (89%)
   2. Moderate—approximate IQ 40 to 55 (6%)
   3. Severe—approximate IQ 25 to 40 (3.5%)
   4. Profound—IQ below 20 (1.5%)
D. Etiology—acquired (12%), inherited (13%), unknown (75%)
E. Signs, symptoms, and clinical manifestations
   1. Variable, depending on etiology and individual circumstances
   2. Unusual difficulty in learning and applying what is learned to issues of daily living
   3. Skull or other craniofacial anomalies may exist
   4. General developmental delays
   5. Other possible manifestations include motor incoordination, intellectual deficiencies, visual or hearing disorders, specific learning disabilities, maladaptive behaviors, emotional disturbances, medical disabilities, and self-injurious behaviors
      a. Microcephaly—small cranium that restricts brain growth
      b. Hydrocephaly—expansion of the cranium from excessive accumulation of cerebrospinal fluid (CSF)
      c. Malformation or asymmetry of growth
      d. Increased seizure risk
F. Oral manifestations
   1. Most oral health problems are not inherent to the disability but are related to extrinsic factors (e.g., neglect by caregivers or lack of coordination leading to poor oral disease control)
   2. Decayed-missing-filled surfaces (DMFS) scores comparable with those of the general population, but the "decayed" component may be higher because of lack of professional treatment (Fig. 19.1)
   3. Higher prevalence of periodontal conditions, probably related to poor oral hygiene and lack of regular care
   4. Higher incidence of malocclusion and deviations in tooth eruption is associated with craniofacial syndromes and growth abnormalities (Figs. 19.2 and 19.3)
   5. Some cases of enamel dysplasia more frequently seen in those with severe mental deficiency resulting from prenatal or perinatal defect or insult
   6. Thick flaccid lips, microglossia, bruxism, tooth anomalies such as microdontia and abnormal eruption patterns
   7. Oral trauma

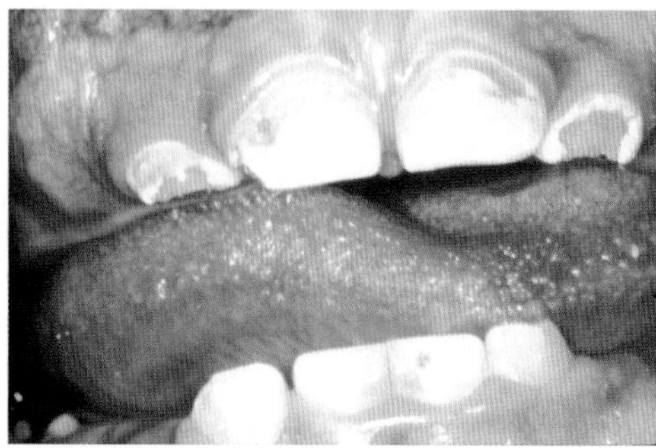

**Fig. 19.1** High incidence of dental caries is common and most likely related to neglect. (From National Oral Health Information Clearinghouse. *Oral Conditions in Children with Special Needs: A Guide for Health Care Providers*. Bethesda, MD: National Institute of Dental and Craniofacial Research; 2011.)

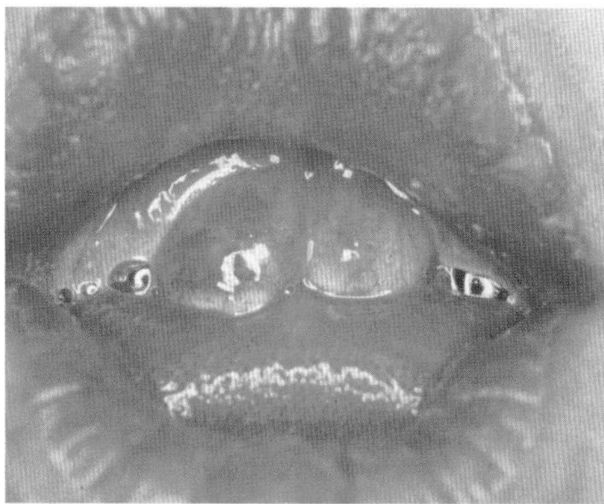

**Fig. 19.2** Delayed tooth eruption is a common oral condition in children with developmental disabilities. (From National Oral Health Information Clearinghouse. *Oral Conditions in Children with Special Needs: A Guide for Health Care Providers*. Bethesda, MD: National Institute of Dental and Craniofacial Research; 2011.)

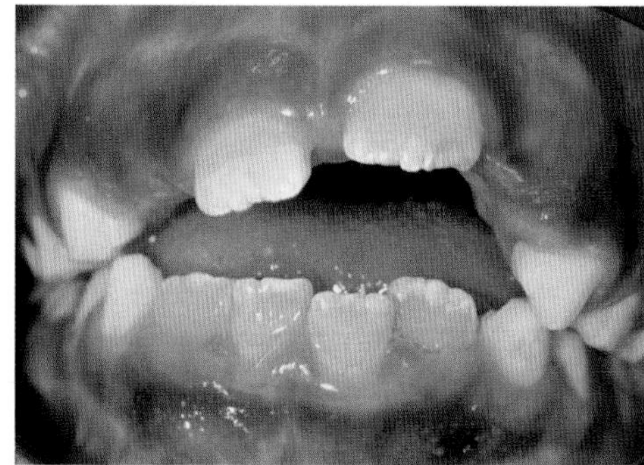

**Fig. 19.3** Malocclusion is a common oral finding in children with developmental disabilities. (From National Oral Health Information Clearinghouse. *Oral Conditions in Children with Special Needs: A Guide for Health Care Providers*. Bethesda, MD: National Institute of Dental and Craniofacial Research; 2011.)

### Fetal Alcohol Spectrum Disorders (FASD)

A. Definition
   1. An umbrella term describing a pattern of malformations caused by maternal alcohol consumption during pregnancy
   2. Characterized by prenatal and postnatal growth deficiency, dysmorphic facial features, and central nervous system (CNS) dysfunction

3. FASD include fetal alcohol syndrome (FAS), alcohol-related neurodevelopmental disorders (ARND), and partial fetal alcohol syndrome (PFAS)

B. Incidence and prevalence
   1. Estimated incidence of FASD is 0.3 to 1.5 per 1000 live births
   2. Leading known preventable cause of mental impairments and birth defects in the United States

C. Signs, symptoms, and clinical manifestations can range from mild to severe
   1. Premature or postnatal (or both) growth retardation—results in short stature, slight build, small head, low body weight
   2. Craniofacial dysmorphia—short eye openings, short upturned nose, smooth philtrum, flat midface, thin upper lip
   3. Nonspecific abnormalities in any organ system, depending on the time of alcohol insult
   4. Wide IQ range, many within the developmental/cognitive-challenged range
   5. Limited ability to read and write, but with minimal comprehension; also language problems
   6. Poor social judgment and socialization skills
   7. Hyperactivity and short attention span
   8. Problems with heart, kidneys, and bones
   9. Skeletal and ear disorders

D. Oral manifestations
   1. The majority of children with developmental and cognitive challenges have oral problems related to tooth eruption, craniofacial malformations, or malpositioning of teeth (usually class II or III malocclusion) (Fig. 19.4)
   2. Some may have V-shaped or cleft palate
   3. Moderate to severe gingivitis is seen

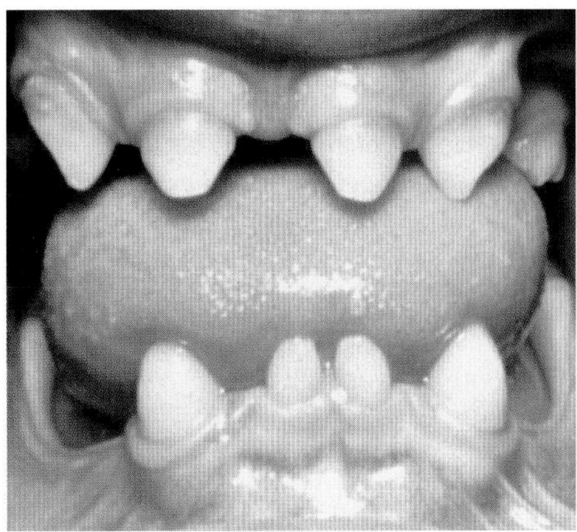

**Fig. 19.4** Tooth anomalies showing variations in eruption patterns and size and shape of the teeth. (From National Oral Health Information Clearinghouse. *Oral Conditions in Children with Special Needs: A Guide for Health Care Providers*. Bethesda, MD: National Institute of Dental and Craniofacial Research; 2011.)

## Down Syndrome

A. Definition and etiology
   1. Mental or intellectual disorder
   2. Associated with an anomaly of chromosome 21 (trisomy 21) in all or some body cells

B. Incidence—most common chromosomal abnormality (1 in 800 live births, but varies with maternal age); approximately 400,000 individuals in the United States affected

C. Signs, symptoms, and clinical manifestations
   1. Mild to profound developmental and cognitive challenges
   2. Poor muscular development, with hyperflexibility and hypotonia during childhood
   3. Short stature, with delay in skeletal maturation
   4. Short neck; extremities with broad stubby fingers
   5. High incidence of congenital heart defects (30% to 50%); language, vision (60%), and hearing problems (75%); risk of leukemia (less than 1%), thyroid problems, and immunologic defects
   6. Abnormal craniofacial features
      a. Small brachycephalic skull
      b. Round flat facies
      c. Small nasomaxillary complex

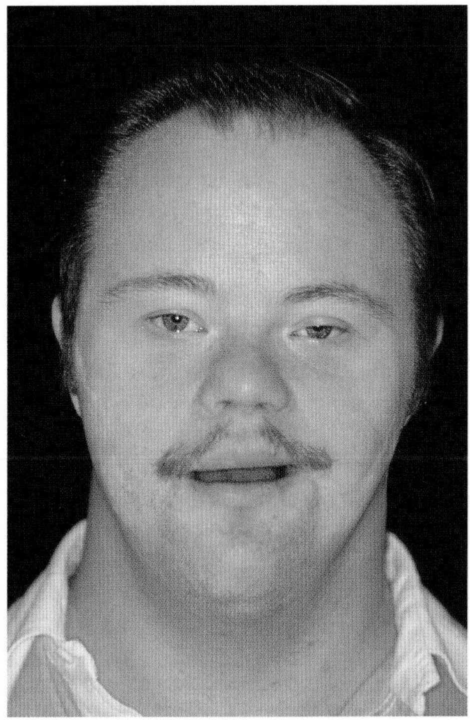

**Fig. 19.5** Common facial characteristics shown in a person with Down syndrome. (From Regezi JA, Sciubba JA, Jordan CK. *Oral Pathology: Clinical Pathologic Correlations*. 7th ed. St. Louis: Elsevier; 2017.)

      d. Ocular hypotelorism (eyes closer together than normal)
      e. Epicanthal folds
      f. Strabismus (convergent eyes)
      g. Simian crease (single transverse palmar crease)
      h. More susceptible to infection because of poor immune response

D. Oral manifestations (Fig. 19.5)
   1. Relative mandibular prognathism as a result of a small nasomaxillary complex
   2. Dry skin and thick, dry, fissured lips
   3. Open-mouth posture, with a protrusive, fissured tongue

4. Hyperplasia of the adenoids and tonsils
5. Altered salivary gland mechanism (decreased flow)
6. Increased susceptibility to severe periodontal disease of early onset, especially in anterior areas; may be related to host immune defects (e.g., periodontitis as manifestation of systemic disease)
7. Delayed eruption of teeth and abnormal tooth development
8. Higher incidence of congenitally missing teeth
9. Small tooth crowns with short crown/root ratio
10. Enamel dysplasia (Fig. 19.6)
11. Malocclusion—anterior open bite or cross-bite, posterior cross-bite, malocclusion common
12. Attrition
13. High palatal vault (Fig. 19.7)

E. Risk of associated conditions—increased risk for congenital cardiovascular defects, leukemia, respiratory conditions, and Alzheimer's disease (AD)

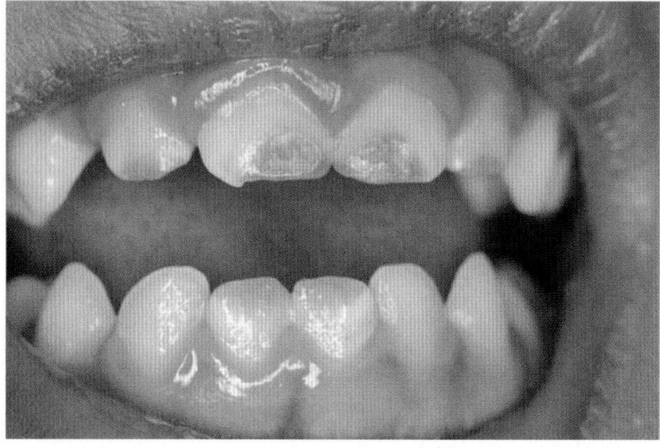

**Fig. 19.6** Discoloration and enamel dysplasia associated with developmental defects. (From Regezi JA, Sciubba JA, Jordan CK. *Oral Pathology: Clinical Pathologic Correlations*. 7th ed. St. Louis: Elsevier; 2017.)

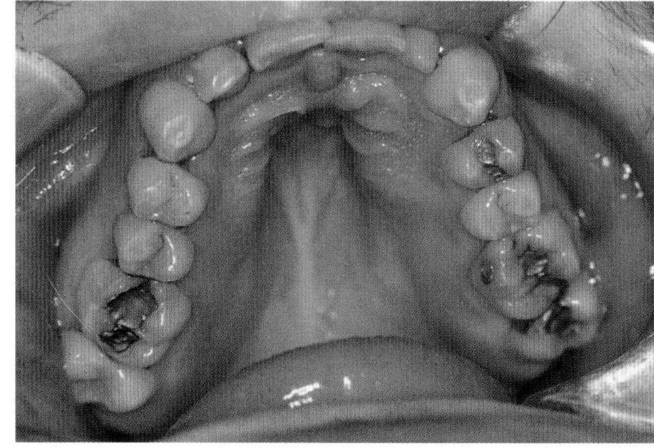

**Fig. 19.7** High-arched palate with decreased width and length. (From Regezi JA, Sciubba JA, Jordan CK. *Oral Pathology: Clinical Pathologic Correlations*. 7th ed. St. Louis: Elsevier; 2017.)

## Autism Spectrum Disorders (ASD)

A. Definition
1. A group of developmental disorders that affect the functioning of the brain, resulting in specific behavioral and communicative difficulties; speech, language and communication, social interaction, sensory impairments, play, and repetition of behaviors are key areas affected
2. Wide range of symptoms and behaviors with considerable individual variation

B. Incidence and prevalence
1. Incidence not completely known; prevalence rate of autism is increasing 10% to 17% annually
2. Unclear if the increase is real or reflects better diagnostic practices
3. Occurs in as many as 1 in 59 children
4. Four times more common in boys (1 in 38 vs. 1 in 152 girls)
5. Appears during the first 3 years of life

C. Signs, symptoms, and clinical manifestations
1. Great variability in expression; no standard type
2. Extreme aloneness; failure to develop eye contact, to cuddle as infants normally do, to develop social relationships, or to perceive others' feelings
3. Language disturbances—repetitious speech, pronoun reversals, lack of ability to use gestures; failure to develop functional speech in 50%
4. Comprehension problems, especially with verbal directions
5. Obsessive about maintaining routines and sameness of the environment (resistance to change)
6. Abnormal response to stimuli; may not respond to pain; or may have constant movement and repetitious activity
7. Sensitivities to sight, hearing, touch, smell, and taste
8. May be aggressive or self-abusive; tolerance to physical contact may be limited

E. Oral manifestations
1. 20% to 25% exhibit bruxism
2. Tongue thrusting common
3. Difficult behaviors, feeding problems, very limited dietary preferences (exclusively pureed foods, no fruits/vegetables, other), and poor cooperation are challenges to dental care
4. Home care measures are exceedingly difficult for many children/parents
5. Oral care may be neglected because of issues with communication, physical limitations, sensory stimulation, and socialization

## Attention Deficit Hyperactivity Disorder (ADHD)

A. Definition
1. Developmental and behavioral disorder affecting specific areas of learning or impulse control that can cause problems in acquiring new skills

B. Controversy over diagnosis and treatment; occurs in 11% to 16% of children
1. Presentation is variable: inattentive, hyperactive, or inattentive/hyperactive types.
2. Impulsivity, cognitive inflexibility, hyperactivity, short attention span, aggression
3. Difficulty with listening, compliance, task completion, work accuracy, and socializing.
4. More than 6.4 million persons have been diagnosed with ADHD
5. More common in boys, 4:1

6. Affects up to 60% of adults who had ADHD in childhood

C. Oral manifestations—none directly associated

## Emotional Disturbance and Mental Illness

A. Definition
1. Any disease or condition affecting the brain that impairs thinking, feeling, behavior, or all of these functions
2. Leading cause of disability in the United States
3. Many suffer from more than one mental disability at any given time

B. Incidence and prevalence
1. Approximately 57.7 million persons in the United States over age 18 affected (26.2% of population)
2. At some point in life, 10% of all adults will need or benefit from some form of mental health intervention
3. Major depression, bipolar disorder, schizophrenia, and obsessive-compulsive disorder are among top 10 leading causes of disability

C. Classification—three common classes:
1. Psychoneuroses—anxiety, depressive, obsessive, or conversion reactions
2. Personality disorders—situational or adjustment reactions
3. Psychoses—schizophrenia

D. Signs, symptoms, and clinical manifestations—depend on the type of disorder
1. Inner tensions create anxiety, frustration, fears, and impulsive behavior
2. Examples of behavior
   a. Translation of fears or anxieties into physical symptoms
   b. Regression to earlier forms of behavior
   c. Displays of hostility or aggression
   d. Withdrawal into fantasy (e.g., daydreaming)
   e. Fear of failure and criticism
   f. Development of substitute fears, phobias, or compulsions

E. Oral manifestations
1. None directly associated
2. May see intraoral trauma resulting from unusual habits or aggressive behavior
3. May have xerostomia as a side effect of medications
4. With compulsive behavior, may have immaculate oral hygiene

## Disorders of Eating

See signs and symptoms of disordered eating in the section on "Energy Balances and Weight Control" in Chapter 12.

A. Definitions
1. Anorexia nervosa, an eating disorder characterized by markedly reduced appetite or total aversion to food;
   a. Psychophysiologic condition characterized by suppression and denial of sensation of hunger
   b. Person may be socially isolated and relatively asexual
   c. Consumption of only 300 to 600 calories per day is common
   d. Often come from middle-class to upper-class families with high parental or societal expectations
   e. Perfectionists, competitive, and overachievers
   f. Deny their emaciated appearance
   g. Diagnosis based on person's refusal to maintain normal body weight for height and age; intense fear of becoming fat despite being underweight; denial of the seriousness of the starvation and a distorted body image
2. Anorexia bulimia, in addition to anorexia purging habit;
   a. Syndrome involving episodic binge eating and purging
   b. Purging involves self-induced vomiting and use of laxatives, diuretics, or enemas
   c. Often occurs after failed attempts to lose weight through dieting
   d. May be of normal weight
   g. Usually outgoing and sexually active
   h. Calories consumed during binging range from 3500 to 20,000
   i. Vomiting episodes may last from 5 to 30 minutes
   j. Diagnosis of bulimia if there are at least two bulimic episodes per week for 3 months
   k. Vitamin deficiencies

B. Incidence and prevalence
1. About 90% are female; 1.1% to 4.5% of the US population have eating disorder in their lifetime; rate is increasing yearly
2. Occurs in 1 in 200 white adolescent females
3. Occurs in 3% to 20% of college students
4. Most common age group is 12 to 35 years; also occurs in older adults
5. From 27% to 42% of persons with anorexia indulge in bulimia
6. Mortality rate of 9%

C. Signs and symptoms
1. Anorexia nervosa
   a. Intense fear of becoming obese; refusal to maintain normal weight
   b. Disturbance of body image
   c. Weight loss of at least 25% of original body weight, not caused by physical illness
   d. Downy growth of body hair (lanugo)
   e. Periods of overactivity
   f. Dry, flaky skin
   g. Lowered blood pressure, body temperature, and pulse
   h. Episodes of bulimia
   i. Complications include cardiac arrhythmia from reduced heart muscle mass and electrolyte imbalance from dehydration
2. Anorexia bulimia
   a. Awareness that eating pattern is abnormal
   b. Depression and self-deprecating thoughts
   c. Repeated attempts to lose weight
   d. Recurrent bingeing (rapid intake of food in a short period), usually high-calorie, easily ingested food
   e. Inconspicuous eating
   f. Termination of episodes by purging with self-induced vomiting, laxatives, diuretics, and enemas

g. Weight fluctuation more than 10 pounds
h. Dehydration
i. Electrolyte imbalance

E. Oral manifestations
1. Esophageal lacerations and chronic sore throat from repeated vomiting
2. Parotid gland swelling and xerostomia
3. Burning sensation in the tongue
4. Perimyolysis (dental erosion), dentinal hypersensitivity, and margination of amalgams from acid erosion of vomiting; lingual surfaces of maxillary incisors most often affected
5. Rampant caries from high consumption of sucrose, xerostomia, and dehydration
6. Irritated soft tissues from vomiting, dehydration, and vitamin deficiencies
7. Dentinal hypersensitivity and vitamin deficiencies

## Alzheimer's Disease (AD)

A. Definition
1. Progressive irreversible brain disorder characterized by intellectual and cognitive disturbance, behavioral changes, and eventually a state of complete dependence
2. Three types:
a. Early onset—diagnosis before age 65
b. Late onset—occurs after age 65
c. Familial—entirely inherited; onset often in the 40s

B. Incidence and prevalence
1. Estimated 5.5 million cases in in Americans over the age of 65 and 200,000 Americans over age 65
2. Estimated 130% increase expected by 2050
3. Two-thirds of Americans with AD are women

C. Signs, symptoms, and clinical manifestations—different parts of the brain affected in varying degrees but reflect neuronal degeneration
1. Early
a. Short-term memory loss
b. Difficulty with activities of daily living
2. Later
a. Memory loss and inability to concentrate, reading problems, poor object recognition
b. Anxiety, irritability, withdrawal, petulance
c. Abnormal sleep patterns
d. Motor abnormalities, including exaggerated reflexes and gait disturbances
e. Apathy, depression
f. Disorientation, lack of judgment and understanding, impulsivity
g. Incontinence

D. Risk factors
1. Age—greatest risk factor
2. Family history
3. Mild cognitive impairment

E. Oral manifestations
1. None specific to the condition
2. Disease states usually are a result of neglect, the aging process, or any accompanying chronic illnesses

## Seizure Disorders

See the section on "Seizures and Convulsive Disorders" in Chapter 21.

A. Definitions
1. Not a disease; the term *seizure disorders* is used to describe symptoms of recurrent or chronic brain dysfunction
2. Characterized by discrete, recurring behavioral manifestations that include disturbances of balance, sensation, behavior, perception, or consciousness
3. Should not be confused with one-time seizures that result from drug overdoses, brain tumors, or other problems
4. Seizure—an episode of cerebral dysfunction produced by abnormal excessive neuronal discharge; not necessarily a recurring condition
5. Convulsion—a broad range of behavioral manifestations, including seizure activity
6. Aura—a specific sensation preceding a seizure, lasting from one to several seconds and manifested as:
7. Status epilepticus
a. Numbness, tingling
b. Unusual smell perception
c. Peculiar sound perception
d. Feeling of nausea or fear
e. Continuous convulsion lasting longer than 5 minutes
f. May lead to death from heart failure, kidney failure, or both
g. Constitutes a medical emergency

B. Incidence and prevalence
1. Affect almost 3.4 million people in the United States
2. About 200,000 new cases of seizure and epilepsy are diagnosed in the United States each year
3. Prevalence is highest among children, with occurrence of 5.2 to 7.3 per 1000 school-age children
4. About 10% of Americans will have at least one seizure in their lifetime

C. Types—can be classified by the origin of the seizure, the cause, or the type of seizure activity

D. Signs, symptoms, and clinical manifestations
1. Generalized tonic-clonic (grand mal)
a. May experience an aura
b. Loss of consciousness
c. Tonic movements (voluntary muscles experience continuous contractions)
d. Clonic movements (intermittent muscular contraction and relaxation)
e. Interruption of respiration and dilation of pupils
f. Loss of bladder or bowel control
g. Seizure activity usually lasts 1 to 3 minutes
h. Lethargy and disorientation follow the return of consciousness
i. May occur any time during the day or only during sleep
2. Generalized absence (petit mal)
a. Transient loss of consciousness
b. May have minor motor movements of the eyes, head, or extremities

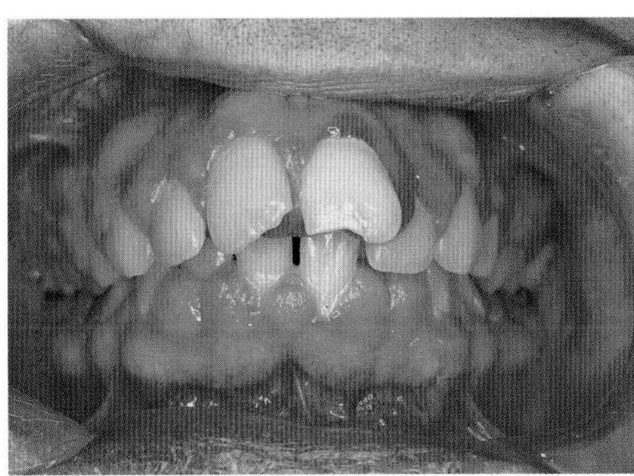

Fig. 19.8 Drug-induced gingival enlargement associated with medication taken to control seizures. (From Regezi JA, Sciubba JA, Jordan CK. *Oral Pathology: Clinical Pathologic Correlations*. 7th ed. St. Louis: Elsevier; 2017.)

c. Lasts 5 to 30 seconds
d. Person may not be aware of having had a seizure

3. Complex partial (psychomotor)
   a. May be preceded by an aura
   b. Transient clouding of the consciousness
   c. Behavioral alterations
   d. Purposeless, repetitive, and stereotypical movements or actions
   e. Changes in affect or perception
   f. May become antisocial
   g. Person usually does not remember the incident
4. Atonic
   a. Type of seizure that consists of a brief lapse in muscle tone
   b. Caused by temporary alterations in brain function
   c. Seizures are brief, usually less than 15 seconds
   d. Originate in childhood and may persist into adulthood

E. Oral manifestations
1. Orofacial trauma—lips, tongue, buccal mucosa, teeth, facial bones, or jawbone
2. Drug-induced gingival enlargement from phenytoin (Fig. 19.8)
   a. More marked in anterior regions and facial surfaces
   b. Does not occur in edentulous areas
   c. Correlated with poor oral hygiene
   d. Characteristically pale, pink, and fibrous
   e. Aesthetic concerns caused by gingival enlargement
   f. Severe gingival enlargement may displace teeth, create malocclusion, and compromise esthetics
   g. Superimposed inflammation occurs from food retention or mouth breathing
   h. Can sometimes be alleviated through meticulous oral hygiene, surgery, or pressure appliances

## Visual Impairment

A. Definitions
1. Visual impairment—when visual acuity in the best eye is no better than 20/200 after correction, or if central or peripheral vision impairment is present
2. Legally blind—visual acuity of less than 20/200 with correction

B. Incidence and prevalence
1. Approximately 0.6 in 1000 persons in the United States is legally or totally blind
2. Visual impairments occur in 12.2 in 1000 persons under age 18
3. About 5 million persons in the United States over age 65 have severe visual impairment
4. Leading cause of vision loss in those 25 to 74 years old is diabetic retinopathy

C. Etiology—congenital, perinatal, postnatal, aging
1. Trauma
2. Disease (infections, inflammation, toxicity)
3. Structural or developmental defects
4. Retrolental fibroplasia—high concentration of oxygen in the incubators of premature infants causes hemorrhage of retinal blood vessels, scarring, and retinal detachment
5. Macular degeneration (loss of central vision)
6. Retinitis pigmentosa—night blindness and loss of peripheral vision
7. Diabetic retinopathy—retinal hemorrhages
8. Glaucoma—failure of liquid in the eye to drain, resulting in increased pressure, pain, and destruction of the optic nerve
9. Cataracts—clouding and opacity of the lens blocking light perception (mainly associated with aging or congenital problems)
   a. Nearsighted
   b. Farsighted
   c. Astigmatism

D. Signs, symptoms, and clinical manifestations
1. Wears glasses or contact lenses
2. Awkward ambulation or bumping into objects
3. Eye pain
4. Constant tearing
5. Unusual squinting or blinking
6. Use of a guide dog or cane
7. Deliberate, slow actions
8. Attention to details and orderliness
9. Cloudy or fuzzy vision
10. Problems with glare
11. Double vision (diplopia)

E. Oral manifestations
1. No particular dental problems; oral hygiene tends to be poor
2. Gingivitis, if the person cannot see the gingiva to monitor gingival health
3. Trauma to the orofacial area if the person experiences frequent accidents or falls

## Hearing Impairment

A. Definitions
1. Hearing impairment—defective but functional hearing
2. Deaf—unable to understand speech, even with the use of an aid
3. Frequency—length of the sound wave (vibrations per second, or cycles per second [cps, hertz]; human range is 16,000 to 30,000 cps/Hz)

**TABLE 19.3 Hearing Loss and Probable Outcomes**

| Classification | Loss (dB) | Hearing Status without Amplification (Hearing Aid) |
|---|---|---|
| Normal range | 0–15 | All speech sounds |
| Slight loss | 15–25 | Hears vowel sounds clearly; may miss unvoiced consonant sounds |
| Mild loss | 25–40 | Hears only louder-voiced speech sounds |
| Moderate loss | 40–65 | Misses most speech at normal conversational level |
| Severe loss | 65–95 | Misses all speech at normal conversational level |
| Profound loss | >95+ | Hears no speech or sounds |

4. Intensity—measured in decibels (dB); human range is 1 to 100 dB

B. Incidence and prevalence
1. 15% of American adults report some hearing issues
2. 66% of those affected are age 65 or older; 1 in 6 persons age 41 to 59 have a hearing impairment
3. Two to three cases of congenital hearing loss in 1000 live births
4. Hearing loss is associated with a number of other disabling conditions
5. Environmental causes are increasing
   a. Cleft palate (90%)
   b. Cerebral palsy (20%)
   c. Down syndrome (70%)

C. Classifications—usually by severity of loss, as measured in decibel loss (Table 19.3)

D. Types of hearing loss (Table 19.4)
1. Conductive hearing loss
2. Sensorineural hearing loss
   a. Injury or disease interferes with organs that conduct sound waves through the outer or middle ear
   b. Usually consistent over the entire range of sound
   c. The person benefits most from the use of a hearing aid (sound conducted by bone)
   d. Speech is soft and low; the person hears own voice louder than that of others
   e. Usually caused by obstruction of the ear canal by cerumen or a foreign object, perforated eardrum, otitis media, otosclerosis, or congenital malformations of the ear
   f. Malfunction of organs that perceive sound (sensory hair cells of inner ear, auditory nerve, auditory center in brain)
   g. Most common causes—aging process (presbycusis), hereditary disease, noise damage, childhood viral infections, skull fractures, intracranial tumors, oxytoxic drugs, and Rh incompatibility
   h. Involves loss of sensitivity and acuity in one or more frequencies (usually higher frequencies and consonants)
   i. If the individual wears a hearing aid, sound is conducted by air
   j. Speech is loud; the person cannot hear own voice

**TABLE 19.4 Description of Hearing Problems**

| Condition | Characteristics |
|---|---|
| Acoustic neurinoma | Benign tumor of the auditory nerve; causes gradual hearing loss, tinnitus, and dizziness |
| Mastoiditis | Inflammation of the air cells of the mastoid |
| Ménière's disease | Condition of the inner ear characterized by hearing loss, tinnitus, and vertigo |
| Otitis media | Inflammation of the middle ear caused by infection |
| Otosclerosis | Disease characterized by formation of spongy bone in bone surrounding the inner ear; results in gradual loss of hearing |
| Presbycusis | Progressive hearing loss that occurs with age |
| Tinnitus | Sensation of sound in the head (e.g., roaring, hissing, buzzing) |
| Transient | Temporary hearing shifts associated with noise exposure |

E. Signs, symptoms, and clinical manifestations
1. May lip-read or focus attention on other facial or nonverbal expressions (speech reading); but can generally only understand 26% to 40% of what is said
2. Speech may be characterized by aberrant modulations, pronunciations, or grammatical structures
3. May use sign language—American Sign Language (ASL) or finger spelling (American or manual alphabet)
4. May turn the head to one side if the loss is unilateral
5. May frequently ask others to repeat phrases, or may provide an unrelated response to a question or comment
6. May not acknowledge having hearing loss

F. Oral manifestations
1. Not generally seen with hearing impairments unless associated with a syndrome (e.g., rubella syndrome)
2. Prematurity or rubella may result in enamel dysplasia
3. Bruxism may be evident

## Cleft Lip or Palate

A. Definition—disturbances in embryologic formation resulting in incomplete closure of the lip, the palatal area, or both

B. Incidence and prevalence
1. About 2650 babies are born with a cleft palate and 4440 with a cleft lip with or without a cleft palate
2. Occurs in 1 in 1000 Caucasian live births in the United States; twice as common in Asian Americans; half as common in African Americans
3. One of the most common congenital malformations of the face and mouth
4. Cleft lip more common in males; cleft palate more common in females
5. One in 2000 babies born with cleft palate, but without cleft lip

C. Classifications of cleft involvement
1. Tip of the uvula
2. Bifid uvula
3. Soft palate
4. Soft and hard palates
5. Unilateral lip and palate (Fig. 19.9)
6. Bilateral lip and palate

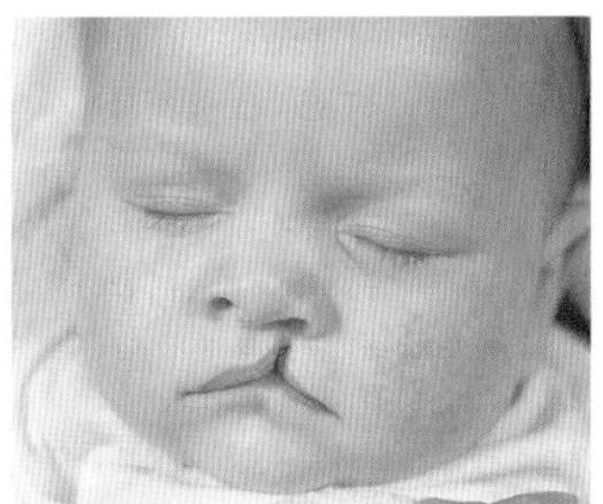

**Fig. 19.9** Cleft lip. (From Regezi JA, Sciubba JA, Jordan CK. *Oral Pathology: Clinical Pathologic Correlations.* 7th ed. St. Louis: Elsevier; 2017.)

D. Signs, symptoms, and associated problems
   1. Orofacial deformities
   2. Ear disease with resultant hearing loss
   3. Speech difficulties are a major disability caused by:
   4. Feeding problems
   5. Predisposition to upper respiratory tract infections
      a. Palatal insufficiency
      b. Missing or malpositioned teeth
      c. Hearing loss
E. Oral manifestations
   1. High incidence of missing or maldeveloped teeth in the line of the cleft, usually affects lateral incisors
   2. Delayed eruption and abnormal tooth development
   3. High incidence of malocclusion resulting from structural defects
   4. Oral-motor dysfunction
   5. Scar tissue from surgery

## Cerebral Palsy

A. Definition—static, nonprogressive neuromuscular condition comprising a series of syndromes that result from damage to the brain
B. Incidence
   1. Approximately 784,000 persons in the United States have some degree of cerebral palsy
   2. About 10,000 babies born each year will develop cerebral palsy; 40% to 50% of children born with cerebral palsy are premature, low birth weight, or both
C. Classification
   1. Motor disorders
   2. Limbs involved
      a. Spasticity (50% to 75%)—slight stimulus causes exaggerated muscle contraction; stiff and jerky movements
      b. Athetosis (15% to 25%)—muscles contract involuntarily; difficulty bringing the body to the upright position
      c. Ataxia (10%)—muscles respond to a stimulus but cannot complete a contraction; low muscle tone and poor coordination
      d. Hypotonia (less than 10%)—unable to respond to a volitional stimulus
      e. Rigidity (less than 10%)—increased initial muscle resistance; gives way with minimal force
      f. Mixed (5% to 20%)—two or more types appearing in the same person

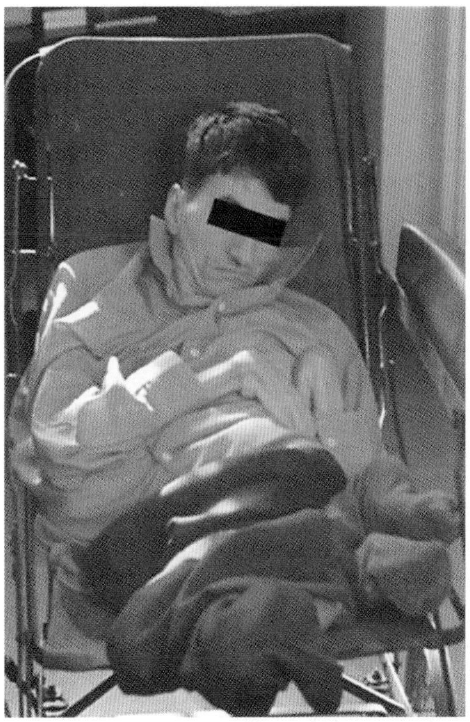

**Fig. 19.10** Person with spastic-type cerebral palsy, in which limbs are in a severely flexed posture. (From Porter SR, et al. *Medicine and Surgery for Dentistry.* Philadelphia: Churchill Livingstone; 1999.)

      g. Monoplegic—one limb
      h. Hemiplegic—both limbs on the same side of the body
      i. Paraplegic—lower limbs
      j. Diplegic—like parts on either side of the body (e.g., both lower limbs, both upper limbs)
      k. Quadriplegic—all four limbs
      l. Triplegic—three limbs
D. Signs, symptoms, and clinical manifestations (Fig. 19.10)
   1. Characterized by paralysis, weakness, muscle spasms, incoordination, or other aberrations of motor function, especially involving voluntary muscles
   2. Joint immobility and contractures increase with age
   3. Retained primitive reflexes (e.g., asymmetrical or symmetrical tonic neck reflex)
   4. Other associated conditions
   5. Wide range of limitations, from mild to totally dependent
      a. Speech and language disorders (60%)
      b. Hearing disorders (20%)
      c. Visual defects (40%)
      d. Developmental and cognitive challenges (40%)
E. Seizures (40%). Oral manifestations—marked variation among individuals
   1. Higher incidence of bruxism (Fig. 19.11), dental caries, enamel dysplasia, malocclusion, and periodontal diseases
   2. Drug-induced gingival enlargement if phenytoin is used
   3. Oral-motor dysfunction (e.g., impaired swallowing), mouth breathing
   4. Temporomandibular joint (TMJ) disorders
   5. Increased gag reflex

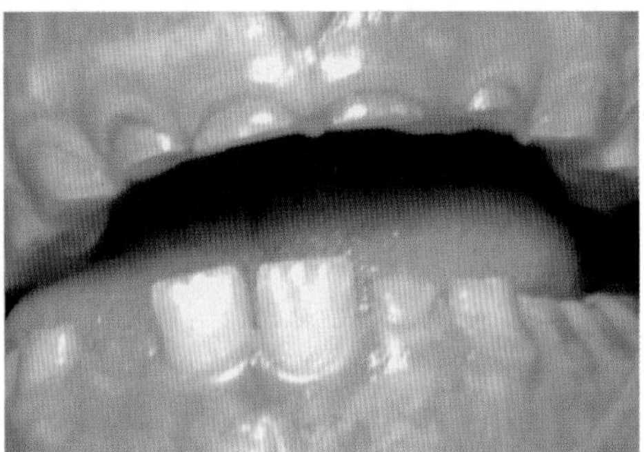

Fig. 19.11 Example of extreme bruxism in a child with a developmental disability. (From National Oral Health Information Clearinghouse. *Oral Conditions in Children with Special Needs: A Guide for Health Care Providers*. Bethesda, MD: National Institute of Dental and Craniofacial Research; 2011.)

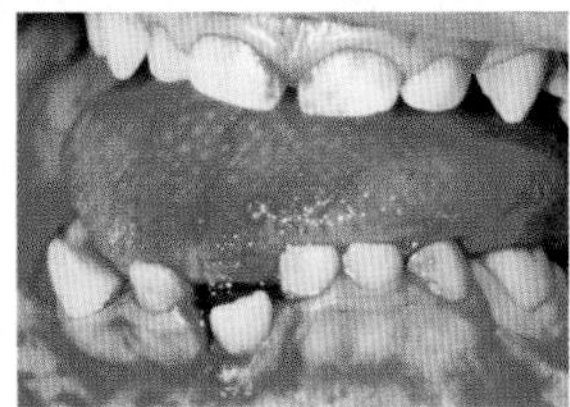

Fig. 19.12 Example of oral trauma. (From National Oral Health Information Clearinghouse. *Oral Conditions in Children with Special Needs: A Guide for Health Care Providers*. Bethesda, MD: National Institute of Dental and Craniofacial Research; 2011.)

6. Drooling
7. Trauma resulting from incoordination and frequent falls (Fig. 19.12)
8. Attrition and possible TMJ disturbances from mouth sticks
9. Increased dental caries as a result of surgery to control saliva and drooling

## Bell's Palsy

A. Definition—paralysis of facial muscles that are innervated by cranial nerve VII (facial nerve)
B. Incidence and prevalence
   1. About 40,000 persons in the United States are affected annually
   2. After age 50; more common in males
C. Signs, symptoms, and clinical manifestations (Fig. 19.13)
   1. Abrupt paralysis without preceding pain
   2. Occurs unilaterally
   3. Corner of the mouth droops, causing drooling
   4. Eyelids will not close; lower eyelid droops; predisposes the eyes to infections
   5. Speech and chewing are difficult
   6. Spontaneous remission may occur in 2 to 8 weeks, or permanent paralysis
E. Oral manifestations—oral-motor difficulties can cause food retention and the potential for increased caries or gingivitis

## Myasthenia Gravis

A. Definition—autoimmune neuromuscular disease characterized by variable weakness or fatigue of striated, voluntary muscles
B. Incidence and prevalence

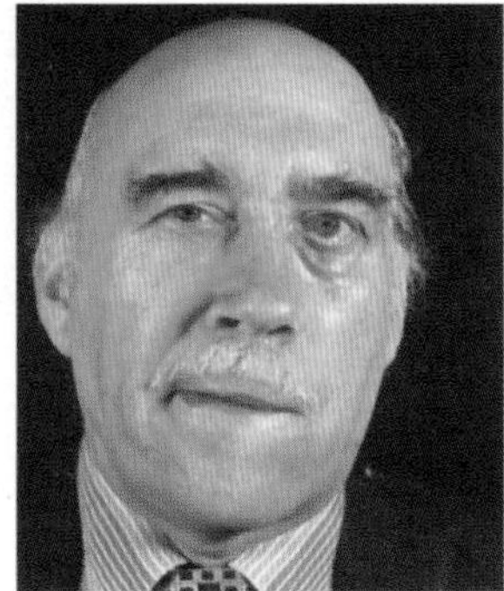

Fig. 19.13 Person with Bell's palsy, in whom the left side of the face is paralyzed. (From Trend P, Swash M, Kennard C. *Neurology: Color Guide*. Edinburgh: Churchill Livingstone; 1998.)

   1. Most often affects women younger than 40
   2. If late onset after 60, men affected more often
   3. Affects approximately 2 in 100,000 persons
C. Signs, symptoms, and clinical manifestations
   1. First symptoms usually affect muscles of the eyes (blurred or double vision, drooping of one or both eyelids, weakness of muscles affecting the eyeball, facial expression, mastication, and swallowing)
   2. Breathing and speech are disturbed (weak, muffled voice)
   3. Fatigue and weakness of muscles vary widely but tend to be worse at the end of the day
   4. Myasthenic crisis—weakness affects muscles that control breathing; usually transient but life threatening
      a. Precipitated by:
      b. Symptoms
         (1) Emotional excitement, stress
         (2) Surgical procedures
         (3) Fatigue or loss of sleep
         (4) Infections
         (5) Unable to clear secretions from the throat
         (6) Impaired breathing; assisted ventilation may be needed
         (7) Double vision
E. Medications that may cause muscle weakness and must therefore be avoided:
   1. β-Adrenergic blockers
   2. D-Penicillamine
   3. Interferon-α
   4. Calcium channel blockers
F. Oral manifestations
   1. Oral-motor dysfunction
   2. Retention of food increases susceptibility to dental caries and periodontal problems
   3. Weakness of masticatory muscles causes the mouth to continuously hang open
   4. Chewing and swallowing difficulties
   5. Furrowed and flaccid appearance of the tongue

## Parkinson's Disease

A. Definition—progressive disorder of the CNS causing loss of postural reflexes, slowness of spontaneous movement, tremors, and muscle rigidity

**TABLE 19.5 Characteristics of Arthritis**

| | Osteoarthritis | Rheumatoid (Adult Type) | Rheumatoid (Juvenile Type) |
|---|---|---|---|
| Etiology | Unknown or from trauma, infection, or joint abnormality | Cause unknown; theories include autoimmunity, hereditary or psychosomatic factors, and infection | Same as adult type |
| Sites affected | Weight-bearing joints (hands, hips, knees, vertebrae) | First affects fingers, hands, and knees; TMJ later | Involves many joints, especially fingers, knees, wrists, vertebrae, and TMJ |
| Signs and symptoms | Pain, aggravated by temperature changes; joint stiffness after inactivity; develops gradually; swelling rare; does not usually limit range of motion | Fatigue, loss of appetite, low-grade fever, migratory joint pain and swelling, stiffness after periods of inactivity, paresthesias, subcutaneous nodules, joint deformities, TMJ involvement, muscle atrophy near joints | Joint enlargement, stiffness, and pain; onset is acute with fever, rash, spleen and lymph node enlargement, tachycardia, and limited oral opening |

*TMJ*, Temporomandibular joint.

B. Incidence and prevalence
   1. Develops between ages 40 and 60
   2. At age 60 or older, 1 in 100 persons affected
   3. Higher incidence in men than in women (2:1)
   4. Approximately 1.5 million persons in the United States affected; 7 to 10 million worldwide
C. Signs, symptoms, and clinical manifestations
   1. Mild, diffuse muscular pain
   2. Tremors of the extremities, occurring mainly at rest
   3. Shuffling, slow gait, with arms held to the side
   4. Slurred, indistinct speech
   5. Staring, mask-like facial expression
   6. Excessive salivation or dryness of mouth (side effects of medications)
   7. Intellect not usually affected
   8. Tremors in the lips, tongue, or neck; difficulty swallowing; can lead to aspiration
   9. Feelings of stiffness and rigidity (particularly of the large joints)
   10. Sensitivity to heat
E. Oral manifestations
   1. Impaired oral-motor functions and home care skills may increase the incidence of dental caries, periodontal disease, and perioral skin irritation
   2. Side effects of medications (e.g., xerostomia) may increase the incidence of dental caries and periodontal disease and negatively affect dental prosthesis retention
   3. Rigidity and tremors can induce orofacial pain, TMJ discomfort, and trauma to soft and hard tissues
   4. Erosion
   5. Oral ulcers
   6. Sialorrhea

## Arthritis

A. Definition
   1. Term used to describe more than 100 disorders that cause pain in the joints and connective tissue
   2. Joint inflammation
   3. The term *polyarthritis* refers to the involvement of many joints
B. Major types (Table 19.5)
   1. Osteoarthritis (affects 22 million US adults)
   2. Rheumatoid (adult type) (affects three million adults)
   3. Rheumatoid (juvenile type)
   4. Others include gout, fibromyalgia, ankylosing spondylitis, lupus
C. Incidence and prevalence: common in all age groups
   1. More than one in five US adults is affected
   2. Affects more than 22% of the US population
   3. Affects 55% of the population age 65 or older
   4. More common in women than men
D. Signs, symptoms, and clinical manifestations—these affect various sites in different ways; most are chronic (see Table 19.5)
E. Oral manifestations
   1. Bruxism and occlusal imbalances
   2. TMJ pain and limited ability to open the mouth
   3. Masking of inflammation by prolonged steroid therapy
   4. Delayed healing and excess bleeding with long-term aspirin therapy
   5. Mucosal ulcerations or secondary oral infections (especially of the gingiva) if gold salts are administered
   6. Monitor need for antibiotic premedication

## Fibromyalgia Syndrome (FMS)

A. Definition—neurosensory disorder characterized by widespread musculoskeletal pain
   1. Pain accompanied by persistent fatigue, sleep disturbances, and memory and mood issues
   2. Most common cause of chronic pain in the United States
B. Incidence and prevalence
   1. FMS can affect any person regardless of age, gender, or ethnicity; however 75% to 90% of those diagnosed are women
   2. Prevalence of fibromyalgia is higher at middle age (30 to 50 years) or over age 50
   3. Worldwide incidence of FMS is 6.88 per 1000 males and 11.28 per 1000 females
C. Signs, symptoms, and clinical manifestations
   1. Widespread pain—exacerbated by physical or emotional stress, nonrestorative sleep, strenuous activity, and changes in weather
   2. Sleep disturbances, including nonrestorative sleep, insomnia, and poor-quality sleep
   3. Fatigue, cognitive deficiency, tenderness on mild palpation
   4. Can result in severe disability and loss of function, making daily tasks, including oral self-care, difficult or unmanageable

D. Oral manifestations
   1. Severe pain when opening; limited opening
   2. TMJ disorder
   3. Burning tongue
   4. Difficulty discerning pain from oral disease from FMS pain
   5. Taste distortion
   6. Xerostomia

## Scleroderma

A. Definition
   1. Group of chronic connective tissue disorders
   2. Autoimmune rheumatic condition with excessive collagen deposition and vascular hyperreactivity and dysfunction
B. Incidence and prevalence
   1. 300,00 cases in United States
   2. Mainly affects women, 4:1 over men, with onset between ages 30 and 50
   3. Approximately 20 per 1 million individuals affected
C. Signs and symptoms
   1. Localized scleroderma affects only the skin—areas of the skin become thickened, hard, and discolored, with hair loss over affected areas
   2. Diffuse scleroderma also harms structures beyond the skin, such as blood vessels, internal organs, and digestive tract
      a. Skin eventually binds with underlying structures, and painful ulcerations occur at the joints
      b. Esophageal dysmotility, renal disease, cardiac dysfunction, and pulmonary disease manifest
      c. Caused from chronic hardening and sclerosis of the connective tissue within these organ systems, with life-threatening consequences
D. Oral manifestations
   1. Limited mouth opening
   2. Fibrosis at the hard and soft palate
   3. Widening of the periodontal ligament space
   4. Mandibular resorption
   5. Trigeminal neuropathy
   6. Increased risk for periodontal disease and caries disease
   7. Xerostomia

## Multiple Sclerosis

A. Definition—chronic degenerative disease of the CNS
   1. Myelin is destroyed through the formation of sclerotic tissue called *plaque*
   2. Nerve impulses to the brain are disrupted or not transmitted
   3. Scattered plaque accumulation causes inflammation and widespread and varied symptoms with periods of exacerbation and remission
B. Incidence and prevalence
   1. Approximately 500,000 persons affected in the United States; more than 2.5 million worldwide
   2. Varies geographically; more common in northern regions

**TABLE 19.6 Symptoms Associated With Lesions in the Central Nervous System**

| Location of Lesions | Possible Symptoms |
|---|---|
| Spinal cord | Numbness |
| | Loss of sensitivity in appendages |
| | Sensitivity to heat |
| | Unsteady gait; muscle stiffness |
| | Loss of strength in the legs |
| | Impaired eye-hand coordination resulting in difficulty in fine motor movements |
| Brainstem | Blurred vision, double vision, or both |
| | Difficulty in swallowing or chewing |
| | Diminished gag reflex |
| | Slurred speech |
| Cerebrum (lesions in the cerebrum usually occur in the later stages of the disease process) | Disruptions in thinking |
| | Euphoria |
| | Depression |
| | Disruptions in behavior |

From Lange BM, Enwistle BM, Lipson LF. *Dental Management of the Handicapped: Approaches for Dental Auxiliaries*. Philadelphia: Lea & Febiger; 1983.

   3. Two to three times more common in women than men
   4. Onset occurs at any age, but usually between 20 and 50
C. Signs and symptoms
   1. Result from the location of lesions (Table 19.6)
   2. Precipitating factors
   3. Periods of remission in some; chronic progression in others
   4. Death is usually the result of an infection
      a. Infections
      b. Stress and emotional trauma
      c. Injury
      d. Heavy exercise and fatigue
      e. Pregnancy
      f. Heat
D. Oral manifestations
   1. Most are the result of poor oral hygiene or the side effects of drugs
   2. Facial pain and TMJ dysfunction and pain
      a. Ulcerations
      b. Xerostomia
      c. Drug-induced gingival enlargement (phenytoin administered for pain)
      d. Trigeminal neuropathy
      e. Facial palsy

## Muscular Dystrophies

A. Definition—group of progressive chronic diseases of the skeletal (striated) muscles characterized by the degeneration of muscle cells with replacement by fat or fibrous tissue
B. Incidence and prevalence
   1. Affects approximately 220,000 persons in the United States
   2. Two-thirds of cases are children; 400 to 600 males are born with this disease each year in the United States
C. Types (Table 19.7)
D. Signs, symptoms, and clinical manifestations—vary by site and type (see Table 19.7)

2. Hypertensive heart disease—sustained elevation of the blood pressure, creating an increased workload for the heart, resulting in left ventricular hypertrophy and in late-stage kidney disease
3. Four hypertension categories (see Table 15.4 in Chapter 15; see the section on "Cardiac Emergencies" in Chapter 21)
   a. Normal—less than 120/80 mm Hg
   b. Elevated —120 to 129 and less than 80 mm Hg
   c. Stage 1—130 to 139 or 80 to 89 mm Hg
   d. Stage 2—140 or higher or 90 or higher mm Hg
   e. Hypertensive crisis—higher than 180 and or /higher than 120 mm Hg

B. Incidence and prevalence
   1. Incidence is increasing, with hypertension affecting approximately one in three (or 74.5 million) persons in the United States; more remain undiagnosed
   2. Prevalence increases with age and is greater in men before age 55 and in women after age 55

C. Signs, symptoms, and clinical manifestations
   1. Early—occipital headache, dizziness, tingling of the extremities, vision changes, tinnitus, dyspnea
   2. Advanced—cardiac enlargement, ischemic heart disease, CHF, renal failure, stroke

D. Oral manifestations
   1. Generally no direct oral manifestations
   2. Facial palsy from some drugs
   3. Oral lesions, taste changes, or xerostomia from drugs
   4. Many side effects and precautions associated with drugs; some calcium channel blockers cause drug-induced gingival enlargement

## Coronary Heart Disease

A. Definition—coronary atherosclerotic heart disease, plaque build-up in coronary arteries causing narrowing of arteries that is symptomatic

B. Incidence and prevalence
   1. Affects 17.6 million persons in the United States; 1 out of 13 Americans over age 18 affected
   2. Leading cause of death after age 40 in men and women
   3. Incidence and severity increase with age; more than 50% who die suddenly have no previous evidence of disease

C. Signs, symptoms, and clinical manifestations
   1. Angina pectoris—transient and reversible oxygen deficiency; classified as stable or unstable
   2. Myocardial infarction (MI)—an infarct or ischemic necrosis caused by a sudden reduction or arrest of blood flow
      a. Pain—crushing or paroxysmal, usually less than 10 minutes; often mistaken for indigestion
      b. Sweating, anxiety, pallor, difficulty breathing
      c. Relieved by administration of nitroglycerin or rest
      d. Pain in the sternum, radiating to the left arm; lasts longer than angina
      e. Not relieved by nitroglycerin
      f. Same symptoms as angina, with nausea and vomiting, palpitations, and lowered blood pressure
      g. Often leads to sudden death from ventricular fibrillation
      h. Symptoms vary between males and females
      i. Women often no chest pain
      j. Women are more likely to have symptoms like nausea, shortness of breath, or pain in their neck, back, or jaw.

D. Oral manifestations
   1. None directly associated
   2. Oral lesions, burning mouth syndrome, lichenoid reactions, or xerostomia may result as a drug side effect
   3. Pain may be radiated to the mandible, palate, or tongue
   4. Drug-induced gingival enlargement may result as a side effect of some calcium channel blockers

## Congestive Heart Failure (CHF)

A. Definition
   1. Represents a symptom complex that involves the failure of one or both ventricles (usually the left ventricle)
   2. Imbalance between the demand placed on the heart and its ability to respond
   3. Results in an inadequate supply of blood and oxygen throughout the body and in congestion of blood within the vascular system

B. Incidence and prevalence
   1. Prevalence is 5.1 million persons; incidence is 550,000 cases each year; incidence 10 per 1000 population after age 65

C. Signs, symptoms, and clinical manifestations
   1. Dyspnea, irregular breathing pattern, coughing, weakness; the person cannot breathe unless sitting up
   2. Swollen ankles late in the day, pitting edema, ascites
   3. Cyanosis, anxiety, fear
   4. Paleness, sweating, cold skin
   5. Decreased urine output
   6. Frothy pink or white sputum
   7. Weak pulse
   8. Confusion from decreased cardiac output, thus decreased oxygen to the brain

D. Oral manifestations
   1. Xerostomia
   2. Gingival bleeding, and petechiae if displaying polycythemia

## CVA, Stroke

A. Definition—sudden loss of brain function resulting from interference with the blood supply to a portion of the brain

B. Incidence and prevalence
   1. Affects 4.6 million persons in the United States, 75% in persons age 66 or older
   2. Third leading cause of death in the United States; leading cause of serious disability
   3. African Americans are at greater risk than Caucasians
   4. Men are at greater risk than women
   5. Likelihood of having a stroke increases with age

C. Signs, symptoms, and clinical manifestations—depend on the area of the brain involved and the extent of damage (Table 19.10)

**TABLE 19.10 Functional Limitations in Stroke (CVA) Victims**

| Right Hemiplegia (L-CVA*) | Left Hemiplegia (R-CVA) |
|---|---|
| Language problems<br>Decreased auditory memory (cannot remember a long series of instructions)<br>Vocabulary problems<br>Slow, cautious, disorganized<br>Anxious | Spatial-perceptual task difficulties—inability to judge distance, size, position, rate of movement, form, and relation of parts to a whole<br>Often thought to be unimpaired because able to speak and understand<br>Visual field cuts; angles, etc. cannot be perceived<br>Cannot use mirrors<br>Cannot sequence tasks, such as toothbrushing<br>Decreased visual memory (loses place when reading)<br>Cannot monitor self (keeps talking even though answered questions already)<br>May neglect left side<br>Tendency to be impulsive and unaware of deficits; spatial-perceptual difficulties are easy to miss |

*CVA,* Cerebrovascular accident.
From Schubert MM, Snow M, Stiefel DJ, *Dental Management of Patients with CNS and Neurologic Impairment: Spinal Cord Injury. DECOD series.* Seattle: University of Washington; 1989.

1. Immediate
2. Residual or chronic
   a. Syncope, headache, chills, convulsions, nausea, and vomiting
   b. Changes in level of consciousness
   c. Transient paresthesias
   d. Mood swing
   e. Paralysis—hemiparesis or localized paralysis
   f. Speech problems and aphasia (reduced capacity for interpretation and formulation of language)
   g. Alterations in reflexes, especially the oral-motor reflexes
   h. Functional disorders of the bladder or bowel
   i. Visual impairments
   j. Seizures

E. D. Oral manifestations
   1. Oral-motor dysfunction
   2. Increased incidence of dental caries or periodontal disease caused by oral-motor problems and poor oral hygiene
   3. Anticoagulant therapy to prevent clot formation creates bleeding issues and physician consults required

## Sickle Cell Disease

A. Definitions
   1. A genetic disease causing a defect of hemoglobin that causes red blood cells to become sickle shaped
   2. Sickle cell trait—individual shows no symptoms unless experiencing abnormally low concentration of oxygen
   3. Sickle cell disease—progressively deteriorating and complex disease with multiple symptoms

B. Incidence and prevalence
   1. Found in African Americans and other nonwhite persons; occurs in both genders
   2. Two million persons in the United States are carriers of the sickle cell trait
   3. Approximately 100,000 persons in the United States have sickle cell disease
   4. About 1 in 1400 Hispanic American children and 1 in 365 African American children are born with sickle cell anemia
   5. Babies do not show symptoms until age 6 months
   6. Hemoglobin gene from both parents; sickle cell anemia is autosomal recessive

C. Signs, symptoms, and clinical manifestations
   1. Adulthood
      a. Can develop enlarged spleen, septicemia, and meningitis
      b. Swelling of the feet and hands, anemia, pallor, tiredness, fever, pneumonia
      c. Severe pain crises affecting the extremities
      d. Stroke occurs in 10% of those affected
      e. Can develop gallstones, enlarged hearts, and lung infarctions
      f. Bones degenerate as a result of repeated sickling
      g. Delayed growth and late puberty
      h. Increased chance for stroke, impaired kidney and liver function with jaundice, and arthritis
      i. Continued pain crises
      j. Hemorrhage in the eye, detached retina
      k. Pain crises—variable in each person
      l. Lung and kidney damage, gallstones
      m. Leg ulcers and bone changes
      n. Infection is a major cause of death and also precipitates crises

E. Oral manifestations
   1. Sore, painful, red tongue
   2. Malocclusion
   3. Loss of taste sensation
   4. Osteoporosis
   5. Decreased radiodensity (ground-glass appearance) with coarse trabecular bone pattern and large marrow spaces
   6. Mucosal pallor; most common
   7. Delayed eruption of teeth
   8. Hypoplastic enamel—pain in the mandible
   9. Bone loss can be significant in children; high degree of periodontitis

## Cancer

A. Definition—abnormal cells that multiply at an abnormally rapid rate, invading and destroying healthy tissue
   1. Metastasis—spread of cancer to distant sites
   2. Invasion—spread of cancer to local sites

B. Incidence and prevalence
   1. Estimated 50,000 new cases of oral cancer per year; about 57% alive after 5 years
   2. About 201 in 100,000 persons will die of cancer each year in the United States
   3. Approximately 75% of all head and neck cancers begin in the oral cavity
   4. The tongue is the most common intraoral location (30%) (Fig. 19.16)

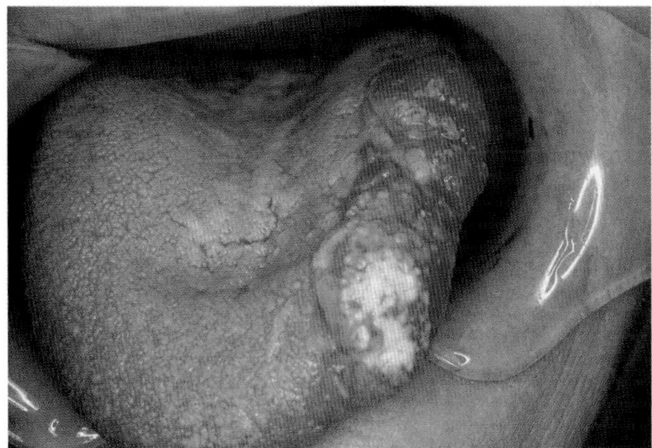

**Fig. 19.16** Squamous cell carcinoma on the lateral border of the tongue. (From Regezi JA, Sciubba JA, Jordan CK. *Oral Pathology: Clinical Pathologic Correlations*. 7th ed. St. Louis: Elsevier; 2017.)

5. Ongoing rise in cases of oropharyngeal cancer linked to human papillomavirus (HPV) infection in both men and women.
6. Cancers caused by HPV 16 respond relatively well to existing treatment modalities, significant survival advantage
7. Oral cancer occurs on the lips (usually the lower lip), inside the mouth, salivary glands, tonsils, on the back of the throat, esophagus, and the tongue and soft tissues of the mouth

C. Warning signs of oral cancer
1. Unexplained swelling, lump, or growth with or without pain
2. White scaly patches or red areas
3. Any sore that does not heal in 2 weeks
4. Unexplained numbness or tingling
5. Difficulty opening mouth or swallowing
6. Prolonged hoarseness

D. Oral manifestations—side effects of treatment and depend on type of cancer and treatment
1. Oral ulcerations and mucositis
2. Candidiasis
3. Anemia
4. Xerostomia/salivary gland problems
5. Radiation caries (Fig. 19.17)
6. Loss of taste
7. Osteoradionecrosis (Fig. 19.18)
8. Tooth sensitivity
9. Muscular dysfunction and trismus
10. Spontaneous gingival bleeding
11. Cosmetic disfigurement
12. Burning, peeling, swelling of tongue

## Leukemia

A. Definition
1. Progressive malignant neoplasms characterized by an overproduction of abnormal leukocytes
2. Abnormal leukocytes displace hematopoietic tissue in the bone marrow, leading to decreased production of platelets, erythrocytes, and normal leukocytes

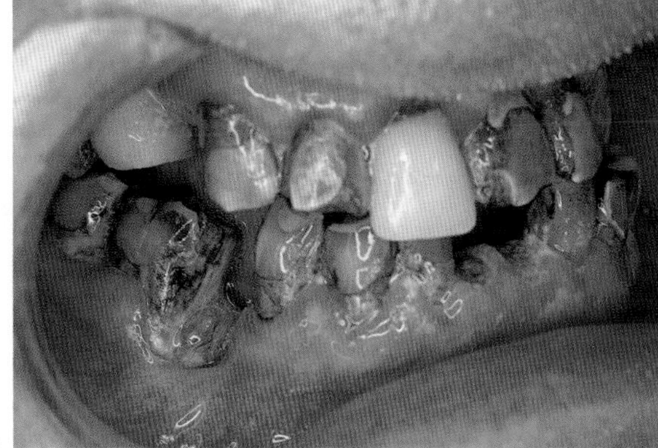


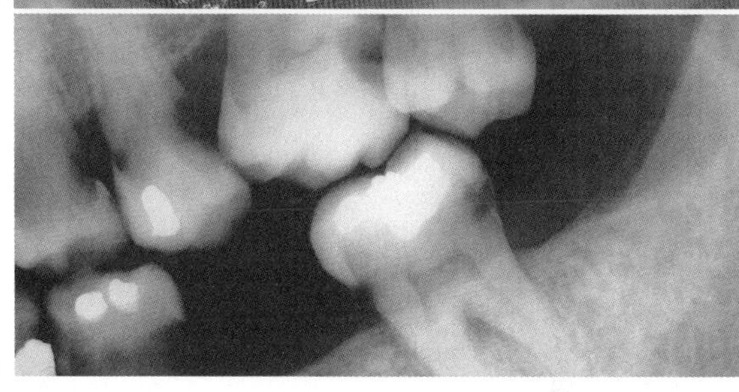


**Fig 19.17** (A) and (B) Radiation-associated cervical caries. (From Regezi JA, Sciubba JA, Jordan CK. *Oral Pathology: Clinical Pathologic Correlations*. 7th ed. St. Louis: Elsevier; 2017.)

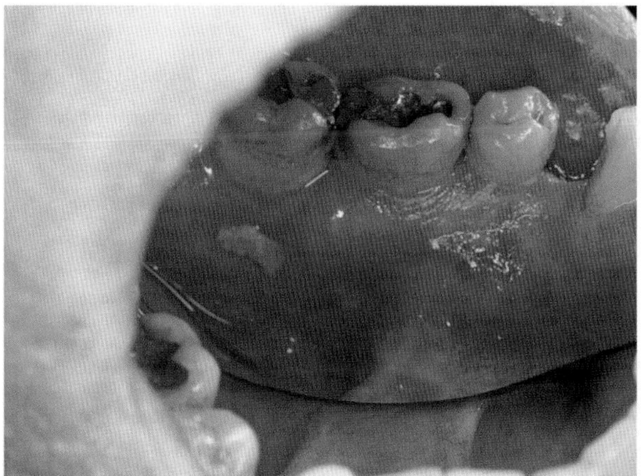

**Fig. 19.18** Osteoradionecrosis of the lingual mandible. (From Regezi JA, Sciubba JA, Jordan CK. *Oral Pathology: Clinical Pathologic Correlations*. 7th ed. St. Louis: Elsevier; 2017.)

B. Classification—chronicity
1. Acute form (A)—large numbers of immature nonspecific leukocytes are produced; accounts for 25% more cases than the chronic form
2. Chronic form (C)—leukocytes are well differentiated and able to mature; but immunologic capacity is decreased

C. Incidence and prevalence
1. Estimated 60,300 new cases each year in the United States
2. About 33% of cancers in children are leukemia
3. Seventh leading cause of cancer death in adults; leading cause of cancer death in children
4. Five-year survival rate is approximately 61%

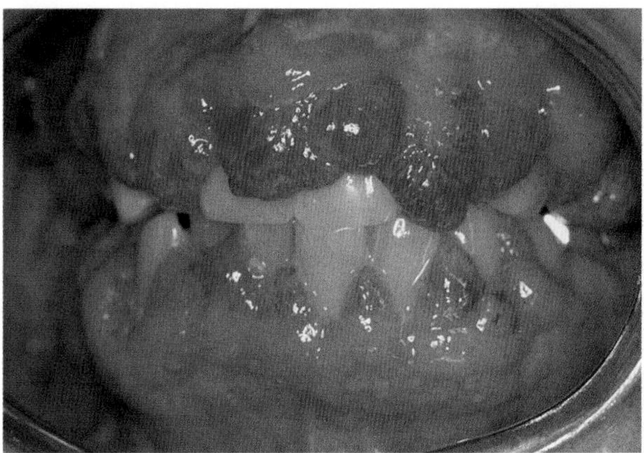

**Fig. 19.19** Gingival conditions associated with monocytic leukemia. (From Regezi JA, Sciubba JA, Jordan CK. *Oral Pathology: Clinical Pathologic Correlations*. 7th ed. St. Louis: Elsevier; 2017.)

D. Signs, symptoms, and clinical manifestations
   1. Acute form appears suddenly and severely; chronic form is insidious
   2. Fatigue, weakness, pallor, weight loss
   3. Ecchymosed skin and nosebleeds
   4. Fever
   5. Headache, nausea, and vomiting
F. Oral manifestations (Fig. 19.19)
   1. Initial
   2. Secondary
   3. Tertiary (treatment effects)
      a. Leukemic infiltrate of the pulp and gingiva
      b. Mucositis, mucosal atrophy, and mucosal pallor
      c. Areas of spontaneous hemorrhage (intermittent oozing) and petechiae
      d. Loss of lamina dura, resorption of alveolar bone, cancellous bone destruction
         (1) Causes pain in teeth
         (2) Enlarged, bluish red, spongy, blunted papilla
         (3) Ulceration and necrosis
      a. Mucosal infections (e.g., *Candida*, *Pseudomonas*) and periapical infections
      b. Necrotizing ulcerative gingivitis
      c. Viral infections
      d. Osteomyelitis
      e. Painful oral ulcerations
      f. Stomatitis
      g. Xerostomia and dental caries
      h. Jaw pain with Bell's palsy
      i. Secondary infections

## Congenital Disorders of Coagulation: Hemophilias

See the section on "Hemophilia" in Chapter 8.

A. Definition—genetic bleeding disorder affecting blood-clotting mechanism
B. Incidence and prevalence
   1. More than 20,000 persons in the United States have hemophilia; 400 births yearly
   2. Hemophilia A accounts for 80% to 85%; hemophilia B for 10% to 15%
   3. About 90% of patients are under age 25
   4. Vast majority of those affected are men
C. Classification
   1. Type
   2. Severity—level of clotting factor (normal level is 50% to 100%)
      a. Hemophilia A (factor VIII deficiency)—1.9 in 10 persons with hemophilia have type A
      b. Hemophilia B (factor IX deficiency)—Christmas disease
      c. Von Willebrand's disease (lack of plasma)—von Willebrand's factor is required for primary hemostasis
      d. Severe—have less than 1% of clotting factor; may bleed spontaneously or from minor trauma
      e. Moderate—have 5% to 25% of clotting factor; hemorrhage only with trauma
      f. Mild—have 25% to 50% of clotting factor; bleed only after severe injury or surgery
D. Clinical manifestations
   1. Bleeding and bruising from minor cuts or pressure
   2. Hemarthroses—bleeding into the soft tissues of joints, leading to pain, swelling, and permanent joint contractures
   3. Renal function is impaired; exposure to hepatitis during transfusions
   4. Intracranial hemorrhages can cause seizures or other neurologic disorders
      a. Ecchymoses and hematomas
      b. Oozing
      c. Intramuscular bleeding causes pain
E. Oral manifestations
   1. Ecchymoses, hematomas, and gingival oozing can be problems
   2. Oral trauma is more evident and can be serious

## Diabetes Mellitus

See the section on "Diabetes Mellitus" in Chapter 21.

A. Definition—hereditary or acquired deficiency of metabolism with:
   1. Inadequate production and action of insulin from the pancreas
   2. Disorders in carbohydrate, protein, and fat metabolism
   3. Body cells unable to use glucose, leading to hyperglycemia
   4. Alternating extremes of hypoglycemia and hyperglycemia found in the person with "brittle" (very poorly controlled) diabetes
B. Incidence and prevalence
   1. Diabetes mellitus affects 30.3 million persons in the United States, with approximately 8 million undiagnosed
   2. Seventh leading cause of death in the United States
   3. Much higher in Hispanic Americans and Native Americans
   4. Approximately 800,000 new cases diagnosed yearly
C. Major types (Table 19.11)
   1. Type 1—insulin dependent
   2. Type 2—noninsulin dependent (92% of cases)
   3. Prediabetes—impaired glucose tolerance; higher than normal levels but not yet diagnostic for diabetes; at risk for atherosclerotic disease (affects 84.1 million Americans)

**TABLE 19.11 Comparison of Type 1 and Type 2 Diabetes Mellitus**

| Characteristic | Type 1 | Type 2 |
|---|---|---|
| Age of onset | Young, usually before or during puberty, but may appear later | Adult, usually after 30 years, but may occur at younger age |
| Body weight | Normal or thin | Obesity is most important risk factor |
| Ethnicity | More common in Caucasians | More common in African Americans, Asian Americans, Hispanic Americans, and Native Americans |
| Hereditary | Yes, but less frequent occurrence in families than type 2 | Much more frequent occurrence in families |
| Lifestyle | Restrictions very difficult for young persons | More frequent in sedentary individuals with high-fat diets |
| Onset of symptoms | Rapid, abrupt symptoms of hyperglycemia | Slow, insidious progression over years |
| Symptoms | Weight loss; weakness; polyuria; polydipsia; polyphagia; blurred vision; mimic flu; frequent/recurrent infections; slow healing; tingling/numb extremities; fatigue; eye/kidney/cardiovascular problems | Any type 1 symptom; kidney/cardiovascular problems |
| Severity | Severe, life-threatening | Early mild but progressively serious |
| Complications | Acute hypoglycemic or hyperglycemic emergencies and chronic long-term complications common | Acute complications rare; chronic long-term complications common |
| Stability | Unstable, difficult and much effort to control | More stable, easier to manage |
| Exogenous insulin required | All | Some |
| Chronic manifestations | Uncommon before 20 years; prevalent and severe by 30 years | Develop slowly at later ages |
| Ketoacidosis | Common | Rare |
| Prevention | None (because of multiple factors) | Prevent or delay with lifestyle changes |

Modified from Wilkins EM. *Clinical Practice of the Dental Hygienist.* 10th ed. Philadelphia: Lippincott Williams & Wilkins; 2009.

**TABLE 19.12 Clinical Manifestations of Diabetes Mellitus**

| Hyperglycemia | Hypoglycemia |
|---|---|
| Polydipsia | Early stage |
| Polyphagia | —Diminished cerebral function |
| Polyuria | —Changes in mood |
| Loss of weight | —Decreased spontaneity |
| Fatigue | —Hunger |
| Headache | —Nausea More severe stage |
| Blurred vision | |
| Nausea and vomiting | —Sweating |
| Tachycardia | —Tachycardia |
| Florid appearance | —Piloerection |
| Hot and dry skin | —Increased anxiety |
| Kussmaul respiration | —Bizarre behavior patterns |
| Mental stupor | —Belligerence |
| Loss of consciousness | —Poor judgment |
| | —Uncooperativeness Later severe stage |
| | |
| | —Unconsciousness |
| | —Seizure activity |
| | —Hypotension |
| | —Hypothermia |

Modified from Malamed SF. *Medical Emergencies in the Dental Office.* 6th ed. St. Louis: Mosby; 2013.

4. Gestational diabetes—occurs in 2% of pregnant women during the second or third trimester; the condition returns to normal after delivery in most cases, but 30% to 40% may develop type 2 diabetes later in life

D. Signs, symptoms, and clinical manifestations (Table 19.12)
   1. Cardinal symptoms are those associated with hyperglycemia
   2. An overdose of insulin or inadequate glucose intake to balance the insulin intake can result in insulin shock (hypoglycemia)
   3. Chronic complications include:
      a. Atherosclerosis and other cardiovascular problems
      b. Renal failure
      c. Motor, sensory, and autonomic neuropathies
      d. Glaucoma and cataracts leading to blindness
      e. Associated with increased incidence of large babies, stillbirths, miscarriages, neonatal deaths, and congenital defects

E. Oral manifestations
   1. Seen more often in persons with uncontrolled diabetes
   2. Delayed wound healing and inability to manage oral infections (e.g., *Candida*), periodontal abscesses
   3. Decreased salivary flow may lead to increased caries; may have parotid gland enlargement
   4. Predisposition to aggressive periodontal disease in both types of diabetes, even in children and adolescents; magenta hue with edematous glassy tissue, enlarged papilla, mobility, alveolar bone loss (Fig. 19.20)
   5. Periodontitis can make blood glucose levels more difficult to control
   6. Poor blood glucose control greatly increases risk for periodontal breakdown, bone loss, and loss of attachment
   7. Children with diabetes may have accelerated tooth eruption and enamel hypoplasia

## Thyroid Disease

A. Definitions: a medical condition that affects the function of the thyroid gland
   1. Hyperthyroidism (thyrotoxicosis)—excess of thyroid hormones in the bloodstream
   2. Graves' disease—type of hyperthyroidism; toxic goiter
   3. Hypothyroidism—inadequate thyroid hormones in the bloodstream
      a. Cretinism—childhood onset (congenital)
      b. Myxedema—adult onset (acquired)

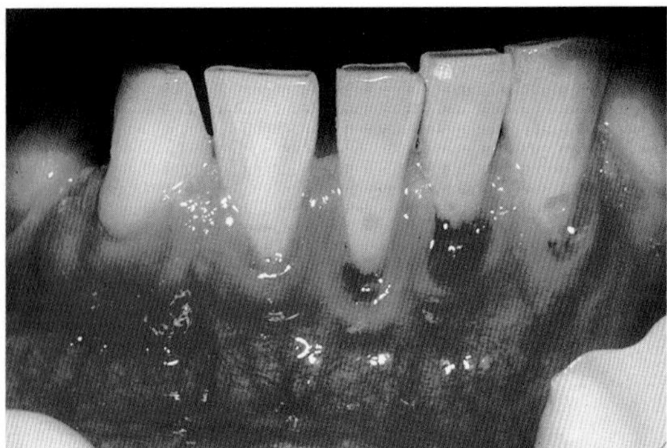

**Fig. 19.20** Gingival tissues exhibiting spontaneous bleeding, inflammation, and edema in an adult patient with diabetes. (From Newman MG, et al. *Carranza's Clinical Periodontology*. 12th ed. St. Louis: Elsevier; 2015.)

B. Incidence and prevalence
   1. Thyroid disease affects 28 million persons in the United States, with up to one-half undiagnosed
   2. Thyroid dysfunction is second most common glandular disorder of the endocrine system
   3. Hyperthyroidism—disease is seven times more common in women; especially manifested during puberty, pregnancy, or menopause
   4. Hypothyroidism
      a. Rare
      b. Myxedema is five times more common in females; most common between ages 30 and 60
      c. Permanent congenital hypothyroidism occurs in 1 in 3500 to 4500 births

C. Signs, symptoms, and clinical manifestations—results of underproduction or overproduction of thyroid hormone (Table 19.13)

D. Oral manifestation(Fig. 19.21 and Table 19.13)
   1. Hyperthyroidism
      a. Increased susceptibility to caries
      b. Periodontal disease
      c. Enlargement of extraglandular thyroid tissue (mainly in the lateral posterior tongue)
      d. Maxillary or mandibular osteoporosis
      e. Accelerated dental eruption
      f. Burning mouth syndrome
      g. Thyroid may be enlarged or noticeably palpable (Graves' disease)
   2. Hypothyroidism
      a. Macroglossia
      b. Dysgeusia
      c. Delayed eruption
      d. Poor periodontal health
      e. Altered tooth morphology
      f. Delayed wound healing

## Chemical Dependency

See the section on "Substance Abuse" in Chapter 11.

A. Definitions
   1. State of psychological or physical dependence (or both) after administration of a drug on a periodic or continuous basis

**TABLE 19.13 Clinical Features of Thyroid Disease**

| HYPOTHYROIDISM | | |
|---|---|---|
| **Cretinism** | **Myxedema** | **Hyperthyroidism** |
| Dwarfism and obesity | Obesity | Weight loss |
| Coarse hair | Hair loss | Fine, friable hair |
| Eyes set apart | Puffy eyelids | Puffy eyelids |
| Muscle weakness | Muscle weakness | Exophthalmos |
| Dry, cold skin | Dry, cold skin | Tremors |
| Decreased sweating | Decreased sweating | Warm, moist skin |
| Cold intolerance | Cold intolerance | Increased sweating |
| Lethargy | Lethargy | Heat intolerance |
| Bradycardia | Bradycardia | Hyperactivity |
| Delayed tooth eruption | | Tachycardia |
| Small jaws and malocclusion | | Accelerated tooth eruption |
| | | Large jaws |
| | | Osteoporosis of alveolar bone |
| | | Rapidly developing dental caries and periodontal disease |

   2. Drug use—when the effects of a drug can be realized with minimal hazard
   3. Drug misuse—when the drug or amount taken makes it more dangerous than necessary to produce the desired effect
   4. Drug abuse—continual misuse of a drug, loss of control over its use, or disruption of family, social, or job responsibilities
   5. Tolerance—use of larger doses of a drug to experience the same effects over time
   6. Recovery—overcoming physical and psychological dependence; commitment to drug-free life

B. Incidence and prevalence
   1. Several drugs or drug categories cause the most concern: cocaine, heroin and other opiates, marijuana, stimulants, barbiturates and other depressants, hallucinogens (psychedelics), tranquilizers, volatile solvents, and other inhalants
   2. Opioids—class of drugs that include the illegal drug heroin, synthetic opioids such as fentanyl, and pain relievers available legally by prescription, such as oxycodone (OxyContin), hydrocodone (Vicodin), codeine, morphine, and many others
      a. High risk of addiction; public health emergency
      b. Overdose crisis; 130 Americans die every day from opioid overdose
   3. Alcohol is a major problem (see next section); 70% of persons in the United States drink at least on a social basis
   4. Nitrous oxide and prescription drug abuse is of concern to dental professionals
   5. Routes of administration—oral ingestion, inhalation, injection, snorting, buccal, suppositories
   6. In the United States, 41.7% of those over age 12 have used illegal drugs at least once

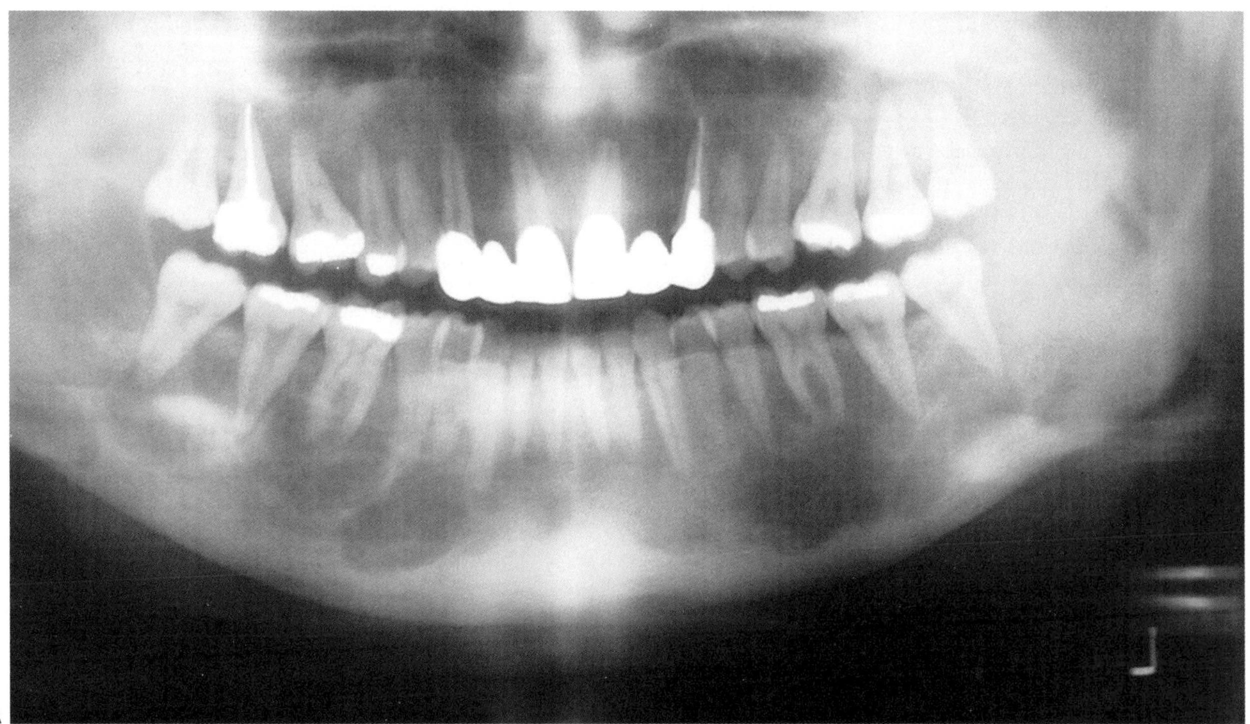

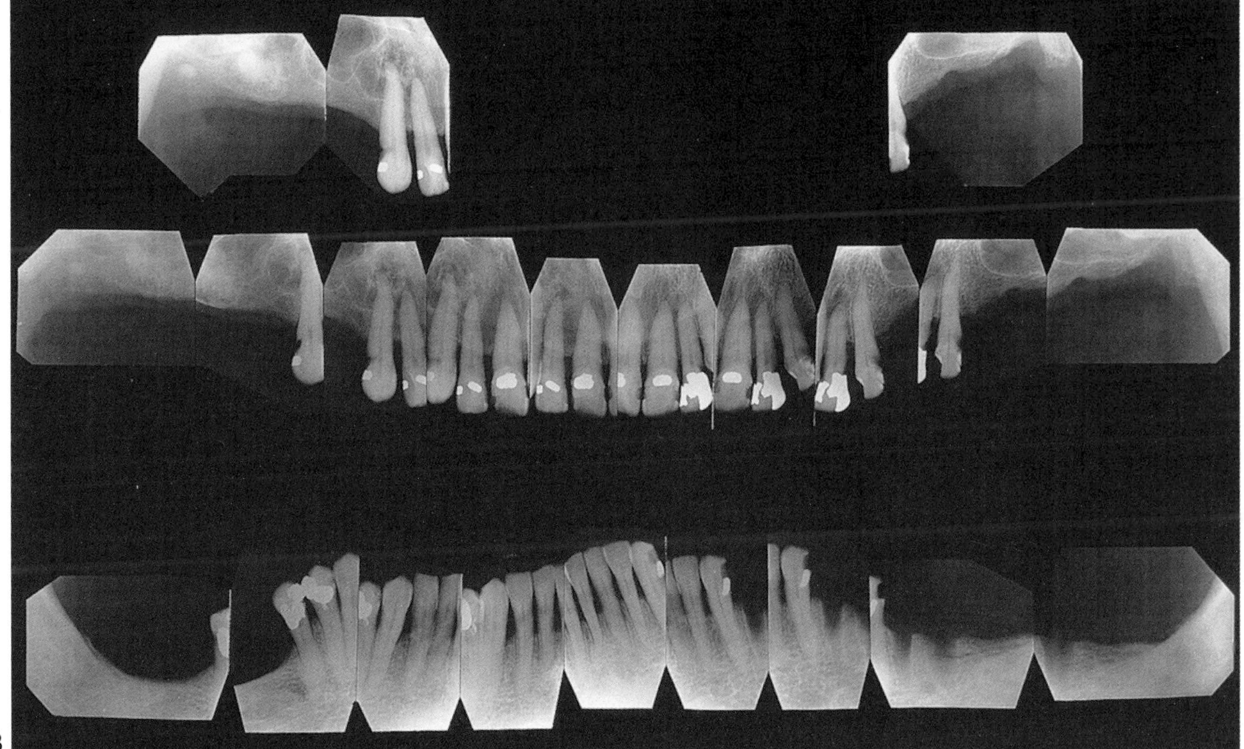

**Fig. 19.21** (A) Radiograph of mandibular radiolucencies associated with hyperparathyroidism. (B) Radiograph of loss of lamina dura associated with hyperparathyroidism. (From Regezi JA, Sciubba JA, Jordan CK. *Oral Pathology: Clinical Pathologic Correlations*. 7th ed. St. Louis: Elsevier; 2017.)

C. Signs and symptoms—vary with the agent involved and route of administration
   1. Affect autonomic, central, and peripheral nervous systems
   2. Drug interactions have additive, inhibitory, and synergistic effects
   3. Duration of effects ranges from 1 hour to many days
   4. Withdrawal symptoms reported for all drug categories except hallucinogens
   5. Common physical and behavioral signs of drug abuse
      a. Needle marks on arms and legs from intravenous (injected) use

b. Constricted, "pinpoint" pupils
c. Having trouble staying awake, or falling asleep at inappropriate times
d. Flushed, itchy skin
e. Withdrawing from social activities that were once enjoyed
f. Sudden and dramatic mood swings that seem out of character
g. Impulsive actions and decision making
h. Engaging in risky activities, such as driving under the influence
i. Visiting multiple doctors in order to obtain more prescriptions

6. Possible effects of some drug categories
a. Narcotics—euphoria, drowsiness, respiratory depression, constricted pupils, nausea
b. Depressants—slurred speech, disorientation, intoxicated behavior
c. Stimulants—alertness, excitation, euphoria, increased pulse rate and blood pressure, insomnia, loss of appetite
d. Hallucinogens—illusions and hallucinations, poor perception of time and distance
e. Marijuana—euphoria, relaxed inhibitions, increased appetite, disoriented behavior

D. Oral manifestations
1. Oral trauma—if the person engages in aggressive behavior or fights or has accidents
2. Xerostomia—if dehydrated
3. Mucosal lesions and leukoplakia from irritants smoked or used orally
4. Increased caries typically seen at the cervical area; periodontal disease prevalent if oral hygiene is neglected or the person consumes high-carbohydrate diet
5. Advanced cervical caries associated with heavy methamphetamine use
6. Tooth abrasion
7. Increased risk for oral and esophageal cancers
8. Reduced tolerance to pain
9. Bruxism

## Chronic Alcohol Use Disorder and Dependence

A. Definition and etiology
1. Chronic impairment in physical, mental, or social functioning caused by frequent ingestion (more than two drinks per day) of alcohol
2. Can become dependent on alcohol ingestion and develop a tolerance to increasing amounts
3. Moderate drinking is up to 1 drink per day for women and up to 2 drinks per day for men
4. Standard alcohol drink defined
a. 12 ounces of regular beer, which is usually about 5% alcohol
b. 5 ounces of wine, which is typically about 12% alcohol
c. 1.5 ounces of distilled spirits, which is about 40% alcohol
5. Binge drinking is five or more alcoholic drinks for males or four or more alcoholic drinks for females on the same occasion on at least 1 day in the past month
6. Genetically transmitted susceptibility to alcoholism
7. Often induced by a psychiatric disorder or stress

B. Incidence and prevalence
1. Estimated 5.1 million persons in United States suffer from alcohol abuse
2. About 1 in 13 US adults abuses alcohol or is an alcoholic (7.42% of persons age 18 and older)
3. Alcohol problems are higher among young adults age 18 to 29
4. Normal activities are maintained by 90%
5. Approximately 80% are heavy smokers

C. Signs, symptoms, and clinical manifestations
1. Alcoholic breath
2. Unexplained tremors
3. Nausea and vomiting, gastrointestinal problems, ulcers
4. Cutaneous lesions (redness, acne, spider angiomas)
5. Edema of the eyelids and other parts of the body
6. Nutritional deficiencies (vitamin B, protein, calcium)

D. Long-term complications
1. Hypertension and other types of heart disease
2. Increased risk for various types of cancers; dehydrating effect of alcohol on cell walls enhances mucosal permeability to other toxins and carcinogens
3. Hepatitis, cirrhosis, hepatocellular carcinoma, and hypoglycemia
4. Interference with secretion of pancreatic enzymes
5. Bleeding tendencies
6. Altered enzyme functioning and malabsorptive syndromes of the small intestine
7. Cancer of mouth, esophagus, larynx, breast, pharynx
8. Irritation of the gastric mucosa leading to bleeding, inflammation, and ulceration
9. FAS (pregnant women)

E. Oral manifestations—increased incidence of:
1. Caries caused by nausea and vomiting, neglected oral hygiene, and xerostomia
2. Missing teeth
3. Periodontal disease caused by an impaired immune system and the effects on white blood cells
4. Glossitis and angular cheilitis from nutritional deficiencies
5. Leukoplakia and oropharyngeal cancer (use of alcohol and tobacco products increases risk of oropharyngeal cancer)
6. Swelling of the parotid glands leads to decreased salivation and increased caries incidence
7. Trauma during inebriated states (accidents or fights)
8. Attrition secondary to bruxism
9. Erosion

## End-Stage Renal Disease; Fifth Stage of Chronic Kidney Disease (CKD)

A. Definition
1. Kidney failure; progressive bilateral deterioration of renal function, resulting in uremia and eventual death
2. Uremia is the toxic condition produced by retention of urinary constituents in the blood

B. Stages of CKD
   1. Stage 1—signs of mild kidney disease but with normal or better glomerular filtration rate (GFR) (greater than 90% kidney function)
   2. Stage 2—signs of mild kidney disease with reduced GFR (indicating 60% to 89% kidney function)
   3. Stage 3—signs of moderate chronic renal insufficiency (where the GFR indicates 40% to 59% kidney function)
   4. Stage 4—signs of severe chronic renal insufficiency (where the GFR indicates 15% to 29% kidney function)
   5. Stage 5—signs of end stage renal failure (where the GFR indicates less than 15% kidney function)
C. Incidence and prevalence
   1. CKD affects approximately 30 million persons in the United States, or 1 in 9 adults; over 5-year period, the number of patients with kidney failure averaged about 90,000 annually
   2. More than 660,000 persons in the United States are being treated for end-stage renal disease; of these, more than 480,000 are patients receiving dialysis and 193,000 have undergone kidney transplantation
   3. More common in Caucasians (62%), followed by African Americans (31.7%), and Hispanic Americans (16%)
D. Signs, symptoms, and clinical manifestations
   1. Mental slowness or depression
   2. Swelling and edema
   3. Muscular hyperactivity
   4. Hyperpigmentation of the skin (brownish yellow)
   5. Anorexia, vomiting, and diarrhea
   6. Anemia
   7. Possible functional defect in factor VIII protein, leading to hemorrhagic episodes
   8. Hypertension, CHF
   9. Kidney transplantation—problems with graft rejection and infection; use steroids, antibiotics, and immunosuppressives such as cyclosporine
      a. Blood runs from the artery to the dialysis machine, is filtered, and then is returned to the vein
      b. Anticoagulant is added to prevent blood clotting
      c. Patient is at risk for acquiring hepatitis B, hepatitis C, and hepatitis D viruses from commercial blood products
      d. Dental treatment 24 hours after dialysis
E. Oral manifestations
   1. Painful oral ulcerations and stomatitis from drugs
   2. Candidiasis or herpetic lesions from immunosuppression
   3. Increased calculus deposits
   4. Anemic mucosa
   5. Oral petechiae and hemorrhage
   6. Ground-glass appearance of alveolar bone caused by leaching of calcium (uremic bone disease)
   7. Bad taste and halitosis from urea in saliva
   8. Enamel hypoplasia
   9. Immunosuppressed patient who has received a transplant may have increased risk for cancer and infections
   10. Drug-influenced gingival enlargement from cyclosporine (an immunosuppressant) or nifedipine (a calcium-channel blocker)
   11. Delayed eruption in primary teeth
   12. Monitor for premedication needs with physician
   13. Schedule appointment 24 hours after dialysis
   14. Xerostomia often a consequence of limited fluid intake allowed

## Older Adults

A. Definition
   1. Age 55 and older
   2. Older/elderly adults age 68 and older
B. Incidence and prevalence
   1. Approximately 13% of the US population age 66 or older; over 52 million persons in United States over age of 65
   2. Fastest-growing segment of population
   3. It is estimated that 20% of US population will be age 65 or older by 2030
   4. About 47% of older adults live in nursing homes; 52% over age of 85
      a. 1% of persons age 65 to 74
      b. 20% of persons age 85 or older
C. Systemic manifestations
   1. Disease response—increased severity, longer course, and slower healing
   2. Decreased metabolism
   3. Reduced elasticity of tissues, diminished reparative ability
   4. Thin, dry, wrinkled skin; delayed healing
   5. Special senses
   6. Musculoskeletal changes
   7. Increase in cardiovascular diseases
   8. 13% of persons age 70 to 74 and 31% of persons age 85 or older have a visual impairment
   9. 26% of persons age 70 to 74 and 49% of persons age 85 or older have a hearing impairment
   10. Osteopenia and osteoporosis
   11. Osteoarthritis
   12. Loss of muscle function and tone
   13. High blood pressure
   14. Coronary heart disease
   15. Valvular disease
D. Common chronic conditions
   1. Arthritis
   2. Hypertension
   3. Cardiovascular disease
   4. Diabetes
E. Oral manifestations
   1. Soft tissues
   2. Hard tissues
      a. Dry, purse-string lips with opening difficulties; angular cheilitis (Fig.19.22)
      b. Capillary fragility, hyperkeratosis of oral mucosa
      c. Fissures, sublingual varicosities, reduced taste from loss of taste buds of tongue
      d. Increased incidence of oral cancer
      e. Abrasion, attrition, dark color of teeth
      f. Root caries
      g. Decreased tooth sensitivity
      h. Decreased pulp chamber size

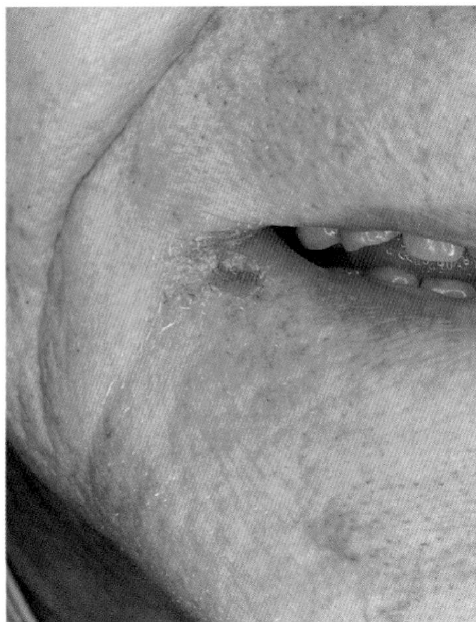

**Fig. 19.22** Angular cheilitis is a common oral finding in older adults because of nutritional deficiencies. (From Ibsen OAC, Phelan JA. *Oral Pathology for the Dental Hygienist*. 6th ed. St. Louis: Elsevier; 2014.)

## OVERALL DENTAL MANAGEMENT CONSIDERATIONS FOR SPECIAL CARE PATIENTS

A. Personal and professional prerequisites (Table 19.14)
   1. Interview the patient in a sensitive manner to gather accurate data; initiate dental hygiene process
   2. Analyze and summarize data in oral or written formats
   3. Use problem-solving skills to develop alternative strategies to manage problems
   4. Evaluate patient and professional goals and progress for appropriateness and effectiveness
   5. Remain current of new conditions, new protocols for medical management, and advances in dental and dental hygiene care
   6. Apply new knowledge or techniques from other areas to dental management of special patients
   7. Apply research principles and techniques to acquire clinical data that serve as the basis for care planning and decision making
   8. Use people "first" language, putting the person before the disability

B. Office management issues
   1. Stress a team concept, with cooperation among members and coordination of information and activities; dental hygiene procedures may require the help of a dental assistant
   2. Identify and anticipate patient needs and problems before initiation of care; use of a previsit questionnaire is helpful (Fig. 19.23)
   3. Obtain informed consent for treatment from the patient or an appropriate representative
   4. Explain office policies, procedures, and philosophy to the patient or guardian before or at the first appointment
   5. Determine financial limitations that may affect care planning or payment procedures
   6. If the patient is unable to receive care in the office because of physical limitations or geographic distance, determine if care can be provided in the home or community setting with portable equipment
   7. If office facilities do not comply with accessibility guidelines, discuss ways to:
      a. Ensure that office layout and environment are not safety hazards or health hazards for some patients
      b. Keep scheduling somewhat flexible to allow for transportation or other problems; block appointments are helpful when dealing with groups
   8. Weigh risk versus benefit of proposed treatment
   9. Make ethical, realistic decisions in treatment planning
   10. Be prepared to implement wheelchair transfers
      a. Assess additional resources available from other sources (e.g., community organizations)
      b. Attempt to provide flexible payment alternatives
      c. Make them physically accessible
      d. Accommodate patient needs, or refer the patient to a provider who can provide access

C. Medical issues
   1. Obtain a health history from the patient or caregiver, with supplemental information from other professionals or agency records
   2. Update the health history at each visit
   3. Because many standard health history forms are inadequate for the multiple conditions and problems of some patients, ask supplemental questions
   4. Obtain specifics regarding medical treatment regimens or other therapies that may affect scheduling or treatment
   5. Obtain names, addresses, and phone numbers for all the patient's physicians who might provide helpful data (e.g., generalist, cardiologist, orthopedist, endocrinologist) with permission to release information
   6. Be particularly alert to the patient's physical status during initial assessment
   7. Monitor vital signs, as indicated
   8. Record all medication information; update at each visit
   9. Note any indications or contraindications to treatment or premedication
   10. Maintain records of all medical advice, prescriptions, or drugs given

D. Treatment adaptations
   1. Demonstrate understanding and acceptance of conditions or problems to the patient and to caregivers or family
   2. Determine which special needs require provider adaptations versus patient adaptations
   3. Demonstrate empathy, not sympathy
   4. Discuss before implementation:
   5. Introduce patients to the oral health care setting gradually by using desensitization, modeling, "show-tell-do," or other methods
   6. Ensure patient comfort in the dental chair through frequent assurance, positioning, and supportive measures as needed (e.g., pillows)

**TABLE 19.14 Dental Management Considerations for Patients With Special Needs**

| Condition | Medical Issues | Barriers to Care | Other Associated Health Issues | Treatment Considerations[a] | Prevention/Education/Health Promotion Issues |
|---|---|---|---|---|---|
| Acquired immuno-deficiency syndrome (AIDS; see Chapters 8 and 9) | Systems involved<br>Degree of impairment<br>Consult with physician<br>Kaposi's sarcoma<br>Treatment regimens<br>Predisposition to multiple opportunistic infections<br>Immunosuppressive medications | Finding dentist who will treat<br>Fear of rejection and discrimination<br>Stigma associated with disease<br>Decreased motivation or depression<br>Limited finances if unemployed, underinsured, or uninsured | Oral infections<br>Debilitated state | Oral infections (e.g., candidiasis): palliation, transmission potential<br>Kaposi's sarcoma: treatment planning<br>Psychological state: communication, motivation<br>Gingivitis should be treated to prevent necrotizing ulcerative periodontitis<br>Povidone-iodine: use with initial debridement with necrotizing ulcerative periodontitis<br>Antibiotic may be needed | Palliative care for oral infections and oral ulceration<br>Increased attention to oral hygiene<br>Daily chlorhexidine rinses<br>Frequent recare<br>Take HIV medicine on schedule<br>Xerostomia management |
| Alzheimer's disease | Multiple medical problems<br>Medications<br>Reduced bowel and bladder control<br>Fatigue from abnormal sleep patterns<br>Wheelchair | Behavior: uncooperative<br>Finances may be limited by disability and medical problems<br>Dependence on others | Oral-motor dysfunction<br>Depression or disorientation leading to oral neglect<br>General motor dysfunction<br>Potential for injury<br>Uncooperative with caregiver | Dental consult as soon as possible after diagnosis<br>Focus on prevention<br>Fluctuating moods and disorientation: short appointments, communication, cooperation, safety<br>Motor problems: oral access, radiographs, stability in chair<br>Memory loss: data collection<br>Never leave unattended<br>May need sedation/antianxiety medications<br>Do not force patient to have treatment | Involve caregivers<br>Involve patient when most lucid and positive<br>Simple and short instructions and frequent repetition<br>Positive reinforcement with a "watch me" technique<br>Frequent continued-care intervals<br>Prevent oral injury<br>Aggressive preventive program<br>Powered oral hygiene aids |
| Arthritis | Medications<br>Degree of impairment<br>Joints affected: pain<br>Joint replacement (premedication may be needed)<br>Potential for adrenal suppression with long-term corticosteroid use | Mobility to and in office<br>Limited finances, if disabled<br>Weakness or fatigue decreases motivation to seek care | General motor impairment<br>Drug-related complications such as prolonged bleeding and bone marrow suppression | Steroid therapy<br>Joint pain: chair position, appointment length<br>Limited oral opening: positioning, instrumentation, radiographs, TMJ assessment<br>Joint replacement: antibiotic premedication<br>Long-term aspirin therapy: prolonged bleeding | Adaptive equipment or assistance is needed<br>Powered oral hygiene aids<br>Counseling about side effects of medications<br>Prevent sources of oral infection<br>Discuss link with inflammation, arthritis and periodontitis<br>Educate on xerostomia management; saliva substitutes, ice chips and drinking water, daily use of xylitol-containing products, fluoride therapy, and calcium phosphate therapy |
| Autism spectrum disorders (ASD) | No major problems unless self-abusive | Behavior<br>Degree of reliance on others<br>Communication, minimal<br>Language skills | Disordered eating or fetishes<br>Resistant behavior | Functional behavioral assessment<br>Schedule when function best<br>Dependence on "routines": procedure sequencing, desensitization appointment<br>Visual pedagogy to prepare for appointment<br>Lack of useful language: communication<br>Learning disabilities and sensitivity to stimuli: communication, limit distractions<br>Avoid light in eyes<br>Cover with lead apron<br>Discuss appropriate behavioral interventions with parent<br>Consider use of nitrous oxide during treatment to manage behavior | Combine verbal and nonverbal communication techniques and positive reinforcers<br>Consider small rewards for appropriate behavior (stickers, etc.) in obtaining compliance<br>Give short, clear instructions directly to child. Give only one instruction at a time<br>Teach toothbrushing as a "motion" rather than a function<br>Avoid metaphors and complex language structures<br>Silver diamine fluoride, Fluoride varnish |

*Continued*

## TABLE 19.14 Dental Management Considerations for Patients With Special Needs—cont'd

| Condition | Medical Issues | Barriers to Care | Other Associated Health Issues | Treatment Considerations[a] | Prevention/Education/Health Promotion Issues |
|---|---|---|---|---|---|
| Bell's palsy | Therapies, especially prednisone<br>Duration of condition<br>Possible surgery to achieve facial symmetry | Language skills<br>Self-image problems | Oral-motor dysfunction anesthesia used or opposite side affected precautions needed | Lack of eye closure: protection of eyes (goggles)<br>Oral-motor dysfunction: protection of airway<br>Corticosteroid therapy | Caution regarding effects of anesthesia<br>Frequent rinsing or toothbrushing for food retention of affected side<br>Antimicrobial mouthrinse daily |
| Bronchial asthma | Type and severity of asthma<br>Frequency and severity of attacks<br>Precipitating factors<br>Treatment regimens<br>History of hospitalizations or status asthmaticus<br>Instruct patient to bring inhalers if used<br>Screen for sensitivity to NSAIDs | Fear of medical and dental environments<br>Allergens in office | No specific risk factors<br>Oral side effects of medications<br>Maxillofacial growth altered with childhood asthma<br>Avoid narcotics and barbiturates due to their histamine releasing properties → bronchospasm and potentiated allergic response.<br>Avoid aspirin, other salicylates and NSAIDS (due to allergies). May provoke a severe exacerbation of bronchoconstriction – use acetaminophen | Anxiety: possible premedication or relaxation techniques<br>Type of asthma, history of attacks<br>Confirm that the patient has taken most recent dose of medication<br>Avoid use of air polisher and ultrasonic scaler<br>Stress-management techniques; may use nitrous oxide in mild to moderate asthmatics after medical consultation but generally contraindicated<br>Anxiety can cause acute exacerbation.<br>Medical emergency preparedness, eliminate allergens<br>Have bronchodilator present/ supplemental oxygen available during treatment in case of acute asthmatic exacerbation.<br>Use of local anesthetic without epinephrine or levonordefrin in some cases;<br>Avoid aspirin-containing medications and NSAIDs | Stress-free environment<br>For xerostomia, recommend a dry-mouth management protocol that includes saliva substitutes, ice chips and drinking water, daily use of xylitol-containing products, fluoride therapy, and calcium phosphate therapy<br>ADA-approved or CDA-recognized antimicrobial mouthrinse daily |
| Cancers | Parts of body affected, treatment regimens, medications and side effects, potential for bleeding and anemia<br>Physician consult regarding need for antibiotic premedication<br>Compromised immunity and low white blood cell counts | Frequent hospitalization or medical appointments<br>Debilitated states<br>Financial burdens<br>Consult oncologist to order blood work 24 hours before oral surgery or other invasive procedures<br>Depression<br>Oral manifestations prevent eating and swallowing; may need tube feeding<br>Dehydration | Side effects of medications<br>Oral infections and ulcerations<br>Metastasis to oral cavity<br>Weakness for self-care | Consult the oncologist before any dental procedure, including prophylaxis<br>Prevention and palliative care for oral infections and ulcerations<br>Postpone treatment if neutrophil count less than 1000/ $mm^3$, or consider prophylactic antibiotics<br>Potential bleeding problem; postpone treatment if platelet count under 75,000 $mm^3$<br>Prompt treatment of dental-related infections<br>Evaluate need for antibiotic premedication<br>Radiation therapy: care before and after<br>"Magic rinse"<br>combination of Lidocaine Benadryl, Maalox, and Nystatin | Increased risk for caries<br>With cues, if bleeding is a problem<br>Fluoride therapy<br>Antimicrobial mouthrinse daily<br>Sodium bicarbonate rinse for palliative care<br>Oral hygiene aids<br>Help with oral care, if needed<br>Monitor removable appliances<br>Frequent maintenance care<br>For xerostomia, recommend a dry-mouth management protocol that includes saliva substitutes, ice chips and drinking water, daily use of xylitol-containing products, fluoride therapy, calcium phosphate therapy, and antifungals, as needed |

| | | | | | |
|---|---|---|---|---|---|
| Cardiac arrhythmias and dysrhythmias | Symptoms<br>Medications and side effects<br>Presence of pacemaker and type | Excessive bleeding if taking blood thinner<br>Avoidance of certain electromagnetic equipment with older pacemakers | No specific risk factors<br>Patient history, symptoms, and palpation of the pulse are the available diagnostic tools | Only treat for preventive measures if stable<br>Advised to take their medication regularly<br>Arrhythmia during treatment, the treatment should be discontinued, supplemental oxygen, patient status closely monitored.<br>Pacemaker: if not shielded, may need to avoid electromagnetic equipment: check with physician<br>Limit epinephrine to less than two carpules of 1:100,000<br>Patient taking digoxin: no epinephrine<br>Blood thinner: INR 3.5 or less<br>Set upright: minimize x-ray exposure<br>Arrhythmia: stress management protocol, drug precautions, bleeding potential from medications | No specific preventive regimens<br>For xerostomia, recommend a dry-mouth management protocol that includes saliva substitutes, ice chips and drinking water, daily use of xylitol-containing products, fluoride therapy, and calcium phosphate therapy |
| Cerebral palsy | Associated disorders<br>Medications<br>Other therapies<br>Respiration impaired?<br>Presence of primitive reflexes<br>Degree of impairment | Communication<br>Transportation if in wheelchair or cannot drive<br>May have limited financial resources<br>Degree of dependence on others for care<br>Mobility issues if in wheelchair<br>Provider attitudes toward condition<br>Self-image problems | Oral-motor dysfunction<br>General motor dysfunction<br>Special diets | Primitive reflexes: patient or clinician position, stability, instrument positioning or fulcrum, oral access, suctioning and amount of water used<br>Treatment based on what patient can tolerate<br>Avoid use of powered instruments<br>Radiographs (few at a time)<br>Wheelchair transfers; calm treatment environment: relaxation needed to avoid muscle spasms<br>Do not force arms and legs in unnatural positions<br>May need sedation or muscle relaxants for extensive treatment<br>Minimize distractions<br>Softly cradle patient's head during treatment | Modified or powered toothbrush<br>Involve caregivers as appropriate<br>Be patient with slowness of responses and progress<br>Use combination of communication methods with consistency and repetition<br>Assess need for adaptive aids for home care<br>Frequent continued care<br>Fluoride therapy, sealants, and antimicrobials if needed<br>Simple, concrete instructions<br>Involuntary movements and safety issues, may need restraints (consent necessary)<br>ADA-approved or CDA-recognized antimicrobial mouthrinse daily |
| Cerebrovascular accident (CVA, stroke) | Type of involvement, degree of limitation<br>Medications and side effects<br>Other therapies | Communication<br>Accessibility if need adaptive equipment or wheelchair<br>Degree of dependence on others | Oral-motor dysfunction<br>Side effects of medications<br>Impaired general motor coordination<br>Dietary inadequacies<br>Transient ischemic attacks<br>Previous stroke, hypertension, cardiac abnormalities, atherosclerosis, diabetes mellitus, elevated blood lipid levels | Dental treatment could precipitate CVA<br>Schedule short, stress-free mid-morning appointments.<br>Monitor blood pressure and heart rate preoperatively and 5 minutes after injection. Should not treat if systolic BP >180 mmHg or if diastolic BP >110 mmHg.<br>Memory and speech impairment: communication, data collection<br>Oral-motor dysfunction or paralysis: radiographs, instrumentation, jaw stability, treatment planning<br>Impaired emotional control: cooperation, communication<br>Evaluate calcifications in carotid artery with panoramic radiographs<br>Short, morning appointments<br>General paralysis: mobility, possible wheelchair transfers, stability in chair<br>Minimize use of epinephrine; limiting epinephrine to 0.04 mg (2 cartridges of 1:100,000 or 4 cartridges of 1:200,000 epinephrine) and levonordefrin to 0.2 mg<br>Avoid elective dental care for 3 to 6 months<br>Potential bleeding problems; obtain INR | Use combination of teaching approaches<br>Reinforce and repeat instructions<br>Frequent continued care<br>Fluoride therapy, if needed<br>ADA-approved or CDA-recognized antimicrobial mouthrinse daily<br>Adaptive aids or supervision for oral care<br>Avoid sensory overload<br>Reorient patient to situation; rinsing difficult or impossible<br>Use one-step instructions<br>Educate about increased CVA risk in patients with periodontitis |

*Continued*

**TABLE 19.14 Dental Management Considerations for Patients With Special Needs—cont'd**

| Condition | Medical Issues | Barriers to Care | Other Associated Health Issues | Treatment Considerations[a] | Prevention/Education/Health Promotion Issues |
|---|---|---|---|---|---|
| Chemical dependency | Obtaining adequate history<br>Types of drugs used<br>Opioid epidemic<br>Treatment interventions<br>Potential for drug interactions or overdose<br>Emotional stability during appointment<br>At risk for AIDS, hepatitis, Bacterial endocarditis<br>Naloxone for opioid overdose | Emotional state<br>Denial of drug problem<br>Demanding requests for use of nitrous oxide or pain medications<br>Disoriented behavior | Neglect personal hygiene<br>Potential for oral trauma<br>Potential drug interaction if local anesthetic with epinephrine is injected into blood vessel | Coordinated care: professional team and family if in treatment program<br>Evaluate for impairment before care<br>Providing provisional restorations and prescription fluoride may be positive first steps so patients build a relationship with the oral health care team.<br>Follow safe prescribing of opioids/drugs<br>Strict guidelines for keeping appointments necessary<br>Avoid local anesthesia with epinephrine for 6 hours after cocaine or methamphetamine use<br>Complete as much treatment as possible per visit<br>Drug use can alter anesthesia effectiveness<br>Naloxone in office for emergencies | Encourage to seek medical care<br>Frequent brushing and flossing<br>Teach oral self-examinations<br>Avoid mouthrinses containing alcohol<br>For xerostomia, recommend a dry-mouth management protocol that includes saliva substitutes, ice chips and drinking water, daily use of xylitol-containing products, fluoride therapy, and calcium phosphate therapy<br>Topical fluoride program |
| Chronic alcohol abuse and dependence | Patient's perception of severity of problem<br>Nutritional deficiencies<br>Chronic complications<br>Degree of liver impairment<br>At risk for tuberculosis | Potential for no-show appointments or intoxication at appointment | Susceptibility to infection<br>Nutritional deficiencies<br>Nausea and vomiting<br>Potential for oral trauma<br>Risk factor for oral cancer; dose response effect | Screen for alcohol consumption<br>Increase risk for oral disease<br>Liver impairment and bleeding potential: pre-appointment laboratory testing, drug metabolism, instrumentation, treatment planning<br>Inebriated states: emergency care, appointment scheduling, treatment planning, data collection<br>Problems with local anesthesia effectiveness<br>Use only alcohol-free medicaments<br>Recommend alcohol-free mouthrinses<br>Increase risk for erosion | Nutritional counseling<br>Frequent continued-care intervals<br>Fluoride therapy and alcohol-free antimicrobials<br>Frequent soft tissue evaluation for oral cancer<br>Counseling regarding oral trauma<br>For xerostomia, recommend a dry-mouth management protocol that includes saliva substitutes, ice chips and drinking water, daily use of xylitol-containing products, fluoride therapy, and calcium phosphate therapy for dental erosion<br>Instill responsibility for oral care<br>Provide alcohol reduction advice<br>Counsel to avoid alcohol prior to premedication |
| Chronic obstructive pulmonary disease (COPD) | Single or coexisting conditions<br>Degree of impairment<br>Medications or need for oxygen<br>Increasing evidence of link between COPD and both gastro-esophageal reflux disease and periodontal disease | Portable oxygen<br>Fear of procedures that impair breathing<br>Patients with severe disease; poor mobility, dyspnea and frequent hospitalization, all of which make regular dental appointments problematic | Side effects of medications<br>Dry mouth and candidiasis | Impaired respiration: upright position, suctioning and coughing, no nitrous oxide–oxygen sedation in severe cases<br>rubber dam, orthopnea<br>Medications: avoid those that depress respiration, $N_2O$-$O_2$ may be used, drug interactions<br>Avoid use of air polisher and ultrasonic scaler<br>Oxygen available for hypoxia | Same as for bronchial asthma<br>Educate periodontal bacteria can be carried into the lung; cause respiratory infection<br>Oral hygiene instruction important.<br>Smoking cessation education as needed |
| Cleft lip or palate | Hearing impairment<br>Upper respiratory tract infections<br>Prosthetic appliances<br>Medications<br>Dietary Issues | Fear of health care providers<br>Self-image problems | Supernumerary tooth, congenitally missing tooth<br>Delayed tooth development morphological anomalies in both deciduous and permanent dentition<br>Delayed eruption of permanent maxillary incisors, microdontia, and abnormal tooth number<br>Oral-motor dysfunction<br>Feeding disorders | Cleft: clear communication<br>Hearing loss and speech difficulties<br>Instrument positioning or fulcruming, suctioning and prevention of aspiration<br>Fear: dental procedures, cooperation | Instruct in cleaning any prosthetic aids<br>Involve caregiver, when necessary<br>Dietary counseling, if needed<br>Fluoride therapy |

| | | | | | |
|---|---|---|---|---|---|
| Congenital disorders of coagulation: hemophilias | Type and severity<br>Frequency and location of bleeds<br>Treatment regimens<br>Joint replacements<br>Hepatitis<br>HIV disease<br>Seizures<br>Inhibitor status<br>Laboratory tests needed | Finding dentist who will treat<br>Resources for emergency care | Potential for oral bleeds<br>Potential to acquire hepatitis, cirrhosis, or AIDS-associated disease with frequent clotting-factor replacement therapy | Bleeding potential: preappointment laboratory tests, surgery, physician consult, clotting-factor replacement therapy, instrumentation, radiographs, use of rubber dam, suctioning, use of aminocaproic acid (Amicar) or tranexamic acid (Cyklokapron)<br>Hepatitis carrier: disease transmission procedures<br>Avoid use of aspirin | Use extra-soft–bristled brush<br>ADA-approved or CDA-recognized antimicrobial mouthrinse daily<br>Counseling regarding first aid for oral trauma<br>Frequent continued-care intervals<br>Educate about role of oral infection and increased bleeding |
| Congenital heart disease | Type and if repaired<br>Extent of limitations<br>Medications<br>Prognosis<br>Need for antibiotic premedication<br>Physician consult | Financial constraints from medical bills<br>Frequent illness<br>Possibly debilitated state<br>Overprotective attitude of parents | Decreased resistance to infections | Bleeding potential in some cases: treatment planning, need for laboratory tests, possible referral to specialist<br>Prophylactic antibiotic premedication, stress management protocols, chair position | Emphasize danger of intraoral infections in terms of aggravating heart condition<br>Frequent continued-care intervals<br>Prevention of infective endocarditis<br>ADA-approved or CDA-recognized antimicrobial mouthrinse daily |
| Congestive heart failure | Same as for severe ischemic or hypertensive heart disease | Drug interactions<br>Mobility<br>Debilitated<br>Labored breathing | Pulmonary congestion and edema<br>Limit use of vasoconstrictor in anesthetics<br>Oxygen available for potential emergency<br>Minimize use of epinephrine; limiting epinephrine to 0.04 mg (two cartridges of 1:100,000 or four cartridges of 1:200,000 epinephrine) and levonordefrin to 0.2 mg | Create stress-free environment<br>Avoid use of air polisher and ultrasonic scaler<br>Prone to nausea and vomiting during oral health care<br>Keep patient upright in dental chair | Frequent continued-care intervals<br>Create stress-free environment<br>ADA-approved or CDA-recognized antimicrobial mouthrinse daily |
| Cystic fibrosis | Degree of impairment and prognosis<br>Dietary changes<br>Treatment regimens<br>Chronic pulmonary disease<br>Abnormal viscous secretions causing damage to major organs, such as lungs, pancreas, and liver | Small stature may cause embarrassment<br>Prognosis may decrease motivation<br>Finances may be limited<br>Short life span | Decreased resistance to infections<br>Pulmonary complications compounded by problems of malabsorption and malnutrition<br>Recurrent attacks of pneumonia, bronchiectasis | Enamel defects, particularly enamel opacities, which can be disfiguring, common<br>Mucus accumulations and impaired breathing: chair position, appointment scheduling and length, coughing, protection of airway, use of rubber dam<br>Avoid use of air polisher and ultrasonic scaler<br>Cooperation and scheduling issues<br>Susceptibility to infections: appointment scheduling<br>Tetracycline staining: esthetics, treatment planning | For xerostomia, recommend protocol that includes saliva substitutes, ice chips and drinking water, daily use of xylitol-containing products, fluoride therapy, and calcium phosphate therapy<br>Frequent oral care because of mouth breathing<br>Low-fat diet<br>Recommend tartar-control products<br>ADA-approved or CDA-recognized antimicrobial mouthrinse daily |
| Developmental and cognitive challenges (formerly called "mental retardation") | Syndrome<br>Associated medical conditions and other disabilities<br>Treatment regimens | Limited financial resources<br>Degree of reliance on others<br>Limited mental ability | Oral-motor dysfunction<br>General incoordination<br>Cariogenic foods and reinforcers<br>Self-abuse<br>Resistant behavior | Pre visit imagery; social stories of appointment<br>Short, midmorning appointments<br>Gagging: radiographs, instrument placement, positioning<br>Consult caregiver for behavioral management approaches<br>Mental impairment: communication, cooperation, stability in chair, limited attention span, minimize distractions<br>Limited finances: alternative treatment plans | "Tell-show-do" approach<br>Simple language<br>Frequent repetition and positive reinforcement<br>Frequent continued-care intervals, minimize distractions<br>Alternatives for snacks and food reinforcers<br>Silver diamine fluoride<br>Chlorhexidine mouthrinses or spray, sealants<br>ADA-approved or CDA-recognized antimicrobial mouthrinse daily |

**TABLE 19.14 Dental Management Considerations for Patients With Special Needs—cont'd**

| Condition | Medical Issues | Barriers to Care | Other Associated Health Issues | Treatment Considerations[a] | Prevention/Education/Health Promotion Issues |
|---|---|---|---|---|---|
| Diabetes mellitus | Type and severity<br>Medication regimens<br>Poor wound healing<br>Dietary regimen<br>Complications<br>Hypertension and other heart conditions<br>Frequency of episodes of hypoglycemia or hyperglycemia | Finding dentist who will treat if have chronic complications | Susceptibility to infections (e.g., oral candidiasis)<br>Decreased salivary flow<br>Recalcitrant periodontal disease<br>Slow healing<br>Complications associated with disturbances in vision and kidney function | Insulin-sugar balance: potential for medical emergency, appointment scheduling, stress management protocol<br>Susceptibility to infection: periodontal maintenance, possible antibiotic premedication<br>Monitor hemoglobin $A_{1c}$ status<br>Avoid elective treatment, if uncontrolled ($HbA_{1c}$ greater than 9) MD consult<br>15 g of oral carbohydrate available for hypoglycemia reaction | 3- to 6-month continued-care intervals<br>Dietary analysis<br>Educate on bi-directional relationship with periodontitis<br>For xerostomia, recommend a protocol that includes saliva substitutes, ice chips and drinking water, daily use of xylitol-containing products, fluoride therapy, and calcium phosphate therapy<br>Need for excellent bacterial biofilm control<br>Antimicrobial mouthrinse daily<br>Minimize stress<br>Control of oral infections<br>Prevention of insulin shock or diabetic coma<br>Role of periodontitis in blood glucose control |
| Disordered eating | Symptoms<br>Amount of weight loss<br>Presence and frequency of bulimia<br>Medical and psychological interventions<br>Eating patterns | Psychological status<br>Denial of symptoms<br>Length of treatment<br>Compliance with appointments | Eating patterns<br>Frequent vomiting<br>Xerostomia<br>Depression<br>Life-threatening risk factors: conflict, life crises, major life changes, need for control and approval | Plan for referral and coordinated care with physicians, nutritionist, and psychologist<br>Carious or eroded teeth: restorations, margination of restorations<br>Anxiety: psychosedation<br>Pit-and-fissure sealants if appropriate<br>Study models to monitor progression of tooth structure loss | Rinsing with sodium bicarbonate after vomiting rather than using toothbrush<br>Neutral-pH sodium fluoride rinses or stannous fluoride gels used daily<br>Frequent continued-care intervals<br>For xerostomia, recommend a dry-mouth management protocol that includes saliva substitutes, ice chips and drinking water, daily use of xylitol-containing products, fluoride therapy, and calcium phosphate therapy<br>ADA-approved or CDA-recognized antimicrobial mouthrinse daily |
| Down syndrome | Possible congenital heart defect (prophylactic antibiotic premedication)<br>Hearing and vision problems<br>Decreased resistance to infection; frequent respiratory infections | Same as for developmental and cognitive challenges | Same as for intellectual and developmental disabilities | Same as for developmental and cognitive challenges plus small oral area: oral access for procedures<br>Hearing and vision disorders: communication<br>Avoid use of powered instruments with respiratory problems | Same as for developmental and cognitive challenges plus stress oral hygiene and periodontal maintenance care |
| Emotional disturbance or mental illness | Medications and potential side effects<br>Psychological causes of reported symptoms or diseases, fears | Limited financial resources in some cases<br>Emotional concerns and fears<br>Disturbed thought processes | Depends on nature of disturbance<br>Inadequate diet or strange food practices<br>Phobias about oral care<br>Self-abuse<br>Side effects of medications | Anxiety, fear, aggression: stability in chair, cooperation, communication, safety for patient and clinician | Reality orientation techniques<br>Possible dietary counseling<br>Involve caregivers<br>Positive reinforcement and repetition<br>For xerostomia, recommend a protocol that includes saliva substitutes, ice chips and drinking water, daily use of xylitol-containing products, fluoride therapy, and calcium phosphate therapy<br>ADA-approved or CDA-recognized antimicrobial mouthrinse daily |

| | | | | | |
|---|---|---|---|---|---|
| End-stage renal disease | Symptoms and severity<br>Hypertension<br>Dialysis?<br>Transplantation?<br>Special diets<br>Need for antibiotic premedication<br>Excretion of drugs<br>Electrolyte and fluid imbalance | Finding dentist who will treat<br>Debilitated condition at times<br>Limited finances<br>Fear of oral health care environment | Susceptibility to oral infection<br>Dietary inadequacies<br>Viral hepatitis<br>Drug-influenced gingival enlargement from cyclosporine | Nephrologist consult<br>Drug interactions<br>Hypertension and kidney failure: monitor vital signs, drug interactions; avoid use of drugs metabolized by the kidney<br>Bleeding tendency: preappointment blood tests, consult with patient's physician<br>Schedule dental treatment the day after dialysis<br>Atrioventricular fistula: consult physician for antibiotic premedication; take blood pressure in arm without fistula<br>Transplants: elective care postponed for 6 months posttransplant<br>Prophylactic antibiotic premedication: amoxicillin and metronidazole | 3- to 6-month continued-care interval because of increased calculus<br>Halitosis<br>Prevent infection<br>Palliative care for oral lesions<br>Daily home fluoride therapy<br>Tartar control dentifrices<br>Chlorhexidine mouthrinses |
| Fetal alcohol spectrum disorders (FASD), fetal alcohol syndrome (FAS) | Which organs affected?<br>Heart<br>Brain<br>Growth deficiency | Family may be dysfunctional<br>Behavioral problems<br>May have mental disabilities | Attention deficit disorders<br>Dental malformations | Behavior and attention: short, structured appointments<br>Family problems: ensure that follow-up care is understood<br>Compliment cooperative behavior | Ensure adequate supervision for oral hygiene care<br>Use same methods as for children with learning disabilities or developmental and cognitive challenges<br>ADA-approved or CDA-recognized antimicrobial mouthrinse daily based on level of cooperation |
| Fibromyalgia syndrome (FMS) | Biophysical issues, fatigue, sleep, depression, stress, cognitive impairments, comorbidities of migraines, Sjögren syndrome, cystitis, chronic fatigue | Muscle pain<br>Discomfort in supine position<br>Decreased platelet formation from large doses of NSAIDs | Side effects of medications<br>Comorbidities: depression, chronic facial muscle pain, migraines, irritable bowel syndrome, fatigue | May not be able to endure long appointments<br>Pain or fatigue in orofacial region limits opening; TMJ pain<br>Chair position: discomfort with supine position<br>Last-minute cancellations due to pain<br>Four-handed dentistry to promote efficacy in time<br>Stress-free appointment<br>Cervical pillows | Dietary counseling<br>Frequent continued care<br>Modified oral care devices<br>Written self-care instructions<br>Xerostomia management<br>Educate on difference between oral pain from FMS and oral disease pain |
| Hearing impairment | Degree of impairment<br>Use interpreter or other assistive devices<br>Functioning of hearing aid | Degree of dependence on others<br>Communication: sign language, lip reading, inaccurate pronunciation | No specific factors | Hearing impairment appointment scheduling,<br>Mobile devices for explanation of procedures<br>Use of normal tone of voice for lip reader, communication, data collection, noise interference, use of hearing aid during appointment<br>Many pretend to hear out of embarrassment<br>Remove mask when talking or use clear face shield because may be lip reader | Determine appropriate communication techniques<br>Provide paper and pencil/computer keyboard or mobile device if desired<br>Involve interpreter if needed<br>Watch facial expressions<br>Demonstrate when possible<br>Make word document with frequently used phrases<br>Use physical models for teaching<br>ADA-approved or CDA-recognized antimicrobial mouthrinse daily |

Continued

**TABLE 19.14 Dental Management Considerations for Patients With Special Needs—cont'd**

| Condition | Medical Issues | Barriers to Care | Other Associated Health Issues | Treatment Considerations[a] | Prevention/Education/Health Promotion Issues |
|---|---|---|---|---|---|
| Hypertensive disease | Vital sign monitoring<br>Physician consult or referral<br>Medications and side effects and other treatment regimens<br>Cause: primary or secondary<br>Predisposing or general risk factors<br>Severity, symptoms<br>Possibility of orthostatic hypotension | Anxiety about oral health care | Side effects of medications<br>Potential for stroke, myocardial infarction, and renal failure<br>Potential for adverse drug interactions between vasoconstrictors and antihypertensive drugs<br>Limit use of vasoconstrictor in anesthetics | Hypertension: stress management protocols, chair position, treatment planning, monitoring vital signs, short appointment<br>Overly stressed: terminate appointment<br>Medications: drug interactions<br>Minimize use of epinephrine; limiting epinephrine to 0.04 mg (two cartridges of 1:100,000 or four cartridges of 1:200,000 epinephrine) and levonordefrin to 0.2 mg<br>Bleeding potential, pain control, xerostomia, gingival enlargement<br>BP 180/110 mm Hg: delay treatment and refer to physician | Counseling regarding reducing general risk factors<br>Palliative care for oral infections from medications<br>For xerostomia, recommend a protocol that includes saliva substitutes, ice chips and drinking water, daily use of xylitol-containing products, fluoride therapy, and calcium phosphate therapy<br>Create stress-free environment<br>Prevent postural hypertension |
| Ischemic heart disease (coronary atherosclerotic heart disease) | Physician consult<br>Angina or myocardial infarction episodes<br>Hospitalizations<br>Medications and side effects<br>Surgery | Possible debilitated state<br>Medical and other expenses<br>Anxiety about dental treatment | Side effect of medications<br>Susceptibility to infections if debilitated<br>Limit use of vasoconstrictor in anesthetics | Heart condition: same considerations as for hypertensive disease and preparation for medical emergency, contraindications to treatment if unstable or recent attack (within 3 to 6 months)<br>Minimize use of epinephrine; limiting epinephrine to 0.04 mg (two cartridges of 1:100,000 or four cartridges of 1:200,000 epinephrine) and levonordefrin to 0.2 mg<br>Medications: same as for hypertensive disease; pain control<br>Aspirin use: bleeding concerns, INR less than 3.6 | Educate on link with periodontitis<br>Counseling on decreasing general risk factors<br>Frequent maintenance visits<br>Create stress-free environment<br>Educate about increased risk for myocardial infarction in patients with periodontitis<br>Antimicrobial mouthrinse daily |
| Learning disabilities, attention deficit hyperactivity disorder (ADHD) | Medications and potential side effects | Depends on type of disability | Depends on disability<br>Oral-motor dysfunction<br>General incoordination<br>Hyperactive behavior | Depends on disability<br>Disorientation/hyperactivity; stability in chair; short appointments; physical contact can be alarming<br>Minimize distractions | Focus on strengths<br>Use combination of teaching approaches<br>Maintain attention through eye contact and physical contact; involve caregiver<br>Consistency important |
| Leukemias | Type<br>Treatment regimens, frequency<br>Presence of anemia<br>Monitor bleeding time<br>Thrombocytopenia and infection<br>Immunosuppression from therapy | Stages of acute disease versus remissions<br>Fear of dental environment | Side effects of chemotherapy or radiation therapy<br>Candidiasis<br>Susceptibility to infections<br>Oral hemorrhage | Bleeding potential: platelet count status needed—avoid treatment if less than 50,000/mm$^3$<br>Appointment scheduling, physician consult, surgical procedures<br>Susceptibility to infections: periodontal maintenance, antibiotic premedication<br>Ideally, provide invasive care before chemotherapy or radiation therapy<br>Acute versus remission stages: treatment planning, appointment scheduling<br>Chemotherapy or radiation therapy: treatment planning<br>Consultation with oncologist | Palliative care for oral lesions<br>Frequent continued-care intervals<br>Fluoride therapy program<br>Involvement of others in care program<br>For xerostomia, recommend a dry-mouth management protocol that includes saliva substitutes, ice chips and drinking water, daily use of xylitol-containing products, fluoride therapy, and calcium phosphate therapy<br>Eliminate potential sources of oral infection<br>Meticulous oral hygiene<br>ADA-approved or CDA-recognized antimicrobial mouthrinse daily |

| | | | | | |
|---|---|---|---|---|---|
| Multiple sclerosis | Medications and side effects<br>Degree of facial pain<br>Degree of impairment<br>Sensitivity to heat | Mobility to and in office, especially if in wheelchair<br>Depression or moodiness<br>Limited finances if disabled | Special diets<br>Side effects of drugs<br>Fine motor coordination problems<br>Oral-motor dysfunction<br>Infection<br>Fatigue, stress, and pain | Weakness and numbness: wheelchair transfer, stability, Schedule appointment at time of day when patient feels best<br>Oral-motor dysfunction: protection of airway<br>Mood changes: communication, acceptance of treatment, cooperation<br>Sensitivity to heat: room temperature<br>Periods of exacerbation or remission: appointment scheduling | Oral care: adaptive equipment or assistance may be needed<br>Suggest weighted glove while brushing if have tremors in hand<br>More frequent rinsing and brushing<br>Fluoride therapy<br>Antimicrobial mouthrinse daily<br>More frequent continued-care intervals to prevent infections<br>Refer for TMD assessment<br>Importance of healthy periodontium: infection can cause exacerbation of multiple sclerosis |
| Muscular dystrophies | Medications<br>Other therapies<br>Type and degree of involvement<br>Prognosis<br>Obesity, scoliosis, or cardiopulmonary involvement? | Depends on type<br>Mobility to and in office, especially if in wheelchair<br>Limited financial resources<br>Weakness and possible decreased life span | Balance issues<br>Oral-motor dysfunction<br>General motor weakness and incoordination<br>Dietary inadequacies<br>Mouth breathing | Facial muscle weakness can interfere with appointment length and self-care<br>Depends on type and degree of involvement<br>Muscle weakness: stability in chair, wheelchair transfers, radiographs, instrumentation, appointment length<br>Oral-motor dysfunction: protection of airway, communication<br>Incoordination: restorative treatment planning and possible emergency care<br>Limited life span: treatment planning, motivation | Frequent continued care<br>More frequent brushing and rinsing<br>Fluoride therapy<br>ADA-approved or CDA-recognized antimicrobial mouthrinse daily<br>Adapted equipment or physical assistance for oral care<br>Powered oral hygiene aids |
| Myasthenia gravis | Medications<br>History of radiation therapy or surgery<br>History of myasthenic crises | Communication<br>Patient may hold chin to help during speaking | Oral-motor dysfunction<br>Choking risk myasthenia crisis from stress | Weakness increases during day: schedule short appointments in morning<br>Drug interaction<br>Amide types of local anesthetics used<br>Oral-motor dysfunction, paralysis, and impaired breathing: protection of airway, use of rubber dam, suctioning, chair position, mouth props<br>Difficulty retaining dentures<br>Be prepared for emergency<br>Avoid use of powered instruments | Frequent continued-care intervals to prevent infection<br>Frequent rinsing or toothbrushing for food retention<br>Fluoride therapy, if needed<br>Modified toothbrush or powered oral hygiene aids<br>ADA-approved or CDA-recognized antimicrobial mouthrinse daily |
| Older adult | Medications and potential side effects<br>Chronic diseases<br>Joint replacements<br>Sensory impairments<br>Reduced disease resistance | Transportation problems<br>Finances may be limited<br>Person may be depressed | Side effects of medications<br>Physical side effects of chronic diseases<br>Anatomical changes of gingiva | Identify side effects of medications<br>Sensory impairments<br>Short appointments in midmorning<br>Increased risk for root caries<br>Assess need for sodium fluoride therapy (home and in office)<br>Assess need for antibiotic premedication | Instruct person about oral cancer self-examination and risk factors<br>Instruct in oral hygiene and modifications of oral hygiene devices<br>For xerostomia, recommend a dry-mouth management protocol that includes saliva substitutes, ice chips and drinking water, daily use of xylitol-containing products, fluoride therapy, and calcium phosphate therapy<br>Make suggestions gradually<br>Antimicrobial mouthrinse daily |

Continued

**TABLE 19.14 Dental Management Considerations for Patients With Special Needs—cont'd**

| Condition | Medical Issues | Barriers to Care | Other Associated Health Issues | Treatment Considerations[a] | Prevention/Education/Health Promotion Issues |
|---|---|---|---|---|---|
| Pregnancy | Trimester<br>Side effects<br>Nutritional status<br>Rise in progesterone levels<br>Significant changes in the immune response | Frequent sickness<br>Physical comfort<br>Nausea and sensitivity to various odors | Possible dietary inadequacies Vulnerability of fetus during first trimester<br>Increased incidence of gingivitis | Fetal sensitivity: avoidance of drugs and elective dental procedures and elective x-ray films; use paralleling techniques for necessary exposures with lead apron on patients front and back<br>Chair position: orthostatic hypotension (turn on left side to alleviate pressure)<br>Safest period to provide routine care is second trimester<br>Short appointments<br>Caution with nitrous oxide; 30 minutes at 50% oxygen | Prenatal counseling<br>Optimal oral hygiene to decrease gingival inflammatory changes<br>Education on relationship among oral biofilm, hormone level, and periodontal disease<br>Education on increased risk for preterm and low-birth-weight delivery in patients who are pregnant and have periodontitis<br>Education on relationship between caries process and gastric acids from vomiting<br>Education on vertical and horizontal disease transmission, care of infant's oral cavity, and causes of early childhood caries (may need to initiate xylitol protocol)<br>Daily home fluoride therapy and sodium bicarbonate mouthrinses (before toothbrushing if episodes of vomiting)<br>Healthy diet<br>Antimicrobial mouthrinse daily |
| Parkinson's disease | Medications and side effects<br>Rigidity of larger muscles<br>Tremors<br>Sensitivity to heat | Mobility to and in office<br>Communication<br>Fall risk high | Oral-motor dysfunction<br>Side effects of drugs<br>Xerostomia<br>Possible inadequate diet<br>Hypersalivation | Tremors: stability, instrumentation, radiographs<br>Sensitivity to heat: temperature of operatory<br>Muscular pain and joint rigidity: chair position, appointment length<br>Slurred speech: communication<br>Schedule appointment when medication has optimal affect (usually 2 to 3 hours after taking)<br>COMT inhibitors have potential to interact adversely with epinephrine Should be limited to concentrations of 1:100,000 in. | Frequent continued care<br>Frequent rinsing and toothbrushing<br>Adaptive equipment or assistance if needed<br>Fluoride therapy<br>Antimicrobial mouthrinse daily |
| Rheumatic fever and heart disease | Residual effects of rheumatic fever | No specific barriers | Rheumatic fever<br>Pharyngeal infection with group A streptococci | Consult with cardiologist<br>Antimicrobial rinse before treatment<br>Stress importance of optimum oral health | Stress oral hygiene to prevent oral infections, self-induced bacteremias/infective endocarditis<br>Antimicrobial mouthrinse daily |
| Scleroderma | Extensive and often rapidly progressive skin indurations as well as involvement of multiple internal organ systems<br>Overall range of motion becomes highly compromised | Mobility<br>Problems with microstomia | May need premedication because of immunosuppressive therapies | Prone to oral disease<br>Early treatment intervention are important complications when implementing dental hygiene care<br>As disease worsens, more problems opening mouth<br>Swallowing problems; avoid powered instruments<br>Four-handed dentistry | Xerostomia management<br>Oral self-care modifications<br>Pediatric toothbrushes for small mouth opening<br>Oral irrigator<br>Frequent continued care<br>Oral stretching exercises |
| Seizure disorders | Medications and side effects<br>Drug induces leukopenia and thrombocytopenia<br>Seizure information<br>Type of disorder<br>Frequency and how well controlled<br>General management<br>History of status epilepticus | Disturbance in self-image<br>Transportation if cannot drive<br>Embarrassment | Side effects of medications<br>Potential for orofacial trauma during seizures | Seizure activity: precipitating factors, treatment planning, appointment scheduling, stability in chair, communication; stop procedures if seizure occurs<br>Avoid NSAIDs and aspirin<br>Replace missing teeth with fixed not removable appliances<br>Drug-influenced gingival enlargement from phenytoin<br>Prolonged bleeding time from valproic acid<br>Assess if medications are taken as prescribed | Optimal oral hygiene and frequent continued-care intervals to control gingival enlargement from phenytoin<br>First-aid instructions for oral trauma<br>Positive reinforcement and self-image building<br>Chlorhexidine mouthrinses or spray<br>For xerostomia, recommend a dry-mouth management protocol that includes saliva substitutes, ice chips and drinking water, daily use of xylitol-containing products, fluoride therapy, and calcium phosphate therapy |

| | | | | | |
|---|---|---|---|---|---|
| Sickle cell disease | Precipitating factors for crises<br>Symptoms and severity<br>Associated conditions<br>Transfusions?<br>Lab tests needed<br>Physician consult regarding need for antibiotic premedication | Periods of pain<br>Debilitated condition at times<br>Fear of dental environment<br>Limited financial resources because of medical bills | Susceptibility to infections<br>Low stress tolerance | Physician consult to determine if stable; Sickle cell crises: emergency care only<br>Susceptibility to infections: periodontal maintenance, physician consult for prophylactic antibiotic premedication<br>Reduce patient stress<br>Avoid medications that depress respiration<br>Limit epinephrine | Dietary counseling<br>Frequent maintenance care because of associated alveolar bone problems and need to control oral infection<br>Involvement of others in patient's care<br>Create a stress-free oral health care environment<br>Emphasis on optimal oral health care behaviors because periodontitis can cause a crisis<br>Antimicrobial mouthrinse daily |
| Spina bifida | Depends on type<br>Similar to spinal injuries<br>Shunt for hydrocephalus (consult physician for antibiotic premedication)<br>Seizure disorders | Depends on type and degree of impairment<br>Similar to spinal injuries<br>Mobility | Similar to spinal injuries, except oral-motor dysfunction not apparent<br>Pulmonary function<br>Craniosyntosis | Similar to spinal injuries, although psychological state not as poor<br>Early morning appointments<br>Latex sensitivity<br>Premedication; hydrocephalus and ventriculoatrial shunts | Learning disabilities influence dental health education methods<br>Powered oral hygiene aids |
| Spinal injuries | Depends on level of injury<br>Medications<br>Respiratory involvement<br>Decubitus ulcers<br>Incontinence and encopresis<br>Contractures<br>Heterotopic ossifications<br>Body temperature regulation<br>Potential for autonomic hyperreflexia<br>Type of adaptive equipment | Mobility to and in office, especially if in wheelchair or on respirator<br>Limited financial resources<br>Psychosocial concerns or depression<br>Poor self-image | Depends on level of injury<br>Oral-motor dysfunction<br>Limited or total dependence on others<br>Special diets | Psychological state: communication, cooperation<br>Spasticity, tremors: stability<br>Paralysis: mobility, wheelchair transfers, stability in chair, length of appointment, graphs<br>Impaired respiration and oral-motor dysfunction: chair position, use of rubber dam, protection of airway, instrumentation<br>Mouth stick appliance | Powered or adaptive equipment or physical assistance needed<br>Fluoride therapy<br>ADA-approved or CDA-recognized antimicrobial mouthrinse daily<br>Emphasize self-care to degree possible |
| Thyroid disease | Type and cause<br>Symptoms and severity<br>Medications<br>Cardiac arrhythmias/dysrhythmias | No specific barriers<br>Swelling of tongue in hypothyroidism may cause difficulty in speech communication | Abnormal dental development<br>Thyroid crisis is life threatening<br>Osteoporosis<br>Medication side effects | Sensitivity to drugs: treatment planning, postoperative instruction, preparation for medical emergency<br>Heat or cold intolerance: room temperature, length of appointment<br>"Thyroid storm" or thyroid crisis precipitated by surgery, infection, trauma, or uncontrolled thyroid disease<br>Exaggerated response to central nervous system depressants | Prevention of infection<br>ADA-approved or CDA-recognized antimicrobial mouthrinse daily<br>Create a stress-free environment |
| Visual impairment | Degree of impairment<br>Sensitivity to light<br>Treated versus untreated conditions | Degree of dependence on others<br>Attitudes and stereotypes about disability and toward guide dogs<br>Physical obstacles to or in office | Difficulty monitoring oral status | Determine level of assistance needed<br>Sight impairment: appointment scheduling, explanation of procedures, communication, positioning of light, mobility in clinic, data collection, noise level<br>Guide dog: role and placement in office<br>Use other senses to connect with patient | Large print with written instructions<br>Braille for oral hygiene pamphlets<br>Demonstrate procedures on finger<br>"Tell-show-do" approach<br>Precede actions with clear verbal descriptions<br>Have patient explore own mouth prior to oral hygiene instructions<br>Involve caregiver when necessary<br>Use audio aids or physical models for teaching<br>ADA-recognized or CDA-recognized antimicrobial mouthrinse daily |

*ADA,* American Dental Association; *CDA,* Canadian Dental Association; *NSAIDs,* nonsteroidal anti-inflammatory drugs; *TMJ,* temporomandibular joint; *TMD,* temporomandibular disorder; *INR,* international normalized ratio.

PatientpatientpatientpatientpatientpatientpatientpatientPatientpatientpatientpatientpatientpatientPatientpatient

[a]Standard precautions for infection control are used at each appointment.

Name________________________________ Telephone____________________

Address______________________________________________________ Age ______

Name and address of contact person (if different) Telephone ____________________

______________________________________________________________________

______________________________________________________________________

______________________________________________________________________

Physician ____________ Specialty ________________ Telephone ____________

Physician ____________ Specialty ________________ Telephone ____________

Medical problems or disabling conditions ______________________________

______________________________________________________________________

Potential barriers:

Transportation ________________________________________________________

Finances ______________________________________________________________

Communication _________________________________________________________

Psychosocial __________________________________________________________

Cultural ______________________________________________________________

Medical _______________________________________________________________

Mobility/stability _____________________________________________________

Other _________________________________________________________________

Scheduling limitations __________________________________________________

Other data ____________________________________________________________

**Fig. 19.23** Previsit questionnaire for gathering preliminary data about individuals with special needs.

7. Explain carefully any need for patient body restraint or stabilization for behavioral or stability purposes to ensure the clinician's safety and the patient's safety while in the chair; Velcro straps similar to safety belts are helpful for stability (Fig. 19.24); ensure the following:
   a. Pharmacologic restraints such as oral, intramuscular, intravenous, or inhalation sedation may be needed;
   b. general anesthesia is sometimes necessary when a patient is not easily stimulated or has partial or complete loss of protective reflexes
9. Be aware that adaptations for specific procedures require problem solving and experimentation among the provider, patient, and caregiver, if appropriate; Fig. 19.25 displays a variety of mouth props
10. Discuss the mechanisms for wheelchair transfers with each patient; preferences and techniques vary
11. Protect the patient's airway through use of a rubber dam, adequate suctioning, and other means; this is of paramount importance because of the frequency of impaired oral reflexes
12. Some pediatric patients' behavior may improve if they bring comfort items such as a stuffed animal or a blanket; asking the caregiver to sit nearby or hold the child's hand may be helpful as well
13. For the most part, keep appointments short and positive
14. Fluoride therapies (varnishes) and antimicrobial rinses are important preventive measures
15. Informed consent issues; patient versus caregiver
16. Stress the importance of good oral health being part of good general health
   a. Behavioral expectations
   b. Overview of the entire care plan
   c. Procedures that will be performed at the appointment
   d. Approximate time required
   e. Communication techniques to be used during the appointment
   f. Obtain informed consent to use these aids

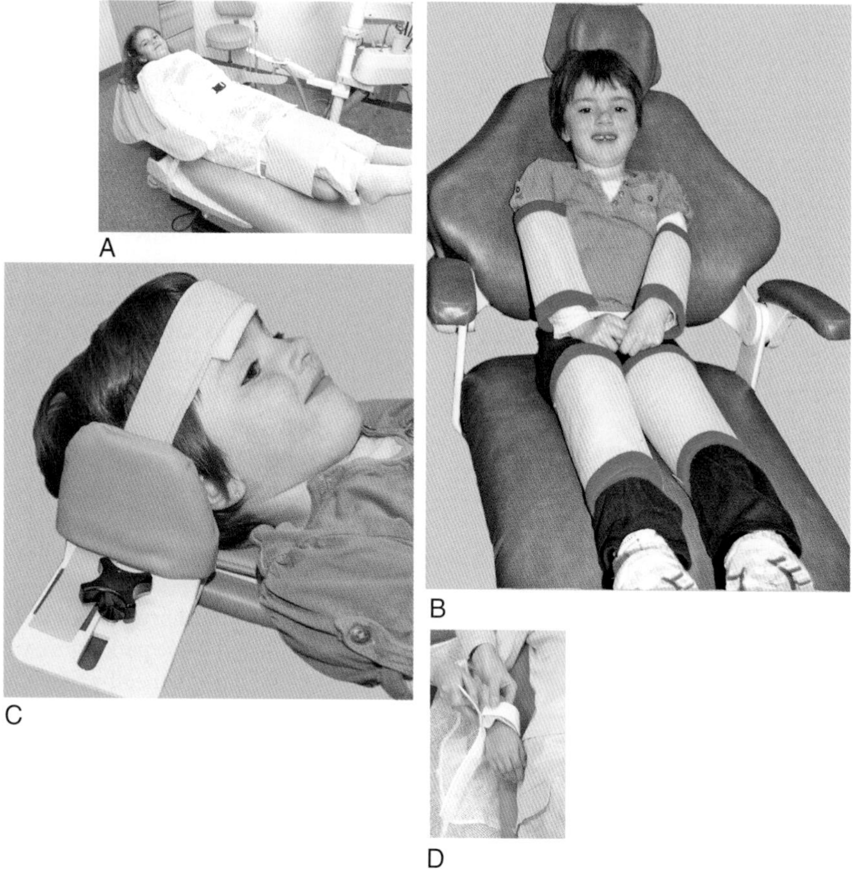


Fig. 19.24 The Rainbow Stabilizing System. (A) Adult on large hinged board. (B) Child with elbow and knee stabilizers that prohibit movement of joints. (C) Head stabilizer. (D) Safety belts for securing the patient safely in the dental chair. (Used with permission from Specialized Care, Hampton, NH.)

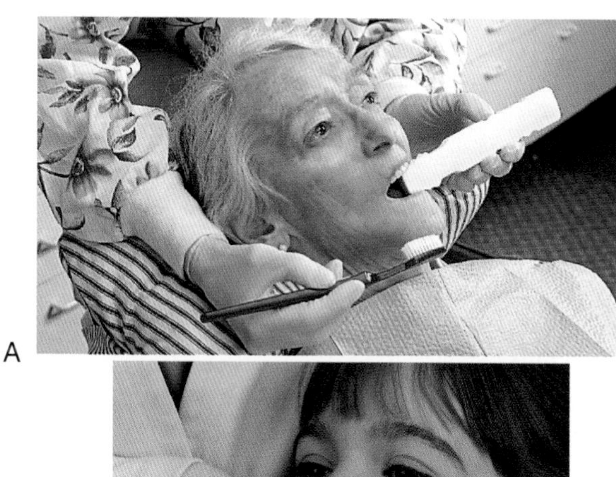

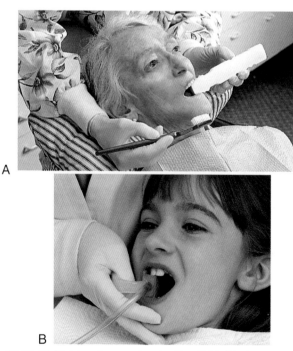


Fig. 19.25 (A) Clinician shown using the OpenWide Disposable Mouth Prop on an adult. (B) Clinician shown using the OpenWide Reusable Mouth Prop that allows for a saliva ejector to be kept in place with the bite block. (Used with permission from Specialized Care, Hampton, NH.)

g. Ensure least restrictive restraint is used
h. Clearly document restraint used
i. Check state regulations to ensure proper compliance

E. Preventive measures
1. Identify risk factors for oral disease to plan preventive programs that:
2. Develop individualized programs to reduce or eliminate the risk factors and increase the protective factors
3. Consider the patient's limitations when recommending home care procedures
4. Provide anticipatory guidance to parents on milestones and preventive measures at each developmental stage
5. Schedule frequent maintenance care appointments
6. Coordinate preventive efforts in the home, school, day care, workplace, or oral health care settings
7. Encourage the establishment of a dental home
   a. Maximize positive health behaviors
   b. Eliminate risk factors
   c. Eliminate existing disease
   d. Inappropriate nursing and feeding habits
   e. Transfer of oral pathogens from mother or caregiver to infant (vertical transmission); usually from sharing food and eating utensils; can also occur among siblings or playmates (horizontal transmission)
   f. Nutritionally inadequate diet
   g. Frequent intake of cariogenic foods

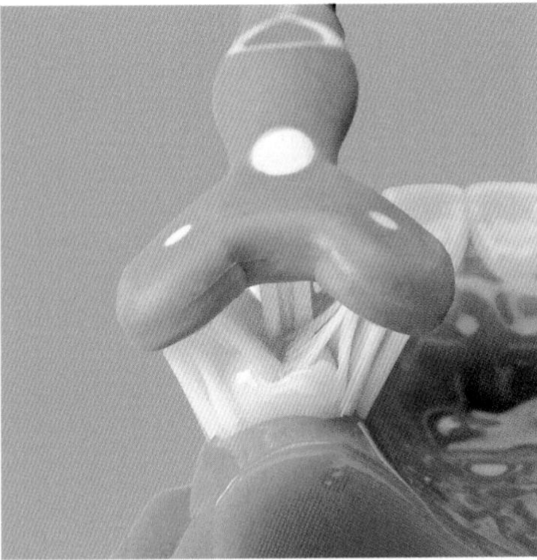

**Fig. 19.26** The Surround Toothbrush has a unique head that surrounds the tooth to clean all surfaces at the same time; ideal aid for caregiver brushing another person's teeth. (Used with permission from Specialized Care, Hampton, NH.)

h. Suboptimal fluoride supplementation
i. Oral-motor dysfunction (e.g., hyperactive gag reflex or impaired tongue control)
j. General motor dysfunction interfering with oral hygiene care
k. Crisis orientation to care
l. Preoccupation with one's disability; depression
m. Previous negative experience with health care
n. Limited income and education
o. Different cultural values and beliefs
p. Problems with fluoride or antimicrobial rinses or disclosing tablets if the patient has oral-motor problems
q. Problems performing the sequence of toothbrushing strokes if the patient has memory or general motor impairment; Fig. 19.26 displays a modified toothbrush for easier accessibility
r. Problems picking up and using a toothbrush and toothpaste if the patient has paralysis or control problems
s. Power toothbrushing and flossing devices can work well, but some patients may respond poorly since they can be frightened by the noise

## WEBSITE INFORMATION AND RESOURCES

| Source | Website Address | Description |
|---|---|---|
| American Academy of Pediatric Dentistry | http://www.aapd.org | Information, education, policies, and guidelines on working with all children, including those with special care needs |
| National Maternal and Child Oral Health Resource Center | http://www.mchoralhealth.org/ | Information on working with children with disabilities |
| National Institute of Dental and Craniofacial Research | http://www.nidcr.nih.gov/health-info | Information, education, and strategies on providing care to patients with special care needs |
| National Institute of Neurological Disorders and Stroke | http://www.ninds.nih.gov | Health information and resources for patients and professionals related to a wide variety of neurologic disorders |
| Special Care Dentistry Association | https://www.scdaonline.org/ | Support related to education on a large range of special care conditions |
| University of Washington; School of Dentistry; Patients with Special Needs | http://dental.washington.edu/oral-medicine/special-needs/patients-with-special-needs/ | Health and dental information for caregivers and professionals related to patients with special care needs |

## CHAPTER 19 REVIEW QUESTIONS

1. The seizure type characterized by purposeless, repetitive movement with a transient clouding of consciousness is termed:
   **a.** Complex partial
   **b.** Generalized absence
   **c.** Generalized tonic-clonic
   **d.** Atonic
2. Each is a common intra oral finding associated with Down syndrome EXCEPT one. Which one is the *exception*?
   **a.** Eyes wider apart than normal
   **b.** Enamel dysplasia
   **c.** Delayed tooth eruption
   **d.** Crossbite
3. The type of hearing loss caused from injury interfering with organs that conduct sound waves through the middle or outer is:
   **a.** Otitis media
   **b.** Presbycusis
   **c.** Mastoiditis
   **d.** Conductive
4. An autoimmune diseases that involve the hardening and tightening of the collagen of the skin and connective tissue defines:
   **a.** Parkinson's disease
   **b.** Scleroderma
   **c.** Trigeminal neuralgia
   **d.** Cerebral palsy
5. Drug-influenced gingival enlargement is often associated with which of the following antiseizure medications?
   **a.** Carbamazepine (Tegretol)
   **b.** Valproic acid (Depakote)

c. Topiramate (Topamax)
d. Phenytoin (Dilantin)

6. Which of the following is an autoimmune neuromuscular disease caused by variable weakness of voluntary muscles?
   a. Myasthenia gravis
   b. Spina bifida
   c. Fibromyalgia
   d. Multiple sclerosis
7. Which of the following is an internal barrier to physical facilities for the person with a disabling condition?
   a. Bathroom with grab-bars by the commode
   b. 28-inch-wide doorways
   c. Nonslip floors
   d. Door with lever-type handles
8. Each of the following is a common oral manifestation in the patient with Down syndrome except one. Which one is the exception?
   a. Delayed eruption patterns
   b. Small tooth crowns with short crown/root ratio
   c. Enamel dysplasia
   d. Low palatal vault
9. Each of the following conditions may cause retention of food and bolus formation except one. Which is the exception?
   a. Myasthenia gravis
   b. Cerebral palsy
   c. Stroke
   d. Fibromyalgia
10. A latex allergy is common in patients with:
   a. Parkinson's disease
   b. Spina bifida
   c. Congenital heart disease
   d. Hypothyroidism
11. Air polishing devices would be *contraindicated* for use in patients with all the following conditions EXCEPT:
   a. Myasthenia gravis
   b. Cystic fibrosis
   c. Seizure disorder
   d. Emphysema
12. A patient with a recent myocardial infarction should postpose elective dental hygiene treatment for:
   a. 2 months
   b. 3 months
   c. 4 months
   d. 6 months
13. The first symptoms of myasthenia gravis usually cause eye weakness and double vision. The disease most commonly affects men in their twenties.
   a. Both statements are TRUE
   b. Both statements are FALSE
   c. The first statement is TRUE; the second statement is FALSE
   d. The first statement is FALSE; the second statement is TRUE
14. Which of the following is the most common classification of cerebral palsy?
   a. Ataxia
   b. Spasticity
   c. Athetosis
   d. Hypotonia
15. Rinse of lidocaine, Benadryl, Maalox, and nystatin, termed "magic rinse," is recommended for symptom treatment of what condition associated with cancer therapy?
   a. Radiation caries
   b. Osteoradionecrosis
   c. Mucositis
   d. Xerostomia
16. Antibiotic premedication would be indicated before dental hygiene treatment for the patient with a history of
   a. Generalized tonic-clonic seizures
   b. Infective endocarditis
   c. Angioplasty and stent placement
   d. Chronic obstructive pulmonary disease (COPD)
17. Lidocaine as a local anesthetic agent is contraindicated in patients with coronary heart disease because the epinephrine found with the lidocaine will predispose the patient to another myocardial infarction.
   a. Both parts of the statement are TRUE
   b. Both parts of the statement are FALSE
   c. The first part of the statement is TRUE, but the second part is FALSE
   d. The first part of the statement is FALSE, but the second part is TRUE
18. In case a patient has an opioid overdose which drug should be used to counteract the effects of the opioid?
   a. Tramadol HCL
   b. Naloxone
   c. Pseudoephedrine
   d. Naproxone
19. Which of the following drugs can be safely used to manage dental pain in a pregnant patient?
   a. Acetaminophen
   b. Naproxen
   c. Ibuprofen
   d. Aspirin
20. A patient on kidney dialysis should have dental hygiene care 4 hours after dialysis treatment since the heparin has reached a threshold of safety.
   a. Both parts of the statement are TRUE
   b. Both parts of the statement are FALSE
   c. The first part of the statement is TRUE, but the second part is FALSE
   d. The first part of the statement is FALSE, but the second part is TRUE
21. An alcoholic patient may have increased bleeding after scaling and root debridement because of:
   a. Chronic swelling of glands
   b. Endocrine imbalances

c. Decreased white blood cell count
d. Pancytopenia

22. Each of the following are hard tissue changes associated with aging EXCEPT one. Which is the EXCEPTION?
a. Root caries
b. Increased tooth sensitivity
c. Dark color of teeth
d. Decreased pulp chamber size

23. Drug-influenced gingival enlargement is commonly associated with all of the following conditions EXCEPT one. Which is the EXCEPTION?
a. Epilepsy/seizure disorder
b. Cerebral palsy
c. Hypertension
d. Bulimia

24. Which condition presents with increased susceptibility for severe aggressive periodontitis?
a. Scleroderma
b. Down syndrome
c. Autism spectrum disorder
d. Myasthenia gravis

25. Radiographically, which condition commonly presents with a ground-glass appearance?
a. Sickle cell disease
b. Parkinson's disease
c. Leukemia
d. Thyroid disease

26. An ultrasonic scaler is typically contraindicated in a patient with
a. Diabetes
b. Cerebral palsy
c. Thyroid disorder
d. Hypertension

27. Which condition is associated with a lower dental caries rate and dental biofilm accumulation with increased calculus?
a. Congenital heart disease
b. Chronic obstructive pulmonary disease
c. Cystic fibrosis
d. Congestive heart failure

28. Common conditions associated with cerebral palsy include all of the following EXCEPT one. Which is the EXCEPTION?
a. Speech and language disorders
b. Seizures
c. Hearing disorders
d. Heart defects

29. Which one of the following is a medical emergency most likely to occur in a patient with diabetes mellitus?
a. Hypoglycemia
b. Anaphylaxis
c. Hyperglycemia
d. Seizure

30. All the following conditions may complicate the patient's ability to perform oral self-care EXCEPT:
a. Scleroderma
b. Parkinson's disease
c. Arthritis
d. Hypothyroidism

31. A powered scaling device would be contraindicated in patients with
a. Hypertensive disease
b. Cystic fibrosis
c. HIV infection
d. Coronary heart disease

32. A chronic immunologic disease in which joint inflammation occurs during periods of remission and exacerbation defines:
a. Tubular sclerosis
b. Graves' disease
c. Rheumatoid arthritis
d. Progressive systemic sclerosis

33. The high incidence of dental caries found in patients with cognitive impairments is likely due to:
a. Oral neglect
b. Swallowing problems
c. Genetic defects
d. Abnormal eruption patterns

34. In which of the following conditions would mouth opening be a potential problem for oral hygiene implementation?
a. Cystic fibrosis
b. Scleroderma
c. Myelomeningocele
d. Addison disease

35. A dental hygiene patient with which condition would need antibiotic premedication prior to scaling?
a. Fibromyalgia
b. Artificial heart valve
c. Chronic obstructive pulmonary disease (COPD)
d. Angioplasty and stent placement

# CASE A

| **SYNOPSIS OF PATIENT HISTORY CASE A** | Age: *35* | **VITAL SIGNS:** |
|---|---|---|
| | Sex: *female* | Blood Pressure: *180/90* |
| | Height: *5 feet 3 inches* | Pulse Rate: *60 bpm* |
| | Weight: *265 pounds* | Respiration Rate: *18 rpm* |

**Chief complaint:**
*My teeth hurt and my gums bleed*

**Medical History**
Under care of a physician: Yes ☒ No ☐

Condition(s):
*epilepsy*
*Seasonal allergy*

Has or had the following conditions:
*Mild mental impairment*
*Cerebral palsy; spastic*
*Hearing impairment*

Current Medications:
*Dilantin 30 mg (Phenytoin)*
*Niravam 5 mg (alprazolam)*
*Zyrtex (Cetirizine HCl) 10 mg*
*Celexa (Citalopram) 5 mg*

1. Smokes or uses tobacco products: Yes ☐ No ☒

**Dental History:**
*Patients' dental visit have been limited; mainly emergency care with extractions. Patient has no memory of having their teeth cleaned or ever receiving self care instructions*

**Social History:**
*Patient lives in a group home with 5 other adults with mental impairments. She works in a sheltered workshop sorting small tools and screws. She wears hearing aids in both ears.*

**Adult clinical examination**

Maxillary – Facial

| | 1 | 2 | 3 | 4 | 5 | 6 | 7 | 8 | 9 | 10 | 11 | 12 | 13 | 14 | 15 | 16 |
|---|---|---|---|---|---|---|---|---|---|---|---|---|---|---|---|---|
| Probe 2 | | | | | | | | | | | | | | | | |
| Probe 1 | X | X | 436 | 535 | 545 | 344 | 434 | 323 | 434 | 343 | 443 | 345 | 524 | 655 | 645 | X |

R

Maxillary – Palatal

| | 1 | 2 | 3 | 4 | 5 | 6 | 7 | 8 | 9 | 10 | 11 | 12 | 13 | 14 | 15 | 16 |
|---|---|---|---|---|---|---|---|---|---|---|---|---|---|---|---|---|
| Probe 1 | X | X | 545 | 654 | 645 | 454 | 434 | 434 | 434 | 434 | 444 | 554 | 645 | 565 | 545 | X |
| Probe 2 | | | | | | | | | | | | | | | | |

Mandibular – Lingual

| | 32 | 31 | 30 | 29 | 28 | 27 | 26 | 25 | 24 | 23 | 22 | 21 | 20 | 19 | 18 | 17 |
|---|---|---|---|---|---|---|---|---|---|---|---|---|---|---|---|---|
| Probe 2 | | | | | | | | | | | | | | | | |
| Probe 1 | X | X | 747 | 747 | 545 | 535 | 434 | 424 | 444 | 444 | 324 | 434 | 545 | 745 | 646 | X |

R

Mandibular – Facial

| | 32 | 31 | 30 | 29 | 28 | 27 | 26 | 25 | 24 | 23 | 22 | 21 | 20 | 19 | 18 | 17 |
|---|---|---|---|---|---|---|---|---|---|---|---|---|---|---|---|---|
| Probe 1 | X | X | 545 | 324 | 545 | 545 | 434 | 434 | 444 | 444 | 456 | 535 | 426 | 635 | 635 | X |
| Probe 2 | | | | | | | | | | | | | | | | |

**CURRENT ORAL HYGIENE STATUS:**
*Generalized bleeding; heavy subgingival calculus*

**SUPPLEMENTAL ORAL EXAMINATION FINDINGS:**
*Mandibular facial anterior areas of 24 and 22 exhibits 4 mm of facial recession*

Clinically visible caries

Clinically missing tooth

△ Furcation

▲ "Through and through" furcation

*Continued*

## CASE A—cont'd

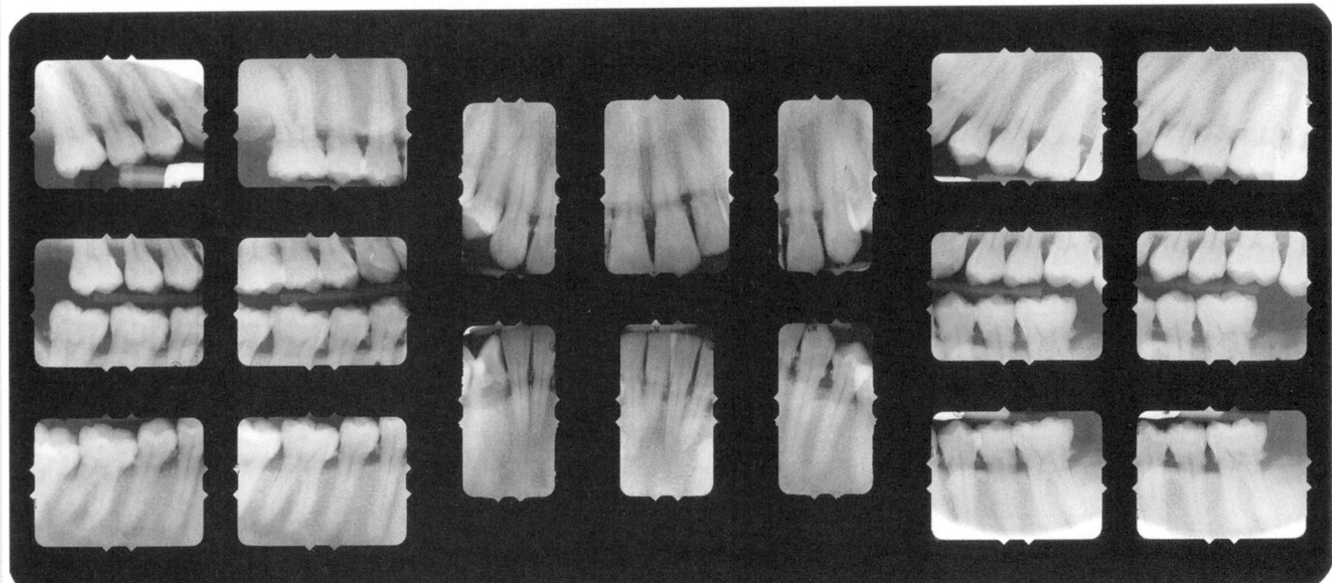

**Fig. 19.27** Full-mouth series.

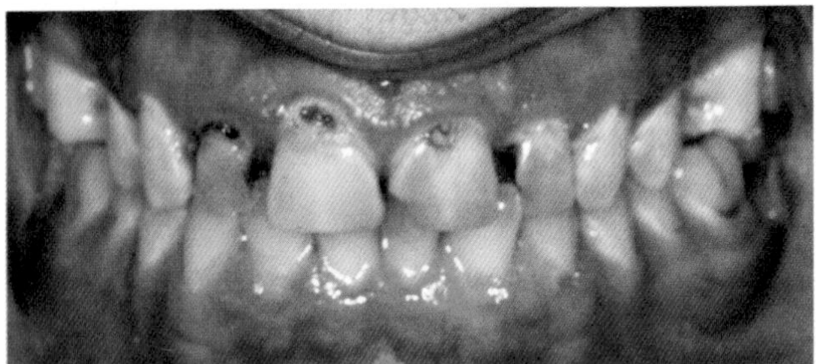

**Fig 19.28** Maxillary anterior teeth.

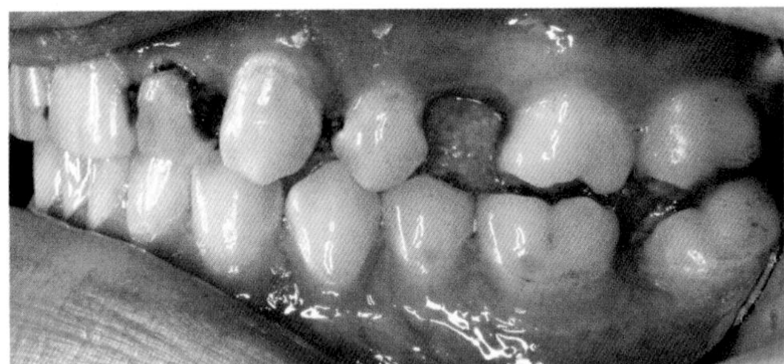

**Fig 19.29** Left lateral teeth.

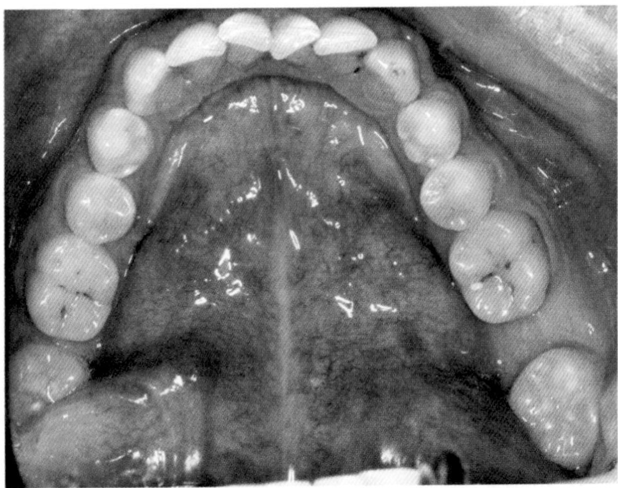

**Fig. 19.30** Mandibular lingual teeth.

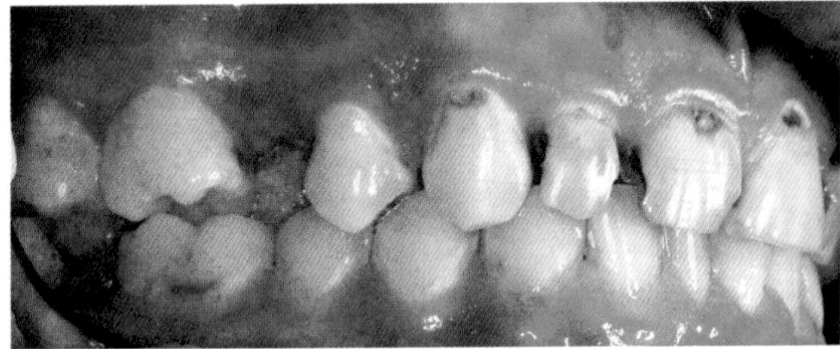

**Fig. 19.31** Right lateral teeth.

## CASE A—cont'd

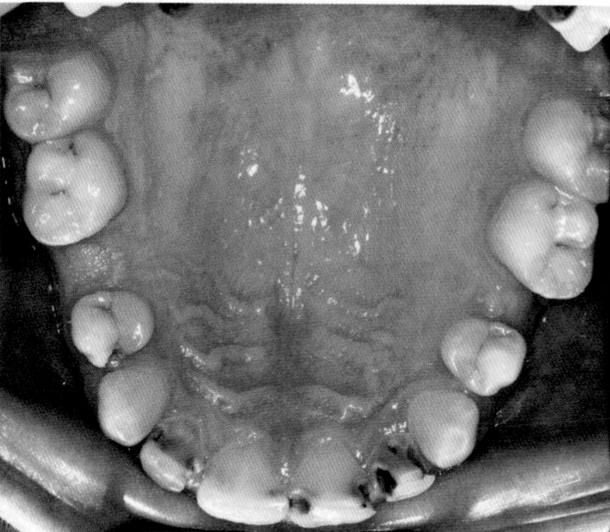

**Fig. 19.32** Maxillary lingual teeth.

Use Case A and Figs. 19.27 through 19.32 to answer questions 36 to 43.

**36.** What G.V. Black classification of caries is found on the facial of tooth #9?
   **a.** Class I
   **b.** Class II
   **c.** Class V
   **d.** Class VI

**37.** A physical restraint might be recommended for safety reason for this patient. Which of the conditions might be a cause for this?
   **a.** Seizures
   **b.** Cerebral palsy spastic
   **c.** Mental impairment
   **d.** Hearing impairment

**38.** As you are working on the patient, she displays a blank, staring look and is nonresponsive for about 30 seconds, but quickly returns to normal. What type of seizure is she experiencing?
   **a.** Generalized tonic-clonic
   **b.** Myoclonic
   **c.** Generalized absence
   **d.** Simple motor partial

**39.** Each of the following would be important when working with this patient with hearing aids except one. Which one is the exception?
   **a.** Exaggerate pronunciations
   **b.** Remove the operator mask during speaking and communication
   **c.** Have patient turn off hearing aids during ultrasonic scaling
   **d.** Turn to the patient when speaking

**40.** What is the technique error associated with the left premolar periapical radiograph?
   **a.** Beam-indicating device alignment
   **b.** Incorrect placement of film-holding device
   **c.** Incorrect KVP setting
   **d.** Incorrect vertical angulation

**41.** All of the following are acceptable approaches for teaching this patient oral self-care EXCEPT:
   **a.** "Show-tell-do" approach
   **b.** Explanation of bone loss using radiographs
   **c.** Demonstration of proper use of disclosing tablets
   **d.** Use of powered toothbrushing techniques

**42.** Which of the following oral rinses would the patient MOST benefit from?
   **a.** Chlorhexidine
   **b.** Povidone-iodine
   **c.** Phenolic-related essential
   **d.** Sodium fluoride

**43.** Which of the patients medications would be a risk factor for drug influenced gingival enlargement?
   **a.** Niravam
   **b.** Zyrtec
   **c.** Dilantin
   **d.** Celexa

## CASE B

| SYNOPSIS OF PATIENT HISTORY CASE B | | VITAL SIGNS: | |
|---|---|---|---|
| Age: | 45 | Blood Pressure: | 170/90 |
| Sex: | male | Pulse Rate: | 60 bpm |
| Height: | 5 feet 8 inches | Respiration Rate: | 16 rpm |
| Weight: | 300 pounds | | |

**Chief complaint:**
*I need my teeth cleaned but I am having issues with keeping my mouth open*

**Dental History:**
*Patients' recent dental visits have been limited; no longer working and lost dental insurance*

**Medical History**
Under care of a physician: Yes ☒ No ☐

Condition(s):
*Type 2 diabetes; HBa1c of 7.5*
*hypertension*
*hyperlipidemia*

Has or had the following conditions:
*Prosthetic heart valve placed as an infant*
*Knee replacement 6 years ago*
*Fibromyalgia*

Current Medications:
*Procardia (Nifedipine)*
*Lipitor (atorvastatin)*
*Metformin (Glucophage)*
*Lyrica (Pregabalin)*

**Social History:**
*Patient lives with his daughter and is on disability; reports drinking 6 to 8 beers nightly*

1. Smokes or uses tobacco products: Yes ☐ No ☒

**Adult clinical examination**

| | 1 | 2 | 3 | 4 | 5 | 6 | 7 | 8 | 9 | 10 | 11 | 12 | 13 | 14 | 15 | 16 |
|---|---|---|---|---|---|---|---|---|---|---|---|---|---|---|---|---|
| Probe 2 (Facial) | | | | | | | | | | | | | | | | |
| Probe 1 (Facial) | 434 | 434 | 423 | X | 324 | 233 | 323 | 323 | 323 | 323 | 424 | 233 | X | 434 | 524 | 535 |
| Probe 1 (Palatal) | 424 | 425 | 425 | X | 424 | 323 | 232 | 323 | 233 | 323 | 323 | 323 | X | 435 | 424 | 535 |
| Probe 2 (Palatal) | | | | | | | | | | | | | | | | |

R

| | 32 | 31 | 30 | 29 | 28 | 27 | 26 | 25 | 24 | 23 | 22 | 21 | 20 | 19 | 18 | 17 |
|---|---|---|---|---|---|---|---|---|---|---|---|---|---|---|---|---|
| Probe 2 (Lingual) | | | | | | | | | | | | | | | | |
| Probe 1 (Lingual) | 525 | X | 525 | 424 | 423 | 324 | 423 | 323 | 222 | 232 | 323 | 423 | 324 | 525 | X | 434 |
| Probe 1 (Facial) | 434 | X | 525 | 424 | 324 | 323 | 323 | 323 | 323 | 323 | 232 | 234 | 323 | 545 | X | 525 |
| Probe 2 (Facial) | | | | | | | | | | | | | | | | |

R

**CURRENT ORAL HYGIENE STATUS:**
*Heavy biofilm; generalized bleeding on probing; moderate calculus*

**SUPPLEMENTAL ORAL EXAMINATION FINDINGS:**
*1 and 16; partially erupted*

Clinically visible caries need to draw in caries on mesial 6 and mesial, facial and distal of 7,8,9,10,11 and mesial of 12

Clinically missing tooth draw in missing teeth

△ Furcation

▲ "Through and through" furcation

## CASE B—cont'd

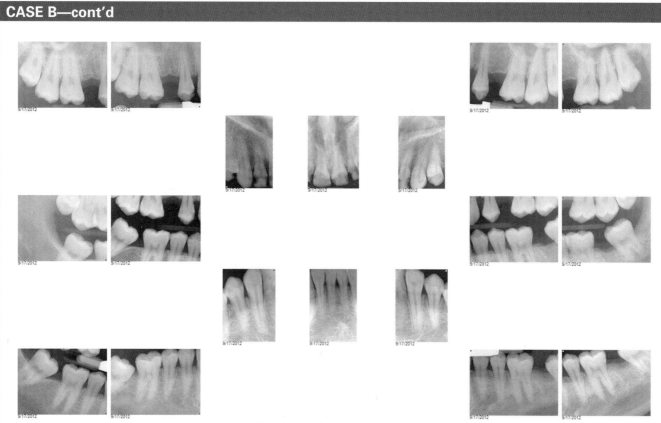

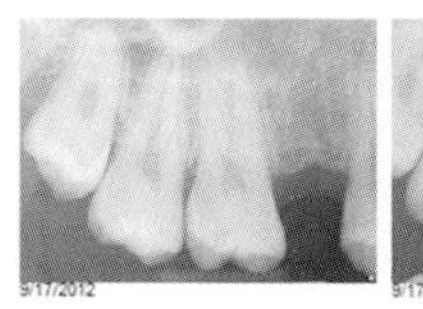
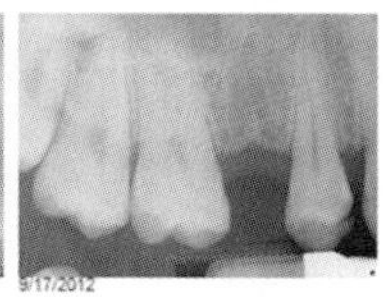
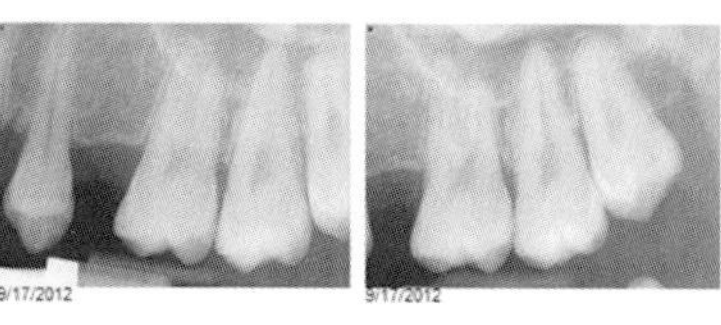
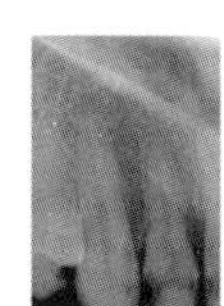
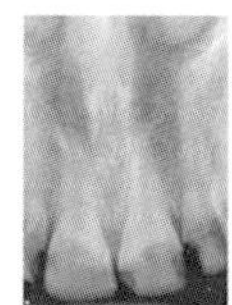
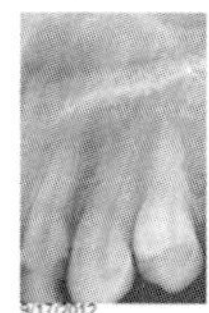
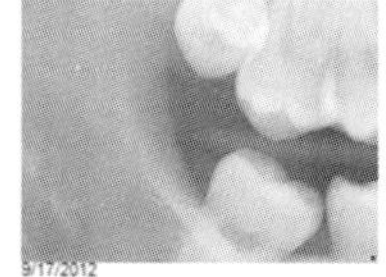
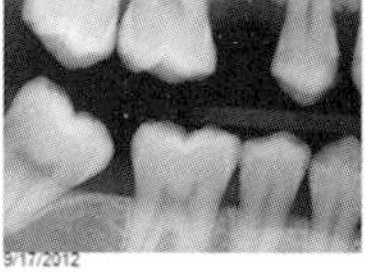
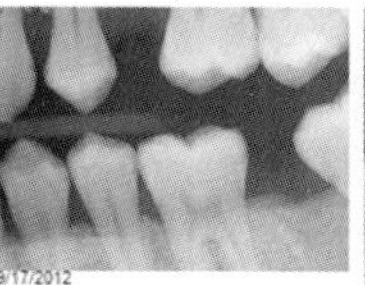
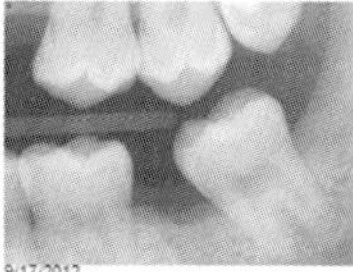
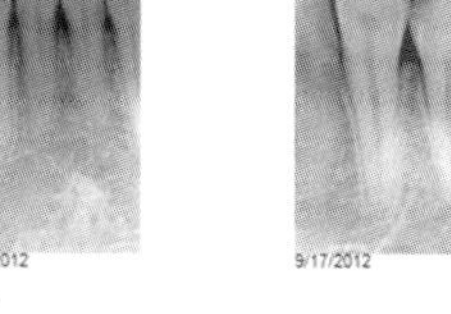
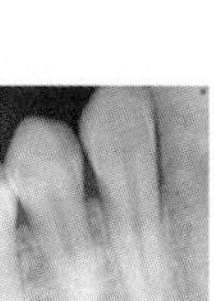
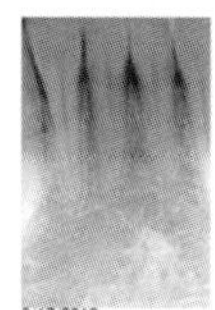
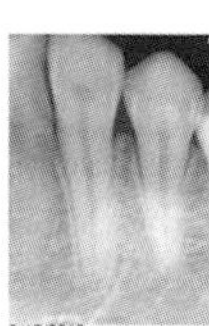
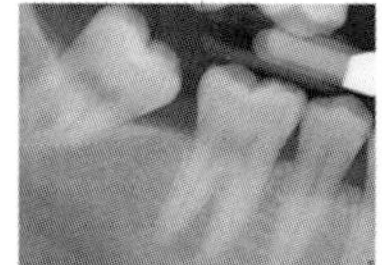
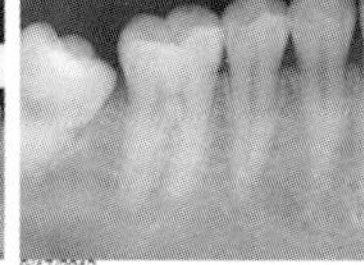
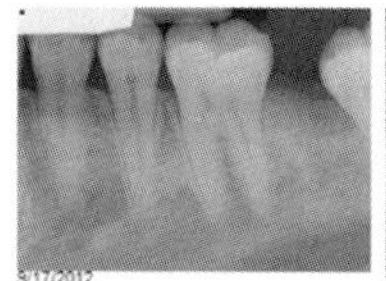
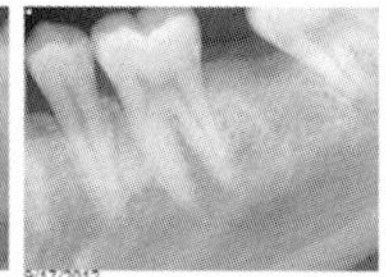

**Fig. 19.33** Full mouth radiographs.

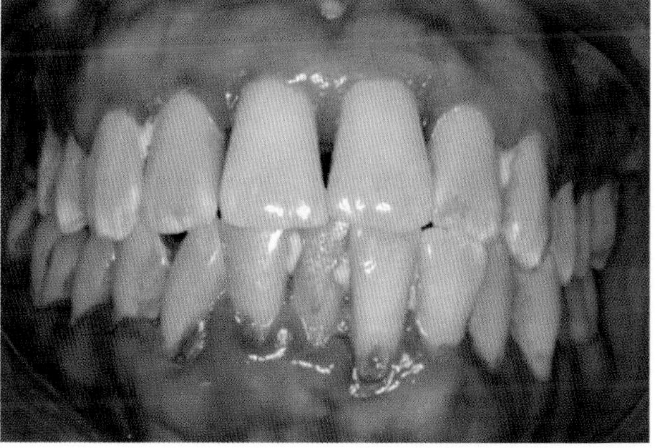

**Fig. 19.34** Anterior teeth.

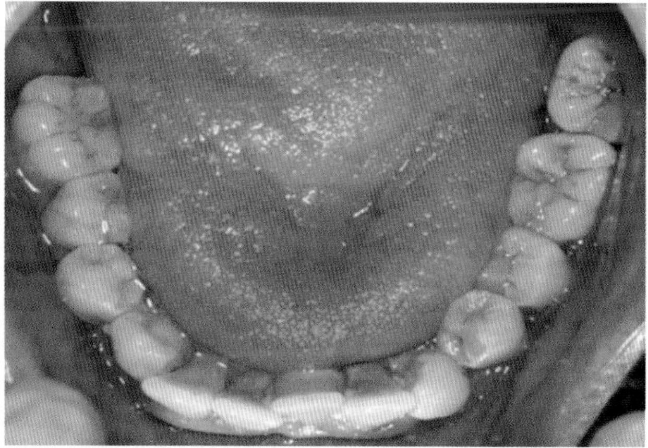

**Fig. 19.35** Lingual teeth.

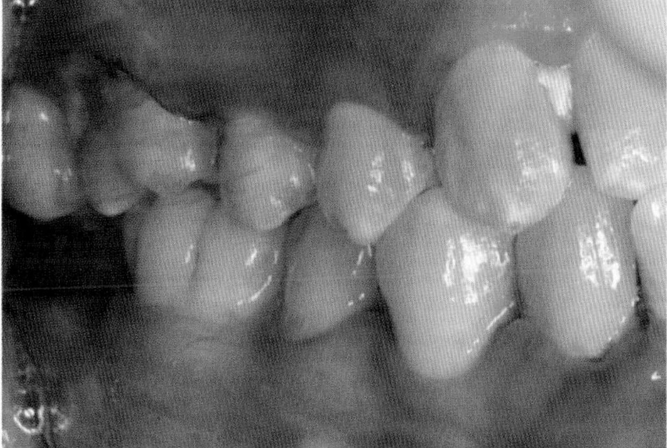

**Fig. 19.36** Right lateral teeth.

*Continued*

CASE B—cont'd

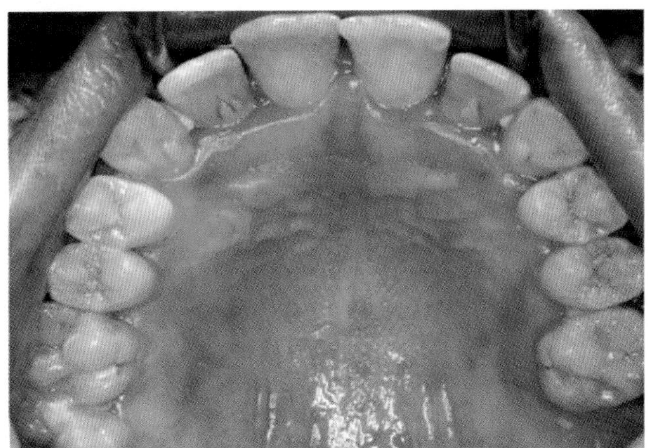

**Fig. 19.37** Maxillary lingual teeth.

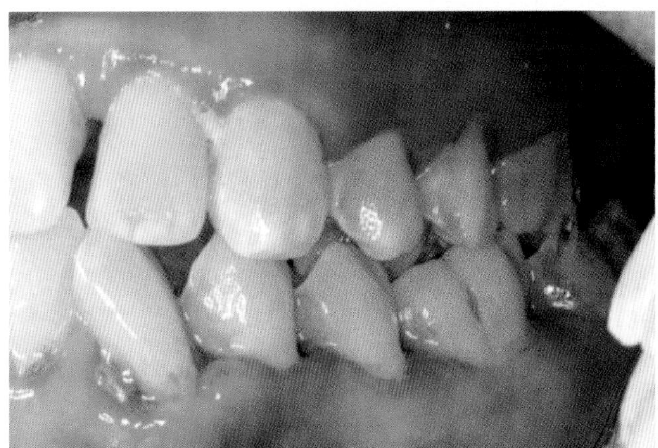

**Fig. 19.38** Left lateral teeth.

Use Case B and Figs. 19.33 through 19.38 to answer questions 44 to 50.

**44.** In which blood pressure category would this patient's reading today be classified?
- **a.** Normal
- **b.** Elevated
- **c.** Stage 1
- **d.** Stage 2

**45.** The apices of the roots are not present on the maxillary right molar view. What is the most likely cause of this error?
- **a.** Incorrect placement of film-holding device
- **b.** Too much horizontal angulation
- **c.** Too little vertical angulation
- **d.** Incorrect KVP causing shadowing

**46.** Which of the patient's conditions is a risk factor for his periodontal disease?
- **a.** Fibromyalgia
- **b.** Hypertension
- **c.** Weight
- **d.** Prosthetic heart valve

**47.** Which of the following medications is the patient taking to help manage the symptoms of fibromyalgia?
- **a.** Metformin
- **b.** Lyrica
- **c.** Procardia
- **d.** Lipitor

**48.** The patient's chief complaint of having jaw-opening problems is most likely related to which of his medical conditions?
- **a.** Diabetes
- **b.** Hyperlipidemia
- **c.** Fibromyalgia syndrome
- **d.** Obesity

**49.** This patient needs premedication. Which of his conditions is the reason?
- **a.** Prosthetic heart valve
- **b.** Hyperlipidemia
- **c.** Hypertension
- **d.** Diabetes

**50.** Which of the following embrasure types best describes the interdental area between teeth #8 and #9? Type
- **a.** I
- **b.** II
- **c.** III
- **d.** IV

Answers and rationales to review questions are available on this text's accompanying Evolve site. See inside front cover for details.

## SUGGESTED READINGS


Alumran A, Almulhim J, Almolhim B, et al. Preparedness and willingness of dental care providers to treat patients with special needs. *Clin Cosmet Investig Dent*. 2018;10:231–236.

Chavez E, Wong L, Suber P, et al. Dental care for geriatrics and special needs populations. *Dent Clin*. 2018;62(2):245–267.

Little JW, Falace DA. *Little and Falace's Dental Management of the Medically Compromised Patient*. 9th ed. St. Louis: Elsevier; 2017.

M. Clinic. Diseases and Conditions. http://www.mayoclinic.org. Accessed 01.25.19.

Moore T. Dental care for patients with special needs. *Decisions in Dentistry*. 2016;2(09):50–53.

National Oral Health Information Clearinghouse. Practical Oral Care for People with Developmental Disabilities. Making a Difference Series. NIH Pub No 04-5193.

New York State GPR Special Care Training Modules; https://www.scdaonline.org/page/EducationModules#:~:text=New%20York%20State%20GPR%20Special%20Care%20Training%20Modules,of%20dental%20treatment%20for%20people%20with%20special%20needs. Accessed Jan 24, 2019.

Odell EW. *Cawson's Essentials of Oral Pathology and Oral Medicine*. 9th ed. Philadelphia: Elsevier; 2017.

20

# Community Oral Health Planning and Practice

*Christine French Beatty*

Assessment, diagnosis, planning, implementation, and evaluation—the dental hygiene process of care—are used in community oral health practice, program development, and outcomes assessment. Community health extends the role of the dental hygienist from a traditional health care setting to the community as a whole. In a sense, the community can be viewed as the patient and the oral care environment as the neighborhood health center, extended care facility, hospital, school, agency, or even country. One of the characteristics of community health is the use of a team approach. Concerns for the oral health of the population has renewed an interest in expanding the roles and responsibilities of dental hygienists in order to increase access to oral health care for underinsured and underserved individuals and groups. Expanding roles in community-based care settings require that the dental hygienist possess the knowledge and skills of public health program development, research and epidemiologic methods, prevention and control of oral diseases, provision and financing of oral health care, and adaptation of care and programs to diverse populations.

## BASIC CONCEPTS

A. Health—community health practice requires a broad view of health that includes the following:
   1. Complete physical, mental, and social well-being; not just the absence of disease or infirmity
   2. Anatomical, physiologic, and psychological integrity
   3. Ability to perform personally valued family, work, and community roles to achieve individual and society goals
   4. Ability to deal with physical, biologic, psychological, and social stress
   5. Freedom from the risk of disease and untimely death
   6. Extent to which an individual or a group is able to realize aspirations and satisfy needs and to change or cope with the environment
   7. Emphasis on social and personal resources as well as physical capabilities

B. Oral health—status of the oral cavity, encompassing all features, normal and abnormal, of the oral, dental, and craniofacial complex

C. Wellness—a dynamic process in which the individual is actively engaged in moving toward fulfillment of his or her human needs and potential; it reflects the following:
   1. A change in the perceptions of health and wellness from the medical model of health care that is treatment oriented
   2. A prevention preference that focuses on the determinants of health and examines the relationships among the host, agent, environment, and preventive strategies
   3. A health promotion orientation aimed at creating an environment that enables individuals to increase control over and improve current and future health status

D. Determinants of health—consist of social and economic factors, the physical environment, the person's individual characteristics and behaviors, availability of health care services, and health care policy; greater emphasis is being placed on impacting social and economic determinants of oral health to increase access to dental care
   1. Many determinants are nonmodifiable
   2. Risk factors are modifiable determinants that can be changed through education, preventive therapies, public health policies, and modifications in the structure of health care delivery

E. Public health—the combination of sciences, skills, and beliefs directed at maintaining and improving the health of all persons by preventing disease, improving the quality of life, and promoting physical and mental health through collective or social actions in the community; characteristics include a collaborative approach, preventing rather than curing disease, dealing with population health rather than individual health, social responsibility for oral health, use of epidemiology and a multifactorial approach to controlling and preventing disease, and application of biostatistics
   1. Aggregate health of a group, community, state, nation, or group of nations
   2. Seen as people's health
   3. Concerned with four broad areas:
      a. Lifestyle, behavior, and culture
      b. Environment
      c. Human biology
      d. Organization of health programs and systems

F. Dental public health—science and art of preventing and controlling oral diseases and promoting oral health through organized community efforts; the form of dental practice that serves the community rather than the individual as the patient; concerned with oral health education of the public, applied dental research, and administration of group oral

**TABLE 20.1 Comparison of Private Dental Practice and Community Oral Health Practice**

| Private Dental Practice | Community Oral Health Practice[a] |
|---|---|
| Individual is the patient | Community group is the patient |
| Assessment of patient's dental, health, pharmacologic, and sociocultural history and oral health status | Survey of community oral health status; situation analysis including assessment of population demographics, culture, mobility, economic resources, and infrastructure |
| Diagnosis of patient's oral health needs | Analysis of survey data to determine the oral health needs of the population |
| Treatment plan based on diagnosis, professional judgment, patient's needs, and priorities | Program plan based on data analysis, community priorities, and resources available |
| Treatment plan initiated; primary dentist may coordinate treatment with other providers (e.g., dental hygienists, specialists) | Program operation implemented by varied, sometimes interdisciplinary, personnel |
| Payment methods determined | Financing throughout process; funds from government (local, state, and federal), philanthropic and/or community agencies |
| Evaluation during treatment, at specific intervals, on completion of treatment, or at all these times | Ongoing and varied evaluation and appraisal conducted in terms of effectiveness, efficiency, appropriateness, and adequacy |
| Documentation of treatment throughout | Report of program outcomes to stakeholders |

[a]Education occurs at all levels to facilitate anticipated outcomes.

health care programs, as well as prevention and control of oral diseases on a community basis; the application of public health and all its characteristics to oral health

G. Community—any group with common traits, shared features, or communal experiences; not strictly defined by traditional geographic boundaries; as broad as a region or a state or as focused as a specific institution or agency, such as a nursing home community, including administrators, staff, residents, and caregivers
H. Community health—generally synonymous with *public health*; full range of health services, environmental and personal, including major activities such as health education of the public and the social context of life as it affects the health of the community; efforts that are organized to promote and restore the health and quality of life of the people; uses a population-based approach for identifying and addressing community-based problems
I. Community oral health—services directed toward developing, reinforcing, and enhancing the oral health status of people, either as individuals or as groups and communities for the purpose of enhancing the oral health of the population
J. Comparison of private oral health care practice to community oral health care practice—the focus of community health is on the population rather than on any individual patient, yet similarities exist between the two in the steps of the process of care (Table 20.1)
K. Access—an individual's or group's ability to obtain appropriate health care services
L. Prevention—primary focus of community oral health is prevention; the wellness model focuses educational and behavioral efforts and programs toward prevention of disease and maintenance of an optimum state of well-being; three levels of prevention:
   1. Primary—prevention of disease before it occurs; for example, placement of dental sealants
   2. Secondary—early disease control, including early identification and prompt treatment before the individual is aware of a problem; for example, restoration of caries identified through a routine dental examination
   3. Tertiary—provision of services that prevent further disability; for example, replacing missing teeth with a partial denture
M. A public health problem is one that meets the following criteria:
   1. Burden of the disease or condition
   2. Prevalence of a risk factor for the disease or condition
   3. Ability of affecting the population as a whole
   4. Seriousness of the problem
   5. Economic or social impact
   6. Public health concern
   7. Political will to address the issue
   8. Availability of resources
   9. Requirement for group action to solve the problem
   10. Availability of current interventions
   11. Cultural appropriateness of the problem
   12. Degree to which it negatively affects *health equity* (attainment of the highest level of health for all people)
N. Public health solution—a solution to a public health problem that is directed to the community at large; preventive strategies possess as many characteristics of an ideal public health solution as possible (Box 20.1)
O. Core functions of public health—nationally identified; form the foundation of all community health activities
   1. Assessment—regular and systematic collection, assembling, and analysis of data related to the health of the population and making the data available for use by

**BOX 20.1 Characteristics of an Ideal Public Health Solution**

1. Safe; not hazardous to life or function
2. Effective in reducing or preventing a targeted disease, condition, or practice
3. Easily and efficiently implemented; minimum compliance required
4. Potency maintained for a substantial time period
5. Attainable regardless of socioeconomic status (SES)
6. Effective immediately upon application
7. Affordable, cost-effective, and within the means of a community

Data from Beatty CF. People's health. In Beatty CF: *Community Oral Health Practice for the Dental Hygienist.* 4th ed. St Louis: Elsevier; 2017: 1–17.

various agencies; for example, oral disease data collected through the National Oral Health Surveillance System

2. Policy development—development of comprehensive public health policies based on scientific evidence; for example, adoption of Healthy People (HP) objectives and the Public Health Service (PHS) recommendations for water fluoridation
3. Assurance—provision of services necessary to achieve agreed-on health goals related to improving the health of the public; for example, provision of services and programs that are publicly funded

P. Governmental levels of public health—each level provides various services, meets different needs of the population, and supports the functions of other levels; for example, the federal departments support state agencies, and local programs are often funded by grants or contracts from the state or federal levels

1. Local—responsible for direct administration of educational resources, preventive care, and patient care programs
2. State—consultation to the local level and other agencies; channels federal and state funds such as Medicaid and Children's Health Insurance Program (CHIP); coordinates programs throughout the state; conducts programs in rural areas that do not have local public health agencies
3. Federal—numerous national public health government agencies are involved in public health issues of national significance; Box 20.2 describes significant agencies and organizations that act as a resource for community programming
4. International—the World Health Organization (WHO) is the best-known and largest international health agency; primarily serves developing countries but also monitors health conditions and establishes programs to coordinate health care throughout the world; the Pan-American Health Organization (PAHO) is the regional office of WHO for the Americas

Q. Key national documents relevant to community oral health programming—classic documents continue to provide a basis to prioritize programs and target specific population groups; newer documents update the vision and strategies for implementation with a broader focus within the medical community; the documents complement each other as they categorize population oral health needs, priorities, and strategies and stress the importance of improving access to oral health care and reducing oral health disparities in the population; based on the three core public health functions of assessment, policy development, and assurance; exemplify public health practice and highlight important achievement in oral health in the United States in the past 20 years

1. See Box 20.3 for significant, relevant past, recent, and future documents
2. HP—a comprehensive list of science-based, 10-year national disease prevention and health promotion objectives in various health topic areas designed to improve the health of all Americans
   a. HP objectives are revised each decade based on outcomes from the previous decade
   b. Developed by a federal interagency workgroup led by the US Department of Health and Human Services (DHHS) with input from various health organizations
   c. Current objectives establish the health agenda for the United States and provide priorities for community programming for the current decade; developmental objectives may be included that as yet have no baseline data source

### BOX 20.2 Federal Governmental Agencies of Interest in Community Oral Health

*Administration for Children and Families* (ACF)—manages the Head Start (HS) program that funds local HS programs that educationally prepare qualified at-risk preschool age children for entry into school.

*Agency for Healthcare Research and Quality* (AHRQ)—supports research to improve the quality of health care, reduce its costs, address patient safety and medical errors, and increase access to care.

*Centers for Disease Control and Prevention* (CDC)—provides expertise, information, tools, and community collaboration to assist agencies with community programming; formulates recommendations for evidence-based practice (e.g., infection control and use of fluoride varnish); develops educational programs for local implementation (e.g., tobacco cessation); provides surveillance data (e.g., water fluoridation); and operates the online Water Fluoridation Reporting System and My Water's Fluoride.

*Centers for Medicare and Medicaid Services* (CMS)—provides oversight for Medicare, the federal portion of Medicaid, the Children's Health Insurance Program (CHIP), and the Health Insurance Marketplace.

*Department of Agriculture* (USDA)—administers the Women, Infants, and Children (WIC) program. Local WIC programs provide nutritional foods, education, screening, and referrals, including for dental care, for eligible women who are pregnant, are breastfeeding, or have young children under age 5 years.

*Department of Defense* (DoD) and *Veterans Administration* (VA)—provide direct care for specific armed services populations.

*Food and Drug Administration* (FDA)—enforces laws to ensure the safety and effectiveness of drugs, biologic products, and medical devices (includes dental).

*Health Resources and Services Administration* (HRSA)—primary agency for improving access to health care for people who are uninsured, isolated, or medically vulnerable through various means, including funding community and school-based health centers, strengthening the health care workforce, building healthy communities, and achieving health equity.

*Indian Health Service* (IHS)—provides direct patient care and community health programming for Native American and Alaska Native populations, with opportunity for maximum tribal involvement in developing and managing the programs.

*National Institutes of Health* (NIH)—conducts epidemiologic research, provides science transfer, and publishes and distributes educational materials. Several institutes are relevant to oral health, such as National Institute of Dental and Craniofacial Research (NIDCR), National Cancer Institute (NCI), and National Institute on Aging (NIA).

*Public Health Service* (PHS)—the primary operating division of the US Department of Health and Human Services (DHHS), responsible for the protection and advancement of the American population's health and safety. Various agencies and programs (e.g., AHRQ, CDC, FDA, HRSA, IHS, NIH) provide activities to advance public health science; provide rapid, effective response to public health crises; and promote leadership and excellence in public health practices. Goals are carried out by the Commissioned Core of health officers led by the Surgeon General, who also staff federal clinics (e.g., in federal prisons, Indian Health Service programs, and some armed services).

Data from Beatty CF. People's health. In Beatty CF: *Community Oral Health Practice for the Dental Hygienist*. 4th ed. St Louis: Elsevier; 2017: 1–17.

## BOX 20.3 Significant Federal Oral Health Initiatives in the United States Since 2000

**Key Points of the Surgeon General's Report *Oral Health in America* (2000)**

- Oral health is essential to general health and well-being.
- General health factors (e.g., tobacco use, diabetes) affect oral health.
- Oral health can be achieved by all Americans.
- Profound and consequential oral health disparities exist.
- Dental public health programs are needed.

**Principle Actions and Implementation Strategies Charged by A National Call to Action to Promote Oral Health (2003)**

- Take specific actions toward optimal oral health.
- Educate the public to change perceptions about oral health.
- Build the science and accelerate the transfer of the science.
- Increase collaborations (partnerships, coalitions).
- Increase workforce diversity, capacity, and flexibility.
- Overcome barriers by replicating effective programs.

**Promoting and Enhancing the Oral Health of the Public: HHS Oral Health Initiative 2010**

- Developed as a coordinated effort of multiple DHHS agencies in response to the realization that many oral health challenges of the 1990's had not been addressed successfully.
- Key message: oral health is integral to overall health.
- Purpose: to improve the nation's oral health by realigning existing resources and creating new activities to maximize outputs.

***Goals:***

- Emphasize oral health promotion and disease prevention.
- Increase access to care.
- Enhance the oral health workforce.
- Eliminate oral health disparities.

***Strategies:***

- Partnership of Office of Head Start and American Academy of Pediatric Dentistry to develop an infrastructure to recruit and support dentists to serve as dental homes for the underserved.
- Collaboration of NIDCR, CDC's DOH, and CDC's National Center for Health Statistics to enhance oral health surveillance.
- Endeavor of the CMS to increase access to dental care in state Medicaid programs by identifying and sharing best practices used successfully by some of these programs.
- Affiliation of DHHS and HRSA administrators to increase the visibility of existing DHHS oral health activities and improve awareness of oral health services available to the public.
- Collaboration of the National Research Council, the Institute of Medicine, the Board on Children, Youth and Families, and the Board on Health Care Services to develop a report on access of vulnerable and underserved groups to oral health care.
- Implementation and expansion of a multidisciplinary Early Childhood Caries Initiative by the IHS Division of Oral Health to promote prevention and early intervention of dental caries in young children by involving other agencies and community partners.
- Support and promotion by NIH of the building of a web-accessible national dental consortium research infrastructure network to facilitate the standardization of dental research.
- Launching of a new Cultural Competency E-Learning Oral Health Continuing Education Program by the Office of Minority Health to target oral health disparities.
- Incorporation of accurate oral health information into educational programs and highlighting of regional oral health activities by the Office on Women's Health to change the perception of the impact of oral health on overall health.

**Advancing Oral Health in America (2011)**

- Described the continuation of the problems of oral disease status and disparities.
- Reinforced the link of oral diseases to complications with medical diseases and conditions.

***Recommendations:***

- Establish high-level accountability.
- Emphasize disease prevention and oral health promotion.
- Improve oral health literacy and cultural competence.
- Reduce oral health disparities.
- Explore new models for payment and delivery of care.
- Enhance the role of nondental health care professionals.
- Expand oral health research and improve data collection.
- Promote collaboration among private and public stakeholders.
- Measure progress toward goals and objectives.
- Advance Healthy People goals and objectives.

**Improving Access to Oral Health Care for Vulnerable and Underserved Populations (2011)**

- Highlighted the problem of oral health disparities.
- Suggested strategies to improve access to oral health care for those who need it the most.

***Recommendations:***

- Integrate oral health care into overall health care.
- Change laws and regulations such as scope of practice.
- Improve dental education in relation to treating diverse populations in various settings.
- Reduce financial and administrative barriers to care.
- Expand capacity of the oral health care system.

**Outcomes of Integration of Oral Health and Primary Care Practice (2014)**

- Developed core clinical oral health competencies for use by primary care medical practitioners to increase oral health care access for safety net populations.
- Designed an infrastructure, payment policies, and evaluation strategies to implement the core clinical oral health competencies in primary care medical practices.

**Reforming America's Healthcare System Through Choice and Competition (2018)**

***Goals:***

- Increase access to care, especially in underserved areas.
- Reduce cost of care.

***Recommendations:***

- Expand scope of practice and eliminate rigid collaborative practice and supervision requirements for dental hygienists and midlevel providers.

*Continued*

**BOX 20.3 Significant Federal Oral Health Initiatives in the United States Since 2000—cont'd**

- Allow direct payment for services to dental hygienists and midlevel providers by private and public insurance carriers and through health reimbursement arrangements for dental benefits.
- Evaluate success of the dental therapy profession relative to increasing access to dental care and reducing costs while still ensuring safe, effective care.
- Consider ways to improve license portability to facilitate movement across state lines and provide interstate telehealth services.

**2020 Surgeon General's Report on Oral Health—commissioned by DHHS in 2018; due to publish in 2020**

***Goals:***
- Present prominent issues affecting oral health.
- Document progress in oral health in the 20 years since the 2000 Surgeon General's Report on Oral Health.
- Identify existing knowledge gaps and articulate a vision for the future.

Data from Department of Health and Human Services, National Institute of Dental and Craniofacial Research: *Oral health in America: A report of the Surgeon General*, Rockville, MD; 2000, https://www.nidcr.nih.gov/research/data-statistics/surgeon-general; Office of the Surgeon General. *A national call to action to promote oral health.* Bethesda, MD: National Institute of Dental and Craniofacial Research, Publication No. 03-5303, ; 2003. https://www.ncbi.nlm.nih.gov/books/NBK47472/; Department of Health and Human Resources: *Promoting and enhancing the oral health of the public: HHS oral health initiative*, 2010, Washington, D.C.; 2010. https://www.hrsa.gov/sites/default/files/oralhealth/hhsinitiative.pdf; Institute of Medicine of the National Academies, Committee on an Oral Health Initiative. *Advancing Oral Health in America*, Washington, D.C.: National Academies Press; 2011. http://www.hrsa.gov/publichealth/clinical/oralhealth/advancingoralhealth.pdf; Institute of Medicine, National Research Council. *Improving access to oral health care for vulnerable and underserved populations.* Washington, D.C.: National Academies Press; 2011. https://www.hrsa.gov/sites/default/files/publichealth/clinical/oralhealth/improvingaccess.pdf; Health Resources and Services Administration. *Integration of oral health and primary care practice.* Rockville, MD, 2014. https://www.hrsa.gov/sites/default/files/hrsa/oralhealth/integrationoforalhealth.pdf; Department of Health and Human Services, Department of the Treasury, Department of Labor. *Reforming America's healthcare system through choice and competition.* Washington, D.C.; December 2018. https://www.hhs.gov/sites/default/files/Reforming-Americas-Healthcare-System-Through-Choice-and-Competition.pdf; Department of Health and Human Services, National Institutes of Health. Notice to announce commission of a Surgeon General's Report on oral health. *Federal Register* 83(145), 35774, Notices; July 27, 2018. https://www.govinfo.gov/content/pkg/FR-2018-07-27/pdf/2018-16096.pdf.

d. HP 2030—provides the health agenda for the decade 2020–2029
   (1) Overarching goals have been established:
      (a) Attain healthy, thriving lives and well-being, free of preventable disease, disability, injury, and premature death
      (b) Eliminate health disparities, achieve health equity, and attain health literacy (Table 20.2) to improve the health and well-being of all
      (c) Create social, physical, and economic environments that promote attaining full potential for health and well-being for all
      (d) Promote healthy development, healthy behaviors and well-being across all life stages
      (e) Engage leadership, key constituents, and the public across multiple sectors to take action and design policies that improve the health and well-being of all
   (2) HP 2030 oral conditions objectives (see Table 20.3)
      (a) Oral conditions are one of the topics by which HP 2030 objectives are organized
      (b) Consists of objectives that represent the health topics oral health (OH), access to health services (AHS), and Nutrition and Weight Status (NWS)
      (c) Some objectives in other HP topics, such as cancer, older adults, tobacco use, and vaccination also relate to oral health (can be viewed on the HP 2030 website at https://health.gov/healthypeople)

R. Roles of the dental hygienist reflect various activities in public health; all should be based on sound scientific information (evidence-based practice [EBP]):
   1. Clinician—provides direct patient care
   2. Educator—uses valid educational theories to present scientific information to individuals and groups to prevent disease and promote oral health
   3. Advocate—promotes change and advances the health of the public through legislation and public policy
   4. Researcher—determines which procedures, products, and programs most effectively promote oral health and prevent disease, and communicates those findings
   5. Administrator—administers and manages programs aimed at promoting oral health
   6. Entrepreneur—creates new enterprises to serve the needs of vulnerable, underserved populations

## EPIDEMIOLOGY

A. Definitions
   1. Epidemiology (Box 20.4)
   2. Applied epidemiology—the application or practice of epidemiology to address public health issues
B. Uses of epidemiology (Box 20.5)
C. Characteristics of epidemiology
   1. Groups rather than individuals are studied
   2. A multifactorial approach is used to study disease (multiple causation); modifiable risk factors are controlled to prevent or influence the disease or condition

**BOX 20.4 Definition of Epidemiology**

Epidemiology is derived from three Greek root words:
- *epi*: upon or among—"upon the body; among the people"
- *demos*: people or district—"demographics"
- *ology*: a branch of knowledge—"the study of"
   1. A branch of medical science that deals with the incidence, distribution, and control of disease in a population
   2. The sum of the factors controlling the presence or absence of a disease or pathogen
   3. The study of the distribution and determinants of disease frequency
   4. Characterized by the use of statistical and research methods to compare groups or defined populations

Data from Dictionary.com, 2019, https://www.dictionary.com/browse/.

**TABLE 20.2 Health Literacy**

| Health literacy: "The degree to which individuals have the capacity to obtain, process, and understand basic health information and services needed to make appropriate health decisions." | |
|---|---|
| What is health literacy?[a] | Health literacy is more than just knowledge about health topics; health literacy involves being able to:<br>- Find health information and health services and process the meaning and usefulness of the information and services<br>- Navigate the health care system, including filling out complex forms, locating providers and services, and making appointments<br>- Share personal information with providers, such as health history and current medications<br>- Engage in self-care and management of chronic disease<br>- Understand mathematical concepts such as probability and risk<br>- Apply numeracy skills such as calculating blood sugar levels, reading nutritional labels, and computing deductibles and copays |
| Why is health literacy important? | Low health literacy is associated with:<br>- Poor health outcomes<br>- Less frequent utilization of preventive services<br>- Higher hospitalization rates<br>- Lower rates of having health insurance<br>- Higher overall health care costs<br>Almost two-thirds of the US population have inadequate health literacy |
| Who is at risk for low health literacy? | Low health literacy is most frequently seen in individuals who are:<br>- Older adults<br>- Racial and ethnic minorities<br>- Less educated, specifically less than a high school diploma or GED; those with lower general literacy and numeracy skills<br>- In lower SES categories<br>- Nonnative English speakers<br>- Medically compromised<br>- Education, language, culture, access to resources, age, and general literacy and numeracy skills are all factors that affect a person's health literacy skills. |
| How is health literacy increased? | Health professionals need to develop skills to:<br>- Understand how to provide useful information and services<br>- Consider which information and services work best for different situations and people so they can act<br>- Use plain language to communicate health information<br>- Convey information in the patient's or client's primary language, using a translator when needed<br>- Verify understanding of what people are explicitly and implicitly asking<br>- Take time to check a patient's or client's recall and comprehension of new concepts<br>- Provide assistance in learning basic numerical skills such as calculating dosages or understanding concepts such as risk<br>- Aid people in finding providers and services and filling out complex forms |

[a]A new definition of health literacy has been proposed for Healthy People 2030 based on research that has shown the need to broaden the definition to include the systems and contexts that can influence a person's health literacy.

Data from *Centers for Disease Control and Prevention.* Health literacy basics. http://www.cdc.gov/healthliteracy/. Accessed 04.25.19 and *Centers for Disease Control and Prevention.* Healthy People 2030 proposes redefining health literacy. https://www.cdc.gov/healthliteracy/healthy-people-2030.html. Accessed 06.26.19.

3. Determinants—risk factors or events that are capable of bringing about a change in health; the various factors that make up the multifactorial approach to a disease or health condition
4. Epidemiologic triad (epidemiologic triangle)—the traditional model of infection or disease causation used to study the occurrence and distribution of disease; includes a susceptible host, an external agent (etiologic agent), an environment that brings the host and agent together so that disease occurs, and a time dimension required for disease to occur; the ongoing interaction among these factors affects disease or health status (Fig. 20.1)
5. Burden of disease—cumulative effect of a broad range of harmful disease consequences on a community; includes the full scope of the health, social, and economic effects of disease
6. Preventive intervention—a strategy to eliminate risk factors and reduce the occurrence of disease

D. General epidemiology concepts—ideas that must be grasped to comprehend epidemiology (Table 20.4)

E. Concepts related to measurement of disease and its distribution
   1. General measurement concepts (Table 20.5)
   2. Surveillance/monitoring
      a. Surveillance—ongoing, constant, systematic observation; use of repeated surveys to analyze and evaluate health data to monitor changes in populations related to disease, conditions, injuries, disabilities, or death trends, for the purpose of program planning; essential feature of epidemiology

**TABLE 20.3 Healthy People 2030 Oral Conditions Objectives**

| Number | Objective | Baseline | Target | Data Sources |
|---|---|---|---|---|
| OH-1 | Reduce the proportion of children and adolescents with lifetime tooth decay experience in their primary or permanent teeth (ages 3–19 years) | 48.4% | 42.9% | National Health and Nutrition Examination Survey (NHANES), Centers for Disease Control and Prevention (CDC)/National Center for Health Statistics (NCHS) |
| OH-2 | Reduce the proportion of children and adolescents with active and currently untreated tooth decay in their primary or permanent teeth (ages 3–19 years) | 13.4% | 10.2% | NHANES, CDC/NCHS |
| OH-3 | Reduce the proportion of adults with active or currently untreated tooth decay (ages 20–74 years) | 22.8% | 17.3% | NHANES, CDC/NCHS |
| OH-4 | Reduce the proportion of older adults with untreated root surface decay (ages ≥75 years) | 29.1% | 20.1% | NHANES, CDC/NCHS |
| OH-5 | Reduce the proportion of adults who have lost all of their natural teeth (ages ≥45 years) | 7.9% | 5.4% | NHANES, CDC/NCHS |
| OH-6 | Reduce the proportion of adults with moderate and severe periodontitis (≥45 years) | 44.5% | 39.3% | NHANES, CDC/NCHS |
| OH-7 | Increase the proportion of oral and pharyngeal cancers detected at the earliest stage | 29.5% | 34.2% | Surveillance, Epidemiology, and End Results Program (SEER); National Institutes of Health (NIH)/National Cancer Institute (NCI) |
| OH-8[a] | Increase the proportion of children, adolescents, and adults who use the oral healthcare system | 43.3% | 45.0% | Medical Expenditure Panel Survey (MEPS), Agency for Healthcare Research and Quality (AHRQ) |
| OH-9[b] | Increase the proportion of low-income youth who have a preventive dental visit (ages 1–17 years) | 78.8% | 82.7% | National Survey of Children's Health (NSCH), Health Resources & Services Administration (HRSA)/Maternal and Child Health Bureau (MCHB) |
| OH-10 | Increase the proportion of children and adolescents years who have received dental sealants on one or more of their primary or permanent molar teeth (ages 3–19 years) | 37.0% | 42.5% | NHANES, CDC/NCHS |
| OH-11[b] | Increase the proportion of persons served by community systems with optimally fluoridated water | 72.8% | 77.1% | Water Fluoridation Reporting System (WFRS), CDC/National Center for Chronic Disease Prevention and Health Promotion (NCCDPHP) |
| OH-D01[c] | Increase the number of states and the District of Columbia that have an oral and craniofacial health surveillance system | N/A | N/A | N/A |
| AHS-02 | Increase the proportion of persons with dental insurance | 54.4% | 59.8% | National Health Interview Survey (NHIS), CDC/NCHS |
| AHS-05 | Reduce the proportion of persons who are unable to obtain or are delayed in obtaining necessary dental care | 4.6% | 4.1% | MEPS, AHRQ |
| NWS-10 | Reduce the consumption of calories from added sugars by persons aged ≥2 years | 13.5% | 11.5% | NHANES, CDC/NCHS |

[a] Proposed Leading Health Indicator; [b] Relates to health equity; [c] Developmental objective.
Data from Department of Health and Human Services: Office of Disease Prevention and Health Promotion. *Healthy People 2030.* https://health.gov/healthypeople/objectives-and-data/browse-objectives; 2020 Accessed 09.03.20; Secretary's Advisory Committee for Healthy People 2030. *Secretary's Advisory Committee on National Health Promotion and Disease Prevention Objectives for 2030: Report #7: Assessment and Recommendations for Proposed Objectives for Healthy People 2030.* https://www.healthypeople.gov/sites/default/files/Report%207_Reviewing%20Assessing%20Set%20of%20HP2030%20Objectives_Formatted%20EO_508_05.21.pdf; 2019 Accessed 03.15.20; National Academy of Sciences. *Leading Health Indicators 2030: Advancing health, equity, and well-being.* https://www.nap.edu/resource/25682/leading-health-indicators-2030-highlights.pdf https://www.nap.edu/resource/25682/leading-health-indicators-2030-highlights.pdf; 2020 Accessed April 2020.

b. National Oral Health Surveillance System (NOHSS)—a collaborative effort between the Centers for Disease Control and Prevention (CDC) Division of Oral Health and the Association of State and Territorial Dental Directors (ASTDD) to track oral health indicators at the national level using a variety of clinical and nonclinical methods (e.g., National Health and Nutrition Examination Survey [NHANES])
c. Tracking of oral health indicators by state requires the involvement of states in the surveillance process; this endeavor continues to be a national emphasis of dental public health (see Table 20.3)
d. Oral health indicators are routinely assessed, based on the current HP objectives; each decade a few specific HP objectives are deemed the leading health indicators, considered to be the most critical to the health of the population at that time
   (1) One of the PH 2030 oral conditions objectives has been proposed as a leading health indicator for this decade: to increase dental utilization (see Table 20.3)

(2) The leading health indicators are scheduled to be released in late 2020 on the HP 2030 website at https://health.gov/healthypeople

e. NHANES—routinely conducted national health surveys carried out by the National Center for Health Statistics of the CDC to monitor the health and nutritional status of US adults and children of all ages; conducted through interviewing and direct physical and dental examinations

(1) Began in the 1960s and has evolved to the current periodic program that focuses on a variety of health and nutrition measurements used to determine the health status of the population and assess progress on HP objectives

(2) Survey examines a nationally representative sample of about 5000 persons each year, located in counties across the US; oral health is one of the areas of diseases and health indictors monitored by NHANES

## EPIDEMIOLOGY AND RESEARCH

A. Evidence-based practice (EBP)

1. Involves the conscientious, explicit, and judicious use of current scientific evidence to inform decisions during

**BOX 20.5 Uses of Epidemiology**

1. To study
   - Describe normal biologic processes
   - Establish a history of disease in a population
   - Measure the distribution of diseases in populations; detect patterns of disease among groups
   - Analyze trends in chronic disease and social epidemiology
   - Identify nondisease entities such as accidents, suicide, or injury
   - Recognize syndromes and precursors
2. To assess
   - Collect data to describe and measure disease or health conditions within a community
   - Identify current public health policies, activities, and health services that relate to disease in the community
3. To identify:
   - Identify risk factors, risk indicators, risk markers, and other determinants of disease such as health literacy
   - Estimate risk of diseases among population groups
   - Detect cause-and-effect relationships of diseases and various factors to help in the diagnostic processes of disease identification, as well as planning of preventive strategies
4. To control
   - Limit causes of diseases, conditions, injury, disability, or death for prevention and/or elimination
   - Contain diseases within the population
5. To plan
   - Develop appropriate health services, public health programs, and policies
   - Design mechanisms to evaluate effectiveness of services, programs, and policies
6. To evaluate
   - Calculate how well public health policies, intervention and preventive strategies, and programs control disease and improve the health status of the population
   - Appraise the appropriateness and utility of health services
7. To research
   - Test hypotheses for the effectiveness of measures to prevent and control disease
   - Determine the success of disease prevention and control measures in populations

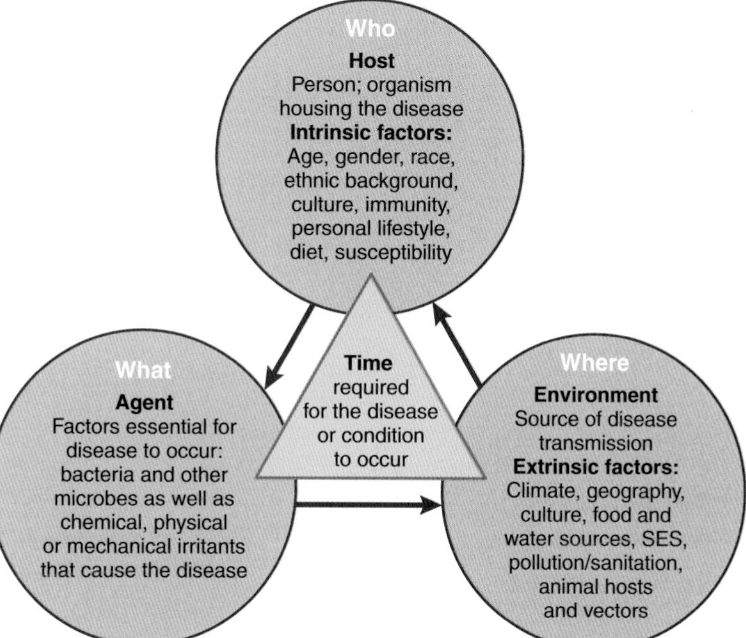


**Fig. 20.1** Epidemiologic triangle. (Data from Centers for Disease Control and Prevention: Bam! Understanding Body & Mind, Classroom Resources for Teachers: Unit 1 CDC Basics: Understanding the epidemiologic triangle through infectious disease working the epidemiologic triangle, September 10, 2020. https://www.cdc.gov/healthyschools/bam/teachers/epi-triangle.html.)

**TABLE 20.4 General Epidemiologic Concepts**

| Term | Definition |
|---|---|
| Acute disease | Beginning abruptly with marked intensity, and then subsiding after a relatively short period; often treatable |
| Chronic disease | Developing slowly and persisting for a long period, often for the remainder of the individual's lifetime |
| Cluster | Aggregate of cases of a disease or other health-related conditions, particularly cancer or birth defect, closely grouped in time or space |
| Endemic | Continuing problem involving normal disease prevalence; the expected number of cases native to a population or geographic area |
| Epidemic | Significantly greater prevalence of a disease than normal (more than the expected frequency); rapid spread of a disease through a population |
| Pandemic | Epidemic that crosses international borders to affect a large proportion of the geographic population of a continent, people, or the world |
| Population at risk | Includes persons in the same community or population group who can acquire a disease or condition |
| Mortality | Death from a disease or condition |
| Morbidity | Presence or extent of disease, injury, or disability in a defined population |
| Status | Current state of a disease or health-related condition in the population |
| Trend | Long-term changes or movements in disease patterns and health-related conditions in the population determined by examining surveillance data |
| Eradication | Elimination of the infectious disease agent through surveillance and containment |
| Socioeconomic status (SES) | Includes education, income, occupation, attitudes, and values and how SES relates to health-associated characteristics in the population |

**TABLE 20.5 Measurement Concepts in Epidemiology**

| Term | Definition |
|---|---|
| Basic screening | Rapid assessment accomplished in a short time by visual detection and providing information about gross dental and oral lesions; accomplished with a tongue blade, dental mirror, and appropriate lighting |
| Epidemiologic examination | Detailed visual tactile assessment; accomplished with dental instruments and a light source, provides more detailed information than basic screening; differs from a clinical examination in that it does not involve a clinical diagnosis that results in a treatment plan |
| Count | The actual number of cases of a disease or condition occurring in a population; simplest measure of a disease or condition; for example, the number of children with a toothache |
| Rate | Expression of disease in a population using a standardized denominator and including a time dimension; allows for valid comparisons; for example, the percentage of people diagnosed with cancer during a specific year, or the percentage of children with caries in 2014 |
| Incidence | Rate of new cases of a disease (number of new cases/population at risk) during or over a specific period; measures how fast a disease is spreading; for example, the number of children with new carious lesions out of the entire school population during the school year |
| Prevalence | Rate of the total number of all existing cases of a disease or health condition in a population measured at a given time, in relation to the number of individuals in the population; expressed as a proportion; can be expressed as a percentage; does not include a time period as incidence does; for example, the percentage of children with untreated caries at the time of a survey |
| Occurrence | General term of frequency of disease; does not distinguish between incidence and prevalence |
| Ratio | Expression of the magnitude of one occurrence of disease exposure in relation to another with a fraction, obtained by dividing one quantity by the other; often compares two rates; for example, if 4% of male and 2% of female infants were born with cleft palate, the ratio of cleft palate in male versus female infants would be 2:1 |
| Prospective | Observations of disease or disease-related factors made forward in time (into the future) |
| Longitudinal | Observations of disease progression made over a long period (appropriate length of time depends on condition being studied) |
| Retrospective | Disease-related data collected in the past; ex post facto, causal comparative, or case control |
| Validity | Accuracy of a measure; produced by measuring what is supposed to be measured |
| Sensitivity | Ability of a test to accurately identify the presence of a disease or condition when disease is, in fact, present |
| Specificity | Ability of a test to accurately identify the absence of a disease or condition when disease is, in fact, not present |
| Predictive value | Ability of a diagnostic test to accurately measure both the presence and the absence of disease |
| Reversal; positive and negative reversals | Change in judgment when measuring the presence of a disease or condition over time; positive reversal is a change of the measurement made in error in a logical direction; negative reversal is a change in an illogical direction |
| Reliability | Consistency or reproducibility of a measurement over time |
| Inter-examiner (rater) reliability | Agreement among two or more examiners as they apply an index or instrument to measure a disease or condition |
| Intra-examiner (rater) reliability | Consistency of a single examiner in applying an index or instrument over time to measure a disease or condition |
| Calibration | Standardization of examiners to increase reliability as they apply epidemiologic measurements |

the care of individual patients and clients in relation to their oral and medical conditions
2. All oral health care must be informed by evidence
3. Scientific evidence alone is not sufficient to make decisions; the clinical expertise of the professional and patient preferences, values, and circumstances are combined with the best available external clinical evidence from a body of rigorous research findings to make EBP decisions (also called evidence-based decision-making; Fig. 20.2)
4. Scientific evidence is ranked according to the design of the research study (Fig. 20.3)
5. EBP relates to the practice of a dental hygienist in all roles and settings, not just clinical; has implications for all aspects of community oral health practice
6. Lifelong learning and access to quality research findings are critical to EBP

B. Research—continual search for new knowledge using the scientific method; systematic and objective inquiry through laboratory, field, and clinical investigations that lead to discovery or revision of knowledge, resulting in improvements in health and health care delivery

C. Scientific method—methods used in any type of research that increase the likelihood that information gathered will be relevant, reliable, and unbiased (Fig. 20.4)

D. Categories of community oral health research
1. Epidemiologic research to determine the presence and distribution of disease in the population and factors that relate to its occurrence in the population
2. Clinical trials and tests of techniques and products to prevent and control disease
3. Research in educational techniques and the behavioral sciences related to oral health education
4. Evaluation of community oral health programs

E. Risk versus causality
1. *Risk* identifies attributes that are associated with a disease, from case-control and cohort studies (Table 20.6);

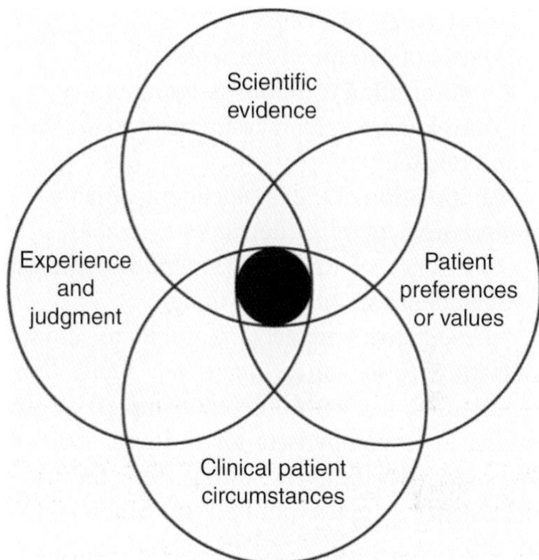


**Fig. 20.2** Evidence-based decision-making used in evidence-based practice. (Data from Forrest JL, Miller SA. Evidence-based decision making. In Bowen DM, Pieren JA. *Darby and Walsh dental Hygiene: Theory and Practice*. 5th ed. Maryland Heights, MO: Elsevier;2020:25-33.)

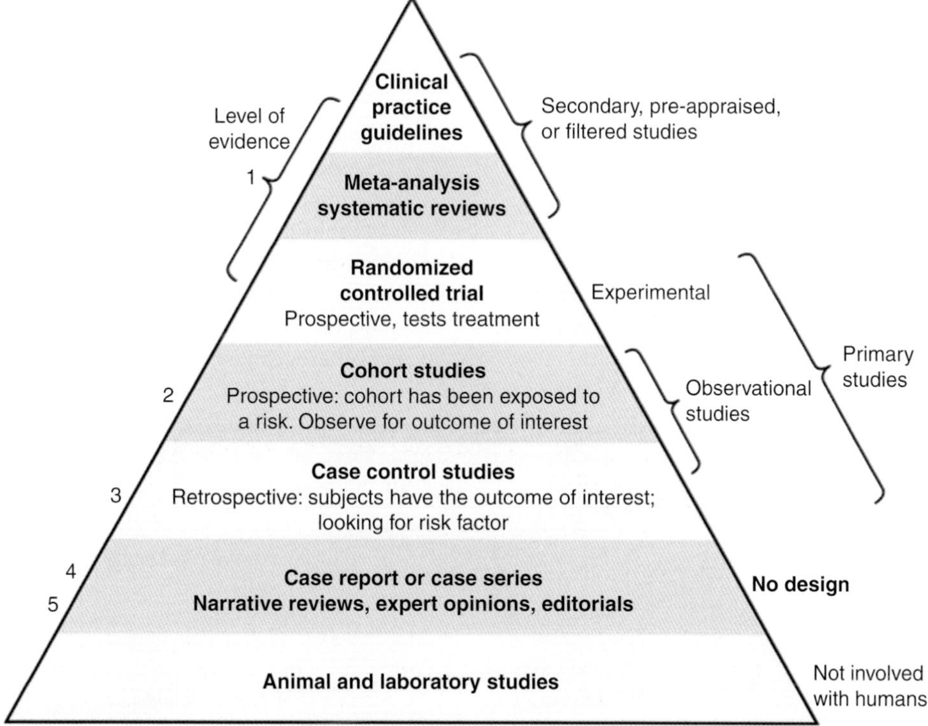


**Fig. 20.3** Hierarchy of research designs and levels of scientific evidence. (Reprinted with permission. Copyright 2012 JL Forrest NCDHRP, National Center for Dental Hygiene Research and Practice. Forrest JL, Miller SA. Evidence-based decision making. In Bowen DM, Pieren JA. *Darby and Walsh dental Hygiene: Theory and Practice*. 5th ed. Maryland Heights, MO: Elsevier; 2020:25-33.)

*causality* identifies factors that have been demonstrated to be causally related
2. Risk is established with analytic studies; causality is established with randomized controlled clinical trials (RCTs); causality can be inferred with high-quality longitudinal analytic studies

F. Three classifications of epidemiologic research (Table 20.7)

G. Experimental research
1. Requirements for an experimental study
   a. Use of a control group
   b. Control of extraneous variables
   c. Randomization (random assignment to groups)
   d. Control of errors in measurement to increase validity and reliability
   e. Manipulation of the independent variable
   f. Measurement of the dependent variable
   g. Occurrence of the independent variable before the dependent variable in the design
2. A representative sample is required to allow for generalization (also called *inference*); replication studies (repeated studies with different samples) are frequently conducted to compensate for the poor generalizability (low external validity) resulting from the use of small convenience samples; multiple-site studies broaden the representation of the population and improve the generalizability of findings
3. Experimental study designs
   a. Pretest/posttest—the dependent variable is measured before and after introducing the independent variable; provides a baseline measure for comparison
   b. Posttest only—the dependent variable is measured only after introducing the independent variable; controls any possible effect of the pretest procedure on the dependent variable
   c. Split-mouth—procedure unique to oral health research in which each side of the mouth receives a different intervention; controls subject-related variables (variables that can change from one research participant to another)
   d. Crossover—each group receives a different intervention or control and, after a period, is switched over to the opposite treatment, with an intervening washout period during which no treatment is given, to eliminate the possibility of the first treatment affecting the second one; controls subject-related variables
   e. Time-series (repeated measures)—design in which the dependent variable is measured several times over a specific period, to determine whether the effect of the independent variable on the dependent variable holds over time
   f. Blind (or masking)—this refers to examiners measuring the dependent variable without knowing the group assignment, to eliminate bias; if *both* examiners and participants are unaware of the group assignments, it is called *double-blind*
   g. Designs can be combined; for example, a study can combine double-blind, pretest/posttest, split-mouth, and repeated-measures designs to test the effectiveness of an antimicrobial to reduce or control periodontal pocket depths over a long period
4. Comparison of clinical trials and epidemiologic surveys (Table 20.8)

H. Hypothesis—a predictive statement of the expected outcome or relationship among variables; answers the research question in a manner that is observable and measurable; hypotheses can exist for all types of epidemiologic studies

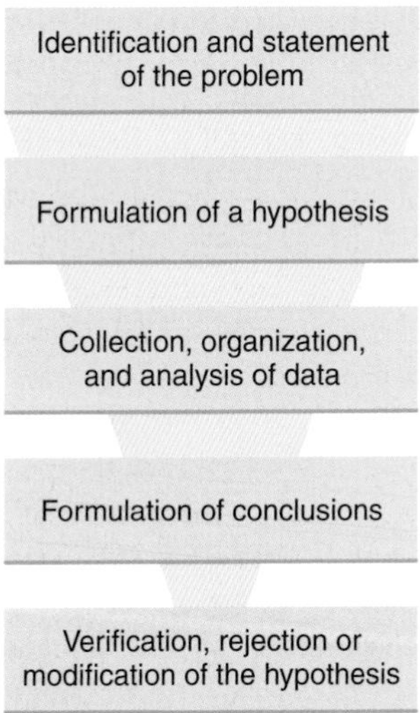

**Fig. 20.4** Steps of the scientific method.

**TABLE 20.6 Types of Risk Attributes**

| Risk Attribute | Modifiable | Type of Analytic Study | Application |
|---|---|---|---|
| Risk factor (strong indication of risk) | Yes | Cohort or case control/retrospective; longitudinal | Causal (cause-and-effect) role is inferred; should be an important consideration in making recommendations to modify it |
| Risk indicator (weaker indication of risk) | Yes | Cross-sectional | Possible causal role; causal role may be incorrectly assumed; should be applied with care when making recommendations |
| Demographic risk factor (also called risk marker or risk predictor) | No | Cross-sectional; case control | No causal role; not important in making individual recommendations to control the factor but indicates greater need to control modifiable risk factors and risk indicators; should be considered when prioritizing target populations for dental public health programs |

Data from Beatty CF, Dickinson C. Oral epidemiology. In Nathe CN, ed. *Dental Public Health and Research.* 4th ed. Upper Saddle River, NJ: Pearson; 2017: 233–262.

**TABLE 20.7 Classifications of Epidemiologic Research**

| Type of Research | Definition | Types of Studies | Classification | Use/Purpose |
|---|---|---|---|---|
| Descriptive | Involves description, documentation, analysis, and interpretation of data to evaluate a current event or situation; does not test a hypothesis | Survey | Cross-sectional | Establish prevalence |
| Analytic (also called observational or developmental) | Encompasses observation of a disease or condition to identify determinants of the disease by showing relationships or associations between diseases and other factors; does not establish cause-and-effect relationship | Cohort: one group observed forward over time; can be compared to a comparison group | Prospective, longitudinal if past data collected over time | Establish incidence; determine risk; infer cause-and-effect relationship (causality) if longitudinal |
| | | Case control: two groups, one with disease (cases) and one without (controls), are compared to identify factors in their history that can be associated with the disease or condition | Retrospective | Examine relationships among variables that cannot be studied prospectively because of ethical concerns about research participants; determine risk |
| | | Cross-sectional: representative cross section of the population (one group, but several subgroups) is observed at one point in time; disease attributes and potential risk attributes are associated | Cross-sectional | Establish prevalence; identify risk indicators and risk predictors; cannot be used to confirm risk factors |
| Experimental | Carefully designed study to test a hypothesis; involves manipulation of the supposed cause or controlling agent and observation of the result | Randomized clinical trial (RCT)—a well-controlled experimental study with humans | Longitudinal | Determine effectiveness of altering a factor or factors to establish causality |
| | | Quasi-experimental—an experimental study that is not well-controlled | | |

Data from Beatty CF, Dickinson C. Oral epidemiology. In Nathe CN, ed. *Dental Public Health and Research*. 4th ed. Upper Saddle River, NJ: Pearson; 2017: 233–262.

1. Null hypothesis—hypothesis that is statistically tested; negative statement of the hypothesis that assumes the absence of statistically significant differences between sample groups; for example, statement that no difference exists in the effectiveness of the two treatments (experimental), or two variables are not associated (nonexperimental)
2. Research hypothesis—also called the *positive* or *alternative hypothesis*; positive statement of the hypothesis is in terms that express the opinion or prediction of the researcher; for example, a statement that a difference exists in the effectiveness of the two treatments (experimental), or two variables are associated (nonexperimental)

I. Variable—a state, condition, concept, construct, or event whose value is free to vary (e.g., health literacy, dental attendance, water fluoridation status, dental caries rate, periodontal status); must be measurable
   1. Independent variable—in an experimental study, the treatment or intervention under study; condition that is manipulated or controlled by the investigator; the experimental variable; the experimental treatment (e.g., a preventive intervention)
   2. Dependent variable—in an experimental study, the dependent variable is a measure of the outcome of manipulating the independent variable; it is measured to observe the effect of the independent variable (e.g., incidence of dental caries)
   3. Nonexperimental studies also measure variables; in analytic studies, the association or relationship of these variables, also called *factors*, is determined
   4. Extraneous variables—uncontrolled variables that may influence the dependent variable and influence (or confound) the outcome, thus interfering with accurate interpretation and producing invalid research results; can be present in all types of research studies

J. Sampling (Table 20.9)
   1. Target population—portion of the population to whom the researcher wants to generalize findings; all members of a specific group who possess a clearly defined set of characteristics
   2. Sample—a portion of a specific population that, if properly selected, can provide meaningful information about the entire population; a sample is examined when the researcher cannot study an entire population; a sample may be random or nonrandom and may be representative or nonrepresentative
   3. Sample size
      a. Large sample, if selected properly:
         (1) Accurately represents a defined population
         (2) Increases the validity and reliability of collected data
         (3) Reduces the standard error of the sample mean
      b. Small sample
         (1) May be necessary, depending on the purpose of the research; for example, a pilot study
         (2) Results from a small sample may not be generalized to target population and lead to inaccurate conclusions when inappropriate for the type of research
         (3) Requires specialized statistics (nonparametrics) for analysis

**TABLE 20.8 Comparison of Clinical Trials and Epidemiologic Surveys**

| | Clinical Trial | Epidemiologic Survey |
|---|---|---|
| Populations | Experimental and control groups are specially constituted from representative samples of appropriate target populations | Naturally occurring samples of target populations are usually studied |
| Sample size | Sample sizes are often small, particularly when "treatments" are more complicated | Fairly large sample sizes are used |
| Time frame | Trials are conducted over a period, usually varying from 1 week to 6 months to several years (e.g., dental caries research), depending on treatment involved and disease or condition measured, to compare treatment outcomes | Surveys are usually cross-sectional in design, measuring only one time; longitudinal designs are used occasionally; surveys can be repeated periodically to show trends |
| Methods | Although assessment methods may include indices, biomedical instruments, or physiologic measures, methods have validity, reliability, and clinical significance | Indices are used for assessment, to establish the disease level of selected populations, and to compare data from different populations and/or at different points in time |
| Data | Data generated from clinical trials are applicable to specific hypothesis testing | Data generated from surveys are used to establish underlying etiologic factors and derive possible preventive methods, leading to the development of hypotheses to be tested by controlled clinical trials |

**TABLE 20.9 Sampling and Group Assignment**

| Type of Sample or Group Assignment | Definition | Result |
|---|---|---|
| Random sample | Study participants are chosen independently of each other, with known opportunity or probability for inclusion; table of random numbers can be used | Increases external validity by controlling differences in study participants; yields a representative sample with a homogeneous population; allows for valid generalization of results to the population (reduced bias) |
| Stratified random sample | Study participants are randomly selected from an existing, known, subdivided population; most representative sample for a heterogeneous population | Results in the sample proportionately and accurately representing the subgroups in the population; yields the most representative sample for a heterogeneous population |
| Systematic random sample | Selection of every *n*th member of the population from a list or file of it; the *n* depends on the size of the sample desired in relation to the population; for example, 10% is every 10th member of the population | Not strictly a random sample; it is considered to be random when the first member of the sample is selected randomly and the list or file is in random order |
| Convenience sample | Study participants are chosen on the basis of availability; used when access to the total population is not feasible for random sample selection | Introduces bias, which reduces validity of the sample and limits the generalizability of study results |
| Judgmental or purposive sample | Study participants are chosen by the researcher or someone else who has knowledge of the population; used when participants are needed that require specific disease levels and/or characteristics | Introduces bias, which reduces validity of the sample and limits the generalizability of study results |
| Experimental group | Sample group in an experimental study whose members are exposed to the experimental variable being studied (receives the independent variable) | Randomization (randomized group assignment) results in equivalent groups to control group differences and control validity of study |
| Control group | Sample group in an experimental study whose members do not receive the experimental treatment (independent variable); receives a placebo, traditional or standard treatment, or no treatment | Provides a comparison group for a stronger study design |

K. Group assignment—experimental and control groups are formed in an experimental study (Table 20.9); randomization of groups is best, to increase validity of the study

L. Pilot study—a trial run to test research design and methodology before initiating a full-scale study; conducted with a small sample; can be applied to any type of research

## EPIDEMIOLOGY OF ORAL DISEASES AND CONDITIONS

A. Role of *Healthy People 2030* objectives
   1. Baseline measures and targets or benchmarks for various oral conditions and preventive strategies are set (see Table 20.3); progress is evaluated throughout the decade in relation to the targets
   2. Disparities in oral health continue to exist; community programs and interventions aimed at reducing oral health disparities remain a high priority

B. Dental caries
   1. Occurrence in the population
      a. Dental caries is the most common chronic disease of children aged 6 to 11 years and adolescents aged 12 to 19 years; it is four times more common than asthma in 14- to 17-year-olds, one of the major reasons for hospitalization of young children, and costly to treat

**TABLE 20.10 Prevalence and Progress of Dental Caries Experience and Untreated Dental Caries in Various Age Groups**

| Age group | Percent With Caries Experience | Progress in Last Decade | Percent With Untreated Caries | Progress in Last Decade |
|---|---|---|---|---|
| 3 to 5 years[1] | 27.9% | Improved | 11.7% | Improved |
| 6 to 9 years[1] | 57.7% | No change | 21.5% | Improved |
| 13 to 15 years[1] | 53.4% | No change | 11.4% | Improved |
| 20 to 34 years[2] | 82.1% | No data | 27.3% | No data |
| 35 to 49 years[2] | 93.6% | No data | — | — |
| 35 to 44 years[1] | — | — | 24.9% | Improved |
| 50 to 64 years[2] | 97.4% | No data | 25.5% | No data |
| 65 to 74 years | 96%[2] | No data | 14.8%[1] | Improved |
| 75 years and older (coronal and root caries)[2] | 96.6% | No data | 19.4% | No data |
| 75 years and older (root caries only)[1] | — | — | 37.9% | No data |

Data from:
[1]U.S. Department of Health and Human Services: Centers for Disease Control and Prevention: National Center for Health Statistics: *Healthy People 2020 midcourse review*, Chapter 32, Oral health, June 18, 2019, https://www.cdc.gov/nchs/data/hpdata2020/HP2020MCR-C32-OH.pdf.
[2]Dye BA, Thornton-Evans G, Li X, Iafolla TJ. *Dental caries and tooth loss in adults in the United States, 2011–2012.* National Center for Health Statistics (NCHS) News Brief No. 197, Centers for Disease Control and Prevention; 2015. https://www.cdc.gov/nchs/products/databriefs/db197.htm.

b. During the last 70 years, substantially declining caries rates in all age groups have been observed in the United States, including lower cumulative caries rates, less severe caries, substantially fewer carious lesions in anterior teeth, and fewer teeth lost as a result of caries; recent years have seen no further substantial reductions in caries rates
c. Dental caries is still widespread and affects all age groups (Table 20.10); average of 90% of people aged 20 to 64 have caries experience; the reduction in caries experience during the last decade in preschool-age children (early childhood caries, or ECC; Table 20.11) is noteworthy because caries increased in this age group in the previous decade
d. Root surface caries rates have increased as a result of the aging population and because older adults are retaining their natural teeth
e. Dental caries prevalence is accompanied by untreated caries in all ages groups (see Table 20.10); the decrease in untreated caries in the last decade is important because the association between low dental utilization and higher rates of caries experience and untreated caries in a population is significant
f. The most commonly occurring type of caries is pit-and-fissure caries, followed by smooth-surface coronal caries and root caries; first and second molars are the most frequently affected teeth

2. Factors that have contributed to the general trend of lower caries rates
   a. Use of fluorides, including water fluoridation, fluoride dentifrices, and other fluoride modalities, is the most significant factor in the long term, primarily reducing smooth-surface caries; widespread use of fluorides has decreased state and regional differences in caries rates
   b. More recently, dental sealants have contributed to reductions in pit-and-fissure caries

**TABLE 20.11 Categorizing Early Childhood Caries[a] (ECC) and Severe Early Childhood Caries (S-ECC)**

| Age (years) | ECC | S-ECC |
|---|---|---|
| Younger than 6 | 1 or more dmfs[b] (cavitated or noncavitated) | |
| Younger than 3 | | Any sign of smooth-surface caries |
| Age 3 | | One or more cavitated, missing (due to caries), or filled smooth surfaces in maxillary anterior teeth OR 4 or more dmfs |
| Age 4 | | One or more cavitated, missing (due to caries), or filled smooth surfaces in maxillary anterior teeth OR five or more dmfs |
| Age 5 | | One or more cavitated, missing (due to caries), or filled smooth surfaces in maxillary anterior teeth OR 6 or more dmfs |

[a]The term early childhood caries replaces previously used terms such as baby-bottle tooth decay, nursing caries, baby-bottle mouth, and baby-bottle caries.
[b]*dmfs,* decayed, missing, and/or filled primary tooth surfaces.
Data from *American Academy of Pediatric Dentistry (AAPD).* Policy on early childhood caries (ECC): classifications, consequences, and preventive strategies. https://www.aapd.org/research/oral-health-policies--recommendations/early-childhood-caries-classifications-consequences-and-preventive-strategies/; 2018 Accessed 07.07.20.

   c. Greater emphasis on preventive care and increased dental utilization also contribute
3. Disparities exist for dental caries and untreated caries (Table 20.12); this has implications for community programming
4. Risk and associated factors vary in the population and form the foundation of public health programs (see Chapter 16 for further discussion of risk factors for caries)

a. Caries is a multifactorial, infectious, transmissible disease
b. Low socioeconomic status (SES) of the family is the most powerful predictor of caries in young children; caries control programs should be targeted especially to low-SES populations
c. Lack of access to water fluoridation is a critical risk factor
d. Health education and health promotion efforts should be directed to preventive measures to reduce the risk factors
   (1) Reduce bacteria with good oral hygiene and antimicrobials
   (2) Reduce the amount and frequency of sugar and other fermentable carbohydrate foods and drinks in the diet
   (3) Routinely use fluorides and other chemotherapeutic measures to increase the resistance of the enamel to acid attack, enhance the protective nature of saliva, and arrest caries
   (4) Place dental sealants to increase the caries resistance of pits and fissures
   (5) Eliminate carious lesions and restore cavitated teeth to eliminate bacteria, improve the individual's ability to remove plaque biofilm, and restore function of teeth

5. Additional risk factors for ECC should be addressed in community programs focused on maternal and child health, especially in lower-SES populations
   a. Transmission of cariogenic bacteria from the parent or caregiver to the young child
   b. Parental risk-related behaviors for ECC include infant feeding practices, whether the infant is breastfed or bottle-fed; delayed weaning from bottle feeding or breastfeeding; allowing a baby to fall asleep with a bottle
   c. High-cariogenic diet, including sugar drinks in the bottle or sippy cup and high sugar levels in other components of the diet
   d. ECC is also more common in situations where childcare is provided by individuals with low oral health literacy or poor understanding of oral disease prevention
6. Other risk and associated factors for root caries to be considered in public health programs
   a. Increases with age because of a greater likelihood of exposed cementum and other risk factors
   b. The increasing age of the population and decreasing tooth loss result in more available root surfaces to become carious
   c. Older adults exhibit greater use of medications that cause xerostomia, in which case saliva loses its protective capacity; multiple medications are especially a major risk factor for this
   d. Increased sugar intake as sense of taste diminishes and eating habits change with age creates a greater risk of caries for older individuals
   e. History of coronal caries and smoking are risk factors for root caries
   f. Diminished manual dexterity may limit oral self-care
7. Further reduction in dental caries and untreated decay continue to be emphasized nationally (see Table 20.3)

C. Dental sealants
   1. Rates of sealed first and second molars have improved each decade of HP; yet, only 4.3% of 3- to 5-year-olds, 37.6% of 6- to 9-year-olds, and 22.2% of 13- to 15-year-olds currently have dental sealants;[1] further increasing these rates among children and adolescents aged 3 to 19 is an important national emphasis for community oral health programs (see Table 20.3)
   2. Disparities exist in the rates of sealants in children (see Table 20.12)
   3. Permanent and deciduous molar teeth of preschool-age, school-age, and adolescent children are targeted in community-based sealant programs
   4. Placement is recommended as soon as possible after tooth eruption

D. Periodontal diseases
   1. Periodontal diseases manifest as different clinical entities, depending on aggressiveness, severity, rate of progression, systemic diseases present, hormonal influences, genetics, and other factors
   2. Prevalence of periodontal diseases (see "Epidemiology of Periodontal Diseases and Related Risks" section in Chapter 14)
      a. Global occurrence
         (1) The presence of some form of periodontal disease is almost universal with over 70% of adults affected
         (2) Most children have signs of gingivitis
         (3) Early periodontal disease in adults is prevalent
         (4) Prevalence of severe periodontitis is in the range of 5% to 15% in almost all countries, regardless of economic development, oral hygiene, or dental care available
         (5) Increased levels of prevalence and severity of periodontal diseases are found in areas of the world where generalized malnutrition is common
         (6) Differences in periodontal disease levels between peoples of developed countries and developing countries are attributed to differences in oral hygiene levels
      b. In the United States, 47.3% of adults aged 45 to 74 years have moderate-to-severe periodontitis;[1] this rate has remained consistent since 2010[1] and represents a decrease since 2000
      c. Variations in data related to the prevalence of periodontal diseases can be attributed to differences in study designs and measurement
   3. Disparities exist for periodontal diseases in the United States (see Table 20.12)
   4. For a discussion of risk and associated factors, see "Epidemiology of Periodontal Diseases and Related Risks" section in Chapter 14
   5. Further reductions in moderate and severe periodontitis are emphasized nationally (Table 20.3)

TABLE 20.12 **Oral Disease Disparities by Age/Gender, Race and Ethnicity, Family Income, Education, Disability, and Dental Attendance**[a]

| Oral Disease | Age/Gender | Race and Ethnicity[b] | Family Income[c] | Education[c] | Disability | Dental Attendance |
|---|---|---|---|---|---|---|
| Dental caries | Higher caries rates in male children compared to female in all age groups (NSS)<br>Higher rates of untreated caries in children of all age groups (NSS in pre-school and school-age children)<br>Slightly higher rates in female adults, possibly because of higher dental care utilization rates<br>Higher rates of untreated caries in male adults and older adults compared to females (SS only for root surface caries in older adults aged 75 and older) | Lower caries rates in non-Hispanic white group in pre-school and school-age children (SS)<br>Lower caries rates in non-Hispanic Black group in teenagers (NSS)<br>Lower rates of untreated caries in non-Hispanic white children of all ages (NSS for teenagers)<br>Lower rates of untreated coronal and root caries in adults and older adults in non-Hispanic white group compared to other racial and ethnic groups | Higher rates of caries in children of all ages from families with lower income level (NSS in school-age group)<br>Higher rates of untreated caries in children of all ages from families with lower income level (SS for pre-school age group only)<br>Lower rates of untreated coronal and root caries in adults and older adults in higher income categories (NSS for older adults) | Higher prevalence of ECC when child care is provided by individuals with low educational level<br>Lower rates of untreated coronal and root caries in adults and older adults with higher educational level (NSS in older adults) | Higher rates of untreated coronal caries in adults and older adults who have disabilities (NSS in older adults) | Higher rates of caries and untreated caries in groups of all ages that have lower rate of dental attendance |
| Dental sealants | Higher rates in school-age and adolescent females compared to males (NSS) | Higher rates in non-Hispanic white school-age children and in Hispanic adolescents compared to other racial and ethnic groups (NSS) | For school-age children, higher rates in children from families with higher income level; for pre-school age and adolescent children, higher rates in children from families with lower income levels (NSS) | ND | ND | Higher rates associated with higher dental attendance |
| Periodontal disease | Higher rates of moderate-to-severe periodontal disease in adult males compared to females<br>Better oral hygiene in women<br>Increasing rates of moderate-to-severe periodontal disease with increasing age; highest in older adults who keep their teeth<br>Very low rates of mild and moderate CAL in children; uncommon in young children | Higher rates of moderate-to-severe periodontal disease in non-white groups | Substantially higher rates and severity with decreasing family income | Substantially higher rates and severity with less education | Higher rates in groups with disabilities | Higher rates in populations with low dental attendance |
| Tooth loss | Higher rates with increasing age<br>Higher rates in adult males compared to females (NSS) | Higher rates in non-white groups | Higher rates in lower income groups | Higher rates in groups with lower educational level | Higher rates in groups with disabilities | Higher rates in groups with lower dental attendance |
| Oral and pharyngeal cancer (OPC) | Higher rates with increasing age; median age of 63 at diagnosis and 67 at death; median age of 54 for human papillomavirus (HPV)-associated OPC<br>Higher OPC and death rates among males; narrowing gender gap, attributed to increased and prolonged use of tobacco products by women | Highest OPC and death rates in non-Hispanic Black group | Lower rates of OPC and higher survival rates among higher SES groups, related to differences in high-risk behaviors<br>Higher rates of HPV-associated OPC in higher SES groups | Lower rates of OPC and higher survival rates among higher SES groups, related to differences in high-risk behaviors<br>Higher rates of HPV-associated OPC in higher SES groups | ND | Lower rates of OPC and higher survival rates in groups with high dental care utilization |

*Continued*

TABLE 20.12 **Oral Disease Disparities by Age/Gender, Race and Ethnicity, Family Income, Education, Disability, and Dental Attendance[a]—cont'd**

| Oral Disease | Age/Gender | Race and Ethnicity[b] | Family Income[c] | Education[c] | Disability | Dental Attendance |
|---|---|---|---|---|---|---|
| Orofacial clefts | More isolated cleft palates in females<br>More facial clefts with or without cleft palate in males | Highest rates in Asian American and Native American populations, with a genetic predisposition suspected to interact with environmental factors<br>Recent studies in the United States found lower rates in Asian American group | ND | ND | ND | ND |
| Malocclusion and orthodontic treatment | ND | Non-Hispanic white group receives more treatment (last reported data were NHANES III, 1998) | Disparities occur in treatment, depending on SES | Disparities occur in treatment, depending on SES | ND | ND |
| TMJD | More common in women<br>More common in younger persons | ND | ND | ND | ND | ND |
| Fluorosis | ND | Higher rates in non-Hispanic white group as a function of SES | Higher rates in higher income group because of excessive use of multiple sources of fluorides | ND | ND | Associated with dental attendance, as a function of SES |

*NSS,* Not statistically significant; *SS,* Statistically significant; *ND,* No differences documented; *ECC,* early childhood caries.
[a]Health literacy is an underlying factor in disparities in the distribution of all oral diseases.
[b]In general, people who are non-Hispanic Black, Hispanic, and American Indian and Alaska Native have the poorest oral health of any racial and ethnic groups in the United States.
[c]In general, populations of low SES (combination of education and educational level) have much greater oral health disparities than higher-SES populations; low SES is the strongest predictor of poor oral health.
Data from Department of Health and Human Services: Centers for Disease Control and Prevention: National Center for Health Statistics (NCHS). *Healthy People 2020 midcourse review,* Chapter 32, Oral health, Hyattsville, MD; 2016, NCHS; https://www.cdc.gov/nchs/data/hpdata2020/HP2020MCR-C32-OH.pdf.
*Centers for Disease Control and Prevention.* Disparities in oral health. http://www.cdc.gov/OralHealth/oral_health_disparities/; 2016 Accessed 07.07.20.
Howlader N, Noone AM, Krapcho M et al, eds: *SEER cancer statistics review, 1975–2016,* Bethesda, MD, National Cancer Institute, Surveillance, Epidemiology, and End Results Program; April 15, 2019. https://seer.cancer.gov/csr/1975_2016/.
*Oral Cancer Foundation. Oral cancer facts.* https://oralcancerfoundation.org/facts/; 2019 Accessed 02.27.19.
*American Speech-Language-Hearing Association.* Cleft lip and palate. https://www.asha.org/PRPSpecificTopic.aspx?folderid=8589942918§ion=Causes; Accessed 06.22.19.
Raut JR, Simeone RM, Tinker SC, Canfield MA, Day RS, Agopian AJ. Proportion of orofacial clefts attributable to recognized risk factors, *Cleft Palate Craniofac J.* 2019; 56:151–158. https://journals.sagepub.com/doi/10.1177/1055665618774019.
Proffit WR, Fields HW, Moray LJ: Prevalence of malocclusion and orthodontic treatment need in the United States: estimates from the NHANES III survey, *Int J Adult Orthodon Orthognath Surg* 1998; 13(2):96–106. https://www.ncbi.nlm.nih.gov/pubmed/9743642.
*National Institute of Dental and Craniofacial Research.* Prevalence of TMJD and its signs and symptoms. https://www.nidcr.nih.gov/research/data-statistics/facial-pain/prevalence; 2018 Accessed 07.07.20.
*Centers for Disease Control and Prevention.* Fluorosis. https://www.cdc.gov/fluoridation/faqs/dental_fluorosis/index.htm; 2019 Accessed 07.07.20.

E. Tooth retention and tooth loss
   1. Rate of complete tooth loss as a result of dental caries or periodontal disease in adults aged 65 to 74 years is 12.9%, representing a significant decrease since 2004
   2. 30.2% of adults aged 45 to 64 years have had no permanent tooth loss as a result of dental caries or periodontal disease, representing a significant increase since 2004
   3. Rates of tooth loss are decreasing despite the aging population because of increased emphasis on preventive dentistry, greater use of fluorides, improved success with periodontal therapy, and higher dental care utilization rates, especially for preventive strategies
   4. Smoking, early tooth loss, poor health, and low level of health literacy are risk factors for edentulism

5. Disparities exist for edentulism and partial tooth loss (see Table 20.12)
6. Reduction of edentulism is emphasized nationally (see Table 20.3)

F. Denture use
1. Current specific data on denture use are unavailable
2. Despite reductions in tooth loss, the number of denture wearers will remain significant because of the aging population; the need will continue for denture fabrication and related patient education and community oral health promotion programs with older adults

G. Oral and pharyngeal cancers (OPC)
1. Occurrence
   a. In the United States, in 2016, an estimated 370,309 people were living with OPC (cancers of the lips, tongue, buccal mucosa, floor of the mouth, and pharynx)[2]
   b. During 2012–2016, the number of new cases per year was 11.3 per 100,000, and the number of deaths from OPC was 2.5 per 100,000 per year; estimates for 2019 are 53,000 new cases of OPC and 10,860 deaths; dramatic increase in the incidence of human papillomavirus (HPV)-associated OPC in the past few decades[2]
   c. OPC account for 3% of all cancers in the United States and 1.84% of all cancer deaths[2]
   d. The 5-year survival rate was 65.3% for 2009–2015, higher than 5 years prior; the mortality rate varies according to the stage of diagnosis; those diagnosed in the earliest stage have an 84.4% 5-year survival rate versus 39.1% for those diagnosed in the latest stage;[2] the proportion of these cancers diagnosed at the earliest stage was 30.9% in 2011, a decrease from 4 years prior[1] ; increasing the number of OPCs detected at the earliest stage is a national emphasis (see Table 20.3)
   e. Occurrence and site distribution within the mouth vary widely in different parts of the world; occurrence is considerably higher in many countries compared to the United States
2. Disparities exist in the distribution of OPC (see Table 20.12)
3. Risk of developing OPC: approximately 1.2% of people will be diagnosed at some point in their lives[2]
4. Causal and risk factors
   a. The establishment of tobacco as a health hazard is one of the greatest public health achievements of the 20th century
   b. HPV is a risk factor for OPC; use of tobacco and alcohol are lower risk factors for HPV-associated OPC
   c. See "Oral Cancer Risk Assessment" section of Chapter 16 for other risk factors

H. Orofacial clefts
1. Orofacial clefts are identified by the CDC as one of the major birth defects
2. The CDC estimates that each year in the United States, 1 in 1574 babies are born with cleft palate (2651 estimated annual cases) and 1 in 940 are born with cleft lip with or without cleft palate (4437 estimated annual cases); cleft lip is more common than cleft palate[3]
3. Risk factors are important in relation to education for prevention; clefts are associated with
   a. Maternal diabetes and thyroid disease
   b. Use of tobacco products during pregnancy
   c. Nutritional deficiencies (e.g., folic acid deficiency)
   d. Alcohol consumption during pregnancy
   e. Use of teratogenic medications (e.g., corticosteroids and medications to treat acne and epilepsy) during pregnancy
   f. Use of drugs of abuse during early stages of pregnancy
   g. Premature birth status
   h. Many occurrences cannot be linked to a direct behavioral link or cause, indicating a genetic cause
4. Prevention is critical because of the high cost of treatment and the potential significant effects on the child
5. In 2014, 39 states in the United States had a system for recording infants and children with cleft lips and cleft palates, and 36 states had a system for referring these children to craniofacial anomaly rehabilitative teams;[1] a successful public health initiative was to increase these numbers over the previous decade and continues to be emphasized nationally (see Table 20.3)
6. Disparities exist for clefts in different population groups in the United States (see Table 20.12)
7. Rates are higher globally, and death rates during the neonatal period are high in poorer countries[4]

I. Malocclusion and orthodontic treatment
1. Although current epidemiologic data are not available for the United States, adequate basic information is available to demonstrate the prevalence of malocclusion and the need for orthodontic care; in general, documentation of the prevalence of malocclusion is increasing worldwide
2. Malocclusions can occur from congenital or acquired crowding of the teeth or jaws, especially as a result of early tooth loss due to caries; prolonged bottle feeding, thumb sucking, and other behaviors during development are also attributed; these causes indicate a need for public health education programs for young mothers regarding feeding practices, the habits of young children, and the need for caries prevention and treatment in order to prevent malocclusion
3. Orthodontic treatment need is a relative concept based on cultural factors and is not comparable between different countries[5]
4. No data are available on differences in distribution of malocclusion among population groups in the United States, but differences occur in frequency of orthodontic treatment (see Table 20.12)

J. Craniofacial injuries and tooth trauma
1. Common dental injuries in children are crown fractures; tooth intrusion, extrusion, and avulsion; and temporomandibular joint injury[6]
2. There is no single risk factor for dental trauma; causes of head and face injuries include accidental falls, assaults, sports-related and recreational activities, bicycle and

automobile collisions, and work-related tasks and projects around the house; sports accidents account for close to one-third of all dental injuries in children; the vast majority of emergency room visits for dental injuries are by children[7]
3. All sporting activities have a risk of dental injury; prevention depends on an understanding of the risk factors
4. The number of injuries can be significantly reduced by requiring the use of protective sports equipment,[7] but few sports have regulations that require their use; health promotion efforts regarding prevention of orofacial injuries should target parents; children, youth, college students, and adults involved in organized sports; coaches; and staff of school and sports organizations that influence policy decisions
5. Most injuries are treated in emergency rooms; education of medical personnel will increase the success of treatment of dental-related injuries

K. Temporomandibular joint and muscle disorder (TMJD)
1. TMJD affects 5% to 12% of people in the United States, is more prevalent in younger persons, and is almost twice as high in women compared to men[8]
2. Possible symptoms include jaw muscle stiffness, limited mobility or locking of the jaw, painful or nonpainful clicking or crepitus in the TMJ, a change in the occlusion, bruxism, sensitive teeth, difficulty chewing, and pain in the jaw joint, muscles of mastication, and in front of the ear;[8] symptoms can be present even when individuals do not perceive a problem
3. Symptoms can be alleviated by eating soft foods, applying ice packs, avoiding extreme jaw movements such as wide yawning and gum chewing, short-term use of over the counter (OTC) or prescription pain and anti-inflammatory medicines, practicing stress-reduction techniques, and use of a stabilization splint (occlusal bite guard); symptoms usually clear with minimal or no treatment; aggressive treatment is rarely recommended[9]
4. Variations in distribution occur according to demographic characteristics (see Table 20.12)

L. Dental fluorosis
1. Description—chronic endemic form of enamel hypoplasia caused by ingesting excessive fluoride during the time of tooth formation in the late secretory to early maturation stage of enamel development; starts for central incisors as early as age 22 months, usually occurs at 24 months, and may occur as late as age 4 years; characterized by retention of enamel proteins and change in enamel matrix structure; defective calcification produces a white, chalky appearance of the enamel that may undergo brown discoloration and change of surface texture in more severe classifications
2. Prevalence of dental fluorosis
   a. Less than one-fourth of the US population exhibit fluorosis, with the vast majority in the classifications "very mild" and "mild"; the prevalence is higher in younger groups; the prevalence of fluorosis in young children may be increasing in the very mild to mild categories as a result of widespread use of fluorides, although it has been suggested that this may be a result of research error[10]
   b. Even children born and raised in optimally fluoridated communities can exhibit mild forms of fluorosis because of excess fluoride consumption from other sources
   c. Occurs in many parts of the world; considered a public health problem in East Africa, India, and Eastern Europe because of the severity; not considered a major public health problem in the United States
   d. Differences occur in the distribution of fluorosis in different groups (see Table 20.12)
3. Causes
   a. Ingesting water with naturally occurring excessive fluoride
      (1) 1 to 2 mg fluoride per liter of water (also referred to as ppm F) results in mild fluorosis; 2 to 4 mg fluoride results in moderate-to-severe fluorosis
      (2) The Environmental Protection Agency (EPA), which is responsible for the safety and quality of water, has set the maximum allowable limit for fluoride at 4 mg per liter of water and a secondary limit at 2 mg fluoride (defluoridation is required at 4 mg F and recommended at 2 mg F)
      (3) Some communities do not have a community water supply; some members of the population depend on well water; fluoride levels of well water vary
   b. Children swallowing excessive amounts of fluoride-containing dentifrices—swallowing or over-enthusiastic use of fluoridated toothpaste by young children is a concern; prudent use is "smear" or "rice-size" amount of toothpaste on the brush for children younger than age 3 years and a "pea-size" amount for children age 3 to 6 years; it is also recommended that toothpaste be placed on the toothbrush by an adult
   c. Inappropriate supplementation with fluoride tablets or fluoride-containing vitamins in children—mild-to-moderate fluorosis is associated with the use of fluoride supplements by children; use tends to be higher in children from higher-SES families
   d. Halo effect of secondary fluoride exposures to fluoride in processed foods and beverages, especially those that vary by water source, can occur even in nonfluoridated areas
      (1) Infant formula that has high fluoride content (e.g., soy formula) should be used in moderation in fluoridated communities; mixing concentrated formulas with fluoridated drinking water can result in excess fluoride consumption
      (2) Fruit juices and drinks with moderate-to-high concentrations of fluoride consumed by children may contribute to fluorosis; in the United States water and processed beverages can provide approximately 75% of a person's fluoride intake
      (3) Some bottled water manufactured in the United States contains an optimal concentration of fluoride, depending on the source of the water

e. Consumption of fluoridated water in combination with other significant dietary sources of fluoride
   (1) Combining systemic fluoride will increase the fluoride level above the optimum and cause fluorosis in children who are still in the stages of enamel development (up to age 8 years); education is needed to inform the public of the need to control early consumption of fluoride
   (2) Care must be taken to control young children inadvertently swallowing other sources of fluoride, such as toothpaste and mouthrinse
4. Prevention of dental fluorosis
   a. The CDC has issued recommendations to reduce the risk of fluorosis (Box 20.6)
   b. Partially because of concerns about the increase in fluorosis in children, in April 2015 the DHHS lowered the recommended amount of F to add to community drinking water (0.7 mg F per liter of water)
   c. Prior to promoting a fluoride modality or combination of modalities, one must consider the group's risk for dental caries, fluoride history, current fluoride sources, and potential for dental fluorosis
   d. Actions and recommendations related to the optimal level of fluoride in drinking water and judicious use of other fluorides are in response to the need to control fluorosis; future assessment will determine the results of current measures to prevent fluorosis

## MEASUREMENT OF DISEASES AND CONDITIONS IN ORAL EPIDEMIOLOGY

A. Dental index—abbreviated measurement tool used for data collection; measures the presence or degree of intensity of a disease or condition in a population; graduated numerical scale with defined upper and lower limits designed to facilitate summarizing or describing a disease or condition in the population, or for comparisons among populations; a higher number on the scale indicates more severe disease or condition; measured by clinical observation with an epidemiologic examination
B. Attributes of an ideal dental index
   1. Validity—accuracy of measuring what is intended to be measured
   2. Reliability—measures consistently at different times; reproducibility, stability of measurement
   3. Utility—clear, simple, and objective
   4. Sensitive to shifts in disease in either direction
   5. Acceptable to the individuals being measured
   6. Quantifiable; amenable to statistical analysis
   7. Clinically significant and meaningful
C. The index may be used to assess disease that is a reversible condition, an irreversible condition, or a combination; therefore, indices are classified as one of the following:
   1. Reversible index—measures a condition that can be reversed (e.g., gingivitis, plaque biofilm, calculus)
   2. Irreversible index—measures a cumulative condition that cannot be reversed (e.g., dental caries, bone loss, fluorosis)
D. Some common dental indices are used in community oral health and oral health research (see Table 20.13)
E. Index selection is determined by the following:
   1. Condition to be assessed, specific to the information of interest or the needs of the patient or community
   2. Age of the population
   3. Purpose of the assessment (e.g., survey or clinical trial)
F. Other approaches to measurement in a population
   1. A disaggregated approach rather than an index is currently used on the NHANES and other surveys to assess periodontal conditions; gingival bleeding, recession, pocket depth, CAL, and calculus as a contributing risk factor are measured
   2. Basic Screening Survey (BSS) for surveillance
      a. A simple screening method currently used with older adults, school-age children, and preschool-age children in national surveys
      b. Includes oral screening (see Table 20.14) and an optional questionnaire
      c. Screeners may be nondental personnel to improve access to the population and reduce cost
      d. Assesses a variety of oral health conditions consistent with the HP oral conditions objectives to monitor the success of these objectives and compare population groups
      e. Efficiently assesses dental caries using dichotomous measures (e.g., yes or no) to assess the absence or presence of untreated dental caries and dental caries experience (at least one decayed, restored, or missing tooth) on a per-person basis, as opposed to using more complex indices
      f. Regardless of condition being measured, results are reported as the following categories to assess need and referral for dental care:
         (1) None—no obvious oral health problem; routine care recommended
         (2) Early—observable oral health problem; early dental care (within several weeks) recommended
         (3) Urgent—signs or symptoms present (e.g., pain, infection, swelling, soft tissue ulceration) of longer than 2 weeks' duration; emergency dental care (within 24 hours) recommended
      g. Useful for screening purposes to assess needs of the priority population for program planning; less useful for measuring success and outcomes of a program; results will underestimate disease prevalence
G. Examiners or raters should use calibrated or standardized observational criteria for an index or the BSS; examiner reliability requires training on the use and interpretation of evaluative criteria and repeated use of the index
   1. Intra-rater (intra-examiner) reliability—each examiner repeats the scoring process using a data collection instrument; extent to which a rater remains consistent within himself or herself
   2. Inter-rater (inter-examiner) reliability—consistency exists between or among examiners; degree to which different raters obtain the same results when using the same data collection instrument

TABLE 20.13 **Common Dental Indices Used in Community Oral Health and Oral Health Research**

| Dental Index | Interpretation |
|---|---|
| **Dental Caries Indices** | |
| *Decayed-Missing-Filled Teeth* (DMFT) *Index*: complex irreversible index used to measure past and present coronal caries experience of a population with permanent teeth<br>*D* indicates a carious tooth<br>*M* indicates a tooth missing as a result of dental caries<br>*F* indicates a filled tooth because of caries<br>*deft Index*: variation of the DMFT; is used to measure observable caries experience in primary teeth; the *d* and *f* symbols are the same as in the DMFT; however, *e* indicates the need for extraction (not extracted), and missing teeth are not considered | DMF and def can be scored on teeth (DMFT and deft) or surfaces (DMFS and defs); scoring on teeth is recommended for survey work, and scoring on surfaces is recommended for clinical trials because it provides more sensitivity even though it has greater variability<br>Total DMF (D + M + F) or dmf indicates cumulative caries experience; D provides information about morbidity and specific treatment needs; F and M provide information about dental utilization<br>Programming needs can be determined by the total score as well as the scores within each category; e.g., high caries experience (DMF or dmf) indicates need for programs to prevent and control caries; high D or d indicates need for treatment programs; high M or m indicates need for education and earlier intervention; high F or f score indicates dental utilization<br>Scores can be compared to evaluate program success; e.g., reduction of D or d and increase in F or f indicates a successful caries treatment program, and marked increase in D or d, DMF or dmf, or both, indicates failure of caries prevention program<br>To control for variability of scoring missing teeth in children at the age of exfoliation, the def index does not score exfoliated or extracted teeth or surfaces, thus possibly underrepresenting caries experience |
| *Root Caries Index* (RCI): method for reporting the severity of root caries (decayed and filled exposed root surfaces) | The index is expressed as a percentage of decayed and filled root surfaces out of the population of at-risk root surfaces (those exposed to the oral environment as a result of gingival recession) |
| **Gingivitis Indices** | |
| *Gingival Index (GI)*: reversible index based on severity of inflammation at the gingival margin; can be used to determine prevalence and severity of gingivitis in epidemiologic surveys as well as individual dentition; often used in controlled clinical trials of preventive or therapeutic agents | Results can be unreliable and difficult to replicate due to subjectivity of criteria (calibration is critical)<br>SCORING CRITERIA:<br>0—Normal gingiva<br>1—Mild inflammation: slight change in color; slight edema; no bleeding on probing<br>2—Moderate inflammation: redness, edema, and glazing; bleeding on probing<br>3—Severe inflammation: marked redness and edema, ulceration; tendency to spontaneous bleeding<br>INTERPRETATION OF GI:<br>0.1 to 1.0: Mild gingivitis<br>1.1 to 2.0: Moderate gingivitis<br>2.1 to 3.0: Severe gingivitis |
| *Sulcus Bleeding Index (SBI)*: complex index designed to detect early symptoms of gingivitis; useful in short-term clinical trials; measured on probing around entire circumference of each tooth | Results can be unreliable due to subjectivity of criteria (calibration is critical)<br>Results are reported by frequency of each score<br>SCORING CRITERIA:<br>0—Healthy appearance of papillary and marginal gingiva; no bleeding on sulcus probing<br>1—Apparently healthy papillary and marginal gingiva showing no change in color and no swelling; bleeding from sulcus on probing<br>2—Bleeding on probing and change of color caused by inflammation; no swelling or microscopic edema<br>3—Bleeding on probing; change in color; slight edematous swelling<br>4—Bleeding on probing; obvious swelling; may have change in color<br>5—Bleeding on probing; spontaneous bleeding; change in color; marked swelling with or without ulceration |
| *Gingival Bleeding Index (GBI)*: simple, easy-to-implement measure of the presence or absence of bleeding (dichotomous measure); measured with the use of floss | Index only provides information about bleeding, not about other parameters of gingivitis<br>Dichotomous measure lacks sensitivity but has good reliability (easy to calibrate)<br>SCORING CRITERIA:<br>Results are reported by frequency of score based on presence (1) or absence (0) of bleeding in each proximal space |
| *Eastman Interdental Bleeding Index (EIBI)*: simple, easy-to-implement measure of the presence or absence of bleeding (dichotomous measure); measured with the use of a triangular interdental stimulator | Index only provides information about bleeding, not about other parameters of gingivitis<br>Dichotomous measure lacks sensitivity but has good reliability (easy to calibrate)<br>SCORING CRITERIA:<br>Results are reported by frequency of score based on presence (1) or absence (0) of bleeding in each proximal space |
| **Periodontal Disease Indices** | |
| *Periodontal Disease Index (PDI)*: used to measure the presence and severity of periodontal disease, combining measures of reversible and irreversible disease within the same index | This index was first to introduce the current method of combining recession and pocket depth to determine clinical attachment loss (CAL; also called loss of attachment [LOA])<br>The six teeth scored by the PDI (numbers 3, 9, 12, 19, 25, and 28), referred to as the Ramfjord teeth (after Dr. Ramfjord, who developed the index), are considered sensitive for partial mouth scoring of periodontal conditions with other indices<br>The PDI is no longer recommended because of the current understanding that gingivitis and periodontitis are two different disease entities; the various components are currently measured separately with other indices or measures |

**TABLE 20.13 Common Dental Indices Used in Community Oral Health and Oral Health Research—cont'd**

| Dental Index | Interpretation |
|---|---|
| *Community Periodontal Index of Treatment Needs (CPITN):* used as part of the Oral Health Surveys by the World Health Organization; facilitates rapid assessment of mean disease status of a population; the Periodontal Screening and Recording (PSR) Index developed by the American Dental Association for use in clinical practice uses the same codes and criteria; pockets are measured with a specially designed, lightweight probe with a 0.5-mm markings, a colored area to denote 3.5-mm to 5.5-mm depth, and a ball tip | Scores are reported as codes in six sextants of the mouth<br>CRITERIA FOR SCORING CODES:<br>*Code 0*—Line at colored area visible; no rough areas, no bleeding<br>*Code 1*—Line at colored area visible with bleeding after probing<br>*Code 2*—Line visible with bleeding and rough areas (calculus)<br>*Code 3*—Colored area only partially visible (> 3.5 mm)<br>*Code 4*—Colored area completely disappears (> 5.5 mm)<br>By code for furcation involvement, mobility, mucogingival problem, marked recession, or all<br>INTERPRETATION OF CODES (Treatment Needs):<br>*Code* 0—Preventive care; biofilm control<br>*Code* 1—Preventive care; biofilm control<br>*Code* 2—Preventive care and calculus removal; biofilm removal<br>*Code* 3—Comprehensive periodontal assessment and treatment plan (TP); counseling regarding TP; biofilm control<br>*Code* 4—Comprehensive periodontal assessment and TP for nonsurgical periodontal therapy; counseling regarding TP; biofilm control |
| *Community Periodontal Index (CPI):* adaptation of the CPITN to measure periodontal status of a community; treatment need codes from the CPITN are eliminated; in contrast to the CPITN, the CPI measures periodontal status, whereas the CPITN reports periodontal treatment needs | Reported as CPI (periodontal status) codes and loss of attachment (LOA) codes<br>SCORING CRITERIA FOR CPI CODES:<br>*Code 0*—Entire colored band visible; healthy periodontal tissues: no bleeding<br>*Code 1*—Entire colored band visible; bleeding on probing<br>*Code 2*—Entire colored band visible; calculus present<br>*Code 3*—Colored band partially hidden: 4-mm to 5-mm pockets<br>*Code 4*—Colored band entirely hidden: > 6-mm pockets<br>If the cemento-enamel junction (CEJ) is visible or the CPI is 4, LOA codes 1 to 4 are used<br>CRITERIA FOR LOA CODES:<br>*Code 0*—0 to 3 mm LOA—CEJ covered by gingival margin and CPI score of 0 to 3<br>*Code 1*—3.5 to 5.5 mm LOA; CEJ within the black band on probe<br>*Code 2*—6 to 8 mm LOA; CEJ between top of black band and 8.5-mm mark on probe<br>*Code 3*—9 to 11 mm LOA; CEJ between 8.5-mm and 11.5-mm marks on probe<br>*Code 4*—LOA > 12 mm; CEJ beyond highest mark (11.5 mm) on probe |
| **Oral Hygiene Indices** | |
| *Simplified Oral Hygiene Index (OHI-S):* reversible index used to measure oral hygiene status; useful to survey oral hygiene in a population; scores six teeth that represent the whole mouth, assessing them separately for debris and calculus, and yielding a DI-S score (debris index–simplified) and a CI-S score (calculus index–simplified), which are combined for the OHI-S score | SCORING CRITERIA FOR DI-S:<br>0—No debris or stain present<br>1—Soft debris covering not more than one-third of exposed tooth surface or presence of extrinsic stains without debris regardless of surface area covered<br>2—Soft debris covering more than one-third but not more than two-thirds of exposed tooth surface<br>3—Soft debris covering more than two-thirds of exposed tooth surface<br>SCORING CRITERIA FOR CI-S:<br>0—No calculus present<br>1—Supragingival calculus covering not more than one-third of exposed tooth surface<br>2—Supragingival calculus covering more than one-third but not more than two-thirds of exposed tooth surface or presence of individual flecks of subgingival calculus around cervical portion of tooth<br>3—Supragingival calculus covering more than two-thirds of exposed tooth surface or a continuous heavy band of subgingival calculus around cervical portion of tooth<br>INTERPRETATION OF OHI-S:<br>0.0 to 1.2: Good oral hygiene<br>1.3 to 3.0: Fair oral hygiene<br>3.1 to 6.0: Poor oral hygiene<br>INTERPRETATION OF DI-S or CI-S:<br>0.0 to 0.6: Good oral hygiene<br>0.7 to 1.8: Fair oral hygiene<br>1.9 to 3.0: Poor oral hygiene |

*Continued*

**TABLE 20.13 Common Dental Indices Used in Community Oral Health and Oral Health Research—cont'd**

| Dental Index | Interpretation |
|---|---|
| *Plaque Index (Pl-I)*: used to assess extent of soft deposits, measuring differences in thickness of debris only at the gingival margin of the tooth surface; useful in longitudinal studies and clinical trials | SCORING CRITERIA:<br>0—No plaque biofilm in gingival area<br>1—Film of plaque biofilm adhering to free gingival margin and adjacent area of tooth; plaque biofilm is noticed only by running probe across tooth surface<br>2—Moderate accumulation of soft deposits within the gingival margin, on adjacent tooth surface, or in both areas that can be seen with the naked eye<br>3—Abundance of soft matter within the gingival pocket, at the gingival margin, or both, and on the adjacent tooth surface<br>INTERPRETATION OF PI-I:<br>0: Excellent<br>0.1 to 0.9: Good<br>1.0 to 1.9: Fair<br>2.0 to 3.0: Poor |
| *Patient Hygiene Performance (PHP)*: provides a simple, quick, overall oral hygiene assessment, scoring disclosed plaque biofilm in five sections of the tooth surface of six representative teeth; scores interproximal areas separately to evaluate interdental cleaning | SCORING CRITERIA:<br>Plaque biofilm is scored as present (1) or absent (0) in each of the five areas; scores are combined for the tooth score or reported separately for evaluation of oral hygiene in specific areas<br>INTERPRETATION OF PHP:<br>0: Excellent<br>0.1 to 1.7: Good<br>1.8 to 3.4: Fair<br>3.5 to 5.0: Poor |
| *Turesky modification of the Quigley-Hein Plaque Index (TPI)*: provides an overall assessment of oral hygiene similar to the OHI-S but more sensitive because (1) the scale has more differentiation at the lower end, (2) all teeth are scored, and (3) disclosant is used; recommended for clinical trials of preventive and therapeutic agents | Teeth are disclosed; all teeth except third molars are evaluated; results can be unreliable because of subjectivity at the lower end of the scale; careful calibration is critical<br>SCORING CRITERIA:<br>Mesial, distal, and middle aspects of buccal and lingual surfaces of all teeth are scored on a scale of 0 to 5<br>0—No plaque biofilm<br>1—Separate flecks of plaque biofilm at the cervical margin<br>2—A thin continuous band of plaque biofilm (up to 1 mm) at the cervical margin<br>3—A band of plaque biofilm wider than 1 mm but covering less than one-third of the tooth surface<br>4—Plaque biofilm covering at least one-third but less than two-thirds of the surface<br>5—Plaque biofilm covering two-thirds or more of the surface |
| *Modified Navy Plaque Index (MNPI)*: provides a detailed assessment of overall oral hygiene as well as effectiveness of interdental cleaning; similar to the PHP with more sensitivity as a result of the surfaces being divided into nine instead of five areas; useful to assess the value of oral health education programs and individuals' oral hygiene practices | Results can be unreliable because of the complexity of the index; requires careful calibration<br>SCORING CRITERIA:<br>Plaque biofilm is scored as present (1) or absent (0) in each of the nine areas; scores are combined for the tooth score or reported separately for evaluation of oral hygiene in specific areas, as follows:<br>Whole mouth (all nine areas)<br>Marginal (mesial, distal, and middle aspects of the marginal area)<br>Approximal (mesial and distal contact areas) |
| *Volpe-Manhold Index (VMI)*: measures extent of supragingival calculus on the lingual surfaces of mandibular anterior teeth for calculus clinical trials | Height of calculus is measured with a probe, which can be reported as a tooth score (possible range of 0 to 15) or whole-mouth score (possible range of 0 to 90)<br>Large range of scores allows for more valid statistical analysis |

TABLE 20.13 **Common Dental Indices Used in Community Oral Health and Oral Health Research—cont'd**

| Dental Index | Interpretation |
|---|---|
| **Fluorosis Indices** | |
| *Dean Fluorosis Index* and *Community Fluorosis Index (CFI)*: Used for survey purposes. Dean developed the classification as categories only, referred to as Dean Fluorosis Index; later numbers ranging from 0 to 4 were added to denote the categories for surveillance purposes, and the index was referred to as the Community Fluorosis Index<br>*Comparison to other fluorosis indices:*<br>The Thylstrup-Fejerskov (TF) fluorosis index and Tooth Surface Index of Fluorosis (TSIF) are based on Dean's categories with expansion of categories to create greater sensitivity for research purposes | An individual is categorized by classification, and prevalence of each category is reported in a population; the CFI of a population is assigned based on the mean of all scores of the study population; a classification of mild or less is not considered a cosmetic problem, and a CFI score of less than 0.6 is not considered a problem for the community<br>SCORING CRITERIA:<br>*Normal (0)*—Enamel presents the usual translucent semivitriform structure; the surface is smooth, glossy, and usually pale creamy white<br>*Questionable (0.5)*—Enamel has slight aberrations from the normal translucency, ranging from a few white flecks to occasional white spots; this classification is used when neither the *Very Mild* nor *Normal* classification is definitively justified<br>*Very mild (1)*—Small, opaque, paper-white areas are scattered irregularly over the tooth but not involving as much as approximately 25% of the tooth surface; frequently included in this classification are teeth showing no more than about 1 to 2 mm of white opacity at the cusp tips of premolars or second molars<br>*Mild (2)*—White opaque areas in the enamel are more extensive but do not involve as much as 50% of the tooth<br>*Moderate (3)*—All enamel surfaces of the teeth are affected, and surfaces subject to attrition show wear; brown stain is frequently a disfiguring feature<br>*Severe (4)*—All enamel surfaces are affected; hypoplasia is so marked that the general form of the tooth may be affected; discrete or confluent pitting is a major diagnostic sign of this classification; brown stains are widespread, and teeth often appear as if corroded<br>SIGNICANCE OF CFI SCORES:<br>0.0 to 0.4: Negative<br>0.4 to 0.6: Borderline<br>0.6 to 1.0: Slight<br>1.0 to 2.0: Medium<br>2.0 to 3.0: Marked<br>3.0 to 4.0: Very marked |

Data from Beatty CF. *Community Oral Health Practice for the Dental Hygienist.* 4th ed. Appendix F St. Louis: Elsevier; 2017.
Newman NG, Takei H. Klokkevold PR, Carranza FA. *Carranza's Clinical Periodontology.* 13th ed. St. Louis: Elsevier Saunders; 2019.
Wilkins EM. *Clinical Practice of the Dental Hygienist.* 12th ed. Philadelphia: Wolters Kluwer; 2017.
*World Health Organization.* Oral health/periodontal/country profiles. http://www.who.int/oral_health/databases/niigata/en/; 2019 Accessed 07.07.20.

H. Potential errors in assessing disease
   1. Errors in sampling technique—use of nonrandomized samples, use of incorrect or inconsistent sampling technique, sample bias and too small sample size can result in a nonrepresentative sample, particularly for subgroups of interest
   2. Errors in collecting and recording data—variation in assessment, lack of calibration, inconsistent or inaccurate data collection by the examiners, known or unknown bias,; intended or unintended misleading or untruthful responses, lack of compliance of participants, incorrect documenting of data by recorders, and inaccurate data entry into the computer
   3. Errors in analyzing data—incorrect computation, incorrect selection of statistical tests, incomplete analysis, and invalid interpretation

# PREVENTING AND CONTROLLING ORAL DISEASES AND CONDITIONS

## Public Health Measures

A. Population-focused strategies to alleviate, reduce, or eliminate a health problem or issue that is an actual or potential cause of morbidity or mortality
B. Selection of strategy is based on the seven characteristics of an effective public health solution (see earlier "Basic Concepts" section); several strategies may be implemented depending on the issue to be addressed
C. Examples of public health measures include tobacco-control policies, vaccination requirements, water fluoridation, adoption of a school-based oral health curriculum, and public funding of dental care

## Measures for Preventing and Controlling Dental Caries

See "Topical Fluorides and Fluoride Varnishes", "Dentifrices and Prophylactic Pastes", "Pit-and-Fissure Sealants", "Caries Management", sections in Chapter 16.

A. Water fluoridation (see Table 20.15)
   1. Adjustment of the natural fluoride concentration to optimal level
      a. Suggested level of F is 0.7 mg F per liter of water as of 2015[11] (same as 0.7 ppm F); this is a nonenforceable recommendation from the DHHS/PHS
      b. In 2014, 74.7% of the US population on public water systems received optimally fluoridated water, an increase from 72.4% in 2008 and representing a

gradual increase over the seven decades of fluoridation; increasing this percentage continues to be an emphasis of dental public health[1] (see Table 20.3)

c. Some states have community fluoridation laws that are enforceable

d. Partial exposure (lower than the recommended F level) provides partial protection

**BOX 20.6 Recommendations to Reduce the Risk of Fluorosis**

- Counsel parents and caregivers regarding the use of fluoride toothpaste by young children, especially those younger than 2 years
- Encourage parents to supervise the use of fluoride toothpaste among children younger than 6 years to reduce swallowing it
- Promote the use of the recommended small amount of toothpaste by young children
- For children younger than 2 years, weigh the risk and benefits of recommending fluoride products, taking into consideration the fluoride level in the community drinking water, other sources of fluoride, and factors likely to affect susceptibility to tooth decay
- Target mouth rinsing and application of high-concentration fluoride products to persons at high risk for dental caries
- Target and judiciously prescribe fluoride supplements according to recommended guidelines
- Know the fluoride concentration in the primary source of drinking water in order to make appropriate recommendations
- Use an alternative source of water for children age 8 years and younger whose primary drinking water contains more than 2 mg F per liter of water
- Label the fluoride concentration of bottled water
- Collaborate with professional health care organizations, public health agencies, and suppliers of oral care products to educate health care professionals and the public
- Identify effective strategies to promote adoption of recommendations for using F

Data from *Centers for Disease Control and Prevention.* Dental fluorosis. http://www.cdc.gov/fluoridation/faqs/dental_fluorosis/#a10. Accessed 03.08.19.

e. Level must be maintained to continue maximum benefits of fluoridation; benefits are lost when fluoridation is discontinued

2. Fluoridation is one of the 10 most effective public health measures of the 20th century; meets the requirements of a public health solution (Box 20.1)
3. Fluoridation does not have specific population targets; it has the potential to reduce disparities by reaching everyone in the community
4. Fluoridation is the most practical form of preventing caries in communities with established community water systems
5. Fluoridation effectively prevents and controls dental caries in children and adults
   a. Is attributed with 20% to 40% caries reduction in the mixed dentition of children (8 to 12 years of age), 15% to 35% caries reduction in the permanent dentition of adolescents (14 to 17 years of age), and 20% to 40% reduction of coronal caries in adults
   b. Benefits both primary and permanent teeth
   c. Primarily prevents smooth surface caries; as overall caries rates in a population are reduced by fluoride, the proportion of pit-and-fissure caries increases, even though the absolute number is reduced
   d. Controls both coronal and root caries in older adults
   e. Helps to control caries resulting from reduced salivary flow caused by medications
   f. Has no known prenatal benefits
   g. Benefits of fluoride accumulate; combination of water fluoridation with topical fluoride provides additional benefits (systemic programs should not be combined to avoid increase in fluorosis in the population)
   h. Fluoride is the most effective means to prevent and control dental caries; a common misconception is that oral hygiene is the most effective means

**TABLE 20.14 Basic Screening Survey Indicators, Revised 2017**

| Preschool Children | School Children | Older Adults |
|---|---|---|
| **Recommended Indicators** | | |
| • Untreated decay<br>• Treated decay<br>• Urgency of need for dental care | • Untreated decay<br>• Treated decay<br>• Dental sealants on permanent molars<br>• Urgency of need for dental care | • Dentures and denture use<br>• Number of natural teeth<br>• Untreated decay<br>• Root fragments<br>• Need for periodontal care<br>• Suspicious soft tissue lesions<br>• Urgency of need for dental care |
| **Optional Indicators** | | |
| • Rampant decay<br>• Number of quadrants with untreated decay<br>• Dental sealants on primary molars<br>• Potentially arrested decay | • Rampant decay<br>• Number of quadrants with untreated decay<br>• Potentially arrested decay | • Functional posterior occlusal contacts<br>• Substantial oral debris<br>• Severe gingival inflammation<br>• Obvious tooth mobility<br>• Severe dry mouth |

Data from Phipps K. *The new & improved children's basic screening survey* (PowerPoint slides), Association of State & Territorial Dental Directors, 2017, https://www.astdd.org/docs/childrens-bss-webinar-ppt-10-12-2017.pdf. Accessed 07.07.20; and *Association of State and Territorial Dental Directors.* Basic screening surveys: An approach to monitoring community oral health: Older adults, 2010. http://www.prevmed.org/wp-content/uploads/2013/11/BSS-SeniorsManual.pdf. Accessed 07.07.20.

**TABLE 20.15 Overview of Fluoride (F) Delivery Modalities**

| Delivery Mechanism | Active Ingredient(s) | Intended Population | Indications for Use |
|---|---|---|---|
| **Professionally Applied Fluoride** | | | |
| Gels, foams, mouthrinses | 2% NaF (920 ppm) *or* 1.23% APF (12,300 ppm) *or* 0.15% $SnF_2$ (1000 ppm) | Any person with an elevated caries risk | APF and $SnF_2$ no longer recommended for general population; may be indicated for high-risk, special-needs groups |
| Varnishes | 5% NaF (22,600 ppm) | Any person with an elevated caries risk | Recommended as a more effective fluoride delivery mechanism due to sustainability in salivary solution |
| Silver diamine fluoride (SDF) | 25% silver (antimicrobial); 38% F (44,800 ppm F) | Individuals who are unable to access dental treatment or cannot tolerate conventional dental care (very young, noncooperative children; frail elderly; persons with intellectual, developmental, or physical disabilities, or with situation anxiety or dental phobias) | Recommended to arrest cavitated carious lesions painlessly and without anesthesia as an interim therapy to control disease process, to be followed up with restoration if necessary to restore form and function of the tooth |
| **Self-Applied Fluoride** | | | |
| OTC dentifrices | 0.243% NaF *or* 0.76% MFP *or* 0.0454% $SnF_2$ All are 1,000 to 1,500 ppm | Ages >2 years Low-to-moderate caries risk, regardless of water fluoridation status | Most important delivery mode for fluoride due to consistent topical exposure; indicated as a preventive agent for all populations, regardless of risk level |
| Fluoride Rx | NaF, $SnF_2$, or APF; concentration % can vary depending on delivery modality and weight of individual | Any person with an elevated caries risk and/or lack of available community water fluoridation | *Children* 0.25-, 0.50-, or 1.0-mg NaF tablets, lozenges, liquids, and vitamin preparations for systemic use generally in children 6 months to 16 years; drops used with infants (see Table 20.16); school programs no longer recommended by CDC because of other multiple sources of F *Adults* 1.1% NaF dentifrice (5000 ppm), 0.5% NaF gel, or 0.15% $SnF_2$ gel prescribed for topical use in individuals age 16 and older |
| **Public Health Fluoride Programs** | | | |
| Community water fluoridation | 0.7 ppm F fluorosilicic acid—also referred to as hydrofluorosilicate (water-based solution), sodium fluorosilicate (dry salt dissolved into solution), or NaF (dry salt dissolved into solution) | Communities at large; municipal water system is required | Most cost-effective and efficient modality for bringing fluoride benefits to all community members regardless of age or SES |
| School water fluoridation | 4.5 times the optimum fluoride concentration | School-age children in nonfluoridated communities, especially in rural areas | No longer emphasized because of increased presence of water fluoridation, multiple other sources of fluoride, and disadvantages of modality |
| School fluoride tablet programs | 1-mg NaF chewable tablet, swished and swallowed | School-age children in unfluoridated communities | No longer emphasized because of increased presence of water fluoridation and other sources of fluoride; can be used in rural areas that have no fluoridation |
| School fluoride mouthrinse programs | 0.05% NaF (230 ppm): daily rinsing 0.2% NaF (920 ppm): weekly rinsing | School-age children in fluoridated and nonfluoridated communities | Limited use today because of increased presence of community water fluoridation; OTC mouthrinses in similar concentrations readily available for at-home use |
| Fluoride varnish programs (see Box 20.9) | 5% NaF (22,600 ppm) | At-risk children and adults, highly recommended for children < 6 years; status of water fluoridation not a consideration | Recommended and widely popular with Head Start and other preschool-age programs as well as in public health well-baby clinics and pediatric medical offices because of effectiveness, minimal risk of ingestion and gagging, and ease of application |
| **Other Fluoride Modalities** | | | |
| Addition of fluoride to salt | 250 ppm NaF | Countries lacking widespread municipal water supplies | Used with food preparation; distribution and equitable population exposure may vary; not used in the United States or Canada |
| Addition of fluoride to milk | ≤ 4 ppm NaF or MFP | School-age children in countries lacking widespread municipal water supplies | Studied in other countries but not used in the United States or Canada due to extensive water fluoridation |

*APF*, acidulated phosphate fluoride; *NaF*, sodium fluoride; *$SnF_2$*, stannous fluoride; *OTC*, over-the-counter; *MFP*, sodium monofluorophosphate

Data from American Academy of Pediatric Dentistry. Fluoride therapy. *Oral health policies and Recommendations (Reference Manual)*. 2018; 40(6), 250–253. https://www.aapd.org/globalassets/media/policies_guidelines/bp_fluoridetherapy.pdf;
*American Dental Association*. Fluoridation facts. https://www.ada.org/en/public-programs/advocating-for-the-public/fluoride-and-fluoridation/fluoridation-facts?utm_source=ADAorg&utm_medium=FLUORotator; 2018 Accessed 07.07.20;
*Association of State and Territorial Dental Directors*. Silver diamine fact sheet. https://www.astdd.org/www/docs/sdf-fact-sheet-09-07-2017.pdf; 2017 Accessed 07.07.20; *Centers for Disease Control and Prevention*. Water fluoridation basics. https://www.cdc.gov/fluoridation/basics/index.htm. Accessed 05.14.19;
*Centers for Disease Control and Prevention*. Water fluoridation guidelines & recommendations. http://www.cdc.gov/fluoridation/guidelines/index.htm/. Accessed 05.14.19; and
*Centers for Disease Control and Prevention*. Water fluoridation additives. https://www.cdc.gov/fluoridation/engineering/wfadditives.htm. Accessed 05.14.19.

6. Indirect benefits of fluoride include fewer missing teeth resulting in improved self-image, less complicated restorative procedures, pain reduction, decreased malocclusion, and decreased periodontal problems related to tooth loss, all of which lead to improved quality of life for the public; indirect benefits also include positive influence on the practice of dentistry and dental hygiene
7. Posteruption benefits—primary benefit of fluoridated water occurs after tooth eruption as a result of topical effects; preeruption effects are minor
   a. Critical period for benefits in children is immediately after tooth eruption so that immature enamel of newly erupted teeth can uptake the fluoride (ages 6 months to 13 years)
   b. Posteruption benefits rely on the fluoride being available in solution (via saliva) at the surface of the tooth; systemic fluoride is released into saliva and is available in saliva and plaque biofilm fluids
   c. Fluoride inhibits demineralization by adsorbing to the carbonated hydroxyapatite crystals, protecting the enamel surface from dissolution by acids
   d. Fluoride enhances remineralization of incipient caries by adsorbing during the continual demineralization-remineralization process; this is the primary action of fluoride for control of dental caries
   e. When fluoridated water is consumed, saliva has a constant fluoride level, making it continually available for uptake by the enamel
   f. Bound fluoride in plaque biofilm is released in response to the lowered pH level and taken up more readily by the demineralized enamel
8. Pre-eruption benefits—once thought to be the primary action, this is now understood to be a minor effect compared with the posteruptive action; fluoride is incorporated into the mineralized tooth structure during the enamel formation of tooth development, replacing hydroxyapatite with fluorapatite
9. Most cost-effective and efficient method of preventing dental caries
   a. Cost of fluoridation varies with the size of the community, water system, labor costs, and chemicals used; smaller communities experience higher costs because equipment and supplies required for smaller water systems are more costly
   b. A community is estimated to save 20 times more than the cost of fluoridation in a year; individuals who drink fluoridated water save an average of $32 per year in treatment costs[12]. The health care system realizes a cost benefit by preventing dental caries rather than having to provide more costly treatment
   c. Fluoridation is compatible with other water treatment processes; quality assurance protocol, including recommended annual training of personnel to prevent spills, is necessary; equipment or machinery used for community water fluoridation resembles that used to add other agents to water systems, facilitating training of water treatment personnel
10. Compounds used for water fluoridation
    a. Any compound that forms fluoride ions in aqueous solution can be used; the selection depends on the number and accessibility of water sources and water quality
    b. Most popular compounds used in fluoridation of water supplies (see Table 20.15)
    c. Fluorosilicic acid—most commonly used and least expensive; it is a byproduct of fertilizer manufacturing, which results in the claim of those opposed to fluoridation that it is a ploy to use waste
11. Extensive research has demonstrated the safety of fluoridation
    a. It is noncarcinogenic (opponents claim it is carcinogenic)
    b. Kidney failure is the only condition that requires consideration; kidney dialysis requires the use of water that is free of minerals and chemicals, including fluoride
    c. No valid research results have linked optimal levels of fluoride to any health problems
    d. It is safe to the fetus; the US Food and Drug Administration (FDA) does not recommend the use of fluoride during pregnancy because no known benefits exist, not because it is considered unsafe
12. Role of government agencies
    a. PHS provides funding through block grants and consultation to states
    b. CDC provides education to the public, delivers training to water operators, monitors water fluoridation as part of the NOHSS (Water Fluoridation Reporting System), and makes water fluoridation data available to the public (My Water's Fluoride)
    c. State oral health departments provide consultation and assistance to counties and cities attempting to fluoridate, training and monitoring for water system operators, and monitoring of water fluoridation within the state
    d. Local governments without state-mandated fluoridation decide whether or not to fluoridate, implement water fluoridation, and pay the ongoing costs of equipment and supplies
13. Legality of fluoridation—courts have upheld the constitutionality of water fluoridation
14. Promotion of water fluoridation
    a. Campaigns are required to initiate fluoridation in communities that are not currently fluoridated and to protect fluoridation in communities that are currently fluoridated
    b. Oral health care professionals are effective advocates for promoting water fluoridation within a community (Box 20.7)
    c. Ongoing education of individuals is required to encourage their continual support of fluoridation; fluoridation continues to be an issue with regard to wider public acceptance
    d. Individuals should be aware of their community water fluoride levels (information is available at My Water's

Fluoride at https://nccd.cdc.gov/doh_mwf/Default/Default.aspx) and of the ways they have benefited from fluoridation in their communities

e. Three methods of implementing fluoridation:
   (1) Administrative decision—a community leader introduces the idea of community water fluoridation through appropriate government channels, and the idea is approved by the appropriate governing body (i.e., water board, public services director, mayor, city council)
   (2) Initiative petition or referendum—allows members of the community to vote for or against fluoridation of the water supply; the referendum should be a last resort to avoid a politically charged situation
   (3) Legislative action—mandate passed by state legislators that requires specified public water supplies to be fluoridated or allows health departments to order public water supplies to be fluoridated under certain conditions; it is generally recommended that the decision to fluoridate be made at the local level, although some states have mandatory fluoridation laws

d. Public attitudes toward water fluoridation are both positive and negative—only 20% of the population are opposed to fluoridation; the majority of Americans support fluoridation; the lack of organization and passivity on the part of the supporters of fluoridation make it easier for well-organized antifluoridationists to block its implementation or adoption

e. Opponents' arguments and use of scare tactics appeal to emotions
   (1) Suggest that water fluoridation is unconstitutional and violates individual freedom of choice
   (2) Create suspicion of government programs, officials, or both
   (3) Allege that fluoridation is overregulation by the government
   (4) Associate fluoridation with concerns about poor health, disease, and aging, based on anecdotal evidence and poorly designed research studies
   (5) Imply that water fluoridation is poisonous and causes health hazards
   (6) Claim that it causes fluorosis when nonfluoridated communities have lower levels of fluorosis than fluoridated communities (invalid interpretation of data)
   (7) Link it to environmental issues, such as addition of unnecessary chemicals to the water
   (8) Incorrectly assert that adults do not benefit from fluoridation, making it inappropriate for appropriation of tax dollars
   (9) Antifluoridationists' organize to oppose new fluoridation campaigns and to have fluoridation cease or removed in communities that are currently fluoridated

f. Strategies used to support water fluoridation

### BOX 20.7 Strategies to Increase Water Fluoridation in the United States

- Develop and implement a plan of action to maintain the efficacy of water fluoridation as a proven public health measure
- Organize and enlist the support of other state and federal organizations that have an influence in guiding the development of health policies bringing about social change
- Effectively translate fluoridation information into the languages of all racial and ethnic groups
- Develop new and innovative strategies to meet the challenge of fluoridation opponents, past and present
- Develop a national clearinghouse for fluoridation materials
- Develop a national surveillance system to collect, analyze, and evaluate risk factor data related to fluorides
- Support legislation to fund community water fluoridation

Data from Department of Health and Human Services: Centers for Disease Control and Prevention: National Center for Health Statistics. *Healthy People 2020 midcourse review*, Chapter 32, Oral health, Hyattsville, Md, 2016. https://www.cdc.gov/nchs/data/hpdata2020/HP2020MCR-C32-OH.pdf; *Association of State & Territorial Dental Directors.* Best practice approach community water fluoridation. https://www.astdd.org/bestpractices/BPAFluoridation.pdf; 2016 Accessed 07.07.20.

   (1) Outcomes from rigorous studies that provide the evidence base for fluoridation
   (2) Knowledge of the community (e.g., past efforts to introduce water fluoridation or discontinue water fluoridation)
   (3) Working with all community leaders, organizations, stakeholders, and members of the community having influence, such as newspaper editors or radio/television personalities; collaboration with other health care professionals
   (4) Creating awareness of the methods, tactics, and nonscientific materials used by fluoridation opponents; recognition of the impact of incorrect information presented in print and electronic media
   (5) Steps to implement a fluoridation campaign (Box 20.8)

g. Value of consuming fluoridated water versus bottled water
   (1) Some bottled water products contain fluoride, depending on the source of the water
   (2) The FDA sets an upper limit for fluoride in bottled water; there is no lower limit
   (3) Manufacturers are not required to indicate the fluoride content on the label unless fluoride has been added
   (4) Bottled water products labeled as de-ionized, purified, demineralized, or distilled contain no or only trace amounts of fluoride

B. Dietary fluoride supplements (see Table 20.15)
   1. Dosage and age recommendations (see Table 20.16)
   2. Other available sources of fluoride should be considered; related factors, such as risk, cooperation, age, and ability of the child, should also be taken into account

**BOX 20.8 Steps to Implement Water Fluoridation in a Local Community to Avoid a Referendum**

1. Form a citizen's community such as "Citizens for Healthy Teeth"; consider hiring a consultant or arrange for consultation from the state dental public health department
2. Know the facts: scientific basis for fluoridation, physiology, effectiveness, safety, cost of fluoridating community, antifluoridationists' tactics, charges and answers, legality of fluoridation, and history of local fluoridation
3. Identify and contact key community leaders to educate them and receive support for the issue
4. Gather endorsements from key community leaders to document support when meeting with the city council
5. Form a broad base of support beyond the dental and medical professions through the committee and endorsements
6. Educate the city council members on the issue, one-on-one, before the issue is brought before council meetings
7. Bring the issue formally before the city council only after support has been received from community leaders and individual council members
8. Attend council meetings to show support of the issue
9. Be prepared to testify at the city council meetings

3. Supplementation is not recommended for children at low risk for caries
4. School-based fluoride supplement programs
   a. Yielded 30% reduction in dental caries
   b. Were cost-effective and efficient
   c. Required parental consent and the need for ongoing cooperation of highly motivated staff and parents made implementation cumbersome
   d. Infrequently used today in the United States except in rural areas without fluoridation; used internationally
5. For children younger than 6 years, the risk of fluorosis should be weighed against the benefit of supplementation; parents should be informed of the possibility of fluorosis[13]
6. Supplements are required daily for effectiveness; at-home use has the disadvantage of dependence on adherence; increased patient adherence may be achieved with combined F-vitamin supplements
7. Controlled daily at-home use results in caries reduction similar to water fluoridation
8. Dietary supplements are not recommended for infants who are breastfed; breast milk contains 0.0004 mg F per liter
9. Prenatal supplementation with fluoride is not recommended, although it is not harmful to the fetus; even though it crosses the placental barrier and enters the fetal circulation, benefits are minor, since mineralization of enamel is not advanced until after birth, and primary benefit of fluoride occurs after tooth eruption

C. Fluoride varnish programs (see Table 20.15)
1. Studies show 45% caries reduction with public health programs
2. Fluoride varnish public health programs have numerous advantages compared to other fluoride modalities (Box 20.9)
3. Child positioning for examination and fluoride varnish application
   a. Knee to knee—infant held by parent in lap, with child's head on parent's knees and child's legs around parent's waist; operator is knee to knee with parent, treating the infant from behind; an alternate is to place infant on an examination table and work from behind
   b. Face to face—young child seated in small school chair; operator is seated directly facing child, tilting child's head back for good visibility; alternative positions are child standing in front of seated operator or operator standing behind seated larger child and working from above
4. Varnish should be reapplied every 3 months in high-risk children and every 6 months in moderate-risk children
5. CDC recommends programs with preschool-age children such as Head Start
6. Educational program with parents and children should be included to increase adherence and address other aspects of caries prevention and control

D. School water fluoridation (see Table 20.15)
1. Still in use in some communities with suboptimal fluoride levels, particularly rural areas where community water fluoridation is impossible; extent of current practice is unknown; no longer recommended by CDC because of disadvantages, expansion of water fluoridation, and increased availability of other sources of fluoride
2. Disadvantages—no benefits until children begin school; exposure occurs only during school year and on school days; benefits only schoolchildren; equipment for these small water systems have logistical problems and greater risk of spills
3. Reduced caries among schoolchildren by approximately 40%
4. Suggested level of fluoride is adjusted (see Table 20.15) to compensate for drinking fluoridated water only when school is in session

E. Fluoridated salt (see Table 20.15)
1. Reduction in caries parallels rates found with water fluoridation
2. Used in some other countries; WHO criteria include the inability to implement water fluoridation, low levels of fluoride in the diet and environment, lack of political will to introduce water fluoridation, centralized salt production, and appropriate package labeling; not used in the United States or Canada

F. Fluoridated milk (see Table 20.15)
1. Consumption of fluoridated milk by children in schools
2. Outcomes of programs in several European countries (not United States or Canada) showed caries protection comparable with water fluoridation at the same concentration; effective but not ideal form of delivery
3. Disadvantages—only provides a single fluoride exposure on school days; requires refrigeration; milk consumption declines with increasing age of child

G. Professionally applied topical fluoride (see Table 20.15)
1. In-office professional application of topical fluoride is the least cost-effective public health fluoride measure

### TABLE 20.16 Dietary Fluoride (F) Supplementation Schedule (in mg F/day[a])

| | CONCENTRATION OF FLUORIDE IN THE WATER | | |
|---|---|---|---|
| Age | < 0.03 mg | 0.3 ppm to > 0.6 mg | > 0.6 mg |
| 0 to 6 months | 0 | 0 | 0 |
| 6 months to 3 years | 0.25 mg | 0 | 0 |
| 3 to 6 years | 0.50 mg | 0.25 mg | 0 |
| 6 to 16 years | 1.0 mg | 0.50 mg | 0 |

This fluoride supplementation schedule was reviewed by the American Dental Association (ADA) and the American Academy of Pediatric Dentistry (AAPD) after the DDHS/PHS guideline for concentration of F in the community water supply was revised in 2015; their decision was to leave the recommended schedule unchanged.

[a]2.2 mg sodium fluoride (NaF) contains 1 mg F ion; .07 ppm, .07 mg/L.

Data from American Academy of Pediatric Dentistry. Guideline on fluoride therapy, *Oral Health Policies and Recommendations (Reference Manual)*. 2018; 40(6), 250–253, http://www.aapd.org/media/Policies_Guidelines/G_FluorideTherapy.pdf; and *American Dental Association*. Fluoride: topical and systemic supplements. https://www.ada.org/en/member-center/oral-health-topics/fluoride-topical-and-systemic-supplements Accessed 05.01.19.

### BOX 20.9 Advantages of Public Health Fluoride Varnish Programs

- No special dental equipment required
- Professional dental cleaning not required before application
- Ease of application
- Dries immediately on contact with saliva
- Safety
- Well tolerated by all; especially convenient for use on infants, young children, and individuals with special needs
- Inexpensive
- Minimal training required for placement; nondental personnel can be trained
- Allows the ability to eat or drink immediately after application
- Prevents and reverses decay
- Shows caries reduction up to 45% compared with 30% to 35% for other fluoride systems
- Recommended for use with children younger than 6 years

Data from American Academy of Pediatric Dentistry. Fluoride therapy. *Oral health policies and Recommendations (Reference Manual)* 2018; 40(6), 250–253. https://www.aapd.org/globalassets/media/policies_guidelines/bp_fluoridetherapy.pdf; and *Centers for Disease Control and Prevention*. Other fluoride products. https://www.cdc.gov/fluoridation/basics/fluoride-products.html. Accessed 03.08.19.

2. Fluoride varnish application is the only type of professionally applied fluoride that is recommended as a public health program
3. Sodium fluoride (NaF), stannous fluoride ($SnF_2$), and acidulated phosphate fluoride (APF) in gel, foam, and mouthrinse forms no longer recommended by CDC as a population-based strategy; may be indicated in high-risk populations in targeted programs such as institutions for high-risk, special-needs groups

H. Fluoride mouthrinses in school-based programs (see Table 20.15)
   1. Widely used at one time; still used in some areas, especially developing countries
   2. Studies indicated 20% to 35% reduction in caries; not cost-effective in combination with systemic fluoride
   3. Although highly successful, use is limited today in the United States because of expansion of water fluoridation and increased availability of other sources of fluoride
   4. Disadvantages—required level of parental compliance and dependence on teachers and school nurses to administer the program

I. Fluoride dentifrices (see Table 20.15)
   1. OTC fluoride dentifrices are the most important fluoride vehicle on a global scale; provide 15% to 30% caries reduction in children without water fluoridation; cost-effective and combine with water fluoridation and other sources of fluoride for increased caries reduction
   2. Use is institutionalized in the United States, Canada, and other developed countries, accounting for over 90% of the market and making distribution as a public health measure unnecessary; public health distribution has value in developing countries where population does not have access to fluoride dentifrices
   3. Prescription fluoride dentifrices only have application for use in high-risk individuals

J. Other chemical therapies (see "Caries Management" section in Chapter 16) Reference is correct
   1. Xylitol
      a. Used in food and snack items as a noncariogenic sweetener; its use may reduce the incidence of dental caries in people with moderate or higher risk, especially children; additional research is needed
      b. Recommended to be used in combination with topical fluorides; fluorides are the first line of defense against dental caries
      c. Some studies have shown that xylitol is superior to other chemical therapies to interrupt the vertical transmission of dental caries from parent or caregiver to infants and the horizontal transmission among siblings; this use is no longer standard practice, and additional research is needed
   2. Chlorhexidine gluconate (CHG)
      a. Effective against *Streptococcus mutans*
      b. CAMBRA (Caries Management by Risk Assessment) recommends its use for caries control by high-risk individuals as a 0.12% CHG rinse for 1 minute daily for 1 week each month; additional research is needed
      c. CHG loses effectiveness in the presence of lauryl sulfate or fluoride ; rinse should be used about 30 minutes after toothbrushing with dentifrices that contain either compound
      d. The American Dental Association (ADA) recommends the use of chlorhexidine-thymol combination varnish to control root caries

K. Silver diamine fluoride (SDF)[14]
   1. An interim caries arresting liquid medicament endorsed by the ADA in 2016 for clinical application to arrest active caries and to prevent and control its progression

2. Noninvasive, painless, and applied quickly
3. Highly effective in arresting dental caries
4. Follow-up required to monitor arrest and permanently restore any cavitation.
5. Especially useful as an intervention for the very young, individuals with disabilities or special health care needs, the frail elderly, and others who cannot tolerate standard treatment because of medical, psychological, or behavioral reasons; also useful in patients who must be stabilized because they have more carious lesions than can be treated conventionally in one visit and for persons with little or no access to dental treatment
6. Dental sealant programs (see "Dental Sealants" in Chapter 16)
   a. Prevent caries in sound and noncavitated pits and fissures; reduce the rate of incipient carious lesions that progress to cavitation
   b. Sealant and F programs are the most beneficial community-based dental disease-prevention programs; sealants are a critical component of caries prevention
   c. Reduce bacteria levels in cavitated lesions 100-fold; reduce lesions with any viable bacteria by 50%
   d. Recommended in both fluoridated and nonfluoridated communities
   e. Use of fluorides in conjunction with sealants is recommended so both smooth surfaces and pit-and-fissure surfaces benefit
   f. Community-based sealant programs are justified for children, adolescents, and young adults, but not for other age groups
   g. Community-based settings include schools, clinics, day care facilities, and community centers; a team approach is necessary for screening and treatment, including necessary support and cooperation from administrators, staff, teachers, parents, caregivers, and volunteers
   h. Prioritizing populations for school-based sealant programs
      (1) Schools are prioritized that have high rates of children from low-SES groups who are at high risk of dental caries, as determined by the percentage of students eligible for free or subsidized lunch programs
      (2) Limited resources require that sealant programs use criteria that include risk of dental caries, availability of care, grade level of the prioritized group (e.g., 2nd and 6th grades), and teeth with deep pits and fissures
      (3) Teeth should be sealed within 6 months of eruption of first and second molars
   i. Cost-effectiveness of community-based sealant programs is a result of the current pattern of dental caries; the vast majority of dental caries in schoolchildren occurs in pits and fissures
   j. Retention rates are
      (1) Comparable for various oral health professionals who place sealants; cost-effectiveness depends on the use of nondentists to place sealants
      (2) Higher with four-handed technique; parent and staff volunteers can be trained to assist
   k. Public and private dental insurance benefits cover sealant application
   l. Educational component is critical for parents and children of the prioritized population to increase adherence to other aspects of caries prevention and control
   m. CDC provides clinical guidelines for sealant use and recommendations for school-based sealant programs (Box 20.10)

L. Caries Management by Risk Assessment (CAMBRA)
   1. Process of dealing with dental caries as an infectious disease by risk assessment and planned interventions or treatment based on that risk (see Chapter 15)
   2. Risk is based on the balance of pathologic factors and protective factors; level of risk is determined by professional judgment of this balance
   3. Prioritizing a population for a community-based program should be done according to the level of risk
      a. Child populations eligible for government programs are at high risk
      b. Children whose parents or caregivers have current or recent caries experience are at moderate-to-high risk, depending on recency of caries experience
      c. Population of any age with current or recent caries experience is at high risk
      d. Children with xerostomia or special-needs status are at high risk
      e. Adults with severe xerostomia are at high-to-extreme risk

## Measures for Preventing and Controlling Periodontal Diseases

A. No parallel to water fluoridation and other fluoride modalities exists for the prevention of periodontal diseases
B. Combination of self-care and treatment methods is required (see "Treatment" and "Postoperative Care" sections in Chapter 14)
C. Addressing periodontal disease at the population level is complicated by the role of genetic factors in destructive periodontal disease
D. Community oral health promotion activities could include the following:
   1. Public education to increase oral health literacy; for example, personal oral hygiene, control of behaviors that increase risk, regular professional oral care, and linking systemic diseases (e.g., diabetes, heart disease, stroke, osteoporosis, stress, respiratory disease) and pregnancy to periodontal health
   2. Tobacco cessation programs and efforts
   3. Support of funding for and promotion of population-based research

## Measures for Preventing and Controlling Other Oral Diseases and Anomalies

A. Oropharyngeal cancers (OPC)
   1. A primary prevention technique for HPV-related OPC is the HPV vaccine (HP 2030 vaccination topic objective)

### BOX 20.10 Recommendations for Sealant Use in Community Oral Health

**Clinical Recommendations**

1. Sealants should be placed on pits and fissures of children's primary teeth when it is determined that the tooth, or the patient, is at risk of experiencing caries.
2. Sealants should be placed on pits and fissures of children's, adolescents', and adults' permanent teeth when it is determined that the tooth, or the patient, is at risk of experiencing caries.
3. Pit-and-fissure sealants should be placed on early (noncavitated) carious lesions in children, adolescents, young adults, and adults to reduce the percentage of lesions that progress.
4. Generally, conditions favor the placement of resin-based versus glass ionomer cement; resin-based sealants are the first choice of material for dental sealants.
5. Use of a bonding agent between the previously acid-etched enamel surface and the sealant material may enhance sealant retention.
6. Use of a bonding agent that excludes acid etching is not recommended.
7. Routine mechanical preparation of enamel before acid etching is not recommended.
8. When possible, a four-handed technique should be used for placement of sealants.
9. The oral health care professional should monitor and reapply sealants as needed to maximize effectiveness.
10. The manufacturer's instructions for sealant placement should be followed.

**Recommendations for School-Based Sealant Programs**

1. Seal pit-and-fissure tooth surfaces that are sound or have noncavitated lesions, prioritizing first and second permanent molars.
2. Unaided visual assessment is adequate prior to sealant placement to differentiate surfaces with the earliest signs of tooth decay from more advanced lesions.
3. Prior to assessment, dry the teeth with a cotton roll, gauze, or, when available, compressed air.
4. An explorer may be used to gently confirm cavitations; do not use a sharp explorer under force.
5. X-ray films are not needed solely for sealant placement.
6. A toothbrush can be used to help clean the tooth surface before acid etching; more complex cleaning methods are not recommended.
7. Use a four-handed technique with an assistant to increase retention.
8. Provide sealants to children even if follow-up examinations for every child cannot be guaranteed.
9. Evaluate sealant retention within 1 year.

Data from Wright JT, Tampi MP, Graham L, et al. Sealants for preventing and arresting pit-and-fissure occlusal caries in primary and permanent molars. *J Am Dent Assoc.* 2016; 147(8), 631–645. https://jada.ada.org/article/S0002-8177(16)30475-5/fulltext; *Centers for Disease Control and Prevention.* School sealant programs. https://www.cdc.gov/oralhealth/dental_sealant_program/school-sealant-programs.htm. Accessed 03.01.18; *National Maternal and Child Oral Health Resource Center.* Seal America: the prevention intervention, 3rd edition, 2016, https://www.mchoralhealth.org/seal/index.php. Accessed 07.07.20.

2. Primary prevention for most OPC is not available; avoiding known risk factors such as alcohol and tobacco is recommended
3. Overall cigarette use in the United States has declined over the last decade; because the use of smokeless tobacco, cigars, e-cigarettes, and hookahs has increased, HP 2030 tobacco use objectives continue to emphasize oral health promotion related to decreasing tobacco use and increasing tobacco cessation counseling by health professionals (see "Tobacco Use Interventions" section of Chapter 16)
   a. A public health initiative has been to promote the provision of tobacco cessation counseling by dentists and dental hygienists; in 2011–2012, 10.5% of patients reported receiving such counseling with disparities by family income; no data are available to determine progress on this initiative since then[1]
   b. Some health insurance policies provide tobacco cessation coverage
4. Importance of school-based tobacco-use prevention programs
   a. Rate of cigarette use among high school students has decreased steadily each year since 1997; use of smokeless tobacco and cigars went down from 2011 to 2018
   b. Even so, 13.9% of high school students reported smoking in 2018 (over 1.1 million students), 21.9% reported the current use of any tobacco product (e-cigarettes, cigars, smokeless tobacco, hookah, pipe tobacco, and/or bidis),[15] and the use of e-cigarettes by high school and middle school youth increased dramatically from 2011 to 2018[16]
   c. Recommendations for education of students—for example, programs and information from the CDC and the American Dental Hygienists' Association (ADHA)
      (1) Focus on restricting social influences and environments that lead to tobacco-use
      (2) Develop and enforce school policy on tobacco-use prevention, control, and cessation
      (3) Provide instruction on short-term and long-term negative physiologic and social influences of tobacco, peer norms regarding tobacco-use, and refusal skills
      (4) Deliver tobacco-use prevention education in K–12th grades; instruction should begin no later than 5th grade, be especially intensive in middle school, and be reinforced in high school
      (5) Offer program-specific training and dialogue scripts to teachers and school nurses
      (6) Involve parents and families in support of school-based programs to prevent tobacco use
      (7) Provide tips, counseling, referral, and support for cessation efforts among students and all school staff who use tobacco; involve other associations and organizations such as parent-teacher associations (PTAs), American Association of Retired Persons (AARP), CDC, ADHA, employers, and health insurers
      (8) Evaluate outcomes of tobacco-use prevention program at regular intervals
5. Secondary prevention consists of early detection (screening) and treatment
   a. Mass screening for oral cancers is costly
   b. Another public health initiative has been to increase OPC examinations by oral health professionals as part of their assessment in the dental office;[1] in 2011–2012, 23.3% of patients reported receiving such an examination

with disparities by family income;[1] although the number of cancer screenings completed in dental offices has increased, the numbers are still very low[17]

6. Other recommended strategies
   a. Focus on populations at risk for use of tobacco products (e.g., little league teams and other youth organizations)
   b. Emphasize health warnings on posters, brochures, websites, products, and public service announcements that warn of hazards
   c. Urge people to regularly visit a professional oral health care provider for examination, advice, and assistance with quitting tobacco use
   d. Provide public education regarding signs and symptoms of oral cancer; promote regular self-examination
   e. Encourage use of QUIT phone lines and other electronic and social media support
   f. Support population-based research efforts and lobbying strategies
   g. Keep abreast of new information on tobacco cessation, such as from ADHA and CDC
   h. Advocate for policies related to controlling the sale and use of tobacco products

B. Orofacial clefts (cleft lip and cleft palate)
   1. Public health programs should emphasize awareness of risk and protective factors during pregnancy (see "Orofacial Clefts" in earlier section "Epidemiology of Oral Diseases and Conditions")
   2. Advocacy for policies related to improvement of surveillance and referral

C. Facial injury or trauma (see "Mouth Protectors [Athletic Mouthguards]" section in Chapter 13)
   1. Oral health education that focuses on preventive behaviors
   2. Increased public attention to the importance of head and facial protection
      a. Headgear and athletic mouth protectors during contact-sports activities
      b. Safety restraints in automobiles
      c. Helmets for bicycling, skateboarding, in-line skating (roller blading), and motorcycle use
      d. Measures to prevent injuries from falls in the home, including good lighting, nonskid flooring materials, and handrails
   3. Emphasis on education of parents, coaches, caregivers, and policy makers
   4. Advocacy for adoption of policies regarding protective equipment-use regulations by schools and sports organization

D. Tooth loss
   1. Oral health education focused on the value of keeping natural teeth and importance of early treatment of caries and periodontal diseases
   2. Advocacy, policies, and programs that improve access to care for underserved populations

E. Problems related to denture use require the following:
   1. Oral health education focused on importance of and techniques used for denture cleanliness and importance of routine examinations for denture wearers
   2. Policies related to denture identification during fabrication
   3. Policies that require oral hygiene care for residents of long-term care facilities
   4. Health promotion programs for caregivers and staff of long-term care facilities to encourage assistance with oral hygiene and denture care for older-adult denture wearers who need assistance

F. Fluorosis
   1. Monitoring of safe water fluoridation practices; training of water treatment personnel
   2. Promotion of policies related to removing excess fluoride from community water supplies
   3. Oral health education of the public and other health professionals related to the safe use of fluorides

## COMMUNITY INTERVENTION

A. Community groups vary—programming principles can be applied to all groups and types of programs; programs may need to be adapted for various priority populations based on culture and other demographic factors

B. Factors to consider in community programming—current health care system, workforce issues, resources, funding, geography, sociocultural background, SES, cultural and political climates, oral health literacy, and determinants of health

C. Community programming uses various strategies
   1. Surveillance at national and state levels
      a. Provides information necessary for public health decision-making
      b. Collects data on health outcomes, risk factors, and intervention strategies
      c. Can link current databases and address identified data gaps
      d. Identifies public health issues requiring immediate action
      e. Measures and monitors trends in the burden of disease
      f. Guides planning, implementation, and evaluation of programs
      g. May influence public policy and allocation of funds
      h. Includes important qualities of surveillance: simplicity, flexibility, data quality, representativeness, and timeliness
   2. Survey
      a. A description of the defined population at a point in time
      b. Can be part of a needs assessment and of surveillance
   3. Needs assessment to identify the following:
      a. Extent and types of assets and challenges in a community
      b. Current system of services and programs available
      c. Extent of needs and resource utilization

D. Roles of dental hygienists in community health planning and practice
   1. Program planner or initiator
   2. Consultant and resource person

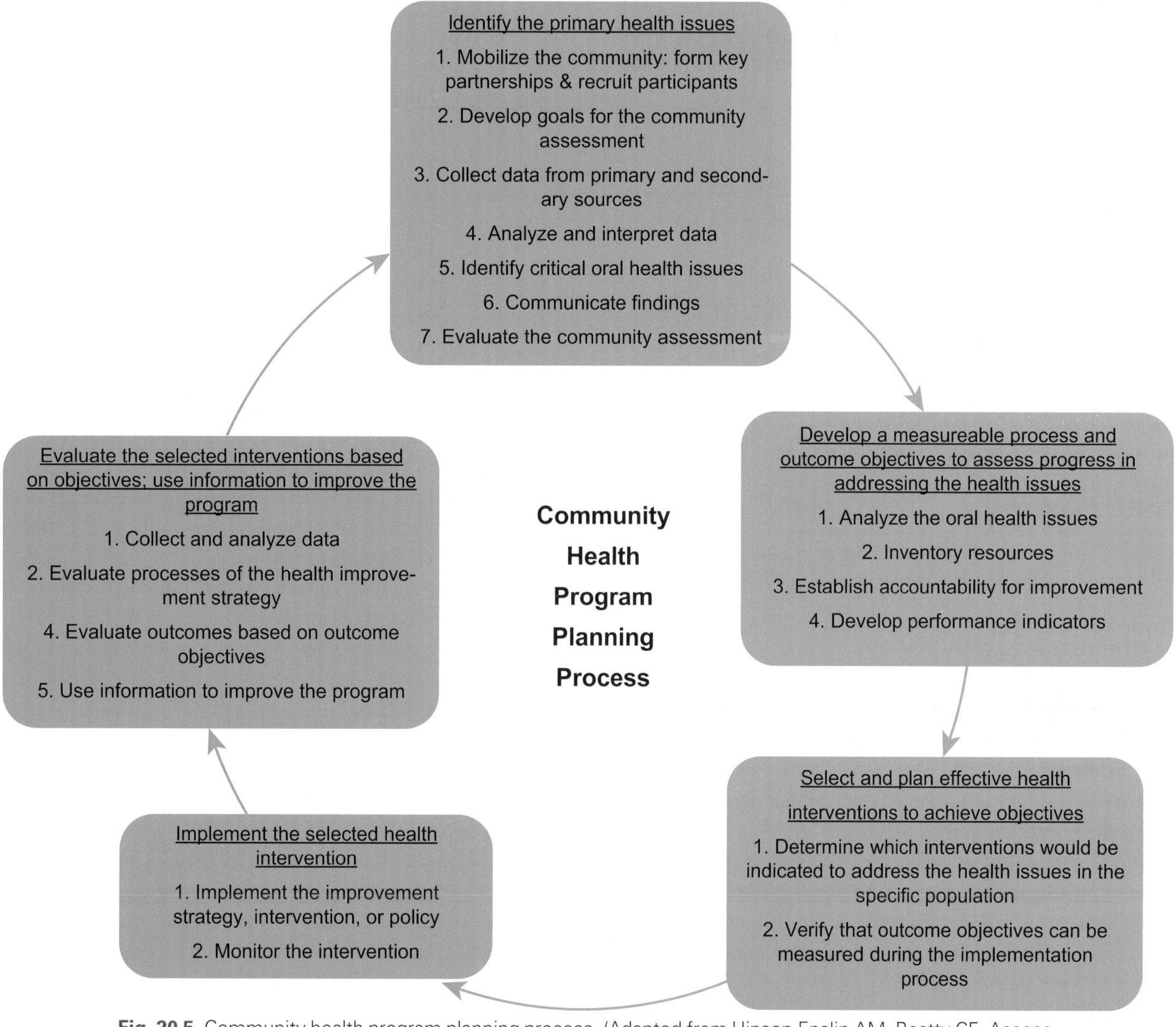


**Fig. 20.5** Community health program planning process. (Adapted from Hinson-Enslin AM, Beatty CF. Assessment for community oral health program planning. In Beatty CF, ed. *Community Oral Health Practice for the Dental Hygienist*. 4th ed. St. Louis: Elsevier; 2017: 50–72)

3. Service provider
4. Administrator or manager of a particular program or division
5. Researcher, including data collection
6. Educator and oral health promotion professional
7. Consumer advocate
8. Politician
9. Trainer—training others (*train the trainer*) to provide services and oral health education is a more efficient use of resources

E. Various program planning models are used, all of which have common steps in the process; generally follow the dental hygiene process of care in a circular approach (Fig. 20.5)
1. Identify primary health issues
2. Develop a measurable process and outcome objectives to assess progress in addressing the health issue
3. Select and plan effective health interventions to help achieve objectives
4. Implement selected health interventions
5. Evaluate selected interventions based on objectives; use information to improve the program

F. Other elements common to community oral health initiatives include education, financing, and formative evaluation

## Assessment and Problem Identification

A. Definition—multifaceted, organized, and systematic approach to identify a priority group and define the extent and severity of the oral health care needs that are present
1. Priority group—group of individuals who are the focus of a particular oral health care service or program; may be identified by health professional or by the community being served
2. Use of a community-oriented primary care philosophy of health planning— focuses on providing care to a defined population, based on their assessed needs, to improve health status by combining primary care and population health[18] (Box 20.11)

B. Data collection
1. Important to complete as part of the needs assessment before planning the intervention

**BOX 20.11 Community-Oriented Primary Care (COPC)**

**Five Principles of COPC**

1. Responsibility for comprehensive care of a defined population
2. Care based on health needs and its determinants
3. Prioritization of those needs to implement health programs
4. Programs that integrate promotion, prevention, and treatment
5. *Community-based participation*

**Requirements of the COPC Process**

1. Defining (geographically, members registered in a practice or as a sociological construct) and characterizing the community to determine health needs, their determinants, and assets
2. Prioritization of identified health problems
3. Detailed assessment of the prioritized condition
4. Development and performance of intervention program
5. Surveillance and evaluation
6. Reassessment of health need

Data from Gofin J, Gofin R, Stimpson JP. Community-oriented primary care (COPC) and the affordable care act: an opportunity to meet the demands of an evolving health care system, *J Prim Care Community Health.* 2015; 6(2):128–133. https://journals.sagepub.com/doi/10.1177/2150131914555908.

2. Develop a community profile of the area where the priority population is located if adequate needs assessment is not available
3. Utilize secondary data if available; collect primary data if secondary data are not available
4. Identify ongoing types of programs or projects
   a. Purpose is to provide oral health services, education, disease prevention, research, or combination
   b. Community individuals and groups responsible for programs and success
   c. Locations or facilities where oral health care activities can occur
   d. Individuals, special equipment (e.g., mobile vans or portable equipment), facilities, coalitions, funding opportunities, and other resources to meet the oral health care needs of the priority population
5. Assess current oral health status and needs
   a. Used to identify the extent and severity of need and in determining project aims and objectives
   b. Three basic approaches to documenting oral health status and needs:
      (1) Identify and use an assessment method to obtain specific data related to the proposed project or program
      (2) Coordinate assessment with an agency or group such as an academic center or community-based agency that is seeking similar data about the priority population
      (3) Secondary data—research and collect secondary data from records of state or local health care agencies, dental or medical programs, and public health or related agencies
6. Various data collection methods can be used (Table 20.17)
   a. Method used is influenced by type of information or data needed
      (1) Baseline data—collected before program implementation; used for problem identification and planning; also used for evaluation by comparing it to outcomes data to evaluate success of program; baseline data are also called *pretest data* in research
      (2) Primary data—new data collected by various techniques (e.g., questionnaire, interview, direct observation, indices, records, documents)
      (3) Secondary data—existing data previously collected by federal or state agencies, public policy organizations, or other sources (e.g., Census Bureau, CDC, National Center for Health Statistics, ADA Health Policy Institute, ADHA)
      (4) Qualitative data—nonnumerical descriptive data such as observations, perceptions, attitudes, and comments made
   b. Multiple data collection methods can be used together based on program goals
   c. Surveys—method used to assess knowledge, oral health status, oral health behavior, interests, values, and attitudes; can be done by use of questionnaire or interview
   d. Oral health surveys—type of survey method used to collect information about oral health, disease status, and treatment needs for planning or monitoring oral health care needs
      (1) Can be accomplished with a clinical examination (primary data) or review of dental records (secondary data)
      (2) Existing survey data may be available for comparisons of the priority group to comparable groups or different geographic regions
         (a) National data from federal agencies responsible for monitoring health and oral health status, such as CDC and NOHSS
         (b) State-level surveillance data available from the CDC, NOHSS, or some state health departments
      (3) ASTDD, CDC, and the Community Toolbox (see Website Information and Resources at the end of the chapter) are resources for guidelines for conducing and reporting results of an oral health survey
      (4) Four types of examinations and inspections are used in oral health surveys to measure dental caries (see Table 20.18); the type used varies according to the index or measurement approach (see Table 20.13 and Table 20.14)
   f. Special considerations are needed in planning oral health surveys
      (1) Cumulative nature of some diseases
      (2) Disease is age related
      (3) Significant percentage of the population is affected
      (4) Irreversible nature of some oral diseases

**TABLE 20.17 Data Collection Methods and Applications**

| Data Collection Method | Instrument | Indications | Advantages | Limitations |
|---|---|---|---|---|
| Direct observation of events, objects, people | Checklist, content analysis, evaluation forms, camera, tape recorder, videotape, thermometer, sphygmomanometer, rating and ranking scales | Used when subject recall may affect accuracy of data collection<br>Used to study behavior<br>Used to study psychomotor activity<br>Used in experimental research | Observations can be made as they occur in the "natural" setting<br>Observations can be made of behaviors that might not be reported by respondents | Time-consuming<br>Difficulty in recording<br>Factors that may interfere with the situation<br>Difficulty in quantification of observations<br>Expensive<br>Observer-respondent interaction |
| Interview; face-to-face or telephone survey | Interview guide (interview schedule) | Used to obtain information on attitudes, beliefs, and opinions<br>Used in a survey<br>Used to gain information on past or present events<br>Face-to-face method that can be used for focus groups or one-on-one | Flexibility<br>Questions can be clarified and explained<br>Complete data can be collected<br>Survey participants do not have to be able to read or write<br>Focus groups have the advantage of interaction among group members to influence each other while discussing and considering ideas and perspectives | Respondents may be inhibited to respond accurately and truthfully<br>Time-consuming<br>Expensive<br>Interviewer may affect the responses<br>Language barriers<br>Focus groups require the use of a skilled facilitator |
| Question-based survey: written or oral | Questionnaire, opinionnaire, email source; asking questions to seek specific information | Used for obtaining information on attitudes, beliefs, and opinions<br>May be used to gain information on present conditions and past events<br>Used to obtain information about existing status<br>Used in planning | Ease of administration<br>Relatively inexpensive<br>Standardization of instructions and questions<br>Economy of time<br>Data can be gathered from a wide geographic area<br>Data can reflect public opinion<br>Vast amount of data can be collected<br>Cross-sectional, generalized statistics can be obtained | Misinterpretation of questions by respondents<br>If written, low return may bias results<br>Superficiality of responses<br>Incomplete data collection<br>Honesty of respondent<br>Control of extraneous variables is lacking |
| Epidemiologic survey, screening survey | Dental indices | Used to study disease patterns in a population<br>Used to evaluate the effectiveness of therapeutic or preventive treatments in a specific geographic area | Vast amount of data can be collected<br>Cross-sectional, generalized statistics can be obtained<br>Data are quantifiable<br>Provides actual measure of health status | Difficulty in determining causation because of complexity of variables<br>Time-consuming<br>Expensive; requires trained and calibrated examiners |
| Records, documents | Reports of legislative bodies and state or city officials, deeds, wills, appointment records, dental charts, report cards | Used to study past events | Unbiased in terms of the investigator<br>Inexpensive<br>No subject-investigator interaction<br>Convenience and economy of time | Incomplete records<br>Accuracy of records may be unknown |

Data from Beatty CF. *Community Oral Health Practice for the Dental Hygienist*. 4th ed. Appendix D-2. St Louis: Elsevier; 2017.

**TABLE 20.18 Types of Caries Examinations and Inspections**

| Type | Description | Advantages | Disadvantages |
|---|---|---|---|
| I | Complete examination—done with mouth mirror and explorer, adequate illumination, thorough radiographic survey, and additional tests as indicated | Comprehensive; designed for comprehensive treatment | Requires extensive time and personnel; expensive |
| II | Limited examination—done with mouth mirror, explorer, adequate illumination, posterior bitewing radiographs, and single periapical radiographs as indicated | Useful when program may include dental treatment for individuals | Requires time, personnel and expense |
| III[a] | Inspection—done with mouth mirror, explorer, and adequate illumination; used in the Basic Screening Survey | Useful in surveys; offers chance to establish rapport and plan motivational strategy for oral health instruction; provides baseline and surveillance data | May be erroneously relied on as an examination; follow-up is required for referral |
| IV[a] | Screening—done with tongue depressor and available illumination | Useful for initial needs assessment in relation to program planning | Identifies only glaring needs for referral; follow-up is required |

[a]Type III and Type IV are the most common methods used in dental public health.

(5) Trends in disease prevalence exist
(6) Common oral diseases exist in all populations; prevalence may be higher in underinsured and uninsured, low-SES, and nonwhite and Hispanic populations
(7) Standard measurements are used to assess many oral diseases (dental indices); subjectivity and potential for error are inherent in use of many dental indices
(8) Surveying requires planning, calibration of examiners, and possibly pilot testing before implementation

C. Development of a community profile
1. Community profile—provides comprehensive information essential in planning a community health program; the rationale is to understand the environment in which the priority population is located
2. Size, location, and type of community dictate the type, amount, and comprehensiveness of information necessary for a community profile
3. General areas for inclusion can consist of:
a. Community overview
(1) Number of individuals in the population and distribution by income, age, education, employment rate, public assistance, health and dental insurance rates, and percentage of population receiving Medicare, Medicaid, or CHIP
(2) Geographic location and boundaries, population setting and density (urban or rural), standard of living, homelessness
(3) Ethnic background, cultural heritage, languages, customs, behaviors, beliefs
(4) Diet, nutritional levels, nutrition programs
(5) Amount, types, and influence of public services and utilities, including transportation schedules, routes, fares, and reliability
(6) Informed-consent procedures and issues related to confidentiality of health records
(7) Distribution of public and private schools and religious or faith-based organizations
(8) Extent and type of community F and sealant programs; fluoridation history
(9) State and local statutes, public health codes, and related administrative rules and regulations
b. Community leadership and organization; political atmosphere
(1) Community, financial, and religious leaders, liaisons, and councils
(2) Community power base for policy formulation
(3) Governance structure (e.g., health council, city government, advisory board, school board, union); political environment
(4) Grassroots individuals with political influence
(5) Educational institutions providing professional education, resources, and support
(6) Attitudes of all these entities toward oral health, acquired through interviews or surveys, is important in terms of whether they will be assets or barriers to the community programming process
c. Financing and funding of health services
(1) Local and state budget allocation procedures for oral health care programs
(2) Funding sources (e.g., federal, state, or local funding; individual or third-party payment; private funds; foundations; grants; endowments)
(3) Mechanism for requesting the necessary funding; the importance of the need for collaborative partners to successfully obtain funding must be determined
d. Facilities, resources, and workforce
(1) Location of space and facilities in the community or institution; US Department of Labor Occupational Safety and Health Administration (OSHA) standard compliance
(2) Availability and adequacy of equipment
(3) Location of medical and health science centers, clinics, community health centers, and dental laboratories; ease of access
(4) Number of licensed practicing dentists, dental hygienists, midlevel dental providers, dental assistants, laboratory technicians, medical personnel, or others experienced in working with the priority population
(5) Consortia of health professionals, facilities, and resources (collaboration is important)
(6) Barriers that limit access of the population to oral health care (e.g., cost, transportation, political climate of community, attitudes of leaders about oral health)
e. Sometimes a community assessment is accomplished for overall community planning before identifying any specific group to target; in this case, population groups previously identified as being at high risk for oral health needs should be included in the community assessment
(1) Preschool-age and school-age children
(2) Intellectually, developmentally, and physically challenged persons
(3) Chronically ill and medically compromised persons
(4) Older adults
(5) Pregnant women and infants
(6) Low-income and minority groups
(7) Residents of inner-city and rural communities

D. Analysis of data
1. Analysis includes organizing, evaluating, and interpreting data
2. Data analysis can range from simple to complex, using simple descriptive tabulations or advanced statistical tests
a. Planner alone can analyze the data
b. Statisticians and epidemiologists can be involved
c. Computers are useful

d. Analysis of qualitative data requires special skills
e. Economic analysis of existing programs, including a cost/benefit ratio

3. After analysis, population needs and priorities can be identified
   a. Formal and informal input is sought through meetings, focus groups, and social media
   b. Input is sought from various stakeholder groups
   c. Community representatives, partners, and advisory groups are consulted
   d. Consumers; political, religious, and financial leaders; and health care professionals may be included
4. An opportunity for dialogue is important to gain support

## Program Planning

A. Definition—organized response to reduce or eliminate one or more problems; organized effort that includes the objective of reducing or eliminating one or more problems, performance of one or more activities, and use of resources
B. Elements of a program plan
   1. Identification of program goals and objectives
   2. Strategies and specific activities to meet objectives, including sequence and individuals responsible
   3. Resources required—facilities, equipment, materials, personnel (employed and volunteer), with consideration of appropriateness, adequacy, effectiveness, and efficiency
   4. Timetables and deadlines clearly outlined, with some flexibility
   5. Projected budget and budget justification
   6. Program promotion and marketing
   7. Identification of strengths, weaknesses/challenges, opportunities, and threats (SWOT/SCOT analysis)
C. Goals and objectives—for each need prioritized, a goal with related objectives must be determined
   1. Goal—broadly based statement of what changes will occur as a result of the program; provides direction
   2. Objectives—specific statements that describe, in a measurable manner, the desired outcomes from program activities
   3. Most activities may deal with immediate goals, but intermediate and long-term goals must also be considered
   4. Objectives are stated in specific, measurable terms; SMART formula for developing objectives provides the necessary components of what, who, where, when, and how much
      a. Specific: clearly states the objectives
      b. Measurable: objectives can be evaluated
      c. Appropriate: taking the identified needs of the priority population into consideration
      d. Realistic or related: objectives that are achievable and related to anticipated outcomes
      e. Time-bound: a timeline is established
D. Program activities
   1. The dynamic, energy-using procedures carried out to achieve program objectives
   2. Can be preventive, educational, treatment-oriented, or research-oriented
E. Promotion or marketing of program
   1. Necessary for participation, recognition, and success of project
   2. Varied promotion techniques
      a. Advisory committee composed of stakeholders (those who have a stake in the outcome of the program) and key leaders from the community
      b. Liaison with related groups
      c. Mass media (television and radio), printed media, banners, billboards, Web-based and special-interest publications and programs
      d. Smaller programs may use posters, flyers, invitations, newsletter announcements, email, and social media
F. Implementation strategy development—steps for implementing the program are outlined before beginning the implementation process
G. Evaluation plan—should be in place before implementing the program to ensure its successful execution

## Implementation

A. Implementation is the process of operationalizing the plan; the implementation strategy is employed to conduct the program
B. During implementation, it is important to monitor the program activities, personnel, equipment, resources, and supplies to ensure smooth program operation
C. Ongoing formative evaluation throughout program implementation provides opportunity to make adjustments as needed; feedback mechanisms from personnel and participants are critical components of this formative evaluation

## Health Education and Health Promotion

See "Concepts of Patient-Centered Education" and "Preventive Care Planning" sections in Chapter 16.

A. Related concepts
   1. Health promotion—a broad concept referring to the process of enabling people and communities to increase their control over determinants of health and therefore improve their own health; includes wide range of strategies that may include policies (e.g., prohibiting the sale of tobacco products to young people), product labeling (e.g., indicating the amount of sugar in a product), strategies to increase access to care, and educational interventions
   2. Health education—the process in which individual patients or clients and groups are encouraged to become responsible for personal oral health and are informed of scientifically based methods for preventing oral diseases
   3. Health continuum—conceptualization of health status as perceived on a continuous scale from optimal health through illness and death
   4. Prevention—health education is one means of primary prevention for both individuals and groups
   5. Theories of health education and health promotion (see Table 20.19)
      a. Approaches to health promotion and health education strategies and interventions should be based on

sound theories in order to result in desired changes in oral health status of individuals and communities
   b. No single theory applies to all situations; theories can be combined to meet the needs of the situation; multidimensional approaches may be more effective for conditions with multiple social, behavioral, and biologic risk factors
   c. These theories can help the professional move individuals through the stages of the learning ladder (progression of learning): unawareness, awareness, self-interest, involvement, action, and habit
   d. Individual models should be used to design community oral health education programs; community models should be used to develop oral health promotion strategies that may include health education
6. Communication skills are critical to the effective implementation of health promotion and health education programs motivational interviewing is essential in community programs that involve one-on-one contact with patients and clients (see Chapter 16)
7. Health education and health promotion programs must demonstrate cultural sensitivity to meet the needs of varied groups within the population; programs should be adapted to the culture of the priority population
8. The health literacy of the priority population must be considered for successful outcomes

B. Goals of health education
   1. Improve knowledge of health topics
   2. Foster motivation for changes in health behaviors
   3. Result in outcomes of changed health behaviors
   4. Ultimately to improve health status

C. Both direct and indirect processes impact oral health education
   1. Formal activities include the deliberate provision of oral health education designed to elicit specific health promotion or disease prevention behaviors
   2. Informal activities and environmental influences can impact the indirect or vicarious acquisition of oral health–related information and motivation that may lead to specific health promotion or disease prevention behaviors

D. Health education and health promotion are often integral parts of community activities; may be directed to:
   1. Other health care professionals
   2. Preschool, elementary, secondary, and college students
   3. Educators
   4. Special population groups and caregivers
   5. Adult and older-adult groups
   6. Institutionalized populations
   7. Diverse population groups recently settled in the community

E. Health education topics cannot be limited to oral hygiene instruction; topics might include:
   1. Preventive measures, such as appropriate use of Fs, sealants, and xylitol
   2. Oral diseases and conditions (e.g., periodontal diseases, malocclusion, OPC, orofacial clefts) and risk factors such as diet, systemic diseases, poor oral self-care behaviors, and infant-feeding practices
   3. Importance of routine assessment, prevention, and treatment
   4. Self-examination techniques
   5. Dental safety and dental emergencies (e.g., use of mouth protectors, procedures for avulsed tooth)
   6. Roles of various health professionals and their interrelationships
   7. Care of the oral cavity and dental prostheses
   8. Careers in dentistry and dental hygiene
   9. Becoming a discriminating dental consumer; oral health care products
   10. Effects of tobacco-use on oral and systemic health
   11. Environmental factors affecting oral health (e.g., occupation-related concerns)
   12. Prenatal and postnatal oral health issues and recommendations; early childhood caries
   13. How to provide oral health care to those unable to care for themselves
   14. Oral and systemic disease links
   15. Topics reflected in current HP objectives (see HP 2030 website at https://health.gov/healthypeople)
   16. Resources for topics are available from government, professional, and health-related sources such as HP, CDC, National Maternal and Child Oral Health Resource Center, ADHA, and ADA

## Methods of Oral Health Education

A. Instructional methods
   1. Lecture—informative talk, prepared beforehand and given to a group; useful to introduce new topics, arouse interest in a subject, or review concepts
      a. Advantages
         (1) Can present many facts and ideas in a short period
         (2) Can convey information to large numbers of individuals
         (3) Preparation takes place before presentation
         (4) Allows instructor to determine aims, content, organization, pace, and direction of presentation
         (5) Integrates diverse materials and highlights various ideas and concepts in an orderly way
         (6) Can use media
         (7) Builds on foundational knowledge in subsequent presentations; allows for gradual development of complex or difficult concepts and theories
      b. Disadvantages
         (1) No active participation by the learner; encourages one-way communication; stifles creativity
         (2) Instructor must have effective writing, speaking, and modeling skills; poor presentation technique is a barrier to learning
         (3) Difficult to monitor student learning; requires a considerable amount of unguided student time outside the classroom
   2. Lecture–demonstration—informative talk that presents information supplemented by a demonstration to

TABLE 20.19 **Health Education and Promotion Theories**

| Theory | Key Points | Application Examples | Limitations |
|---|---|---|---|
| **Individual Theories** | | | |
| Health belief model (HBM) | Underlying foundation: when individuals have accurate information, they will make better health choices<br>Four health perceptions (beliefs) accepted in order:<br>- Susceptibility to disease (risk)<br>- Seriousness of disease<br>- Effectiveness of intervention to control disease<br>- Possibility of overcoming barriers (self-efficacy) | Presentations that provide health information<br>Providing individuals with brochures and handouts of health information<br>Most knowledge-based oral health education programs are based on HBM | Just knowledge is not enough: information is essential but not sufficient<br>Does not provide tools needed for behavior change to occur<br>Behavior change is not so linear |
| Trans-theoretical model (stages of change) | State of readiness is required to change; follows step-by-step, orderly process of change through predictable stages:<br>- Precontemplation—no intention to change behavior within next 6 months<br>- Contemplation—intending to change behavior in foreseeable future (within 6 months)<br>- Preparation—taking small steps toward making change within 30 days<br>- Action—recent change in behavior and intending to keep moving forward<br>- Maintenance—having sustained behavior change for more than 6 months, intending to keep moving forward, and working to prevent relapse to earlier stages<br>- Termination—no longer having desire to return to unhealthy behavior and being certain of not relapsing | Assessing individual's state of readiness and position in the stages, then adapting education to the appropriate stage<br>Smoking cessation programs are based on stages of change<br>Useful for any health education strategy that involves progression through the stages, e.g., adoption of flossing behavior and reducing sugar in the diet | Behavior change is not so linear; relapsing to an earlier stage and starting over are common<br>Research shows more success in immediate change (early stages) than in long-term change (maintenance and termination stages)<br>Continual motivation required to encourage movement forward after relapse |
| Theory of reasoned action | People make rational decisions based on behavioral intention; person's intent to change is strongest predictor of action<br>Behavioral intention is affected by one's personal behavioral beliefs and attitudes and social norms | Focus on or establishment of social norms for desired oral health behavior (e.g., children brushing at school, mother brushing with child, authority figures expressing concern for oral health, parents' smoking behavior, appealing to social acceptability for teens)<br>Soliciting behavioral intentions (e.g., to stop smoking on specific quit date) | Does not deal with factual information<br>Focuses only on the emotional aspects and motivation of behavior |
| Social cognitive theory (SCT) | Knowledge, behavior, and environment act in a reciprocal (circular) manner to continually affect each other (multidimensional) and increase self-control over personal actions<br>Self-efficacy is belief that personal actions affect outcomes and predict health status<br>Self-efficacy is acquired through enactive attainment, verbal persuasion, observational learning, behavioral capability, and reinforcements | Using small successes to motivate behavior change, (e.g., praise for increased frequency of flossing)<br>Counseling that failure is part of the learning process<br>Using credible role models to tie learning to someone else's experience<br>Providing ongoing counseling<br>Reinforcing behavior<br>Encouraging self-initiated rewards and incentives<br>Personally modeling desired oral health behaviors and outcomes | Not a step-by-step model; considered "sloppy"<br>Self-efficacy varies for different health conditions |
| Locus of control (LOC) | Perception of personal control over health status:<br>- Internal LOC: personal actions determine health status<br>- External LOC: others strongly influence health decisions and health status; can negate positive influence of knowledge<br>- One's LOC tends to relate to all health issues | Counseling that focuses on individual's personal power over health decisions and health status | Perceptions can be deeply ingrained and emotionally driven |
| Sense of coherence (SOC) | Extent to which one has confidence that one's environment is predictable and that things will work out as well as can reasonably be expected; application to health is based on concept that disease is a continuum; stressors and tension (problems) move one along the continuum toward disease; individuals develop resources to reduce or manage stressors to move along the continuum toward health; resources consist of heredity, knowledge, finances, physical resources, friends, family, faith, etc., that help one view problems as manageable (have resources to cope), understandable (make sense), and meaningful (willing to use or spend resources to manage stressors); higher SOC is associated with better oral health | Helping people identify resources that are available to manage the stressors that relate to their oral health such as dental insurance; source of accurate information, trusted oral health care provider, access to healthy food, belief that oral health is important<br>Focus on motivation | Cognitive, perceptual, and social model; does not include a focus on expanding knowledge of factual oral health information<br>Time-consuming to implement |

*Continued*

**TABLE 20.19 Health Education and Promotion Theories—cont'd**

| Theory | Key Points | Application Examples | Limitations |
|---|---|---|---|
| **Community Theories** | | | |
| Community organization | Represents several theories that describe how community groups are assisted in identifying common problems or goals, mobilizing resources, and implementing strategies to reach the goals they have set collectively<br>Accomplished through empowerment, community competence, participation and relevance, issue selection, and critical consciousness | Involvement of staff, parents, students, patients, clients, community members and leaders, and other stakeholders in the program planning process of a school-based or community-based oral health program or clinic<br>Involvement of a broad-base of community leaders (e.g., in a fluoridation campaign) | Requires time and effort to identify key influencers and involve the members of the community |
| Diffusion of innovation | Addresses how new ideas, products, practices, and services spread within a society<br>Diffusion process consists of a spread of planned efforts to make the innovation become routine, taking into account the society's communication channels and social system<br>Strategies are planned that address the characteristics of the innovation: relative advantage, compatibility, complexity, triability, and observability | Adoption of sealants, fluoride varnish, CAMBRA, and other innovative dental procedures by our society, including the profession<br>The dental profession's level of acceptance of innovative workforce models and an expanded scope of practice for dental hygienists in relation to increasing access to oral health care | Requires a complex and comprehensive approach |
| Organizational change theory | A wide variety of forces make an organization resistant to change; these forces include how it operates, and its structure, culture and control systems<br>A wide variety of forces also push an organization toward change; these include changing of tasks and the environment of the organization<br>These two sets of forces always oppose each other; for an organization to change, it is necessary to find ways to increase the forces for change, decrease the resistance of change, or do both at the same time | Reorganizing the structure of the health system in the nation<br>Reorganizing a community-based clinic to meet the changing needs of the population it serves<br>Reorganizing a professional organization to influence its members in the direction of meeting population needs<br>Reorganizing a health care profession to increase its focus on access to care and social needs of the population served | Theory relates to the infrastructure of community oral health practice, not to health promotion<br>Requires a complex and comprehensive approach<br>Requires time and effort to change an organization |

*CAMBRA,* caries management by risk assessment.
Data from Isman B: Health promotion and health communication. In Beatty CF: *Community oral health practice for the dental hygienist,* ed 4, 2017, St Louis, Elsevier; and Nathe CN: *Dental public health & research,* ed. 8. Upper Saddle River, NJ, Pearson; 2017: 210–227.

reinforce learning; can be used to introduce information and to demonstrate skills or techniques to supplement information
   a. Advantages
      (1) Illustrates information visually
      (2) Sets forth information in a complete format
      (3) Allows for concentration of attention and economical use of time
      (4) Useful for reinforcing material
      (5) May use models, computer-generated presentation, slides, videotapes, or other teaching tools; technology may allow larger number of participants to view a demonstration (e.g., viewing computer monitors)
   b. Disadvantages
      (1) Difficult for large groups to see a demonstration unless appropriate technology is used
      (2) Requires careful preparation for success; requires adequate equipment and facilities
3. Discussion—group activity in which the student and teacher define a problem and seek a solution; an interaction between teachers and students to promote divergent thinking where closure is not expected; promotes understanding and clarification of concepts, ideas, and feelings; includes use of questions by the leader to stimulate interaction
   a. Advantages
      (1) Allows interaction among participants
      (2) Provides two-way communication between the group leader and members
      (3) Encourages individuals to contribute to the discussion
      (4) Engages participants in problem solving (higher-order learning)
      (5) Encourages teamwork, tolerance of divergent opinions, and development of interpersonal skills
      (6) Assists leader in directing the learning experience
      (7) Can be focused on both cognitive and affective learning
   b. Disadvantages
      (1) Strong personalities can influence a group
      (2) Poor discussion leader may contribute to failure of the discussion
      (3) Nothing may be achieved; discussion may go in many directions without closure
      (4) May not be profitable if group members do not have appropriate background
4. Discovery learning—uses a less direct questioning format to prod the learner into using logic or common sense to discover ideas or concepts; useful to build on foundational knowledge and introduce new concepts

a. Advantages
   (1) Requires learner involvement
   (2) Requires application of knowledge (higher-level learning)
   (3) Promotes critical thinking; motivates student to discover the "right answer"; several answers may be plausible
b. Disadvantages
   (1) May be interpreted as guessing
   (2) Learner needs guidance so correct information is concluded

5. Brainstorming—free sharing of ideas generated by unstructured group interaction; may have a well-defined, clearly stated problem to address; ideas recorded for future discussion but never analyzed for merit during session; useful for group identification of an issue or problem
   a. Advantages
      (1) Useful for youth and adult groups
      (2) Encourages creativity
      (3) Encourages application of knowledge
      (4) Encourages contribution by all participants with no fear of a "wrong answer"
      (5) Encourages people to build on others' ideas
   b. Disadvantages
      (1) Group dynamic may be influenced by stronger personalities
      (2) Needs to be carefully managed so the purpose is not lost
      (3) Not useful for actual sharing of information, just for problem identification or issue clarification
6. Web-based learning—uses a computer to present information in a method that can be interactive; includes use of the monitor to present photos, animation, video, print, and sound for lecture–demonstration and cases, discussion groups, online testing, and other online teaching methods
   a. Advantages
      (1) Provides an alternative medium to present information
      (2) Accessible at all times if learner has access to a computer
      (3) Can be updated
      (4) Provides enhanced printed material
      (5) Provides ready access to wealth of resources on the Internet
   b. Disadvantages
      (1) Some older adults and institutionalized persons may not have computer skills or access to appropriate technology
      (2) Cost of equipment and linkages
7. Cooperative and collaborative learning activities—occur both inside and outside the classroom or learning environment, such as group activities and projects
8. Additional options
   a. Field trips; virtual field trips
   b. Panel discussions and debates
   c. Problem-solving assignment
   d. Symposium reporting
   e. Distance learning
   f. Computer simulations and modeling
   g. Library research
   h. Independent study
9. General principles for selection of oral health instructional methods
   a. Oral health education should be focused on education and intervention, stressing skill acquisition and adoption of risk-reducing behaviors (evidence-based)
   b. Oral health education is more successful when characterized by active involvement of participants
   c. A combination of teaching techniques should be used for best results to meet the needs of various learning styles and keep the interest of the audience
   d. Various techniques are more suitable for different topics and for different age groups

B. Selection of media—vehicles of communication
   1. Criteria for selection of media for instruction
      a. Some priority populations may not have access to specific equipment, computers, or the internet
      b. Mass media can be used to create awareness
      c. Material must be presented at a convenient time for the majority of participants
      d. Media must be directed at participants' level of understanding
      e. Size of participant group may affect the appropriateness of different types of media
      f. Availability and familiarity with the operation of the educational technology are necessary
      g. Environments vary in their conduciveness to the use of media and technology
   2. Educational aids
      a. Printed materials (e.g., pamphlets, books)
      b. Photos, overheads, charts, posters, models, puppets, mobiles
      c. Electronic, computer-generated presentations, slides, videotapes, CD-ROMs, DVDs
      d. Boards—story, flannel, bulletin, magnetic
      e. Science experiments
      f. Computer-generated media
      g. Mass media—useful to increase awareness; not as useful to motivate change of health behaviors
      h. Radio and television (including cable)
      i. Newspaper and magazine
      j. Billboards
      k. Advertisements
      l. Distance education technologies (e.g., internet, computerized instruction, Web-based tutorials, telecommunications, teleconferencing, iPods, discussion boards)
      m. Social media
   3. General principles for evaluation and selection of media
      a. Specific purpose—arouse interest, provide information, develop attitudes, change behavior
      b. Accuracy and relevancy
      c. Based on scientific principles and rigorous research (evidence-based)

   d. Target audience—appropriateness (reading level, use of pictures), attractiveness, audience appeal, gender and racially inclusive, culturally sensitive
   e. Complexity of information and readability
   f. Physical properties—illustrations, color, continuity, and style

## Characteristics of Different Types of Learners

A. Groups of learners share commonalities; all groups are made up of individuals, so care must be taken not to generalize indiscriminately

B. Characteristics of adult learners
   1. Goal orientation and relevancy orientation; need to know the reason to learn something
   2. Driven by intrinsic motivation to learn
   3. Interested in the immediacy of its application
   4. Bring knowledge and experience to the learning situation
   5. Come to the learning situation ready to learn
   6. Possibly shy and apprehensive; do not respond as quickly as children do
   7. Used to an authority system and can take direction
   8. Enjoy a fun, warm, friendly and humorous learning environment
   9. Respond well to personal attention, compliments, and reinforcement
   10. Value being treated as equals; are put off if "talked down to," embarrassed, humiliated, or kept waiting
   11. Are social; like to share stories and get to know each other
   12. Prefer hands-on, practical, tangible, orderly, and predictable activities that include active involvement
   13. Need a focus on transference of information (ability to use information in a new setting)

C. Suggestions for oral health education programs for low-literacy learners
   1. Assess level of knowledge
   2. Provide new information, building on and relating to what is already known
   3. Have meaningful interactions; ask questions related to responses
   4. Provide information through familiar and uncomplicated modes; use television, DVDs, radio, personal experience, demonstration, and oral explanation
   5. Provide explicit information that is relevant to current needs
   6. Limit the amount of information taught at one time
   7. Limit written materials; use basic terminology; maintain a 5th-grade level, especially for written materials

D. Characteristics of young children as learners
   1. Have undeveloped intrinsic motivation; respond to reinforcement and behavior modification
   2. Have limited attention and concentration spans; a variety of activities are required to maintain attention
   3. Have undeveloped problem-solving skills
   4. Have a weak memory; repetition is required
   5. Have limited life and learning experience; tend to accept information being presented at face value
   6. Use concrete reasoning; are unable to understand abstract concepts; learning is better with hands-on and visual activities related to the tangible, such as demonstration and practice
   7. Very young children are unable to read and write; lessons must use pictures
   8. Have varied interests at different ages, based on their physical and emotional development and life experiences
   9. Motivations are current interests and needs (e.g., young children's need for approval by teacher; adolescents' need for peer acceptance)
   10. Respond well to oral health education geared to current level of development (e.g., tooth eruption, orthodontic treatment)
   11. Do not possess fine motor coordination skills; recommended oral hygiene methods must be age appropriate (e.g., method of brushing, flossing)
   12. Possess a social nature and interest in sharing stories when asked questions
   13. Show lack of self-control; classroom management is required to control behavior

## Oral Health Education Plan Development

A. Health education plan (lesson plan)—organization of topics, goals, objectives, learning experiences, and evaluation plan in relation to a central theme or problem; provides educators with an organized approach, which is vital in dynamic teaching for both student and teacher; includes all the elements of a program plan previously described

B. Assessment of needs—learner needs, oral health status, interests, and developmental level; teaching environment; availability of media; resources available to support the lesson; previous oral health learning experiences and current oral health knowledge and behavior

C. Prioritization of the learning needs of the audience to determine the purpose, aim, and rationale of the lesson

D. Planning the lesson
   1. Goals—one or two recommended; general, broad statements of direction for the lesson
   2. Instructional objectives—statements that describe the intended outcomes, aims, or products of instruction; what a successful learner is able to do at the end of instruction; expected behavior; should be precise and measurable; useful for guiding instruction and evaluation; components of an effective, precise instructional objective include
      a. Performance—what a learner is expected to be able to do or demonstrate when the instructional event ends, using a verb that denotes an observable behavior or action; for example, "The patient will demonstrate the modified Bass toothbrushing technique"
      b. Conditions—the important conditions (if any) under which the performance is to occur; for example, "Given a soft-bristled toothbrush, the patient will demonstrate the modified Bass toothbrushing technique on all tooth surfaces and on the tongue"
      c. Criterion—the criterion of acceptable performance; a description of how well the learner must perform

to be considered acceptable; for example, "Given a soft-bristled toothbrush, the patient will use the modified Bass toothbrushing technique to remove all clinically visible plaque biofilm, as measured by the Plaque Index"
3. Identifying teaching strategies and learning experiences—should be based on the objectives and on the principles of learning and strategy selection previously explained earlier
4. Identifying materials and media needed based on criteria described earlier; identifying resources for materials; allowing preparation time
5. Identifying and arranging for equipment required to present lesson
6. Planning follow-up activities and materials, such as handouts to send home to parents or caregivers

E. Implementing the lesson
1. Introduction, main activity or activities, closure or conclusion, and follow-up activities
2. Considering the learning needs of the audience during presentation
3. Preparing and practicing beforehand to control anxiety
4. Flexibility and adjustment of plans as needed

F. Evaluation of learning outcomes—should relate to objectives and to pretest and assessment procedures to provide basis for comparison; used for changes in future lessons and self-development as an educator

### Health Education and Promotion Programs in the School Setting

A. The program should focus on a combination of strategies and efforts to reach parents, students, school personnel, and the community
B. Programs in school settings have the potential to reach significant numbers of participants
C. The school environment supports learning and reinforcement, ideally through an integrated curriculum, not isolated instances
D. The school program should be comprehensive, including efforts directed at improving the environment, providing education, and providing or promoting services (e.g., referrals, school-based sealant and F programs)
E. Teachers can serve as role models
F. Success is enhanced by identifying responsible individual(s) (decision makers), involving parents for reinforcement at home, using community resources and personnel (e.g., agencies, other oral health care professionals), and evaluating and revising the program when appropriate
G. The primary role of the dental hygienist is to be a resource, train teachers, work with the various groups to enhance the overall program, and manage and support the program, not to provide all the classroom instruction

## PROGRAM EVALUATION

### General Principles

A. Program evaluation is a key element of community oral health programs; should take place at all stages; consists of both formative and summative evaluation
1. Formative evaluation—ongoing evaluation during the program to assess processes; can lead to revisions to improve program success
2. Summative evaluation—evaluation of outcomes based on program objectives; provides comparison to needs assessment (baseline) data to determine success of the program

B. Program evaluation is applied research; research methods are used (see earlier sections "Epidemiology and Research" and "Measurement of Diseases and Conditions in Oral Epidemiology")
C. Points to evaluate
1. Quality of program and personnel (formative)
2. Progress and effectiveness of activities—identify problems and solutions to assist in revisions and modifications to meet goals and objectives (formative)
3. Perceptions, attitudes, and participation of recipients of program (formative)
4. Systematic and regular evaluation of goals and objectives by using specific measurement instruments; outcomes assessment (summative)
5. Health status indicators of recipients of program (summative)

### Use of Statistics

A. Data—numbers collected from measurements or counts
1. Continuous data—numerical data capable of being any value along a continuum (e.g., periodontal probe readings, blood pressure, time, temperature); can be expressed meaningfully as a fraction
2. Discrete data—numerical variables or data that are counted only in terms of whole numbers (e.g., number of individuals examined, number of children who had teeth sealed)
3. Categorical data—division of data into categories with no numeric representation (e.g., SES, ethnic group membership, gender, school attended, grade in school)
4. Dichotomous data—categorical variable with only two groups (e.g., male/female, yes/no, bleeding/no bleeding)

B. Scales of measurement—data fall in one of four scales:
1. Nominal scale—observations belong to mutually exclusive classes or categories (e.g., political party, smoking status, place of residence, gender)
2. Ordinal scale—classes or categories that have ranking of characteristics in some empirical order (e.g., Likert scales such as strongly disagree, disagree, agree, and strongly agree for patient satisfaction and other measures; most dental indices; periodontal classification; SES)
3. Interval scale—measurement scale characterized by equal intervals along the scale; has no absolute zero (e.g., Fahrenheit temperature scale) ; not useful in oral health research
4. Ratio scale—measurement scale characterized by equal intervals along the scale and the presence of an absolute zero (e.g., age; decayed, missing, and filled tooth count [DMFT]; number of sealants; test scores); most dental indices are treated as ratio data

C. Statistics—science that describes, summarizes, analyzes, and interprets numerical data

1. Statistic—numerical characteristic of a sample derived from the data collected
2. Parameter—numerical characteristic of a population

D. Descriptive statistics—statistics used to describe and summarize data numerically (Box 20.12)
   1. Measures of central tendency—used to describe what is typical (the midpoint) in the data gathered (mean, median, mode)
   2. Measures of dispersion—used to describe variability of scores in a distribution (range, standard deviation [SD])

E. Correlation statistics—statistical measure for determining the strength of the linear relationship between two or more variables; used to associate variables and determine risk in analytic studies; correlation does not establish causality (Box 20.12)

F. Summary presentation of descriptive and correlation statistics
   1. Frequency distribution table—table that summarizes the frequencies of data in the distribution; data are entered into a frequency distribution table before creating a graph
   2. Bar graph (or bar chart)—two-dimensional diagram used pictorially to display data that are discrete in nature, regardless of scale of measurement; bars do not touch
   3. Histogram—type of bar graph used to represent interval-scaled or ratio-scaled variables that are continuous in nature; bars touch each other
   4. Frequency polygon—line graph used to represent data that are continuous in nature; a histogram and a frequency polygon can be used to represent the same data; a frequency polygon can be easier to read than a histogram when more than one distribution is presented for comparison
   5. Polygon—line graph that does not represent frequency data; for example, a line graph showing the progression of a Plaque Index score over time in a repeated-measures experimental study (this example would also be called a time series graph)
   6. Pie graph (or pie chart)—used to display parts of a whole
   7. Scattergram (or scatter plot)—graph in which scores are plotted to show the relationship or association of two variables; visually shows the relationship represented by a correlation statistic
   8. Advantages of tables and graphs—provide a neat and organized way to present data, facilitate understanding and analysis of data at a glance, expedite review of data, enable comparisons, and ease recall of data

G. Distributions of data (Fig. 20.6)
   1. Normal (bell) curve—symmetrical distribution of scores in which the mean, median, and mode have the same value, and the scores fall within a standard relationship to the mean (SD)
      a. 68% of the scores fall between + 1 and − 1 SD of the mean
      b. 95% of the scores fall between + 2 and − 2 SD of the mean
      c. 99% of the scores fall between + 3 and − 3 SD of the mean
   2. Skewed distribution—one in which the distribution is asymmetrical
      a. Positive skew—mean has a higher value than the median and mode; bulk of the scores are at the lower end of the distribution, and tail of the curve is at the higher end
      b. Negative skew—mean has a lower value than the median and mode; bulk of the scores are at the higher end of the distribution, and tail of the curve is at the lower end

H. Inferential statistics—branch of statistics used to infer research findings from the sample to the target population; used to test hypotheses, make inferences to the target population, and provide evidence of causality (see Box 20.12)
   1. Parametric statistics—inferential statistics that require the following assumptions about the population parameters:
      a. Data are interval or ratio scaled; dental indices are treated as ratio scaled even though many are ordinal scaled
      b. Population from which the data are taken is normally distributed (bell curve)
      c. Sample is large (i.e., $n \geq 30$) and randomized
   2. Nonparametric statistics—inferential statistics used when the population parameters do not meet the assumptions required for parametric statistics
      a. Required if data are nominal or ordinal in nature
      b. Population from whom the sample is drawn does not have a normal distribution (has a skewed curve), or distribution is unknown
      c. Required with continuous data if sample size is small or skewed

I. Hypothesis testing
   1. Definition—formal decision-making process of testing a hypothesis using statistical significance and inference, followed by interpreting the statistical results
   2. Null hypothesis is tested statistically to make the statistical decision
      a. Retaining the null hypothesis is equivalent to rejecting the research or alternative hypothesis
      b. Rejection of the null hypothesis is equivalent to the acceptance of the research or alternative hypothesis
      c. Failure to accept (rejecting) the null hypothesis implies accepting the research or alternative hypothesis
   3. Statistical significance—according to the probability established by the level of significance, the obtained result is less likely to be a chance occurrence and more likely the result of the independent variable
   4. Probability level ($p$ value)—researcher's acceptable odds for determining the operation of chance factors in producing the obtained research result; the cutoff point used to reject or accept the null hypothesis; also known as *significance level* and *alpha value*
      a. Small $p$ values indicate rare chance occurrences that lead to the rejection of the null hypothesis and provide more confidence that the statistical decision is correct
      b. Large $p$ values indicate that chance occurrences are more likely to account for the result

## BOX 20.12 Common Statistics in Community Oral Health

### Descriptive Statistics

*Mean*—the arithmetic average; the sum of the values divided by the number of items
- Incorporates the value of each score
- Affected by extreme scores
- Used with interval or ratio data

*Median*—midpoint of a distribution, with 50% of the scores falling above it and 50% below it; scores of distribution are arranged in either ascending or descending order to locate the midpoint
- When the total number of scores is odd, the median is the middle score
- When the total number of scores is even, the two middle scores are added, then divided by 2
- Median can be a decimal
- Not affected by extreme scores
- Can be used with ordinal data; can be used with ratio data to avoid effect of extreme scores

*Mode*—the most frequently occurring score in a distribution
- Distribution may be unimodal, bimodal, multi-modal, or have no mode
- Can be used with nominal data

*Range*—the spread between the highest and the lowest scores in a distribution
- Easily determined
- Somewhat unreliable because it is determined by only two scores of the distribution
- Can be used with ordinal and higher data

*Standard deviation* (SD)—the positive square root of the variance
- The greater the dispersion or spread of scores around the mean of the distribution, the higher the value of the SD and variance
- A small SD indicates that the distribution of scores is clustered closely around the mean; a large SD indicates that scores are dispersed widely around the mean

### Correlation Statistics

- Correlation coefficient, *r*, ranging from + 1.0 to − 1.0; the sign indicates the direction of the correlation, and the number indicates the strength of the correlation
- Interpretation of correlation coefficient

1. Direction of relationship
   - Positive—value of one variable increases as the value of the second also increases (e.g., presence of plaque biofilm and gingivitis); expressed as a positive number
   - Negative—inverse relationship between two variables; as the value of one increases, the other decreases, and vice versa (e.g., fluoride exposure and dental caries); expressed as a negative number
2. Strength, regardless of direction of relationship
   - Very high: $r = 0.9$ to 1.0 (+ or −)
   - High: $r = 0.70$ to 0.89 (+ or −)
   - Moderate: $r = 0.50$ to 0.69 (+ or −)
   - Weak: $r = 0.26$ to 0.49 (+ or −)
   - Little if any: $r = 0$ to 0.25 (+ or −)

### Inferential Statistics

#### *Parametric Inferential Statistics*

- *t* test—determines if a statistically significant difference exists between two mean scores
- *t* test for independent samples—data are from two sample groups drawn independently from a population (two independent groups); commonly known as *Student's t test*
- *t* test for dependent samples—data are from two samples that are related (two groups that are matched for relevant variables or pretest and posttest from one group); also known as *t test for correlated samples* and *paired t test*; more sensitive than the *t* test for independent samples because groups are paired, eliminating a possible source of variance
- Analysis of variance (ANOVA)—used to analyze differences among three or more mean scores; used to examine the effects of two or more independent variables simultaneously within the same research design and to determine interactions among the variables in multiple sample groups
  - *F* ratio—value that results when ANOVA is computed
  - Result communicates if a difference exists somewhere among the mean scores; follow-up statistics are used to determine exactly where the difference lies
  - Variations of ANOVA include ANCOVA (analysis of covariance) to control for extraneous variables in a study design and MANOVA (multivariate analysis of variance), which is used when multiple dependent variables are measured

#### *Nonparametric Inferential Statistics*

- Chi-square test—used to determine if a statistically significant difference exists between frequencies of data (versus comparing mean scores as is done with parametrics); used with nominal data from two or more distributions with more than 5 scores in each one; has different versions for special applications
  - One version is used with a single distribution of data to determine whether or not a significant difference exists between the observed number of cases within designated categories and the expected number of cases within designated categories according to the hypothesis (goodness of fit)
  - Another version is used with two data sets to test the differences in the distributions of data (versus the differences in the mean scores)
  - Another version is used to test the statistical significance of a correlation coefficient result
- Other similar nonparametric statistics exist to test differences of data distributions that represent ordinal data, come from groups with more than five in each one, come from more than two groups, or a combination

Data from Beatty CF, Beatty CE. Biostatistics. In Nathe CN: *Dental Public Health and Research.* 4th ed. Upper Saddle River, NJ: Pearson; 2017: 210–232.

c. Maximum *p* value to reject the null hypothesis in oral health research is typically 0.05; *p* values of 0.01 and 0.001 indicate greater statistical significance
   (1) If the probability is 0.05 or less, the results obtained are reported as statistically significant
   (2) A probability result of greater than 0.05 ($p > 0.05$) indicates results are not statistically significant

5. Inferential statistics are used to test the hypothesis
6. Which test statistic is appropriate to use to make the statistical decision depends on the size of the sample, the number of samples, the type of data, and other factors (see assumptions in the previous discussion of inferential statistics and Box 20.12)
7. Because statistical decision-making is based on probability (chance), errors may occur (Table 20.20)
   a. Type I error—based on statistical results, the researcher rejects the null hypothesis and concludes that a statistically significant difference exists when, in fact, no true difference is present; rejecting a null hypothesis that is true

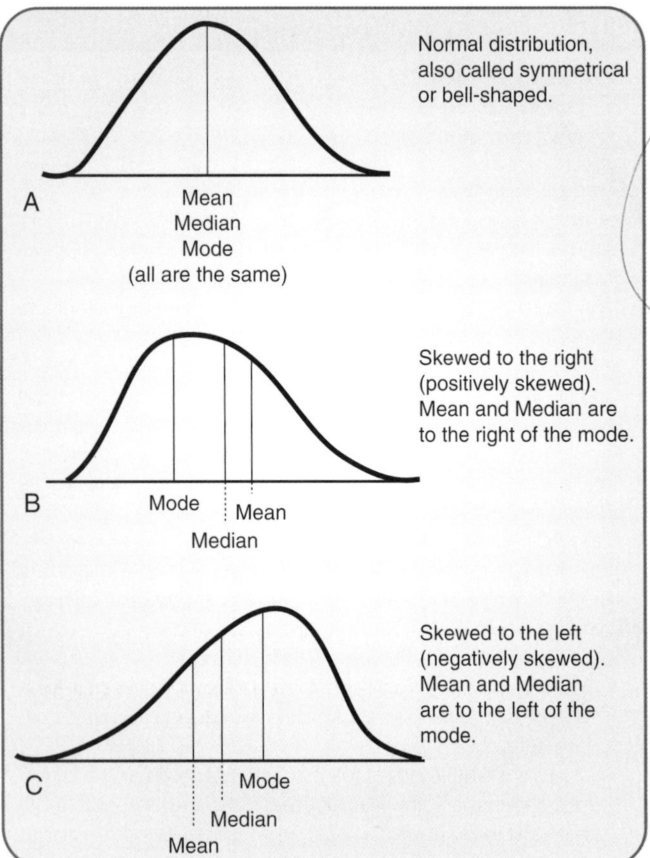


**Fig. 20.6** Distribution curves. (From Beatty CF, Hinson-Enslin AM. Applied research. In Beatty CF, ed. *Community Oral Health Practice for the Dental Hygienist*. 4th ed. St. Louis: Elsevier; 2017:177-209.)

b. Type II error—the researcher concludes that no statistically significant difference exists and accepts the null hypothesis when, in fact, a significant difference does exist; accepting a null hypothesis that is false

c. The p value is set to control the acceptable rate of error, which depends on the clinical importance or significance of the question being researched

(1) Type I errors lead to unwarranted change; for example, a research participant could receive ineffective treatment

(2) Type II errors maintain status quo; for example, a research participant could miss out on treatment that could have been helpful or even lifesaving

d. The potential for error is the reason why multiple studies are critical for evidence-based decision-making

J. Clinical significance

1. Statistical decision-making is not the sole means by which research findings are interpreted and applied; findings may have statistical significance without having clinical significance

2. Practical implications of research may or may not be inherent in research results; statistical significance does not necessarily indicate that results are important or meaningful; for example, the free gingival margin may have a statistically significant resorption of 1.0 mm, while the pocket depth is still 6.0 mm, so the resorption may not be meaningful in the overall periodontal outcome

**TABLE 20.20 Errors Related to the Statistical Decision About the Null Hypothesis**

| | NULL HYPOTHESIS IS | |
|---|---|---|
| **Null hypothesis is actually** | **Accepted** | **Not Accepted** |
| True | No error | Type I α (alpha) error |
| False | Type II β (beta) error | No error |

Data from Beatty CF, Hinson-Enslin AM: Applied research. In Beatty CF: *Community oral health practice for the dental hygienist*, 4th ed. St Louis, Elsevier; 2017: 177–209.

## Evaluating Professional Literature

A. Professional responsibility includes keeping current with new developments for evidence-based decision-making

B. Reviewing and studying the professional literature is important for the contemporary dental hygienist in all roles

1. It is necessary before and during community programming

2. It provides an impetus and evidence base for various types of community activities

3. Journal articles, particularly randomized clinical trials, systematic reviews, and meta-analyses, as well as standards of practice and clinical guidelines, serve as a source of current information for evidence-based decision-making

C. Reviewing the professional literature is a valuable means of professional development

D. Scientific writing should be comprehensible for the average reader who is knowledgeable about the general area

E. Professional literature should be evaluated to ascertain the validity of results (Box 20.13)

# PROVISION OF ORAL HEALTH CARE

## Diverse Modes of Dental Practice in the United States

A. Dental care is delivered via a complex, fragmented system of care that consists of diverse modes of dental practice and multiple sources of funding (see Table 20.21)

B. Community oral health programs generally remain small, understaffed, and underfunded, with great variation in capacity to meet oral health needs

1. Public health recommendations include making changes to the public health infrastructure to improve capacity and increase utilization

2. Recommendations related to infrastructure and capacity include the following:

a. Using oral health professionals with public health training to direct community oral health programs

b. Increasing the number of health centers that have an oral health component that provides primary and secondary preventive services

c. Increasing state-based oral and craniofacial surveillance, including of cleft lip and cleft palate

**BOX 20.13 Criteria for Evaluating the Professional Literature**

1. Overall description of the article
   - Concise and descriptive title
   - Descriptive abstract
2. Reputable and refereed journal
   - Editorial review board in place
   - Peer review of articles before publication
   - Affiliation with a learned society, professional group, specialty group, or reputable scientific publisher
   - Not a "popular" magazine sponsored by a cause or published by a commercial firm
   - Concisely written articles, using a scientific style
3. Currency of data published
   - Represents current knowledge, not outdated by more recent research
   - General guide of 5 years
4. Qualified author
   - Appropriate credentials to have knowledge of the topic
   - Expertise in a particular area supported by current or past position
   - Satisfactory reputation for well-conducted research
   - No affiliation with a commercial firm if the report is of product research
5. Funding of research
   - Evidence of finances and facilities to support the research if the article reports research results
   - No conflict of interest represented
6. References
   - Comprehensive, accurate, and reputable
   - Appropriate number of current references, according to the topic (older references may be indicated for historical purposes or because they are considered classic)
7. Clear, accurate, and complete description of the research problem
   - Clear purposes of the study
   - Inclusion of a thorough review of the literature
   - Adequate operational definitions of important terms and concepts
   - Adequate and clear statement of the hypotheses or objectives that follow directly from the problem statement

**Methods**

1. Adequate description of the research design
2. Appropriate for the type of study (descriptive, analytic, and experimental studies require different methods)
3. Adequate description of the characteristics of the population sampled and an outline of the allocation of groups if a clinical trial
4. Adequate description of the sampling techniques
5. Lack of bias in the selection or assignment of objects or persons in the sample
6. Control of variables that might influence the results
7. Evidence of comparability of experimental and control groups
8. Evidence of control of bias
9. Discussion of the limitations of the study design
10. Use of tests and instruments that reasonably measure the factors under study
    - Use of valid and reliable measures (evidence of reliability is provided)
    - Control of conditions in which measurements are made
    - Control and reporting of the reliability of the examiners
    - Appropriate duration of the study
11. Data analysis
    - Inclusion of all the factors needed to test the hypotheses or achieve the objectives
    - Use of appropriate statistical tests
    - Description of general-purpose computer programs used for data analysis
    - Presentation of statistical results of hypotheses testing
    - Clear presentation of findings
    - Clear, easy-to-understand, and titled data tables and figures
    - Straightforward presentation of data
12. Discussion to highlight significant issues from the research
    - Interpretation of results
    - Clear discussion of the importance or clinical significance of the findings
    - Explanation of the strengths and limitations of the study
    - Report of any treatment or study complications and adverse effects
    - Discussion of the relationship of the results to previous studies
    - Discussion of the implications for practice or the profession
13. Conclusions
    - Clear
    - Supported by methods and findings

Data from Beatty CF, Hinson-Enslin AM. Applied research. In Beatty CF: *Community Oral Health Practice for the Dental Hygienist*. St Louis: Elsevier; 2017, and Nathe CN. *Dental Public Health and Research*. 4th ed. Upper Saddle River, NJ: Pearson; 2017: 177–209.

d. Increasing and diversifying funding of oral health programs
e. Placing oral health programs and components within an organizational structure to maximize visibility, communication, coordination, leadership, and productivity

## Oral Health Care Workforce

A. Types—dentist, dental assistant, dental hygienist, expanded-function dental hygienist and assistant, dental laboratory technician, denturist, other emerging midlevel practitioners in some states such as the dental therapist or dental therapist/hygienist
B. Supply and distribution of dentists in the United States
   1. Supply is traditionally measured with a dentist-to-population ratio—not always an accurate reflection of supply because of location, population involved, community need, demand for dental services, travel time to an available dentist, number of Medicaid/CHIP providers, and trends in use of other oral health care personnel to provide dental treatment services[19]
   2. The number of active dentists was projected to decline through 2020, influenced by retirement patterns and smaller annual number of graduates;[20] however, in 2018, 199,486 dentists were working in dentistry, with a ratio of 61.0 dentists per 100,000 population, higher than any year since 2001, partially as a result of higher age at retirement[21] and an increase in dental school graduates annually over the last decade;[22] this trend is projected to continue
   3. Dental school enrollment
      a. As of 2017, there were 66 US dental schools, located in 36 states, the Commonwealth of Puerto Rico, and the District of Columbia, representing a significant increase from 56 dental schools in 2007[23]

TABLE 20.21 **Modes of Dental Practice**

| Practice Setting | Population Served | Financing | Utilization Patterns | Advantages | Disadvantages | Oral Health Personnel |
|---|---|---|---|---|---|---|
| Private practice (solo or group) | Mid- to high-level SES patients<br>Tend to be located in areas of economic opportunity and desirable locations | Third-party private dental insurance<br>Fee-for-service systems<br>Some discounted-fee programs | Higher SES and dental insurance are associated with greater utilization of dental services (see Table 20.12)<br>Greater demand for esthetic services | Flexibility for patients and providers<br>Providers determine practice philosophy<br>Inherent economic incentive to be efficient<br>Groups compared to solo have availability during nontraditional hours, e more varied services, quality assurance via built-in peer review and consultation, and availability of emergency care from partners | Serves limited population<br>Difficult to monitor quality assurance | Single or multiple dentists and hygienists<br>Limited experience to date with incorporation of midlevel providers into this model |
| Corporately managed dental practice (e.g., dental service organizations) | Low-level to mid-level SES patients<br>May be located in urban or suburban areas | Third-party private dental insurance<br>Public financing via Medicaid and CHIP<br>Some discounted-fee programs | Greater utilization by children and adolescents up to age 21 (Medicaid and CHIP coverage)<br>Higher rate of racial minority groups that correlates with SES | Nontraditional hours<br>Convenient locations<br>Dentists are employees rather than owners<br>Corporate benefits often available to employees<br>Multiple payment options | Practice decisions usually made by corporate administrators<br>Quality of care may suffer from focus on profit over patient care | Multiple dentists and hygienists<br>No evidence of incorporation of midlevel providers into this model, but has been suggested[a] |
| Hospital dental clinic | Specific, medically compromised patient populations<br>Located in or near public or private hospital facilities, military bases, Indian reservations | Public and private financing combined<br>Medicaid/CHIP<br>From patient and hospital funding sources | Special populations such as children who are medically compromised or have other disabilities; cancer patients; veterans<br>Dental services often mandatory before medical procedures or surgery | Accessible to hospital patients who are unable to travel elsewhere<br>Resources, personnel specifically oriented toward patients' special needs<br>Utilize extensive quality assurance programs | Limited to hospital population, and in some cases, family members<br>May require extensive travel for outpatients | Variety of providers, including dental/dental hygiene students, residents<br>Strong inter-professional collaborative practice (IPP) component<br>Student participation often as service learning<br>Federally funded clinics may use USPHS, NHSC, or military personnel |
| Community-based clinics | Lower-SES patients<br>Located in nontraditional settings in urban or rural areas<br>May serve specific populations, e.g. migrant farm workers, Indian reservation, prison population<br>School-based clinics serve high-risk schoolchildren | Public and private financing combined via Medicaid/CHIP, grants, donations, and patient fees<br>Some are faith based with funding from related faith organization<br>May utilize a sliding-fee scale based on income | Increased utilization of services among low-SES groups because of affordability and accessibility<br>For school-based clinics, increased utilization by children and adolescents | Ease of access<br>Affordable care<br>Providers are often bilingual and often share the same cultural background<br>Services may be deeply discounted, sometimes free | State practice acts may limit locations for some providers (RDHs, ADHPs, DHTs)<br>Consistent financing may be difficult | Variety of providers, including midlevel providers<br>Often includes strong IPP component<br>Student participation often as service learning<br>Federally funded clinics may use USPHS, NHSC, or military personnel |
| Mobile clinics | Lower-SES populations<br>Located in nontraditional settings, urban or rural areas<br>High-risk school children<br>Populations with limited mobility and transportation<br>Patients in institutions or homebound, e.g., long-term care facilities | Public and private financing combined via grants, donations, and patient fees<br>Medicaid/CHIP | Increased utilization of services for populations with poor access to care (homebound, long-term care facilities, homeless)<br>Increased utilization for school-age children | Portability of care<br>Increased flexibility with scheduling, delivering care<br>Services may be deeply discounted, sometimes free | State practice acts may limit locations for some providers (RDHs, ADHPs, DHTs)<br>Quality assurance measures may or may not be in place<br>Consistent financing may be difficult<br>Services may be limited | Variety of providers, including mid-level providers<br>Student participation often as a service learning opportunity |

**TABLE 20.21 Modes of Dental Practice—cont'd**

| Practice Setting | Population Served | Financing | Utilization Patterns | Advantages | Disadvantages | Oral Health Personnel |
|---|---|---|---|---|---|---|
| Dental/dental hygiene educational clinics | Low-SES to mid-SES patients<br>Located in educational institutions in or near metropolitan or urban areas | Public and private financing combined<br>From patient and institutional funding sources | Increases utilization of services among lower-SES populations due to affordability of care<br>Provide a safety net for lower-SES populations | High quality of care resulting from close oversight by institution<br>Extensive quality assurance program | Limited flexibility with scheduling<br>Lengthy appointments<br>Multiple appointments often required<br>Extensive travel required by most patients because of location | Dental and dental hygiene students and residents<br>Faculty clinic may or may not be available |

[a]Cain K. 'Corporate dentistry'—defined. *Dentistry IQ*, April 7, 2016, https://www.dentistryiq.com/practice-management/industry/article/16366546/corporate-dentistrydefined

b. There were 25,010 dental students enrolled in 2018, and 6238 dentists graduated in 2017,[22] also representing a significant increase since 2004[23]

4. The dental profession has recognized the need to develop programs to resolve the problem of uneven distribution of dentists, which exists for various reasons
   a. Dentists have freedom to choose their practice location and tend to locate in areas of economic opportunity, high demand for services, and desirable environments; most are drawn to suburban areas rather than rural and urban areas
   b. Location of dental schools provides an abundant number of dentists in some areas and few in other areas; not all states have a dental school
   c. Increased portability of license from state to state is needed to be able to relocate easily in response to geographic population shifts that result in changes in areas of high demand; a national dental licensing examination would provide greater portability
5. The dental profession has recognized the need to increase underrepresented minorities in the oral health care professions
   a. Women in the dental profession
      (1) Women are underrepresented; 32.3% of dentists were female in 2018[21]
      (2) The number of women graduating from dental schools has gradually increased; in 2018, for the first time, the number of female first-time dental school enrollees was almost 4% higher than the number of males[22]
      (3) There is a need to evaluate the effect of this increasing shift of gender on the values, caring quality, patient orientation, and practice models of dentistry, as well as the number and distribution needed to meet the needs of the population[24]
   b. Ethnic diversity of the dental profession
      (1) A continuing need exists to increase it to impact access, health equity, and health care quality for minority populations; current policies aimed at doing so have not had a significant impact[25]
      (2) The ethnic/racial make-up of the population is estimated by the US Census Bureau to be the following: 76.5% non-Hispanic white, 18.3% Hispanic or Latino, 13.4% black or African American, and 5.9% Asian American; in relation to the population, the profession is overrepresented by white dentists (20% more) and Asian American dentists (three times more) and underrepresented by black, Hispanic, and other racial/ethnic group dentists (approximately three times less);[26] dental student graduation of underrepresented groups has increased significantly over the past 10 years[26]
   c. Various federal agencies and organizations support diversification of the oral health care professions workforce through scholarships, repayment programs, and other incentives[27]
6. Inadequate supply and maldistribution of dental personnel can result in designation as a *dental health professional shortage area* (dental health HPSA), as defined by the federal government
   a. Based on population-to-provider ratio (4000–5000:1, depending on the level of dental needs);[28] also considered are access to care according to distance and time, access to fluoridated water, and incomes at *federal poverty level* (income defined annually as poverty level by the federal government for qualification for government programs)[29]
   b. As of the end of 2019, over 56 million people were living in 6782 dental health HPSAs; and the number of practitioners needed to achieve the recommended dentist/population ratio was 9951;[28] these data represent an increase in the number of shortage areas, the number of people living in shortage areas, and the shortage of dentists
   c. Dental health HPSA designation qualifies a community for special government programs
   d. The federal government provides incentives for oral health professionals to locate in communities designated as dental health HPSAs
7. Projections of future adequacy of supply of dentists
   a. The per capita supply of dentists is projected to increase through 2037 even after adjusting for

factors that limit productivity in relation to changes in expected age and gender of the dental workforce[30]

b. However, according to HRSA and ADA, these increases will not be sufficient to meet the increasing population demands for dental care[23,31]

C. Supply of dental hygiene personnel in the United States

1. About 211,600 dental hygienists were employed in the United States in 2018,[32] with a projected increase of 20% from 2016 to 2026;[33] approximately 6700 dental hygienists graduate annually[34]

2. In 2018, there were 364 accredited dental hygiene programs in the United States offering a certificate, associate's or bachelor's degree,[35] reflecting a 9% increase in number of programs since 2014; there are 56 degree completion programs[36] and 19 master's degree programs in dental hygiene and related disciplines[37]

3. More dental hygienists than dentists have graduated every year since 1991, and the difference has increased each year; projections are that this trend will continue[31]

4. Gender and racial/ethnic group representation among dental hygienists

a. Primarily women—95.6% of dental hygienists in 2017 were female[38]

b. In relation to the population, the profession is overrepresented by white dental hygienists and underrepresented by all other racial/ethnic groups[38]—72.5% enrolled in 2012 were non-Hispanic white

5. Projections of future supply of dental hygienists

a. HRSA projects a surplus of dental hygienists in some states by 2025[31]

b. Surplus may be offset in some states as they continue to expand the scope of dental hygiene practice, expand practice settings, and require less supervision in order to meet the increasing demand for greater access to dental care at a more affordable cost[31]

c. Future surplus of dental hygienists can offset the future shortage of dentists in a state as long as the above-mentioned changes occur in the dental hygiene profession within that state[31]

D. Impact of the dental hygiene profession on oral health of the population—as an organized profession, dental hygiene has sought to help meet the oral health care needs of the population and improve access to care in the following ways:

1. Promoting higher levels of education within dental hygiene, such as baccalaureate, master's, and doctoral degree preparation

2. Establishing the dental hygienist as a primary care provider

3. Expanding the scope of practice for the dental hygi enist

a. Although it continues to expand nationally,[39] a vastly varying scope of practice exists from one state to another[40] with some states still having a very narrow scope of practice (e.g., five states still do not allow administration of local anesthesia by dental hygienists)[41]

b. Expanding the dental hygiene scope of practice within a state is associated with improved oral health of the population of that state[39]

4. Seeking direct reimbursement of dental hygienists and midlevel dental practitioners; in 2019, 18 states recognized and reimbursed dental hygienists as Medicaid providers[42]

5. Developing and supporting the advancement of new, nontraditional practice models, such as collaborative and independent practice as well as dental hygiene–based midlevel providers, to improve access to care for underserved populations and better meet the needs of community oral health care practice[43](see Table 20.22)

6. Advocating for states to allow dental hygienists to provide direct care to patients in at least one practice setting in the community without a dentist present (direct access)—as of 2018, 42 states allow for direct access; many of these states were authorized within the last 10 years, and many of them have collaborative dental hygiene practice models under various names that allow for unsupervised practice of dental hygiene[44]

E. Midlevel dental providers in the United States

1. The concept of midlevel providers in dentistry has become a reality in the United States[43] (see Table 20.22)

a. As of 2019, 11 states have authorized dental therapists who function as midlevel providers[43]

b. The first state to benefit from dental therapists was Alaska; the Alaska dental health aide therapist was authorized in 2004; the next state to authorize dental therapy did so in 2009, the next in 2014; nine states authorized it between 2016 and 2019, and eight additional states were pursuing dental therapy in 2019[45]

c. The fast progress of midlevel providers in the last few years marks a new era in dentistry in which the crisis of inadequate access to dental care is being addressed seriously

2. Midlevel providers and other alternative practice models are able to increase access to quality, cost-effective care for underserved population groups who do not have access to the traditional dental office, as well as expand access to dental care in dental Health HPSAs, especially in rural areas;[45,46]

3. Some midlevel providers are dentistry-based, whereas others are dental hygiene-based; ADHA promotes the value of the dental hygiene–based model to build on the foundation of dental hygiene education and practice experience;[43] others have criticized the dental hygiene-based model based on it lengthening the training and substituting rather than adding an oral health care provider[47]

4. Dental hygiene therapy in the United States has also been criticized for its focus on treating adults as well as children and its implementation in private offices[47]

5. As of 2014 more than 14,000 dental therapists practice in more than 54 countries, including Canada, New Zealand, Australia, and the United Kingdom,[48] providing high quality, cost-effective care and improving access to care in those countries, in some cases for over 80 years[49]

F. Other innovative nontraditional practice models

1. Interprofessional collaborative practice (IPP)[50]

a. Dentistry and dental hygiene are exploring IPP as a way to expand and enhance access to care

b. Recommended by public health experts

TABLE 20.22 **Nontraditional Oral Health Care Personnel and Mid-level Providers**

| Models | Practice Settings | Status | Supervision | Education/ Qualifications | Scope of Services |
|---|---|---|---|---|---|
| Community dental health coordinator (CDHC) | Community health centers: clinics, schools, churches, senior citizen centers, Head Start and other community programs in dental health professional shortage areas (dental health HPSAs) | Developed by ADA; meeting or exceeding expectations based on evaluation by ADA; CDHCs are working in 40 states, and ADA is seeking opportunities to expand the program nationwide | Direct supervision; assists practicing dentist in triage of patients, addressing social, environmental, and health literacy issues | 18-month training program at institutions in 30 states<br>CDHC comes from the community, thus is accepted by the community and understands the culture of the community | Advocacy role to address social barriers to utilization of dental care: providing education, interviewing and counseling patients to enroll in government-funded dental programs, providing social support, and offering limited preventive services |
| Dental health aide therapist (DHAT) | Community health center clinics in rural Alaska villages | Developed by the Alaska Native Tribal Health Consortium in 2003 for implementation with Alaska Native population<br>Approved in Washington state in 2017 and Montana in 2019 and being considered by other states with American Indian populations | General supervision; partners with dentist via teledentistry, including real-time video and radiologic oversight; refers to a dentist as needed | 2-year training program<br>Comes from the community served to better address social barriers to dental care utilization | Considered a mid-level provider; based on dentist's diagnosis and treatment plan, performs restorations, pulpotomies, prophylaxis, basic extractions, preventive services, and referral to dentist for care beyond DHAT's scope |
| Dental therapist (DT),[a] dental hygiene therapist (DHT),[b] and advanced dental therapist (ADT)[a] | Settings that serve low-income, uninsured, and underserved populations, DHSAs | DT and ADT established in 2009 in Minnesota (MN);<br>Similar programs approved in seven other states through 2019<br>Accreditation standards adopted by Commission on Dental Accreditation in 2015 | Indirect supervision of DT in MN; direct supervision of DHT in ME; ADT can practice unsupervised in MN under collaborative agreement with a dentist<br>Programs can vary slightly from state to state | DHT: advanced training after licensure as dental hygienist in Maine<br>ADT: MS or MDT awarded; graduates must practice as DT for 2000 hours and pass an examination to be certified as ADT<br>Programs can vary slightly from state to state | Considered midlevel providers; broad range of basic preventive and restorative treatment, minor surgical care, pain control; similar scope of practice for all levels<br>Programs can vary slightly from state to state |
| Independent practice for dental hygienists (IPDH) | Personal private offices, community settings | Very few states have independent practice | Unsupervised | Licensed to practice dental hygiene; varying hours of clinical dental hygiene experience | Traditional scope of dental hygiene practice authorized in that state |
| Collaborative, affiliated, alternative, public health, or extended care practice of dental hygiene (various names in different states) | Private dental offices, facilities and institutions, schools, homebound, community centers, public health clinics, DHSAs, serving low–SES, underserved populations | Numerous states | Unsupervised; for consultation, referral, and emergencies, must have collaborative agreement with a dentist on file with the state dental board; in some states, patient must have a current referral from a dentist or physician | Licensed dental hygienist; various years or hours of clinical dental hygiene experience in different states; BS degree in some states; additional education and training in some states | Traditional scope of dental hygiene practice authorized in that state |

*BS,* Bachelor of Science; *MS,* Master of Science.
[a]Dentistry-based dental therapist/midlevel provider.
[b]Dental hygiene based dental therapist/midlevel provider.
Data from *American Dental Association Action for Dental Health*: About CDHCs, n.d., http://www.ada.org/en/public-programs/action-for-dental-health/community-dental-health-coordinators. Accessed 07.14.19; *American Dental Hygienists' Association*. Expanding access through dental therapy. https://www.adha.org/resources-docs/Expanding_Access_to_Dental_Therapy.pdf. Accessed 07.07.20; American Dental Hygienists' Association: *Bills into law 2017*, July 2017, https://www.adha.org/resources-docs/75110_Bills_Signed_Into_Law.pdf. Accessed 09.10.20; Beek MV, Davidson J: *Dental therapists at work in other countries and states*, November 8, 2016, Mackinac Center for Public Policy (Policy Brief), https://www.mackinac.org/22946; *Minnesota Dental Therapy Association*. Scope of practice. n.d., http://www.mndta.org/what-we-do. Accessed 07.14.19; *University of Minnesota School of Dentistry*. Dental therapy http://www.dentistry.umn.edu/programs-admissions/dental-therapy/index.htm; 2018 Accessed 07.07.20; and Wahowiak L. Dental health therapists bringing oral health care to U.S. tribal communities: opening up access, *Nation's Health*. 2016; 46(5):1–25. http://thenationshealth.aphapublications.org/content/46/5/1.2.

c. IPP competencies and expanded interprofessional collaborative education (IPE) have the potential to improve health of populations and reduce cost of care
2. Arguments have been made to increase the scope of practice of medical practitioners to increase access to dental care; others argue against this because of legal, regulatory, and training barriers[51]

G. Workforce issues should continue to be analyzed and adjustments made on the basis of retirement patterns of practicing dentists, availability of oral health care personnel, productivity improvement, population and economic growth, demand for and financing of dental care, new models of midlevel oral health care practitioners, and the potential for medical practitioners to deliver oral health care services[23]

## FINANCING ORAL HEALTH CARE

A. Oral health care financing in the United States is complex because of the dual involvement of the corporate sector and the public sector, as well as the presence of varied and multiple mechanisms of payment, sources of payment, types of insurance plans, and providers of insurance plans

B. This pluralistic system results in greater emphasis on individual responsibility for oral health care

C. The Patient Protection and Affordable Care Act (ACA; also referred to as Obamacare) expanded dental coverage for children and selected groups of adults through Medicaid and state exchanges; some believe that the new benefits are not sufficiently comprehensive or affordable[52]

D. Overall spending for dental services and out-of-pocket spending have continued to increase[53] and are forecasted to increase even more over the next 8 years[54]

### Mechanisms of Payment for Dental Care

A. Payment by the individual or fee-for-service—two-party system consisting of the provider and patient (see Table 20.23)

B. Third-party payment—also called *insurance*
1. Payment for health care services by some agency other than the patient or client (e.g., insurance company, employer, government agency); designed to improve access to care and increase utilization
2. The dentist and the patient are the first and second parties; the administrator is the third party (also known as the *carrier, insurer, underwriter,* or *administrative agent*) and may collect premiums, assume the financial risk, pay claims, and provide administrative services
3. Third-party plans can be private (a private insurance company or employer) or public (government program such as Medicaid, Medicare, or CHIP)
4. The purchaser of a private plan can be an organized private group (e.g., union, employer) or a government agency
5. Reimbursement for services occurs by a variety of mechanisms (see Table 20.23)
6. Mechanisms are used by third-party carriers to minimize (control) costs by discouraging overuse and protecting the third-party payer's ability to continue in business (see Table 20.23)

C. Different types of insurance (benefits) plans—although frequently referred to as "dental insurance," *benefits plan* is a more accurate term because, unlike medical insurance, it does not truly represent the concept of insurance; specific types of dental benefits plans fall into two categories, fee-for-service and managed care (see Table 20.24)
1. Fee-for-service—traditional system that provides freedom-of-choice arrangements under which patients are not limited in their selection of providers (called *open panel*), control of treatment decisions are maintained by the provider and beneficiary, and the provider is paid for each service rendered according to the fees established by the provider[55]
2. Managed care—cost-containment systems that restrict the type, level, and frequency of treatment; limit the patient's freedom of choice to select a provider with financial benefits to use only certain providers; and control the level of reimbursement for services[56]
   a. Applies one or all of the following to the financing and delivery of health care
      (1) Arrangements with selected providers to furnish services to members (called *closed panel*)
      (2) Defined criteria for the selection of dental care providers
      (3) Significant financial incentives for members to use contracted providers
      (4) Procedures associated with the plan, subject to limitations and exclusions
      (5) Formal programs to monitor the amount and quality of services (i.e., utilization review and quality assurance)
      (6) Providers are compensated in a predetermined form (e.g., fixed amount per program member, fixed amount per service)
   b. Has resulted from the escalating costs of health care, the need to minimize those costs, and the need to improve access to care for a large segment of the population without traditional dental insurance (benefits)
   c. Although initially not well-received by organized dentistry, managed care plans are becoming more common
   d. Views on managed care applied to dental care vary
      (1) Managed dental care has not yet evolved to the extent of managed medical care[56]
      (2) Dental professionals have continued to express concern about closed-panel third-party approaches because patients are denied freedom of choice of dentists[57]
      (3) An argument against the closed-panel approach relates to the quality of care provided, although charges of poor quality have not been substantiated
      (4) Publicly funded insurance is often administered through managed care programs (see Table 20.24)
      (5) Managed care is expected to increase because of the need to control the cost of dental care nationwide and because of greater governmental involvement in financing dental care
      (6) Dental hygienists may contribute significantly in a managed care model because of the emphasis on prevention and on cost savings

**TABLE 20.23 Mechanisms of Payment for Oral Health Care and Methods Used to Minimize Costs**

| Mechanism | Description |
|---|---|
| **Individual Payment Methods** | |
| Fee-for-service | Traditional two-party arrangement in which fee is set for a service and patient is charged for service performed; declining method of payment as third-party payment becomes more prevalent |
| Barter system | The provider and patient negotiate payment by exchanging goods or services without using money; still evident in some rural areas and developing countries |
| Encounter fee | A set fee each time a patient has a treatment encounter (comes in for treatment), regardless of the services provided; used by community programs as a discounted fee for patients with no dental insurance |
| **Third-Party Reimbursement Methods** | |
| Usual, customary, and reasonable (UCR) fee | Third-party payment generally based on an average of fees for the area; varies by geographic area and population size, and from carrier to carrier; most commonly used payment method in dentistry |
| Discounted fee | Third-party system in which fees lower than the area UCR are agreed to by a provider for members of a specifically identified group (students, older adults) or participants in a prepaid group; becoming more common in dentistry |
| Fee schedule | List of charges set by the third-party payer and agreed to by the provider who enrolls as a provider; provider is reimbursed by the third-party payer and cannot charge more; system used by Medicaid/CHIP |
| Table of allowances | List of covered services with an assigned dollar amount set by the third-party payer; providers are reimbursed by the third-party payer and can charge patients the difference between their fees and the fees set by the table of allowances |
| Capitation | A form of contracted care in which a provider receives a fixed payment from a third-party payer in exchange for all or most care needed by a group of patients during the contract period; method used by health maintenance organizations (HMOs); designed to increase preventive care; payment is made to the provider regardless of use by enrollees; effectiveness is in question; not typically used in dentistry |
| Direct reimbursement | Beneficiaries (patients) are reimbursed by the employer or benefits administrator (e.g., insurance company) for a specified percentage of dental expenses on presentation of evidence of expenses |
| **Methods Used to Minimize Costs** | |
| Co-payment | Patient pays a fixed amount at each visit, and the remainder of the fee is covered by the third party; the purpose is to discourage overuse |
| Coinsurance | Similar to co-payment, but it is a percentage rather than a fixed amount; used by most dental insurance plans |
| Deductible | Patient must pay a required amount as an out-of-pocket expense before the insurance plan will pay |
| Preexisting conditions | Coverage is restricted for dental conditions that are present before enrollment in the plan |
| Annual limits (maximum coverage) | Insurance plan will pay only up to a specific dollar limit each year, can be based on individual or family maximums |
| Waiting period | Patient must wait specified length of time before coverage begins |
| Use of UCR | There is no universally accepted method for determining the UCR fee schedule; may vary a great deal among plans, even when the plans operate in the same area |

Data from *American Dental Association*. Typical dental plan benefits and limitations. https://success.ada.org/en/dental-benefits/typical-dental-plan-benefits-and-limitations, accessed 09.10.20.

(7) It has been suggested that managed care will result in tying reimbursement to outcomes of treatment[56]

## Providers of Dental Benefits Plans

A. The variety of providers of dental benefits plans adds to the complexity of the pluralistic system of payment for dental care in the United States
B. The types of providers that offer different types of plans are explained in Table 20.24

## Public Financing of Dental Care

A. Primarily addresses the needs of low-income persons
   1. The percentage of the population living in poverty in 2017 was 12.3%, slightly lower than the previous 2 years[58];
   2. The poverty rate of children under age 18 years in 2017 continued to be considerably higher than other age groups; the rate was 17.5%, representing one-third of all Americans living in poverty[59]
   3. There is less poverty among the non-Hispanic white population, especially in contrast to the Hispanic, non-Hispanic black, and American Indian/Alaska Native populations[59]poverty rates vary by geographic region and metropolitan status[58]
   4. The significance of poverty rates in the population is that low-SES groups experience a greater number of factors that are associated with poor health (determinants of health) and generally have poorer oral health status
B. Problems with public financing
   1. Fragmented; difficult to find and utilize resources
   2. Medicaid has been plagued by changing eligibility requirements, limitation of services, low allowable fees paid, delays in payment for services, and dentists' refusal to treat Medicaid patients
   3. Poor enrollment of dentists as providers—reasons given include low reimbursement rates, missed appointments by Medicaid patients, difficult treatment issues, too much bureaucratic paperwork, reluctance to have patients from low-SES

**TABLE 20.24 Dental Insurance (Benefits) Plans**

| Type of Plan | Provider | Description |
|---|---|---|
| **Fee-for-Service** | | |
| Indemnity dental benefits plan | For-profit, commercial insurance companies | Traditional plan; patient can visit any provider (freedom of choice) and provider is free to set fees; includes deductible, coinsurance, and maximums; company reimburses patient or provider based on UCR; patient is responsible for difference between benefit paid and fee charged; may include a prepayment review and require preauthorization; most expensive form of insurance |
| Direct reimbursement | Employers | Not a true insurance plan; self-funded plan that reimburses patients according to dollars spent rather than type of treatment; administrator (can be employer) pays patient percentage of actual treatments received, saving the cost of the middleman; allows freedom of choice and autonomy of decision-making about treatment; may eliminate claim forms and administrative processing by dental offices |
| **Managed Care** | | |
| Preferred provider organization (PPO) | Health service and dental service corporations (not for profit), commercial insurance companies (for profit) | Regular indemnity insurance combined with a network of dentists under contract to the insurance company to provide services for set fees below the average; patient can visit a dentist outside the PPO and pay the difference (amount above the discounted fee); includes co-insurance, deductible, and maximum coverage; insurance company reimburses patient or dentist accepts payment directly from insurance company; less costly than traditional indemnity plan |
| Exclusive provider organization (EPO) | Same as PPO | A closed panel variation of a PPO; does not cover out-of-network care; can severely limit access to care |
| Dental health maintenance organization (DHMO) (prepaid plan) | Health service and dental service corporations; commercial insurance companies; prepaid, large group practices | Patients must use one dentist or facility (plan does not pay if they go outside the HMO); includes copayment and possibly maximums but no deductibles; uses capitation; usually lowest-cost program; uncommon for dental benefits; dentists frequently limit number of HMO patients to offset loss of income |
| Point of service plan | Same as DHMO | Variation of DHMO; patient may go out of network and be reimbursed based on a low table of allowances that reflects reduced benefits |
| Dental discount plan | Employers, provider organizations; organization of corporate clinics | Providers join the plan by paying a fee and agreeing to offer discounted fees, then are listed as a member provider (way of recruiting patients); patients join the plan by paying a fee, receive a list of providers who are on the plan and a card to present to the member provider, and pay deeply discounted fees to member providers; not "true" insurance; no deductibles, no annual limits, no copayments, no paperwork for the patient or dentist for reimbursement, and no pre-qualifications; more employers are providing this type of plan |
| Table or schedule of allowances plan | Same as PPO | Indemnity plan that pays a set dollar amount for each procedure and patient pays the difference; may also be a variation of a PPO that limits contracted dentists to a maximum allowable charge |
| Individual practice association (IPA) | Association of independent dental providers | More of a business arrangement than a dental benefits plan; organization contracts with independent dentists to provide services to DHMO patients for discounted fees or through capitation arrangement |

Data from *American Dental Association. Types of dental plans.* https://success.ada.org/en/dental-benefits/dental-plan-overview. Accessed 07.02.19; *American Dental Association.* Typical dental plan benefits and limitations. https://success.ada.org/en/dental-benefits/typical-dental-plan-benefits-and-limitations. Accessed 07.02.19.

groups in the reception room with other patients, and preference to provide charity care rather than Medicaid services

4. Many children who qualify are not enrolled in Medicaid/CHIP
5. Overall quality of care provided may continue to be affected by the limitations and complexity of public and publicly subsidized private insurance, the lack of transparency in dental coverage in various policies making its purchase and use confusing to consumers,[60] and the increased burden placed on providers accepting publicly funded insurance programs
6. Increases in public dental benefits will not necessarily bring about a proportional increase in dental utilization[52]

C. Strategies to address problems with public financing
   1. Recent increases in the services allowed and fees reimbursed by Medicaid—still severely lag behind dentist fees and reimbursement rates from private dental insurance[61]
   2. Recent public health department initiatives to increase the number of Medicaid/CHIP dental providers[61]—in 2015 the proportion of dentists enrolled as Medicaid/CHIP providers increased to 38%[62]
   3. Increase in population with Medicaid dental benefits—recent policies under the ACA increased the availability of public financing for dental care to all children from low-income families and to low-income adults;[61,62] because of the complexity of benefits plans, dental insurance coverage for children has not expanded as much as expected[52]
   4. Development of midlevel dental providers—makes available a workforce that can provide dental care at a lower cost to society

D. Medicaid/CHIP—most public expenditures for dental care are from Medicaid or CHIP (see Table 20.25)
   1. In 2018, more than 36 million children were enrolled in Medicaid and 9.2 million in CHIP; this is a marked increase in the number of children enrolled in Medicaid and CHIP and a significant reduction in the rate of uninsured children since passage of the ACA in 2010[63]

2. In 2017, 14.9 million additional adults were enrolled in Medicaid as a result of the ACA;[64] in 2018, 25 states, including the District of Columbia, provided at least limited dental benefits to adults[62]
3. Utilization rates for children enrolled in Medicaid are lower than for children on private dental benefits; utilization rates of children on Medicaid increased from 2006 to 2016[62]
4. Nonelderly adult Medicaid beneficiaries who reside in nursing homes and those with intellectual/developmental disabilities have higher dental utilization rates than the general Medicaid population[65]
5. Adult utilization of Medicaid benefits is associated with the comprehensiveness of a state's dental benefits package[65]
6. It is uncertain how health policies under the Trump administration will affect enrollment in Medicaid and CHIP[52,66]

E. Federal and state programs (see Table 20.25)
F. Local programs
   1. Funded through a variety of sources, including local health department funds; federally funded programs; national, state, and local foundations; faith-based organizations; and other local sources of funding (see Table 20.25)
   2. Collaboration must occur among public health agencies, nongovernmental organizations (NGOs), dental and dental hygiene associations and educational programs, community agencies, and volunteer groups to fund local community oral health care programs
G. Involvement of the federal government in health care financing has increased steadily, especially since 1965
   1. Dental care has continued to be a small part, at best
   2. Demand for services for the low-income population has increased at a time when available services are declining
   3. Obamacare increased federal government involvement, and it may change under Trump health policies[52]
   4. It is expected that future oral health care financing will continue the current varied and complex financing systems and pubic coverage for a large proportion of the population, primarily low-income and special-needs groups

## NEED FOR, DEMAND FOR, AND UTILIZATION OF DENTAL SERVICES

A. Definition of terms (see Table 20.26)
B. Current dental care utilization
   1. Primary indicator of access to dental care is the proportion of children, adolescents, and adults who use the oral health care system (see Table 20.3)
   2. Status of this indicator shows an increase from 2010 to 2017 (see Table 20.27); this increase in dental care utilization is across all age groups, racial/ethnic groups, income levels, geographic regions, and categories of metropolitan statistical area
   3. An important emphasis of dental public health nationally is to continue working toward further increases in use of the oral health care system by all ages and in preventive dental visits by low-income youth (see Table 20.3)
   4. Other indicators reported by CDC also show growth in the use of the oral health care system (see Table 20.28), indicating an increase in access to care compared to the previous decade
   5. Dental public health officials recommended that teeth cleaning in women during the 12 months before the most recent pregnancy be added by the NOHSS as an indicator of the use of dental care and a preventive behavior to be monitored;[67] no data are available yet from the CDC, but Delta Dental Plans Association released data in 2016 that demonstrated an increase in visits to the dentist by pregnant women in 2016 (63%) compared to 2015 (57.5%)[68]
   6. Data are limited to date on outcomes of increased services and oral health resulting from increased numbers of children and adults enrolled in Medicaid and CHIP
C. Emergency-department (ED) use as a safety net for preventable dental conditions
   1. This utilization pattern is low, but it has increased over the past several years and is costly to hospitals and society[65]
   2. In most cases, dental-related needs could be addressed in community settings and don't require the ED; very few ED visits for dental services result in admittance to the hospital[65]
   3. The need has been highlighted to find ways to encourage the utilization of preventive dental care services in the community for a better, more cost-effective outcome[65]
   4. The following factors are associated with ED use for dental care by adult Medicaid patients:[65]
      a. Of the four major ethnic/racial groups, Hispanic individuals have the lowest rate of ED use, and white individuals have the highest rate, primarily related to SES and community factors
      b. Individuals with intellectual/developmental disabilities have the lowest rate of ED use
      c. Nonelderly adult nursing home residents have a lower rate of ED use
      d. Communities with more dentists per residents have a higher rate of outpatient use and a lower rate of ED use
      e. Individuals in rural areas show greater use of the ED than those in urban areas
D. Patterns of dental care utilization
   1. Gender—females continue to have more dental visits than males[69]
   2. Age—higher utilization rates for children than adults and older adults; increase in utilization for all ages; marked increase in utilization by older adults with rate now slightly greater than that of adults[69] (see Table 20.27)
   3. Race and ethnicity—utilization varies for racial and ethnic groups, mostly as a function of SES and culture; in 2017, for the first time, utilization by children and adolescents was highest for the American Indian or Alaska Native only population, compared with the white only, Black or African American only, Asian only, and Islander only groups, presumably because of the utilization of dental therapists by IHS in this population; utilization continued to be highest in the white only population for adults and older adults[69]

**TABLE 20.25 Public and Other Funding of Oral Health Programs**

| Program | Description |
|---|---|
| **Reimbursement to Providers for Services Provided** | |
| Medicaid | Title XIX amendment of the Social Security Act passed in 1965; federal insurance program to provide access to health care to low-income and other special groups, for example, children of lawfully admitted immigrants, newborn children without insurance, children under Child Protective Services, and disabled individuals; funded via a partnership of federal and state governments; administered by the state; eligibility, designated expenditures, and authorized services vary from state to state<br>Dental care became mandatory for children under the ACA; all states must provide oral health care services to Medicaid-eligible children as specified by the Early and Periodic Screening, Diagnosis, and Treatment (EPSDT) program (medical, dental, and vision care are mandatory), and dental care is required in all health care insurance policies as an essential health benefit; providers must enroll; patients must be enrolled in Medicaid and can only seek care from Medicaid providers; source of funding for local philanthropic, educational, and community programs that bill Medicaid for services provided to Medicaid beneficiaries |
| Children's Health Insurance Program (CHIP) | Joint federal-state program created by the Social Security Act in 1997, giving each state permission to offer health insurance to children up to age 19 from families with incomes above Medicaid level but too low to afford health insurance (up to 200% to 250% of federal poverty level); all states participate; state can establish the CHIP program as an extension of the Medicaid program or as a separate state program; jointly funded by state and federal governments; state administers program and determines eligibility requirements and available services; benefits must be at least equivalent to those provided under Medicaid; program varies from state to state<br>Covers dental as well as medical care; all states provide CHIP coverage for dental benefits as required by the ACA; copayments and coinsurance for certain treatments vary from state to state; patients must be enrolled in CHIP and use a CHIP provider |
| Medicare | Title XVIII amendment of the Social Security Act passed in 1965; federal insurance program to pay medical bills for insured persons age 65 years and older and certain disabled individuals; administered by the Centers for Medicare and Medicaid Services (CMS); no income limitations<br>Dental care coverage is limited to services that have medical implications; federal legislation was introduced in 2019 to include dental care, hearing aids, and eyeglasses |
| **Publicly Funded Programs** | |
| Indian Health Service (IHS) | Federal funding of hospitals and clinics on reservations and in urban areas that serve Native Americans and Alaska Natives who are members of federally recognized tribes; IHS clinics are staffed by PHS officers; also pays for contracted care through private dental offices and collaborates with other agencies to provide community oral health programs on Indian reservations |
| Public Health Service (PHS) | Federal funding of PHS officers who provide dental care for US Coast Guard, federal prisons, and IHS facilities as well as selective defined groups such as migrant and seasonal farmworkers and homeless persons |
| Community Health Center Fund | Federal funding established by the Affordable Care Act (ACA) for expansion of local community-based health centers and clinics, to be used in combination with state funding |
| School-Based Health Center Capital (SBHC) Program | Federal funding established by the ACA for expansion of school-based health centers and clinics, to be used in combination with state funding |
| Maternal and Child Health Services | Federal funding from HRSA for comprehensive prenatal care for women and primary and preventive care for children; health and supportive services for special needs children; funding comes to the state via *block grants* |
| Women, Infants and Children (WIC) program | Federal funding of supplementation of food, health care referrals (including dental), and nutritional education for low-income pregnant women, mothers of infants and young children, and infants and children at nutritional risk; administered through the Department of Agriculture |
| Head Start program | Federal funding of oral health screening, oral hygiene activities, and weekly oral health curricula for children in Head Start, which is the federal preschool child development program administered by the Administration for Children and Families |
| Tricare (formerly Civilian Health and Medical Program of the Uniformed Services [CHAMPUS]) | Health care services for military personnel and dependents; also provides a voluntary dental benefits program; requires participants to pay part of premiums |
| Children with Special Health Care Needs Program | Federal and state funding of treatments for children who require health care and related services beyond what they generally require; this can include children with conditions such as cystic fibrosis, HIV/AIDS, cerebral palsy, and Down Syndrome, and can cover such dental needs as craniofacial deformities and cleft lip and palate |
| Ryan White HIV/AIDS Program | Provides varied health care and support services, including dental care for people living with HIV |
| Other federal governmental agencies | Responsible for the provision of dental services and oral health education to specific population groups, such as military personnel and their dependents, disadvantaged groups, and incarcerated persons; staffed by PHS officers; examples are Department of Defense (DoD); Department of Veterans Affairs (VA); Department of Justice, Bureau of Prisons (BoP); DHHS Health Resources and Services Administration (HRSA) |
| State programs | Vary from state to state; use state funds to provide care to particular populations; primarily provide programs to support health education and health promotion at state and local levels through health departments; treatment programs are provided for state institutions such as state prisons and residential facilities for intellectually challenged individuals |

**TABLE 20.25 Public and Other Funding of Oral Health Programs—cont'd**

| Program | Description |
|---|---|
| **Other Funding of Community-Based Programs** | |
| Faith-based programs | Clinics and school oral health programs operated by churches and other faith-based institutions (e.g. San José Clinic, a ministry of the Archdiocese of Galveston-Houston [Texas]), partially funded by the United Way and staffed by volunteers from the Greater Houston dental hygiene and dental societies |
| Community clinics | Funded by local or national foundations (e.g., International College of Dentists U.S.A. Section), civic organizations (e.g., Kiwanis Club), and community resources (e.g., United Way) |
| Programs operated by organized dental hygiene and dentistry | Head Start varnish programs and school- and community-based sealant programs operated by ADHA constituents and components; Give Kids a Smile (free dental care events) sponsored by the ADA Foundation) |
| Programs operated by non-profit organizations | Special Smiles (screening and oral hygiene education for Special Olympics athletes) operated by Special Olympics; Donated Dental Services (direct dental care), Donated Orthodontic Services (direct orthodontic care), Campaign of Concern (preventive education services and screening in facilities for developmentally challenged individuals), and Dental House Calls (homebound dental care), all operated by Dental Lifeline Network for qualified individuals |
| Programs operated by corporations | Bright Smiles, Bright Futures (mobile-dental-van screenings and oral health education in schools) sponsored by Colgate; Delta Dental Community Care Foundation (funds state and local community oral health programs and dental clinics) sponsored by Delta Dental |

Data from Yarbrough C, Reusch C. Progress to build on: Recent trends in dental coverage access (blog), *Teeth Matter*, Children's Dental Health Project October 18, 2018. https://www.cdhp.org/blog/557-progress-to-build-on-recent-trends-on-dental-coverage-access Accessed 09.10.20; Children's Dental Health Project. How the Affordable Care Act moved oral health forward. *Teeth Matter (Blog)*, March 23, 2018. https://www.cdhp.org/blog/502-how-the-affordable-care-act-moved-oral-health-forward Accessed 09.10.20; *National Committee to Preserve Social Security & Medicare*. Expanding Medicare to provide dental, vision, and hearing care. https://www.ncpssm.org/documents/medicare-policy-papers/expanding-medicare-to-provide-dental-vision-and-hearing-care/ Accessed 04.26.19; *Indian Health Service, Division of Oral Health*. ECC program spotlight archive. https://www.ihs.gov/medicalprograms/doh/index.cfm?fuseaction=ecc.archive Accessed 07.07.20; U.S. Public Health Service. About us. https://www.usphs.gov/about-us Accessed 09.10.20; Rosenbaum S. The community health center fund: What's at risk? *Milbank Quarterly*, October 2017. https://www.milbank.org/quarterly/articles/community-health-center-fund-whats-risk/ Accessed 09.10.20; *Health Resources & Services Administration*. FY 2019 School-based health center capital program. https://bphc.hrsa.gov/programopportunities/fundingopportunities/sbhcc/ Accessed 07.07.20; *Health Resources & Services Administration*. Find Maternal & Child Health Bureau funding. https://mchb.hrsa.gov/find-funding Accessed 09.10.20; *U.S. Department of Agriculture*. Special Supplemental Nutrition Program for Women, Infants, and Children (WIC). https://www.fns.usda.gov/wic Accessed 07.07.20; *Office of Head Start:* Head Start programs, February 11, 2019, https://www.acf.hhs.gov/ohs/about/head-start Accessed 09.10.20; *Military.com*. Tricare dental plan benefits and coverage. https://www.military.com/benefits/tricare/dental/tricare-dental-plan-benefits-and-coverage.html Accessed 07.07.20; *Health Resources & Services Administration*. Children with special health care needs. https://mchb.hrsa.gov/maternal-child-health-topics/children-and-youth-special-health-needs Accessed 07.07.20; *Health Resources & Services Administration*. About the Ryan White HIV/AIDS program. https://hab.hrsa.gov/about-ryan-white-hivaids-program/about-ryan-white-hivaids-program Accessed 07.07.20; *Association of State & Territorial Dental Directors*. Proven and promising best practices for state and community oral health programs. https://www.astdd.org/best-practices/ Accessed 07.07.20; *San José Clinic*. 2019 annual report. https://www.sanjoseclinic.orgreports-stastics Accessed 09.10.20; *International College of Dentists*, USA Section Foundation. Welcome to the foundation. https://www.usa-icd.org/foundation/ Accessed 09.10.20; *American Dental Association*. About Give Kids a Smile. https://www.ada.org/en/public-programs/give-kids-a-smile/about-give-kids-a-smile Accessed 09.10.20; *Special Olympics*. Special Smiles. https://www.specialolympics.org/tag/special-smiles Accessed 07.07.20; Dental Lifeline Network. *Our programs*. https://dentallifeline.org/about-us/our-programs/ Accessed 07.07.20; *Colgate*. Bright Smiles, Bright Futures. https://www.colgate.com/en-us/bright-smiles-bright-futures Accessed 07.07.20; and *Delta Dental*. Delta Dental Community Care Foundation. https://www1.deltadentalins.com/about/foundation.html Accessed 09.10.20.

a. Disparities are less for utilization of preventive dental services by low-income children and adolescents who are more likely to have dental benefits than other age groups[69]
b. Culture and SES are associated with health literacy, which affects health decisions (see Table 20.2)
c. The Hispanic or Latino and the Black or African American groups have lower utilization rates than the white only group in upper income brackets; in the lowest income bracket, white only children and adolescents have the lowest utilization rates and white only adults and older adults have the highest utilization rates[69]

4. Geographic location—utilization of dental care is lower in rural communities (both farm and nonfarm) than urban areas, especially in adults and older adults;[69] suburban populations are the most frequent users
5. Region—utilization rates differ among states; the South continues to have lower utilization in all age groups[69]

## Factors That Influence Dental Care Utilization and Oral Health Behaviors

A. Increase in public awareness of health and oral health, influenced by the following:
   1. New technologies such as telehealth, bioinformatics, and virtual reality
   2. Databases specifying the human, animal, and microbial genomes
   3. Strong emphasis on evidence-informed approaches to health care delivery
   4. Increased emphasis on oral health literacy

**TABLE 20.26 Terminology Related to Utilization**

| Term | Definition/Description |
|---|---|
| Demand | Volume and types of health care services that an individual or population desires to consume at some price level; measured by self-report surveys<br>*Effective demand*—desire for care and ability to obtain care (patient or community has access to care)<br>*Potential demand*—desire for care and inability to obtain care (patient or community lacks access to care) |
| Need | *Normative need*—expressed in terms of a population or individual; includes specific needs professionally determined through individual or community-based clinical assessment procedures<br>*Perceived need* or *felt need*—identified by the patient or the community through self-report surveys and interviews; can differ from normative need; health education is required to help a patient or community adjust perceived need to match normative need |
| Utilization | Proportion of the population who use dental services over a period; volume and types of services actually consumed; typically measured by dental attendance rates during the year |

Data from Dickinson C, Beatty CF. Measuring oral health status and progress. In Beatty CF: *Community oral health practice for the dental hygienist*, ed 4. St Louis, Elsevier; 2017: 73–103.

**TABLE 20.27 Percentage of Persons With a Dental Visit in the Past Year, 2010 and 2017**

| Age Group | 2010 | 2017 | Percent increase |
|---|---|---|---|
| 2 years and older | 64.7 | 68.7 | 6.2 |
| 2 to 17 years | 78.9 | 84.9 | 7.2 |
| 18 to 64 years | 61.1 | 64.0 | 5.4 |
| 65 years and older | 57.7 | 65.6 | 11.4 |

Data from *Centers for Disease Control and Prevention. National Center for Health Statistics*: Oral and dental health: Dental visits: Health, United States 2018, Table 37. https://www.cdc.gov/nchs/fastats/dental.htm; 2019 Accessed 09.11.20.

B. A person's level of adopting the wellness paradigm versus the health-disease paradigm

C. Compliance with recommendations varies as a result of the following:

1. Beliefs—trust placed in a provider, health custom, or system of health care because of acceptance that something is true; personal or cultural beliefs about illness and wellness may influence health behaviors
2. Attitudes—patterns of mental views based on judgments of likes and dislikes (about health care systems, providers, or utilization); established because of prior experience; in 2016 and 2017, close to half of Americans expressed a desire to see the dentist more often[70]
3. Values—the importance or worth placed on health care and health practices; beliefs, attitudes, and values are all interrelated and affect each other; although difficult, beliefs, attitudes, and values related to oral health care and health practices can be changed over time through development of rapport, communication, persuasion, education, and new experiences
4. Beliefs, attitudes, and values are influenced by health literacy

D. Access to dental insurance benefits—those with benefits are more likely to utilize care, and the type of dental benefits is associated with utilization

1. In 2016, 77% of the US population had dental benefits, representing a 35% increase from 10 years prior;[71] approximately one-third of them had publicly funded dental benefits, and two-thirds had some form of private dental insurance, in contrast to 14% on publicly funded benefits and 86% on private dental insurance 10 years prior;[71]
2. Coverage varies by age; in 2015, about 10% of children, one-third of adults, and two-thirds of older adults had no benefits[72]
3. Of those who have dental benefits, a greater percentage have private dental coverage (about 33% more children and eight times more adults) compared to public insurance (e.g., Medicaid, CHIP);[72] because the majority of dental benefits are private, a higher rate of coverage is associated with higher income levels
4. More than twice as many people were on publicly funded benefits in 2016 compared to 2014;[71] this increase primarily represents the low-income adults that qualified for Medicaid through the ACA[52] the number of children with public insurance did not increase as dramatically as expected during this same period[52]
5. The ACA has expanded dental coverage for the population
   a. Dental services must be included in health insurance as *essential health benefit*[73]
   b. Medicaid dental coverage of low-income adults has increased since the availability of Medicaid for this population[71] (see earlier "Medicaid/CHIP" section)
   c. Dependent dental coverage for young adults was expanded through age 26; early outcomes have shown increased utilization of restorative care but not of preventive care for this population group[74]
   d. The process of purchasing dental health insurance has become more complex with government-subsidized insurance and increased choices[60]
6. Parents have two options to purchase dental benefits for their children
   a. Dental coverage folded into health insurance[75]
   b. Dental coverage through a dental insurance–only policy[75]
   c. The cost-effectiveness of each option depends on the treatment needs of the child[75]
7. The problem of unmet dental needs of older adults, especially those with lower income and lack of access to dental insurance, is getting more attention; a proposal to expand Medicare to include dental benefits has been discussed for several years and a bill was introduced in 2019[76]

**TABLE 20.28 Status and Trends of Other Current Indicators of Access to Care**

| Indicator | Status and Improvement |
|---|---|
| Proportion of low-income children and adolescents aged 2–18 who received preventive dental services in the past year | Increased from 30.2% in 2007 to 34.6% in 2012 |
| Proportion of school-based health centers with an oral health component that included the following: | From 2007–2008 to 2010–2011: |
| • Dental sealants | • Increased from 17.1% to 24.4% |
| • Dental care | • Increased from 6.4% to 9.1% |
| • Topical fluoride | • Increased from 20.6% to 33.1% |
| Proportion of Federally Qualified Health Centers (FQHCs) with an oral health care program | Decreased from 75% in 2007 to 71.4% in 2014 |
| Proportion of local health departments that have oral health prevention or care programs | 25.8% in 2008; no current data to indicate degree of change |
| Proportion of patients at Federally Qualified Health Centers (FQHCs) who received dental services | Increased from 17.5% in 2007 to 20.9% in 2014 |

Data from *Department of Health and Human Services: Centers for Disease Control and Prevention.* National Center for Health Statistics: Healthy People 2020 midcourse review. Chapter 32, Oral health, June 5, 2018. https://www.cdc.gov/nchs/healthy_people/hp2020/hp2020_midcourse_review.htm. Accessed 07.07.20.

8. Dental insurance coverage influences the types of services used; concerns exist about insurance companies and government agencies dictating the care provided based on guidelines for payment

E. Barriers to dental care utilization—factors that block or prevent access or ability to seek care or adopt healthy behaviors, thus reducing dental utilization; must be addressed to increase utilization within a population
1. Cost-related barriers—main barriers relate to affordability[77]
   a. Services not affordable
   b. Dental insurance benefits issues
      (1) Coverage limited or not available (see previous discussion on access); not wanting to spend money out of pocket
      (2) Continuing lack of providers available to individuals with Medicaid/CHIP coverage[77]
      (3) A narrow insurance company definition of "medically necessary dental care" that sets limits on oral health care services available to many insured patients
   c. Lost wage resulting from time away from work; more critical than the perceived need for services
2. Barriers not related to cost
   a. Lack of time
   b. Lack of perceived need
   c. Access to care difficult or impossible
   d. Availability of providers (e.g., office hours, distribution of personnel, distance to travel)
   e. Types of services needed not being available because of practitioners' lack of skill or interest
   f. Geographic isolation
   g. Nonambulatory status (e.g., homebound or institutionalized)
   h. Lack of public transportation
   i. Values, attitudes, and beliefs
   j. Low health literacy
   k. Unfavorable view of dental personnel—lack of cultural sensitivity
3. The *safety net* provides access by overcoming some of these barriers—consists of institutions and programs that provide dental care and services for low-income, medically underserved, immigrant, racial/ethnic, rural, and other populations that otherwise have limited or no access to dental care; examples are hospital emergency rooms, dental and dental hygiene educational program clinics, and community clinics funded by federal or foundation grants
4. Social and psychological barriers
   a. Low value placed on dental care and facial appearance related to the oral cavity
   b. Unpleasant prior experience resulting in anxiety
   c. Emotional factors such as fear of dental care
5. Cultural barriers
   a. Language—patient unable to find a provider who speaks his or her language or a qualified interpreter
   b. History and tradition—no importance given to dental care in the client's culture
   c. Basic cultural beliefs about general and oral health, illness, disease, and health care model
   d. Failure to understand that a missed appointment can be costly and disruptive
   e. Difficulty in understanding the recommendations for dental care or dietary changes
   f. Inadequate number of oral health care providers from minority groups

## Shifts in Dental Care Utilization Patterns

A. Reported increase in examinations, preventive services, extractions, implants, and esthetic dentistry and slight decline in dentures
1. Resulting partially from the changing demographics of the population; persons over age 65 are the fastest-growing segment of the US population and have higher tooth retention rates, resulting in their increased utilization of dental services; dentate individuals are more likely than edentulous individuals to visit the dentist
2. Each generation demands a different variety of services; older populations focus on restoration, periodontal treatment, prosthetics, and control and treatment of root caries; middle-age persons need some restorative and periodontal services or orthodontic services; children need more primary prevention and orthodontic services

B. Prevention
1. General interest in prevention has caused an increase in preventive dentistry services

2. The success of preventive interventions affects the types of future services required

C. The American society's interest in appearance and esthetics influences demand for restorative options, cosmetic dentistry, orthodontics, periodontal services, and dental implants

D. Increases in Medicaid/CHIP coverage for children and adults have impacted the shift of services

E. Continued increased utilization is expected as a result of the ACA

F. Increase in utilization and reduction of disparities in oral health care services require a multipronged approach
   1. This includes oral health literacy of the population, improved access to care for underserved populations, increased demand for preventive oral health care, and reduction of barriers to oral health care
   2. Various interventions are needed that address all the core functions of public health, assessment, policy development, and assurance, using evidence-based approaches to health education, health promotion, and provision of services

## ORAL HEALTH CARE CHALLENGES AFFECTING COMMUNITY ORAL HEALTH PRACTICE

A. Continuing significant burden of oral diseases and disorders in the US population in the 21st century
   1. Striking disparities in dental diseases and conditions, depending on income levels; unprecedented changes in demography and patterns of diseases and disorders
   2. Effect of unintentional injuries on craniofacial tissues
   3. Increases in systemic conditions that are associated with oral diseases and that compromise oral health
   4. Prevalence of tobacco-related oral diseases beginning in adolescence
   5. Increased prevalence of oral cancer among young adults associated with more common sexual practices in adolescents and young adults
   6. Significant caries prevalence and rates of untreated caries in all age groups
   7. Significant loss of school and work hours each year because of dental-related illnesses
   8. Progressive and cumulative nature of oral diseases that become more complex over time

B. Trends in oral health care delivery
   1. Continuing trend of low dental attendance, although utilization increases each year
   2. Emphasis on increasing access to care for underserved population to decrease oral health disparities
   3. Greater awareness of the need to provide dental benefits for older adults
   4. Changes in health care financing, including greater involvement of public financing
   5. Increase in the cost of oral healthcare
   6. Lower utilization of dental services by those on public insurance compared to private insurance
   7. Potential for increased utilization because of the aging population, combined with changes in oral disease patterns and a decline in total tooth loss in older adults
   8. Continuing low rates of detecting oral cancer at early stages, low numbers of oral cancer screening completed in dental offices, and low rates of tobacco-cessation counseling in the dental office
   9. Broadening treatment options due to an emphasis on esthetics, adult orthodontics, and dental implants
   10. Changes in science, technology, and therapeutics; availability of new biomaterials and biotechnology
   11. Access to multiple information systems, including the Internet, computer-assisted technology, telehealth care, and distance education technology
   12. Access to genetic information that will influence assessment of risk factors and care planning
   13. A philosophy of "best practices," that is, determining which treatment will work for which patients and under what circumstances; an evidence-based approach to dental and dental hygiene care based on risk assessment
   14. Paradigm shift to a treatment model that focuses on nonsurgical, noninvasive, biologic, and pharmacologic interventions that are guided by genetics and risk assessment, requiring a shift in oral health care education, teaching, and outcome methodologies and a greater focus on lifelong learning for oral health care personnel
   15. Greater emphasis on the use of validated health education, health promotion, and organizational theories for individual and community-based oral health education and promotion
   16. Coordination and collaboration of dental care and medical care (IPP and IPE)
   17. Greater orientation of the current society in general on oral disease prevention
   18. An increase in the complexity of the oral health care delivery system because of the numerous, multifaceted arrangements for delivering services and financing care, the changes in supply and distribution of provider personnel, and the varying state laws regarding scope of practice and supervision for dental assistants, dental hygienists, and midlevel dental personnel

C. Redirected focus of dental personnel
   1. Identify individuals currently not seeking care; for example, special population groups and low-income and minority individuals
   2. Increase access to and availability of care; for example, vary office hours, offer care in nontraditional settings, improve payment and financing mechanisms, continue to explore the use of midlevel practitioners, and support low-income patients in identifying resources for oral health care
   3. Increase awareness of available dental services among those who do not seek dental care
   4. Develop creative solutions to meet increasing demands for dental care personnel during a period of natural

retirement of an older dental profession, continuing shortage of dentists, increasing numbers and increased educational levels of dental hygienists, and emergence of midlevel oral health care practitioners

5. Educate the public with an evidence-based focus on periodontal disease, dental caries, oral cancer, tobacco cessation, systemic health–oral health connection, and preventive interventions
6. Implement health promotion strategies designed to change oral health behaviors that have the potential to improve oral health
7. Encourage professional lifelong learning to address current scientific understanding of oral diseases, the changing oral health care needs of the population, cultural competence and sensitivity, and technologies to assess and treat populations
8. Develop an understanding within the oral health professions about the demographic and ethnic changes in the population; cultivate cultural sensitivity and competence, and apply strategies to improve health literacy
9. Recognize dentistry's changing role, with an emphasis on diagnostic skills and evaluation
10. Accept dental hygienists' changing role as more autonomous, interdependent practitioners and as collaborators with other members of the oral health care team as well as interdisciplinary health care teams (IPP)
11. Employ appropriate oral health care personnel; recognize the capabilities of all team members to increase access to care, and be aware that the current litigious society demands skilled practitioners and high-quality services
12. Make changes in oral health care delivery and oral health promotion that address the current status of oral health and recommendations made by relevant national agency reports (e.g., increase OPC screening and tobacco-cessation counseling in the dental office, focus on dental caries prevention and control, implement school-based tobacco education programs)
13. Incorporate scientific evidence into all aspects of oral health care practice
14. Strengthen the infrastructure of the oral health care delivery system of the nation
15. Use innovative collaborations and partnerships to promote oral health and solve oral health problems
16. Focus on local community needs
17. Develop multiple skills to function in many roles, with multidisciplinary approaches, and in diverse care delivery environments

D. Recommendations to reduce disparities in oral health and oral health care
   1. Through research, identify biomarkers that will facilitate early detection and diagnosis of disease
   2. Conduct epidemiologic studies of populations to establish baselines for the incidence and prevalence of specific oral health problems and to assist in tracking, reducing, or eliminating identified health disparities
   3. Conduct RCTs to provide an evidence base for the effective prevention and management of health disparities
   4. Carry out population-based research to understand the basis of health disparities
   5. Place a high priority on efforts to reduce widespread disparities in oral health status and access to care
   6. Increase measures to ensure oral health and access to care for children by correcting inadequate government policies, such as increasing Medicaid funding, increasing the number of Medicaid and CHIP dentist providers, implementing school sealant and F varnish programs, fluoridating water supplies, and protecting the current status of fluoridated water supplies
   7. Emphasize research and community oral health promotion programs that will result in decreasing incidence and prevalence rates of oral diseases and conditions for the entire population, as well as special emphasis on populations at high risk for these conditions
   8. Restructure oral health care professional education programs to meet the critical requirement of preparing a workforce that is qualified in public health principles and practice
   9. Incorporate a focus on serving all Americans, regardless of SES, gender, and ethnic or racial group representation, into the recruitment of students and faculty, design and implementation of curricula, conduct of research, provision of services, and participation in community outreach

## ETHICAL AND LEGAL ISSUES

See Box 20.14.

## BOX 20.14 Ethical/Legal Issues Related to Community Oral Health*

### General Ethical Issues

- Application to community as the "patient"
- Weighing the needs of the individual and the community
- Application of principles of social justice, common good, human dignity, confidentiality, informed consent, nonmaleficence, beneficence, integrity and totality, competence and capacity, autonomy, and surrogacy to community oral health practice
- Encompassing professionalism, personal and professional ethics, and the role of the profession and the educational system in the context of the greater society

### Ethical Practices in Action

- Focus by educational institutions to develop skilled, ethically and socially sensitive graduates committed to their professional obligation to community education and service
- Development and implementation of community-based models of education and service that may include alumni participation, local professional society participation, or both
- Commitment of educational institutions to incorporate community outreach activities as part of the professional curriculum; emphasis on a multidisciplinary approach with other health care students and providers (IPE)
- Reinforcement of a lifelong commitment to the professional codes of ethics (ADHA, ADA) that suggest an ethical obligation to community oral health and well-being
- Development of strategies to develop cultural and linguistic competence through lifelong learning
- Expansion of minority representation in the profession
- Education of students about the career opportunities in federal, state, and local public health agencies and in other community organizations that provide oral health care services to various population groups (e.g., IHS, VA, local hospitals)
- Developing mechanisms that encourage and support a perspective of social responsibility
- Identification and development of mechanisms, such as scholarships and payback programs, to encourage minority and other health care providers to serve underserved populations
- Increasing knowledge and awareness of community oral health issues, best practices, skills, and resources by obtaining information from journals, conferences, seminars, websites, and other means
- Promotion of evidence-based decision-making in relation to all aspects of community oral health practice, including scientific bases for disease control and prevention, as well as application of tested theories of organization, health promotion, and health education
- Setting standards of ethical conduct that reflects social responsibility to the community through oral health promotion, education, and practice
- Focusing of individual practitioners on social responsibility in their dental hygiene practice
- Serving on advisory boards to community oral health programs
- Volunteering in community service activities sponsored by local professional societies, educational institutions, and community organizations
- Participating in, encouraging the development of, and organizing community outreach events through private offices of employment
- Commitment to lifelong learning and evidence-based practice in relation to community oral health practice as well as clinical practice
- Providing leadership in the solution of local public health problems to improve the oral health of the local community

### Legal Issues

- Effect of varying state laws related to scope of practice and supervision on the ability of various personnel to participate fully in community programs
- Emergence of midlevel practitioner-models of practice in some states; resulting differences among states in the ability to address access-to-care issues within the state and on a national level

* Refer to Chapter 22 for discussion of ethical principles.

## WEBSITE INFORMATION AND RESOURCES

| Source | Website Address | Description |
|---|---|---|
| American Dental Hygienists' Association | http://adha.org | Data on the profession; information about careers in public health, midlevel providers, professional changes that relate to access to care, and advocacy |
| Association of State and Territorial Dental Directors | http://www.astdd.org | Access to state and territorial public health agencies of the United States, US territories, and the District of Columbia; engaged in legislative, scientific, educational, and programmatic issues and activities on behalf of public health; provides best practices for current, effective community oral health programming |
| Centers for Disease Prevention and Control | https://www.cdc.gov/ | Variety of resources for information, data, and statistics on oral health topics useful for community programming; includes links to *Oral Health in America: A Report of the Surgeon General,* current Healthy People website (history and development, objectives, baseline measures, target outcomes, suggestions for interventions and resources, and methods to measure outcomes), and various other resources |
| Community Toolbox | https://ctb.ku.edu/en | Consists of 46 chapters that provide practical, step-by-step guidance in skills for assessing, planning, taking action, evaluating, and sustaining community oral health programming efforts. |
| National Maternal and Child Oral Health Resource Center | http://www.mchoral-health.org/ | A variety of resources to develop community oral health programs for young children, including publications, "how-to" guides, toolboxes, Head Start information, and grants |

## CHAPTER 20 REVIEW QUESTIONS

Answers and rationales to review questions are available on this text's accompanying Evolve site. See inside front cover for details.

### CASE A

You have been employed as a public health dental hygienist in a local health department to provide educational presentations for the participants in the Women, Infants, and Children (WIC) program in a nonfluoridated community. One of your first assignments is to present an educational program on basic oral health practices for culturally diverse pregnant teens in an alternative high school and a fluoride varnish program for their children who are cared for during the school day at a school-based day care facility. General consent forms are on file at the school for the children to participate in special activities. The ethnic group representation of this population is 15% Hispanic American, 5% African American, 75% non-Hispanic white, and 5% Asian American. The first session with the teen mothers is an informational session about the program to explain how it can benefit them and their children. The success of the fluoride varnish program is evaluated by tracking the number of children who receive fluoride varnish the recommended number of times during the school year. An outbreak of the flu prevented attendance of the mothers and their children for a period of time, which had a significant effect on this outcome. The state allows unsupervised collaborative practice by the dental hygienist.

***Use Case A to answer questions 1 to 5.***

1. Which of the following is a required action for the program targeted to the children?
   - **a.** Dental examination by the dentist prior to applying fluoride varnish
   - **b.** Phone call to each mother to describe the program
   - **c.** Presence of a dentist while the children receive treatment by the dental hygienist
   - **d.** Written informed consent form signed by the mother of each participating child
2. Which of the following terms BEST communicates the situation described in relation to the flu?
   - **a.** Endemic
   - **b.** Epidemic
   - **c.** Occurrence
   - **d.** Pandemic
3. The same educational materials used in this school could be used also with teen mothers in additional alternative high schools in other geographic locations of the city. The cultural diversity of the population of this program represents the cultural diversity of the general US population.
   - **a.** Both statements are TRUE
   - **b.** Both statements are FALSE
   - **c.** The first statement is TRUE; the second statement is FALSE
   - **d.** The first statement is FALSE; the second statement is TRUE
4. Which index would be the MOST appropriate one to use to determine the rate of pregnancy gingivitis in this population?
   - **a.** CPI
   - **b.** CPITN
   - **c.** GI
   - **d.** PDI
   - **e.** PSR
5. Which of the following would be MOST appropriate to explain during the informational session?
   - **a.** Benefits of community water fluoridation
   - **b.** Effective oral hygiene procedures for the mothers and their children
   - **c.** Introduction to early childhood caries
   - **d.** Making healthy food choices

### CASE B

The Activities Director of the Vintage Apartments, which provide federally-subsidized housing for older adults, contacts the local dental hygiene society to provide a seminar on oral health and conduct oral cancer screenings for the purpose of improving the oral health of the residents. The facility has a population of 150 well residents between ages 65 and 89. All of them possess mobility, and about half of them drive and have a car. In addition, a local nonprofit organization provides transportation for older adults in the community. Two public health hygienists complete an assessment of the population. The findings include the following: only 10% have dental insurance, mean OHI-S of 2.3, mean GI of 1.5, mean SBI of 3.5, mean DMFT of 8.2 with a mean D of 3.0, mean RCI of 21.3% (5.1/24) with a mean of 3.5 unfilled or untreated carious root surfaces, and over 50% report signs and symptoms of xerostomia. In addition, an oral cancer screening is accomplished with a tongue blade and available light. Data analysis reveals a correlation coefficient of $r = -0.62$ for the relationship between untreated dental caries and dental insurance coverage. About 70% of the residents report failure to visit the dentist as frequently as they desire because of financial barriers, and 40% have no dental home. The Society has a budget for community oral health that can be used to support the program.

***Use Case B to answer questions 6 to 11.***

6. What assessment classification is used to screen this population for oral cancer?
   - **a.** Type I
   - **b.** Type II
   - **c.** Type III
   - **d.** Type IV
7. The correlation between untreated dental caries and dental insurance coverage demonstrates a moderate negative relationship. The interpretation of this result is that the lack of dental insurance causes the lack of treatment.
   - **a.** Both statements are TRUE
   - **b.** Both statements are FALSE
   - **c.** The first statement is TRUE; the second statement is FALSE
   - **d.** The first statement is FALSE; the second statement is TRUE
8. According to the results of the assessment, how many teeth are affected by root caries experience?
   - **a.** 3.5
   - **b.** 5.1
   - **c.** 6.5
   - **d.** 8.6

9. All of the following are indicated by the assessment results EXCEPT one. Which one is the EXCEPTION?
   a. Assistance in identifying local safety net clinics
   b. Daily use of a high-concentration fluoride dentifrice
   c. Educational presentation on basic oral hygiene
   d. Dental health fair held at the apartments
   e. Referral for restorative treatment
10. What is the BEST measure of the success of this program?
   a. Improved oral health indicators of the residents
   b. Improved oral hygiene of the residents
   c. Increased availability of oral hygiene supplies for use by the residents
   d. Increased health literacy of the residents
   e. Support of apartment management for the program
11. What is the average level of oral hygiene demonstrated by this population?
   a. Excellent
   b. Good
   c. Fair
   d. Poor

## CASE C

The human resources director of an urban county hospital is alarmed by the rising cost of employee health insurance premiums related to tobacco-associated health conditions. The administrator charges the occupational health director, a dental hygienist, with addressing the issue of employee tobacco consumption. The dental hygienist conducts an employee tobacco usage survey as part of the program planning process. Analysis of the survey reveals mean cigarette usage per day of 4.6 for administrators, 19.6 for clerical support staff, 10.6 for nurses, 6.2 for physicians, and 19.8 for allied health technicians. Standard deviation is 2.2 cigarettes for all groups. Cigarette packs are known to contain 20 cigarettes. Data analysis results in a $p$ value of 0.15 for the difference in cigarette usage by the clerical support staff and the allied health technicians, and $p$ values ranging from 0.01 to 0.04 when comparing the usage by these two groups to the usage by all other groups.

*Use Case C to answer questions 12 to 16.*

12. What is the first step that should be accomplished to conduct this program?
   a. Develop a lesson plan for an educational session on the effects of tobacco
   b. Meet with the people involved to discuss program goals and objectives
   c. Research available resources for planning a tobacco cessation program
   d. Select teaching strategies for an educational program
   e. Write a grant to support the program
13. Which group should be targeted FIRST with an intervention?
   a. Allied health technicians
   b. Allied health technicians and clerical staff
   c. Hospital administrators
   d. Hospital patients
   e. All the staff groups are equally important and should be targeted at the same time
14. Which of the following is the BEST instructional objective for this initiative?
   a. After completing the educational program, participants will understand the harmful effects of tobacco and how they contribute to oral and systemic diseases and conditions.
   b. Ninety percent of the staff will voluntarily participate in the program during the first month of availability.
   c. On completion of the educational program, staff members will be able to correctly identify 80% of the harmful ingredients in tobacco.
   d. Participants will be able to list recommended methods to control cravings that can lead to failure.
15. Which step of the community health program planning process is represented by this survey?
   a. Develop a measurable process and outcome objectives to assess progress in addressing the health issue
   b. Evaluate selected interventions based on objectives; use information to improve the program
   c. Identify primary health issues
   d. Implement selected health interventions
   e. Select and plan effective health interventions to help achieve objectives
16. The data reported from the survey represent ratio data. A pie chart is the most appropriate graphic representation of these results.
   a. Both statements are TRUE
   b. Both statements are FALSE
   c. The first statement is TRUE; the second statement is FALSE
   d. The first statement is FALSE; the second statement is TRUE

## CASE D

The director of a local nursing home has contracted with a public health dental hygienist to design an oral health protocol for the 300 residents. Currently, a registered nurse performs the intake oral examination. The majority of the residents require assistance with daily hygiene practices. The caregivers report that the residents have severe halitosis, trouble eating, and frequently lose their removable partial dentures. The dental hygienist observes that the caregivers are neglecting daily oral hygiene care and are not conducting oral cancer screenings routinely. Thus, the dental hygienist determines to carry out oral hygiene and oral cancer screening of all residents and introduce an educational component for the facility's caregivers and interested family members. Students from the local dental hygiene educational program are recruited to assist with the educational program. The caregivers' knowledge is measured prior to and a week following the educational program with a multiple choice test; these measures are compared to evaluate change in knowledge. The caregivers' ability to conduct oral cancer screening is evaluated weekly for several weeks after the educational program. One measure of the success of the program will be to screen the residents again one year later to discover any lesions that have not been identified during the year. If the data reveal any such lesions, the dental hygienist plans to work with the director of nursing to establish a new protocol for routine oral cancer screening by the registered nurses on staff.

*Use Case D to answer questions 17 to 22.*

17. Which of the following is an effective teaching strategy to raise the caregivers' compliance in this situation?

a. Demonstrate to them the proper oral hygiene procedures
b. Provide a lecture presentation on the importance of oral hygiene
c. Show them pictures of good oral health versus oral disease
d. Provide training on how to maintain their own personal oral hygiene

18. Which statistic is BEST to determine the statistical significance of the change in knowledge?
    a. Analysis of variance (ANOVA)
    b. Chi-square
    c. Correlation coefficient
    d. The *t* test
19. What type of data is being collected by the screening?
    a. Qualitative and primary
    b. Qualitative and secondary
    c. Quantitative and primary
    d. Quantitative and secondary
20. What is the BEST method for evaluating the caregivers' ability to conduct oral cancer screening in this program?
    a. Administer a weekly written test over the cancer screening procedure
    b. Interview the residents about the caregivers' technique
    c. Observe the caregivers conducting oral cancer screening
    d. Survey the family members about the caregivers' technique
21. Which term BEST describes the extent of oral cancer lesions found at the 1-year evaluation?
    a. Count
    b. Incidence
    c. Prevalence
    d. Proportion
    e. Rate
22. Which core public health function is exemplified by the potential solution if the outcomes of the training in oral cancer screening are not successful?
    a. Assessment
    b. Assurance
    c. Policy development
    d. Prevention

## CASE E

A high dental caries rate has been reported by the school nurses in Head Start children in the county on the basis of the rate of toothaches and absences. The families are primarily Hispanic and East Indian migrant farmworkers. They reside in predominantly rural settings with individual well-water supplies. Most of the children are enrolled in Medicaid, but the closest providers are at a dental clinic that is part of a federally qualified health center a 1-hour drive away. At an informational meeting, the Head Start dental health coordinator introduces the goal of the program to the Head Start family advocates. A team of dental hygiene students from the local college is asked to design a comprehensive program to address the problem of dental caries in this population. They begin by collecting baseline data using the deft, OHI-S, and GI on a sample of the children. They randomly select the first child from each class list and then select every fourth child from the lists to produce a 25% sample. The results included a high level of S-ECC and a DI-S score of 1.8.

*Use Case E to answer questions 23 to 28.*

23. Which of the following agencies would be the BEST resource for program planning for this population?
    a. Centers for Medicare and Medicaid
    b. Health Resources and Services Administration
    c. National Maternal and Child Oral Health Resource Center
    d. Public Health Service
24. Which of the following is indicated by the second component of the caries index used for the assessment?
    a. Decayed surface
    b. Decayed tooth
    c. Tooth that has been extracted because of decay
    d. Tooth that has naturally exfoliated
    e. Tooth that needs to be extracted because of the severity of decay
25. What is the MOST important cultural factor to consider when planning an intervention for this population?
    a. Age
    b. Educational level
    c. Ethnic background
    d. Health literacy
26. All of the following preventive programs are indicated for this priority population EXCEPT one. Which one is the EXCEPTION?
    a. At-school brushing program
    b. School-based fluoride varnish program
    c. School-based oral health education
    d. School-based sealant programs
    e. Water fluoridation
27. All of the following would be appropriate sources of funding to meet the oral health needs of this community EXCEPT one. Which one is the EXCEPTION?
    a. Head Start grant
    b. Health Resources and Services Administration grant
    c. Medicare
    d. Medicaid
    e. Private funding from a state foundation
28. What sampling technique is used for the assessment?
    a. Convenience sampling
    b. Judgmental or purposive sampling
    c. Random sampling
    d. Stratified random sampling
    e. Systematic sampling

## CASE F

Dental hygiene students from a local program visit a geriatric day care called Camp Sunshine to implement a service learning project. These older adults are functionally independent, although they are medically compromised. Under faculty supervision, the students screen the participants to measure denture cleanliness and teach them how to clean their dentures daily. The goals are to improve their oral health by cleaning their dentures or partial dentures, increase their awareness of the need for daily oral care, and empower them to clean their dentures. The students compute the mean scores of the denture cleanliness measure for future evaluation of the program outcomes. The educational program consists of three weekly visits to teach and provide practice in various aspects of denture care. During the

## CASE F—CONT'D

first weekly lesson, the students use motivational interviewing to identify the clients' current practices, beliefs, attitudes, and intentions regarding daily denture cleaning. The students use this information to plan individualized instruction for each client. The students return 3 months after completing the denture cleaning instruction to measure denture cleanliness to evaluate the success of the program. At the end of the program, the students prepare a final report for the facility director in which they communicate the successful outcomes of the program and propose funding of supplies by Camp Sunshine to continue the program in the future.

***Use Case F to answer questions 29 to 33.***

29. Which role of the dental hygienist is illustrated by this activity?
    a. Advocate
    b. Clinician
    c. Educator
    d. Educator and clinician
    e. Researcher
30. Which of the following is an ethical responsibility of the students and faculty who are implementing this program?
    a. Communicate oral findings to the staff of the facility
    b. Prepare a formal report of findings to submit to the health department
    c. Prepare a manuscript describing the program for publication in the college newsletter
    d. Refer participants who have suspicious lesions identified during the program
    e. Take the denture back to the dental hygiene clinic to clean them more thoroughly
31. Which health education theory is MOST reflected by the strategies used in the education program?
    a. Health belief model
    b. Locus of control
    c. Social cognitive theory
    d. Theory of reasoned action
32. What is the BEST way for the student to provide the final report?
    a. Discuss the results at a meeting with the facility director in which they propose future funding for the program
    b. Include a few paragraphs in a written report that describe the statistical analysis of the pretest and posttest denture cleanliness data
    c. Include in a written report a list of the participants with their baseline and posttest denture cleanliness scores
    d. Include tables and graphs in a written report to summarize the pretest and posttest denture cleanliness data
33. What type of study is represented by the 3-month evaluation of denture cleanliness?
    a. Case-control
    b. Correlational
    c. Crossover
    d. Pretest/posttest
    e. Time-series

## CASE G

A committee was formed to plan and operate a comprehensive school-based oral disease prevention program targeted to an inner-city public elementary school. The local dental hygiene society serves on this committee along with a faith-based organization involved in health care for this population, members of the school administration and the parent-teacher organization, and other stakeholders. The school serves a low-income population, and 75% of the children qualify to participate in the school lunch program. The community water supply is not fluoridated; the natural fluoride content is 0.3 mg fluoride per liter of water. A public health hygienist screens the children in preschool through grade 5 annually. Data for 2019 indicate a 22% urgent decay rate across all ages. Further assessment reveals that many of the children do not see a dentist following the referral from the screening. Fluoride varnish is applied in conjunction with sealant application in 3- and 4-year-olds and in grades 2 and 5. In addition, fluoride varnish application is scheduled to assure that all children in all grades have access to four applications annually. Oral health education is conducted for all grades. Finally, the team has explored the option of conducting a campaign to achieve water fluoridation in the community.

***Use Case G to answer questions 34 to 39.***

34. What is the primary factor in the community profile that is the basis for targeting this school with this comprehensive program?
    a. Cultural diversity of the population
    b. Fluoridation status of the community
    c. Inner-city location of the school
    d. Low dental attendance
    e. Percent of children on the school lunch program
35. What method of measuring caries is being used to identify the decay rate each year?
    a. Basic Screening Survey (BSS)
    b. Deft
    c. DMFT
    d. RCI
36. How much additional fluoride (F) is required to bring the F concentration of the community water supply to the optimal level?
    a. 0.4 mg F per liter of water
    b. 0.7 mg F per liter of water
    c. 0.4 to 0.9 mg per liter of water
    d. 1 mg F per liter of water
37. Which of the following should be done FIRST in relation to pursuing a fluoridation campaign?
    a. Contact key community leaders to obtain a broad base of support for fluoridation
    b. Organize a massive community education program about the benefits and safety of fluoridation
    c. Schedule a referendum to allow the citizens to express their opinion about fluoridation
    d. Testify before the city council to convince them to fluoridate the water supply
38. Which theory of health promotion is exemplified by this program?
    a. Community organization
    b. Diffusion of innovation
    c. Organizational change
    d. Sense of coherence

39. Which of the following programs would be appropriate to add?
   a. School-based fluoridated milk program
   b. School-based fluoride rinse program
   c. School-based fluoride tablet program
   d. School water fluoridation

## CASE H

A dental hygiene Public Health Service–commissioned core officer is assigned to an Indian Health Service (IHS) clinic to improve the oral care of pregnant women in an American Indian rural community with a population of 26,000. Approximately 30% of the pregnant women in this population develop gestational diabetes. An interprofessional collaborative practice approach is used in the clinic. When a woman first sees the physician in the clinic for prenatal care, she meets with a dental therapist for oral health education, including personal oral hygiene care. She is also referred to the dental clinic for a dental examination and dental hygiene treatment. Only 25% of the patients referred during the previous 6 months complied with the dental referral, scheduled an appointment, and received treatment. The community is not classified a "dental manpower shortage area" because of the staffing of this clinic and the existence of this program. A survey of the pregnant women served by this clinic reveals that the women do not realize their risk for diabetes, are unaware of the relationship between oral health status and diabetes, and do not understand the benefits of oral health care in relation to their overall health and the health of their babies. For the purpose of discussing the problem and possible solutions, the dental hygienist arranges a meeting of the medical clinic director, the dental clinic director, the medicine man of the Indian tribe, and a dental clinic staff member who is a member of the tribe. This team sets a goal of doubling the rate of compliance with the dental referral to 35% within 6 months.

***Use Case H to answer questions 40 to 44.***

40. Which of the following is the BEST intervention to implement first?
   a. Develop written educational materials for distribution during prenatal visits
   b. Document the oral condition of the pregnant women who have complied and received a dental examination
   c. Implement an oral health screening during the prenatal care visits
   d. Mail cards to remind the referred pregnant women to schedule an appointment for a dental examination
   e. Plan an educational presentation for the pregnant women on the relationship of oral health, systemic health, and the risks and consequences of diabetes
41. Which health education theory is indicated as the foundation for an oral health education intervention to meet the goal of this program?
   a. Health belief model
   b. Learning ladder
   c. Transtheoretical model (stages of change theory)
   d. Wellness model
42. In this situation, lack of compliance with the dental referral is most likely the result of which of the following factors?
   a. Cost of dental care
   b. Lack of available appointments
   c. Low dentist-to-population ratio
   d. Low health literacy
43. The involvement of the dental therapist during the prenatal visit and the dental referral by the medical clinic exemplify which characteristic of public health?
   a. Application of biostatistics to analyze population health problems
   b. Community rather than the individual as the patient
   c. Multidisciplinary team approach to solving public health problems
   d. Social responsibility for oral health
44. What is the BEST teaching method for the psychomotor learning in this program?
   a. Demonstration
   b. Guided practice
   c. Motivational interviewing
   d. Video presentation

## CASE I

Dental hygiene students conduct a study to compare the effectiveness of two nonalcohol mouthrinses, a 0.02% NaF rinse (Listerine Total Care Zero Alcohol) and a 0.07% CPC rinse (Crest Pro Health), in controlling plaque biofilm and gingivitis. A sample of 136 healthy adult volunteers is taken from the university dental hygiene clinic. Only dentate adults with no to mild periodontitis are accepted to participate in the study. The study participants are qualified for inclusion in the study by their plaque biofilm forming potential and presence of mild gingivitis. Two groups are formed, and each participant receives the mouthrinse randomly assigned to him or her. Examiners are unaware of the formula used by each participant. Two examiners are calibrated in the use of the PI-I and GI to measure plaque biofilm and gingivitis at baseline, 2 months, and 4 months. During group assignment the groups are matched for baseline PI-I scores to ensure that the two groups have equivalent oral hygiene.

***Use Case I to answer questions 45 to 50.***

45. What type of study is this?
   a. Analytic
   b. Descriptive
   c. Experimental
   d. Quasi-experimental
46. What is the purpose of matching the groups for baseline oral hygiene scores?
   a. Control an extraneous variable
   b. Control reliability of the oral hygiene measurements
   c. Decrease the necessary length of the study
   d. Improve generalizability of the results of the study
47. The application of the PI-I in this study is an example of which step in the scientific method?
   a. Collection, organization, and analysis of data
   b. Formulation of a hypothesis
   c. Identification and statement of the problem
   d. Verification, rejection, or modification of the hypothesis
48. Which of the following is a statement of the research hypothesis for this study?
   a. Neither mouthrinse is effective in controlling plaque biofilm and gingivitis.
   b. Plaque biofilm and gingivitis are strongly associated.
   c. The 0.02% NaF mouthrinse and the 0.07% CPC mouthrinse differ in the ability to control plaque biofilm and gingivitis.

d. There is no difference between the ability of the 0.02% NaF mouthrinse and the 0.07% CPC mouthrinse to control plaque biofilm and gingivitis.
e. Which controls plaque biofilm and gingivitis better, the 0.02% NaF mouthrinse or the 0.07% CPC mouthrinse?

49. What study design is reflected by the methods of this research study?
a. Correlational
b. Double-blind
c. Posttest only
d. Split-mouth
e. Time-series

50. Which of the following is controlled by the procedure used by the examiners in preparation to measure the dependent variables?
a. Inter-examiner reliability
b. Intra-examiner reliability
c. Inter-examiner variability
d. Intra-examiner variability

## CASE J

The administrator of a community group home for intellectually disabled adults located in a suburban area has received multiple complaints from the attending caregivers regarding the residents' oral health. Limited manual dexterity abilities of the residents requires that they receive assistance with oral hygiene routines; yet complaints of severe resident halitosis and bleeding during normal oral hygiene routines have made the caregivers reluctant to provide assistance. The 16 residents are 25 to 52 years old. Frustrated by a lack of staff compliance, the group home administrator contacts the local county public health dental hygienist, knowing that the county health department has a grant for oral care for this population. After gathering basic demographic information, the dental hygienist makes a visit to the home to assess the problem. She screens the residents using the Pl-I and GI to determine the extent of the problem.

***Use Case J to answer questions 51 to 56.***

51. What is the BEST way for the dental hygienist to assess the caregivers' attitudes, opinions, and beliefs about the problem?
a. Conduct a focus group with the caregivers
b. Measure the plaque biofilm and gingivitis scores of residents over time
c. Observe the caregivers as they provide oral hygiene procedures for residents
d. Perform an oral health survey with the residents

52. Which characteristic of a public health problem is LEAST evident in the description of this problem?
a. Burden of disease
b. Group action required to solve the problem
c. Impact on health equity
d. Social impact

53. What necessary component of a community profile is not described for this population?
a. Age
b. Ethnicity
c. Gender
d. Source of program funding

54. Which of the following is the LEAST efficient use of the dental hygienist in this situation?
a. Conduct an oral health survey to determine the oral health status of the residents
b. Conduct a focus group with the staff to ascertain their perception of the problem
c. Meet with the group home administrator to determine her goals
d. Present an in-service training program for the staff of the group home
e. Provide regular oral hygiene care for the residents

55. Which dental index would be MOST appropriate to evaluate the improvement in oral hygiene resulting from strategies introduced in this program?
a. OHI-S
b. PHP
c. Pl-I
d. Turesky modification of the Quigley-Hein Plaque index
e. Any of the above would be acceptable

56. Which of the following resources would be best to review to help align a program for this group with current national health priorities?
a. Oral Health in America: A Report of the Surgeon General
b. Community Toolbox
c. Improving Access to Oral Health Care for Vulnerable and Underserved Populations
d. Healthy People 2030
e. American Association on Intellectual and Developmental Disabilities website

## REFERENCES


1. Department of Health and Human Services. *Centers for Disease Control and Prevention: National Center for Health Statistics. Healthy People 2020 Midcourse Review*; 2019. https://www.cdc.gov/nchs/healthy_people/hp2020/hp2020_midcourse_review.htm. Accessed July 07, 2019.
2. National Cancer Institute. *Surveillance, Epidemiology, and End Results (SEER) Program. Cancer Stat Facts: Oral Cavity and Pharynx Cancer*; 2016. http://seer.cancer.gov/statfacts/html/oralcav.html. Accessed July 11, 2019.
3. Centers for Disease Control and Prevention. *Data and Statistics on Birth Defects*; 2018. https://www.cdc.gov/ncbddd/birthdefects/data.html. Accessed 07.12.19.
4. World Health Organization. *Oral Health*; 2018. https://www.who.int/news-room/fact-sheets/detail/oral-health. Accessed June 23, 2019.
5. Agarwal SS, Chopra SS, Jayan B, Verma MM. Epidemiology in orthodontics—a literature review. *Orthod Cyber J*. 2013:11e. https://www.researchgate.net/publication/261708766_Epidemiology_in_Orthodontics_A_Literature_Review; 2013. Accessed July 12, 2019.
6. Young EJ, Macias CR, Stephens L. Common dental injury management in athletes. *Sports Health*. 2015;7(3):250–255. https://dx.doi.org/10.1177/1941738113486077. Accessed June 23, 2019.
7. American Academy of Pediatric Dentistry. Policy on prevention of sports-related orofacial injuries. *Oral Health Policies and Recommen-*

*dations (Reference Manual)*. 2018;40(6):86–91. http://www.aapd.org/media/Policies_Guidelines/P_Sports.pdf. Accessed June 23, 2019.
8. National Institute of Dental and Craniofacial Research. *Prevalence of TMJD and its Signs and Symptoms*; 2018. https://www.nidcr.nih.gov/research/data-statistics/facial-pain/prevalence. Accessed July 12, 2019.
9. National Institute of Dental and Craniofacial Research. TMJ (temporomandibular joint and muscle disorders). *http://www.nidcr.nih.gov/oralhealth/topics/tmj/*. Accessed June 23, 2019.
10. National Center for Health Statistics. Data Quality Evaluation of the Dental Fluorosis Clinical Assessment Data from the National Health and Nutrition Examination Survey, 1999–2004 and 2011–2016: Data Evaluation and Methods Research. *Vital and Health Statistics*; 2019. Series 2(183). https://www.cdc.gov/nchs/data/series/sr_02/sr02_183-508.pdf. Accessed June 23, 2019.
11. Department of Health and Human Services. Public health service recommendation for fluoride concentration in drinking water for prevention of dental caries. *Fed Regist*. May 1, 2015. https://www.federalregister.gov/documents/2015/05/01/2015-10201/public-health-service-recommendation-for-fluoride-concentration-in-drinking-water-for-prevention-of. Accessed June 23, 2019.
12. O'Connell J, Rockell J, Ouellet J, Tomar SL, Maas W. Costs and savings associated with community water fluoridation in the United States. *Health Aff*. December 2016;35(12). Oral Health & More. https://www.healthaffairs.org/doi/abs/10.1377/hlthaff.2016.0881. Accessed July 12, 2019.
13. Centers for Disease Control and Prevention. *Other Fluoride Products*; 2019. https://www.cdc.gov/fluoridation/basics/fluoride-products.html. Accessed June 23, 2019.
14. Illinois Department of Public Health. *Public Health Intervention: Use of Silver Diamine Fluoride for Arresting Dental Caries*; 2017. http://www.dph.illinois.gov/sites/default/files/publications/publicationsohpmsdf-guidance_0.pdf. Accessed June 23, 2019.
15. Campaign for Tobacco-Free Kids. *Tobacco Use Among Youth*; 2019. https://www.tobaccofreekids.org/assets/factsheets/0002.pdf. Accessed June 24, 2019.
16. Centers for Disease Control and Prevention. Youth and Tobacco Use. https://www.cdc.gov/tobacco/data_statistics/fact_sheets/youth_data/tobacco_use/index.htm. Accessed June 24, 2019.
17. Boechler A. The importance of oral cancer screening in the dental practice. *DPR*. September 18, 2015:2e. http://www.dentalproductsreport.com/dental/article/importance-oral-cancer-screening-dental-practice?page=0,1. Accessed July 12, 2019.
18. Gofin J, Gofin R, Stimpson JP. Community-oriented primary care (COPC) and the affordable care act: an opportunity to meet the demands of an evolving health care system. *J Prim Care Community Health*. 2015;6(2):128–133. https://journals.sagepub.com/doi/10.1177/2150131914555908. Accessed July 12, 2019.
19. Vujicic M. A new way to measure geographic access to dentists in North Carolina. *N C Med J*. 2017;78(6): 391–302. https://dx.doi.org/10.18043/ncm.78.6.391. Accessed June 29, 2919.
20. Valachovic RW. *Current Demographics and Future Trends of the Dentist Workforce: The Dental Workforce. Dentists, the U.S. Oral Health Workforce in the Coming Decade*. Institute of Medicine Workshop; 2009. https://www.ncbi.nlm.nih.gov/books/NBK219663/. Accessed July 12, 2019.
21. American Dental Association. Health Policy Institute. Workforce. https://www.ada.org/en/science-research/health-policy-institute/dental-statistics/workforce. Accessed July 11, 2019.
22. American Dental Education Association. Applicants, Enrollees and Graduates. https://www.adea.org/data/students/. Accessed July 11, 2019.
23. American Dental Education Association. Educational Institutions. https://www.adea.org/data/EdInstitutions/. Accessed July 05, 2019.
24. Finnery DS. Women: the changing face of dentistry. *J Calif Dent Assoc*. 2017;45(1):15–16. https://www.cda.org/Portals/0/journal/journal_012017.pdf. Accessed June 30, 2019.
25. Mertz EA, Wides C, Kottek A, Calvo JM, Gates PE. Underrepresented minority dentists: quantifying their numbers and characterizing the communities they serve. *Health Aff (Millwood)*. 2016;35(12):2190–2199. https://www.ncbi.nlm.nih.gov/pmc/articles/PMC5364808/. Accessed June 30, 2019.
26. American Dental Association, Health Policy Institute. *Racial and Ethnic Diversity Among Dentists in the U.S. (Infographic)*; 2016. https://www.ada.org/~/media/ADA/Science%20and%20Research/HPI/Files/HPIgraphic_1117_6.pdf?la=en. Accessed July 12, 2019.
27. American Dental Education Association. *State and Federal Loan Forgiveness Programs*; November 2018. file:///C:/Users/Admin/AppData/Local/Temp/2018%20ADEA%20Summary%20of%20Loan%20Forgiveness%20Programs-1.pdf. Accessed July 12, 2019.
28. Kaiser Family Foundation. Dental care health professional shortage areas (HPSAs). *September 30*, 2019. https://www.kff.org/other/state-indicator/dental-care-health-professional-shortage-areas-hpsas/?currentTimeframe=0&sortModel=%7B%22colId%22:%22Location%22,%22sort%22:%22asc%22%7D. Accessed September 11, 2020.
29. Health Resources and Services Administration. Shortage designation scoring criteria. https://bhw.hrsa.gov/shortage-designation/hpsa-process; May 2020. Accessed September 11, 2020.
30. Munson B. Vujicic M *Supply of full-time equivalent dentists in the U.S. expected to increase steadily (Research brief)*. American Dental Association, Health Policy Institute; July 2018. https://www.ada.org/~/media/ADA/Science%20and%20Research/HPI/Files/HPIBrief_0718_1.pdf?la=en. Accessed June 29, 2019.
31. Health Resources and Services Administration. *National and State-Level Projections of Dentists and Dental Hygienists in the U.S., 2012–2025*; 2015. https://bhw.hrsa.gov/sites/default/files/bhw/nchwa/projections/nationalstatelevelprojectionsdentists.pdf. Accessed July 01, 2019.
32. Bureau of Labor Statistics. *Occupational Employment and Wages*; May 2017. Dental hygienists https://www.bls.gov/oes/2017/may/oes292021.htm; 2018. Accessed June 30, 2019.
33. Bureau of Labor Statistics. *Occupational Outlook Handbook: Dental Hygienists: Job Outlook*; 2019. https://www.bls.gov/ooh/healthcare/dental-hygienists.htm. Accessed July 12, 2019.
34. American Dental Hygienists' Association. *Facts about the Dental hygiene Workforce in the United States*; 2019. https://www.adha.org/resources-docs/75118_Facts_About_the_Dental_Hygiene_Workforce.pdf. Accessed June 30, 2019.
35. American Dental Hygienists' Association. *Entry-level Dental hygiene Programs*; 2018. https://www.adha.org/resources-docs/71617_Entry_Level_Schools_By_States.pdf. Accessed 07.01.19.
36. American Dental Hygienists' Association. *Degree Completion Dental hygiene Programs*; 2017. https://www.adha.org/resources-docs/71618_Degree_Completion_Programspdf. Accessed July 01, 2019.

37. American Dental Hygienists' Association. *Master of Science in Dental hygiene (MSDH) and Master's/doctoral Degree in Related Disciplines*; 2019. https://www.adha.org/resources-docs/71619_MSDH_Programs.pdf. Accessed July 01, 2019.
38. *Data USA. Dental Hygienists*; 2017. https://datausa.io/profile/soc/292021. Accessed July 01, 2019.
39. Langelier M, Continelli T, Moore J, Baker B, Surdu S. Expanded scopes of practice for dental hygienists associated with improved oral health outcomes for adults. *Health Aff.* 2016;35(12). https://www.healthaffairs.org/doi/10.1377/hlthaff.2016.0807. Accessed July 2, 2019.
40. Oral Health Workforce Research Center. *Variation in Dental hygiene Scope of Practice by State*. University of Albany SUNY, School of Public Health; 2019. http://www.oralhealthworkforce.org/resources/variation-in-dental-hygiene-scope-of-practice-by-state/. Accessed July 02, 2019.
41. American Dental Hygienists' Association. *Local Anesthesia Administration by Dental Hygienists – State Chart*; 2018. https://www.adha.org/resources-docs/7514_Local_Anesthesia_Requirements_by_State.pdf. Accessed July 02, 2019.
42. American Dental Hygienists' Association. *Reimbursement*; 2019. https://www.adha.org/reimbursement. Accessed July 01, 2019.
43. American Dental Hygienists' Association. *Expanding Access to Care through Dental Therapy*; 2019. https://www.adha.org/resources-docs/Expanding_Access_to_Dental_Therapy.pdf. Accessed July 11, 2019.
44. American Dental Hygienists' Association. *Direct Access States*; 2019. https://www.adha.org/resources-docs/7513_Direct_Access_to_Care_from_DH.pdf. Accessed July 01, 2019.
45. PEW Charitable Trusts. *5 Dental Therapy FAQs*; 2019. https://www.pewtrusts.org/en/research-and-analysis/articles/2016/04/5-dental-therapy-faqs. Accessed July 11, 2019.
46. Minnesota Department of Health. *Dental Therapy Toolkit: A Resource for Potential Employers*; 2017. https://www.health.state.mn.us/facilities/ruralhealth/emerging/dt/docs/2017dttool.pdf. Accessed July 01, 2019.
47. Nash DA, Mathu-Muhu KR, Friedman JW. The dental therapist trend in the United States: a critique of current trends. *J Public Health Dent.* 2018;78:127–133. https://onlinelibrary.wiley.com/doi/full/10.1111/jphd.12252. Accessed July 1, 2019.
48. Friedman JW, Mathu-Muju KR. Dental therapists: improving access to oral health care for underserved children. *Am J Public Health.* 2014;10(6):1005–1009. https://www.ncbi.nlm.nih.gov/pmc/articles/PMC4062028/. Accessed July 1, 2019.
49. Wahowiak L. Dental health therapists bringing oral health care to US tribal communities: opening up access. *Nation's Health.* 2016;46(5):1–25. http://thenationshealth.aphapublications.org/content/46/5/1.2. Accessed July 1, 2019.
50. Interprofessional Education Collaborative. *Core Competencies for Interprofessional Collaborative Practice: 2016 Update*; 2016. https://www.unthsc.edu/interprofessional-education/wp-content/uploads/sites/33/Core-Competencies-for-Interprofessional-Collaborative-Practice.pdf. Accessed July 12, 2019.
51. Manski RJ, Hoffmann D, Rowthorn V. Increasing access to dental and medical care by allowing greater flexibility in scope of practice. *Am J Public Health.* 2015;105(9):1755–1762. https://www.ncbi.nlm.nih.gov/pmc/articles/PMC4539795/. Accessed July 10, 2019.
52. Health Affairs, Vujicic M. *Obamacare, Trumpcare, and Your Mouth*; 2017. https://www.healthaffairs.org/do/10.1377/hblog20170113.058329/full/. Accessed July 04, 2019.
53. American Dental Association Health Policy Institute. U.S. dental expenditures, 2017 update (Power Point). https://www.ada.org/~/media/ADA/Science%20and%20Research/HPI/Files/HPIBrief_1217_1.pdf?la=en; 2017. Accessed July 12, 2019.
54. Centers for Medicare & Medicaid Services. *Projected: NHE Projections 2019-2028: Table 8 Dental Service Expenditures*; 2020. https://www.cms.gov/research-statistics-data-and-systems/statistics-trends-and-reports/nationalhealthexpenddata/nationalhealthaccountsprojected.html. Accessed September 11, 2020.
55. American Dental Association. Types of Dental Plans. https://success.ada.org/en/dental-benefits/dental-plan-overview. Accessed July 02, 2019.
56. Berg JH. Managed care plans in dental practice: a commentary. *Decisions in Dentistry*. February 13, 2019. https://decisionsindentistry.com/article/managed-care-plans-in-dental-practice/. Accessed July 12, 2019.
57. Gregory V. Closed panel dental benefits (letter). *ADA News*. May 18, 2015. https://www.ada.org/en/publications/ada-news/viewpoint/letters-to-the-editor/2015/may/closed-panel-dental-benefits. Accessed July 11, 2019.
58. U.S. Census Bureau. *Income and Poverty in the United States: 2017*; 2019. https://www.census.gov/library/publications/2018/demo/p60-263.html. Accessed July 2, 2019.
59. Children's Defense Fund. *Child Poverty in America 2017: National Analysis*; 2018. https://www.childrensdefense.org/wp-content/uploads/2018/09/Child-Poverty-in-America-2017-National-Fact-Sheet.pdf. Accessed July 03, 2019.
60. Reusch C. *How the Affordable Care Act Moved Oral Health Forward (Blog), Teeth Matter, Children's Dental Health Project*; March 23, 2018. https://www.cdhp.org/blog/502-how-the-affordable-care-act-moved-oral-health-forward. Accessed July 4, 2019.
61. Gupta N, Yarbrough C, Vujicic M, Blatz A, Harrison B. *Medicaid Fee-For-Service Reimbursement Rates for Child and Adult Dental Care Services for All States, 2016 (Research Brief)*. American Dental Association, Health Policy Institute; April 2017. https://www.ada.org/~/media/ADA/Science%20and%20Research/HPI/Files/HPIBrief_0417_1.pdf?la=en. Accessed July 7, 2019.
62. American Dental Association. *Health Policy Institute*. Dental Benefits and Medicaid. https://www.ada.org/en/science-research/health-policy-institute/dental-statistics/dental-benefits-and-medicaid. Accessed July 11, 2019.
63. Medicaid.gov. Medicaid CHIP Enrollment Data. https://www.medicaid.gov/medicaid/program-information/medicaid-and-chip-enrollment-data/index.html. Accessed July 04, 2019.
64. Medicaid and CHIP Payment Access Commission. *Medicaid Enrollment Changes Following the ACA*; 2018. https://www.macpac.gov/subtopic/medicaid-enrollment-changes-following-the-aca/. Accessed July 04, 2019.
65. Chazin S, Glover A. *Examining Oral Health Care Utilization and Expenditures for Low-Income Adults (Databrief). Faces of Medicaid.* Center for Health Care Strategies, Inc.; November 2017. https://www.chcs.org/media/FOM-Oral-Health_111617.pdf. Accessed July 6, 2019.
66. Garvin J. ADA to Congress: prioritize oral health care in ACA reform. *ADA News. March.* 2017;8. https://www.ada.org/en/publications/ada-news/2017-archive/march/ada-to-congress-prioritize-oral-health-in-aca-reform. Accessed July 4, 2019.
67. Oh J, Graff R, Hayes D, Phipps K. *Revision to the National Oral Health Surveillance System (NOHSS) Indicators (Position Statement 15-CD-01)*. Council of State and Territorial Epidemiologists; 2015. https://cdn.ymaws.com/www.cste.org/resource/resmgr/2015PS/2015PSFinal/15-CD-01-ALL.pdf. Accessed September 11, 2020.
68. Manchir M. Survey: more pregnant women in U.S. visiting a dentist, *ADA News*. https://www.ada.org/en/publications/ada-news/2016-archive/may/survey-more-pregnant-women-in-us-visiting-a-dentist; May 16, 2016. Accessed July 6, 2019.

69. Centers for Disease Control and Prevention. National Center for Health Statistics. *Oral and Dental Health: Dental Visits: Health, United States 2018, Table 37*; 2019. https://www.cdc.gov/nchs/fastats/dental.htm. Accessed September 9, 2020.
70. American Dental Association. Survey: more Americans want to visit the dentist, *ADA News*. March 21, 2018. https://www.ada.org/en/publications/ada-news/2018-archive/march/survey-more-americans-want-to-visit-the-dentist. Accessed July 7, 2019.
71. National Association of Dental Plans. *Who Has Dental Benefits Today?*; 2019. https://www.nadp.org/Dental_Benefits_Basics/Dental_BB_1.aspx. Accessed July 10, 2019.
72. American Dental Association. *Dental Benefits Coverage in the U.S*; 2015. https://www.ada.org/~/media/ADA/Science%20and%20Research/HPI/Files/HPIgraphic_1117_3.pdf?la=en. Accessed July 10, 2019.
73. National Association of Dental Plans. *Dental Benefits Basics: Impact of PPACA on Dental Benefits*; 2019. https://www.nadp.org/Dental_Benefits_Basics/dental_bb_12. Accessed July 07, 2019.
74. Shane DM, Wehby G. The impact of the Affordable Care Act's dependent coverage mandate on use of dental treatments and preventive services. *Med Care*. 2017;55(9):841–847. https://www.ncbi.nlm.nih.gov/pmc/articles/PMC5568688/. Accessed July 9, 2019.
75. National Association of Dental Plans. *Dental Benefits Basics. Dental Benefits Choices for Children: One Size Does Not Fit All*; 2019. https://www.nadp.org/docs/default-source/gr-documents/dental-benefit-choices-for-children_5-5-15_v14-2.pdf?sfvrsn=2. Accessed July 10, 2019.
76. National Committee to Preserve Social Security & Medicare. *Expanding Medicare to Provide Dental, Hearing, and Vision Care*; 2019. https://www.ncpssm.org/documents/medicare-policy-papers/expanding-medicare-to-provide-dental-vision-and-hearing-care/. Accessed July 09, 2019.
77. Gupta N, Vujicic M. *Main Barriers to Getting Needed Dental All Relate to Affordability (Research Brief)*. American Dental Association, Health Policy Institute; April 2019. http://www.ada.org/~/media/ADA/Science%20and%20Research/HPI/Files/HPIBrief_0419_1.pdf. Accessed July 11, 2019.


## SUGGESTED READINGS


Beatty CF. *Community Oral Health Practice for the Dental Hygienist*. 5th ed. Maryland Heights, MO: Elsevier; 2021.

Department of Health and Human Services, Department of the Treasury, Department of Labor. *Reforming America's Healthcare System through Choice and Competition*; December 2018. https://www.hhs.gov/sites/default/files/Reforming-Americas-Healthcare-System-Through-Choice-and-Competition.pdf Accessed September 11, 2020.

Department of Health and Human Services: Office of Disease Prevention and Health Promotion. *Healthy People 2030*; 2020. https://health.gov/healthypeople. Accessed September 12, 2020.

Featherston JDB, Rechmann JP, Zellmer IH. Dental caries management by risk assessment. In: Bowen DM, Pieren JA. *Darby and Walsh Dental Hygiene Theory and Practice*. 8th ed. Maryland Heights, MO: Elsevier; 2020: 265–284.

Nathe CN. *Dental Public Health and Research*. 4th ed. Upper Saddle River, NJ: Pearson; 2017.

American Association for Community Dental Programs, National Maternal and Child Oral Health Resource Center. A Guide for Developing and Enhancing Community Oral Health Programs. http://www.aacdp.com/guide/. Accessed September 10, 2020.

21

# Medical Emergencies

*Leslie Koberna*

Dental hygienists must prevent and effectively manage medical emergencies that occur in the health care environment. The ability to recognize signs and symptoms of medical disorders, prevent further complications through appropriate interventions, and manage a medical emergency is essential.

## GENERAL CONSIDERATIONS[1–3]

A. Medical emergency occurs when a patient experiences an unforeseen, immediate, health-related difficulty that is potentially life threatening
B. A medical emergency requires prompt recognition and action by the dental team to maintain the patient's health and, at times, the patient's life
C. The dental hygienist's legal responsibilities are to:
   1. Provide timely, quality care according to current standards of practice
      a. Be prepared to manage medical emergencies and adverse events in a health care environment
      b. Understand they may be held liable if they lack knowledge and training in medical emergency management
      c. Keep current in medical emergency management, including basic life support (BLS)
   2. Maintain complete records of medical emergencies in the health care setting
      a. Thorough documentation must describe the onset and management of the emergency, the patient's vital signs, the nature of the treatment performed and the patient's response, the type and dose of drugs administered, and the time when treatment was provided
      b. Thorough and complete records of medical emergencies are an important component of continuous quality improvement and protection for the oral health care team in the event of legal action
      c. Obtain informed consent for dental care

## MEDICAL HISTORY[1–3]

A. Reviewing a patient's health history is the first step in preventing a medical emergency
B. A thorough health history, taken at the first appointment and updated at each subsequent appointment, reveals conditions that predispose a patient to medical complications
C. Information obtained from the health history is used to modify the patient's care plan and reduce the risk of a medical complication or emergency in the oral health care setting
D. It may indicate the necessity for the dentist or dental hygienist to consult with the patient's physician prior to beginning treatment
E. Vital signs are taken to provide information regarding the patient's health status
F. Careful appointment planning, stress reduction protocol, good patient rapport, and prescribed stress-reducing medication (identified through the medical history) may lessen the risk of a stress-induced medical emergency

## VITAL SIGNS[1–5,6]

### Basic Concepts

A. Vital signs refer to numerical values given to blood pressure, body temperature, pulse rate, and respiration rate
B. Vital signs and a health history are used to determine a patient's fitness to undergo oral health care procedures
C. Abnormal values and significant findings should be brought to the attention of the dentist, the patient, and the patient's physician
D. Vital sign values should be taken for each new patient, at each recall appointment, and more frequently for patients with hypertension and other cardiac diseases
E. Vital signs should be compared to the baseline readings and monitored during an emergency; vital signs should be taken every 5 minutes during emergencies
F. Vital signs should be recorded in the patient's chart

### Blood Pressure

A. Definitions
   1. Blood pressure (BP)—the force exerted by blood on the walls of the blood vessels during the contraction and relaxation of the heart; BP depends on the heart's contractile force, peripheral vascular resistance, and vascular volume
      a. BP may increase with age or in response to exercise, stress, certain medications, smoking, and illness
      b. BP is recorded as millimeters of mercury (mm Hg), with the systolic pressure over the diastolic pressure; systolic (mm Hg)/diastolic (mm Hg)

2. Systolic pressure—the force exerted during ventricular contraction (heartbeat); the highest pressure in the cardiac cycle; the first sound of the heartbeat heard through the stethoscope
3. Diastolic pressure—the resting pressure, which occurs during ventricular relaxation (heart rest); the lowest pressure of the cardiac cycle; the last distinct sound heard through the stethoscope
4. Pulse pressure— the difference between systolic and diastolic pressure
5. Korotkoff sounds—the beats heard through the stethoscope caused by blood passing through the varying degree of artery obstruction as pressure is released from the Sphygmomanometer
6. Hypertension—sustained, abnormally high BP
7. Hypotension—sustained, abnormally low BP

B. Blood pressure values
   1. Children—BP values vary based on age, height, and gender
   2. BP classifications and recommended management regimen for adults
      a. Normal - BP reading is < 120/80 mm Hg; BP should be checked every 2 years
      b. Elevated—systolic reading is 120-129 mm Hg and the diastolic reading is < 80 mm Hg; BP should be rechecked once a year and lifestyle changes should be encouraged
      c. Stage I hypertension—systolic reading is 130-139 mm Hg or diastolic reading is 80-89 mm Hg; patient should be referred to physician for evaluation; local anesthesia with epinephrine should be limited to .54mg epinephrine (3 carpules 1:100:000).
      d. Stage II hypertension—systolic reading is ≥ 140 mm Hg or diastolic reading ≥ 90 mm Hg; medical evaluation before dental treatment recommended; local anesthesia with epinephrine should be limited to .54 mg epinephrine (3 carpules 1:100,000)
      e. Hypertensive crisis - Systolic reading is > 180 mm Hg and/or diastolic reading > 120 mm Hg; transport to ER immediately even if patient is asymptomatic

C. Equipment for measuring blood pressure
   1. Sphygmomanometer—an inflatable cuff and pressure gauge used to measure BP
   2. Stethoscope—an instrument used to listen to the sounds of the blood as it passes through the brachial artery (Figs. 21.1 and 21.2)
      a. Cuff size affects BP reading:
         (1) Bladder too small-increases readings
         (2) Bladder too large-decreases readings
      b. Exception: obese patient- may need to use regular adult bladder with cuff placed below the antecubital fossa; this will result in a systolic reading only

## Body Temperature

A. Normal oral temperature for both adults and children ranges from 97.6°F to 99.6°F (36.1°C to 37.5°C); the rectal and tympanic temperature readings are 1°F higher and the axillary and forehead temperature readings are 1°F lower than the oral temperature reading

B. Values above 99.6°F indicate a fever

C. Values higher than 101°F may indicate an active disease process

D. Body temperature elevation may be caused by exercise, ingestion of hot food or drink, smoking, or a pathologic condition

E. Body temperature may be decreased because of starvation or shock

F. Body temperature varies during the day

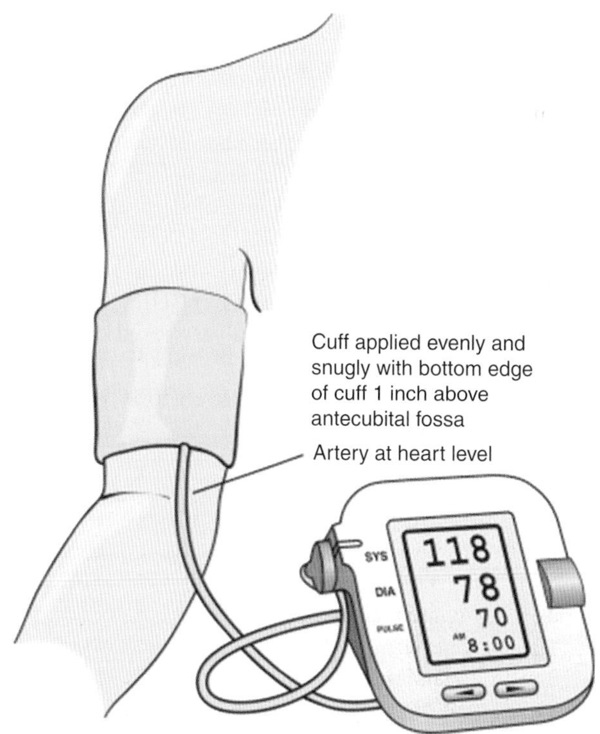


**Fig. 21.1** Proper placement of the blood pressure cuff. (Redrawn from Burch GE, DePasquale NP. *Primer of Clinical Measurement of Blood Pressure*. St. Louis: Mosby; 1962.)

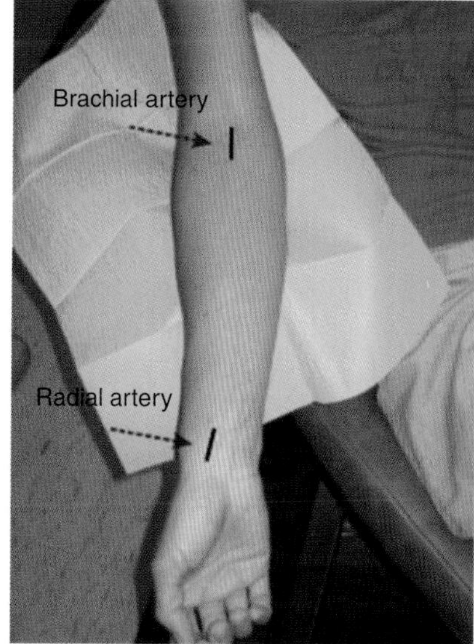


**Fig. 21.2** Location of the brachial and radial arteries. (From Malamed S. *Medical Emergencies in the Dental Office*. 7th ed. St Louis: Mosby Elsevier; 2015.)

1. Lower in the morning
2. Higher in the afternoon

G. Fever or pyrexia is an abnormal elevation in body temperature

## Pulse

A. Definition and basic concepts
   1. Pulse—the force of the blood through an artery created by contraction of the heart; each contraction creates a wave of blood that can be felt by gently pressing a superficial artery against underlying tissue
   2. Pulse is evaluated by rate (fast, slow), rhythm (regular, irregular), and quality (full or strong, thready or weak)
   3. Pulse rate is measured in heartbeats per minute (beats/min)
   4. Pulse rate may increase because of exercise, certain drugs, anxiety, heat, eating, or disease
   5. Pulse rate may decrease because of sleep, certain drugs, fasting, or disease
B. Heart rate
   1. Heart rates of infants and children ten and under are more rapid than adult rates and vary based on age, gender, and size
   2. Normal heart rates for children age 1 to 10 years—60 to 140 beats/min
   3. Normal heart rates for children older than 10 years and adults—60 to 100 beats/min
      a. Bradycardia—less than 60 beats/min
      b. Tachycardia—greater than 100 beats/min
C. Heart rhythm
   1. Normal beats occur at consistent intervals
   2. Irregular, dysrhythmic, arrhythmic beats occur at uneven intervals
   3. Detect pulse for 1 minute to determine beat rhythm
D. Determining the pulse rate
   1. Sites used for determining pulse rates (Fig. 21.3)
      a. Brachial pulse—located on the medial aspect of the antecubital fossa of the elbow

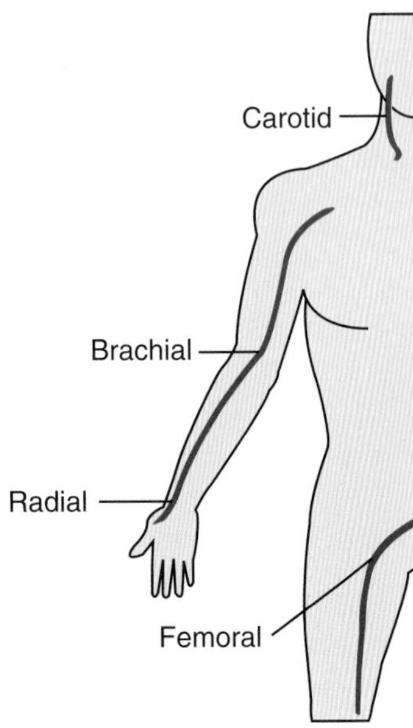


**Fig 21.3** Location of pulse points.

      b. Radial pulse—located on the lateral aspect of the wrist (thumb side) on the ventral surface
      c. Carotid pulse—located in the neck groove, just anterior to the sternocleidomastoid muscle
      d. Femoral pulse—located on the medial aspect of the upper thigh
   2. In emergency situations, the carotid pulse (which indicates that blood is flowing to the brain) is monitored
      a. Care is required in carotid palpation because vagal stimulation may occur, resulting in a decrease in BP or syncope
      b. It is important to palpate only one carotid artery at a time because one or both arteries may be partially occluded
   3. In nonemergency situations, the brachial or the radial pulse is monitored

## Respiration Rate

A. Definitions and basic concepts
   1. Respiration is the inspiration and expiration of air by the body
   2. Respiration rate is the number of breaths per minute; counted by the rise and fall of the chest
   3. Assessment of respiration requires evaluation of depth (shallow, deep), rhythm (regular, irregular), rate, quality (labored, easy), breathing sounds (wet/noisy, clear), and patient position
B. Factors that affect respiration
   1. Respiration rate may be increased as a result of exercise, pain, certain drugs, anxiety, shock, or disease
   2. Respiration rate may be decreased as a result of sleep, certain drugs, or disease
C. Respiration rate ranges
   1. Normal
      a. Resting adult—12 to 16 respirations per minute
      b. Teens to adults—12 to 20 respirations per minute
      c. Older children—15 to 25 respirations/min
      d. Preschool children—20 to 25 respirations/min
   2. Hypopnea—lower than normal, shallow
   3. Tachypnea—above normal, rapid
   4. Apnea—absence of respirations

# EMERGENCY KIT AND PREPARATON PROCEDURES[2]

A. A basic medical emergency kit accessible to all treatment areas should be maintained and be readily available for use
   1. Staff should be familiar with the content of the kit and its location
   2. An emergency kit should contain only the emergency medications the dentist and staff are trained to use (Table 21.1 to Table 21.4)
B. Emergency preparation
   1. Each member of the dental team should be current in BLS (cardiopulmonary resuscitation), including the use of an automated external defibrillator (AED), and should be trained to recognize and manage common medical emergencies

**TABLE 21.1 Medications Typically Supplied With Basic Medical Emergency Kit***

| Drug | Route | Indication | Comments |
|---|---|---|---|
| Oxygen | Inhaled (nasal cannula, face mask, bag-valve-mask) | Respiratory distress, cardiac disease | Do not use in hyperventilation |
| Nitroglycerin | Sublingual | Angina pectoris | No more than three doses in 15 minutes; may cause a drop in blood pressure |
| Epinephrine pen | Subcutaneous | Acute allergic reaction; acute bronchospasm (asthma) | — |
| Bronchodilator (e.g., albuterol) | Inhaled | Bronchospasm (asthma) | — |
| Antihistamine (e.g., diphenhydramine) | Oral | Allergic reaction | May cause drowsiness in adults; may excite children |
| Glucose (nondiet soft drink; glucose tablet, honey sticks) | Oral | Hypoglycemia | — |
| Aspirin | Oral (chewable) | Analgesic, antipyretic, anti-inflammatory | Potentiates bleeding problems |

*The drugs and equipment available in the dental office should reflect the training of the dentist and the staff. Only drugs and equipment that the dentist, the dental hygienist, and the staff are trained to use should be included in the medical emergency kit.

**TABLE 21.2 Recommended Emergency Drugs for Pediatric Office**

| Drug (brand name) | Indication | Availability | Recommended for Kit |
|---|---|---|---|
| Epinephrine (Adrenalin) | Anaphylaxis | 1:1000 (adult) (0.3 mg/dose) | 1 preloaded syringe + 3 × 1 mL ampules of 1:1000 |
| Epinephrine (Adrenalin) | Anaphylaxis | 1:2000 (pediatric)(0.15 mg/dose) | 1 preloaded syringe + 3 × 1 mL ampules of 1:1000 |
| Diphenhydramine HCl (Benadryl) | Mild allergy | 50 mg/mL | 2–3 × 1 mL ampules of 50 mg/mL |
| Oxygen | All emergencies | "E" cylinder + delivery devices | Minimum 1, preferably 2, "E" cylinders |
| Albuterol (Proventil, Ventolin) | Bronchospasm | Metered aerosol inhaler | 1 aerosol inhaler |
| Sugar | Hypoglycemia | Orange juice, Insta-Glucose | 12-ounce bottle of orange juice and/or 1 tube of Insta-Glucose |
| Aspirin | Suspected myocardial infarction | 325-mg powdered aspirin | 1–2 packets of powdered aspirin |
| Nitroglycerin | Angina pectoris | 0.4 mg sublingual tablets | 1 bottle 0.4 mg Nitrostat tablets |

(From Malamed S: *Medical Emergencies in the Dental Office*. 7th ed. St Louis: Mosby Elsevier; 2015.)

2. Each oral health care team member should have delegated responsibilities in the event of a medical emergency; simulations ensure each individual understands their role should a medical emergency arise

## EMERGENCY CARE[1,2,4,6–11]

A. Definitions and basic concepts
   1. Stress reduction protocol
      a. Establish good patient rapport
      b. Create a low-stress environment
      c. Possibly administer pretreatment medication
      d. Administer pain control
      e. Assess patient's anxiety level
   2. Steps for emergency procedures:
      a. Although not stated, dental treatment is discontinued at the onset of all emergencies
      b. Positioning: unless specifically noted, positioning for a conscious patient is based on patient preference, usually upright or semi-Fowler's (semi-upright with patient's head and back at 30-45 degrees); unconscious patients are placed in the supine position with feet slightly elevated
      c. C-A-B: must check for and maintain the following
         (1) Circulation: ensure heartbeat

**TABLE 21.3 Antidotal Drugs**

| Drug | Indication | Availability | Recommended for Kit |
|---|---|---|---|
| Flumazenil (Romazicon) | Benzodiazepine antagonist | 0.1 mg/mL | 1 × 10 mL multidose vial |
| Naloxone (Narcan) | Opioid antagonist | 0.4 mg/mL | 2 × 1 mL ampule of 0.4 mg/mL |

(From Malamed S: *Medical Emergencies in the Dental Office*. 7th ed. St Louis: Mosby Elsevier; 2015.)

**TABLE 21.4 Dental Office Emergency Equipment**

| Device | Availability | Recommended for Kit |
|---|---|---|
| Automated external defibrillator (AED) | Many | 1 AED (pediatric AEDs are available)[9] |
| Face masks | Various sizes for children and adults | Several pediatric masks + adult mask |
| Disposable syringes and needles | 2-mL syringe with 20-gauge needle | 2–3 sterile, disposable syringes |
| Spacer for bronchodilator inhaler | Various manufacturers | 1 spacer |

(From Malamed S: *Medical Emergencies in the Dental Office*. 7th ed. St Louis: Mosby Elsevier; 2015.)

(2) Airway: must be open to allow for respirations
(3) Breathing: ensure breathing

d. Definitive care (specific to each emergency; the procedure followed once C-A-B has been provided for)

3. Cardiopulmonary resuscitation (CPR)—BLS technique with the goal of providing oxygen to the brain, heart, and other vital organs until definitive medical treatment can be given; CPR requires assessment and basic skills in the management of the airway, breathing, and circulation
4. Emergency medical system (EMS) —a coordinated community system that uses communication, transportation, prevention, education, trained personnel, emergency medical facilities, and other elements in providing emergency medical care
5. Respiratory arrest—sudden cessation of breathing
6. Cardiac arrest—sudden, unexpected cessation of the heartbeat and circulation
7. Clinical death—cessation of the activity of the heart and of breathing; may be reversible through life support measures, especially if initiated within 4 to 6 minutes, or may progress to biologic death
8. Biologic death—permanent cellular damage, particularly of the oxygen-sensitive brain cells, resulting from an inadequate supply of oxygen

B. Administering basic life support—cardiopulmonary resuscitation

1. The steps in CPR are known as Circulation-Airway-Breathing (C-A-B):
   a. First step in CPR: Circulation—assess circulation and provide cardiac support by external cardiac compressions and defibrillation
   b. Second step in CPR: Airway—assess airway and establish clear air passage
   c. Third step in CPR: Breathing—assess breathing and provide respiration through rescue breathing
2. Performing CPR
   a. Determine the patient's level of consciousness
   b. Activate the emergency response system immediately for an adult; for child-perform 5 cycles of compressions before leaving child to contact EMS
   c. Attain an automated external defibrillator (AED)
   d. Place patient in supine position with feet elevated
   e. Check pulse for less than 10 seconds; use carotid artery for adults, femoral artery for children ages 1 to 12, and brachial artery for infants
   f. If pulse is not present
      (1) Begin compressions for 1 cycle
         (a) Adult—administer 30 compressions at rate of 100-120 beats per minute and depress sternum 2 inches (5cm) - 2.4 inches (6cm) for each compression
         (b) Child (1 year to puberty)—administer 30 compressions at rate of 100-120 per minute and depress sternum 1/3 depth of anterposterior depth of chest (about 2 inches) with one or two hands for each compression
         (c) Infant (under 1 year)—administer 30 compressions at rate of 100-120 per minute and depress sternum 1/3 depth of anterposterior depth of chest (about ½ inches) using 2 fingers between nipples for each compression
      (2) Give 2 breaths: Trained healthcare workers perform 30 compressions to 2 breaths. If rescuer is ACLS trained, an endotracheal intubation can be performed to administer positive pressure oxygen
      (3) Defibrillator: use AED immediately, within 3-5 minutes of cardiac arrest
      (4) Administer epinephrine 1 mg or 0.1mg/ml IV/IO for an adult; pediatric dose 0.01 mg/kg; administer IV/IO; administered every 3-5 minutes
      (5) Begin sequence CPR (30 compressions/2 breaths for adults and children over 11 years; 15:2 for infants and children up to 11 years) for 2 minutes; then use AED; then administer epinephrine
      (6) Repeat sequence until pulse and respiration are detected (determined by AED) (Figure 21.4)
   g. If pulse is present—Perform rescue breathing
      (1) Adults administer 1 breath every 5-6 seconds at a rate of 10-12 breaths/minute
      (2) Infants and children administer 1 breath every 3 seconds at a rate of 20 breaths/minute
3. Basic life support in late pregnancy
   a. Oxygen demands increase during pregnancy
   b. Functional residual capacity of the lungs is decreased because of the upward displacement of the diaphragm; as a result, oxygen reserve is compromised and cardiac output is decreased by 25% when the pregnant woman is in the supine position, To help alleviate the effects of the supine position on circulation, the uterus should be shifted toward the left side by placing a wedge under the right hip
   c. Aspiration caused by delayed gastric emptying is a concern
   d. Chest compressions for CPR should be performed higher than usual on the sternum, just above the center of the sternum, to accommodate the upward displacement of the diaphragm

C. Automated external defibrillator (AED)

1. A computerized device that analyzes cardiac rhythms and delivers an electric shock to the heart when appropriate; manual defibrillators and pediatric-capable AEDs are the preferred devices to be used on infants and children age 1 to 8 years
2. If available, an AED should be used as soon as possible in the CPR sequence, since early defibrillation increases the chances of survival for victims of sudden cardiac arrest
3. Considerations when using an AED
   a. Patient should be kept dry
   b. Defibrillator pads should be placed at least 1 inch to the side of implanted pacemakers, not over the implanted pacemaker
   c. Transdermal medication patches in the area should be removed before placing the AED

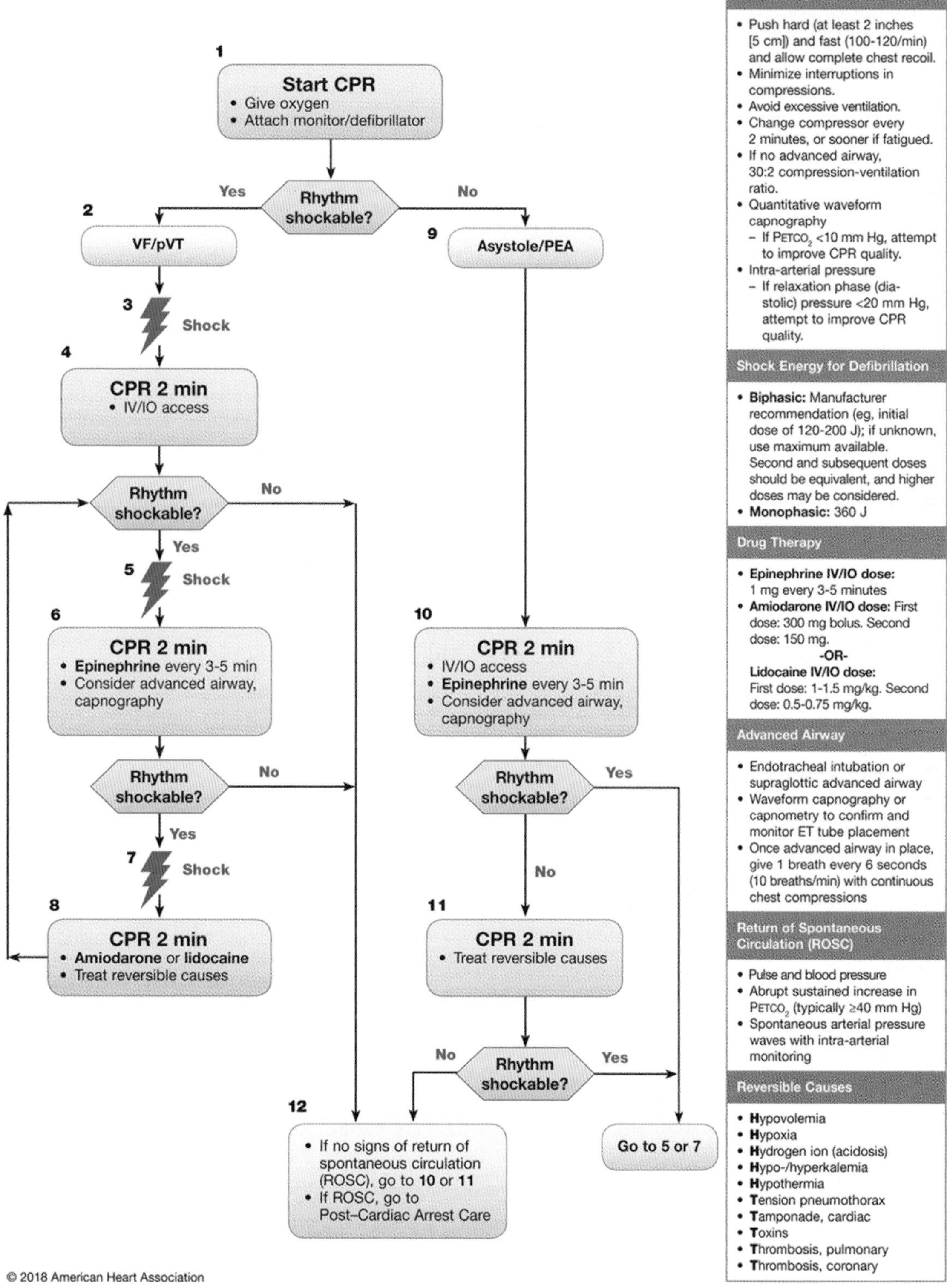


**Fig. 21.4** Figure of American Heart Associate Algorithm 2015. (From: https://eccguidelines.heart.org/wp-content/uploads/2018/10/ACLS-Cardiac-Arrest-Algorithm-2018.png)

## Administration of Oxygen

A. Basic concepts
   1. During a medical emergency, the body's increased need for oxygen, or its diminished ability to obtain or use oxygen, may call for the administration of a higher concentration of oxygen than exists in regular air
   2. Indications for oxygen administration include syncope, cardiac problems, and respiratory difficulties (with the exception of hyperventilation)

B. Equipment—a portable oxygen unit consists of an oxygen tank (an E cylinder is recommended), regulator, tubing, a self-inflating resuscitation bag with mask or a positive-pressure demand valve

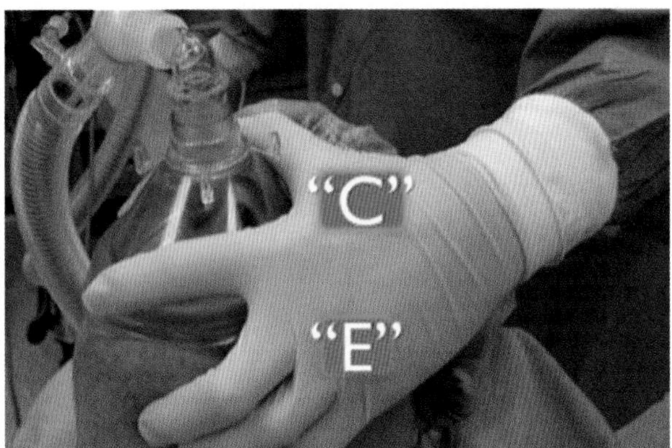

**Fig. 21.5** Proper placement of face mask. To secure mask, fingers and thumb should form the letters "C" and "E" (From Malamed S. *Medical Emergencies in the Dental Office.* 7th ed. St Louis: Mosby Elsevier; 2015.)

C. Oxygen flow for rescue breathing in the event of respiratory or cardiac arrest is 10-15 L/minute, 5-6 L/minute for definitive care during an emergency except for acute pulmonary edema which is 10 L/minute, and below 5 L/minute for preventive care
D. Place an unconscious patient in the supine position; a conscious patient can be seated in a comfortable position for administration of oxygen (Fig. 21.5)

## MANAGEMENT OF MEDICAL EMERGENCIES

### Obstructed Airway[2,6,7]

A. Basic concepts for conscious patients
   1. An obstructed airway occurs when an object or foreign body prevents exchange of air during breathing
   2. Foreign body obstruction may occur when eating, when unconscious (the tongue may block the pharynx), during resuscitation (aspiration of vomitus or blood), or during other events
B. Mild airway obstruction
   1. Patients with mild airway obstruction can cough forcefully
   2. Management—encourage spontaneous coughing and deep breathing
C. Severe airway obstruction with poor air exchange
   1. Patients experiencing severe airway obstruction may exhibit a weak cough, cyanosis, high-pitched sounds, increased difficulty breathing; may be unable to speak or breathe, clutching at the neck
   2. Management
      a. Patient is conscious:
         (1) Position: standing or sitting position
         (2) C-A-B:
            (a) Assess CAB and perform BLS as needed
            (b) To open the airway when there is severe foreign body airway obstruction
               [1] Adults and children: Perform 5 back blows and 5 Subdiaphragmatic abdominal thrusts (Heimlich maneuver) for severe foreign body airway obstruction; Heimlich maneuver is sufficient if rescuer is unfamiliar with back blows
               [2] Infants: Perform back blows and chest thrusts
               [3] Blind finger-sweep is never performed
               [4] For women in their last trimester of pregnancy or for obese patients, chest thrusts rather than abdominal thrusts are recommended for severe foreign body airway obstruction
               [5] Repeat sequence until object is removed or patient becomes unconscious
      b. Patient is unconscious
         (1) Position: Supine
         (2) Summon EMS
         (3) C-A-B: Assess and perform BLS as needed
            (a) Circulation: begin compressions if no pulse
            (b) Airway: quick check for clear airway, no longer than 10 seconds
            (c) Breathing: 2 rescue breaths
            (d) Repeat CAB sequence, if necessary
         (4) Definitive care:
            (a) Administer oxygen if possible
            (b) Monitor vital signs

### Unconsciousness[1,2,4,6]

A. Definitions and basic concepts
   1. Unconsciousness—the inability to respond to stimuli, make purposeful movements, or gain awareness of events taking place
   2. Levels of unconsciousness range from syncope (transient, simple fainting) to coma (prolonged, deep unconsciousness)
B. Causes and treatment
   1. Caused by diminished blood supply to the brain or cerebral hypoxia (inadequate cerebral circulation), altered quality of blood flow to the brain (metabolic disorder), central nervous system (CNS) disorder, or emotional disturbance
   2. Common causes in the dental setting are fear, anxiety, impaired physical status, stress, reaction to drugs
   3. Treatment is aimed at increasing the amount of oxygenated blood received by the brain
C. Preventing loss of consciousness
   1. Obtain a complete health history
   2. Evaluate vital signs
   3. Determine patient's dental stress level
   4. Treatment for the anxious patient
      a. Stress reduction protocol
      b. Premedication
      c. Pain management
D. Managing unconsciousness
   1. Position: Supine with feet slightly elevated
   2. Circulation: check carotid pulse (circulation)
   3. Airway: check airway
   4. Breathing: check breathing
      a. Respiratory arrest but strong pulse: perform rescue breathing

b. Positive pressure oxygen preferred over rescue breathing—administer oxygen at a flow rate of 10-15 liters/minute; administer at rate of 10-12 breaths/min for adults; 12-20 breaths/minute for infants and children.
5. Definitive: assess vital signs; if breathing on own-administer oxygen at a rate of 5-6 liters/minute

## Vasodepressor Syncope, Vasovagal Syncope (Fainting)[1–3,6]

A. Definition
  1. Sudden, transient loss of consciousness
  2. During third trimester of pregnancy—Known as supine hypotensive pregnancy syndrome
B. Causes
  1. Decreased cerebral function resulting from impaired circulation or altered metabolism
  2. Psychogenic factors—anxiety, fear, pain, sight of blood
  3. Nonpsychogenic factors—hypoglycemia, position change, heat, pain
C. Preventing syncope
  1. Obtain a complete health history to determine previous syncopal episodes, dental stress level, illness, if patient has eaten, and other pertinent information
  2. Follow stress reduction protocol
  3. Patients who "feel faint" should be placed in the supine position
D. Signs and symptoms—three stages of syncope:
  1. Presyncope stage—Patient reports feeling of warmth in neck and face, not feeling well, weakness and nausea, lightheadedness, and tingling in the toes and fingers; observation of pallor or gray color of skin, dilated pupils, piloerection, hypotension, and tachycardia
  2. Syncope stage—Patient exhibits flaccid muscles, impaired consciousness, pallor, weak slow pulse, shallow breathing; unconsciousness of less than 5 minutes
  3. Postsyncope stage—Patient wakens and may report feeling weak and disoriented. BP and pulse rate return to normal
E. Managing syncope
  1. Presyncope
    a. Position: Supine with feet slightly elevated; in most cases, this will prevent syncope
    b. Definitive care:
      (1) Administer oxygen
      (2) Consider postponing treatment
  2. Syncope
    a. Position:
      (1) Supine position with legs slightly elevated
      (2) Last trimester of pregnancy-lower patient to supine and turn on left side; place a wedge under the right hip to support the patient
      (3) Positioning must be done immediately; permanent damage or death can occur if the patient is not placed in supine position immediately
    b. C-A-B: Assess and perform BLS as needed
    c. Definitive care:
      (1) Administer oxygen; 5-6 L/minute
      (2) Monitor vital signs
      (3) Place blanket over the patient to keep patient warm
      (4) Administer aeromatic ammonia to increase breathing and muscular movement
      (5) Administer sugar
      (6) Administer atropine if bradycardia persists
      (7) Contact EMS if recovery delayed
  3. Postsyncope
    a. Position: Once recovered, supine position and rest for a time sufficient to prevent another episode
    b. Definitive care:
      (1) Administer glucose (soft drink or orange juice) for associated hypoglycemia (optional)
      (2) Determine cause of the syncope
      (3) Someone should accompany patient home
      (4) Possible referral to physician

## Orthostatic Hypotension or Postural Hypertension[1,2,6]

A. Definition—sudden drop in systolic BP of at least 20 mm Hg caused by a change in body position
B. Causes
  1. Sudden change from the supine to sitting or from sitting to standing position
  2. Prolonged bed rest, medications, prolonged standing, pregnancy, and age can affect the body's ability to adjust quickly to the impact of gravity on the cardiovascular system as body position changes
  3. Addison's disease
  4. Exhaustion and starvation
C. Signs and symptoms: lightheadedness, blurred or darkened vision, nausea, pallor, syncope, and sweating
D. Prevention
  1. Raise the patient slowly from the supine to the upright position
  2. Have the patient slowly change from the sitting position to the standing position
E. Management of the emergency
  1. Position: supine with feet slightly elevated
  2. C-A-B: Assess and provide BLS as needed
  3. Definitive care:
    a. Administer oxygen if needed
    b. Monitor vital signs
    c. Raise the patient slowly; provide assistance
    d. Contact EMS for delayed recovery

## Shock[1–3,6]

A. Definition—the circulatory system does not adequately circulate blood through body tissues, resulting in a lack of oxygen in the cells
B. The patient experiencing shock may complain of thirst, restlessness, or anxiety
  1. May exhibit low BP; rapid, weak pulse; shallow, rapid respiratory rate
  2. Skin may be pale, cool, and clammy
  3. In severe cases, the victim may go into a coma

C. Management procedures for shock
  1. Position: Supine position with feet slightly elevated
  2. Contact EMS
  3. Initiate CAB
  4. Definitive care:
    a. Administer oxygen
    b. Monitor vital signs
    c. Additional definitive treatment based on type of shock

D. Types of shock
  1. Hypovolemic shock—the most common type of shock
    a. Cause—severe hemorrhage or dehydration leading to inadequate blood volume or venous return
    b. Signs and symptoms—dehydration, rapid thready pulse, cool clammy skin, decreased urine output, confusion, weakness, pallor
    c. Management—follow procedures listed earlier for shock
  2. Distributive shock or vasogenic shock—three types: anaphylactic, septic, neurogenic
    a. Anaphylactic shock
      (1) Cause—acute allergic reaction; release of histamine results in sudden vasodilation throughout the body and bronchoconstriction
      (2) Signs and symptoms—bronchoconstriction, difficulty in breathing, hypotension, respiratory arrest
      (3) Management—follow procedures listed earlier for shock; in addition:
        (a) administer epinephrine intermuscular (IM) left lateral thigh is best location: adult dose - .3 ml 1:1,000; child 33-65 lbs .15 ml 1:1000 – should be in preloaded syringe; second dose within 5 minutes if not responding; additional doses every 5-10 minutes if needed
        (b) Administer histamine blockers once patient responds to epinephrine
        (c) Administer corticosteroids
    b. Septic shock
      (1) Cause—infectious agent produces an acute systemic infection that prevents blood flow to the cells, tissues, and organs; often fatal; toxic shock syndrome is an example of septic shock
      (2) Signs and symptoms—fever, vasodilation, increased cardiac output; tissue edema, pink and warm skin; hypotension; restlessness and anxiety; tachycardia; thirst; eventual respiratory failure
      (3) Management—follow procedures previously listed for shock; in addition, administer intravenous (IV) fluids and antimicrobial therapy; patient may need surgery
    c. Neurogenic shock
      (1) Cause—psychological or neurologic disorder or injury to the brainstem or spinal cord from disease, drugs, or trauma; causes loss of sympathetic nerve activity, impairing nerve impulses to the blood vessels, which in turn prevents vasoconstriction
      (2) Signs and symptoms—hypotension, bradycardia, peripheral vasodilation
      (3) Management—follow procedures previously listed for shock; in addition, administer phenylephrine or dopamine and epinephrine
  3. Cardiogenic shock
    a. Cause—inadequate cardiac output to peripheral organs and tissues; common causes are myocardial infarction (MI), cardiac arrhythmias, and heart failure; occurs approximately 10 hours after an MI
    b. Signs and symptoms—hypotension, rapid weak pulse, cold clammy skin, peripheral cyanosis, chest pain, shortness of breath, reduced urine output, confusion
    c. Management—follow procedures listed earlier for shock; in addition, administer IV fluids and medications to restore heart rate and blood pressure (beta blockers, vasodilators, and positive inotropes)
  4. Obstructive shock
    a. Cause—obstruction of blood flow peripheral to the heart, as in arterial stenosis and pulmonary embolism; obstructive shock prevents the heart from beating
    b. Signs and symptoms—severe hypotension and dyspnea
    c. Management—follow procedures listed earlier for shock; in addition, remove or correct obstruction and administer IV fluids with caution

## Asthma[1,2,6]

A. Definition—chronic inflammatory disease of the airway that causes reversible airway obstruction from hyperresponsiveness to stimuli, resulting in episodes of dyspnea, wheezing, and coughing

B. Types and causes
  1. Extrinsic or allergic asthma—caused by allergens outside the body (i.e., airborne, such as dust, foods, and drugs); bronchospasms occur within minutes of exposure
  2. Intrinsic asthma (also known as nonallergic, idiopathic, or infective asthma)—caused by nonallergic factors such as respiratory infections, psychological and physiologic stress, physical exertion, and/or environmental factors
  3. Additional categories in some textbooks include exercise-induced, drug-induced, and infectious asthma
  4. Signs and symptoms—onset of a productive or a nonproductive cough, dyspnea (shortness of breath), tachypnea (increased respiratory rate), tachycardia (increased heart rate), anxiety and agitation, wheezing, cyanosis, chest tightening, nostril flaring, flushing; occurs most often at night

D. Prevention of the emergency
  1. Identify patients at risk through thorough health history taking
  2. Ask probing questions related to asthma
  3. Implement stress reduction protocol
  4. Have the patient take a prophylactic dose of bronchodilator before the appointment
  5. Encourage patients with asthma to bring their inhalers to all dental appointments

E. Management of an emergency related to asthma
   1. Position: Sitting upright
   2. Initiate CAB
   3. Definitive care:
      a. Have the patient administer their own prescribed medications (bronchodilators); if not available, use bronchodilator from office emergency kit: have patient take two breaths; repeat in 5 minutes if episode continues; maximum 3 doses of 2 puffs each dose
      b. Administer oxygen if the episode continues – 5 to 6 L/min.
      c. Activate the EMS if the episode continues
      d. Severe asthmatic episode, not responding to bronchodilator, or unresponsive patient – administer epinephrine 1:1000 (0.3 mL) IM; repeat in 5 minutes if episode continues; children 33-65 pounds receive 0.15 mg dose
      e. IV glucocorticosteroid administration is optional

## Hyperventilation[2]

A. Definition—rapid breathing; often the result of pain, anxiety, or drugs; rapid breathing causes an excessive elimination of carbon dioxide, which results in respiratory alkalosis
B. Prevention of the emergency—implement stress reduction protocol
C. Signs and symptoms—tingling or numbness of extremities, giddiness, lightheadedness, dizziness, confusion, cold hands, heart palpitations, rapid respirations (25-30 breaths/min), rapid pulse
D. Management of the emergency related to hyperventilation
   1. Position: Sitting upright
   2. C-A-B: Assess and perform BLS as needed
      a. Breathing: Have the patient cup hands over mouth and nose and breathe slowly and deeply (only 4-6 breaths/min)
      b. patient could also breathe into an $O_2$ mask with oxygen turned off
   3. Definitive care:
      a. Calm the patient
      b. Oxygen should **NOT** be administered

## Cardiac Emergencies[1,2,6]

A. Cardiac emergencies have many causes and require immediate, definitive medical treatment
B. Cardiac arrest is a sudden, unexpected cessation of cardiac activity; unless CPR is promptly performed to maintain the heart's function and EMS contacted, biologic death may result; use of an AED increases chances of survival
C. Causes and pathophysiology
   1. Coronary disease and cardiac emergencies may result from a change in the heart's function (arrhythmia, hypertrophy, ischemia), blood vessels (atherosclerosis, arteriosclerosis), blood volume change (shock, hemorrhage), or blood composition (anemia)
   2. A cardiac emergency may be caused by accidents (electric shock, drowning, trauma, asphyxiation) or coronary disease
D. Prevention
   1. Identify patients at risk by taking a thorough health history
   2. Recognize signs and symptoms (see below)
   3. Promptly refer the patient to a physician
   4. If coronary symptoms develop in the dental office, rapid access to EMS is indicated
E. Cardiovascular diseases
   1. Hypertension—persistent BP elevation indicates the heart is working harder to supply blood through the arteries; the probability of a CVA (stroke), MI, congestive heart failure, and kidney disease may be increased because of a consistently elevated blood pressure
      a. Signs and symptoms—may include headaches, dizziness, or no symptoms; consistent, elevated blood pressure readings
      b. Prevention of medical emergencies—for recommendations regarding treating patients with elevated BP, see earlier discussion under the section "Blood Pressure"
   2. Angina pectoris—a transient (temporary) ischemia (lack of oxygenated blood) of the myocardium (heart muscle), usually manifested by chest pain or discomfort; angina occurs because the heart requires more oxygen than the amount produced
      a. Signs and symptoms
         (1) Sudden onset of a dull chest pain or discomfort that may be described as a constant pressing, crushing, burning, or squeezing sensation
         (2) Pain may radiate to the shoulders (left is most common), arms, neck, mandible, or epigastrium
         (3) Pain is reproducible and predictable and may last 1 to 10 minutes
         (4) Pain may be precipitated by exertion, emotional stress, cold weather, or a heavy meal and may be accompanied by weakness and shortness of breath
         (5) Patient may appear apprehensive, have labored breathing, or is sweating
         (6) Heart rate and blood pressure are elevated
      b. Prevention
         (1) Schedule short, late-morning or early-afternoon appointments
         (2) Take a thorough health history, identifying patients with angina; discuss questions related to the angina episodes, cause, length of episode, medication, effectiveness of medication, frequency of episodes, and usual symptoms
         (3) Dismiss patients with unstable angina (pain is increasing in duration, intensity, and frequency) and refer to a physician
         (4) Place the patient's nitroglycerin medication within easy reach of the clinician and patient to use in the event of an emergency
         (5) Use stress reduction protocol
         (6) Monitor vital signs
         (7) Administer low-flow oxygen during appointment

(8) Administer local anesthetic for pain control when needed (maximum of 2 carpules local anesthesia with 1:100,000 epinephrine, not to exceed 0.04 mg epinephrine)
(9) Administer nitrous oxide–oxygen ($N_2O$-$O_2$) to provide psychosedation
(10) Dismiss the patient if they shows signs of fatigue, sweating, anxiety, or fidgeting

c. Management of an emergency
(1) If the patient has no history of angina, follow the procedures listed under myocardial infarction
(2) Position: comfortable position for patient
(3) C-A-B: Assess and perform BLS as needed
(4) Definitive
(a) Administer nitroglycerin
[1] A patient's own nitroglycerin is preferred; if not available use nitroglycerin from office emergency kit
[2] Administer 1 nitroglycerin tablet (0.4 mg) or 1 to 2 metered sprays (0.3-0.6 mg) every 5 minutes; do not exceed three doses within 15-minutes
[3] Patient's discomfort should lessen within 2 to 4 minutes
[4] If patient's discomfort has not decreased significantly after first dose, second dose should come from the office emergency kit
[5] Nitroglycerin should NOT be taken if the patient exhibits hypotension
(b) Administer oxygen - 5-6 L/min
(c) Monitor the patient's vital signs
(d) Activate EMS and administer 325 mg aspirin (tablet is chewed or powder form is mixed in water) if pain is not relieved within 10 minutes, or the patient requests EMS, or the pain returns
(e) If pain is relieved by rest and nitroglycerin, encourage rest, discontinue oral health services for that appointment, and refer the patient for further evaluation by a physician
(f) Treatment should be modified for the next visit to alleviate the patient's stress

3. Myocardial infarction (MI)—a diminished or interrupted supply of oxygenated blood to the heart that causes death (necrosis) of part of the heart muscle, resulting in impaired heart function and diminished cardiac output; if a large area of the heart is affected, the heart may be unable to function and may stop beating (cardiac arrest)

a. Signs and symptoms
(1) Chest pain, often described as a "crushing pressure," is the classic symptom of an MI; the pain often radiates to the arm (most frequently the left arm), neck, or mandible; the pain intensifies and lasts for more than 15 to 20 minutes; nitroglycerin, rest, and changing positions do not alleviate the pain
(2) Patient may have an ashen-gray appearance and may exhibit a cold sweat, nausea, vomiting, dyspnea, dizziness, weakness, and the feeling of impending doom
(3) Vital signs most often present as a weak, thready, rapid pulse; low BP; and rapid, shallow respirations
(4) Women do not always present with chest pain but rather may experience more vague warning signs, such as fatigue, nausea, vomiting, dizziness, breathlessness, back pain, or deep throbbing in the left or right bicep or forearm
(5) A patient who is developing signs of acute pulmonary edema will begin to have a slight dry cough; this will develop into a paroxysmal nocturnal dyspnea, asthmatic-type wheezing, pallor, sweating, frothy blood-tinged sputum, tachypnea, dyspnea, and a feeling of suffocation

b. Prevention for patients who have had a previous MI
(1) Take a thorough health history to identify patients at risk
(2) Patients who have had a previous MI should have vital signs checked at the start and at the end of each appointment
(3) Implement stress reduction protocol
(4) Administer oxygen at a flow rate of 3 to 5 L/min
(5) Administer $N_2O$-$O_2$ sedation to decrease the patient's stress
(6) Maintain adequate pain control through administration of local anesthesia with 1:100,000 epinephrine; contraindicated if taking propanolol
(7) Keep appointments short, and dismiss the patient if he or she begins to appear anxious and is showing signs of increased stress
(8) Do not treat a patient for the first 30 days after an MI
(9) Refer patients to their physician if they appear unable to handle the stress of a dental appointment

c. Management of an emergency
(1) Immediately activate the EMS if:
(a) Patient does not have a history of angina
(b) Patient with history of angina is experiencing chest pains different than normal
(c) Patient requests the EMS
(2) Position: conscious patient according to patient preference; sitting upright preferred; unconscious in supine with feet slightly elevated
(3) C-A-B: Assess and perform BLS as needed
(4) Definitive care:
(a) Monitor the patient's vital signs (BP, heart rate/rhythm, respirations) every 5 minutes
(b) Administer oxygen at a flow rate of 5 to 6 L/min
(c) Administer nitroglycerin unless the patient exhibits hypotension (systolic BP $< 90$ mm Hg or $< 30$ mm Hg below baseline); administer 1 nitroglycerin tablet; pain should decrease within 2 to 4 minutes if angina is the cause of the pain; pain will continue or return if the cause is an MI

(d) Administer uncoated aspirin (325 mg) to prevent thrombus formation
(e) Initiate EMS, if needed

4. Congestive heart failure (CHF)—results when the heart is unable to pump an adequate amount of blood to meet the body's demands; precipitating factors include hypertension, coronary artery disease (CAD), congenital and valvular heart disease, toxins, inflammatory disorders, and endocrinopathies
   a. Signs and symptoms
      (1) Weakness, anxiety, shortness of breath, unexplained sudden weight gain, cough, and swelling of the ankles, edema, cyanosis, elevated BP, narrowed pulse pressure, tachycardia, increased respiratory rate, and prominent jugular veins
      (2) Left ventricular failure causes respiratory distress with accompanying signs of weakness, fatigue, and dyspnea
      (3) Right ventricular failure causes venous congestion with accompanying signs of cyanosis, coolness in the extremities, peripheral edema, and prominent jugular veins
   b. Prevention of an emergency
      (1) Identify patients at risk through a thorough health history
      (2) Refer patients with symptomatic CHF (experience CHF symptoms during normal activities) for a medical consultation before elective dental care; patients who are asymptomatic and do not experience CHF symptoms during normal exertion may be seen for dental treatment
      (3) Implement stress reduction protocol
      (4) Administer low-flow oxygen at a rate of 3 to 5 L/min
      (5) Position so that the patient is comfortable, generally upright or semi-Fowler; if the patient has orthopnea (inability to breath when reclined), refer for a medical evaluation
      (6) Watch for signs of acute pulmonary edema (see signs and symptoms under myocardial infarction discussion)
   c. Management of acute pulmonary edema (can occur with MI, CHF, and thyroid storm)
      (1) Contact EMS
      (2) Position: if conscious, position according to patient preference; if unconscious place in supine position with feet slightly elevated
      (3) C-A-B: Assess and perform BLS as needed
      (4) Definitive care:
         (a) Calm the patient
         (b) Administer oxygen at a high flow rate of 10 L/min
         (c) Monitor vital signs every 5 minutes (BP, heart rate/rhythm, respirations)
         (d) Perform a bloodless phlebotomy if symptoms of acute pulmonary edema are present—BP cuffs are used as tourniquets on three extremities (below shoulders and below the groin), always leaving one of the extremities without a cuff; the cuffs are inflated for 5 to 10 minutes, removed, and are then rotated between the extremities
         (e) Administer 2 or 3 nitroglycerin tablets or sprays every 5 to 10 minutes unless the patient is hypotensive

5. Cardiac arrest or sudden cardiac death (SCD)—the unexpected cessation of heart and lung functions as a result of an electrical malfunction of the heart
   a. Cardiac arrest is cardiopulmonary collapse caused by ventricular fibrillation, CAD, respiratory arrest, shock, drugs, arrhythmias, accidents, or anaphylaxis; some sources consider cardiac arrest and SCD to be the same, whereas other sources consider them to be different
   b. Signs and symptoms
      (1) Loss of consciousness; no pulse, BP, or respirations (clinical death)
      (2) Signs and symptoms of impending SCD are chest pain, cough, shortness of breath, fainting, dizziness, palpitations, and fatigue
      (3) 25% of those who experience SCD or cardiac arrest will have no signs or symptoms
   c. Management of the emergency
      (1) Activate EMS
      (2) Position: supine
      (3) Begin CAB and Defibrillation
         (a) Circulation: Check pulse for 10 seconds: 100-120 compressions/minute; give 30 compressions if no pulse
         (b) Airway: establish airway
         (c) Breathing: give two breaths after every 30 compressions
         (d) Defibrillate: use AED if available
      (4) Definitive care: Continue CAB and defibrillation until the EMS arrives

## ALLERGIC REACTIONS[1,2,6]

A. Allergic reactions occur from a wide range of physiologic responses caused by hypersensitivity to an allergen

B. Causes
   1. Allergic responses may be evoked by drugs, pollens, foods, chemicals, insect bites, or other factors
   2. When the body comes into contact with these substances, an antigen-antibody reaction occurs and results in an inappropriate response by the body's immune system

C. Preventing allergic reactions
   1. A thorough health history should reveal a previous history of allergic reactions to drugs or materials used in dental therapeutics
   2. Ask the patient who has a prior history of an allergic reaction to describe its type and severity
   3. Refer the patient with a suspected allergy for evaluation by a physician

D. Types of allergic reactions
  1. Delayed allergic reactions
    a. Signs and symptoms include skin manifestations such as erythema (redness), urticaria (hives), and angioedema (swelling) or respiratory reactions (respiratory distress, wheezing, dyspnea, angioedema) that occur hours or even days after contact with an allergen
    b. Treatment of delayed allergic reactions
      (1) C-A-B: Assess and perform BLS as needed
      (2) Definitive care:
        (a) Administer antihistamine and/or oxygen if allergic reaction is severe
        (b) If the reaction persists, the patient should be accompanied to a physician; if a delayed reaction becomes severe, epinephrine may be administered
        (c) If epinephrine is administered, EMS should be contacted
  2. Immediate allergic nonanaphylactic reaction and anaphylaxis
    a. Immediate allergic reactions occur within 60 minutes of exposure to the antigen and are characterized by urticarial reactions (hives), abdominal cramps, diarrhea, nausea, angioedema, rhinitis (inflamed mucous membranes of the nose), respiratory distress (bronchospasms, dyspnea), cyanosis, and cardiovascular changes, including hypotension, rapid weak pulse, tachycardia, and arrhythmias, which may progress to cardiovascular collapse
    b. Types of immediate allergic reactions
      (1) Food allergies irritate the gastrointestinal tract
      (2) Bronchospasms affect the respiratory tract
      (3) Urticarial reactions affect the skin
      (4) Anaphylactic reactions can be localized (i.e. laryngeal edema) or generalized
    c. Treatment for immediate nonanaphylactic reactions
      (1) Position: hypotensive patient in supine with feet slightly elevated
      (2) C-A-B: Assess and perform BLS as needed
      (3) Definitive care:
        (a) Monitor vital signs every 5 minutes
        (b) Administer an antihistamine and oxygen
        (c) If the patient exhibits signs of cardiovascular or respiratory distress, or if the heart rate, respirations, or BP change, administer epinephrine and contact EMS
    d. Treatment for bronchospasms
      (1) Position: sitting upright
      (2) CAB: Assess
      (3) Summon EMS
      (4) Definitive care:
        (a) Calm the patient
        (b) Administer a bronchodilator
        (c) Administer an antihistamine
    e. Treatment of laryngeal edema
      (1) Position: according to patient preference, generally sitting upright
      (2) C-A-B: Assess and perform BLS as needed; continue to monitor airway
      (3) Contact EMS
      (4) Definitive care:
        (a) Administer 0.3 mL of 1:1000 epinephrine IM; repeat in 3 to 5 minutes if needed
        (b) Administer oxygen
        (c) Administer histamine blocker (diphenhydramine)
    f. Treatment for generalized anaphylaxis
      (1) Position: supine position with feet slightly elevated if hypotensive or unconscious
      (2) CAB: Implement
      (3) Summon EMS
      (4) Definitive care:
        (a) Administer 0.3 mL 1:1000 epinephrine in a preloaded syringe IM; administer a second dose if condition does not improve within 5 minutes; an additional dose can be administered at 5- to 10-minute intervals depending on cardiovascular response
        (b) Administer oxygen at a rate of 5 to 6 L/min
        (c) Administer antihistamine, 50 mg of diphenhydramine, intramuscularly (IM), or intravenously (IV)
        (d) Administer corticosteroid, 100 mg of hydrocortisone, subcutaneously (SC), IM, or IV, once the patient has improved
        (e) Perform CPR as needed
        (f) An insufficient dose of medication could cause anaphylaxis to return within 3 to 10 hours, known as biphasic anaphylaxis; advise patient of this possibility

## Drug-Related Emergencies and Poisoning[1,2,4,6]

### Basic Concepts

A. Drug-related emergencies include allergic response (see above), overdose, psychogenic response (syncope or hyperventilation), idiosyncratic reaction, drug interactions, and complications in a patient who is chemically dependent
B. A thorough health history should reveal the patient's drug allergies, previous adverse reactions, or chemical dependency; these agents, materials, and drugs must be avoided during dental and dental hygiene care

### Specific Reactions

A. Local anesthetic—result of psychogenic or allergic response, toxic overdose, or chemical intoxication
  1. Psychogenic response—usually manifests as syncope or hyperventilation; generally the result of fear of the injection rather than a reaction to the local anesthetic agent; syncope and hyperventilation should be managed according to the criteria described earlier in related sections
  2. Allergic reactions—occur more often with ester-type anesthetics (procaine); very rare and should be managed by the criteria established under the previous section on "Allergic Reactions"

3. Toxic overdoses—result from delayed biotransformation or elimination of the agent, excess total dose, or IV injection of the agent
   a. Prevention—must consider the following when administering local anesthesia
      (1) patient factors such as age, weight, and predisposing medical conditions
      (2) drug factors such as amount, rate of injection, and type of anesthetic used must be considered when administering local anesthesia
   b. Signs and symptoms: headache, dizziness, disorientation, very talkative, agitated, anxious, confused, slurred speech, facial muscle twitching, convulsions, and elevated BP, heart rate, and respiratory rate; with moderate to high levels of local anesthetic, the patient may have seizures, lose consciousness, and undergo respiratory arrest
   c. A mild overdose reaction generally occurs within 5 to 30 minutes of the injection
   d. Steps to manage a toxic overdose
      (1) Position: comfortable for patient
      (2) C-A-B: Assess and perform BLS as needed
      (3) Definitive care:
         (a) Administer oxygen
         (b) Ask patient to hyperventilate to lower arterial carbon dioxide tension ($Paco_2$) levels to lower the risk of a seizure
         (c) Monitor vital signs every 5 minutes until the patient has recovered
         (d) Administer anticonvulsant drug if needed
         (e) Summon EMS if needed
         (f) After recovery, the patient should be assessed by a physician or hospital
   e. Steps to manage seizure or unconsciousness associated with an anesthetic overdose reaction or a severe overdose reaction (signs and symptoms occur during or immediately after administration of anesthetic):
      (1) Position: supine position
      (2) Summon EMS (if unconscious patient regains consciousness once patient is put in supine, EMS may not be needed)
      (3) C-A-B: Assess and perform BLS as needed; may need head tilt, chin lift
      (4) Definitive care:
         (a) Protect patient from injury
         (b) Administer oxygen
         (c) Monitor the patient's vital signs every 5 minutes
         (d) Administer an anticonvulsant IV (benzodiazepine, midazolam or diazepam); if an anticonvulsant has been administered, EMS should be contacted
         (e) Follow seizure management protocol, once anticonvulsant has been administered, patient will experience more severe postictal period
            [1] CAB- begin chest compressions if pulse absent, maintain airway
            [2] Administer oxygen
            [3] Monitor vitals
            [4] May need supportive therapy administered by ACLS trained rescuer; vasopressor to elevate blood pressure or atropine to increase heart rate
4. Chemically dependent patient
   a. Prevention --identify the chemically dependent patient and adjust the dental treatment accordingly
   b. Cocaine-intoxicated patient
      (1) Do not administer anesthetic containing epinephrine within 6 hours of cocaine use
      (2) If cardiac arrest occurs after administration of an anesthetic containing epinephrine, follow the management procedures listed earlier for cardiac arrest (SCD)
   c. Methamphetamine use—patient should not be seen within 24 hours of drug administration
   d. Steps to manage a toxic overdose
      (1) Position: Supine with feet slightly elevated
      (2) C-A-B: Assess and perform BLS as needed
      (3) Definitive:
         (a) Summon EMS
         (b) Administer oxygen
         (c) Monitor vital signs every 5 minutes until the patient has recovered
         (d) Establish IV line if trained
         (e) Administer naloxone if opioid overdose; flumazenil for benzodiazepine overdose; there are no antidotal drugs for other sedative-hypnotic drug overdoses, including barbiturates

B. Fluoride poisoning
1. Some oral health care products contain enough fluoride to be hazardous, especially to children
   a. 1 ounce of topical fluoride gel or one 8-ounce tube of fluoridated toothpaste could be life threatening to a small child
   b. A lethal dose of fluoride for a child is 500 to 1000 mg, depending on the child's weight and size
2. Signs and symptoms of fluoride overdose
   a. Nausea, abdominal pain, excessive salivation, thirst, vomiting, and diarrhea within 30 minutes of ingestion
   b. Burning sensation in the oral cavity and a sore tongue may also be present
   c. In severe cases, muscle cramping, bronchospasm, and cardiac arrest may occur
3. Treatment of acute fluoride poisoning (for adults and children age 6 years and older)
   a. Administer ipecac syrup to induce vomiting (only if patient has a gag reflex, is conscious, and is not convulsing)
   b. Administer milk or 1% calcium gluconate or calcium chloride PO
   c. Activate EMS
   d. Implement CAB

C. $N_2O$-$O_2$ oversedation
1. Signs and symptoms—lethargy
2. Management of emergency

a. Increase $O_2$ intake and decrease $N_2O$ intake
b. C-A-B: Assess and perform BLS as needed

## Cerebrovascular Accident (CVA)[2,4,6]

A. CVA, or stroke, results when the supply of oxygen to the brain cells is disrupted by ischemia, infarction, or hemorrhage of the cerebral blood vessels; co-contributing factors include tobacco use, hypertension, diabetes mellitus, and coronary artery disease
B. Prevention
  1. Take a thorough health history, and evaluate vital signs to help identify patients at risk for a CVA
  2. Do not alter anticoagulant medication before dental care for post-CVA patients
  3. Post-CVA patients should not be seen for at least 6 months after CVA or transient ischemic attack (TIA)
  4. Post-CVA patients with systolic readings above 160 mm Hg and diastolic readings above 95 mm Hg should be referred to their physician for an immediate consultation and should not be seen for dental treatment
  5. Stress reduction protocol should be followed
    a. Appointments should be short and scheduled for midmorning
    b. $N_2O$-$O_2$ can be administered; a pulse oximeter should be used to monitor oxygen saturation ($So_2$) levels
    c. Light oral sedation (benzodiazepines) can be administered; central nervous system (CNS) suppressants should not be taken
    d. Pain control should be monitored; a local anesthetic with 1:100,000 or 1:200,000 epinephrine can be given in limited amounts
C. Signs and symptoms
  1. A patient could experience sudden weakness on one side (hemiparesis), difficulty of speech, temporary loss of vision (especially in one eye), unexplained dizziness, altered level of consciousness, shortness of breath, nausea, sudden severe headache, and confusion
  2. A patient experiencing CVA may have an elevated BP and cardiac arrhythmias (irregular heartbeats);
D. Treatment
  1. Conscious patient
    a. Position: Semi-Fowler's position or sitting upright
    b. Activate EMS
    c. C-A-B: Assess; ensure airway, breathing, and pulse
    d. Definitive care:
      (1) Monitor the patient's vital signs every 5 minutes (heart rate, rhythm, BP, oxygenation)
      (2) Administer oxygen
      (3) Do not administer CNS depressants
      (4) Administer acetaminophen for pain; Do not administer aspirin
  2. Unconscious patient
    a. Activate EMS
    b. Position: Supine position with feet slightly elevated unless BP is noticeably elevated, in which case, place in the semi-Fowler position
    c. C-A-B: Assess and perform BLS as needed
    d. Definitive care: Continue to monitor the vital signs (heart rate, rhythm, BP, respirations)
E. Transient ischemic attacks (TIAs)
  1. TIAs, or "mini-strokes," can present with similar symptoms as a stroke; however, the patient recovers within 10 minutes
  2. Because of a high risk for future strokes, a TIA requires immediate referral to a physician for preventive treatment

## Seizures and Convulsive Disorders[1,2,6]

A. Seizures and convulsive disorders are the result of changes in brain function
  1. Seizures—characterized by alterations in consciousness, motor function, and sensory perceptions; usually have a rapid onset and brief duration (1 to 3 minutes)
  2. Convulsions—involuntary contractions of the voluntary muscles
  3. Epilepsy or seizure disorder—condition characterized by recurrent seizures and convulsions
B. Preventing seizures
  1. A thorough health history should identify an individual with a history of seizures or convulsive disorders
  2. Questions should be asked that address causes, type, and severity of seizure and the aura the patient experiences prior to a seizure
  3. If a patient has a history of seizures, prescribed medications to control seizures should be taken before the dental appointment
  4. Short appointments scheduled early in the day may reduce the likelihood of a seizure in the oral health care setting
  5. Administration of $N_2O$-$O_2$ with at least 20% oxygen is recommended for the apprehensive patient with seizure disorders
  6. Benzodiazepines for oral conscious sedation may also be effective for seizure prone patients who are less apprehensive
  7. Administration of local anesthesia is the most likely cause of a seizure in a nonepileptic patient in the dental setting; care should be taken in the administration, dose, and type of anesthesia administered
  8. Alcohol can precipitate a seizure; therefore a patient who has a history of seizures should not be seen for dental care if alcohol has been consumed
C. Types of seizures
  1. Convulsive—generalized tonic-clonic (grand mal) seizure
    a. Signs and symptoms include an aura (change in taste, smell, or sight precedes the seizure), loss of consciousness (may be several minutes), an epileptic cry (sudden expulsion of air through glottis), involuntary tonic-clonic muscle contractions, altered breathing, and sometimes involuntary defecation or urination
    b. After the seizure, respirations should spontaneously return, muscles relax, and consciousness returns; the person may have a headache or muscle aches and may be drowsy or disoriented

2. Nonconvulsive—absence (petit mal) seizure
   a. Signs and symptoms are sudden momentary loss of awareness without loss of postural tone and a blank stare for up to 90 seconds, although the individual may twitch or blink
   b. The person is usually unaware of the seizure
3. Complex partial (psychomotor) seizure—signs and symptoms may include an aura, purposeless movements, and loss of awareness lasting for only a few minutes

D. Management of seizure
1. Convulsive seizure (Grand mal)— three phases:
   a. Prodromal phase - marked by subtle changes in mood
      (1) Seizure will occur within several minutes or hours, prepare for seizure
      (2) If noticed, postpone treatment
   b. Preictal—marked by the presence of an aura; the beginning of the seizure
      (1) Prepare for the seizure
      (2) Position: Supine with legs elevated
      (3) Remove all dental equipment and removable appliances from the patient's mouth
      (4) Clear the area of all sharp and dangerous objects
   c. Ictal phase—the tonic-clonic phase of the seizure
      (1) Position: supine with feet elevated
      (2) C-A-B: Assess and perform BLS as needed
         (a) Assess and establish airway - head tilt, chin lift may be needed-this may be done by adjusting the headrest on the dental chair
         (b) Suction buccal vestibule if needed
      (3) Definitive care:
         (a) Consider activating EMS
         (b) Prevent injury
            [1] Remove all objects that could harm the patient
            [2] Lightly restrain the patient to protect from injury
            [3] Do not place any objects in the mouth
            [4] Protect the patient's head, if needed, by placing a soft item under the head
         (c) Monitor vital signs
   d. Postictal phase—most dangerous phase of the seizure; the body experiences a generalized depression that affects the central nervous, respiratory, and cardiovascular systems; death can occur during this phase
      (1) Position: Keep in supine with feet slightly elevated
      (2) C-A-B: Continue to assess and perform BLS as needed
      (3) Definitive:
         (a) Monitor vital signs every 5 minutes (BP, respirations, heart rate)
         (b) Administer oxygen at a flow rate of 5 to 6 L/min
         (c) Reassure the patient when consciousness returns
         (d) Allow the patient to recover-may take 2 hours
         (e) Assess the patient to send home, to physician, or to hospital
2. Status epilepticus
   a. Grand mal (tonic-clonic) seizure that lasts longer than 5 minutes
   b. Contact EMS if not already contacted
   c. Assess CAB and perform BLS as needed
   d. Administer anticonvulsant drug IV and 50% dextrose IV
   e. Once seizure ceases, administer oxygen at a flow rate of 5 to 6 L/min
3. Nonconvulsive seizure in the oral health care setting
   a. Position: according to patient comfort
   b. Assess CAB and perform BLS as needed
   c. Closely observe the patient
   d. Reassure the patient when the seizure has concluded
   e. Discharge the patient when he or she has recovered
   f. If the seizure lasts longer than 5 minutes, contact EMS

## Diabetes Mellitus[1,2,6]

A. Definition—characterized by elevated levels of blood glucose resulting from an impaired ability to produce or use the hormone insulin

B. Four types of diabetes
1. Type 1, or insulin-dependent, diabetes mellitus usually occurs in children and young adults; more likely to precipitate a diabetic emergency known as ketoacidosis or diabetic coma; primarily hereditary or genetic
2. Type 2, or non–insulin-dependent, diabetes mellitus usually occurs in adulthood; rarely results in an emergency situation; patients may become insulin dependent; a milder form of diabetes than type 1
3. Gestational diabetes occurs during pregnancy
4. Impaired glucose tolerance, also known as prediabetes; patients at risk for developing diabetes and cardiovascular disease

C. Emergencies related to diabetes may result from two different situations:
1. Hypoglycemia: Patient has too much insulin (hyperinsulinism), resulting in hypoglycemia (low blood sugar)
   a. Blood glucose levels are < 50 mg/dL in adults; <40 mg/dL in children; or symptoms present; normal glucose levels are 100-120 in adults; 100-180 in children
   b. Typical causes are increased insulin dosage, missed meal, vomiting, or excessive exercise
   c. Can lead to insulin shock
2. Hyperglycemia: Patient has inadequate insulin, resulting in hyperglycemia (high blood sugar)
   a. Blood glucose levels are above 250 mg/dL
   b. Can lead to ketoacidosis and diabetic coma
   c. Occurs most often with type 1 diabetes from inadequate insulin levels, infection, or MI
   d. Can occur with type 2 diabetes from stress, epinephrine therapy, or medication

e. Emergency situations develop slowly and generally take more than 48 hours from the onset of signs and symptoms

D. Prevention
1. A thorough health history is essential to prevent diabetic emergencies in the oral health care setting; factors to determine when taking the health history include the type and severity of diabetes and the patient's medications and their frequency, duration, and dosage; medical consultation may be necessary
2. Patients whose diabetes is not under control or who exhibit the signs and symptoms listed next should postpone elective dental and dental hygiene care
3. Establish that the patient's medications have been taken according to prescriptions, and the patient has eaten meals according to schedule on the day of the appointment
4. Minimize the patient's stress and anxiety in the dental office
5. Appointments should be scheduled to ensure the patient is rested and the patient's meal and medication schedules are not interrupted; morning appointments are best, 1 to 1½ hours after breakfast

E. Signs and symptoms
1. Patients with uncontrolled diabetes may be experiencing xerostomia, infection, poor healing, increased incidence and severity of caries, candidiasis, gingivitis, periodontal disease, periapical abscesses, or burning mouth syndrome
2. Signs and symptoms of hypoglycemia may occur suddenly or gradually; patients experience an altered state of consciousness (confusion, anxiousness, incoherence, uncooperative or bizarre behavior), hunger, headache, pale moist skin, hyperthermia, dizziness, weakness, trembling, tonic-clonic movements, normal or depressed respirations, hypotension or loss of consciousness; if left untreated, will lead to coma and death
3. Signs and symptoms of hyperglycemia in conscious patients experiencing diabetic ketoacidosis or impending diabetic coma include the "classic" signs of polydipsia (excessive thirst), polyuria (excessive urination), polyphagia (excessive hunger), nausea, vomiting, dry flushed skin, deep and rapid respirations (Kussmaul respirations or air hunger), weak and rapid pulse, and a "fruity" breath odor; blurred vision, hypotension, and unconsciousness may follow; if left untreated, will lead to coma and death

F. Management of the emergency
1. Regardless of the cause of the emergency, a diabetic patient is treated based on consciousness or unconsciousness, not on hyperglycemia or hypoglycemia; **all diabetic emergencies are treated based on the assumption the emergency is hypoglycemia**
2. Treatment for the conscious patient
   a. Position: based on patient comfort
   b. C-A-B: Assess and perform BLS as needed
   c. Definitive care:
      (1) Administer oral carbohydrates and sugars (orange juice, candy bar, soft drink), 3 to 4 ounces every 5 to 10 minutes
      (2) Observe for 1 hour before dismissing patient
3. Treatment for the unconscious patient
   a. Position: supine position with feet slightly elevated
   b. C-A-B: Assess and perform BLS as needed, pulse may be weak
   c. Activate EMS
   d. Definitive
      (1) Administer oxygen, 5 to 6 L/min flow rate
      (2) Administer 5% dextrose IV, or glucagon 1 mg IM; administer 0.5 mg of 1:1000 epinephrine if dextrose or glucagon is not available
      (3) Monitor vital signs every 5 minutes

## Acute Adrenal Insufficiency, or Adrenal Crisis[2,6]

A. Definition
1. Adrenal crisis is a life-threatening situation
2. Patients having adrenal insufficiency may go into cardiac arrest or shock

B. Causes
1. Acute adrenal insufficiency (adrenal crisis) occurs when the adrenal gland is unable to produce enough cortisol to enable the body to respond to a stressful situation, either physical or psychological
2. In the dental office, stress from surgical procedures or severe anxiety of dental and dental hygiene care can cause acute adrenal insufficiency
3. Results from:
   a. Abrupt withdrawal of exogenous administration of glucocorticosteroids
   b. Primary adrenal insufficiency (Addison's disease)
   c. Secondary adrenal insufficiency -- occurs when the body is unable to produce cortisol because of prolonged exogenous glucocorticosteroid use; the body cannot meet the increased demand for cortisol during a time of stress

C. Prevention—patients who are extremely anxious or who will be undergoing surgical procedures and who are at risk for adrenal suppression should be given two to four times their normal dose of glucocorticosteroids on the day of the appointment

D. Signs and symptoms
1. Patients will exhibit confusion; weakness; lethargy; abdominal, lower back, and leg pain; extreme fatigue; wet, clammy skin; headache; nausea; and vomiting
2. The cardiovascular system will deteriorate; pulse may be rapid and weak; the patient may develop hypotension, followed by shock-like symptoms and unconsciousness or coma

E. Management of emergency
1. Activate the EMS
2. Position: varies
   a. According to patient comfort if conscious and not showing signs of hypotension (confused, wet, clammy)

b. Supine with feet slightly elevated if unconscious or showing signs of hypotension
3. C-A-B: implement; confirm pulse, open and maintain airway, confirm breathing
4. Definitive care:
   a. Monitor vital signs every 5 minutes (BP, heart rate)
   b. Administer high-flow oxygen at rate of 5-6 L/min
   c. Administer 100 mg of glucocorticosteroid or 4 mg of dexamethasone IV
   d. May need to also administer a vasopressor drug (epinephrine 1:1000, 0.05 mL) if patient is unconscious
   e. Transport to hospital via EMS

### Thyroid Storm or Thyrotoxic Crisis[1-3]

A. Definition
   1. Advanced stage of thyrotoxicosis
   2. Thyroid storm is a life-threatening situation
   3. If untreated leads to pulmonary edema, coma, cardiac arrest, death
B. Causes
   1. Uncontrolled hyperthyroidism
   2. Body is unable to respond to physiological stress: trauma surgery, infection, fear
   3. Undiagnosed thyroid disease, excessive thyroid hormone or treatment
C. Prevention
   1. Physical exam—check vital signs, head and neck exam will reveal swelling or goiter
   2. Limit use of local anesthetics with vasoconstrictors
   3. Consult with physician if acute oral infection is present in patient taking thyroid hormone
D. Signs and symptoms: anxiety; tremors; abdominal pain; nausea; vomiting; diarrhea; high fever >102°F; high blood pressure ≥ 180/110; widened pulse pressure; tachycardia; diaphoresis; warm, moist skin; restlessness; delirium; pulmonary edema
E. Management of emergency
   1. Activate EMS
   2. Position: seated upright if conscious; supine with feet slightly elevated if unconscious
   3. C-A-B: Assess and perform BLS as needed
   4. Definitive care:
      a. Monitor vital signs every 5 minutes
      b. Administer oxygen; 5 to 6 L/min
      c. Cover with cooling blanket
      d. Administer 100 mg of glucocorticosteroid
      e. Administer IV infusion hypertonic glucose
      f. Transport to hospital via EMS

### Aspirated Materials[2]

A. Dental materials and instruments may be aspirated into the oropharynx and trachea during oral health care because of the patient's position, diminished responses caused by drugs, and diminished "oral awareness" caused by local anesthesia
B. Prevention - use of a rubber dam or oral packing can prevent the aspiration of dental materials during many dental procedures
C. Treatment:
   1. Aspiration into oropharynx area -- lower the back of the chair, and place patient on his or her side with patient's head hanging off the chair, using gravity to help dislodge the object; encourage coughing
   2. Aspiration into the trachea -- activate the EMS; manage as mild or severe obstruction; the patient may want to sit upright to facilitate breathing and coughing
   3. Swallowed object – escort patient for medical evaluation; a chest x-ray film may be indicated to rule out aspiration into a lung

## CONCLUSION

This chapter is only an approximate guideline for some common medical emergencies encountered in dental hygiene practice. Dental professionals should use standard operating protocols to manage emergencies and review or practice them regularly. Please consult current textbooks and journals for detailed information, and refer to the American Heart Association and American Red Cross for current protocol and training in BLS, ACLS, and EMS (see "Website Information and Resources").

### WEBSITE INFORMATION AND RESOURCES

| Source | Website Address | Description |
|---|---|---|
| eMedicine, Inc. | http://emedicine.medscape.com/emergency_medicine | Medical emergency reference |
| American Academy of Family Physicians | www.aafp.org | Health topic search and health information handouts and links to health-related sites; search under patient care |
| American Heart Association | http://www.heart.org | resources related to heart diseases |
| American Heart Association | https://eccguidelines.heart.org | Link to ECC guidelines which contain AHA updates |
| Nemours Center for Children's Health Media | www.kidshealth.org | First-aid and safety section; also contains articles and fact sheets on a variety of health topics |
| Medline Plus Encyclopedia | http://www.nlm.nih.gov/medlineplus/encyclopedia.html | Links to A.D.A.M Medical Encyclopedia with over 4,000 articles |
| | http://www.nlm.nih.gov/medlineplus/ | Link to many health related topics |
| Mayo Clinic | https://www.mayoclinic.org/diseases-conditions | Link to Mayo Clinic's comprehensive guide of health-related topics |

## CHAPTER 21 REVIEW QUESTIONS

Answers and rationales to review questions are available on this textbook's accompanying Evolve site. See inside front cover for details.

1. Your patient has congestive heart failure. While working on the maxillary arch, you notice your patient has a slight dry cough and is beginning to wheeze. He coughs into a tissue, and you notice his sputum is frothy and tinged with blood, and he develops dyspnea. First, you realize your patient is experiencing acute pulmonary edema. Second, you should immediately contact EMS, implement CAB, calm your patient, administer oxygen, and perform a bloodless phlebotomy.
   - **a.** Both statements are TRUE
   - **b.** Both statements are FALSE
   - **c.** The first statement is TRUE; the second statement is FALSE
   - **d.** The first statement is FALSE; the second statement is TRUE
2. Which of the following flow rates settings would you use to administer oxygen during an emergency involving acute pulmonary edema?
   - **a.** 10–15 L/minute
   - **b.** 10 L/minute
   - **c.** 5–6 L/minute
   - **d.** Below 5 L/minute
3. The use of local anesthesia can increase the risk of aspiration of a dental material. If oral pharyngeal aspiration occurs, the patient's chair back should be lowered to the supine position with the patient placed on their side with their head hanging off the chair.
   - **a.** Both statements are TRUE
   - **b.** Both statement are FALSE
   - **c.** The first statement is TRUE; the second statement is FALSE
   - **d.** The first statement is FALSE; the second statement is TRUE
4. The key to preventing aspiration of a dental material is to:
   - **a.** Lay patient on their left side
   - **b.** Lay patient on their right side
   - **c.** Use a rubber dam
   - **d.** Keep patient in semi-Fowler's position
5. In the event of a stressful situation, acute adrenal insufficiency can occur if the body does not produce enough ____________ to handle the stressful situation.
   - **a.** Glucagon
   - **b.** Glucose
   - **c.** Oxygenated blood
   - **d.** Cortisol
6. Which of the following occurs when the body is unable to produce or use insulin?
   - **a.** Acute adrenal insufficiency
   - **b.** Diabetes Mellitus
   - **c.** Hypoglycemia
   - **d.** Thyroid storm
7. Your patient is 34 years old and was just diagnosed with diabetes mellitus. The doctor has put her on a diet regimen to help control the diabetes. Which type of diabetes does your patient have?
   - **a.** Impaired glucose tolerance
   - **b.** Gestational diabetes
   - **c.** Type I
   - **d.** Type 2
8. Your patient is exhibiting the following signs and symptoms: poor healing and frequent infections, increased caries, gingivitis, increased pocket depths, and complains of a burning mouth. Your patient most likely has:
   - **a.** Acute adrenal insufficiency
   - **b.** Septic shock
   - **c.** Cocaine abuse
   - **d.** Diabetes mellitus
9. Your patient is beginning to get confused and anxious as you ask her questions. She is beginning to look pale, when you touch her skin, it is moist. She is complaining of a headache and she is hungry. Which of the following is she most likely experiencing?
   - **a.** Hypoglycemia
   - **b.** Hyperglycemia
   - **c.** Adrenal insufficiency
   - **d.** Preictal phase of a seizure
10. Oxygen is administered during which phase of a convulsive seizure?
    - **a.** Ictal
    - **b.** Preictal
    - **c.** Postictal
    - **d.** All of the above
11. The aura appears during which phase of a convulsive seizure?
    - **a.** Tonic
    - **b.** Clonic
    - **c.** Postictal
    - **d.** Preictal
12. Your patient's blood pressure is 181/104. The patient is feeling great. Her dental appointment is the third stop of her full schedule this day. She is scheduled for her six month routine oral prophylaxis appointment. Which of the following should you do?
    - **a.** Repeat her BP in 5 minutes, if her BP is still high, complete her care today and then recommend she see her physician
    - **b.** Repeat her BP in 5 minutes, if her BP is still elevated, reschedule her appointment and recommend she see her physician
    - **c.** Recommend she go immediately to her physician or the ER
    - **d.** Contact EMS and have her transported to the ER via EMS
13. Which of the following persons has Stage II hypertension?
    - **a.** 132/79
    - **b.** 167/110
    - **c.** 128/79
    - **d.** 184/105

14. Unconscious patients are placed in the upright position. Improper position causes cerebral hypoxia or diminished blood supply to the brain from inadequate circulation.
   a. Both statements are TRUE
   b. Both the statements are FALSE
   c. The first statement is TRUE; the second statement is FALSE
   d. The first statement is FALSE; the second statement is TRUE
15. Your adult patient is turning blue, emitting high-pitched sounds, is unable to speak, and is holding her throat. If you are properly trained, which of the following should you perform *first*?
   a. Chest compressions
   b. Back blows
   c. Subdiaphragmatic abdominal thrusts
   d. Chest thrusts
16. Your patient's son was stung by a wasp as they passed the flowers in front of your office. He is crying and appears to have difficulty breathing. His blood pressure is dropping. What medical emergency is the boy most likely experiencing?
   a. Asthma
   b. Seizure
   c. Anaphylactic shock
   d. Syncope
17. Which of the following should you do for the above emergency involving a young boy stung by a bee?
   a. Contact EMS, administer oxygen, dispense diphenhydramine
   b. Contact EMS, administer epinephrine, administer oxygen
   c. Dismiss patient and instruct her to take her son to the doctor
   d. Give her son a cold compress and begin your patient's appointment
18. Which type of shock can occur from a disease that causes injury to the spinal cord?
   a. Hypovolemic
   b. Obstructive
   c. Septic
   d. Neurogenic
19. Your patient does not feel well. She complains of being anxious, restless, and thirsty. Upon examination your find she has a fever, she is puffy and her skin appears warm and pink in color. Her blood pressure is lower than normal, and her heart rate is up. She also thinks she may have a bladder infection. Which type of shock is your patient most likely experiencing?
   a. Septic
   b. Hypovolemic
   c. Obstructive
   d. Cardiogenic
20. Your elderly patient has been in the supine position for 45 minutes. When you raise the chair, your patient becomes pale, her heart is beating faster, she feels nauseous, and feels like she is going to pass out. Your patient is experiencing:
   a. Syncope
   b. Orthostatic hypertension
   c. Hypoglycemia
   d. Cardiogenic shock
21. Your patient indicates on the medical history he has asthma. While reviewing his medical history, he discloses that he has problems each spring because of pollen. He usually uses his inhaler 1 to 2 times a month, but this week he has had to use it more often because of the high pollen count. His inhaler dissipates the asthma attack. He has not used his inhaler today. Which of the following would be the best to do for your patient in order to prevent an emergency?
   a. Dismiss your patient until the pollen count lowers
   b. Have him put the inhaler on the counter for easy access in case of an attack
   c. Take two puffs from his inhaler
   d. Create a stress free environment
22. What dose of oxygen should usually be administered during the definitive stage of a medical emergency?
   a. 2–3 L/min
   b. 5–6 L/min
   c. 7–9 L/min
   d. 10–15 L/min
23. When administering a bronchodilator, what is the frequency and the maximum number of doses (2 puffs per dose) that can be administered to an adult?
   a. 2 doses; 5 minutes apart
   b. 2 doses; 10 minutes apart
   c. 3 doses; 5 minutes apart
   d. 4 doses; 5 minutes apart
24. Your patient is hyperventilating, you should have your patient breath into their cupped hands at a rate of 8 breaths/minute. Administer oxygen once the patient is breathing normally,
   a. Both statements are TRUE
   b. Both statements are FALSE
   c. The first statement is TRUE; the second statement is FALSE
   d. The first statement is FALSE; the second statement is TRUE
25. A transient ischemia of the myocardium is the definition for which of the following:
   a. Myocardial infarction
   b. Angina pectoris
   c. Congestive heart failure
   d. Transient ischemic attacks
26. When performing rescue breathing, how many breaths per minute should be given on an adult?
   a. 8–10/minute
   b. 10–12/minute
   c. 12–17/minute
   d. 20/minute
27. When is an AED used?
   a. Acute adrenal insufficiency
   b. Syncope
   c. Cardiac arrest
   d. Orthostatic hypotension

28. An oral temperature of 99.7°F indicates:
   a. Below normal oral temperature
   b. Normal oral temperature
   c. Normal high oral temperature
   d. Fever
29. Normal pulse rates for children are:
   a. 30–60 beats/minute
   b. 60–80 beats/minute
   c. 80–120 beats/minute
   d. 60–100 beats/minute
30. The best artery on an adult to take a pulse rate during an emergency is:
   a. Brachial
   b. Radial
   c. Carotid
   d. Femoral
31. Which of the following will help relieve a patient's stress in the dental office?
   a. Prescribe prophylaxis medication
   b. Help your patient feel relaxed and at home
   c. Administer nitrous oxide-oxygen sedation
   d. All of the above
32. During emergencies, except respiratory and cardiac arrest, and acute pulmonary edema, oxygen is administered at a rate of:
   a. 3–4 L/minute
   b. 5–6 L/minute
   c. 10 L/minute
   d. 10–15 L/minute
33. Which type of asthma can be caused by respiratory infections?
   a. Allergic
   b. Extrinsic
   c. Intrinsic
   d. Exercise induced
34. When the onset of an asthma attack begins, the patient should take two puffs from his bronchodilator. The patient should be placed in the supine position until breathing returns to normal.
   a. Both statements are TRUE
   b. Both statements are FALSE
   c. The first statement is TRUE; the second statement is FALSE
   d. The first statement is FALSE; the second statement is TRUE
35. In the event that a severe asthmatic attack in an adult patient is not alleviated following several administrations of the bronchodilator, what should be administered?
   a. Epinephrine 1:1000; 0.15 ml
   b. Epinephrine 1:1000; 0.3 ml
   c. Epinephrine 1:50,000; 0.2 mg
   d. Hydrocortisone sodium succinate, 100–200 mg IV
36. It would be best to schedule a patient with a history of angina in the early morning or late afternoon. For pain control, an anesthetic with 1:50,000 epinephrine should be used.
   a. Both statements are TRUE
   b. Both statements are FALSE
   c. The first statement is TRUE; the second statement is FALSE
   d. The first statement is FALSE; the second statement is TRUE
37. If your patient is complaining of chest pains and has not had them before, you should follow the emergency protocol for which of the following?
   a. Angina
   b. Cardiac arrest
   c. Myocardial infarction
   d. Gastrointestinal upset
38. It is warm outside, your patient just rushed to get to the appointment on time and reports having chest pains. Your patient has a history of angina. Which of the following should you do?
   a. Administer the office nitroglycerin tablets
   b. Administer the office nitrolingual spray
   c. Have your patient take his own nitroglycerin tablets
   d. Call EMS
39. Nitroglycerin tablets or spray can be administered every three minutes within a 15 minute period. A maximum of 5 doses can be administered.
   a. Both statement are TRUE
   b. Both statement are FALSE
   c. The first statement is TRUE; the second statement is FALSE
   d. The first statement is FALSE; the second statement is TRUE
40. How long does it take for patient discomfort to diminish following administration of an effective dose of nitroglycerin?
   a. Immediately
   b. 2–4 minutes
   c. 5–7 minutes
   d. 9–10 minutes
41. EMS should be contacted if the pain has not been relieved within 10 minutes following administration of nitroglycerin, or the pain returns, or the patient requests EMS be contacted. Aspirin should be administered.
   a. Both statements are TRUE
   b. Both statement are FALSE
   c. The first statement is TRUE; the second statement is FALSE
   d. The first statement is FALSE; the second statement is TRUE
42. Your patient has gained weight since you last saw him four months ago. He is short of breath, his ankles are swollen, his hands were cold when you shook hands, his color is bluish, and you notice his jugular vein is distended. What is the most likely cause of your patient's signs and symptoms?
   a. Myocardial infarction
   b. Adrenal insufficiency
   c. Right ventricular failure
   d. Left ventricular failure
43. The incidence of angina in dental offices decreased with the advent of sit down dentistry. Supine position decreases the incidence of an emergency.

a. Both statements are TRUE
b. Both statements are FALSE
c. The first statement TRUE; the second is FALSE
d. The first statement is FALSE; the second if TRUE

44. Local anesthetic was administered. Your patient begins to complain of a headache and dizziness. She seems disoriented, confused, and is more talkative. Her BP and heart rate have increased. Which of the following should you do?
a. Have your patient hyperventilate
b. Place your patient in the supine position
c. Administer benzodiazepine
d. Administer glucose

45. Your patient has indicated he used cocaine 4 hours ago, it is safe to use local anesthetic containing epinephrine on your patient. Anesthetic containing epinephrine can be administered after 3 hours following cocaine use.
a. Both statements are TRUE
b. Both statements are FALSE
c. The first statement is TRUE; the second statement is FALSE
d. The first statement FALSE; the second statement is TRUE

46. If an opioid overdose is suspected, which of the following should be administered?
a. Naloxone
b. Flumazenil
c. Atropine
d. Nothing can be administered for opioid overdose

47. A patient who experienced a heart attack or myocardial infarction cannot be seen for routine dental care for the first 3 months following the incident. A patient who experienced a stroke or TIA must wait 6 months before being seen for routine dental care.
a. Both statements are TRUE
b. Both statements are FALSE
c. The first statement is TRUE; the second statement is FALSE
d. The first statement is FALSE; the second statement is TRUE

48. In a dental office, the most likely cause of a seizure in a non-epileptic patient is the administration of local anesthesia. It is important to record the dose and type of anesthesia administered.
a. Both statements are TRUE
b. Both statements are FALSE
c. The first statement is TRUE; the second statement is FALSE
d. The first statement is FALSE; the second statement is TRUE

49. Which of the following should you administer when hyperglycemia is suspected?
a. Glucose
b. Cortisol
c. Atropine
d. Insulin

## CASE A: MALE PATIENT WITH PTSD

| | |
|---|---|
| Age | 28 years old |
| Sex | Male |
| Height | 6′0″ |
| Weight | 170 lb. /77.111 kg |
| B/P | 127/84 |
| Pulse | 80 |
| Respiration rate | 15 |
| Chief complaint | "His gums hurt really bad", gums are swollen |
| Medical history | Under care of a physician; has never been hospitalized; being treated for PTSD |
| Dental history | Last had teeth cleaned in the military 17 months ago. While in the military, he had his teeth cleaned once per year when stationed in the United States. He reports he has not brushed his teeth much since leaving the military, but does when he leaves the house. |
| Current medications | Paxil |
| Social history | Unemployed, discharged from the military 6 months ago; served nine years in the military; two tours in Afghanistan; single; lives with parents and a younger brother; reclusive; appears anxious; is sweating; doesn't want to be at the dental office; has no insurance; parents are paying for his dental visit and he is embarrassed by his living arrangements. When parents made the appointment for him, they indicated he was deathly afraid of going to the dentist. |
| Smoking | Yes; 2 packs a day |

**Scenario:**

Patient presents with disheveled appearance, polite but not talkative; it is difficult to get more than a yes/no response from him. He indicates he does not like going to the dentist. He only came because his mouth really hurts. He appears very anxious and on guard, and startles easily. He has a history of anxiety which began during his first tour in Afghanistan. He has been under the care of a physician for PTSD for the last two years. He is not always good about taking his medicine and he forgot to take it before he came for his appointment this morning. He smokes two packs of cigarettes a day and drinks two cups of coffee each morning. He was running late this morning, so he did not have either.

***Use Case A to answer questions 50 to 59.***

50. Based on the current blood pressure classifications from the American College of Cardiology and the American Heart Association (2017), what is your patient's blood pressure classification?
a. Normal
b. Elevated
c. Stage I hypertension
d. Stage II hypertension

51. Based on your patient's blood pressure classification, what is your patient's recommended management regimen?
a. Check blood pressure every year

b. Dental treatment can be performed, limit use of epinephrine, refer your patient to his physician for evaluation
c. Refer him for a medical evaluation prior to dental treatment; limit use of epinephrine
d. Transport to the ER

52. Your patient's baseline heart rate is considered:
a. Low
b. Normal
c. High

53. Your patient's baseline respiration rate is considered to be:
a. Normal
b. Hypopnea
c. Tachypnea
d. Apnea

54. As you begin to probe, you notice your patient is clutching the chair, his knuckles are white. He begins to pale and his pupils become dilated. He complains that his heart is racing, he feels nauseous, light-headed, and complains that his fingers are tingling. Which of the following is your patient experiencing?
a. Angina
b. Orthostatic hypotension
c. Presyncope
d. Cardiac arrest

55. Which of the following should you do first for this patient?
a. Place your patient in supine position with legs slightly elevated
b. Place your patient in the semi-Fowler's position
c. Administer oxygen
d. Administer aromatic ammonia

56. Which of the following is the second step in managing an emergency that you should perform for your unconscious patient?
a. Administer oxygen
b. Monitor vital signs
c. Place your patient in supine position with legs slightly elevated
d. Assess C-A-B

57. If you do not place your patient in the proper position, what can occur?
a. It makes no difference
b. A longer recovery time
c. Permanent damage or death

58. During late presyncope and syncope, your patient's blood pressure will?
a. Increase
b. Decrease
c. Stay the same

59. Which of the following would NOT be given to your patient as definitive treatment during postsyncope:
a. Nitroglycerine
b. Glucose
c. Atropine
d. Ammonia ampule

## CASE B: MALE PATIENT WITH CROHN'S DISEASE

| | |
|---|---|
| Age | 20 years old |
| Sex | Male |
| Height | 5'11" |
| Weight | 135 lbs./61.235 kg |
| B/P | 96/62 |
| Pulse | 95 |
| Respiration rate | 16 |
| Chief complaint | "Gums are bleeding and his jaw hurts" |
| Medical history | Under the care of a physician; Hospitalized one year ago; Crohn's Disease diagnosed one year ago during a colonoscopy performed in a hospital; experiences abdominal cramps after eating, recently lost 10 pounds; patient does not smoke. |
| Dental history | Extensive orthodontic treatment including a palatal expander, head gear, and braces. Currently has a lingual bar. He sees the dentist regularly but missed the last dental visit because of work. He claims to brush 3 times a day, but biofilm is generalized. |
| Current medications | Prednisone 20 mg/day, Asacol |
| Social history | He is a full time student and has a part time job at a law firm. This semester he is interning with the state court of appeals, working Saturdays and evenings at the law firm, and study for the LSAT. He is studying every free moment in order to do well on the exam to get into a prestigious law school. He is too busy to go out for or fix a meal. He snacks when he is hungry. |

***Use Case B to answer question 60 to 68.***

60. Your patient appears tired, stressed, and anxious. While in your chair, he seems to be getting confused, appears lethargic, complains of stomach cramping and nausea. His pulse is rapid and weak. What is the most likely cause of your patient's signs and symptoms?
a. Anaphylactic shock
b. Acute adrenal insufficiency
c. Allergic reaction
d. Thyroid storm

61. You rescheduled your patient until he received medical clearance. Prior to him having his wisdom teeth removed, which of the following should you do in preparation for his appointment.
a. Plan to administer nitrous oxide-oxygen sedation
b. Prescribe a sedative
c. Increase his glucocorticosteroid dose by 2–4 times the day of his appointment
d. Prescribe a prophylactic antibiotic

62. Your patient is at risk of acute adrenal insufficiency during each appointment because he has Crohn's disease. Crohn's disease affect the body's production of cortisol.
a. Both statements are TRUE
b. Both statements are FALSE
c. The first statement is TRUE; the second statement is FALSE
d. The first statement is FALSE; the second statement is TRUE

63. One of the classic signs indicating acute adrenal insufficiency is a seizure. If not treated in time, acute adrenal insufficiency may result in cardiac arrest.
   a. Both statements are TRUE
   b. Both statements are FALSE
   c. The first statement is TRUE; the second statement is FALSE
   d. The first statement is FALSE; the second statement is TRUE
64. During the emergency your conscious patient should be placed in which of the following positions?
   a. Patient's choice
   b. Sitting Upright
   c. Semi-Fowler's
   d. Supine with feet slightly elevated
65. Definitive treatment for your patient includes all of the following EXCEPT:
   a. Oxygen
   b. Glucocorticosteroid
   c. Atropine
   d. Epinephrine
66. Your patient's baseline blood pressure is considered:
   a. Normal
   b. Elevated
   c. Stage I hypertension
   d. Stage II hypertension
67. What is your patient's blood pressure most likely to do during an acute adrenal insufficiency episode?
   a. Decrease
   b. Remain the same
   c. Increase
68. Stress reduction techniques would be beneficial during each appointment. Establishing good patient rapport, creating a low-stress environment, and assessing your patient's anxiety level are part of the protocol.
   a. Both statements are TRUE
   b. Both statements are FALSE
   c. The first statement is TRUE; the second statement is FALSE
   d. The first statement is FALSE; the second statement is TRUE

## REFERENCES

1. Grimes E. *Medical Emergencies: Essentials for the Dental Professional*. 2nd ed. Boston: Pearson; 2014.
2. Malamed S. *Medical Emergencies in the Dental Office*. 7th ed. St Louis: Mosby Elsevier; 2015.
3. Pickett F, Gurenlian J. *Preventing Medical Emergencies: Use of the Medical History*. 3rd ed. Baltimore: Wolters Kluwer Health; 2015.
4. Sangrik L. In: Pulkrabek K, ed. *Medical Emergencies in the Dental Office Response Guide*. American Dental Association; 2018.
5. *New ACC/AHA High Blood Pressure Guidelines Lower Definition of Hypertension, American College of Cardiology*; November 2, 2017. Retrieved April 29, 2019 from https://www.acc.org/latest-in-cardiology/articles/2017/11/08/11/47/mon-5pm-bp-guideline-aha-2017.
6. Little J, Miller C, Nelson R. *Dental Management of the Medically Compromised Patient*. 9th ed. St Louis: Elsevier; 2018.
7. American Red Cross. *CPR/AED for Professional Rescuers: Participants Handbook*; 2017. Retrieved April 29, 2019 from https://www.redcross.org/content/dam/redcross/uncategorized/6/CPro_PM_digital.pdf.
8. American Heart Association. *AHA Guidelines Update for CPR and ECC*; 2015. Retrieved April 29, 2019 from https://www.cercp.org/images/stories/recursos/Guias%202015/Guidelines-RCP-AHA-2015-Full.pdf.
9. American Heart Association. Adult Cardiac Arrest Algorithm 2018 Update. Retrieved April 29, 2019 from https://eccguidelines.heart.org/wp-content/uploads/2018/10/ACLS-Cardiac-Arrest-Algorithm-2018.png.
10. American Heart Association. Pediatric Cardiac Arrest Algorithm 2018 Update. Retrieved April 29, 2019 from https://eccguidelines.heart.org/wp-content/uploads/2015/09/PALS-Cardiac-Arrest-Algorithm-2018.png.
11. American Heart Association. Part 12: Pediatric Advanced Life Support. Retrieved April 29, 2019 from https://eccguidelines.heart.org/wp-content/themes/eccstaging/dompdf-master/pdffiles/part-12-pediatric-advanced-life-support.pdf.

22

# Ethical and Legal Issues

*Vickie Kimbrough*

Dental hygienists make decisions that are influenced by laws and ethics. At times, these decisions are clear and at other times they are not, and create ethical dilemmas for oral health providers. Dental hygienists must be cognizant of the laws governing the employer-employee relationship and influencing the responsibilities and rights of the parties involved. Understanding and applying legal and ethical principles protects the provider (dental hygienist), the patient, the employer, and the employee. This chapter reviews the laws and ethics most closely associated with the dental hygiene profession.*

## ETHICAL CONSIDERATIONS

A. Definitions
   1. Ethics—the science of human behavior; correlate motives and attitudes with moral actions and values
   2. Professional ethics—rules or standards governing conduct of members of a profession
   3. Bioethics—ethical and moral implication of new biologic discoveries and biomedical advances

B. Ethical theories
   1. Are the foundation of ethical analysis; explain moral principles
   2. Provide a basis for ethical rule, policy development, or both
   3. Assist in the resolution of ethical dilemmas

C. Three major theories
   1. Teleologic/utilitarian ethics (John Stuart Mill)—comprise rules for conduct based on consequences of action; an action is considered right or wrong on the basis of its usefulness; useful actions bring about the greatest good for the greatest number of individuals
      a. Act utilitarianism—examines a situation and determines which course of action will bring about the greatest happiness or least harm and suffering to an individual regardless of personal feelings or societal constraints such as laws
      b. Rule utilitarianism—searches for the greatest happiness and seeks public agreement to define nature of happiness; considers the law and fairness; an action is considered right if it conforms to a rule; the rule should have positive results in a wide range of situations
   2. Deontologic ethics (Immanuel Kant)—focus on the morality of the act rather than the situation or consequences of actions; one would say, "It's the principle of the thing"; a person's intention, not the consequences of the action, is key; three important elements: applied universally to all individuals, unconditional, and demand an action
      a. Act deontology—based on personal moral values of the individual making the decision and considers the ethical principles involved in an action in light of the circumstances; for example, avoid the truth if it is harmful
      b. Rule deontology—based on the belief that certain standards for ethical decisions are of greater value than an individual's moral values; considers the principles and rules in general as they apply to types of actions
   3. Virtue ethics (Aristotle and Plato)—focus on character traits and excellence of character; evaluate ethical dilemma by asking, "Is this what a virtuous person would do?"
   4. Other theories
      a. Situational ethics—course of action determined by:
         (1) The unique characteristics of each individual
         (2) The relationship between the health care provider and the patient
         (3) The most humanistic action in a given circumstance
      b. Principalism—focuses on ethical principles, including autonomy, veracity, beneficence, nonmaleficence, and justice
      c. Professional codes of ethics—designed in a rule-making format; may include aspirational statements, usually directs decision making among professionals more than ethical theories

D. Universal Ethical Principles
   1. Veracity—truthfulness; mutual responsibility for the patient and the provider; for example, the patient must be truthful to receive appropriate care, and the provider must provide truthful information so that the patient can exercise his or her autonomy
   2. Autonomy—personal liberty; individuals are free to make decisions regarding their own health; respect for the individual autonomy of others is basic to the health care provider–patient relationship; informed consent and informed refusal is basic to autonomy (see discussion on informed consent later in this chapter)

*Vickie J. Kimbrough and the publisher acknowledge the past contribution of Pamela Zarkowski to this chapter.

3. Beneficence—the provider's duty is a commitment to the health and welfare of the patient above all other considerations; duty to prevent or remove harm and promote good
4. Nonmaleficence—the provider's duty not to use the treatment to injure or wrong the patient; inflict no harm
5. Fidelity (role fidelity)—health care providers are required to provide services within the scope of their practice; ethics require that health care providers practice within the constraints of the role assumed within the health care environment; the provider is expected to follow through with commitments
6. Confidentiality—based on an individual's right to privacy; for example, a patient has the right to expect all his or her medical records and communications to be kept confidential
7. Justice—fair and equitable treatment of patients

## PROFESSIONALISM

### Defining a Profession

A. Characteristics of a profession
   1. Special advanced education or preparation
   2. Identifiable membership
   3. Community service orientation
   4. Promotion of a body of knowledge in the field (research and theory development)
   5. Autonomy of practice
   6. Self-regulation
   7. The recognized authority with societal sanction
   8. Primarily intellectual nature of the work
   9. Adherence to a code of ethics
B. Code of ethics
   1. Historical evidence traced to guidelines outlining the duties of physicians
   2. Early evidence included oaths and rabbinic and Christian sources
   3. Common themes include:
      a. Respecting autonomy
      b. Preventing harm
      c. Protecting confidentiality
   4. Hippocratic Oath—fifth century BCE; statement of principles guiding the professional conduct of physicians
      a. Interpreted to advocate, "Above all, do no harm," or "First, do no harm"
      b. Protected the rights of the patients
      c. Required physicians to maintain patient confidentiality
      d. Placed needs of patient above those of society
      e. Placed an obligation on physicians to teach the next generation of physicians
   5. Ethical codes for health care professionals continue to be evaluated and revised to reflect:
      a. Current practice issues
      b. Protections for population groups that are subjects in research investigations
      c. Identification of impaired health care providers
      d. Professional responsibilities
      e. Use of social media
   6. Common elements of codes
      a. Self-imposed—the health care professional self-assesses and determines compliance; range of sanctions from a professional organization or licensing agency for lack of compliance
      b. Set rules governing behavior—the professional uses them as a framework for action
      c. Serving to protect the public—on the basis of ethical principles that support actions to benefit the patient and prevent harm
      d. Striving to enhance the profession—adherence to code characterizes a profession
      e. Providing a framework for ethical decision making
   7. American Dental Hygienist's Association (ADHA) Code of Ethics and the Canadian Dental Hygienists Association (CDHA) Code of Ethics
      a. Identify and describe ethical principles to guide the oral health care provider
      b. State the obligations and responsibilities of the dental hygienist
         (1) Personal and professional obligations and responsibilities
         (2) Obligations and responsibilities to the public and the scientific community
   8. Codes of Ethics—compare all codes
      a. For the ADHA's Code of Ethics, visit the website at https://www.adha.org/resources-docs/ADHA_Code_of_Ethics.pdf (also see Appendix C)
      b. For the California Dental Hygienist Association's (CDHA) Code of Ethics, visit the website at https://www.cdha.ca/cdha/The_Profession_folder/Resources_folder/Code_of_Ethics_folder/CDHA/The_Profession/Resources/Ethics_Corner.aspx?hkey=136b1f06-5743-47d6-904f-98d048eefabf
      c. For the American Dental Association's Code of Professional Responsibility and Conduct (revised April 2012), visit the website at https://www.ada.org/en/about-the-ada/principles-of-ethics-code-of-professional-conduct
   9. Patient's Bill of Rights—outlines patient expectations and provides guidelines for provider conduct; the patient has the right to:
      a. Respectful, competent, and considerate care, irrespective of ethnicity, gender, national origin, age, or disability
      b. Receive current, accurate, and complete information regarding diagnosis, treatment, and prognosis
      c. Receive information necessary to give informed consent or informed refusal before treatment; be informed of the consequences of refusing treatment
      d. Confidentiality regarding all communications, consultations, and records except when permission has been granted to submit this information to others
      e. Obtain information relating to the credentials of all providers rendering services

f. Reasonable continuity of care
g. Examine and receive accurate copies of professional services and fees
h. Receive treatment from health care professionals who act within the limits of their professional licenses (scope of practice) and adhere to the standard of care in delivering services

10. Types of professional credentials
 a. Licensure—state regulation of professionals
  (1) Granted by a state agency or board
  (2) Limits practice to:
   (a) Responsibilities and behaviors prescribed by law in the state practice act in the United States or determined by the provincial practice act in Canada
   (b) Responsibilities and behaviors delineated by rules and regulations
  (3) Authorized practice by professionals meeting specified qualifications
  (4) Failure to meet responsibilities and expected behaviors may result in fines, suspension, or removal of license
  (5) Status of provider's license available to public; may indicate current license status (e.g., active, pending, suspended)
  (6) The purpose is to protect the public from unqualified or unethical providers
 b. Registration—qualified professionals listed in a directory
  (1) Dental hygiene is a self-regulated profession in most Canadian provinces, and registration is a provincial responsibility (e.g., College of Dental Hygienists of Ontario http://cdho.org/cdho-home
  (2) A certificate of registration to practice is issued only to those who meet established standards of qualification and practice
 c. Certification—state or national recognition
  (1) Recognition by a nongovernmental agency (e.g., a professional association)
  (2) Identification of professionals who have met specified qualifications

## ETHICAL ISSUES IN PUBLIC POLICY

A. Ethical issues and public policy
 1. Distributive justice—fair allocation of resources involved
  a. Macro-allocation of resources—based on public needs (e.g., water fluoridation)
  b. Micro-allocation of resources—based on individual needs (e.g., fluoride varnish treatment)
 2. Distributive justice or allocation of scarce resources—determination of who should receive treatment when all cannot be treated; services may be allocated on basis of:
  a. Equity—all persons receive equal treatment
  b. Need—treatment allocated on the basis of prioritized needs
  c. Effort—treatment allocated to those who have earned it
  d. Contribution—treatment allocated to those who are making a contribution to society
  e. Merit—treatment allocated to those who are most deserving
 3. Influenced by principles of human dignity and human rights and contributing to the common good
 4. Current health policy debates
  a. Question of whether public health funds should be used for:
   (1) Financial assistance and care of the disadvantaged or seniors
   (2) Financial assistance and care for undocumented immigrants
   (3) Financial support for victims of:
    (a) Acute or chronic diseases
    (b) Personal choices (e.g., tobacco use, risky lifestyle)
   (4) Provision of health care services
    (a) Appropriate range of services provided
    (b) Impact of public versus private funding on the:
     [1] Consumer and taxpayer
     [2] Provider
     [3] Third-party payer
     [4] Government (local, state, federal, or all)
    (c) Concerns about authority in treatment decisions
    (d) Tele–health care
    (e) Expanded scope of practice for midlevel providers
    (f) Delegation of responsibility to non-health providers
  b. Research
   (1) Identification of appropriate decision makers to identify and prioritize research agendas, especially for controversial topics (e.g., stem cell research)
   (2) Identification of sources of financial support (e.g., what proportion of the national budget should be allocated to health care and research)

B. Public policy
 1. A system of plans of action, regulatory measures, laws, and funding priorities concerning a specific topic or issue
 2. Promulgated by a governmental entity or its representatives
 3. Public policy is typically embodied in constitutions, legislative acts, and judicial decisions

C. Creating public health policy
 1. Goal—assessment of a variety of actions and consequences to solve identified societal problem
 2. Action—a decision by all members of society or their elected representatives (e.g., public vote vs. state legislature passing statute regarding mandatory use of seat belts)

TABLE 22.1 **Differentiating Between Ethics and Law**

| | Ethics | Law |
|---|---|---|
| Definition | Individual interpretation of the nature of right and wrong and rules of conduct | Rules and regulations by which society is governed set forth in a formal and legally binding manner |
| Source | Internalized; individual nature and beliefs | Externalized rules and regulations of society |
| Emphasis | Individual moral behavior for the good of the individual within society | Social behaviors that are good for society as a whole |
| Conduct | Motives and reasons why the individual behaves the way he or she does | Overt conduct of the individual; what a person actually did or failed to do |
| Sanctions | Professional organization—expulsion from the organization | Judicial and administrative bodies—criminal sanctions such as fines and imprisonment imposed by the courts; civil sanctions such as monetary damages imposed by the courts; disciplinary sanctions such as fines, license suspension, or license revocation by a board of dentistry |

3. Analysis—determining which policy among alternatives best achieves the goal, how policy should be implemented, or how to evaluate what is currently being done

D. Policy makers—usually legislators, members of executive branch of government, and government officials who write regulations

E. Policy analysts—provide policy makers with information required to determine the impact of past and current public policies; determine whether new policy should be implemented or present policy or no policy should continue

F. Examples of community-based programs requiring public policy analysis
1. Federal or state partnerships to provide oral health services
2. Fluoridation initiatives (e.g., community water fluoridation and school fluoride programs)
3. Caries prevention programs such as dental sealant or fluoride varnish programs in public health settings
4. Provision and funding of oral health care services by nondental personnel

G. Policy makers may seek input from professionals or professional associations; health-related professional associations frequently hire lobbyists to influence government policy makers

H. Distinctions between ethics and law
1. Laws are societal mandates, whereas ethics are professionally based
2. Ethical principles and legal doctrine are related
   a. Ethical principles integral to federal and state legislation that is enacted
      (1) Obligation to obtain informed consent (patient autonomy)
      (2) Health Insurance Portability and Accountability Act (HIPAA) regulations (confidentiality)
      (3) Discrimination protections for patients with specific disease states such as human immunodeficiency virus (HIV) infection (justice)
      (4) Tort regulation (nonmaleficence)
      (5) Occupational Safety and Health Administration (OSHA) regulations (beneficence)
   b. Ethical issues inherent in the litigation of cases
3. Ethical duties are usually greater than legal duties; for example, a health care provider who is acquitted in civil or criminal court after being charged with illegal conduct did not necessarily act ethically
4. Compliance with the law sometimes mandates unethical conduct—health care providers are ethically and legally bound to keep confidential all patient communications and records; however, the law makes exceptions and requires disclosure to appropriate authorities in specific situations (e.g., in cases of suspected child or elder abuse or threats of inflicting bodily harm to another person or self)
5. Personal values not necessarily congruent with professional ethics or the law—under law, individuals have a right to control their own bodies; this includes the right to refuse medical or dental treatment; health care providers must honor this right despite their own personal values
6. Differentiating between ethics and law (Table 22.1)

## LEGAL CONCEPTS

A. Law defined
1. Rules and regulations that govern society
2. Reflects society's attitudes, mores, and needs; therefore, law is constantly changing to meet the requirements and expectations of society

B. Sources of law
1. United States Constitutional law
   a. Constitutional law—supreme law of the land; both state and federal laws must be consistent with the U.S. Constitution
   b. The U.S. Constitution establishes the organization of the federal government and places limitations on the federal government through the Bill of Rights (first 10 amendments to the U.S. Constitution)
   c. Delineates the specific powers of the federal government to the:
      (1) Executive branch (Office of the President)
      (2) Legislative branch (U.S. Congress)
      (3) Judicial branch (U.S. Supreme Court)
   d. Powers not specifically granted to the federal government are the powers of state government

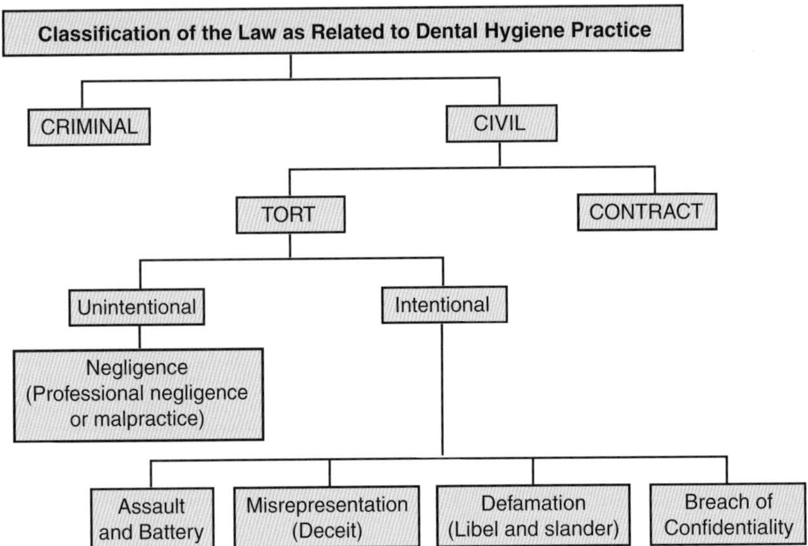

**Fig 22.1** Classifications of law as it relates to dental hygiene practice.

   e. Each state has its own constitution that grants powers and places limitations on the powers of the state government
2. Statutory law
   a. Laws made by the legislative branch of government (federal, state, and local governments)
   b. State dental practice acts are examples of statutory laws
3. Administrative law
   a. Administrative agencies are given the authority to oversee the specific laws or statutes to ensure that the intent of the law is enforced
   b. Administrative laws are the results of decisions of administrative agencies; for example, state boards of dentistry and the College of Dental Hygienists of Ontario implement rules and regulations to enforce the law
   c. Administrative agencies may conduct investigations and hearings and may issue decisions that suspend or revoke the license of a dentist, dental hygienist, or dental assistant; decisions of administrative agencies may be appealed through the state court system to determine whether:
      (1) The agency complied with the regulation
      (2) Evidence supports the agency's decision
      (3) The agency exceeded its authority
      (4) The delegation of power to the agency was proper
      (5) The agency followed proper procedures
      (6) The agency acted in an arbitrary or capricious manner
4. Judicial law
   a. Determined by courts (state, provincial, and federal), which interpret legal issues in dispute
   b. *Stare decisis*[1] (Latin, meaning "let the decision stand")—doctrine of law whereby the court will base its decision on previous case law (a prior case with similar facts); the previous case must be from the same jurisdiction (state); emphasizes the importance of legal precedent
   c. Landmark decisions—court decision that departs from precedent; for example, new technology may require different conclusions based on the same facts
   d. *Res judicata*[1] (Latin, meaning "a thing or matter settled by judgment")—legal doctrine that applies when a legal ruling has been made by a competent court of jurisdiction, and no appeals are possible; prevents parties from taking the same issues to different courts

C. Classifications of law (Fig. 22.1)
1. Common law and civil law—two concepts of legal thought, one from England (common law) and one from Europe (civil law)
   a. Common law—general principles derived from decisions in case law using the concept of precedent
   b. Civil law—civil code system developed by legislature, based on rules and regulations; enforced through the court system and protects the legal rights of private persons
   c. Level of proof—preponderance of evidence; the greater weight of the evidence required in a civil (noncriminal) lawsuit for jury or judge without a jury to decide in favor of one side or the other
2. Criminal law—relates to acts considered offensive to society as a whole
   a. Classifications of crimes
      (1) Misdemeanors—usually involve fines of less than $1000 or imprisonment for less than 1 year, or both; examples include vandalism, trespassing, and reckless driving
      (2) Felonies—serious crime; usually involve punishment ranging from fines of more than $1000 or imprisonment of more than 1 year (or both); receiving a death sentence depending on the crime committed and the jurisdiction (state); examples include robbery, illegal drug use or sale, and battery

b. Certain violations of law may be considered both criminal and civil; for example, if a patient loses his or her life resulting from gross negligence of a dental hygienist, the estate of the deceased person could bring civil charges such as wrongful death against the hygienist, and the state may bring criminal action such as manslaughter against the hygienist
c. Level of proof—"beyond a reasonable doubt" required to determine innocence or guilt in a criminal case; the level of certainty a jury must have to find a defendant guilty of a crime

D. Primary individuals involved in a lawsuit
1. Plaintiff—party bringing the lawsuit
2. Defendant—party against whom the lawsuit is filed
3. Attorney—individual serving as an advocate for either the plaintiff or the defendant
4. Expert witness—explains specialized information to jurors; possesses appropriate credentials and expertise
5. Lay witness—testifies as to facts for judge and jury
6. Dental hygienist as a witness (lay or expert)
a. Expert qualifications based on education, licensure or certification, experience, and publications
b. Expertise to testify as to standard of care for dental hygiene
c. Familiarity with the state or provincial dental practice act
d. Knowledgeable about all records (written or electronic) relating to the controversy
e. Knowledge of office, agency, or institutional policy and procedure where (and at the time) the incident occurred
7. Cannot be lay witness if named in lawsuit

E. Due process and equal protection
1. Due process—protects the public from arbitrary actions of the state; the law must apply to all persons equally; elements of due process
a. The law, as applied, must be reasonable and definite
b. Fair procedures must be followed in enforcing the law; for example, the state may not arbitrarily take away a license to practice dental hygiene; the hygienist must first be given notice of the violation, a hearing, and an opportunity to respond before license revocation or suspension is imposed
2. Equal protection—equal protection clause of the Fourteenth Amendment to the U.S. Constitution protects individuals from state action; states may not enforce laws based solely on classification of persons such as race, age, gender, religion, national origin, or disability

F. Judicial process
1. Questions of law or fact—usually the jury determines what is fact from the evidence admitted by the court; the judge determines questions of law
2. Jurisdiction of the courts—authority of the court to determine the controversy; for example, the bankruptcy court may not hear divorce cases
3. State courts
a. Trial courts—courts with trial jurisdiction; usually handle cases such as traffic, probate, family matters, arraignments for felonies, small claims, juvenile, and criminal misdemeanors
b. Appellate courts—courts with trial, appellate, civil, and criminal jurisdiction; usually with a monetary restriction (plaintiff must request a fair minimum amount)
c. State supreme court—appellate jurisdiction only
4. Federal courts
a. Federal district courts—courts with trial jurisdiction; hear only matters that involve federal law or parties with diversity of citizenship (residents of different states)
b. U.S. Courts of Appeal—courts with appellate jurisdiction only
c. U.S. Supreme Court—court with appellate jurisdiction only; decisions cannot be overturned by any other court (state or federal); decisions can only be changed by new congressional legislation or subsequent Supreme Court decisions

G. Statute of limitations
1. Each state (or province) has a statute (law) that delineates specific periods within which a lawsuit must be filed after the event that caused the action; after that period, the right to initiate a lawsuit is lost
2. In tort actions, time may be measured from the time of the injury or harm or may be measured from when the plaintiff discovers the injury; periods vary from state to state

H. Case law—case law comprises the decisions, or the interpretations made by judges while deciding on the legal issues before them which are considered common law or as an aid for interpretation of a law in subsequent cases with similar conditions; case law is used by attorneys to support their views to favor their clients; it also influences the decisions of the judges; it is public record (occasionally court records are sealed)
1. Citations—references to legal authority that provide key information about the case; for example, in the following citation, *Edwards v Penn. Dental Examining Board,* 454, A2d 218 (1983): Edwards is the plaintiff (party bringing the lawsuit), the Dental Board is the defendant (party against whom the lawsuit is filed), 454 is the volume number of A2d (second series of the Atlantic Regional Reporter); 218 is the page number; and 1983 is the year the case was decided

## CIVIL LAW AND THE DENTAL HYGIENIST

A. A lawsuit can be filed against an oral health care provider in two areas of civil law:
1. Contract violation
2. Tort violation

B. Contract law[1]—a contract is an agreement between two or more consenting and competent parties to do or not to do a legal act for which sufficient consideration exists; breach of contract occurs if either party fails to comply with the terms of the contractual obligations

1. Two methods to create a contract:
   a. Implied contract through signs, inaction, or silence; also called *apparent*
   b. Express contract entered through oral or written communication
2. The contract exists between a patient and a health care provider when the patient agrees to a specific treatment
3. Contractual responsibilities of the provider to the patient
   a. Possess proper license and certification
   b. Exercise reasonable skill, care, and judgment in diagnosis and treatment
   c. Use standard drugs, materials, and techniques
   d. Complete the treatment in a reasonable time
   e. Never abandon the patient
   f. Complete procedures consented to by the patient
   g. Provide adequate instructions
   h. Refer appropriately
   i. Maintain confidentiality and patient privacy
   j. Maintain an appropriate level of knowledge and skill
   k. Practice within the scope of practice; never exceed the defined scope
   l. Maintain accurate records
   m. Comply with all laws regulating practice
   n. Practice in a manner consistent with a code of ethics
4. Contractual obligations of the patient
   a. Pay a reasonable fee in a reasonable time
   b. Cooperate in care
   c. Keep appointments
   d. Provide accurate history and information
   e. Follow instructions
   f. Keep the dental provider aware of status
   g. Follow home care instructions
5. Patient-practitioner relationship—contractual; both are free to enter or decline the relationship; a practitioner may decline to undertake treatment of a patient unless the practitioner has agreed to treat the patient by participating in a specific dental insurance plan or the practitioner is employed by another who makes treatment decisions; if the practitioner offers services to the public, he or she may not refuse to treat patients because of race, color, gender, religion, national origin, disability, or any other basis that would constitute invidious discrimination; being bound to the code of ethics assumes a preexisting relationship between the patient and practitioner
6. Termination of the patient-practitioner relationship may be by:
   a. The patient
   b. The practitioner, after giving the patient notice and an opportunity to secure an alternative source of future treatment
7. Abandonment[1]—failure of a health care professional to provide services after the professional has established a relationship with the patient; duty to the patient to complete all treatment started; patients may be dismissed from future treatment

C. Tort law[1]—deals with civil wrongs committed against a person or a person's property; wrongful conduct

1. Unintentional torts
   a. Negligence and malpractice
      (1) Negligence—failure to use such care as a reasonable person would use under similar circumstances
      (2) Malpractice—wrongful acts of professional persons; usually failure to meet the standard of care or failure to foresee consequences that one with his or her particular skills and education should foresee
   b. Elements of negligence or malpractice, which must be shown in order for a lawsuit to go forward
      (1) Duty owed to the patient (the plaintiff)
      (2) Breach of the duty by the professional or the defendant
      (3) Harm to the patient (the plaintiff)
      (4) Causation—harm must be caused by breach of duty; foreseeability, that is, the event may reasonably be expected to cause the result
   c. Standard of care—the degree of care that a reasonably prudent professional should exercise; minimum requirements of acceptable patient care; for example, practicing within the rules and regulations of the state or provincial dental practice act
   d. Damages (awarded to the defendant; to restore injured party)
      (1) Special damages—actual expenses
      (2) Nominal damages—at the court's discretion (could be $1)
      (3) General damages—part of harm; difficult to determine (e.g., can include pain and suffering)
      (4) Contract damages—for breach of contract
      (5) Punitive damages—to punish deliberately wrongful conduct (usually not covered by liability insurance)
      (6) States may place a cap on the maximum allowable damages that can be paid
   e. *Res ipsa loquitur*[1] (Latin, meaning "the thing speaks for itself")—legal doctrine that permits the plaintiff to prove negligence or malpractice without proving fault; no expert testimony required if the plaintiff shows a particular result occurred and would not have occurred except for someone's negligence
      (1) The type of injury does not occur unless negligence has occurred
      (2) The injury is caused by something or someone under exclusive control of defendant
      (3) The injury was not caused by plaintiff by contributing to own injury in any manner (no contributory negligence)
   f. Defenses to unintentional torts (protect defendant from liability)—not limited to, but include:
      (1) Statute of limitations—time limit for initiating lawsuit has passed
      (2) Comparative or contributory negligence—injured party is held responsible for a portion or all of the injury (states or provinces differ regarding degree of responsibility)

(3) Release—signed during the settlement of claim to prevent future claims
(4) Immunity—protection from prosecution; for example, the action may fall within a state's Good Samaritan law
(5) Defense of fact—no causation exists

2. Intentional tort—an act must be willful; the defendant must have intended to cause the harm or injury; the act must have been a substantial factor in bringing about the injury
   a. Assault—any action that places one in fear of bodily harm (e.g., threatening behaviors)
   b. Battery—intentional infliction of offensive or harmful bodily contact; unwanted touching
   c. Defamation—communication to a third person of an untrue statement about another person
      (1) Libel—written defamation (e.g., untrue or unflattering statement entered into a patient's record)
      (2) Slander—spoken defamation (e.g., discussing an employer in a derogatory manner while dining in a restaurant and being overheard by a third person)
   d. Invasion of privacy—protects one's right to privacy
      (1) Intrusion on seclusion—invasion of a private place or affairs of another; must be highly offensive to a reasonable person
      (2) Appropriation—use of another's name or likeness for financial gain (e.g., unauthorized photographs of dental patients used in a research article or textbook)
      (3) Publicity of private life—publicizing details of another person's private life; must be highly offensive to a reasonable person; health care professionals must not disclose a patient's information without written authorization (e.g., no disclosure of patient information over the phone or via email or to patient's relatives, including spouse or friends)
      (4) False light—putting another person before the public eye in a false light; highly offensive to a reasonable person
   e. Infliction of mental distress—outrageous conduct that causes emotional distress; behavior must be beyond standards of rudeness; behavior was intended to cause mental distress and actually did cause mental distress (e.g., publicly revealing patient's nonpayment; notifying neighbors or relatives of nonpayment)
   f. Fraud or intentional misrepresentation—intentional perversion of truth (misrepresentation) for the purpose of gaining another person's trust and reliance whereby that person suffers harm or loss as a result of trusting and relying (e.g., never guarantee treatment outcomes)
   g. Interference with advantageous relations—generally prevents an individual from interfering with the gainful employment of another; name and definitions may vary from state to state; giving a former employee a poor reference is not a basis for this tort
   h. Wrongful discharge—illegal termination of an employee; most dental hygienists are hired without employment contracts and are employees-at-will; they can be fired for any reason except:
      (1) If reason for firing was against federal and/or state anti-discrimination laws (e.g., pregnancy of employee)
      (2) If firing is against public policy (e.g., sexual harassment or "whistleblower" cases)
      (3) Office policy and procedures (oral and written) may be considered an implied employment contract (e.g., office manual must address the issue in controversy)
   i. Defenses against intentional torts are not limited to, but include:
      (1) Statute of limitations—whether the time limit for initiating lawsuit has passed
      (2) Privilege—person making the statement has the duty to do so; for example, dental hygienists are often required by state law to report cases of suspected child abuse; in that case, they are not held legally liable for doing so
      (3) Disclosure statutes (state and federal)—permit access to patient records by specific individuals or agencies without patient consent (e.g., workers' compensation statutes allow for such access to patient information if a claim is filed)
      (4) Consent—oral, implied by law (e.g., during emergencies, when a patient is not capable of consent) or apparent (e.g., patient sits in dental chair and opens mouth for an examination)
      (5) Self-defense or defense of others—behavior is justified to protect self or others from harm; if force is necessary, one may use only the amount of force necessary for protection (reasonable force)
      (6) Necessity—allows personal property to be confiscated (e.g., weapon)

3. Informed consent—from concept of battery and individual rights to make choices regarding own body
   a. Content—legal requirements vary from state to state; in general, a patient must have information that a reasonable person would find material in making a decision regarding treatment
   b. Patient should be told in a language or format that the patient can understand
   c. Specifically, patient must be informed of:
      (1) Diagnosis
      (2) Proposed treatment and benefits
      (3) Risks regarding proposed treatment and chances of success
      (4) Alternative forms of treatment; and benefits; risks associated with the alternatives offered
      (5) Prognosis if treatment is refused
      (6) Provided with an opportunity to ask questions
      (7) Needs to sign a consent form indicating that the patient fully understands the information provided (minimum to no technical language on form, or explanation provided if technical language is used)

d. Competency of consent
   (1) Patient must be of legal age and mentally competent (able to understand material facts)
   (2) Consent must be based on knowledge and understanding and voluntary (cannot force someone to consent to a procedure)
   (3) Minors and incompetent adults
      (a) Parents or legal guardian must sign for a child; children of divorced parents may have specific requirements for consent related to divorce decree
      (b) Emancipated minor (individual is not a legal adult; most states define adult as 18 years or older) may sign for themselves; teenager can obtain emancipation by:
         [1] Proving independence from parental control to the court; legal process involved
         [2] Being legally married
         [3] Enlisting in one of the U.S. Armed Forces
      (c) Legal guardians or health care decision maker must sign for incompetent adults

e. Informed refusal[2,3]—patient may refuse treatment; to refuse
   (1) Patient must be provided with same type information as provided informed consent; include general and oral health risks
   (2) Documentation of refusal, including information provided to patient, must be placed in the patient's record
   (3) Patient, operator, and witness signature recommended

D. Dental practice acts
1. Statutes regulating the dental professions; in all legal jurisdictions (e.g., states and the District of Columbia or provinces)
2. Enacted by state or provincial legislature; grant authority to a board of dentistry (board of dental examiners or other administrative agency) to adopt rules and regulations for dentistry, dental hygiene, and dental assisting and for dental laboratory technologists and denturists
   a. Rules and regulations must be consistent with the statute
   b. A board may not waive provisions unless specifically authorized to do so by statute
3. Practice acts are enacted to protect the public; boards of dentistry or other agencies grant licenses to individuals to engage in a specific profession after demonstrating a minimal level of competence to perform the responsibilities required of the profession
4. Composition of dental boards—usually elected or appointed officials
   a. Dentists
   b. Dental hygienists
   c. Consumers
   d. Others (e.g., lawyers, dental assistants, denturists)
5. Board duties
   a. Regulate applications for licensure
   b. Implement mechanisms for measuring competence of applicants, that is, credentials, examinations, mandatory continuing education or other certifications
   c. Implement mechanisms for investigating complaints made against practitioners
   d. Grant and revoke licenses
   e. Draft laws pertaining to the dental professions for the legislature
   f. Design rules and regulations pertaining to the dental professions
   g. Monitor educational standards
   h. Monitor other procedures related to licensure (e.g., licensure renewal, continuing education requirements)
6. Elements of dental practice act (vary from jurisdiction to jurisdiction)
   a. Requirements for licensure and renewal to show minimum competence
      (1) Minimum age and education
      (2) Character references
      (3) Examinations (regional, written) required
      (4) Continuing education requirements for relicensure
      (5) Evidence of specific requirements (e.g., current CPR certification)
      (6) Exemptions—"grandfather" clauses (e.g., licensure of dental hygienists trained in jurisdictions where preceptorship is legal)
      (7) Provisions for licensure across jurisdictions
         (a) Reciprocity—agreements between states for recognition of licensure from another state
         (b) Endorsement—granting of licensure if the applicant is licensed in another state and can present specific documents or credentials, and the states' requirements were the same or similar
         (c) Licensure by examination—when no reciprocity or endorsement is granted by states
         (d) Licensure by waiver—when a step toward licensure can be omitted (e.g., waiver of the clinical examination requirement)
      (8) Disciplinary action—boards have this authority with the power to enforce licensure requirements
         (a) License revocation or refusal to renew
         (b) License suspension
         (c) Probation
         (d) Reprimand—public or private
   b. Requirements for practice—defines scope of practice, that is, legally permissible tasks or procedures
      (1) List regulations—many states have a list of legal tasks delegated to dental hygienists
      (2) Open provision—some states have a general statement of what cannot be delegated; tasks delegated are at the discretion of the supervising dentist
   c. Legally problematic areas (scope of practice)

(1) If a negligent act presents a scope-of-practice issue, a dental hygienist's actions should be within the scope of practice for the particular jurisdiction; procedures billed to the insurance company must be performed by the appropriately licensed professional, or the state insurance board also could take action
(2) When the standard of care changes or increases because of the type of procedure performed or the addition of a legally recognized duty; for example, a dental hygienist administering a local anesthetic agent would be held to the same standard of care as a comparably trained professional such as a dentist
(3) When issues arise relating to use of new technology that may not yet be addressed in the dental practice act (e.g., use of lasers to fuse deep pits and fissures)
(4) Wide variations exist from state to state in the scope of dental hygiene practice; for example, practicing in a new jurisdiction where the dental practice act is more restrictive does not always allow the dental hygienist to deliver the treatment he or she was trained to perform or is competent to provide in another jurisdiction

d. Supervision (varies from state to state, and province to province)
(1) General supervision and assignment—licensed dentist authorizes the procedures on the basis of his or her diagnosis and treatment plan; need not be physically present when procedures are performed; some states require that the dentist or a designated dentist be available for consultation, if needed
(2) Indirect or close supervision—licensed dentist authorizes procedures and remains in dental facility while procedures are being performed
(3) Direct and immediate supervision—licensed dentist diagnoses the condition to be treated, authorizes procedures to be performed, and remains on premises while treatment is being performed, before the patient is dismissed; some states do not require a dentist to approve the work before dismissal
(4) Personal supervision—licensed dentist provides a service for a patient and authorizes an auxiliary to aid treatment by concurrently performing supportive procedures
(5) Unsupervised practice—services may be performed by a licensed dental hygienist without the supervision of a licensed dentist
(6) States are diverse in requirements for dental hygienists
(a) Forty-seven states allow general supervision, which does not require that a dentist be physically present during traditional dental hygiene procedures in offices
(b) Forty-two states allow direct access, which means that the dental hygienist can initiate treatment on the basis of his or her assessment of a patient's needs without the specific authorization of a dentist to treat the patient and without the presence of a dentist and can maintain a provider-patient relationship (Box 22.1 and Fig. 22.2)
(c) Forty-five states permit dental hygienists to administer a local anesthetic agent (Table 22.2 and Fig. 22.3); all states except Oregon require the administration of a local anesthetic agent to be completed under direct supervision
(d) Thirty-three states and Washington D.C. permit dental hygienists to administer nitrous oxide–oxygen ($N_2O$-$O_2$) analgesia (Fig. 22.4)
(e) Thirty-eight states allow dental hygienists to perform some types of restorative procedures (Table 22.3)

7. State dental hygiene committee
   a. Nineteen states have dental hygiene committees. One state has a dental hygiene board.
   b. These agencies assist in varying degrees in the regulation of dental hygiene practice (Box 22.2)
8. Alabama dental hygiene practice and education
   a. The state practice act allows only direct supervision of dental hygienists
   b. Prohibits performance of restorative functions by dental hygienists
   c. Prohibits administration of $N_2O$-$O_2$ analgesia by a dental hygienist
   d. Has unique educational and licensing procedures for dental hygienists
      (1) Alabama Dental Hygiene Program, since 1919
      (2) Only such preceptorship program in the United States
      (3) Eligibility—1-year employment as a dental assistant, followed by an educational program that includes basic science and clinical theory
      (4) Dentists are "preceptors," who provide on-the-job training in the dental office
      (5) Program replaces formal dental hygiene education from an accredited academic program; graduates are not eligible to take the National Board Dental Hygiene Examination; therefore, their practice is limited to Alabama
      (6) Graduates are not eligible for membership in the American Dental Hygienists Association
9. Updating dental practice acts
   a. Revision or amendments made by state legislatures
   b. Sunset laws—set review of the entire act at a fixed interval (e.g., every 7 years, to keep act updated and relevant to society); if not completed by legislature by designated date or if found to no longer serve its function to society, the act will automatically expire (thus the term *sunset*)

## BOX 22.1 Direct Access States

From the American Dental Hygienists Association, 2020. https://www.adha.org/resources-docs/7513_Direct_Access_to_Care_from_DH.pdf

The American Dental Hygienists' Association (ADHA) defines direct access as the ability of a dental hygienist to initiate treatment based on their assessment of a patient's needs without the specific authorization of a dentist, treat the patient without the presence of a dentist, and maintain a provider-patient relationship (ADHA Policy Manual, 13-15).

**Alaska 2008**
***Sec. 08.32.115***
*Collaborative Agreement:*

Dental hygienist may provide services according to the terms of a collaborative agreement. The dentist's presence, diagnosis or treatment plan are not required unless specified by agreement. Care under the agreement can be provided in settings outside of the "usual place of practice" (i.e. private dental office).

*Requirements:* Dental hygienist must have minimum of 4,000 hours of clinical experience within preceding 5 years. Agreement must be approved by state board of dental examiners. Dentists are limited to 5 or fewer collaborative agreements.

*Provider Services:* Agreement can authorize nearly the entire dental hygiene scope of practice (patient education, prophylaxis, sealants, radiographs, etc.).

**Arizona 2004/2015/ 2019**
***Sec. 32-1281, 32-1289***
*Affiliated Practice Agreement:*

Dental hygienist with a written affiliated practice agreement may perform dental hygiene services in specified settings outside the private dental office. The written agreement must be submitted to state board of dental examiners. The affiliated practice dental hygienist shall consult with the affiliated practice dentist before initiating further treatment on patients who have not been seen by a dentist within 12 months of the initial treatment by the dental hygienist.

*Requirements:* Dental hygienist must have held an active license for at least 5 years and be actively engaged in dental hygiene practice for at least five hundred hours in each of the 2 years immediately preceding the affiliated practice relationship. Alternatively, dental hygienist who holds a bachelor's degree in dental hygiene, an active license for at least 3 years and is actively engaged in dental hygiene practice for at least 500 hours in each of the 2 years preceding the affiliated practice relationship, may also quality for affiliated practice. In addition, dental hygienist must successfully complete 12 hours of specified continuing education that hold a current certificate in basic cardiopulmonary resuscitation.

*Provider Services:* The agreement must outline practice settings and services provided. The full dental hygiene scope is permitted with the exception of root planing, nitrous oxide and the use of local anesthesia unless under specified circumstances. After taking an accredited course and exam the dental hygienist will also be able to: place, contour and finish restorations, cement prefabricated crowns and place interim therapeutic restorations.

**Arizona 2006**
***Sec. 32-1289***

Dental hygienist employed by or working under contract or as a volunteer for a public health agency or institution or a public or private school authority before an examination by a dentist may screen patients and apply topical fluoride without entering into an affiliated practice relationship pursuant to this section.

**Arkansas 2010**
***Sec. 17-82-7***
*Collaborative Agreement:*

Dental hygienist with a Collaborative Care permit I or II who has entered into a collaborative agreement may perform dental hygiene services on children, senior citizens age 65 and older, and persons with developmental disabilities in long-term care facilities, free clinics, hospitals, head start programs, residence of homebound patients, local health units, schools, community health centers, state and county correctional institutions. Dental hygienist must have written agreement with no more than one dentist.

*Requirements*: Must have malpractice insurance. Collaborative Care Permit I: Dental hygienist must have 1,200 hours of clinical practice experience, or have taught dental hygiene courses for 2 of the proceeding 3 years. Collaborative Care Permit II: Dental hygienist must have 1,800 hours of clinical practice experience or taught dental hygiene courses for 2 of the proceeding 3 years and has completed 6 hours of continued education courses.

*Provider Services:* Collaborative Care Permit I may provide prophylaxis, fluoride treatments, sealants, dental hygiene instruction, assessment and other services in scope if delegated by consulting dentist to children in public settings without supervision or prior examination.

Collaborative Care Permit II may provide prophylaxis, fluoride treatments, sealants, dental hygiene instruction, assessment, and other services in scope if delegated by the consulting dentist to children, senior citizens, and persons with developmental disabilities in public settings without supervision or prior examination.

**California 1998**
***Sec. 1922-1931***
*Registered Dental Hygienist in Alternative Practice (RDHAP):*

RDHAP may provide services to a patient without obtaining written verification that the patient has been examined by a dentist or physician. If the RDHAP provides services to a patient 18 months or more after the first date that he or she provides services, the RDHAP shall obtain written verification that the patient has been examined by a dentist or physician.

Once licensed, the RDHAP may practice as: an employee of a dentist; an employee of another RDHAP; as an independent contractor; as a sole proprietor of an alternative dental hygiene practice; as an employee of a primary care clinic or specialty clinic; as an employee of a clinic owned or operated by a public hospital or health system; or as an employee of a clinic owned and operated by a hospital that maintains the primary contract with a county under the California welfare code. Allowed practice settings include: residences of the homebound; schools; residential facilities and other institutions; hospitals; or dental health professional shortage areas.

*Requirements:* Must hold a current and active California license as a dental hygienist; have been engaged in clinical practice as a dental hygienist for a minimum of 2,000 hours during the immediately preceding 36 months (in California or another state); possess a bachelor's degree or an equivalent of 120 semester units; complete 150 hours of an approved educational RDHAP program; and pass a written examination.

*Provider Services:* All services permitted under general supervision, including prophylaxis, root planing, pit and fissure sealants, charting and examination of soft tissue.

**California 2002**
***Sec. 1911***

Dental hygienist may provide screening, apply fluorides and sealants without supervision in government created or administered public health programs.

**Colorado 1987**
***Sec. 12-35-124***
*Unsupervised Practice:*

There is no requirement that a dentist must authorize or supervise most dental hygiene services. Dental hygienist may also own a dental hygiene practice.

*Requirements*: None.

## BOX 22.1 Direct Access States—cont'd

*Provider Services:* Dental hygienist can provide dental hygiene diagnosis, radiographs, remove deposits, accretions, and stains, curettage without anesthesia, apply fluorides and other recognized preventive agents, topical anesthetic, oral inspection and charting. Local anesthesia requires general supervision.

**Connecticut 1999**
***Sec. 20-126l***
*Public Health Dental Hygienist:*
Dental hygienist with 2 years of experience may practice without supervision in institutions, public health facilities, group homes and schools.

*Requirements:* Dental hygienist must have at least 2 years of experience.

*Provider Services:* Dental hygienist can provide oral prophylaxis, remove deposits, accretions and stains, root planing, sealants, assessment, treatment planning and evaluation.

**Florida 2011**
***Sec. 466.003, 466.024***
Dental hygienist may provide services without the physical presence, prior examination, or authorization of a dentist, provided that a dentist or physician gives medical clearance prior to performance of a prophylaxis in "health access settings." A dentist must examine a patient within 13 months following a prophylaxis and an exam must take place before additional oral services may be performed.

Health access settings are: a program of the Department of Children and Family Services, the Department of Health, the Department of Juvenile Justice, a nonprofit community health center centers, a Head Start centers, a federally-qualified health center, a school-based prevention program or a clinic operated by an accredited dental or dental hygiene program.

*Requirements:* Dental hygienist must maintain liability insurance.

*Provider Services:* Dental charting, take vital signs, record histories, apply sealants and fluorides (including varnish) and perform prophylaxis.

The setting operating the program may bill a third party for reimbursement.

**Georgia 2017**
***Article 3 of Chapter 11 of Title 43***
*General Supervision:*
The requirement of direct supervision shall not apply to the performance of licensed dental hygienists providing dental screenings in settings which include: schools, hospitals and clinics, state, county, local, and federal public health programs, federally qualified health centers, volunteer community health settings, senior centers, and family violence shelters.

*Requirements:* Dental hygienist shall have at least two years of experience in the practice of dental hygiene, shall be in compliance with continuing education and cardiopulmonary resuscitation certification requirements and shall be licensed in good standing.

*Provider Services:* Licensed dental hygienists may apply topical fluoride and perform the application of sealants and oral prophylaxis under general supervision in certain designated settings.

**Idaho 2004**
***Sec. 54-903, 54-904***
*Extended Access Endorsement (EAE):*
Dental hygienist can provide services in hospitals, long term care facilities, public health facilities, health or migrant clinics or other board-approved settings, if the dentist affiliated with authorizes services.

*Requirements:* Dental hygienist must be an employee of the facility or obtain extended care permit. EAE requires 1,000 hours experience in last 2 years.

*Provider Services:* As determined by authorizing dentist.

**Illinois 2015**
***225 ILCS 25/18.1***
*Public Health Dental Hygienist:*
A dental hygienist may treat patients in specified public health settings without a dentist first examining the patient and being present during treatment, who are Medicaid-eligible or uninsured and with household incomes not greater that 200% of the federal poverty level.

*Requirements:* A licensed dental hygienist must have 2 years of full-time clinical experience or an equivalent of 4,000 hours of clinical experience and have completed 42 hours of additional course work in areas specific to public health dentistry. The dental hygienist must also practice pursuant to a written public health supervision agreement with a dentist.

*Provider Services:* Dental hygienist may provide prophylactic cleanings, apply fluoride, place sealants, and take radiographs. Additional services may be prescribed by the Illinois Department of Financial and Professional Regulation.

**Indiana 2018**
*Sec. 1. IC 25-13-1-10 Access Practice Agreement:*
A dental hygienist may provide preventive dental hygiene services directly to a patient without a prior examination, presence, or authorization of a dentist. A dental hygienist may practice in any setting or facility that is documented in the dental hygienist's access practice agreement.

*Requirements:*
- Professional licensure
- Has at least 2,000 documented clinical hours of dental hygiene services during 2 years of active practice under the direct supervision of a dentist
- Obtains a national provider identifier number
- Enters into an access practice agreement with a licensed dentist
- Maintains liability insurance
- Before providing dental hygiene services to a patient under an access practice agreement, the dental hygienist has obtained a signed consent form

*Provider Services:* Dental hygienist may provide preventive dental hygiene services as outlined in the access practice agreement.

**Iowa 2004**
***Rule 650-10.5 (153)***
*Public Health Dental Hygienist:*
Dental hygienist may administer care based on standing orders and a written agreement with a dentist. Services can be administered in schools, Head Start settings, nursing facilities, federally-qualified health centers, public health vans, free clinics, community centers and public health programs.

*Requirements:* Dental hygienist must have 3 years of clinical experience and must submit an annual report to the state department of health noting the number of patients treated/services administered.

*Provider Services:* All services in the dental hygiene scope (except local anesthesia and nitrous) may be provided once to each patient. The supervising dentist must specify a period of time in which an examination by a dentist must occur prior to the dental hygienist rendering further dental hygiene services. However, this requirement does not apply to educational services, assessments, screenings and fluoride if specified in the supervision agreement.

**Kansas 2003/2012**
***Sec. 65-1456***
*Extended Care Permit I, II & III (ECP):*
Dental hygienist may practice without the prior authorization of a dentist if the dental hygienist has an agreement with sponsoring dentist. Examples of settings are schools, Head Start programs, state correctional institutions, local health departments, indigent care clinics, and in adult care homes, hospital long term units, or at the home of homebound persons on medical assistance. The ECP I permit authorizes treatment on children in various limited access categories,

*Continued*

## BOX 22.1 Direct Access States—cont'd

while the EPT II permit is for seniors and persons with developmental disabilities. ECP III permit authorizes dental hygienists to treat a wider range of patients, including underserved children, seniors and developmentally disabled adults and to provide more services than ECP I and II.

*Requirements:* Dental hygienist must have 1,200 clinical hours or 2 years teaching in last 3 years for ECP I; 1,600 hours or 2 years teaching in last 3 years plus 6 hour course for ECP II. Dental hygienist must also carry liability insurance and must be paid by dentist or facility. ECP III requires 2,000 hours clinical experience plus 18 clock hour board approved course. Dentist can monitor a maximum of 5 practices.

*Provider Services:* ECP I and II provide prophylaxis, fluoride treatments, dental hygiene instruction, assessment of the patient's need for further treatment by a dentist, and other services if delegated by the sponsoring dentist. ECP III can additionally provide atraumatic restorative technique, adjustment and soft reline of dentures, smoothing sharp tooth with handpiece, local anesthesia in setting where medical services available, extraction of mobile teeth.

**Kentucky 2010**
***Sec. 313.040***
***Volunteer Community Health Settings:***

A dental hygienist may provide the services listed below without the supervision of a dentist in volunteer community health settings.

*Provider Services:* Dental hygienist can provide dental hygiene instruction, nutritional counseling, oral screening with subsequent referral to a dentist, fluoride application, demonstration of oral hygiene technique, and sealants.

**Kentucky 2010**
***201 KAR 8:562***
***Public Health Dental Hygienist:***

A public health dental hygienist shall perform dental hygiene services under the supervision of the governing board of health. Settings are limited to local health departments, public or private educational institutions with affiliation agreement, contracted mobile dental health programs, and public or private institutions under the jurisdiction of a federal, state, or local agency.

*Requirements*: Dental hygienist must have 2 years and 3,000 hours of experience. During each renewal period, complete a 3 hour course approved by the board on the identification and prevention of potential medical emergencies, as well as 5 hours of other CE in area of public health or public dental health. A dental hygienist authorized to practice as a public health dental hygienist shall receive a certificate from the board indicating their registration. Prior to performing services, must receive informed consent from patient. The patient must be in the ASA Patient Physical Status Classification of ASA I or ASA II, meaning a normal healthy patient or a patient with mild systemic disease.

*Provider services*: Limited to preventative services.

**Maine 2001**
***Rule 02 313 Chap. 2. Sec. 3 Public Health Dental Hygienist:***

Dental hygienist may provide services in a public or private school, hospital or other nontraditional practice setting under a public health supervision status granted by the dental board on a case-by-case basis. The dental hygienist may perform services rendered under general supervision. The dentist should have specific standing orders and procedures to be carried out, although the dentist need not be present when the services have been provided.

A written plan for referral or an agreement for follow-up shall be provided by the public health hygienist recording all conditions that should be called to the attention of the dentist. The supervising dentist shall review a summary report at the completion of the program or once a year.

*Requirements*: A dental hygienist must apply to the board to practice providing such information the board deems necessary. The board must take into consideration whether the program will fulfill an unmet need, whether a supervising dentist is available and that the appropriate public health guidelines and standards of care can be met and followed.

*Provider Services:* All services that can be provided under general supervision. Dentist's diagnosis for sealants is not needed in public health or school sealant programs.

**Maine 2008/2015/2017**
***32 §18345 & 18375***
***Independent Practice Dental Hygienist:***

Independent practice dental hygienist means an individual licensed to practice independent dental hygiene without supervision of a dentist. However, a written practice agreement is required when engaging in the taking of dental radiographs pursuant to Chapter 16 of the Board's rules.

*Requirements*: Verification of 2,000 work hours of clinical practice. For purposes of meeting the clinical practice requirements, the applicant's hours in a private dental practice or nonprofit setting under the supervision of a dentist may be included as well as the applicant's hours as a public health dental hygienist or, prior to July 29, 2016, as a dental hygienist with public health supervision status.

*Provider Services:* An independent practice dental hygienist may perform only the following duties without supervision by a dentist:

- Interview patients and record complete medical and dental histories;
- Take and record the vital signs of blood pressure, pulse and temperature;
- Perform oral inspections, recording all conditions that should be called to the attention of a dentist;
- Perform complete periodontal and dental restorative charting;
- Perform all procedures necessary for a complete prophylaxis, including root planing;
- Apply fluoride to control caries;
- Apply desensitizing agents to teeth;
- Apply topical anesthetics;
- Apply sealants;
- Smooth and polish amalgam restorations, limited to slow-speed application only;
- Take impressions for athletic mouth guards and custom fluoride trays;
- Place and remove rubber dams;
- Place temporary restorations in compliance with the protocol adopted by the board;
- Apply topical antimicrobials, including fluoride but excluding antibiotics, for the purposes of bacterial reduction, caries control and desensitization in the oral cavity. The independent practice dental hygienist shall follow current manufacturer's instructions in the use of these medicaments;
- Expose and process radiographs, including but not limited to vertical and horizontal bitewing films, periapical films, panoramic images and full-mouth series, under protocols developed by the board as long as the independent practice dental hygienist has a written agreement with a licensed dentist that provides that the dentist is available to interpret all dental radiographs within 21 days from the date the radiograph is taken and that the dentist will sign a radiographic review and findings form; and
- Prescribe, dispense or administer anticavity toothpastes or topical gels with 1.1% or less sodium fluoride and oral rinses with 0.05%, 0.2%, 0.44% or 0.5% sodium fluoride, as well as chlorhexidine gluconate oral rinse. For the purposes of this paragraph, "topical" includes superficial and intraoral application.

**Maryland 2010/2014/2019 (effective 10/1/19)**
***Md. Health Occupations Code Ann. § 4-308 General Supervision:***

Dental hygienist may practice under the general supervision of a dentist in a nursing home, assisted living program, medical office, and a group home or adult day care center. A dental hygienist practicing under the general supervision of a licensed dentist in these facilities shall have a written agreement with the supervising dentist that clearly sets forth the terms and conditions under which the dental hygienist may practice.

## BOX 22.1 Direct Access States—cont'd

*Requirements:* Dental hygienist must hold an active license, hold a current certificate evidencing Health Care Provider Level C Proficiency, or its equivalent, in cardiopulmonary resuscitation, have at least 3,000 hours of active clinical practice in direct patient care, and ensure that the facility where the dental hygienist will practice under general supervision has:

- A written medical emergency plan in place;
- equipment, including portable equipment and appropriate armamentarium, available for the appropriate delivery of dental hygiene services, unless the dental hygienist provides the equipment; and
- Adequate safeguards to protect the patient's health and safety.

*Provider Services:* Initial appointment is limited to dental hygiene tasks and procedures including toothbrush prophylaxis, application of fluoride, dental hygiene instruction, full mouth debridement, and other duties as may be delegated, verbally or in writing, by the supervising dentist.

**Massachusetts 2009 Chap. 112, Sec. 51.**
***Public Health Dental Hygienist:***
Dental hygienist may provide services without the supervision of a dentist in public health settings including, and not limited to, hospitals, medical facilities, schools and community clinics. Prior to providing services, a public health dental hygienist must have a written collaborative agreement with a local or state government agency or institution, or licensed dentist that states the level of communication with the dental hygienist to ensure patient health and safety. Public health dental hygienists shall provide patients with a written referral to a dentist and an assessment of further dental needs.

*Requirements:* Dental hygienist must have at least 3 years of full-time clinical experience practicing in a public health setting and any other training deemed appropriate by the department of health.

*Provider Services:* Dental hygienist can provide full scope of dental hygiene practice services allowed under general supervision in the private office, including prophylaxis, root planing, curettage, sealants and fluoride.

**Michigan 2005**
***Sec. 333.16625***
*PA 161 Dental Hygienist:*
Dental hygienist with grantee status can practice in a public or nonprofit entity, or a school or nursing home that administers a program of dental care to a dentally underserved population. Collaborating dentist need not be present for or authorize treatment, but dental hygienist must have continuous availability of direct communication with a dentist to establish emergency protocol and review patient records.

*Requirements:* Dental hygienist must apply to the state department of community health for designation as grantee health agency.

*Provider Services:* Dental hygienist can provide full scope of dental hygiene services allowed under general supervision, including prophylaxis, sealants, and fluoride treatments.

**Minnesota 2001/2017**
***Sec. 150A. 10, Subd. 1a Collaborative Practice:***
A Collaborative practice dental hygienist may be employed or retained by a health care facility, program, or nonprofit organization to perform the dental hygiene services without the patient first being examined by a licensed dentist. Practice setting can be a hospital; nursing home; home health agency; group home serving the elderly, disabled, or juveniles; state-operated facility licensed by the commissioner of human services or the commissioner of corrections; and federal, state, or local public health facility, community clinic, tribal clinic, school authority, Head Start program, or nonprofit organization that serves individuals who are uninsured or who are Minnesota health care public program recipients

*Requirements:* Has entered into a collaborative agreement with a licensed dentist that designates authorization for the services provided by the dental hygienist and has documented completion of a course on medical emergencies within each continuing education cycle.

*Provider Services:*

- Complete prophylaxis to include scaling, root planing, and polishing of restorations;
- Preliminary charting of the oral cavity and surrounding structures to include case histories, perform initial and periodic examinations and assessments to determine periodontal status, and formulate a dental hygiene treatment plan in coordination with a dentist's treatment plan;
- Dietary analysis, salivary analysis, and preparation of smears for dental health purposes;
- Etch appropriate enamel surfaces, application and adjustment of pit and fissure sealants;
- Removal of excess bond material from orthodontic appliances;
- Replacement, cementation, and adjustment of intact temporary restorations extraorally or intraorally;
- Removal of marginal overhangs;
- Make referrals to dentists, physicians, and other practitioners in consultation with a dentist;
- Administer local anesthesia. Before administering local anesthesia, a dental hygienist must have successfully completed a didactic and clinical program sponsored by a dental or dental hygiene school accredited by the commission on dental accreditation, resulting in the dental hygienist becoming clinically competent in the administration of local anesthesia;
- Administer nitrous oxide inhalation analgesia; and
- Obtain informed consent, according for treatments authorized by the supervising dentist pursuant to the dental hygienist's scope of practice.

**Missouri 2001**
***Sec. 332.311.2***
*Public Health Dental Hygienist:*
Dental hygienist may provide services without supervision in public health settings to Medicaid-eligible children and can be directly reimbursed.

*Requirements:* Dental hygienist must have 3 years of experience.

*Provider Services:* Dental hygienist can provide oral prophylaxis, sealants and fluorides.

**Montana 2003/2017**
***Sec. 37-4-405***
*Public Health Dental Hygienist/Limited Access Permit (LAP):*
Public Health Supervision means the provision of limited dental hygiene preventative services without the prior authorization or presence of a licensed dentist in a public health facility which includes: federally qualified health centers; federally funded community health centers, migrant health care centers, or programs for health services for the homeless; nursing homes; extended care facilities; home health agencies; group homes for the elderly, disabled, and youth; head start programs; migrant worker facilities; local public health clinics and facilities; public institutions under the department of public health and human services; mobile public health clinics; and other public health facilities and programs identified by the Montana Dental Board.

*Requirements:* A dental hygienist practicing under public health supervision shall obtain a limited access permit from the board. The board shall issue a limited access permit (LAP) to a Montana licensed dental hygienist who:

- Possesses an active, unrestricted Montana dental hygiene license;
- Certifies that the dental hygienist has actively practiced either:
  - o 2400 clinical hours over the last three years; or
  - o A career total of 3000 hours, with a minimum of 350 hours in each of the last two years;
- Provides the name of the applicant's current liability insurance carrier, policy number, and expiration date;

Continued

## BOX 22.1 Direct Access States—cont'd

- Provides the name and address of the public health facility or facilities where the applicant intends to provide services under a LAP;
- Provides certificates of attendance of completion of 12 additional continuing education credits for the three-year cycle immediately preceding LAP application; and
- Submits a completed application and pays all appropriate fees.

*Provider Services:* A licensed dental hygienist practicing under public health supervision may provide dental hygiene preventative services that include removal of deposits and stains from the surfaces of teeth, the application of topical fluoride, polishing restorations, root planing, placing of sealants, oral cancer screening, exposing radiographs, and charting of services provided, and prescriptive authority limited to fluoride agents, topical oral anesthetic agents, and nonsystemic oral antimicrobials.

**Nebraska 2007**
***Sec. 38-1130***
***Public Health Dental Hygienist:***
The Department of Health may authorize an unsupervised dental hygienist to provide services in a public health setting or a health care or related facility.

*Requirements:* Dental hygienist must have 3,000 hours experience in at least 4 of last 5 years. Dental hygienist must also have professional liability insurance.

*Provider Services:* Dental hygienist can perform prophylaxis for a healthy child, pulp vitality testing and preventive measures including fluorides and sealants.

**New Hampshire 1993 Rule 302.02(d), 402.01(d) Public Health Supervision:**
Dental hygienist may treat patients in a school, hospital, institution or residence of a homebound patient. Supervising dentist must authorize dental hygienist to provide services but need not be present for care.

*Requirements*: None.

*Provider Services:* Dental hygienist can provide instruction in oral hygiene, topical fluorides, prophylaxis, assess medical/dental history, periodontal probing/charting, and sealants.

**New Hampshire 2012**
***Sec. 317-A:21-e***
***Certified Public Health Dental Hygienist:***
Dental hygienist may practice in a school, hospital, or other institution, or for a homebound person without the dentist having to be present, provided the dentist has reviewed the records once in a 12-month period. Dental Hygienists may perform any procedure that is within the scope of practice that has been authorized under public health supervision.

*Requirements:* Any dental hygienist shall be considered qualified as a certified public health dental hygienist after obtaining a bachelor's degree in dental hygiene with a minimum of 6 semester hours in community dental health; obtaining a master's degree in public health; or after successfully completing specified courses and successful completion of an examination by the course provider.

*Provider Services:* Dental hygienist can perform radiographic imaging limited to bite wings, and occlusal and periapical radiography and provide nutritional counseling for the control of dental disease.

**New Mexico 1999/2011**
***Sec. 16.5.17***
***Collaborative Practice:***
Dental hygienist can practice in any setting with collaborative agreement and can own or manage a collaborative dental hygiene practice. Dental hygienist must enter into a written agreement with one or more collaborative dentist(s) which must contain protocols for care. Dental hygienist must refer patients for annual dental exam.

*Requirements:* Dental hygienist must have 2,400 hours of active practice in preceding 18 months or 3,000 hours in 2 of the past 3 years. Dentists may not collaborate with more than 3 dental hygienists.

*Provider Services:* Collaborative practice dental hygienist can provide a dental hygiene assessment, radiographs, prophylaxis, fluoride treatments, assessment for and application of sealants, root planing, and may prescribe and administer and dispense topically applied fluoride and antimicrobials, depending on the specific services allowed in agreement with collaborating a dentist.

**New Mexico 2007**
***Sec. 61-5A-4-C***
No supervision required for any dental hygienist to apply topical fluorides and remineralization agents in public and community medical facilities, schools, hospitals, long-term care facilities and such other settings as the board may determine.

**New York 2005 Rules Sec. 61.9 General Supervision:**
General supervision means that a supervising dentist is available for consultation, diagnosis and evaluation, has authorized the dental hygienist to perform the services, and exercises that degree of supervision appropriate to the circumstances.

*Provider Services:* The following services may be performed under the general supervision of a licensed dentist:

- Removing calcareous deposits, accretions and stains, including scaling and planing of exposed root surfaces indicated for a complete prophylaxis;
- Applying topical agents indicated for a complete dental prophylaxis;
- Removing excess cement from surfaces of the teeth;
- Providing patient education and counseling relating to the improvement of oral health;
- Taking and exposing dental radiographs;
- Performing topical anticariogenic agent applications, including but not limited to topical fluoride applications, and performing topical anesthetic applications;
- Polishing teeth, including existing restorations;
- Taking and assessing medical history including the measuring and recording of vital signs as an aid to diagnosis by the dentist and to assist the dental hygienist in providing dental hygiene services;
- Performing dental and/or periodontal assessments as an aid to diagnosis by the dentist and to assist the dental hygienist in providing dental hygiene services;
- Applying pit and fissure sealants;
- Applying desensitizing agents to the teeth;
- Placing and removing temporary restorations;
- Making assessments of the oral and maxillofacial area as an aid to diagnosis by the dentist;
- Taking impressions for study casts. Study casts shall mean only such casts as will be used for purposes of diagnosis and treatment planning by the dentist and for the purposes of patient education; and Providing dental health care case management and care coordination services.

**New York 2013**
***Sec. 6606***
***Collaborative Practice:***
A collaborative arrangement is an agreement between a registered dental hygienist working for a hospital and a licensed and registered dentist who has a formal relationship with the same hospital.

*Requirements:* A registered dental hygienist providing services pursuant to a collaborative arrangement shall:

- Only provide those services that may be provided under general supervision as specified in subdivision (b) of this section, provided that the physical presence of the collaborating dentist is not required for the provision of such services;
- Instruct individuals to visit a licensed dentist for comprehensive examination or treatment;

## BOX 22.1 Direct Access States—cont'd

- Possess and maintain certification in cardiopulmonary resuscitation in accordance with the requirements for dentists set forth in section 61.19 of this part and the following:
  - At the time of his or her registration renewal, the dental hygienist shall attest to having met the cardiopulmonary resuscitation requirement or attest to meeting the requirements for exemption as defined in clause (b) of this subparagraph.
  - A dental hygienist may be granted an exemption to the cardiopulmonary resuscitation requirement if he or she is physically incapable of complying with the requirements of this subparagraph. Documentation of such incapacity shall include a written statement by a licensed physician describing the dental hygienist's physical incapacity. The dental hygienist shall also submit an application to the department for exemption which verifies that another individual will maintain certification and be present at the location where the dental hygienist provides dental hygiene services, pursuant to a collaborative arrangement, while the dental hygienist is treating patients.
  - Each dental hygienist shall maintain for review by the department records of compliance with the cardiopulmonary resuscitation certification requirement, including the dental hygienist's cardiopulmonary resuscitation certification card; and
- Provide collaborative services only pursuant to a written agreement that is maintained in the practice setting of the dental hygienist and collaborating dentist.

*Provider Services:* The following services may be performed pursuant to a collaborative arrangement:

- Removing calcareous deposits, accretions and stains, including scaling and planing of exposed root surfaces indicated for a complete prophylaxis;
- Applying topical agents indicated for a complete dental prophylaxis;
- Removing excess cement from surfaces of the teeth;
- Providing patient education and counseling relating to the improvement of oral health;
- Taking and exposing dental radiographs;
- Performing topical anticariogenic agent applications, including but not limited to topical fluoride applications, and performing topical anesthetic applications;
- Polishing teeth, including existing restorations;
- Taking and assessing medical history including the measuring and recording of vital signs as an aid to diagnosis by the dentist and to assist the dental hygienist in providing dental hygiene services;
- Performing dental and/or periodontal assessments as an aid to diagnosis by the dentist and to assist the dental hygienist in providing dental hygiene services;
- Applying pit and fissure sealants;
- Applying desensitizing agents to the teeth;
- Placing and removing temporary restorations;
- Making assessments of the oral and maxillofacial area as an aid to diagnosis by the dentist;
- Taking impressions for study casts. Study casts shall mean only such casts as will be used for purposes of diagnosis and treatment planning by the dentist and for the purposes of patient education; and Providing dental health care case management and care coordination services.

### Nevada 1998

***Sec. 631.287***

***Public Health Dental Hygienist:***

Dental hygienist may obtain approval to work as public health dental hygienists in schools, community centers, hospitals, nursing homes and such other locations as the state dental health officer deems appropriate without supervision.

*Requirements*: Special endorsement from the dental board. Submissions of protocol to describe the methods a dental hygienist will use to provide services.

*Provider Services:* May provide most hygiene services and may administer local anesthesia and nitrous oxide in a facility with certain equipment and dentist authorization.

### Ohio 2010/2014/2017

***Sec. 4715.363***

***Oral Health Access Supervision Permit Program:***

Dental hygienist who possess an oral health access supervision permit may provide dental hygiene services through a written agreement with a dentist in public health settings including, and not limited to a health care facility, state correctional institution, residential facility, school, shelter for victims of domestic abuse or runaways, foster home, non-profit clinic, dispensary or mobile dental clinic.

Prior to providing services, a dental hygienist with an oral health access supervision permit must have a written agreement with a dentist, who possesses an oral health supervision permit, that states the dentist has evaluated the dental hygienist's skills and the dentist has reviewed and evaluated the patient's health history. The dentist need not be present or examine the patient before the dental hygienist may provide care. The collaborating dentist must perform a clinical evaluation of the patient before the dental hygienist may provide subsequent care. The evaluation may be done using electronic communication.

*Requirements:* One year and a minimum of 1,500 hours of clinical experience, minimum of 24 continuing education credits during the two years prior to apply for the oral health access supervision permit including an eight hour course as required by the board.

*Provider Services:* Prophylactic, preventive and other procedures a dentist can delegate to a dental hygienist except definitive root planing, definitive subgingival curettage, administration of local anesthesia and other procedures specified in rules adopted by the board.

### Ohio 2013

***Sec. 4715.22***

The requirement for a dentist to perform an examination and diagnose a patient prior to the patient receiving dental hygiene services through a program operated by a school district or other specified entity does not apply when the only services to be provided are the placement of pit and fissure sealants.

### Oklahoma 2003

***Sec. 328.34***

***General Supervision:***

Dental hygienist may provide services outside of the private dental office for a patient not examined by the dentist. Dentist must authorize care in writing.

*Requirements:* Dental hygienist must have at least 2 years of experience.

*Provider Services:* Most dental hygiene services, including sealants, fluorides, and prophylaxis, to a patient one time prior to a dental exam.

### Oregon 1997

***Sec. 680.200, Rule 818-035-0065 Limited Access Permit (LAP):***

Dental hygienists who have obtained a limited access permit (LAP) may initiate unsupervised services for patients in a variety of limited access settings such as extended care facilities, facilities for the mentally ill or disabled, correctional facilities, schools and preschools, medical offices or offices operated or staffed by a nurse practitioner midwives or physicians assistants, and job training centers. Dental hygienist must refer the patient annually to a licensed dentist available to treat the patient.

*Requirements:* Dental hygienist must have 2,500 hours of supervised dental hygiene practice and complete 40 hours of board-approved courses in an accredited dental hygiene program or completed a course of study approved by the board that includes at least 500 hours of dental hygiene practice on limited access patients while under direct faculty supervision. Dental hygienist must also have liability insurance.

Continued

## BOX 22.1 Direct Access States—cont'd

*Provider Services:* LAP dental hygienists can provide all dental hygiene services, except several (local anesthesia, pit and fissure sealants, denture relines, temporary restorations, radiographs and nitrous oxide) which must be supervised by a dentist. Dental hygienist may prescribe fluorides and assess the need for sealants.

**Oregon 2011 Sec. 680.205**
***Expanded Practice Dental Hygienist (EPDH)***
Replaces Limited Access Permit. Adds services to patients below federal poverty level and other settings approved by the board to EPDH practice settings. Adds limited prescriptive authority, local anesthesia, temporary restorations and dental assessments to unsupervised EPDH scope if EPDH has agreement with a dentist. Requires insurance reimbursement of EPDHs.

**Pennsylvania 2007**
***Sec. 2 (Definitions), Sec. 11.9***
*Public Health Dental Hygiene Practitioner:*
Dental hygienists who are certified as public health dental hygiene practitioners may provide care in a variety of public health settings without the supervision or prior authorization of a dentist.

*Requirements:* Dental hygienist must have 3,600 hours experience and liability insurance. Dental hygienist must also complete 5 hours of continuing education in public health during each licensure period.

*Provider Services:* Dental hygienist may perform educational, preventive, therapeutic and intra-oral procedures which the hygienist is educated to perform and which require the hygienist's professional competence and skill.

**Rhode Island 2006 Sec. 5-31.1-6.1 General Supervision:**
Dental hygienists working under a dentist's general supervision can initiate dental hygiene treatment to residents of nursing facilities. Dental hygienists working in nursing facilities can treat patients, regardless of whether or not the patient is a patient of record, as long as documentation of services administered is maintained and necessary referrals for follow-up treatment are made.

*Requirements*: None.

*Provider Services:* Dental hygienist can initiate dental hygiene services, including oral health screening assessments, prophylaxis, fluoride treatments, charting, and other duties delegable under general supervision.

**Rhode Island 2015**
***Sec. 5-31.1-39***
*Public Health Hygienists:*
Any public health dental hygienist may perform dental hygiene procedures in a public health setting, without the immediate or direct supervision or direction of a dentist. Public health settings includes, but are not limited to, residences of the homebound, schools, nursing home and long-term care facilities, clinics, hospitals, medical facilities or community health centers.

*Requirements:* A public health dental hygienist shall enter into a written collaborative agreement with a local or state government agency or institution or with a licensed dentist. Any public health dental hygienist shall provide to the patient or to the patient's legal guardian a consent form to be signed by the patient or legal guardian. The consent form shall also inform the patient or legal guardian that the patient should obtain a dental examination by a dentist within ninety days after undergoing a procedure.

*Provider Services:* Any procedure or service that is within the dental hygiene scope of practice that has been authorized and adopted by board as a delegable procedure for a dental hygienist under general supervision in a private practice setting.

**South Carolina 2003**
***Sec. 40-15-110 (A) (10) General Supervision:***
Dental hygienist employed by, or contacted through, the Department of Health and Environment Control may provide services under general supervision that does not require prior examination by a dentist in settings such as schools or nursing homes.

*Requirements:* Dental hygienist must carry professional liability insurance.

*Provider Services:* Dental hygienist employed by, or contacted through, the Department of Health and Environment Control may provide prophylaxis, fluorides, and sealants.

**South Dakota 2011**
***Rules 20:43:10***
Dental hygienist may provide preventive and therapeutic services under collaborative supervision of a dentist in a school, nursing facility, Head Start program, non-profit mobile dental clinic, community health center or government program.

*Requirements:* Dental hygienist must possess a license to practice in the state and have 3 years of clinical practice in dental hygiene and a minimum of 4,000 practice hours. A minimum of 2,000 of those hours must have been completed within 2 of the 3 years preceding application. Dental hygienist must have a written collaborative agreement with a dentist and satisfactorily demonstrate knowledge of medical and dental emergencies and their management, infection control, pharmacology, disease transmission, management of early childhood caries and management of special needs population.

*Provider Services*: Any services that can be provided under general supervision.

**Tennessee 2013**
***Sec. 63-5-109***
Dental hygienist may apply dental sealants or topical fluoride to the teeth of individuals in a setting under the direction of a state or local health department, without requiring an evaluation by a dentist prior to such application, under a protocol established by the state or a metropolitan health department.

**Texas 2001**
***Sec. 262.1515 General Supervision:***
Dental hygienist may provide services for up to 6 months without dentist seeing the patient. Services may be performed in school-based health center, nursing facility or community health center. Dental hygienist must refer the patient to a dentist following treatment and may not perform a second set of services until the patient has been examined by a dentist.

*Requirements:* Dental hygienist must have at least 2 years of experience.

*Provider Services:* No limitations. Dentist must authorize services in writing.

**Utah 2015**
***Sec. 58-69-801***
*Public Health Dental Hygienist:*
A dental hygienist may treat patients in specified public health settings pursuant to a written agreement with a dentist. The settings include a homebound patient's residence, a school, a nursing home, an assisted living facility, a community health center, a federally qualified health center and a mobile dental health program that employees a dentist.

*Requirements:* Must be a licensed Utah dental hygienist and have a written agreement with a collaborating dentist. The agreement provides that the dental hygienist shall refer a patient with a dental need beyond the dental hygienist's scope of practice to a dentist. Each patient must complete an informed consent form that provides that treatment by a dental hygienist is not a substitute for a dental examination by a dentist.

*Provider Services:* All general supervision preventive functions in scope of practice. Local anesthesia and nitrous oxide administration are not permitted.

**Vermont 2008/2019**
***§ 582 & 624***
*Public-Health Hygienists:*
Dental hygienist may provide services in out-of-office settings under general supervision agreement with a dentist, including residences, schools, nursing

## BOX 22.1 Direct Access States—cont'd

home and long-term care facilities, clinics, hospitals, medical facilities, community health centers licensed or approved by the Department of Health, Head Start programs, and other locations deemed appropriate. The agreement authorizes the dental hygienist to provide services, agreed to between the dentist and the dental hygienist. The agreement does not require physical presence of the dentist but it stipulates that the supervising dentist review all patient records.

*Requirements:* Dental hygienist must have 3 years licensed clinical practice experience.

*Provider Services:* Dental hygienist can provide sealants, fluoride varnish, prophylaxis and radiographs. Periodontal maintenance is allowable to patients with mild periodontitis.

### Virginia 2009/2016/2017/2019

***Sec. 54.1-2722 Remote Supervision:***

Remote Supervision means that a supervising dentist is accessible and available for communication and consultation with a dental hygienist during the delivery of dental hygiene services, but such dentist may not have conducted an initial examination of the patients who are to be seen and treated by the dental hygienist and may not be present with the dental hygienist when dental hygiene services are being provided.

*Requirements:* Complete a continuing education course designed to develop the competencies needed to provide care under remote supervision offered by an accredited dental education program or from a continuing education provider approved by the Board and have at least two years of clinical experience, consisting of at least 2,500 hours of clinical experience. A dental hygienist practicing under remote supervision shall have professional liability insurance with policy limits acceptable to the supervising dentist. A dental hygienist shall only practice under remote supervision at a federally qualified health center; charitable safety net facility; free clinic; long-term care facility; elementary or secondary school; Head Start program; mobile dentistry program for adults with developmental disabilities operated by DBHDS; or women, infants, and children (WIC) program.

*Provider Services:*

A dental hygienist practicing under remote supervision may:

- Obtain a patient's treatment history and consent;
- Perform an oral assessment;
- Perform scaling and polishing;
- Perform all educational and preventative services;
- Take x-rays as ordered by the supervising dentist or consistent with a standing order;
- Maintain appropriate documentation in the patient's chart;
- Administer topical oral fluorides, topical oral anesthetics, topical and directly applied antimicrobial agents for treatment of periodontal pocket lesions, and any other Schedule VI topical drug approved by the Board of Dentistry under an oral or written order or a standing protocol issued by a dentist or a doctor of medicine or osteopathic medicine; and
- Perform any other service ordered by the supervising dentist or required by statute or board regulation.

No dental hygienist practicing under remote supervision shall administer local anesthetic or nitrous oxide. After conducting an initial oral assessment of a patient, a dental hygienist practicing under remote supervision may provide further dental hygiene services following a written practice protocol developed and provided by the supervising dentist.

### Washington 1984/2009

***Sec. 18.29.056***

*Unsupervised and Off-Site Supervision:*

Dental hygienist may be employed, retained or contracted by health care facilities to perform authorized dental hygiene services without supervision, provided the dental hygienist refers patient to a dentist for dental planning and treatment.

Health care facilities are limited to hospitals; nursing homes; home health agencies; group homes serving the elderly, individuals with disabilities and juveniles; state operated institutions under the jurisdiction of the department of social and health services or the department of corrections; and federal, state, and local public health facilities, state or federally funded community and migrant health centers and tribal clinics. Specifically in senior centers, dental hygienist may provide limited dental hygiene services with under the "off-site supervision" of a dentist.

*Requirements:* Dental hygienist must have 2 years clinical experience within the last 5 year with a dentist. Written practice plan required in certain settings.

*Provider Services:* Dental hygienist may provide prophylaxis, application of typical preventive or prophylactic agents, polishing and smoothing restorations root planing and curettage.

### Washington 2001

***Sec. 18.29.220***

*Public Health Dental Hygienist:*

Dental hygienist who is school endorsed may assess for and apply sealants and fluoride varnishes and perform prophylaxis in community-based sealant programs carried out in schools.

*Requirements:* Sealant/Fluoride Varnish Endorsement from Department of Health. Dental hygienist must submit data to the Department of Health concerning patient demographics, treatment, reimbursement and referrals.

### West Virginia 2008

***Sec. 5-1-8.5***

*Public Health Dental Hygienist:*

Dental hygienist may provide care in hospitals, schools, correctional facilities, jails, community clinics, long-term care facilities, nursing homes, home health agencies, group homes, state institutions under the Department of Health and Human Resources, public health facilities, homebound settings and accredited dental hygiene education programs. Dentist must authorize dental hygienist to provide care but need not be present or have previously seen patient.

*Requirements:* Dental hygienist must have 2 years and 3,000 hours of clinical experience and take six additional continuing education hours. Dental hygienist and dentist must submit annual written report of care to state board of dental examiners.

*Provider Services:* Dental hygienist can provide patient education, nutritional counseling, oral screening with referral to dentist, apply fluoride, sealants, and offer a complete prophylaxis (pursuant to a collaborative agreement or written order.)

### Wisconsin 2007/2017

***Sec. 447.06***

In settings other than a dental office, the authorization and presence of a licensed dentist is not required for the practice of dental hygiene. Under prior law, the authorization and presence of a licensed dentist was required in most cases. in addition to a dental office setting, a dental hygienist may practice dental hygiene in any of the following settings, in accordance with conditions specified in the statutes:

- Federal, state, county, or municipal correctional or detention facilities and facilities established to provide care for terminally ill patients;
- Charitable institutions open to the general public or members of a religious sect or order;
- Nonprofit home health care agencies;
- Nonprofit dental care programs serving primarily indigent, economically disadvantaged, or migrant worker populations;
- Nursing homes, community-based residential facilities, and hospitals.
- Facilities that are primarily operated for the purpose of providing outpatient medical services;
- Adult family homes;

Continued

## BOX 22.1 Direct Access States—cont'd

- Adult day care centers; and
- Community rehabilitation programs. Community rehabilitation program is defined to mean a nonprofit entity or governmental agency providing vocational rehabilitation services to disabled individuals to maximize the employment opportunities of such individuals.

*Requirements*: None

*Provider Services:* Dental hygienist can provide prophylaxis, root planing, screening, treatment planning, sealants and delegable duties.

**Wyoming 2017**

***Rules Chapter 7, Section 5(c)***

***Public Health Dental Hygienist:***

The Wyoming Dental Board adopted regulations allowing the public to directly access limited dental hygiene services from a Public Health Dental Hygienist. A public health dental hygienist may provide public health services at facilities to include, but not limited to:

- federally funded health centers and clinics
- nursing homes
- extended care facilities
- home health agencies
- group homes for the elderly, disabled and youth
- public health offices
- Women, Infants, and Children (WIC)
- Head Start programs
- child development programs
- early intervention programs
- migrant work facilities
- free clinics
- health fairs
- public and private schools
- state and county correctional institutions
- community school-based prevention programs
- public health vans

*Requirements:* The public health hygienist must submit a Collaboration Agreement with a Wyoming licensed dentist. The hygienist must have a current Wyoming dental hygienist license with a minimum of two years clinical experience. Lastly, the dental hygienist must carry liability insurance.

*Provider Services:* Public health services solely consist of prophylaxis, fluoride varnishes, oral health education, and dental screenings. These services can be provided by the hygienist without prior authorization of the dentist. All patients seen shall be referred to a dentist annually.

From www.adha.org (https://www.adha.org/resources-docs/7513_Direct_Access_to_Care_from_DH.pdf). Revised January 2020. This document is intended for informational purposes only and does not constitute a legal opinion regarding dental practice in any state. To verify any information, please contact your state's dental board.

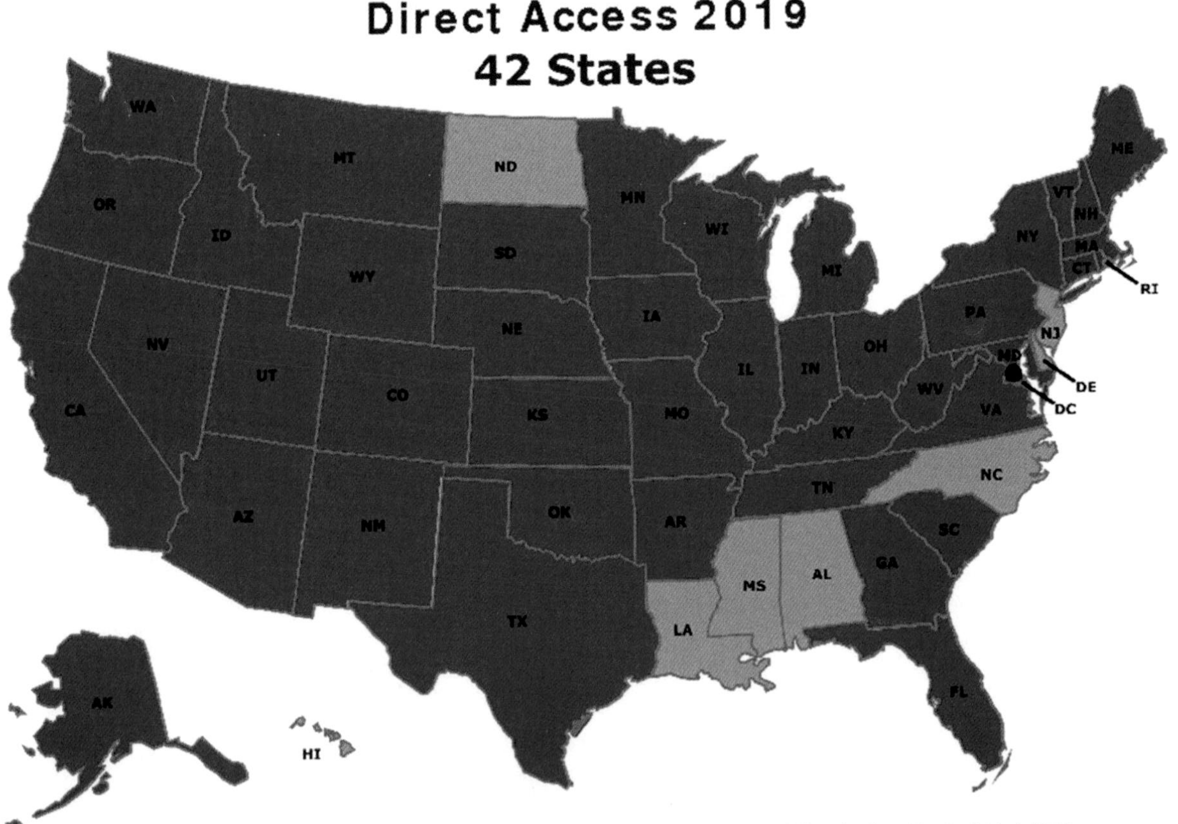

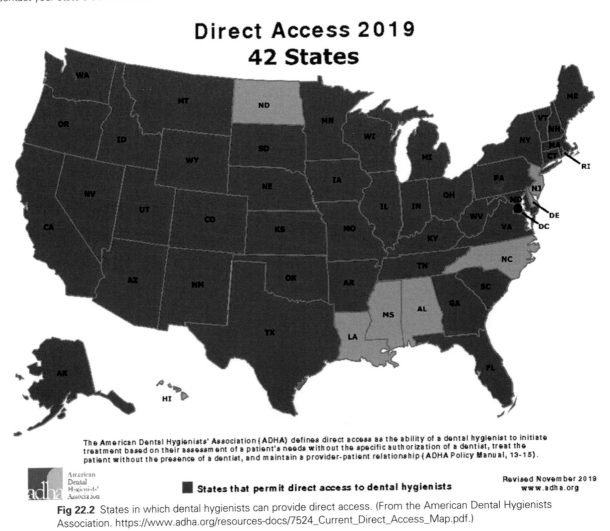

**Fig 22.2** States in which dental hygienists can provide direct access. (From the American Dental Hygienists Association. https://www.adha.org/resources-docs/7524_Current_Direct_Access_Map.pdf.)

**TABLE 22.2 Local Anesthesia Administration by Dental Hygienists: State Chart**

| State & Year Implemented | Supervision Required | Block and/or Infiltration | Education Required | Exam Required | Authorized by Statute or Rule | Legal Requirements for Local Anesthesia Courses |
|---|---|---|---|---|---|---|
| AL 2018 | Direct | Infiltration | Board Approved | No | Statute | 32 hrs |
| AK 1981 | General | Both | Specific | Yes – WREB | Statute | 16 hrs didactic; 6 hrs clinical; 8 hrs lab |
| AZ 1976 | General | Both | Accredited | Yes – WREB | Statute | 36 hrs; 9 types of injections |
| AR 1995 | Direct | Both | Accredited/ Board Approved | No | Statute | 16 hrs didactic; 12 hrs clinical |
| CA 1976 | Direct | Both | Course taken as part of a DH program/approved by the Dental Hygiene Committee of CA | No | Rules | At least 15 hrs didactic; pre-clinical & clinical;14 injection sites |
| CO 1977 | General | Both | Accredited | No | Statute | 12 hrs didactic; 12 hrs clinical |
| CT 2005 | Direct | Both | Accredited | No | Statute | 20 hrs didactic; 8 hrs clinical |
| DC 2004 | Direct | Both | Board Approved | No | Rules | 20 hrs didactic; 12 hrs clinical |
| FL 2012 | Direct | Both | Accredited/ Board Approved | No | Statute | 30 hrs didactic; 30 hrs clinical |
| HI 1987 | Direct | Both | Accredited | Yes – Exam given by course | Statute | 39 hrs didactic and clinical; 50 injections |
| ID 1975 | General | Both | Accredited | Yes – Board approval | Statute | No |
| IL 2000 | Direct | Both | Accredited | No | Statute | 24 hrs didactic; 8 hrs clinical |
| IN 2008 | Direct | Both | Accredited | Yes – CDCA Local anesthesia exam or equivalent state or regional exam | Rules | 15 hrs didactic; 14 hrs clinical; permit required |
| IA 1998 | Direct | Both | Accredited | No | Rules | No |
| KS 1993 | Direct | Both | Accredited/Board Approved | No | Statute | 12 hrs |
| KY 2002 | Direct | Both | Accredited/Board Approved | Yes – Written exam given by course | Statute | 32 hrs didactic; 12 hours clinical |
| LA 1998 | Direct | Both | Accredited | Yes – Board approved | Rules | 72 hrs; Minimum of 20 injections |
| ME 1997 | Direct | Both | Accredited | Yes – Board adminis-tered | Rules | 40 hrs; minimum of 50 injections |
| MD 2009 | Direct | Both | Accredited/Board Approved | Yes – NERB | Rules | 20 hrs didactic; 8 hrs clinical |
| MA 2004 | Direct | Both | Accredited | Yes – NERB written exam by NERB | Statute | 35 hrs; No less than 12 hrs clinical |
| MI 2002 | Direct | Both | Accredited | Yes – state or regional board- administered written exam (NERB) | Statute | 15 hrs didactic; 14 hrs clinical |
| MN 1995 | General | Both | Accredited | No | Rules | No |
| MO 1973 | Indirect | Both | Accredited/Board Approved | No | Rules | No |
| MT 1985 | Direct | Both | Accredited | Yes – WREB | Statute | No |
| NE 1995 | Direct | Both | Board Approved | No | Statute | 12 hrs didactic; 12 hrs clini-cal; 10 types of injections |
| NV 1982 | Direct/General | Both | Accredited/Board Approved | No | Rules | No |
| NH 2002 | Direct | Both | Accredited | Yes – NERB local anesthesia exam | Statute | 20 hrs didactic; 12 hrs clinical |
| NJ 2008 | Direct | Both | Accredited/Board Approved | Yes – NERB local anesthesia | Rules | 20 hrs didactic; 12 hrs clinical; Minimum of 20 hrs monitored administration of local anesthesia |
| NM 1972 | Direct/General | Both | Accredited/Board Approved | Yes – WREB | Statute | 24 hrs didactic; 10 hrs clinical |

*Continued*

**TABLE 22.2 Local Anesthesia Administration by Dental Hygienists: State Chart—cont'd**

| State & Year Implemented | Supervision Required | Block and/or Infiltration | Education Required | Exam Required | Authorized by Statute or Rule | Legal Requirements for Local Anesthesia Courses |
|---|---|---|---|---|---|---|
| NY 2001 | Direct | Infiltration | Accredited | No | Statute | 30 hrs didactic; 15 hrs clinical & Lab |
| ND 2003 | Direct | Both | Accredited | No | Rules | Course must include clinical and didactic components, but there are no specific hourly requirement |
| OH 2006 | Direct | Both | Accredited | Yes – Written regional or state exam | Statute | 15 hrs didactic; 14 hrs clinical |
| OK 1980 | Direct | Both | Board Approved | No – Exam given by course | Rules | 20.5 hrs |
| OR 1975 | General/ Unsupervised | Both | Accredited/Board Approved | No | Rules | No |
| PA 2009 | Direct | Both | Accredited/Board Approved | No | Rules | 30 hrs didactic and Clinical permit, must renew |
| RI 2005 | Direct | Both | Accredited | Yes – NERB | Statute | 20 hrs didactic; 12 hrs clinical |
| SC 1995 | Direct | Infiltration | Board Approved | Yes – Board | Statute | No |
| SD 1992 | Direct | Both | Accredited/Board Approved | No | Statute | No |
| TN 2004 | Direct | Both | Accredited/Board Approved | No | Rules | 24 hrs didactic; 8 hrs clinical |
| UT 1983 | Direct | Both | Accredited | Yes – WREB | Statute | No |
| VT 1993 | Direct | Both | Accredited | Yes – Board Administered | Statute | 24 hrs |
| VA 2006 | Direct | Both (Only on patients over 18) | Accredited | Yes — accredited program; Board of another jurisdiction accepted | Statute | 36 hrs didactic-clinical |
| WA 1971 | General | Both | Board Approved | Yes - WREB | Statute | 10 injections |
| WI 1998 | Indirect | Both | Accredited | No | Statute | 10 hrs didactic; 11 hrs clinical |
| WV 2003 | Direct | Both | Board Approved | NERB local anesthesia exam or equivalent state or regional exam | Statute | 12 hrs didactic; 15 hrs clinical |
| WY 1991 | Direct | Both | Board Approved | Yes | Rules | None |

From www.adha.org (https://www.adha.org/resources-docs/7514_Local_Anesthesia_Requirements_by_State.pdf). Revised June 2018. This document is intended for informational purposes only and does not constitute a legal opinion regarding dental practice in any state.

10. Due process requirements for disciplinary action—if a complaint is filed against a professional, with the licensing board, the licensee has a right to:
    a. Receive a clear statement of charges
    b. Question opposing witnesses
    c. Produce witnesses and give testimony (answer charges)
    d. The services of an attorney
    e. Receive a firm conclusion based on the evidence
    f. Contest the board's decision at a court of law
    g. If these rights are not provided, the board's decision could be reversed by a court of law
11. Practicing without a license—penalties vary from state to state
    a. Criminal charges—usually result in a fine or imprisonment, or both
    b. Civil suits—may be filed for monetary damages by individuals who have been harmed
    c. Criminal or civil actions, or both, may be brought against the unlicensed person
12. Reporting professional violations—failure to report a violation is grounds for disciplinary action; failure to report is considered unprofessional conduct; reporting a violation requires the following:
    a. Facts must be documented in writing with complete description of violation

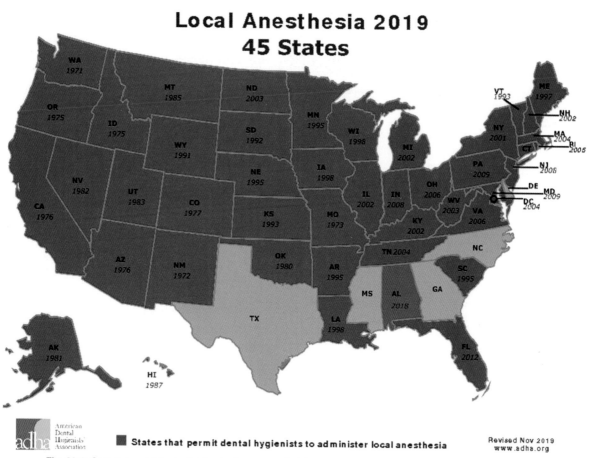


**Fig 22.3** States in which dental hygienists can administer local anesthesia. (From the American Dental Hygienists Association. http://www.adha.org/resources-docs/7521_Local_Anesthesia_by_State.pdf.)

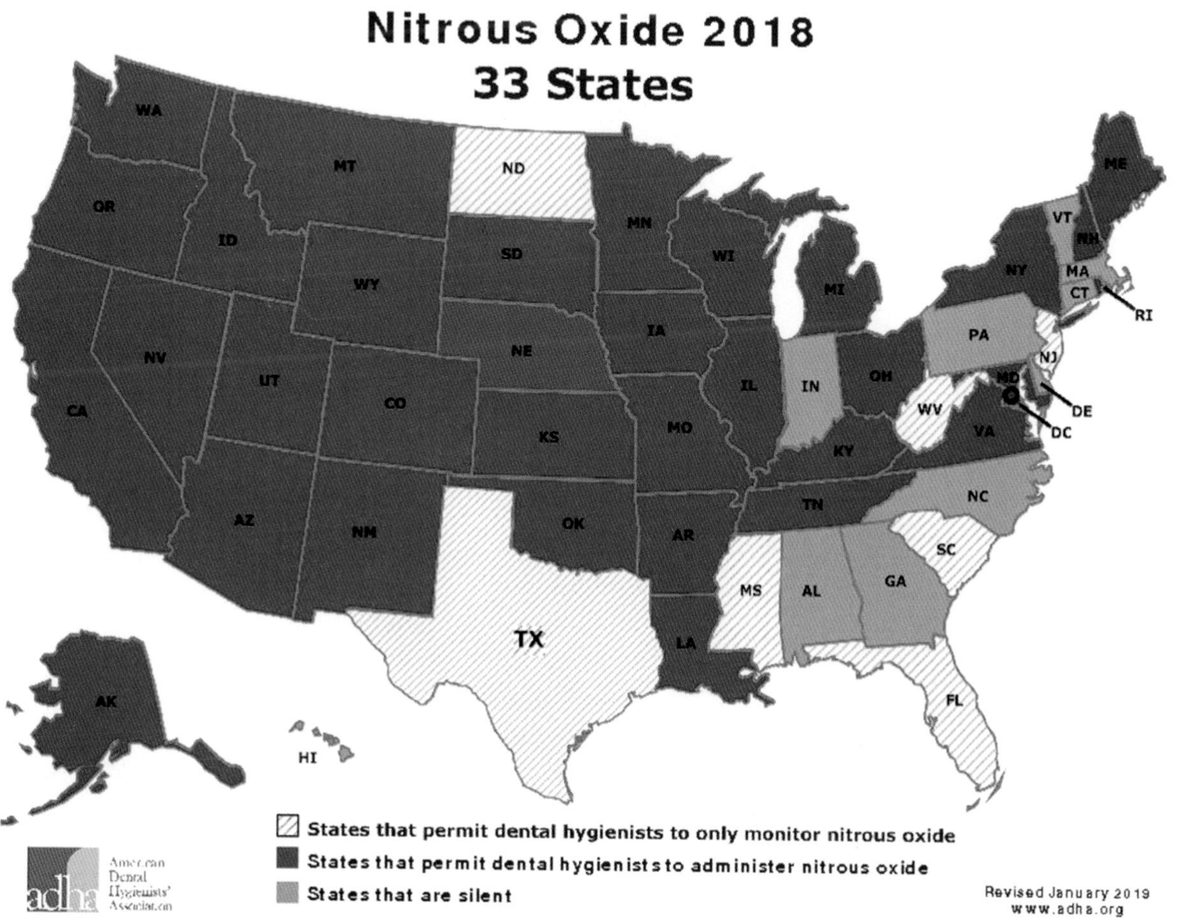


**Fig 22.4** States in which dental hygienists can administer nitrous oxide–oxygen analgesia. (From the American Dental Hygienists Association. http://www.adha.org/resources-docs/7522_Nitrous_Oxide_by_State.pdf.)

**TABLE 22.3 Dental Hygienists Restorative Duties by State**

| State | Apply Cavity-Liners and Bases | Place/Remove Temporary Restorations | Place/Remove Temporary Crowns | Place/Carve/Finish Amalgam Restoration | Place & Finish Composite Resin Silicate Restoration | Requirements |
|---|---|---|---|---|---|---|
| AL | Allowed* | Allowed* | Place Only* | Prohibited | Prohibited | |
| AK | | | | Allowed* | Allowed* | Board Approved Course WREB or Equivalent Exam |
| AZ | | Place* | | | | |
| AR | | | | Prohibited | Prohibited | Program |
| CA | Allowed** | Allowed** | Allowed** | Allowed* Requires RDAEF License | Allowed* Requires RDAEF License | |
| CO | | Allowed | | | | |
| CT | | Prohibited | | Prohibited | Prohibited | |
| DE | | Prohibited | Prohibited | Prohibited | Prohibited | |
| DC | Prohibited | Allowed | | Prohibited | Prohibited | |
| FL | Allowed | Allowed | Allowed | Prohibited | Prohibited | |
| GA | Allowed* | | Allowed* | | | |
| HI | | | | Prohibited | Prohibited | |
| ID | Allowed* | | Place Only* | Allowed | Allowed | Restorative Endorsement. WREB or Equivalent Restorative Exam. |
| IL | | | | Prohibited | Prohibited | |
| IN | | | | | | |
| IA | Allowed* | Allowed* | | | | |
| KS | | | | | | |
| KY | Allowed* | | Allowed* | Allowed* | Allowed* | Proof of competency. |
| LA | | | | Prohibited | Prohibited | |
| ME | | Allowed | Allowed* | Allowed* | Allowed* | Board approved EFDA program |
| MD | | Allowed | Allowed | Prohibited | Prohibited | |
| MA | Prohibited | Remove Only* | Allowed* | Prohibited | Prohibited | |
| MI | Allowed* | Allowed* | Allowed | Allowed* | | Registered Dental Assistant took approved course |
| MN | | Allowed* | Allowed* | Allowed | Allowed* | Board approved course to place/adjust permanent restorations |
| | | MN also permits RDH to place, contour, and adjust glass ionomer | | | | |
| MS | | | | | | |
| MO | | Allowed* | | Allowed* | Place Only* | Proof of Competency |
| MT | | Allowed* | | Prohibited | Prohibited | |
| NE | | | | Prohibited | Prohibited | |
| NV | | Place Only | Allowed | | | |
| NH | Allowed | Allowed | Allowed* | Place | | Expanded Duty Course |
| NJ | | Allowed* | | | | |
| NM | | Allowed | Allowed | Allowed | Allowed | EFDA Certification |
| NY | | Allowed* | | Allowed* | Allowed* | Approved Course |

**TABLE 22.3 Dental Hygienists Restorative Duties by State—cont'd**

| State | Apply Cavity-Liners and Bases | Place/Remove Temporary Restorations | Place/Remove Temporary Crowns | Place/Carve/Finish Amalgam Restoration | Place & Finish Composite Resin Silicate Restoration | Requirements |
|---|---|---|---|---|---|---|
| NC | Allowed* | Place Only* | | | | |
| ND | Prohibited | Allowed* | Allowed | Allowed | Allowed | Board approved course, WREB or Equivalent Exam, Restorative function component of the DANB-certified restorative functions dental assistant examination |
| OH | | Allowed* | | Place Only | Place Only | |
| OK | | Place Only | | | | |
| OR | Allowed | Place Only | Allowed | Allowed | Allowed* | Board approved course, WREB or Equivalent Exam, Restorative Function Endorsement. |
| PA | Allowed* | | | Allowed* | Allowed* | |
| RI | | Allowed | | Prohibited | Prohibited | |
| SC | | Place Only* | | Prohibited | Prohibited | |
| SD | | Place Only | | Prohibited | Prohibited | |
| TN | Allowed | Allowed | | Place Only | | Restorative Function Permit |
| TX | Prohibited | Prohibited | Prohibited | Prohibited | Prohibited | |
| UT | | | | | | |
| VT | | | | | | Trainings expanded function |
| VA | | | | | | |
| WA | | Allowed* | Allowed* | Allowed* | Allowed* | Restorative services in curriculum of WA DH programs. WREB restorative required for dental hygiene license. |
| WV | Allowed* | Allowed* | Allowed | | | |
| WI | | Place Only | | | | Replacement of temporary restorations in emergency situations only. |
| WY | | Place Only | | Allowed (with EP Certificate) | Allowed (with EP certificate) | Expanded function certificate no longer offered, but existing certificates honored. |

*Can do services by virtue of inclusion in dental assistants' Scope of Practice licensed prior to 2006.
**Allowed for an RDH, RDHEF, or RDHA
From www.adha.org (https://www.adha.org/resources-docs/7516_Restorative_Duties_by_State.pdf). Revised April 2016. This document is intended for informational purposes only and does not constitute a legal opinion regarding dental practice in any state.

b. Report must list other witnesses and patients involved, if applicable

13. National Practitioner Data Bank (NPDB)
    a. Created by the U.S. Department of Health and Human Services (DHHS) in 1990
    b. Purpose—electronic repository that collects information on adverse licensure actions, certain actions restricting clinical privileges, and professional society membership actions taken against physicians, dentists, and other practitioners

## BOX 22.2 Dental Hygiene Participation in Regulation

The following states have dental hygiene advisory committees or varying degrees of self regulation for dental hygienists.

### Arizona

The Arizona Dental Hygiene Committee consists of one dentist and one dental hygienist from the board, plus four additional dental hygienists and one public member. The committee serves as a forum for discussion of dental hygiene issues and advises the board on rules and proposed statute changes concerning dental hygiene education, regulation and practice. In addition, the committee evaluates CE classes for expanded functions and monitors dental hygienists' compliance with CE requirements.

### California

The Dental Hygiene Board of California is a self-regulating dental hygiene board. The board members are appointed by the Governor, except as noted. The board consists of four dental hygienists, 4 public members (two appointed by the Governor and two by the Legislature) and one dentist. The responsibilities of DHBC include issuing, reviewing, and revoking licenses as well as developing and administering examinations. Additional functions include adopting regulations, determining fees and continuing education requirements for all hygiene licensure categories.

### Connecticut

Connecticut is unique because dental hygiene is directly under the Department of Public Health. Although there is no standing dental hygiene committee the department director has the ability to appoint an ad hoc committee of dental hygienists, if there is a need to address rules or disciplinary matters.

### Delaware

Delaware's Advisory Committee is appointed by the governor and consists of three dental hygienists. The committee writes the examination for dental hygiene licensure (in conjunction with the dental board). In addition, the committee votes with the board on issues of dental hygiene licensure by credentials, disciplinary decisions, continuing education requirements for dental hygiene licensure, disciplinary action involving dental hygienists and issues involving the policy and practice of dental hygiene but not the scope of practice.

### Florida

Florida has both dental hygiene and dental assisting councils. The dental hygiene council is composed of four dental hygienists, one of whom sits on the board, and one dentist member of the board. The council is expected to develop all dental hygiene rules to submit to the board for its approval.

### Georgia

Georgia has a Dental Hygiene Committee. This committee is comprised of a dentist and a dental hygienist.

### Iowa

Beginning in 1999, both dental hygienists on the dental board and one of the dentists became a dental hygiene committee of the board. This committee has the power to make all rules pertaining to dental hygiene. The board is required to adopt those rules and enforce the committee rules.

### Maine

Maine has a Subcommittee on Dental Hygienists. The subcommittee consists of five members: one dental hygienist who is a member of the board; two dental hygienists appointed by the governor; two dentists who are members of the board and appointed by the president of the board. The duties of the subcommittee are to perform an initial review of all applications for licensure as a dental hygienist, submissions relating to continuing education of dental hygienists, and all submissions relating to public health supervision status of dental hygienists.

### Maryland

Maryland's committee consists of three dental hygienists, one dentist, and one public member, all of whom are full voting members of the dental board. The committee was created during a sunset review as a compromise to the creation of a separate dental hygiene regulatory board. According to statute, all matters pertaining to dental hygiene must first be brought to the committee for its review and recommendation.

### Michigan

This six member committee, comprised of two dental hygienists and two dentists, one dental assistant and one public member, considers matters related to the dental hygiene profession and makes recommendations to the full board of dentistry. All members of the committee are voting members on the board. The existence of the committee is not mandated by state rules or statutes, but instead is a committee appointed by the chairperson of the board.

### Missouri

A five member advisory commission, composed of the dental hygienist on the dental board and four dental hygienists appointed by the governor was created by the state legislature in 2001. The commission makes recommendations to the board concerning dental hygiene practice, licensure, examinations, discipline and educational requirements.

### Montana

In 2002, the board assigned both dental hygienist members and one dentist member to be a standing committee to consider and address dental hygiene issues in a timely fashion. The committee formulates specific recommendations to bring to the entire board for action.

### Nevada

Legislation in 2003 added a third dental hygienist to the board who, together with a dentist appointed by the board, constitute a dental hygiene committee that formulates recommendations on dental hygiene rules for the board.

### New Hampshire

The New Hampshire Dental Hygienists' Committee is a five member advisory committee, comprised of one dental hygienist member of the board, one dentist member of the board and three addition dental hygienist members appointed by the governor. The Dental Hygienists' Committee proposes rules concerning the practice, discipline, education, examination, and licensure of dental hygienists. The rules proposed by the committee may be accepted by the Board of Dental Examiners for adoption.

### New Mexico

New Mexico has a Board of Dental Health Care comprised of five dentists, two dental hygienists and two public members. There is a dental hygiene committee comprised of five dental hygienists, two public members and two dentists. The committee selects two of its dental hygiene members to serve as the dental hygienists on the board. The board's public members and two of its dentist members are the dentist and public members of the committee. The committee adopts all the rules pertaining to dental hygiene and is also responsible for the discipline of dental hygienists. The board enforces the dental hygiene committee's rules.

### Oklahoma

The Dental Hygiene Advisory Committee is comprised of the current dental hygienist on the Oklahoma dental board, and four additional dental hygienists appointed by the board.

### Oregon

Under its authority to create standing committees, the Oregon dental board has appointed a dental hygiene committee to advise the board concerning dental hygiene issues.

**BOX 22.2 Dental Hygiene Participation in Regulation—cont'd**

**Rhode Island**

Dental Hygiene Licensing, Dental Hygiene Disciplinary and Public Health Licensure committees exist in Rhode Island. The Board Chair appoints three members of the board, one of whom is a licensed dentist, one of whom is a public member, and one of whom is a licensed dental hygienist, to serve as an examining committee for applicants applying for licensure as dental hygienists. The examining committee for dental hygienists shall recommend to the full board, which shall recommend to the director, applicants for licensure to practice dental hygiene who meet the requirements for licensure.

**Texas**

In 1995, a dental hygiene advisory committee, comprised of three dental hygienists and two public members appointed by the governor and one dentist appointed by the board, was established.

**Washington**

The state of Washington has a uniform disciplinary code which applies to all health professions and creates the regulatory bodies to implement each practice act. Dentistry and dental hygiene have separate practice acts. Dentists are regulated by the Dental Quality Assurance Commission (an independent dental board with no dental hygiene members). Dental hygienists are regulated by the Department of Health, but the statute requires that the department develop rules and definitions to implement the dental hygienist act in consultation with the Dental Hygiene Examining Committee. The committee is comprised of three dental hygienists and one public member appointed by the department.

From www.adha.org (https://www.adha.org/resources-docs/75111_Self_Regulation_by_State.pdf). Revised February 2019. This document is intended for informational purposes only and does not constitute a legal opinion regarding dental practice in any state. To verify any information, please contact your state's dental board.

c. Medical and dental regulatory boards are required to report certain actions taken against licensees
d. Health care entities such as hospitals are required to report certain disciplinary action taken against staff members
e. Licensees are not required to report incidents
f. Access to data bank information
   (1) Individuals, who may request their own record
   (2) State licensing boards
   (3) Researchers, health care entities (e.g., hospitals, nursing homes)
   (4) Professional societies
   (5) Attorneys
g. The law prohibits the release of information in the NPDB to the public

14. Health Care Integrity and Protection Data Bank (HIPDB)
   a. Combats fraud and abuse in health insurance and health care delivery
   b. Flagging system used to alert users
   c. Intended to augment, not replace, traditional forms of review and investigation, serving as an important supplement to a review of a practitioner's, providers, or supplier's past actions

## DENTAL RECORDS AND RECORD KEEPING

A. Purpose of dental records
   1. Provides all privileged parties with information; method of communication with dental and other medical providers
   2. Tool for quality assessment and management
   3. Documents assessment findings, treatment, care provided, and outcomes
   4. Serves as an important document in third-party relationships
   5. Provides evidence of compliance with state record-keeping requirements
   6. Resource in forensic identification
   7. Reference in litigation and provides information for the patient and provider
   8. Useful in research

B. Written record management
   1. Adheres to state dental practice or state medical records guidelines, if required
   2. Legible and written in black ink or ballpoint, not pencil
   3. Corrections and additions clearly explained
   4. Deletions noted by single line through entry
   5. Signed and initialed by appropriate operator

C. Electronic dental records
   1. Same record-keeping principles as for paper records
   2. System should include protections from tampering
   3. Courts accept as documentation

D. Patient records—must be clear, complete, and accurate and include:
   1. Patient identification data—patient's name, address, employment, home and cell telephone numbers, Social Security number or patient record number, birth date, emergency contact, physician's name and phone number, insurance information; legal guardian information, if appropriate
   2. Consent forms—informed consent and informed refusal
   3. Health, pharmacologic, and dental histories, updated at each visit, signed and dated by the patient and oral health care professional
   4. Referrals—referrals made to other professionals, reports of tests, or reports from other providers
   5. Clinical observations—intraoral and extraoral examination results, findings of pathology, periodontal evaluation, radiographs, study models, diagnostic photographs
   6. Progress or treatment notes—chronologic notation of treatment, pretreatment procedures, unusual incidents or circumstances, diagnosis and care plans, oral hygiene recommendations, patient noncompliance, postoperative instructions, telephone conversations with the patient or other health care providers, medications taken or prescribed with dosage, patient's missed or canceled appointments
   7. Failure to maintain or store dental records for a specified period may violate state dental practice acts; considered medical malpractice in some jurisdictions in a court of law

8. Records also include radiographs, photographs, and models
9. State regulations or statutes may delineate specific costs for duplication of records

E. Confidentiality—patient confidentiality is protected by federal and state laws; state laws often regulate the disclosure of substance abuse, mental health history, human immunodeficiency virus/acquired immunodeficiency syndrome (HIV/AIDS) status; improper disclosure can result in liability for breach of fiduciary duty, breach of implied contract, or invasion of privacy
   1. Health Insurance Portability and Accountability Act (HIPAA)
      a. Purpose—this federal act allows employees to move their health insurance when changing jobs and is in place to develop standards for health information, provide greater safeguards regarding privacy of protected health information (PHI), and reduce health care fraud and abuse
      b. Protects health information by establishing transaction standards for the exchange of health information, security standards, and privacy standards for the use and disclosure of individually identifiable health information (IIHI)
      c. PHI includes all individually identifiable health information that is:
         (1) Sent or stored in any form
         (2) Identifies the patient or can be used to identify the patient
         (3) Created or received by a covered entity
         (4) About the patient's past, present, or future treatment and payment for services
      d. Three major areas addressed relating to requirements for privacy and confidentiality of health information (effective April 14, 2003)
         (1) Privacy standards
            (a) Patient notification of privacy policies of office or institution
            (b) Written acknowledgment of receipt of notice of privacy policies
            (c) Written and signed authorization and consent
         (2) Patient's rights
            (a) Right to inspect and copy confidential health care information
            (b) Right to amend confidential information in the patient record
            (c) Right to obtain a list of disclosures of PHI
            (d) Right to confidential communication
            (e) Right to complain to the practice, to the DHHS Secretary, or to both
         (3) Administrative requirements
            (a) Develop policies, procedures, and documentation
            (b) Provide notice of privacy policy to patients
            (c) Designate a privacy officer and a contact person to receive complaints
            (d) Implement complaint systems
            (e) Provide training for employees
            (f) Execute business associate contracts
            (g) Mitigate any breach of confidentiality
   2. Exceptions to nondisclosure of patient information—original patient records should never be released
      a. Patient consent—with written authorization only, specifying name of the patient, name of the person authorized to disclose the information, amount and type of information to be released, name of the person or entity to receive the information, the date information is to be released, the date authorization expires, and the patient's signature
      b. Relevant copies of a patient's medical records may be released to the court where the patient's medical condition is put in issue by filing a lawsuit[4]
      c. Duty to disclose—state reporting statutes may require release of patient information (e.g., in cases of child or elder abuse); state statutes identify health care providers who are obligated by law to report suspected cases of abuse; statutes also provide immunity from civil liability for health care providers involved in reporting suspected abuse, unless it can be proved that a false report had been made, and the person knew that the report was false; access statutes allow for release of patient information with no patient authorization required (e.g., workers' compensation statutes)
   3. PHI in electronic form is sometimes referred to as ePHI, which can include patient information in an email, in an electronic file, or on a CD or memory stick
   4. Health Information Technology for Economic and Clinical Health (HITECH); enacted as part of the American Recovery and Reinvestment Act of 2009; signed into law on February 17, 2009
      a. Expands HIPAA's privacy and security provisions
      b. Requires covered entities to provide notice of any breaches or unauthorized disclosures of PHI

## EMPLOYER AND EMPLOYEE RIGHTS AND RESPONSIBILITIES

A. Employment
   1. Employer—person, business, or organization that hires and compensates one or more workers; engages the services of an individual
   2. Employee—person who is hired to provide services to a company on a regular basis in exchange for compensation
   3. Status
      a. At will; individual can be hired or terminated without notice
         (1) Employees without a contract
         (2) Should a dispute arise relating to termination of employment, courts often examine the office policy and procedure manual in determining an implied contract

b. Contract—a legally binding agreement between two or more parties
   (1) Elements (to be enforced by a court)
      (a) Offer—one party proposes a bargain
      (b) Acceptance—the other party agrees to the proposed bargain
      (c) Consideration—one party gives up something of value, and the other party makes a promise in exchange for that something of value
      (d) Mutuality—parties must reach an agreement or understanding
      (e) Legal capacity—all parties must have legal capacity (i.e., must be the age of majority and mentally competent)
   (2) Contract must be for a lawful purpose
   (3) Breach of contract—failure of performance of a contractual agreement by one or more parties
      (a) Remedies for breach of contract
         [1] Specific performance (the court requires performance of the contract)
         [2] Monetary damage
         [3] Injunctions (the court orders a party to refrain from specific behavior)
   (4) Employment contracts (Box 22.3)
      (a) Define duties and responsibilities of the position; location and hours
      (b) Define salary and benefits
      (c) Describe notice and termination requirements
      (d) Provide written description of understanding between the parties

4. Independent practitioner—one who provides services directly to the public; dental hygienists who perform as independent practitioners may do so only in a state where it is allowed by the dental practice act; a dental hygienist as an independent practitioner must follow the state's (province's) dental practice act and regulations (Box 22.4)
5. Independent contractor—contracted by another person, company, or agency to produce a certain result, but not subject to the control of the employer and may do the work in a manner he or she selects; a dental hygienist as an independent contractor must follow both Internal Revenue Service (IRS) rules and the state's dental practice act and regulations
6. Vicarious liability—one party is responsible for another's action; *respondeat superior* (Latin, meaning "let the master answer"), an employer is legally responsible for the wrongs committed by an employee acting within the scope of his or her employment; dentist employer may be held responsible for negligent acts of a dental hygienist
   a. Vicarious liability or negligent retention may shield a dental hygienist from liability in tort cases
   b. Dental hygienists are liable for their actions
7. Negligent hiring and retention—employer can be held liable for acts or omissions of employees if the patient can show that the employee was incompetent and the employer knew or should have known

B. Employment laws—offer protections for employer and employee
   1. Equal Employment Opportunity Commission (EEOC)—enforces federal laws passed to prevent discrimination in the workplace; investigates complaints and assists an individual or the Department of Justice in bringing a lawsuit
   2. Title VII of the Civil Rights Act of 1964—forbids discrimination against employees by federal, state, and local governments, by employers with 15 or more employees, and by labor organizations, if the basis of discrimination is race, color, national origin, religion, or gender

### BOX 22.3 Employment Contract Terms

An employment contract describes the conditions of employment, including wages, hours, and type of work. Depending on the level of employment, the responsibility of the new employee, and the nature of the business, the conditions of employment should be detailed regarding the following elements:

Parties, including the name of the employer and the entity and the name of the employee
Time and place: hours of employment and location
Duties: general and specific, scope of practice, if appropriate
Term and conditions of employment
Compensation, including salary, bonus pay, vacation, sick leave, continuing education policies and reimbursement, and professional memberships
Benefits, including disability, medical, life insurance, and retirement plan
Termination provisions

### BOX 22.4 Independent Practice

There is virtually no legal guidance—even in the laws of states which allow it—about what "independent practice" means. If one equates it with other health practices, one would expect that the practice is a business entity that can be sold to another, can be directly reimbursed for services, and has patients of record.

Four states that have specific authorization in the practice act law allowing a hygienist to own a dental hygiene practice: Colorado (any hygienist), Maine (hygienists licensed as independent dental hygiene practitioners), New Mexico (hygienists in collaborative practice) and California (RDHAPs, registered dental hygienists in alternative practice). In several other states, including Washington and Oregon, where dental hygienists may practice with no or little supervision in various types of settings outside the dental office, dental hygienists do own dental hygiene businesses.

If you are interested in what business ownership options are available in a state other than these, you need to review the practice laws to see whether there is an actual or implied prohibition. Some state practice acts specify or strongly imply that a dental hygienist must be employed or must be an independent contractor. Others define owning, operating, or managing a dental practice as the practice of dentistry.

Keep in mind that supervision issues are different from worker status (employee vs. independent contractor) and business option issues. Supervision concerns the degree of oversight of patient treatment that the practice law requires. Even owners of dental hygiene practices in Colorado and Maine must have an agreement with a dentist to provide supervision for some services; New Mexico practitioners need to practice in an agreed protocol with a collaborating dentist, and patients of California RDHAPs need a prescription from a dentist or physician to obtain dental hygiene services.

3. Civil Rights Act of 1991—expanded rights under federal anti-discrimination law
4. Sexual harassment—"unwelcome sexual conduct that is a term of employment"[5] is considered sexual discrimination and is prohibited under Title VII
   a. *Quid pro quo* (Latin, meaning "something for something") sexual harassment[6] criteria
      (1) The employee was in a "protected group" (a subordinate position)
      (2) The employee encountered unwelcome sexual advances or requests for sexual favors
      (3) Conduct was sexually motivated (e.g., hostile acts toward an individual because of his or her gender)
      (4) Harassment must affect a "tangible aspect of the job," such as salary, benefits, and promotions
   b. Hostile work environment as sexual harassment criteria—"verbal or physical conduct of a sexual nature that has the purpose or effect of creating an intimidating, hostile, or offensive work environment"[7]
      (1) Created by the words or conduct of an employer, colleague, vendor, or patient
      (2) Examples
         (a) Unwanted touching
         (b) Suggestive comments about one's appearance
         (c) Display of sexually suggestive objects or pictures
         (d) Use of diminutive terms such as "honey" or "cutey"
      (3) Employer has legal duty to take action to stop or prevent sexual harassment
      (4) Sexual harassment may occur between members of the opposite sex or members of the same sex
5. Age Discrimination in Employment Act of 1967 (ADEA)—forbids discrimination against persons over age 40 by federal, state, and local governments and by employers with 20 or more employees
6. Equal Pay Act of 1963 (EPA)—illegal to pay lower wage to employees of one gender if the jobs have equal responsibility, working conditions, requirements for mental or physical effort, and requirements in experience, education, or training
7. Uniformed Services Employment and Reemployment Rights Act of 1994 protects civilian job rights and benefits for veterans and members of Reserve components
8. Occupational Safety and Health Act of 1970 (OSHA)—see Chapter 10
   a. The dental profession must comply with all General Industry standards[8] of primary importance to the dental practice, such as OSHA's Bloodborne Pathogens Standard (1991)
   b. Requirements for employers—employers must:
      (1) Identify employees at risk
      (2) Provide personal protective equipment to employees (e.g., gloves, protective eyewear, masks)
      (3) Provide hepatitis B vaccinations to employees
      (4) Provide safety needles for the workplace
      (5) Provide puncture-proof containers for sharps
      (6) Ensure that standard precautions are practiced in the work environment
      (7) Provide prompt treatment to employees who have needlestick or other exposures (includes immediate medical screening and follow-up treatment)
      (8) Provide annual employee education relating to bloodborne diseases
   c. OSHA amended the Bloodborne Pathogens Standard[6] (2001)—stricter requirements to prevent needlesticks and other exposures to blood (http://www.osha.gov/SLTC/bloodbornepathogens/); employers covered by the standards must:
      (1) Provide safety needles
      (2) Maintain a log of needlestick or other injuries to employees
      (3) Enlist the assistance of employees who provide direct patient care to prevent needlestick and other exposures by seeking input regarding equipment selection and work practices
      (4) State OSHA laws—if a state has a health and safety law that meets or exceeds federal OSHA standards, enforcement of the law is assumed by the state rather than by a federal agency
      (5) Twenty-five states, Puerto Rico, and the Virgin Islands have OSHA-approved state plans that cover public and private sector employees; five states have plans that cover only public sector employees; and the states have adopted their own standards and enforcement policies; for the most part, these states adopt standards that are identical to federal OSHA; however, some states have adopted different standards applicable to this topic or may have different enforcement policies; contact state agency for copy of the safety and health standards (State plans, see https://www.osha.gov/dcsp/osp/index.html)
9. Family and Medical Leave Act of 1993 (FMLA)—protects job security for women and men by allowing unpaid leave for medical reasons (e.g., care of a child, spouse, or parent; birth; adoption; or serious illness); updated January 19, 2009, to include military family leave entitlements
10. Pregnancy Discrimination Act of 1978 (PDA)—protects rights of pregnant women in the workplace; maternity-related medical conditions must be treated as all other medical conditions
    a. FMLA and Americans with Disabilities Act (ADA) both require an employer to grant medical leave to an employee in certain circumstances; FMLA and Title VII both have requirements governing leave for pregnancy and pregnancy-related conditions
    b. FMLA covers private employers with 50 or more employees within a 75-mile radius of the workplace; ADA and Title VII cover private employers with 15 or more employees; only those private employers with 50 or more employees are covered concurrently by FMLA, ADA, and Title VII
    c. State and local government employers are covered by ADA and FMLA, regardless of the number of employees; state and local government employers are covered by Title VII, but only if they have 15 or more employees

11. Americans with Disabilities Act (ADA of 1990)—prohibits discrimination against qualified applicants and employees on basis of disability
    a. Must be a mental or physical impairment that substantially limits one or more of the major life activities
    b. Disabilities include visual and hearing impairments, epilepsy, HIV-positive status, and AIDS
    c. Employer must make reasonable accommodations for employee
    d. Updated by the ADA Amendments Act of 2008 and expanded list of major life activities protected by the Act https://www.eeoc.gov/laws/statutes/adaaa.cfm
12. Fair Employment Statutes—many federal employment laws apply to workplaces with as many as 50 employees (e.g., FMLA); therefore, most do not apply to dentistry; most states have passed statutes that enhance these federal laws; each state's statutes differ; contact specific state's attorney general for information
13. Workers' compensation: insurance program regulated by each state's insurance commission; employer must purchase insurance through an insurance company to protect employees should they become seriously ill or injured as a result of conditions in the workplace; programs vary from state to state; employees are covered on first date of employment, and benefits include medical expenses and income

## RISK MANAGEMENT AND AVOIDING LITIGATION

A. Concepts
  1. Risk management—clinical and administrative activities undertaken to identify, evaluate, and reduce the risk of injury to patients, staff, and visitors
  2. Risk assessment
    a. Evaluation of personnel, policies, and protocol to identify and address risk factors
    b. Strategies
      (1) Personnel evaluations; conducted by employer or peer review
      (2) Office audits
        (a) Review and updating of staff handbook
        (b) Assessment of policies related to patient care (e.g., record keeping, referral policies, documentation)
        (c) Evaluation of equipment (e.g., condition)
        (d) Protocol reviews (e.g., accident protocol)
        (e) Personnel assessment (e.g., current licenses, communication style)
    c. Identified risks are addressed and remedied
B. Individual risk management
  1. Maintain a current license and certifications, if required (e.g., CPR certification)
    a. Be knowledgeable of state dental practice act and statutes or guidelines impacting health care providers
    b. Comply with state guidelines, federal guidelines, or both for infection control, record keeping, reporting requirements, confidentiality, and other specified mandates
  2. Obtain membership in a professional association such as ADHA or CDHA that provides legal updates through various publications
  3. Provide evidence-informed care in all aspects of patient care activities
  4. Maintain competence by participation in continuing education; continuing education is mandatory in 47 states; from a legal perspective, it is advisable to document current competency with tasks routinely performed and those within the scope of practice
  5. Possess knowledge of legally protected employee rights and responsibilities
    a. Use legal or state or federal resources that provide guidance
    b. Document in detail any incidents occurring in the workplace
    c. Seek legal advice, if necessary
  6. Purchase professional liability insurance; keep the policy current
    a. Policy classifications
      (1) Occurrence-based policy—covers injuries arising out of incidents that occurred during the time the insurance was in effect, even if cancelled at a later date
      (2) Claims-made policy—covers injuries occurring and reported during the period in which the policy premiums are paid and in force
    b. Declaration—states policyholder's personal data and limits of liability coverage (dollar figure for each claim and aggregate for policy period)
    c. Exclusions—liabilities not covered by policy; usually injuries resulting from criminal behavior, those involving alcohol or drug abuse on the part of health care provider, or cases involving practice beyond the scope of one's license
    d. Injuries covered—listed in policy (e.g., bodily injury, defamation, invasion of privacy)
    e. Supplemental coverage—lost earnings
    f. Conditions—subrogation of rights, policyholder's right to hire counsel versus insurance company's right to retain counsel
      (1) Policyholder's interest and insurance company's interest may be in conflict
      (2) A conflict of interest could also arise if a health care provider relies on the employer's insurance for liability coverage; protection is broader with an individual policy; an employer's policy provides coverage only when acting within the scope of employment; if the health care provider (by his or her action or failure to act) was liable for the patient's injury, the employer (or his or her insurance company) may bring an indemnity claim and recover a portion of dollar amount awarded by the court to the patient
C. Professional risk management
  1. Maintain knowledge of professional and legal responsibilities related to the provision of oral health care services

2. Be familiar with and adhere to the professional code of ethics
3. Maintain a professional and respectful relationship with employers, colleagues, and patients
4. Provide accurate and appropriate communication to patients, verbally and in writing; poor record keeping can contribute to a poor outcome in a lawsuit
5. Maintain confidentiality—obtain proper written authorization from the patient before release of any patient information; ensure that any disclosure is covered by a reporting or access law and is appropriately followed
6. Document informed consent or informed refusal in patient record before treatment
7. Ensure that all progress notes and patient records are complete, accurate, factual, legible, unaltered, and promptly recorded; failure to do so is considered malpractice; a patient's record may be obtained by an opposing party in a lawsuit
8. Be familiar with professional guidelines and practice standards
9. Remain up-to-date on state or provincial dental hygiene practice acts and regulations

Answers and rationales to review questions are available on this text's accompanying Evolve site. See inside front cover for details.

## WEBSITE INFORMATION AND RESOURCES

| Legal Resources | Website Address | Description |
|---|---|---|
| Find Law | https://www.findlaw.com/ | Provides resources to learn about the law, find a lawyer, and find answers to legal questions and legal forms |
| 9to5 National Office | 9 to5 National Headquarters<br>207 E. Buffalo Street, Suite 211<br>Milwaukee, WI 53202<br>T: (414) 274-0925<br>Fax: (414) 272-2870<br>http://www.9to5.org | National organization dedicated to putting working women's issues on the public agenda; 9to5's constituents are low-wage women, women in traditionally female jobs, and those who have experienced any form of discrimination; committed to, among other objectives, eliminating workplace discrimination through educating women about legal rights on the job, monitoring enforcement agencies, and expanding anti-discrimination laws |
| American Dental Hygienists Association | 444 N. Michigan Avenue, Suite 3400<br>Chicago, IL 60611<br>T: 312-440-8900<br>https://www.adha.org/ | Largest professional association representing dental hygienists |
| National Practitioner Data Bank and Health Care Integrity and Protection Data Bank | http://www.npdb.hrsa.gov/ | U.S. Department of Health and Human Services (DHHS), Health Resources and Services Administration (HRSA), Bureau of Health Professions (BHPr), Division of Practitioner Data Banks (DPDB) is responsible for the management of the National Practitioner Data Bank and the Health Care Integrity and Protection Data Bank |
| U.S. Equal Employment Opportunity Commission | http://www.eeoc.gov/contact/index.cfm<br>Charge filing process 1-800-669-4000, email: info@eeoc.gov | Responsible for enforcing federal laws that make it illegal to discriminate against a job applicant or an employee because of the person's race, color, religion, gender (including pregnancy), national origin, age (40 or older), disability or genetic information; it is also illegal to discriminate against a person because the person complained about discrimination, filed a charge of discrimination, or participated in an employment discrimination investigation or lawsuit<br>Work is conducted at the headquarters and at 53 field offices throughout the United States |
| Occupational Safety and Health Administration<br>Seeking legal advice from a qualified attorney is also recommended; the State Bar Association provides referrals to an attorney for legal services in a particular location | 200 Constitution Avenue NW<br>Washington, DC 20210<br>T: 1.800.321.OSHA (6742)<br>https://www.osha.gov/ | Ensures safe and healthful working conditions for working persons by setting and enforcing standards and by providing training, outreach, education, and assistance |

| Ethics Resources | Website Address | Description |
|---|---|---|
| Center for Health Policy and Ethics, Creighton University Medical Center | https://www.creighton.edu/program/health-care-ethics-ms | A multi-disciplinary group of scholars dedicated to the study and teaching of ethical dimensions of health care and health policy; also offer round tables, lectures, and courses |
| Center for Law, Ethics and Health, University of Michigan School of Public Health | https://sph.umich.edu/findings/fall2010/place/collaboration.cfm?abbr=cleh | An interdisciplinary research center to examine the influence of law and ethics on the health care and public health system; provides publications and other resources |
| Berman Bioethics Institute, Johns Hopkins University | https://bioethics.jhu.edu/ | Provides education, conducts research, and provides leadership for the understanding of ethical issues in health care; trains mentors and future leaders in the field of bioethics, health and science |

## CHAPTER 22 REVIEW QUESTIONS

1. The dentist and dental hygienist have reviewed a new patient's medical history. The patient has not identified any health issues or reported taking any medications. When speaking with the patient, the dental hygienist, observes dilated pupils. This causes concern regarding the patient's responses on the health history. Which of the following ethical principles may have been violated by the patient?
   a. Beneficence
   b. Justice
   c. Veracity
   d. Autonomy
2. A newly licensed dental hygienist accepted a position in an office with a newly licensed dentist. The dentist recently bought the practice where patients have been established for over 20 years. The dentist explains that all dental hygiene appointments are being reduced to 30 minutes and assisted dental hygiene will be implemented. Which ethical principle should the new dental hygienist be concerned about?
   a. Nonmaleficence
   b. Fairness
   c. Scope of practice
   d. Utility—good for all
3. Dental insurance companies contact dental offices every day seeking patient information regarding insurance claims and payments. Patient records are private and protected information. In order to provide health-related information to such requests, which of the following ethical principles should guide the decision-making process of dental office staff?
   a. Autonomy
   b. Justice
   c. Respecting patient privacy
   d. Non-maleficence
   e. Veracity
4. Some states have a dental hygiene board or committee that oversee the practice of dental hygiene. This includes education, licensing, disciplinary matters, and scope of practice. This type of oversight indicates an obligation to:
   a. Ensure legal and ethical practice
   b. Guide and monitor scope of education
   c. Protect consumers (public members)
   d. Only A and C are correct
   e. All of the above are correct
5. A patient has received dental hygiene services in an office for 10 years. The dental hygienist has determined that the patient should be referred to a periodontist after probing and assessing patient data. The dentist reviews and examines the patient, and tells the dental hygienist to schedule the patient with the office in six months, versus referring. Which of the following best describes this situation?
   a. A difference in philosophy
   b. A potential of causing harm
   c. Failure of informed consent
   d. Justice
6. A patient was sent to the hospital as a result of dental treatment after his 10 AM appointment. The state dental practice act mandates the dentist to report such situation within seven days of the incident. The time limit established refers to which type legal oversight?
   a. Law that governs state administrative agencies
   b. Laws to protect the public, properties and privacy
   c. Laws limiting when lawsuits can be filed
   d. Laws and guidelines protecting the provider
7. A dental hygiene student has completed a course requirement that includes photos of a patient treated in clinic. After presenting the case in class, the student posted the photos on social media and identified the patient by name. When the patient visited her regular dental office, the dental hygienist reported she saw the photos on social media. Which of the following violations did the student commit?
   a. Beneficence
   b. Paternalism
   c. Integrity
   d. Informed consent
   e. Implied contract
8. Family G has twins who are now 17-years old. Twin A has driven Twin B to his dental hygiene appointment. As this is the third dental appointment based on the treatment plan, the dentist has decided an additional restoration is needed. Twin A gives permission to complete the additional restoration because Twin B is a special needs patient. Which of the following ethical principles is Twin A following?
   a. Parentalism
   b. Autonomy
   c. Nonmaleficence (do no harm)
   d. Expressed consent
9. A state's dental practice act has been revised and now mandates all providers take one hour of continuing education in ethics during each license renewal period. This type of action by the dental board falls within:
   a. Protecting the public
   b. Authority to revoke licenses
   c. Continued education to support competence
   d. Authority to grant licensing
10. The dentist is on vacation for the next two weeks and has asked the dental hygienists to continue working while she is away. Patients scheduled have a treatment plan and do not require local anesthesia. Which type of supervision governs the dental hygienist?
   a. Direct supervision
   b. Indirect supervision
   c. General supervision
   d. Unsuperv.ised supervision
11. A dental hygienist relocates to a new state and is working as a dental assistant until a dental hygiene license can be approved. The dentist asks him to remove calculus with an ultrasonic scaler. Which of the following is a consequence if the dental hygienist agrees to the dentists' request?
   a. Violation of tort law

b. Practicing without a license
c. Breach of contract
d. A civil and/ or criminal lawsuit
e. Both B and D

12. A dental hygienist is terminated from the practice she has worked with for seven years. Extremely upset, she submits a blog post to the local online newspaper where it is determined many of her accusations were false. This situation falls under tort law. What is the violation described?
a. Equity
b. Libel
c. Slander
d. Defamation

13. Summer wildfires claimed the lives of 16 people in a small Northwestern town. Local and state officials requested dental records from two offices in order to positively identify the victims. Both offices have agreed to submit records. Which of the following functions do the dental records satisfy?
a. Documentation as an exhibit in a lawsuit
b. Forensic data for analysis
c. Sharing private information among all providers
d. Information addressing quality control of patient records to avoid risk management issues.

14. Mr. A attends a city council meeting and provides public comment which are complaints about his dental hygienist and the office where she is employed. The dental hygienist is negatively affected by the comments during the city council meeting and several patients leave the practice. Which of the following intentional torts does this BEST describe?
a. Miscommunication
b. Battery
c. Libel
d. Slander

15. Sam RDH is employed in a pediatric dental office. His extraoral assessment indicates potential abuse. The dentist does not agree and will not report the findings. Sam decides he must report his suspicions to authorities and begins the process. Which of the following ethical concepts does Sam's actions BEST follow?
a. Rule deontology—standards are of greater value than personal morals
b. Virtue ethics—acting virtuous based on excellent character
c. Act Deontology—personal morals influence decision based on circumstances
d. Situational ethics—course of action is determined by the circumstances

16. Which of the following guides the obligation for dental professionals to report suspected abuse or violence against other persons, essentially patients under their care?
a. Laws regarding utility—good for all
b. HIPAA regulations
c. Practice Act laws regarding mandated reporting
d. All of the above

17. A patient has signed an informed consent regarding quadrant periodontal therapy. The dental hygienist explained the treatment, alternatives, risks and outcomes and the patient had no questions. Which of the following ethical principles applied to the patients' action?
a. Beneficence
b. Justice
c. Autonomy
d. Veracity

18. Students at DH University are collaborating with local dental and medical professionals in a research project targeting at-risk teens. The results will be published in a peer-reviewed journal next year. Which of the following best describes the project, overall?
a. Peer review
b. Contribution to evidence-based research and outcomes
c. Volunteering for community-based activities
d. Following codes of ethics for community service

19. Which of the following best describes the function of a 'Patient Bill of Rights'?
a. Scope of practice for dental professionals
b. The dental hygiene treatment plan
c. Patient services and procedures
d. Patient expectations of their providers

20. One of the earliest guiding principles for medical providers was the Hippocratic Oath. Its primary purpose was focused on 'doing no harm'. Which of the following ethical terms is defined as 'doing no harm'?
a. Veracity
b. Justice
c. Beneficence
d. Nonmaleficence
e. Autonomy

21. Sanctions for actions and behaviors of licensed dental professionals violating practice laws falls under the duties of the dental or dental hygiene board/committee. This is due to:
a. The codes of ethics guiding the professions
b. Lack of federal oversight
c. The duty of state boards/committees to protect the public
d. State and national associations mandating scope of practice

22. The Governor has increased funding to the State Public Health Department to expand a statewide sealant program. Each county was consulted on how to best implement the expansion. It was determined that children enrolled in federally funded preschool programs would receive sealants. Which ethical principle did the county officials exercise to reach their decision?
a. Prioritization of needs
b. The individual's contribution to society
c. Equal services for all in community
d. Individuals most deserving get the services

23. A co-worker alleges professional misconduct against the dental hygienist in the office and has filed charges. The state board conducts a hearing presided by an Administrative

Law Judge. The dental hygienist had the opportunity to hear the full allegations and provide responses. These actions BEST demonstrate:
a. Right to communicate one's ideas and opinions
b. Illegal activity based on protected classifications (e.g., gender, race)
c. Written and untrue statements
d. Protecting a person from discrimination

24. A dental hygiene student is hired in an office during summer while waiting to finish his last year of the program. The associate dentist was scheduled to provide a dental cleaning for a child patient at 4 o'clock, and the office manager scheduled a dental emergency patient at the same time. The dentist directs the dental hygiene student to do a "quick" polishing so he/she can attend to the emergency patient.
The dentists' action falls under which area of jurisprudence?
a. Administrative law; prohibiting non-licensed persons from performing services as defined in a practice act
b. Failure to understand the duties for office employees
c. Professional negligence; failure to perform a clinical action
d. Case law; formulated by judge or determined by the court

25. After working 30 years with the same dental office, the 62-year old dental hygienist is terminated. The practice has changed over the last five years with younger personnel, including new dental associates. The dental hygienist believes she was terminated because of age. Which federal regulation legally protects the dental hygienist?
a. Occupational Safety and Health Act
b. Civil Rights Act of 1964
c. Age Discrimination Act
d. The State Dental Practice Act

26. Mr. S is a new patient to the practice. General and dental health assessments are taken by the dentist and dental hygienist as a team. However, each agree that the patient's case presents numerous challenges the practice cannot accommodate. Mr. S is told the [practice cannot accept him as a patient and is recommended to seek another provider. Which of the following best describes the situation?
a. Careful risk management
b. Breach of contract
c. No obligation to treat patients barring discriminatory reasons
d. Abandonment

27. Dental hygienists relocate to a new state each day. A new license is required as the dental practice act is different in each state. The application may ask if the applicant has ever been convicted of a felony. Which answer best describes a felony?
a. Violating the scope of practice
b. A misdemeanor
c. A civil rights violation
d. A crime punishable by death or imprisonment

28. Dental hygiene care provided in a similar manner by two different practitioners in different offices and different states is best described as:
a. Informed consent
b. Standard of care
c. Harm avoidance
d. Risk management

29. The "at-will" employment agreement between the dentist and a dental hygienist is best described by which of the following:
a. An agreement where the employee can be hired or fired without cause
b. Insurance protecting professionals in case of lawsuits
c. Insurance that provides wage replacement in case of work-related injuries
d. The willingness of the dental hygienist to work for the dentist

30. In 2009, HIPAA was expanded and required notification to consumers when and if a security breach affecting private information had occurred. Which of the following identifies the HIPAA expansion mandate?
a. Occupational Health and Safety Act
b. Affordable Health Care Act
c. Health Information Technology Economical and Clinical Health Act
d. Medical Record Protection Act

31. Patients along with the dentist or other persons in the practice can sue dental hygienists. A good practice in defense of lawsuits is to:
a. Complete required continuing education courses
b. Carry malpractice insurance
c. Understand employee rights
d. Join the professional organization

32. All patients have the right to review his or her dental chart and receive copies upon request. Which of the following legal regulations allows for this?
a. Patient Bill of Rights
b. Fraud Avoidance
c. Health Insurance Portability and Accountability Act (HIPPA)
d. U.S. Legislative Patient Act

33. Mr. H was treated in the dental office, and was given a prescription for antibiotics and informed to take them for the next ten days. Two weeks after the dental treatment, Mr. H was taken to the hospital due to a serious infection. The dental office is sued, yet the judge determined that the patient was responsible for the injury. Which of the following concepts applies?
a. Informed consent
b. Duty of care
c. Contributory negligence
d. Technical battery

34. The majority of states allow the administration of local anesthetics by dental hygienists. Generally this requires direct supervision of the dentist. Which if the following best describes direct supervision?
a. The ability to contact the dentist by cell phone
b. Dentist is present in the office during the procedure
c. Dentist remains in the operatory during the procedure
d. Dentist views the procedure via telehealth communications

35. Dr. M completes a comprehensive dental examination on new patient. Dr. M develops the treatment plan and the patient signs the informed consent. Dr. M smiles and nods, then proceeds to make the next appointment. Which of the following contractual foundation is best described?
   a. Written contract through verbal communication
   b. Implied contract through nonverbal actions
   c. Ethical obligation to complete treatment on an established patient
   d. Contract between insured parties
36. During a review of a patient's chart, the dental hygienist notices that an entry dated one week ago stated an incorrect number of sites for antimicrobial product used during treatment. From a legal standpoint, how can the dental hygienist correct the chart entry?
   a. Use white out on the chart and enter the correct information
   b. Date and enter the correct information on a separate line below the original (incorrect) entry.
   c. Use a pen to draw a line through the original entry and make the correction
   d. Leave the chart as is without corrections
37. When a patient agrees to the dental hygiene treatment plan and signs the informed consent, the patient's responsibilities include all the following EXCEPT:
   a. Maintaining a 6-month recare visit
   b. Providing accurate information on the medical history; following all post-operative instructions
   c. Payment for services rendered
   d. Keeping all scheduled appointments
38. To maintain licensure, it is recommended that dental hygienists adopt risk management strategies. All of the following are best strategies EXCEPT:
   a. Maintaining current licenses and certifications
   b. Using evidence-based research to support treatment plans and standard of care
   c. Purchasing liability insurance
   d. Accepting consequences of one's own decisions
39. Carlos is having sealants placed on all four first molars. Carlos is 6 years old and his chart indicates difficulty with managing his behavior during dental treatment. The dental hygienist and the dental assistant decide to tie his hands to the chair arms at the beginning of the appointment in order to keep him from moving around. During the appointment, Carlos keeps moving his head away from the dental hygienist, so the assistant decides to hold his chin in place so he can't move his head. Only two of the sealants could be placed as Carlos was difficult to manage. When he goes back to the reception area, his mother is visibly upset when she sees red marks on his chin and wrists. She asks the assistant, "What happened to my son? Which of the following might the mother accuse the dental assistant?
   a. Failure to follow standard of care
   b. Loss of patient's rights
   c. Intentional or harmful physical contact
   d. Actions that resulted in threat or harm
40. A new associate dentist has joined Dr. Thompson's practice. The computer in the staff lounge is used by everyone to check emails and order supplies. Dr. Thompson's staff is diversified in gender and ethnicity. The new dentist shares many of the jokes from his emails with staff members when they are in lounge at the same time, yet most are crude and inappropriate for the workplace. Which of the following best describes the workplace violation?
   a. Sexual harassment
   b. American w/ Disabilities Act
   c. The state dental practice act
   d. Affirmative action
41. The dental hygienist is providing root planing services on a patient, and a composite restoration on #30 chips in the distal area, but the dental hygienist does not inform the patient. Two days later the patient calls and complains the filling is 'gone', and the tooth is painful. The chart notes do not indicate the composite chipped. Which intentional tort was committed by the dental hygienist?
   a. Malpractice
   b. Breach of contract
   c. Technical battery
   d. Negligence
42. Dr. Monroe has been providing services to Susan for the past six months. Dr. Monroe has opted to discontinue treatment as a result of many disagreements with Susan over the approved treatment plan. In order for the patient to be terminated by the practice, which of the following is required?
   a. Two week notice must be given in writing to the patient so another dentist can be found
   b. The office must inform the patient in writing
   c. The patient must be informed by the office manager via telephone
   d. The patient must be referred to a new dentist
43. A dental hygienist and dentist are accused of a criminal violation against a patient. A trial took place, and the jury is instructed to make their decision based on one of the following:
   a. Proof must be beyond a reasonable doubt
   b. Jurors must agree, unanimously
   c. The state dental board has the burden of proof
   d. Punitive damages must be awarded to the victim
44. When presenting the treatment plan and obtaining informed consent from her patient, the dental hygienist discusses diagnosis, risks and benefits, and treatment outcomes. The patient asks questions and is provided answers. Which aspect of the informed consent is missing?
   a. Payment plan options
   b. A witness to the signatures
   c. Treatment options
   d. Pretreatment photographs
45. Tammy, the RDH, has many days at work where she speaks so loudly that others in the office can hear the conversation, including other patients. On this occasion, she is about to administer local anesthesia, and has become irritated with the patient. Tammy is animatedly waving the syringe over the patient with the needle uncapped. The patient may choose to accuse Tammy of which of the following torts?

a. Violation of personal rights
b. Battery
c. Assault
d. Negligence

**46.** A dental hygiene was on trial for negligence. The judge instructs the jury on how to analyze the case and what level of proof the jury has to consider when making their determination of guilt or innocence. What is required to convict the dental hygienist?
a. Information presented during the trial that proves or disproves the allegation
b. Unanimous agreement of the jurors
c. Overwhelming evidence
d. Injury to the patient

**47.** A patient is allowed to refuse treatment despite the benefits to his/her oral health. All the of the following are key items to the informed refusal except one. Which is the exception?
a. A verbal refusal is a legal agreement
b. Treatment alternatives with risks and benefits
c. Documenting the reasons the patient refuses treatment
d. Signatures of the dentist/dental hygienist and patient

**48.** The dental hygienist has been providing dental hygiene care for Mrs. G over the past 20 years. The new associate dentist has determined Mrs. G requires one new crown and needs to have two others replaced. Mrs. G is concerned after all these years and asks the dental hygienist if the treatment is truly necessary. What ethical principle should guide the dental hygienist?
a. Commitment to the patient's well-being
b. Veracity
c. Justice
d. Commitment to the dental hygiene profession

**49.** A 15-year old patient has mandibular first molars in linguoversion making it difficult to keep clean between dental hygiene appointments. The patient asks the dentist to speak to his parents about orthodontics. The parents do not believe orthodontics is required and refuse the treatment. All the following apply to this case except one. Which is the exception?
a. Insurance coverage
b. Evidence-based research during case presentation
c. Fidelity
d. Beneficence

**50.** Dental hygienists use critical thinking skills in order to determine the best pathway in an ethical situation. What is the first step in the decision-making process that can guide the best outcome in ethical situations?
a. Gather facts
b. List alternatives
c. Identify the problem
d. Evaluate the action

## REFERENCES AND LEGAL CITATIONS

1. Garner BA. *Black's Law Dictionary*. Vol. 11. Thomas Reuters; 2019.
2. *564 NE 2d 1017*. Norwood Hospital V Munoz; 1991.
3. Thor v superior court, 855 P2d 375, 21 cal. *Rept. 2d*. 1993;357.
4. H. v Lewis, 141F.DR (Dev Rev) 107, 109, n5.
5. 729 CRF, } 1604.11(a).
6. 29 CRF 1910.1030. Occupational exposure to bloodborne Pathogens, needlestick and other sharps injuries. Final rule. *Fed Reg*. January 18, 2001;66:5317–5325.
7. Harris v F. Sys. Inc.; 1993. 510 US 17.
8. 29 CRF 1910.

## SUGGESTED READING

American Dental Hygienists Association. *Standards for Clinical Dental Hygiene Practice*. Chicago: ADHA; 2016. 2016 https://www.adha.org/resources-docs/2016-Revised-Standards-for-Clinical-Dental-Hygiene-Practice.pdf.

American Dental Hygienists Association. *Bylaws—codes of Ethics*. Chicago: ADHA; 2010. 2010 http://www.adha.org/resources-docs/7611_Bylaws_and_Code_of_Ethics.pdf. Accessed October 15, 2019.

Beemsterboer PL. *Ethics and Law in Dental Hygiene*. 2nd ed. St Louis: Saunders; 2010.

Canadian Dental Hygienists Association. *Codes of Ethics, 2002*. Ontario: CDHA; 2002. http://cdho.org/docs/default-source/pdfs/reference/code-of-ethics/codeofethics_pocketmanual.pdf?sfvrsn=735f83a0_10. Accessed April 16, 2019.

Darby ML, Walsh MM. *Dental Hygiene Theory and Practice*. 4th ed. St Louis: Saunders; 2014.

# A APPENDIX

# Medical Terminology

## PREFIXES

**a-, ab-, abs-** From; away; departing from normal
**ad-** Addition to; toward; nearness
**amb-, ambi-** Both; ambidextrous, having the ability to work effectively with either hand
**amphi-** On both sides
**ampho-** Both
**an-** Negative; without or not
**ana-** Upper, away from
**andro-** Signifying man; human
**ant-, anti-** Against
**ante-, antero-** Front; before
**bili-** Pertaining to bile
**brady-** Slow
**brom-, bromo-** A stench
**broncho-** Pertaining to the bronchi
**cac-** Bad
**cardi-, cardio-** Pertaining to the heart
**cata-** Down or downward
**cervico-** Pertaining to the neck
**circa-** About
**circum-** Around
**co-** With or together
**con-** Together with
**contra-** Opposite; against
**demi-** Half
**di-** Twice
**dia-** Through
**dialy-** To separate
**en-** In
**end-, endo-, ento-** Inward; within
**ep-, epi-** On; in addition to
**ex-** Out; away from
**exo-** Without; outside of
**extra-** Outside of; in addition to
**fibro-** Pertaining to fibers
**gaster-, gastr-, gastro-** Pertaining to the stomach
**hemi-** Half
**hemo-** Pertaining to the blood
**hepat-, hepatico-, hepato-** Pertaining to the liver
**heter-, hetero-** Denoting other; relationship to another
**homeo-** Denoting likeness or resemblance
**homo-** Denoting sameness
**hyal-, hyalo-** Transparent
**hyper-** Above; excessive; beyond
**hypo-** Below; less than
**ideo-** Pertaining to mental images
**idio-** Denoting relationship to one's self or to something separate and distinct
**in-** Not; in; inside; within; also intensive action
**infra-** Below
**inter-** In the midst; between
**intra-** Within
**intro-** In or into
**iso-** Equal or alike
**juxta-** Of close proximity
**karyo-** Pertaining to a cell's nucleus
**kypho-** Humped
**laryngo-** Pertaining to the larynx
**medi-** Middle
**myelo-** Pertaining to the spinal cord or bone marrow
**omni-** All
**ovari-, ovario-** Pertaining to the ovary
**per-** Through; by means of
**peri-** Around; about
**post-** Behind or after
**postero-** Pertaining to the posterior
**pre-** Before
**pro-** Before, in front of
**pseudo-** False
**re-** Back; again (contrary)
**retro-** Backward
**semi-** Half
**steato-** Fatty
**sub-** Under; near
**syn-** Joined together
**trans-** Across; over
**un-** Not; reversal

## SUFFIXES

**-able, -ible, -ble** The power to be
**-ad** Toward; in the direction of
**-aemia, -emia** Pertaining to blood
**-age** Put in motion; to do
**-agra** Denoting a seizure; severe pain
**-algia** Denoting pain
**-ase** Forms the name of an enzyme
**-blast** Designates a cell or a structure
**-cele** Denoting a swelling
**-centesis** Denoting a puncture
**-ectomy** A cutting out
**-esthesia** Denoting sensation

**-facient** That which makes or causes
**-gene, -genesis, -genetic, -genic** Denoting production; origin
**-gog, -gogue** To make flow
**-gram** A tracing; a mark
**-graph** A writing; a record
**-iasis** Denoting a condition or pathologic state
**-id** Denoting shape or resemblance
**-ite** Of the nature of
**-itis** Denoting inflammation
**-logia** Denoting discourse, science, or study of
**-oid** Denoting form or resemblance
**-oma** Denoting a tumor
**-osis** Denoting a morbid process
**-ostomosis, -ostomy, -stomy** Denoting an outlet; to furnish with an opening or mouth
**-plasty** Denoting molding or shaping
**-rhaphy** Denoting suturing or stitching
**-rhea** Denoting a flow or discharge
**-rrhagia** Denoting a discharge; usually bleeding
**-scope, -scopy** Generally an instrument for viewing
**-tomy** Denoting a cutting operation
**-trophy** Denoting a relationship to nourishment

## COMBINING FORMS

**aer-, aero-** Denoting air or gas
**alge-, algesi-, algo-** Pertaining to pain
**allo-** Other; differing from the normal
**anomalo-** Denoting irregularity
**arthro-** Pertaining to a joint or joints
**brevi-** Short
**celio-** Denoting the abdomen
**centro-** Center
**cheil-, cheilo-** Denoting the lip
**chol-, chole-, cholo-** Pertaining to bile
**chondr-, chondri-** Pertaining to cartilage
**chrom-, chromo-** Pertaining to color
**cole-, coleo-** Denoting a sheath
**colp-, colpo-** Pertaining to the vagina
**cranio-** Pertaining to the cranium of the skull
**crymo-, cryo-** Denoting cold
**crypt-** To hide; a pit
**cyano-** Dark blue
**cyclo-** Pertaining to a cycle
**cysto-** Pertaining to a sac or cyst
**cyto-** Denoting a cell
**dacryo-** Pertaining to the lacrimal glands
**dactylo-** Pertaining to digits
**dent-, dento-** Pertaining to teeth
**derma-, dermat-** Pertaining to skin
**desmo-** Pertaining to a bond or ligament
**dextro-** Right
**diplo-** Double; twofold
**dorsi-, dorso-** Pertaining to the back
**duodeno-** Pertaining to the duodenum
**electro-** Pertaining to electricity
**encephalo-** Denoting the brain
**entero-** Pertaining to the intestines
**episio-** Pertaining to the vulva
**eso-** Inward
**esthesio-** Pertaining to feeling or sensation
**facio-** Pertaining to the face
**gangli-, ganglio-** Pertaining to a ganglion
**geno-** Pertaining to reproduction
**gero-, geronto-** Denoting old age
**giganto-** Huge
**gingivo-** Pertaining to the gingiva or gum
**gloss-, glosso-** Pertaining to the tongue
**gluco-** Denoting sweetness
**glyco-** Pertaining to sugar
**gnath-, gnatho-** Denoting the jaw
**gon-** Denoting a seed
**grapho-** Denoting writing
**hapt-, hapte-, hapto-** Pertaining to touch or a seizure
**helo-** Pertaining to a nail or callus
**hist-, histio-, histo-** Pertaining to tissue
**holo-** Pertaining to the whole
**hydr-, hydro-** Denoting water
**hygro-** Denoting moisture
**hyl-, hyle-, hylo-** Denoting matter or material
**ileo-, ilio-** Pertaining to the ileum
**ipsi-** Denoting self
**irido-** Pertaining to a colored circle
**iso-** Equal
**jejuno-** Pertaining to the jejunum
**kerato-** Pertaining to the cornea
**kino-** Denoting movement
**labio-** Pertaining to the lips
**lacto-** Pertaining to milk
**laparo-** Pertaining to the loin or flank
**latero-** Pertaining to the side
**leido-, leio-** Smooth
**leuk-, leuko-** Denoting deficiency of color
**lip-, lipo-** Pertaining to fat
**litho-** Denoting a calculus
**macr-, macro-** Large; long
**mast-, masto-** Pertaining to the breast
**meg-, mega-** Great; large
**meli-** Sweet
**meningo-** Denoting membranes; covering the brain and the spinal cord
**micr-, micro-** Small in size or extent
**mono-** One
**morpho-** Pertaining to form
**multi-** Many
**my-, myo-** Pertaining to muscle
**myc-, mycet-** Denoting a fungus
**myringo-** Denoting the tympanic membrane or the eardrum
**myx-, myxo-** Pertaining to mucus
**narco-** Denoting stupor
**naso-** Pertaining to the nose
**necro-** Denoting death

**neo-** New
**nephr-, nephro-** Denoting the kidney
**normo-** Normal or usual
**oculo-** Denoting the eye
**odyno-** Denoting pain
**oleo-** Denoting oil
**onco-** Denoting a swelling or mass
**onycho-** Pertaining to the nails
**oo-** Denoting an egg
**opisth-, opistho-** Backward
**ophthal-, ophthalmo-** Pertaining to the eye
**optico-** Pertaining to the eye or vision
**orchi-, orcho-** Pertaining to the testes
**oro-** Pertaining to the mouth
**ortho-** Straight; right
**oscillo-** Denoting oscillation
**osteo-** Pertaining to the bones
**ot-, oto-** Denoting an egg
**palato-** Denoting the palate
**patho-** Denoting disease
**pedia-, pedo-** Denoting a child
**perineo-** Combining form for the region between the anus and the scrotum or vulva
**phago-** Denoting a relationship to eating
**pharyngo-** Pertaining to the pharynx
**phleb-, phlebo-** Denoting the veins
**phon-, phono-** Denoting sound
**phot-, photo-** Pertaining to light
**phren-** Pertaining to the mind
**picr-, picro-** Bitter
**pilo-** Denoting hair
**plasmo-** Pertaining to plasma or the substance of a cell
**pneuma-, pneumono-, pneumoto-** Denoting air or gas
**pod-, podo-** Denoting the foot
**poly-** Many
**proct-, procto-** Denoting the anus and rectum
**psych-, psycho-** Pertaining to the mind
**ptyalo-** Denoting saliva
**pubio-, pubo-** Denoting the pubic region
**pulmo-** Denoting the lung
**pupillo-** Denoting the pupil
**py-, pyo-** Denoting pus
**pyel-, pyelo-** Denoting the pelvis
**pyloro-** Pertaining to the pylorus
**recto-** Denoting the rectum
**rhin-, rhino-** Denoting the nose
**salpingo-** Denoting a tube, specifically the fallopian tube
**schizo-** Split
**sclero-** Denoting hardness
**scoto-** Pertaining to darkness
**sero-** Pertaining to serum
**sialo-** Pertaining to saliva or the salivary glands
**sidero-** Denoting iron
**sinistro-** Left
**somato-** Denoting the body
**somni-** Denoting sleep
**spasmo-** Denoting a spasm
**spermato-, spermo-** Denoting sperm
**sphero-** Denoting a sphere; round
**sphygmo-** Denoting a pulse
**splen-, spleno-** Denoting the spleen
**staphyl-, staphylo-** Resembling a bunch of grapes
**steno-** Narrow; short
**sterco-** Denoting feces
**steth-, stetho-** Pertaining to the chest
**stomato-** Denoting the mouth
**sym-, syn-** With; along
**tacho-, tachy-** Swift
**tarso-** Pertaining to the flat of the foot
**terato-** Denoting a marvel, prodigy, or monster
**thoraco-** Pertaining to the chest
**thrombo-** Denoting a clot of blood
**toxico-, toxo-** Denoting poison
**tracheo-** Denoting the trachea
**trichi-, tricho-** Denoting hair
**ur-, uro-, urono-** Pertaining to urine
**varico-** Denoting a twisting or swelling
**vaso-** Denoting a vessel
**veno-** Denoting a vein
**ventri-, ventro-** Denoting the abdomen
**vertebro-** Pertaining to the vertebra
**vesico-** Denoting the bladder
**viscero-** Denoting the organs of the body
**vivi-** Denoting alive
**xantho-** Denoting yellow
**xero-** Denoting dryness

## TERMINOLOGY FREQUENTLY USED TO DESIGNATE BODY PARTS OR ORGANS

**anus** Anal, ano-
**arm** Brachial, brachio-
**blood** Hem-, hemat-
**chest** Thoracic, thorax
**ear** Auricle, oto-
**eye** Ocular, oculo-, ophthalmo-
**foot** Pedal, ped-, - pod
**gallbladder** Chole-, chol-
**head** Cephalic, cephalo-
**heart** Cardium, cardiac, cardio-
**intestines** Cecum, colon, duodenum, ileum, jejunum
**kidney** Renal, nephric, nephro-
**lip** Cheil-
**liver** Hepatic, hepato-
**lungs** Pulmonary, pulmonic, pneumo-
**mouth** Oral, os, stoma, stomat-
**muscle** Myo-
**neck** Cervix, cervical, cervico-
**penis** Penile
**rectum** Rectal
**skin** Derma, integumentum
**stomach** Gastric, gastro-
**testicle** Orchio-, orchi-, orchido-
**urinary bladder** Cysti-, cysto-
**uterus** Hystero-, metra
**vagina** Vulvo, vaginal

# APPENDIX B

# Professional Organizations of Interest to Dental Hygienists

**Academy of General Dentistry**
560 W. Lake Street, Sixth Floor
Chicago, IL 60661
Phone: (888) 243–3368
Fax: (312) 335–3443
http://www.agd.org
**American Academy of Pediatric Dentistry**
211 E. Chicago Avenue, Suite 1600
Chicago, IL 60611
Phone: (312) 337–2169
Fax: (312) 337–6329
http://www.aapd.org
**American Association for Dental Research**
1619 Duke Street
Alexandria, VA 22314
Phone: (703) 548–0066
Fax: (703) 548–1883
http://www.aadronline.org
**American Association of Public Health Dentistry**
3085 Stevenson Drive, Suite 200
Springfield, IL 62703
Phone: (217) 529–6941
Fax: (217) 529–9120
http://www.aaphd.org
**American Dental Association**
211 E. Chicago Avenue
Chicago, IL 60611
Phone: (312) 440–2500
Fax: (312) 440–2800
http://www.ada.org
**American Dental Education Association**
655 K Street, NW, Suite 800
Washington, DC 20001
Phone: (202) 289–7201
Fax: (202) 289–7204
http://www.adea.org
**American Dental Hygienists Association**
444 N. Michigan Avenue, Suite 3400
Chicago, IL 60611
Phone: (312) 440–8900
http://www.adha.org
**American Public Health Association**
800 I Street NW
Washington, DC 20001
Phone: (202) 777–2742
Fax: (202) 777–2534
http://www.apha.org
**Association of Schools of Allied Health Professions**
122 C Street, NW, Suite 650
Washington, DC 20001
Phone: (202) 237–6481
Fax: (202) 237–6485
http://www.asahp.org
**Canadian Dental Association**
1815 Alta Vista Drive
Ottawa, Ontario
Canada K1G 3Y6
Phone: (613) 523–1770
Fax: (613) 523–7736
http://www.cda-adc.ca/
**Canadian Dental Hygienists Association**
1122 Wellington Street W
Ottawa, Ontario
Canada K1Y 2Y7
Phone: (613) 224–5515 or (800) 267–5235
Fax: (613) 224–7283
http://www.cdha.ca
**Canadian Public Health Association**
404–1525 Carling Avenue
Ottawa, Ontario
Canada K1Z 8R9
Phone: (613) 725–3769
Fax: (613) 725–9826
http://www.cpha.ca
**Centers for Disease Control and Prevention**
1600 Clifton Road
Atlanta, GA 30329
Phone: (800) 232–4636 or (888) 232–6348
http://www.cdc.gov
**FDI World Dental Federation**
Avenue Louis Casaï 51
P.O. Box 3
1216 Geneve-Cointrin
Switzerland
Phone: 41 22 560 81 50
Fax: 41 22 560 81 40
http://www.fdiworldental.org

**Hispanic Dental Association**
401 Penn Street
Third Floor, Washington Suite
Reading, PA 19601
Phone: (855) 337-9992
http://www.hdassoc.org

**International Association for Dental Research**
1619 Duke Street
Alexandria, VA 22314
Phone: (703) 548–0066
Fax: (703) 548–1883
http://www.iadr.com

**International Association for Disability and Oral Health**
Spoorstraat 94
6591 GV Gennep
Netherlands
http://www.iadh.org

**International Federation of Dental Hygienists**
100 South Washington Street
Rockville, MD 20850
Phone: (240) 778–6790
Fax: (240) 778–6112
http://www.ifdh.org

**National Center for Dental Hygiene Research & Practice**
USC School of Dentistry
925 W. 34th Street
Los Angeles, CA 90089
Phone: (213) 740–8669
Fax: (213) 740–1072
http://www.usc.edu/hsc/dental/dhnet/

**National Dental Hygienists' Association/National Dental Association**
5506 Connecticut Avenue, NW Suite 24-25
Washington, DC 20015
Phone: (202) 244-7555
http://www.ndaonline.org

**Special Care Dentistry Association**
Special Care Dentistry Association
2800 West Higgins Rd.
Suite 440
Hoffman Estates, IL 60169
Phone: (312) 527–6764
Fax: (84) 885-8393
http://www.scdaonline.org

**World Health Organization**
Avenue Appia 20
1211 Geneva 27
Switzerland
Phone: 41 22 791 21 11
Fax: 41 22 791 31 11
http://www.who.int

2b. in the case of clients who lack the capacity for informed choice, actively involve and promote informed choice on the part of the client's substitute decision-makers, involving the client to the extent of the client's capacity
2c. honor the client's informed choices, including refusal of treatment, and regard informed choice as a precondition of treatment
2d. do not rely upon coercion or manipulative tactics in assisting the client to make informed choices
2e. recommend or provide only those services they believe are necessary for the client's oral health or as consistent with the client's informed choice.
Note: Critical elements of informed choice include disclosure (i.e., revealing pertinent information, including risks and benefits); willingness (i.e., the choice is not coerced or manipulated); and capacity (i.e., the cognitive capacity to understand and process the relevant information). "Informed choice" encompasses what is sometimes referred to as "informed consent."

## Principle III: Privacy and Confidentiality

Privacy pertains to the individual's right to decide the conditions under which others will be permitted access to his or her personal life or information. Confidentiality is the duty to hold secret any information acquired in the professional relationship. Dental hygienists respect the privacy of clients and hold in confidence information disclosed to them, subject to certain narrowly defined exceptions.

### Standards for Principle III

Dental hygienists:
3a. demonstrate regard for the privacy of their clients
3b. hold confidential any information acquired in the professional relationship and do not use or disclose it to others without the client's express consent, except:
3b.i as required by law
3b.ii as required by the policy of the practice environment (e.g., quality assurance)
3b.iii in an emergency situation
3b.iv in cases where disclosure is necessary to prevent serious harm to others
3b.v to the guardian or substitute decision-maker of a client, in these cases, disclose to others only as much information as is necessary to accomplish the purpose for the disclosure
3c. may infer the client's consent for disclosure to others directly involved in delivering and administering services to the client, provided there is no reason to believe the client would not give express consent if asked
3d. obtain the client's express consent to use or share information about the client for the purpose of teaching or research
3e. inform their clients in advance of treatment about how they will use or share their information, in particular about any uses or sharing that may occur without the client's express consent
3f. promote practices, policies, and information systems that are designed to respect client privacy and confidentiality.

## Principle IV: Accountability

Accountability pertains to the acceptance of responsibility for one's actions and omissions in light of relevant principles, standards, laws, and regulations and the potential to self-evaluate and to be evaluated accordingly. Dental hygienists practise competently in conformity with relevant principles, standards, laws and regulations, and accept responsibility for their behaviour and decisions in the professional context.

### Standards for Principle IV

Dental hygienists:
4a. accept responsibility for knowing and acting consistently with the principles, standards, laws and regulations under which they are accountable
4b. accept responsibility for providing safe, quality, competent care including, but not limited to, addressing issues in the practice environment within their capacity that may hinder or impede the provision of such care
4c. take appropriate action to ensure first and foremost the client's safety and quality of care when they suspect unethical or incompetent care
4d. practise within the bounds of their competence, scope of practice, personal and/or professional limitations, and refer clients requiring care outside these bounds
4e. inform the dental hygiene regulatory body when an injury, dependency, infection, condition, or any other serious incapacity has immediately affected, or may affect over time, their continuing ability to practise safely and competently
4f. promote workplace practices and policies that facilitate professional practice in accordance with the principles, standards, laws and regulations under which they are accountable.

## Principle V: Professionalism

Professionalism is the commitment to use and advance professional knowledge and skills to serve the client and the public good. Dental hygienists express their professional commitment individually in their practice and communally through their professional associations and regulatory bodies.

### Standards for Principle V

Dental hygienists:
5a. uphold the principles and standards of the profession before clients, colleagues, and others
5b. maintain and advance their knowledge and skills in dental hygiene through continuing education and the quality of the care they provide through ongoing self-evaluation and quality assurance
5c. advance general knowledge and skills in the field of oral health by supporting, participating in, or conducting ethically approved research
5d. participate in professional activities such as meetings, committee work, peer review, and participation in public forums to promote oral health
5e. participate in mentoring, education, and dissemination of knowledge and skills in oral health care

5f. support the work of their professional associations and regulatory bodies to promote oral health and professional practice
5g. inform potential employers about the principles, standards, laws and regulations to which they are accountable and determine whether employment conditions facilitate professional practice accordingly
5h. collaborate with colleagues in a cooperative, constructive, and respectful manner toward the primary end of providing safe, competent, fair, quality care to clients
5i. communicate the nature and costs of professional services fairly and accurately.

## APPENDIX A: ETHICAL CHALLENGES/ PROBLEMS

No code of ethics can be expected to resolve definitively all ethical challenges or problems that may arise in practice. The analysis below is intended to help dental hygienists understand the nature of ethical challenges or problems and thereby better resolve them.

Ethical challenges or problems faced by practicing dental hygienists tend to fall into the categories of ethical violations, ethical dilemmas, and ethical distress.

Ethical violations: when dental hygienists fail to meet or neglect their specific ethical responsibilities as expressed in the Code's standards. An example would be a dental hygienist who recommends unnecessary treatment in order to achieve personal gain at the expense of the client.

Ethical dilemmas: when one or more ethical principles conflict either with other ethical principle(s) or with self-interest(s) and no apparent course of action will satisfy both sides of the dilemma. An example would be a client with a hip prosthesis who may refuse to be premedicated prior to receiving invasive dental treatment. In this case, the principle of autonomy conflicts with the principle of beneficence.

Ethical distress: when dental hygienists experience constraints or limitations in relation to which they are or feel powerless and which compromise their ability to practise in full accordance with their professional principles or standards. An example would be a dental hygienist who is expected by the employer to complete dental hygiene treatment in a length of time insufficient to render quality care or to provide an acceptable level of infection control.

This Code is a useful guide in helping dental hygienists to identify, work through, and put into words ethical issues in light of their responsibilities as articulated in the Code's principles and standards, and to decide on an ethically responsible course of action. It is important to realize that some challenges or problems are perceived to be primarily ethical in nature when, in fact, they arise less from conflicting principles than from poor communication or lack of information. Reflecting on a perceived challenge or problem in light of the Code can help determine to what extent the problem or challenge is truly rooted in conflicting ethical principles, and to what extent it can be resolved by improved communication or by new information.

The Code provides clear direction for avoiding ethical violations. When a course of action is mandated by a standard in the Code or by a principle where there exists no opposing principle, ethical conduct requires that course of action.

In the case of ethical dilemmas and ethical distress, the Code cannot always provide a clear direction. The resolution of dilemmas often depends on the specific circumstances of the case in question. Total satisfaction by all parties involved may not be achieved. Resolution may also depend on which opposing ethical principle is considered to be more important, a matter on which reasonable people may disagree. Ethical distress often arises in situations where the dental hygienist is significantly limited by factors beyond his or her immediate control that may not be resolvable in the specific context.

In all cases, dental hygienists are accountable for how they conduct themselves in professional practice. Even in situations of ethical dilemma or distress where the Code does not prescribe a specific course of action, the hygienist can be expected to give account of his or her chosen action in light of the principles and standards expressed in the Code. Ultimately, dental hygienists must reconcile their actions with their consciences in caring for clients.

## APPENDIX B: REPORTING SUSPECTED INCOMPETENCE OR UNETHICAL CONDUCT

The first consideration of the dental hygienist who suspects incompetence or unethical conduct in colleagues or associates is the welfare of present clients and/or potential harm to future clients. Adherence to the following guidelines could be helpful:

1. First, confirm the facts of the situation.
2. Ensure you are familiar with existing protocols in the practice setting for reporting incidents, incompetence, or unethical care and follow those protocols.
3. Document and report issues that cannot be resolved within the practice setting and report to the appropriate authority or regulatory body.

The dental hygienist who attempts to protect clients threatened by incompetent or unethical conduct should not be placed in jeopardy (e.g., loss of employment). Colleagues and professional organizations are morally obligated to support dental hygienists who fulfil their ethical obligations under the Code.

## APPENDIX C: DECISION—PROCEDURE

### Guidance Regarding the Process for Resolving Ethical Challenges

Ethical problems or challenges arise in a variety of contexts and require thoughtful analysis and careful judgment. The following guide may be useful to assist dental hygienists faced with an ethical challenge, recognizing that other stakeholders may need to be involved in resolving the matter. Talking with or getting advice from others at any step on the way to a decision can be very helpful.

1. Identify in a preliminary way the nature of the challenge or problem. What is the issue? What kind of issue is it? What ethical principles are at stake?

2. Become suitably informed and gather information (e.g., talk to others to find out the facts; research relevant policy statements) relevant to the challenge or problem, including:
   a. Factual information about the situation. What has happened? What is the sequence of events?
   b. Applicable policies, laws or regulations. Does a workplace policy address the issue? What does the Code say? What does law or regulation say?
   c. Who are the relevant stakeholders? How do they view the situation?
3. Clarify and elaborate the challenge or problem after getting this information. Now that you are better informe: What is the issue? What ethical principles are at stake? What stakeholders need to be consulted or involved in resolving the challenge or problem?
4. Identify various options for actions, recognizing that the best option may not be obvious at first and realizing it may require creativity or imagination.
5. Assess the various options in light of applicable policy, law or regulation, being as clear as possible in your mind of the pluses and minuses of each option as assessed in this light.
6. Decide on a course of action, mindful of how you would justify or defend your decision in light of the applicable policy, law or regulation, if you are called to account.
7. Implement your decision as thoughtfully and sensitively as possible, communicating a willingness to explain or justify the reasons for taking it.
8. Assess the consequences of your decision. Evaluate the process you used to arrive at the decision and the decision itself in light of those consequences. Did things turn out as you thought they would? Would you do the same thing again? What went wrong? Or, what went right?

In all of this, bear in mind that reasonable people can disagree about what is the right thing to do when faced with an ethical challenge or problem. If you cannot be certain whether you have made the right decision, you can at least have some assurance that you came to your decision in a responsible way. The test for this is whether you are able to defend your decision in light of relevant laws, principles, and regulations, and to defend the process by which you came to your decision. Reference to the above guidelines will help in this.

In addition, there is a very rich literature on ethics that can be very helpful for thinking through ethical challenges and problems in dental hygiene or for ongoing professional education and development.

Dental hygienists may also find it useful to familiarize themselves with various ethical theories, which tend to guide or orient ethical thinking along different lines. The main ethical theories current today are briefly described below:

- Deontology guides ethical thinking in terms of duties and rights, which the philosopher Immanuel Kant grounds in the fundamental imperative to act in relation to others according to principles that apply universally to all people, and that one would also wish for others to apply in their actions in relation to oneself
- Utilitarianism guides ethical thinking in terms of harms and benefits, which the philosopher J.S. Mill grounds in the fundamental imperative to promote the greatest good for the greatest number
- The ethic of care guides ethical thinking in terms of preserving and enhancing relationships and service to others. This theory derives from the work of Carol Gilligan, who found in her research that this style of ethical thinking tends to be more associated with females than with males
- Virtue ethics guides ethical thinking in terms of habits of acting and assesses actions in terms of virtues and vices of character. This theory derives from the work of the philosopher Aristotle, who emphasized that ethics cannot be reduced to rules or formulas and held that the person of good character (the "good man") is the ultimate standard of right and wrong and should be emulated by others as a role model
- Feminist ethics guides ethical thinking in terms of sensitivity to the power or political dimension of human interaction. The philosopher Susan Sherwin grounds feminist ethics in the allegiance to those who are oppressed, vulnerable, or disadvantaged and the imperative to improve their situation.

This is by no means a complete listing of ethical theories, nor is the richness of these theories captured in the condensed descriptions given. Moreover, considerable controversy exists not only among these theories but also among adherents of each theory.[1]

## REFERENCES

American Dental Hygienists Association. *Code of ethics for dental hygienists.* Chicago: ADHA; 1995, 2019.

Canadian Dental Assistants Association. *CDAA code of ethics.* Ottawa: CDAA; 2000.

Canadian Dental Association. *Code of ethics.* Ottawa: CDA; August 1991.

Canadian Dental Hygienists Association. *Code of ethics.* Ottawa: CDHA; July 2012.

Canadian Dental Hygienists Association. *Dental hygiene: client's bill of rights.* Ottawa: CDHA; October 2001.

Canadian Medical Association. *Code of ethics of the Canadian Medical Association.* Ottawa: CMA; 1997.

Canadian Nurses Association. *Code of ethics for registered nurses.* Ottawa: CNA; March 1997.

College of Dental Hygienists of British Columbia. *Code of ethics.* Victoria: CDHBC; March 1, 1995.

Canadian Dental Hygienists Association 1122 Wellington Street Ottawa, ON K1Y 2Y7Telephone (613) 224-5515 or (800) 267-5235Fax (613) 224-7283.

www.cdha.ca.

---

[1]Reprinted with permission from the American Dental Hygienists' Association homepage (www.adha.org).

# Index

*Note*: Page numbers followed by *b* indicate boxes, *f* indicate figures, and *t* indicate tables.

**O**

## S